Case-Smith's

# Occupational Therapy *for* Children *and* Adolescents

NINTH EDITION

# Case-Smith's Occupational Therapy *for* Children *and* Adolescents

**Jane Clifford O'Brien,** PhD, OTR, FAOTA
Professor, Occupational Therapy, Retired
North Waterboro, ME, United States

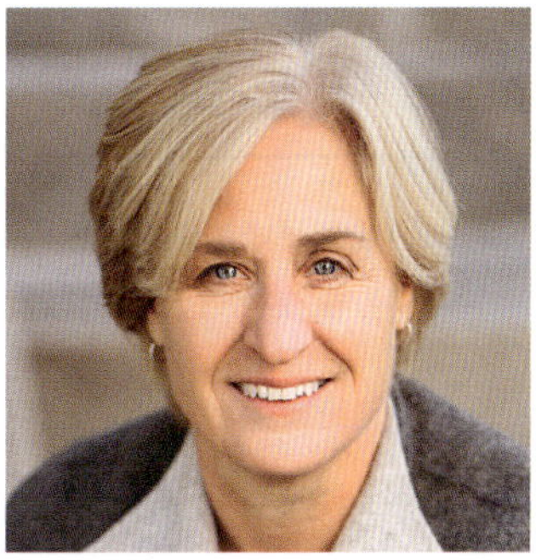

**Heather Miller Kuhaneck,** PhD, OTR/L, FAOTA
Professor of Occupational Therapy
Department of Recreation, Tourism, and Sports Management
Southern Connecticut State University
New Haven, CT, United States

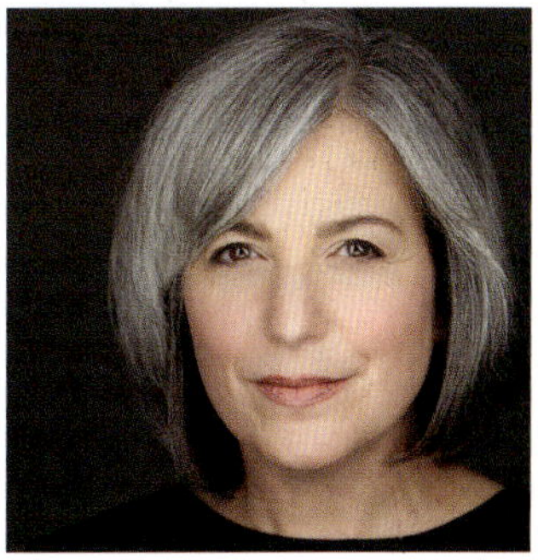

ELSEVIER

Elsevier
3251 Riverport Lane
St. Louis, Missouri 63043

CASE-SMITH'S OCCUPATIONAL THERAPY FOR CHILDREN AND ADOLESCENTS, NINTH EDITION
ISBN: 978-0-443-11021-4



*Content Strategist*: Laura Klein
*Content Development Manager*: Meghan Andress
*Content Development Specialist*: Erika Ninsin
*Publishing Services Manager*: Deepthi Unni
*Senior Project Manager*: Kamatchi Madhavan
*Design Direction*: Ryan Cook

Printed in India

Last digit is the print number: 9 8 7 6 5 4 3 2 1

# CONTRIBUTORS

**Renee M. Allen, MS OTR/L, MSW/L**
Early Intervention Liaison
Early Head Start-Developmental Services
Ability Connection Colorado
Aurora, Colorado;
Owner
ROOTS Pediatric Occupational Therapy
Denver, Colorado
United States

**Susan Bazyk, PhD, FAOTA**
Professor Emerita
School of Health Sciences
Cleveland State University
Cleveland, Ohio;
Director
Every Moment Counts, LLC
Cleveland, Ohio
United States

**Melissa "Missy" Bell, OTR, CDRS, LDI**
Occupational Therapy Driver Rehabilitation Specialist
Outpatient Occupational Therapy/Adaptive Driving Program
St. David's Medical Center/Rehabilitation Hospital
Austin, Texas;
Owner/Operator
Safe Driving & Rehabilitation, LLC
Austin, Texas
United States

**Patricia L. Bowyer, EdD, MS, OTR, FAOTA**
Professor
Department of Occupational Therapy
Houston Center
Texas Woman's University
Houston, Texas
United States

**Susan Cahill, PhD, OTR/L, FAOTA**
Director of Evidence-based Practice
American Occupational Therapy Association
Bethesda, Maryland
United States

**Kaitlyn Carmichael, PhD, MSc**
Researcher
School of Occupational Therapy
Western University
London, Ontario
Canada

**Theresa Carlson Carroll, OTD, OTR/L, CLA**
Clinical Associate Professor
Occupational Therapy
Valparaiso University
Valparaiso, Indiana
United States

**Jana Cason, DHSc, OTR/L, FNAP, FAOTA**
Professor
Doctor of Occupational Therapy Program
Hawai'i Pacific University
Honolulu, Hawaii
United States

**Megan C. Chang, PhD, MS, OTR/L, FAOTA**
Professor
Occupational Therapy
San Jose State University
San Jose, California
United States

**Gloria Frolek Clark, PhD, OT/L, BCP, SCSS, FAOTA**
Owner
Gloria Frolek Clark LLC
Occupational Therapy
Adel, Iowa
United States

**Patricia C. Coker-Bolt, PhD, OTR/L, FNAP, FAOTA**
Professor
Doctor of Occupational Therapy
Hawai'i Pacific University
Honolulu, Hawaii;
Professor Emeritus
Division of Occupational Therapy
Medical University of South Carolina
Charleston, South Carolina
United States

**Katherine Dimitropoulou, OTR/L, PhD**
Assistant Professor
Rehabilitation & Regenerative Medicine, Occupational Therapy Programs, Vagelos College of Physicians & Surgeons
Columbia University
New York, New York
United States

**Jenny Marie Dorich, PhD, OTR/L, MBA, CHT**
Assistant Professor
Department of Orthopaedic Surgery
University of Cincinnati College of Medicine
Cincinnati, Ohio;
Assistant Professor
Division of Occupational Therapy and Physical Therapy
Cincinnati Children's Hosptial Medical Center
Cincinnati, Ohio;
Assistant Professor
College of Health Sciences
University of Cincinnati
Cincinnati, Ohio
United States

**Patricia Fingerhut, PhD, OTR**
Professor and Chair
Department of Occupational Therapy
School of Health Professions
University of Texas Medical Branch at Galveston
Galveston, Texas
United States

**Tara J. Glennon, EdD, OTR/L, FAOTA**
Professor of Occupational Therapy
Department of Occupational Therapy
Quinnipiac University
Hamden, Connecticut
United States

**Sandy Hanebrink, OTR/L, CLP, FAOTA, PLY**
Executive Director
Touch the Future Inc
Anderson, South Carolina
United States

**Karen Harpster, PhD, OTR/L**
Associate Professor
Director of Occupational Therapy Research
Division of Patient Services Research
Cincinnati Children's Hospital Medical Center
Cincinnati, Ohio;
Associate Professor
Department of Pediatrics
University of Cincinnati
Cincinnati, Ohio
United States

**Claudia List Hilton, PhD, MBA, OTR, FAOTA**
Professor
Occupational Therapy
University of Texas Medical Branch
Galveston, Texas
United States

**Carole K. Ivey, PhD, OTR/L, FAOTA**
Associate Professor and Chair
Department of Occupational Therapy
Virginia Commonwealth University
Richmond, Virginia
United States

**Leslie Jackson, OTD, MEd, OT/L, FAOTA**
Associate Professor & Program Director and Chairperson
Occupational Therapy
Drake University
Des Moines, Iowa
United States

**Jean S. Koketsu, OTD, OTR/L**
Occupational Therapist
Department of Rehabilitation
On Lok PACE
San Jose, California;
Lecturer
Department of Occupational Therapy
San Jose State University
San Jose, California
United States

**Kimberly Korth, MEd, OTR**
Occupational Therapist
The Children's Hospital Colorado
Denver, Colorado
United States

**Heather Miller Kuhaneck, PhD, OTR/L, FAOTA**
Professor
Occupational Therapy
Department of Recreation, Tourism, and Sports Management
Southern Connecticut State University
New Haven, Connecticut
United States

**Jane Loscheider, OTD, OTR/L, ATP, CLT**
Assistant Professor
Occupational Therapy
University of North Dakota
Grand Forks, North Dakota;
Occupational Therapist
Altru Health System
Grand Forks, North Dakota
United States

**Cheryl B. Lucas, EdD, OTR/L, LNHA, CLA**
Clinical Associate Professor
Assistant Director, Occupational Therapy Program
Department of Rehabilitation Science
University at Buffalo
Buffalo, New York;
Owner and Founder
CBL Consulting and Training, LLC
Worcester, Massachusetts
United States

**Helen Lynch, PhD, MSc, Dip Montessori, Dip OT**
Senior Lecturer
Occupational Science and Occupational Therapy
University College Cork
Cork, Ireland;
P4play Co-ordinator
P4play
Europe

**Zoe Mailloux, OTD, OTR/L, FAOTA**
Adjunct Associate Professor
Occupational Therapy
Thomas Jefferson University
Redondo Beach, California
United States

**Angela Mandich, PhD, MSc OT**
Associate Professor
School of Occupational Therapy
Western University
London, Ontario
Canada

**Nancy Creskoff Maune, BS**
Occupational Therapist
Occupational Therapy
Children's Hospital Colorado
Aurora, Colorado
United States

**Teresa A. May-Benson, ScD., OTR/L, FAOTA**
Owner
TMB Educational Enterprises, LLC
Norristown, Pennsylvania
United States

**Alice Moore, PhD, MSc OT, BSc (Hons.) OT**
Research and Impact Lead
The Crann Centre
Cork, Ireland

**Said Nafai, OTD, CLT, CAPS**
President
Occupational Therapy
Occupational Therapy Association of Morocco
Kenitra
Morocco

**Jane Clifford O'Brien, PhD, OTR, FAOTA**
Professor
Occupational Therapy
Retired
North Waterboro, Maine
United States

**Kyle H. O'Brien, PhD, DHSc, MSOT, MSW, OTR/L, LCSW**
Associate Professor
Department of Recreation, Tourism, & Sport Management
Southern Connecticut State University
New Haven, Connecticut;
Founding Academic Fieldwork Coordinator
Graduate Occupational Therapy Program
Southern Connecticut State University
New Haven, Connecticut;
Director of Health Science
Southern Connecticut State University
New Haven, Connecticut
United States

**Mim Ochsenbein, MSW, OTR/L**
Owner and Therapist
Treatment and Consultation
Potential Therapy, LLC
Denver, Utah;
Adjunct Instructor
Department of EL OTD Program
Rocky Mountain University
Provo, Colorado;
Adjunct instructor
Department of MOT Program
Rocky Mountain University
Provo, Utah
United States

**Meira L. Orentlicher, PhD, OTR/L, FAOTA, CRA**
Director of Research and Faculty Scholarship
School of Health Sciences
Touro University
New York, New York;
Professor & Associate Chairperson for Research and Scholarship
Occupational Therapy
Touro University
New York, New York
United States

**Andrew C. Persch, PhD, OTR/L, BCP, FAOTA**
Associate Professor
Occupational Therapy
Colorado State University
Fort Collins, Colorado
United States

**Beth Pfeiffer, PhD, OTR/L**
Professor
Health and Rehabilitation Sciences
Temple University
Philadelphia, Pennsylvania
United States

**Aimee Piller, PhD, OTR/L, BCP, FAOTA**
Director
Therapy
Piller Child Development, LLC
Phoenix, Arizona
United States

**Evguenia Sergeevna Popova, PhD, OTR/L**
Assistant Professor
Occupational Therapy
Rush University
Chicago, Illinois
United States

**Karen Ratcliff, PhD**
Associate Professor
Department of Occupational Therapy
University of Texas Medical Branch at Galveston
Galveston, Texas
United States

**Pamela Richardson, PhD, OTR/L, FAOTA**
Associate Dean
College of Applied Sciences and Arts
San José State University
San José, California
United States

**Mitchell Scheiman, OD, PhD**
Associate Dean of Research
Research
Pennsylvania College of Optometry at Drexel University
Elkins Park, Pennsylvania;
Professor
Optometry
Pennsylvania College of Optometry at Drexel University
Elkins Park, Pennsylvania
United States

**Elizabeth Koss Schmidt, PhD, OTR/L**
Director of Research, Assistant Professor
Department of Occupational Therapy
Lincoln Memorial University
Knoxville, Tennessee
United States

**Judith Weenink Schoonover, MEd, OTR/L, ATP, FAOTA**
Independent Contractor
Holland, Michigan
United States

**Jayne Tyson Shepherd, MS, OTR/L, FAOTA**
Professor Emeritus
Occupational Therapy
Virginia Commonwealth University
Richmond, Virginia;
Occupational Therapist
Rural Infant Services Program
Middle Peninsula and Northern Neck Behavioral Health
Saluda, Virginia
United States

**Natasha Smet, OTD, OTR/L, ADHD-RSP, FAOTA**
Founder and CEO
Occupational Therapist
Natasha Smet OT, LLC
Phoenix, Arizona;
Associate Professor and Academic Fieldwork Coordinator
Occupational Therapy
University of Western States
Portland, Oregon;
Higher Education Leadership PhD Student
School of Education
Colorado State University
Fort Collins, Colorado
United States

**Jenn Soros, PhD, OTR/L**
Assistant Professor
Department of Occupational Therapy
Cleveland State University
Cleveland, Ohio
United States

**Susan L. Spitzer, PhD, OTR/L**
Owner/Director
Occupational Therapy
Private Practice
Pasadena, California
United States

**Elizabeth W. Stevens-Nafai, MS OTR/L, CLT**
Elizabeth W. Stevens-Nafai
Occupational Therapy
Worcester Public Schools
Worcester, Massachusetts
United States

**Ashley Stoffel, OTD, OTR/L, FAOTA, FNAP**
Clinical Professor
Department of Occupational Therapy
University of Illinois Chicago
Chicago, Illinois
United States

**Yvonne Swinth, PhD, OTR/L, FAOTA**
Professor
School of Occupational Therapy
University of Puget Sound
Tacoma, Washington
United States

**Renee Taylor, MA, PhD**
Professor
Department of Occupational Therapy
University of Illinois at Chicago
Chicago, Illinois
United States

**L. Diane Parham Trigg, PhD, OTR, FAOTA**
Professor Emerita
Occupational Therapy Graduate Program, Department of Pediatrics
University of New Mexico
Albuquerque, New Mexico
United States

**Jolien van den Houten, MHPE, BScOT**
OT Lecturer
Ergotherapie Nederland
jolien.vandenhouten.OT
Utrecht, Utrecht
Netherlands

**Vivian Villegas, OTD, OTR/L**
Research Specialist
Department of Occupational Therapy
University of Illinois Chicago
Chicago, Illinois;
Occupational Therapist
Easterseals Academy-Chicago
Chicago, Illinois
United States

**Renee Watling, PhD, OTR/L, FAOTA**
Professor, MSOT and OTD Program Director, Chair
School of Occupational Therapy
University of Puget Sound
Tacoma, Washington;
Clinical Assistant Professor
Department of Rehabilitation Medicine
University of Washington
Seattle, Washington
United States

**Elisa Wern, MEd, OTR/L, ATP**
Lead Therapist and Local AT Specialist
ESE & Student Services
Alachua County Public Schools
Gainesville, Florida;
Owner
AT & OT Consulting and Coaching
Gainesville, Florida
United States

**Colleen Cameron Whiting, OTD, OTR/L**
Assistant Professor
Department of Occupational Therapy
Johnson & Wales University
Providence, Rhode Island
United States

**Jessie Wilson, PhD, OT Reg. (Ont.)**
Assistant Professor
School of Occupational Therapy
Western University
London, Ontario
Canada

**Jarrett Wolske, OTD, OTR/L**
Coordiantor of Accommodations
Access and Disability Services
McHenry County College
Crystal Lake, Illinois
United States

# PREFACE

## ORGANIZATION

The current edition is organized into six sections to assist the reader in understanding the background and foundational knowledge and skills needed to practice occupational therapy with children and then to help readers apply these concepts in practice in evaluation and intervention. Section I (Chapters 1–8) describes foundational knowledge for occupational therapy for children and youth beginning with an overview of the occupational therapy process in pediatric practice and outlining essential concepts. This leads to chapters emphasizing the use of creativity in practice, knowledge and skills for working with families, and strategies to embrace diversity when working with children and families. A review of the common conditions seen in children and the settings where pediatric occupational therapists work is followed by documentation requirements and billing practices. This section ends with a chapter exploring the developmental trajectories of childhood.

The second section (Chapters 9 and 10) focuses on the ability to evaluate and assess children and adolescents, write goals, measure outcomes, and document progress from intervention. This section begins with a new, comprehensive chapter that combines information about evaluation and assessment from all the areas of pediatric practice and across all occupations. Each chapter author contributed expertise to this expanded chapter. This is followed by a chapter that discusses interpreting results, goal writing, and measuring outcomes.

Section III (Chapters 11–21) highlights intervention methods to address feeding and eating, resting and sleeping, activities of daily living, instrumental activities of daily living, education, play, leisure, social participation, sexuality, driving and community mobility, and work.

Sections IV and V emphasize targeted approaches to intervention that may be used to address many occupations. Section IV (Chapters 22 and 23) describes strategies to empower families and the use of telehealth, whereas Section V (Chapters 24–34) describes approaches to address social-emotional learning and challenging behaviors. Chapters within this section also examine cognitive-based, sensory (including Ayres Sensory Integration® and other sensory-related approaches), and motor-based approaches. Specific chapters address intervention to address fine motor skills, visual and visual information processing, mobility, hand impairments, and assistive technology.

The sixth and final section of the book provides resources to apply concepts in practice. This section includes a chapter illustrating the professional reasoning process in various practice settings. Each case includes a description of the practitioner's thought process to help readers expand their professional reasoning. Appendix A provides a thorough listing of the assessment tools often used by occupational therapists in pediatrics. Appendix B lists resources to support learning that are available on the Ebooks+ website. Appendix C summarizes the case examples from the book so that readers can apply concepts to a variety of cases to enhance their understanding and apply concepts in practice. Faculty may use this matrix to add to student learning opportunities.

## DISTINCTIVE FEATURES

Section I chapters provide foundation material to set the stage for the remainder of the chapters. Section II provides extensive information on evaluation and goal setting that are essential to effective intervention planning. It may be beneficial to read these sections before Sections III, IV, V, and VI.

Each chapter presents current research-based information that can guide practitioners in making optimal decisions in their practice with children. Each chapter begins with key questions to guide reading. The key questions highlight the focus of the chapter. Case examples reinforce key concepts and are designed to help the reader integrate the material. Authors use tables, boxes, and figures to emphasize important points. Chapters conclude with a summary section that briefly answers the key questions posed at the beginning of the chapter.

## ANCILLARY MATERIALS

The *Case-Smith's Occupational Therapy for Children and Adolescents* text includes an enhanced e-book—free with print purchase—that provides learning aids and tools which can be accessed by registering at eBooks.Health.Elsevier.com with the scratch- off access code that comes with each NEW print textbook. The site provides additional materials to reinforce student learning and apply concepts in practice. Materials support student learning so that students can be more prepared for class, perform better on exams, and succeed in coursework. Instructor resources can be found on the Evolve site.

Each chapter includes:

- Multiple choice questions with rationale for answers
- Additional case examples with guiding questions
- Video clips with guiding questions to reinforce chapter concepts
- A glossary
- Other content to support the chapter (such as handouts, forms, and evidence-based tables)

Please visit eBooks.Health.Elsevier.com to access these additional resources.

# ACKNOWLEDGMENTS

First, we acknowledge the authors who contributed their time and expertise and devoted themselves to the idea of "paying it forward" to educate the next cohort of occupational therapy students. This book could not have happened without all of you! Many people contributed (or were in) videos, cases, photos, and myriad things that a text of this size requires to come alive for students and engage them in their learning. These contributions are interspersed throughout the book and in the online learning materials. We appreciate the willingness of practitioners, parents, and children to have their stories, photos, or videos included in this text. For the sake of privacy and anonymity, the names of children highlighted in the case examples, photos, and videos have been changed.

The dedicated staff at Elsevier were instrumental in developing and completing this textbook. Their attention to detail, gentle reminders, creativity, and professionalism in producing a high-quality textbook and ancillary materials are commendable. Thank you to Laura Klein (Content Strategist), Erika Ninsin (Content Development Strategist), and Kamatchi Madhavan (Senior Project Manager).

Jane Clifford O'Brien would like to thank her family—Mike, Scott, Alison, and Molly—for their continual support and encouragement. Thank you to my colleagues, students, and especially the children and families who provided inspiration for the material, and Heather Miller Kuhaneck for her expertise, support, and ability to keep the process fun. I am grateful to my friends and family, who made the work of editing this text possible by providing needed breaks for CrossFit, outdoor activities, spa days, travel, and chats.

JOB

For Heather Miller Kuhaneck, the work of editing a text of this size would not be possible without the unwavering support of her husband Shayne, her family and friends, and her coworkers (all of whom suffer somewhat from her disengagement from her real life while she has her head stuck in a laptop). To Jane, thank you for being an exceptional coeditor and partner. Your willingness to jump in, dividing and conquering as we work through the process, and your good humor no matter what makes it manageable and enjoyable. To all of my "peeps," I am eternally grateful for all you do and for tolerating all we were not able to do while I was otherwise busy. To Shayne, as always, you are my rock!

HMK

Thank you to the following individuals who assisted us on this edition.

Renee Allen
Michelle Atanu
Susan Bazyk
Jana Cason
Julia Chiapetta
Patricia Fingerhut
Charlotte Gould
Haleigh Gould
Michael Gould
Adam Griffin
Jessica Gutierrez
Debi Hinnerfeld
Kaitlin Ibara
Lorinda Jackson
Leslie Jackson
Jean Koketsu
Kirsten Lansier
Carol Lambdin-Pattavina
Alexandra Loukas
Austin Loukas
Jacob Loukas
Carol Loukas
Kathryn Loukas
Chelsea Maziarz
Kyle O'Brien
Sandy Hanebrink
Jyoti Heiple
Kathryn MacLeay
Stephanie Madonna
Nancy Maune
Said Nafai
Brenin Nixon
Molly O'Brien
Angela Notaristefano Olujimi
Evgenia Popova
Jenny Presgraves
Karen Ratcliff
Renee Reel
Luke Riley
Maureen Riley
Krysta Rives
Gabrielle Rives
Danielle Robbins
Gabrielle Robbins
Michelle Rodriquez
Lauren Shain
Patricia Schaefer
Natasha Smet
Zara Smet
Ethan Serpas
Kim Serpas
Caroline Stevens
Elizabeth Stevens-Nafai
Isaiah Stevenson
Kirk Stromberg
Erin Tobitsch
Patricia Tomsic
Elizabeth Tontini-L'heureux
Vivian Villegas
Brooks Weldner
Syndey Bast Weldner
Colleen Whiting
Eli Wilcox
Maria Wolford

*Dr. Jane Case-Smith was a soft-spoken, thoughtful, and a brilliant scholar, who believed strongly in using science as a foundation for intervention, while never overlooking the art of therapy. Her ability to integrate these two important aspects of occupational therapy will forever influence the profession and help many children and their families participate in daily occupations.*

*Jane valued people, consistently striving to foster relationships with her colleagues, coauthors, and the families she served. She mentored numerous students, practitioners, and colleagues and her legacy exists in those who carry on the work she loved, including this text.*

*For the prior edition, the text was renamed to honor Jane's years of commitment and her stewardship, foresight, and rigor as the amount of occupational therapy pediatric content grew substantially and the importance of documenting evidence-based practice became increasingly evident. This text now carries her name, and we again dedicate this edition to her.*

*Jane, we miss you, think of you daily, and we are continually amazed and awed by all you did for the profession of occupational therapy. Much has changed in our profession as reflected in this current text and we hope you would continue to be proud of this work.*

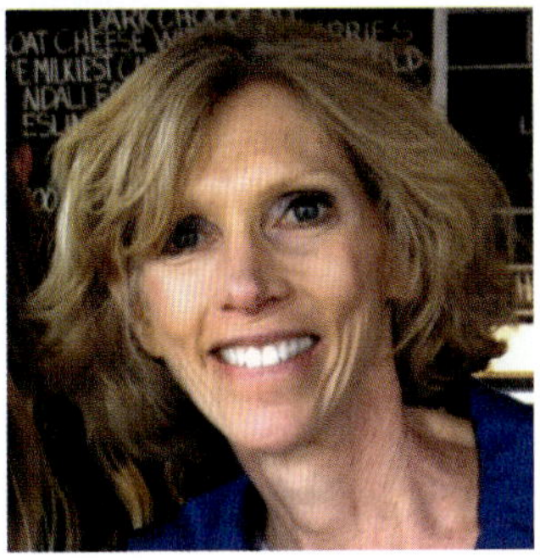

# CONTENTS

# VIDEO TABLE OF CONTENTS

The videos include video descriptions of the cases with leading questions that can be found on the enhanced e-book to reinforce chapter content.

# 1

# The Occupational Therapy Process in Pediatrics: Overview of Essential Concepts

*Heather Miller Kuhaneck, Jane Clifford O'Brien, and Kyle O'Brien*

## GUIDING QUESTIONS

1. What is pediatric occupational therapy practice?
2. What is the process of occupational therapy in pediatrics?
3. What are essential concepts of pediatric practice?

## KEY TERMS

Child centered
Childhood
Cultural humility
Family centered
Growth mindset
Interprofessional practice
Just-right challenge
Occupational engagement
Occupational identity
Occupational therapy assistant
Professional reasoning
Self-efficacy
Self-determination
Strengths-based approaches
Therapeutic relationship

## INTRODUCTION

Occupational therapists and occupational therapy assistants (referred to as occupational therapy practitioners in this text) work with people across the lifespan from birth to older adulthood. No matter the age of the client, occupational therapy professionals share the same philosophy, engage in the same processes, and possess the same overall belief system in relation to human beings and the value of engaging in one's desired occupations. One primary philosophical assumption of occupational therapy as a profession is that "people of all ages and abilities require occupation to grow and thrive; in pursuing occupation, humans express the totality of their being, a mind–body–spirit union. Because human existence could not otherwise be, humankind is, in essence, occupational by nature." (Hooper & Wood, 2019, p. 46). Occupational therapy practitioners believe that occupation both brings meaning to and has the power to influence the health of human beings (AOTA, 2020a). The diverse experiences and contexts of occupation across a person's life trajectory are unique. Occupations are meaningful, goal directed and purposeful, provide personal satisfaction, occur over time, may or may not be observed by others, and occur within the contexts of daily life (AOTA, 2020a). They may be completed with others, and as such are called co-occupations.

Occupations include activities of daily living, instrumental activities of daily living, health management, rest and sleep, education, work, play, leisure, and social participation (AOTA, 2020a). These conceptualizations of occupation, however, have been developed, described, and explored primarily in Western cultures and may not fully adapt to or fit with other cultural views and experiences (Whalley Hammell, 2015). To understand how children and families engage in occupations based on their values, beliefs, culture, expectations, routines, and experiences, occupational therapy practitioners engage in conversation and collaborate with children and families to support valued occupations.

This text is devoted specifically to childhood and pediatric occupational therapy practice. Each chapter highlights a specific area or aspect of practice with children and youth to provide readers with detailed information about established current occupational therapy practices informed by evidence, to guide professional reasoning and decision-making. This initial chapter provides an overview of key features of occupational therapy practice during childhood and highlights essential concepts that are presented across multiple chapters.

### What Is Pediatric Occupational Therapy Practice?

Pediatric practice refers to occupational therapy provided to clients in childhood (infants, toddlers, children, and youth) and ends with the period of adulthood. Both childhood and adulthood are socially and culturally defined constructs. In the United States, childhood is commonly considered to be between birth and age 18 years, when a child officially becomes an adult in the eyes of many laws. Adulthood is legally defined as the age of majority, which is defined by the states. However, many adult tasks are allowed at different ages in different states, so the definitions of childhood and adulthood may be blurred. Adult activities are often considered driving, voting, military enlistment, marriage, work, and the use of legal substances such as alcohol and cigarettes. Some of these adult activities are allowed in youth as young as 14–16 years of age and others not until 21 years. Although biologically adulthood begins with puberty, even puberty occurs at different ages for different individuals. And if one considers skeletal development, the last bone to develop occurs at about 25 years

(Smithsonian, 2018). Therefore, childhood and adulthood may overlap in varied ways.

There are large numbers of occupational therapists in pediatric practice. The recent practice analysis by the National Board for Certification in Occupational Therapy (NBCOT, 2018) suggests that 20% of occupational therapists work in this practice area. Of those responding, 15% specified that they worked in the school system (NBCOT, 2018).

Ideally, pediatric occupational therapy practice assists children in engaging in childhood roles in a meaningful and satisfying way and preparing for and attaining adult roles. The varied developmental levels of the clients require a different focus of intervention at times, from other areas of practice. Pediatric practice is also influenced, as are other areas of practice, by a variety of contextual issues such as family engagement, laws, and funding concerns. There are also options for varied models of service delivery in pediatric occupational therapy, some that are used less often in other areas of occupational therapy practice.

## Developmental Impact on the Focus of Intervention

The balance of engagement in varied occupations shifts and changes across the lifespan. In pediatric practice, especially with children as opposed to youth, the occupational therapy practitioner may find themself concerned with play and education rather than work, for example. Working on co-occupations may also be very common in pediatric occupational therapy, where the client, for example an infant, may require the assistance of a caregiver to engage in occupations, such as feeding, dressing, and bathing. Fig. 1.1 shows a parent engaged in the co-occupation of feeding her infant.

A child's level of participation can be influenced by an adult's behavior, affect, attention, engagement, and language use (Pesch et al., 2018; Ryan et al., 2016; Zaidman-Zait et al., 2014). Adult playfulness may enhance a child's attitude, approach, and engagement (i.e., playfulness) (Pinchover, 2017). Therefore, in pediatric practice, the occupational therapy practitioner may need to be playful and creative, as well as immersed in the activity with the child, to gain the child's active engagement in therapeutic activities (Kuhaneck & Spitzer, 2023). Fig. 1.2A and B show a practitioner playfully emoting as the child "works with tools." The practitioner learns how to communicate with children and youth at an appropriate level for their development (PBS, 2018; Traub, 2016) and in ways that encourage interest, curiosity, and a desire to participate in daily activities and occupations.

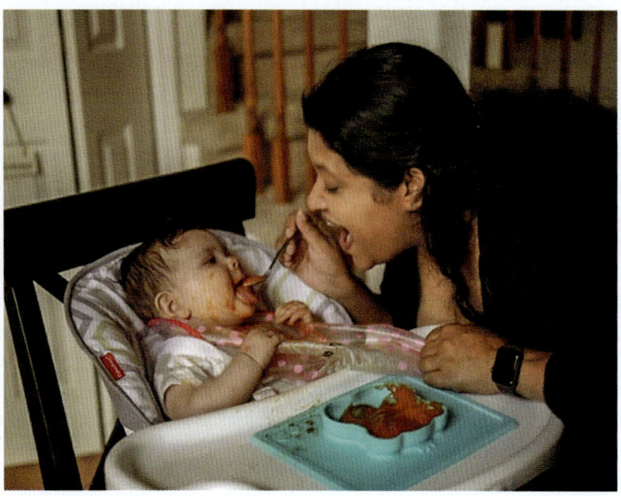

**Fig. 1.1** Occupational therapists may work on co-occupations such as infant feeding.

## Families

Pediatric occupational therapy practitioners work with and manage interactions with various family members, including parents, guardians, grandparents, siblings, and often other extended family members. Although all occupational therapy practitioners consider the life stage of their clients, the rapid changes in child development that occur during early childhood create an additional facet for managing pediatric assessment and intervention. Similarly, although all occupational therapy practitioners consider the client's family members and the familial impact of a client's disability, practitioners working with children and youth must also consider the stage of development the family is in, and support parents or primary caregivers in understanding their child's diagnosis, health management, behaviors, strengths, and challenges (Cadwgan & Goodwin, 2018; Cahill & Beisbier, 2020).

Occupational therapy practitioners working with children and youth must balance and navigate conflicts between the occupational needs and desires of their clients who are minors with those of their parents and other adults who influence them and may attempt to exercise control of their access to specific occupations. They may also need to navigate the differences in opinion regarding a child's capabilities, as parents and children do not always agree on their assessment of the child's ability level (Hemmingsson et al., 2017). Furthermore, young children or children with developmental, cognitive, or language impairments may have difficulty communicating their desires and contributing fully to decisions regarding their intervention plan. Consequently, pediatric occupational therapy practitioners often act as "detectives" to uncover a child's preferred or favored occupation. They watch and observe children closely to understand their style, preferences, motivations, and strengths.

## Legal Influence

For many occupational therapy practitioners the boundaries of "pediatric" practice are defined by law. The Individuals with Disabilities Education Improvement Act of 2004 (IDEA), for example, states that services for individuals receiving special education, end at 21 years of age. The American Occupational Therapy Association (AOTA) also typically ends "pediatric" practice at 21 (Cahill & Beisbier, 2020). Occupational therapy practice with children and youth is also influenced by US policies related to specific settings that pediatric practitioners work in, such as hospitals, early intervention settings, homes, and schools. The laws that apply to occupational therapy practice with infants to children 3 years of age (early intervention) and school age may differ from the laws that influence practice with adult clients. The laws often place different boundaries around occupational therapy practice by specifying the role of the occupational therapy practitioner within that policy's implementation. Additionally, these unique practice settings influence the structure of the teams with whom pediatric occupational therapy practitioners work. For example, since the large majority of pediatric occupational therapists work in public schools, they often collaborate with teachers, school psychologists, administrators, aides, other professionals (e.g., speech therapists, physical therapists, nurses), and parents.

## Funding

Funding issues for occupational therapy for children differ from those for older or working adults. For example, over 9 million children receive funding for their healthcare through the Children's Health Insurance Program (CHIP) (Centers for Medicaid and Medicare Services, 2020). Children may also receive funding for occupational therapy services from Medicaid, or from their caregiver's employer-sponsored insurance. Under Medicaid, occupational therapy is an optional program funded as determined by each state. The variability of insurance coverage for occupational therapy services among funding sources (e.g., employer-sponsored insurance or CHIP) from state to state influences affordability and accessibility to occupational therapy services. Families in poverty-impacted communities may not have consistent access to occupational therapy services for their children.

### Service Delivery Methods in Pediatric Practice

There are a variety of possible service delivery models and methods for pediatric occupational therapy, and choices about service delivery often vary by practice setting. In direct service provision, the child is seen by the occupational therapy practitioner either individually or in a group. In consultation models, the child receives indirect service through the practitioner's collaboration and communication with another professional, such as a teacher. Additional indirect services include advocating on behalf of the client. While the delivery model of telehealth practice has always been an option for rural areas and communities where healthcare services are less accessible, its use emerged and became a more widespread model of service delivery throughout the COVID-19 pandemic that began in 2020. The benefits of its adoption for pediatric occupational therapy services suggest that it will likely continue to be a sought-after option (Camden & Silva, 2021; Hoel et al., 2021). Fig. 1.3 show a telehealth activity for children. Telehealth models are often provided through collaboration, consultation, or coaching, but throughout the pandemic, direct service was also provided in this fashion (Önal et al., 2021). Further adoption and growth will require the profession to create and implement informed practices (Little et al., 2021) and to further document its effectiveness (Baratta-Ziska et al., 2021; Proffitt et al., 2021). See Chapter 6 on settings and Chapter 23 for more information regarding telehealth.

## THE OCCUPATIONAL THERAPY PROCESS IN PEDIATRICS

The occupational therapy process progresses from referral and evaluation, to the creation of an intervention plan (if appropriate),

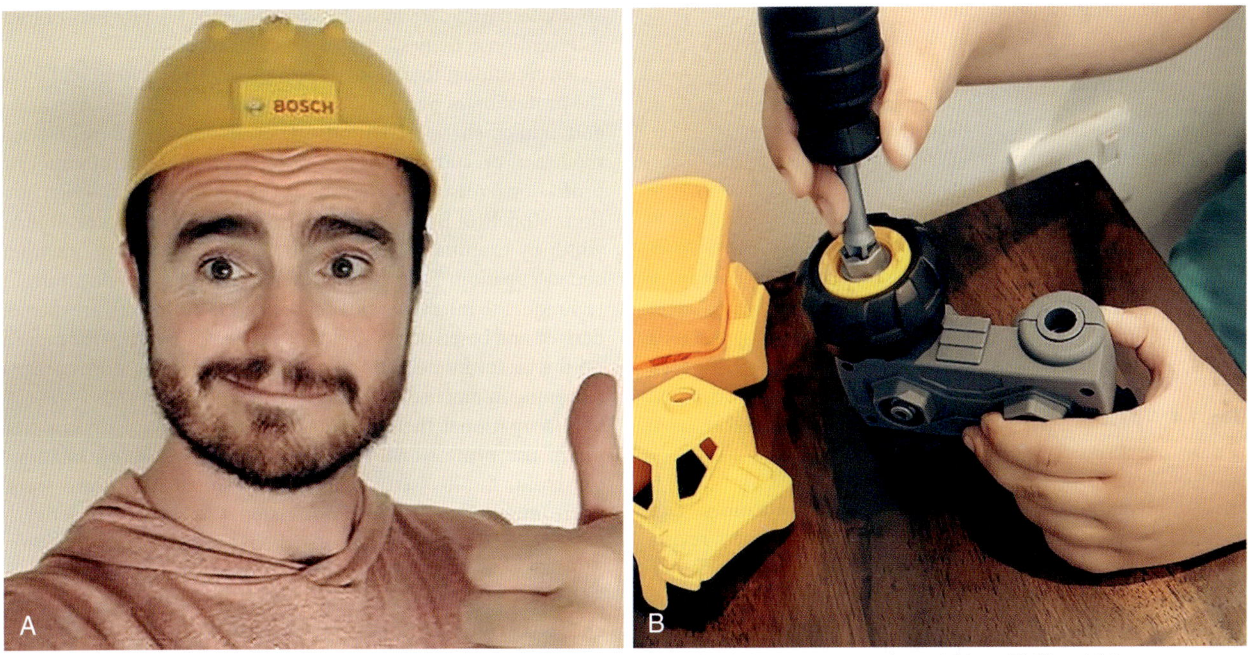
BOSCH
A
B

**Fig. 1.2** (A) Being willing to play and be silly can help with children's engagement in activities. (B) The child uses tools during the playful activity.

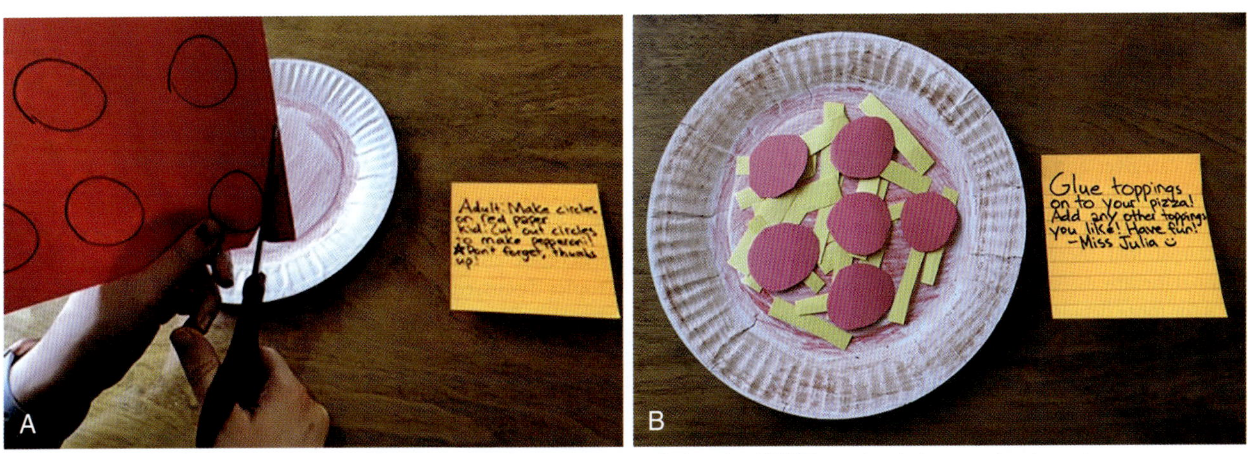
Adult: Make circles on red paper
Kid: Cut out circles to make pepperoni!
★Don't forget, thumbs up!
Glue toppings on to your pizza! Add any other toppings you like! Have fun!
-Miss Julia ☺
A
B

**Fig. 1.3** (A) Telehealth models became more prevalent during the COVID pandemic but require therapists and caregivers to prepare. (B) Sending craft kits to children promotes novelty in the session.

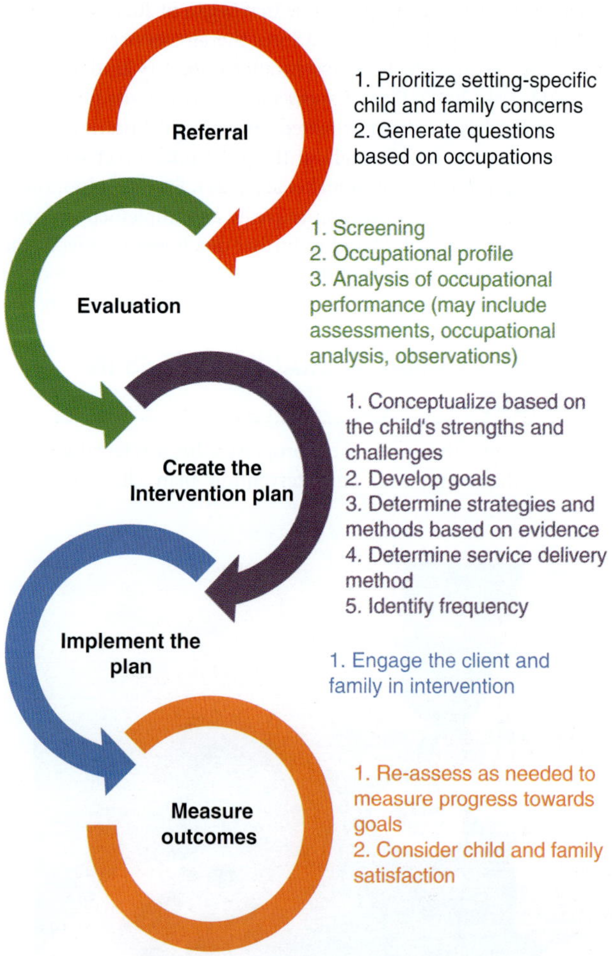


**Fig. 1.4** A description of the occupational therapy process.

implementation of the plan, and measurement of outcomes. Fig. 1.4 illustrates the process. Occupational therapy practitioners revisit the steps in the process often. For example, as practitioners gather new information during intervention, they may decide to further assess a specific area, revise goals, change the intervention priorities or approach, or make additional referrals. The occupational therapy process is dynamic so that the practitioner can adjust and address the child's strengths and challenges over time. See Case Example 1.1 for an overview of the OT process.

Occupational therapists receive referrals from physicians, healthcare professionals, teachers, parents, and caregivers. They follow the guidelines of their state licensure laws and worksite policies when receiving referrals. Once the occupational therapist receives a referral, they begin the evaluation process by gathering information and interviewing the caregiver and child if possible, creating an occupational profile, observing the child's occupational performance, and administering assessments to identify the child's strengths and challenges. While occupational therapists are responsible for the evaluation, occupational therapy assistants may contribute to the evaluation. (See Chapter 9 for more details on the evaluation process.)

They engage in **professional reasoning** (also referred to as clinical reasoning or therapeutic reasoning) as they make decisions, prioritize, and synthesize the information from multiple sources to create meaningful intervention plans for children and their families. Professional reasoning includes integrating knowledge from theory, research evidence, clinical practice, along with client and family information, and it requires practitioners reflect and assess their decisions throughout the process. Fig. 1.5 provides an overview of the professional reasoning process. See Chapter 35 for more information.

Throughout the process, occupational therapy practitioners consider the family, culture, setting, and environmental influences on the child's occupational engagement. Occupational therapists working with children and youth use knowledge of occupational therapy philosophy, conditions, development, neurology, psychology, and information from occupation-centered models of practice and frames of reference to structure the evaluation (O'Brien, 2023).

Following the evaluation, occupational therapists synthesize all the information to create intervention plans to enable children to participate in meaningful activities by (1) providing interventions to enhance performance; (2) recommending activity adaptations, accommodations, and environmental modifications; (3) consulting, coaching, and educating children on ways to participate in their desired roles; and (4) advocating for services or occupational opportunities. Occupational therapy practitioners use multiple approaches to support the child's ability to participate in daily activities. Box 1.1 provides examples of intervention activities.

Occupational therapists rely on theory from within and outside of the profession of occupational therapy to evaluate children and youth and implement interventions. They use both occupation-centered models of practice and frames of reference as underpinnings of their professional reasoning to structure the evaluation and design intervention. Models of practice provide a structure to evaluate children and youth by examining the interactions between person, environment, and occupation. Frames of reference provide specific strategies and techniques to intervene with children and youth. Both are theoretically derived and based on research evidence. See Chapter 9 for more details on the use of models and frames of reference to inform professional reasoning in practice.

Occupational therapy practitioners working with children and youth use professional reasoning to synthesize information from the child, family, setting, interprofessional healthcare team, and environment, along with professional theory, knowledge, experience, and research to create client-centered intervention plans. They use evidence to guide the process and inform intervention planning. They gather information throughout the process to influence goals, interventions, and approaches. They collaborate with the child and family and include them in all aspects of service delivery by engaging them in shared decision-making. Occupational therapy practitioners engage in child- and family-centered practice to help children and youth achieve important and meaningful goals. This requires practitioners to work collaboratively and communicate clearly with team members. They document services regularly and communicate with clients, family, and team members to benefit children and youth.

## ESSENTIAL CONCEPTS IN PEDIATRIC OCCUPATIONAL THERAPY PRACTICE

There are components of pediatric practice that cross many of the topics discussed in the following chapters of this text. These components, referred to as essential concepts, are ideas, philosophies, methods, or strategies that are important within all pediatric settings and areas of focus of intervention, makeup of teams, or the experiences of the individual practitioner. These essential concepts are discussed in the following section and embedded throughout the chapters of this book.

## CASE EXAMPLE 1.1 OCCUPATIONAL THERAPY PROCESS FOR EARLY INTERVENTION

**Referral**

Miracle is a 3-month old infant who was born at 30 weeks' gestation to a 16-year-old single mother. Miracle was hospitalized for 4 weeks, where she received occupational therapy for issues related to feeding. She was referred by the neonatologist for follow up at the High-Risk Clinic.

**Screening**

The occupational therapist completed a screening that included an interview with the mother (occupational profile) and a quick developmental screening. Based on findings from the screening, the therapist recommended that Miracle receive a more thorough occupational therapy evaluation of feeding/eating, motor, and cognitive development, in order to provide education and support to the mother.

**Evaluation**

The occupational therapist completed an in-depth evaluation of the infant's development by completing the Hawaii Early Learning Profile (HELP), which provides age ranges for development of fine and gross motor, social, self-care, language, and cognition. The HELP also provides a visual display of the infant's progress and specific activities for the parent to address. The therapist thought that the HELP could provide the mother information on child development and the mother noted that she wanted more information. The therapist also completed an observation of the child's motor, sensory, behaviors, and feeding, and a medical record review.

**Interpretation and Goal Setting**

The occupational therapist noted Miracle's strengths as motor abilities to reach, take a bottle, smile, and indicate her wants. Her mother is curious, asks and responds to questions, and has support from her mother and several friends. Miracle shows difficulty maintaining a strong suck–swallow–breathe pattern and takes frequent breaks during bottle feeding. She is gaining weight at a slow rate and is in the low percentage for her corrected age. Miracle was born prematurely and is at risk for developmental delays. Together, the therapist and mother collaborated on the following goals for Miracle.

1. Within 3 months (6 months corrected age), Miracle will achieve developmental milestones within corrected age expectations (as measured by HELP) for motor, social, and self-help.
2. Within 2 weeks (3.5 months corrected age), Miracle will consume 4 oz from the bottle within 10 min.
3. Within 4 weeks (4 months corrected age), Miracle will establish a sleep–wake routine.

**Intervention**

Occupational therapy intervention consisted of establishing daily routines to support feeding, play, and rest routines; developing Miracle's suck–swallow–breathe coordination for feeding; and promoting self-soothing strategies and play, cognitive, and social development. The therapist coached and advised Miracle's mother on strategies to promote infant development and validated her efforts. As new issues arose, such as Miracle's sporadic sleep schedule, the therapist and parent created strategies to establish daily patterns and problem-solved methods to support routines. They discussed each week's progress and adjusted methods as needed. This family-centered collaborative approach empowered Miracle's mother as a parent.

**Monitoring Progress**

They used the HELP, weight gain, and food intake to measure Miracle's progress in therapy. As Miracle progressed they promoted new motor, social, cognitive skills. The therapist monitored her progress weekly as they engaged in play and feeding activities. For example, they made note of her motor abilities as well as her ability to self-soothe, indicate her wants, make choices, and interact. They reflected each week on Miracle's activities and problem-solved together to decide when to gather new information and how that affected the intervention process.

**Discharge**

Miracle made progress on her feeding/eating and met her goals within 3 months of therapy. She achieved her developmental milestones (as measured by the HELP) within age expectations by 1 year of age (corrected age). At this time, Miracle was discharged from early intervention services and scheduled for a screening in 6 months.

## Occupational Engagement

The focus of occupational therapy intervention is to enable children to engage in occupations in a way that makes sense for them. Occupational engagement refers to the ability to participate and complete the tasks and activities associated with the routine that fulfills one's desired roles within the natural context. For example, a child gets dressed, puts his shoes on, and grabs his backpack from the hallway before running out to the school bus. These tasks and activities are part of his daily routine and essential to his role as family member. The tasks may differ from other children, whose families may engage in alternate morning routines. In this case, the child is engaged in his occupation of belonging to his particular family. A child engaging in eating his birthday cake with his family is shown in Fig. 1.6.

Occupational therapy practitioners use occupation as both the goal of intervention and as the tool or method to reach the goals. The art of therapy involves creating intervention that focuses on occupational engagement outcomes by promoting the child's strengths, while also addressing factors that may be interfering with the child's participation. Occupational therapy practitioners working with children and youth may decide to adapt the occupation or environment so that the child may engage along with peers in the natural setting. They may decide to work on the child's performance challenges in therapy as well.

Occupational therapy approaches that address holistic, meaningful, and goal-oriented activities are more effective than interventions targeting specific parts or components of activities (Kreider et al., 2014; Pfeiffer et al., 2018; Rodger & Polatajko, 2017). The use of occupation-centered approaches for children is supported by research and by theories of motor control and motor learning (Cano-De-La-Cuerda et al., 2015). Holistic activities with multiple steps and a meaningful goal (vs. repetition of activity components) and use of the actual objects elicit the child's full engagement and participation. Repeating a single component (e.g., squeeze the Play-Doh or place pennies in a can) has minimal therapeutic value. By engaging in an activity with a meaningful goal and emphasis on the process (e.g., cooking or an art project), children use multiple systems and organize their performance around that goal. If a game requires that a preschool child attend to a peer, wait for their turn, and correctly place a game piece, the child develops attention needed to participate in circle time or a family meal. Approaches that acknowledge the importance of engaging children in meaningful, purposeful activities to harness their motivation and full efforts result in improved motor, cognitive, and social performance (see Chapter 29).

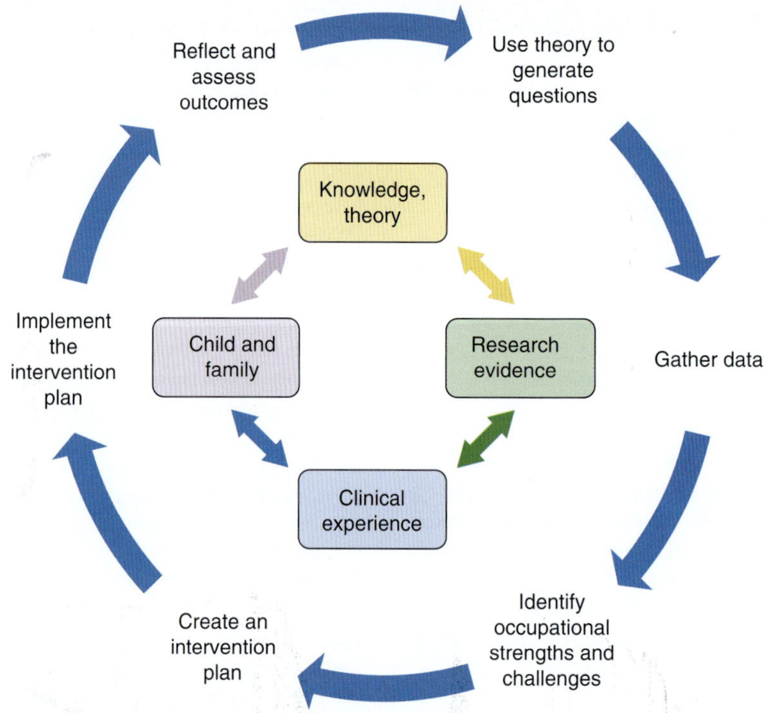


**Fig. 1.5** Professional reasoning process. (Adapted from Patnaude, M. E. (2023). Student success: Therapeutic reasoning progress. In Jane Clifford O'Brien, M. E. Patnaude, & T. G. Reidy (Eds.), *Therapeutic reasoning in occupational therapy: How to develop critical thinking for practice* (p. 8). Elsevier.)

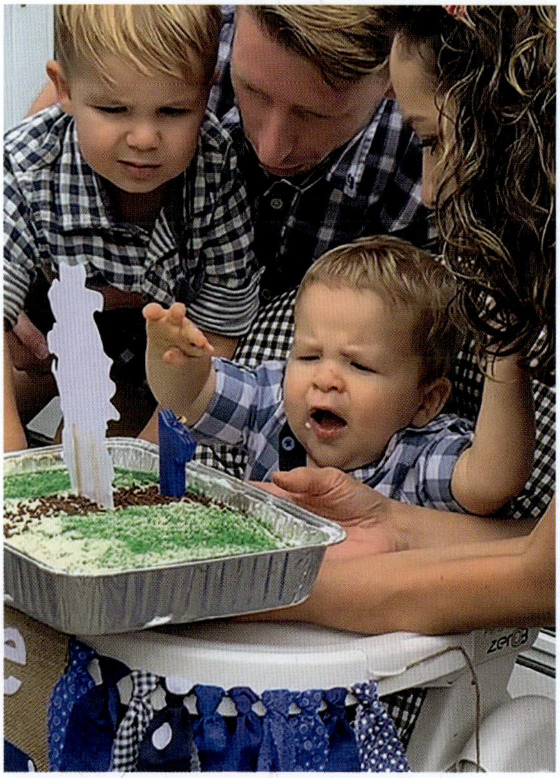

**Fig. 1.6** Occupational therapy supports child engagement in the typical routines of a family.

## Cultural Humility

Pediatric occupational therapy practitioners often work with families and children from different backgrounds or cultures than their own. They use information about the family's culture, values, beliefs, customs, roles, habits, and routines to determine valued occupations and priorities. For example, parents differ in their expectations of their children regarding behaviors, feeding, dressing, school, work, and social participation. Understanding the families' structure, goals, expectations, and routines helps the practitioners develop a therapeutic relationship to benefit the child and family. Occupational therapy practitioners working with children and families learn from each other, which requires respect, active listening, and nonjudgmental actions. Having an awareness of cultural values and beliefs, and knowledge and understanding of varied cultures (i.e., cultural competence), and one's own cultural point of view can be important; however, practitioners must demonstrate cultural humility in practice (Lekas et al., 2020).

**Cultural humility** refers to "the ability to maintain an interpersonal stance that is other oriented (or open to the other) in relation to aspects of cultural identity that are most important to the [person]" (Hook et al., 2013, p. 2). Three components of cultural humility are important to occupational therapy practitioners.

1. Commitment to lifelong learning, self-evaluation, and a humble boldness to enable self-critique with an openness to change and growth (Tervalon & Murray-Garcia, 1998)
2. Recognition of the role of power in healthcare interactions and desire to fix or alter imbalances of power (Agner, 2020)
3. Partnering with those who advocate for others to create systems change

By engaging in self-evaluation of their own biases and positions, occupational therapy practitioners practice lifelong learning and demonstrate willingness to change. Occupational therapy practitioners recognize the potential power imbalance in the provision of health care and work alter imbalances. For example, they acknowledge that parents are the most knowledgeable experts about their own children.

## BOX 1.1 Examples of Occupational Therapy Intervention Activities

**Sample Intervention Activities**

**Interventions to enhance performance:** Activities that facilitate the child's skills and ability through repetition.

- *Self-feeding:* Games to pick up spoons, hold objects, scoop sand, pick up small foods
- *Dressing:* Pretend games to put on costumes, dress up, playing with a variety of hats, treasure boxes full of fasteners
- *Bathing:* Water play, bubbles, play in sprinklers, washing hands prior to snacks, washing dolls or toy animals
- *Hygiene/grooming:* Makeup games, "hair styling"
- *Fine motor:* Finger plays and craft games, playing the keyboard or musical instruments, grasping toys, writing, coloring, paint by numbers, spinning tops, toys to sort, popsicle sticks construction
- *Gross motor:* Dance party, crawling like animals, tag, outdoor games, climbing, swinging, obstacle courses
- *Oral motor:* Bubbles, making silly noises, singing, imitating funny faces, kazoos, harmonicas, recorders
- *Sensory:* Shaving cream play, making things with different textures (e.g., sandpaper, cotton balls, satin), slime, water tables, playing in the sprinkler, sandcastles, balance games, hop when you hear a noise, smelly games, I Spy, Where's Waldo?
- *Social participation:* Games to take turns, sharing items, partner games, such as team treasure hunts together, ball games, cat's cradle string games, jump ropes, playing games to learn about each other, such as icebreakers

**Activity adaptations:** Making changes to how activities are completed so that children can participate in their desired activities.

- *Cognitive:* Simplify directions, provide visual instructions, prepare activity to eliminate difficult steps for child, allow child more time or adapted materials to allow them to succeed, provide cues (e.g., visual cues, verbal cues) to assist child
- *Social:* Change activities to support social interactions, provide opportunities for a child to interact with an older child in one-on-one situations to learn behaviors, keep initial activities short with minimal social requirements (such as playing catch), engage children in social activities with products, such as playing a game where each team must find three objects. Engage a child in social activities they enjoy or design them using the child's interests (e.g., a sport, hobby, or object the child likes).
- *Fine motor:* Change the fine motor manipulation or handling requirements by providing different equipment (such as adapted handled scissors, crayons, or pencils). Use built-up handles, lighter weighted objects, and change activities so a child who has fine motor challenges can be successful. For example, a school-age child may use a computer keyboard instead of a pencil for writing at times. Change dressing requirements by providing children with pull-up pants or loose t-shirts (to eliminate some fine motor requirements).
- *Mobility:* Finding mobility devices that suit the child's needs (such as scooters, wheelchairs). Engaging the child in obstacle courses and training activities so they can effectively maneuver as desired. Providing the child with multiple types of equipment options so they can engage in activities in a variety of positions (such as sitting, standing, side lying).

**Consulting, coaching, educating:** Supporting children by consulting, educating, or coaching others to understand the child's unique situation. Supporting the child's ability to engage in desired occupations by coaching and educating them.

- Consulting with others on how to support children in school, home, and community
- Educating others on child's strengths and challenges (and ways to support child to do those things they want to do)
- Coaching others and children on strategies to engage in meaningful activities
- Educating children on how to engage in desired activities with their unique strengths and challenges
- Consulting with children and family as challenges arise to problem-solve solutions together

**Advocating:** Identifying the child and family's needs and seeking ways to support them.

- Advocating for wheelchair-accessible classrooms and buildings, paths in the community
- Securing equipment for children
- Creating or finding training and support systems (such as parent support groups) for children and families
- Finding opportunities for social and leisure activities for children of all abilities (such as dance classes at all levels)
- Knowing resources available to children and families and helping them access them

Occupational therapy practitioners showing cultural humility acknowledge, identify, and support changes in systems that are unfair or biased against children and families. This may include practices whereby funding sources limit needed services for children. They engage in advocacy at many levels to ensure that children receive equal occupational opportunities. For example, they may advocate for technology, environmental modifications, or academic accommodations to support a child's ability to participate in daily activities with peers. Please also see Chapter 4 on embracing diversity in practice. Understanding the beliefs, values, habits, routines, and family structure is essential for engaging in child- and family-centered occupational therapy practice.

### Child- and Family-Centered Practice

Occupational therapy practitioners enable children to participate in occupations that are meaningful to them and allow them to engage with others. In child-centered practice, children are given choices to the extent that they are able to participate in making them. Children participate in decision-making and occupational therapy practitioners use activities that are meaningful and preferred by the child, knowing that they engage the child's efforts. Occupational therapy practitioners following child-centered practice value and respect children by asking for their perceptions, including them in goal setting, listening to their feedback, and planning activities for which the child prefers.

**Child-centered practice** is an approach that often includes asking children questions as part of the initial evaluation process. For example, the practitioner may ask children to complete a self-report questionnaire (e.g., the Child Occupational Self Assessment) indicating activities they feel they are "good" at and identifying activities that they find challenging. Children as young as 5 may be able to complete self-report measures (Conijn et al., 2020; Varni et al., 2007). However, because children are minors and not yet completely responsible for their own health care, occupational therapy practitioners must also engage in family-centered practices.

**Family-centered practice** involves understanding the family environment, expectations, and goals. Occupational therapy practitioners work closely with family members to support their children in doing meaningful activities within their environment. They celebrate the family's success and encourage family members to engage in the

## BOX 1.2 Family-Centered Activities

**Family-Centered Activities**

The following examples of activities were specifically designed to allow children to be a part of their family and to participate fully. Each example allowed the occupational therapy practitioner to work with the child on the performance skills required to engage in the activities. Each activity was created based on the family's routines and expectations.

*Baking with Grammy*: When informed that Grammy was visiting and she liked to bake, the practitioner found a simple recipe that the child could make with Grammy. They practiced the skills in the therapy session. The child was able to match the ingredients with the pictures and directions.

*Dancing with Big Sister:* The practitioner and child (a 5-year-old boy) practiced a variety of simple dance moves so the child could show his 7-year-old sister. They added music and simple routines (such as holding hands at certain points or reaching toward the sky). Over the weekend, the child and his sister practiced the moves. The child was excited to tell the practitioner about which dances they liked the best and work on new routines.

*Morning Routine:* A 10-year-old child had difficulty with her family's morning routine. The practitioner worked with the child to develop a plan, schedule, and practice each step during the therapy sessions. Together, they streamlined tasks to minimize the amount that the child needed to complete. For example, the child decided to pick out their clothes the night before and have breakfast "to-go" style. After discussing options with the parents, they also decided to wake the child up 15 min before everyone else so they could have uninterrupted morning time.

therapy process. For example, a father built a child-sized prone stander for his son. The practitioner used the prone stander in the next session with the child and praised the construction and child-friendly design. The father was proud he provided a much-needed piece of equipment to benefit his child; the child enjoyed standing and playing; and the practitioner incorporated standing activities as part of the home program. Box 1.2 provides some examples of family-centered activities. Case Example 1.2 provides an example of focusing on important family concerns when creating intervention. Chapters 4 and 22 expand upon family-centered care.

Occupational therapists (in collaboration with occupational therapy assistants) create goals and interventions that reinforce the family's culture, roles, and routines to ensure carryover and support the child and family. They do this by listening to parents and children and considering their views on feeding, play, leisure, academics, and social participation when designing intervention. They respond to the family's views, roles, time, and structure when creating home programs. They support the child's engagement in their family and community (such as community sports and play as shown in Fig. 1.7). The unique family situations may result in creative intervention that is reinforced by the family structure.

## CASE EXAMPLE 1.2 JAMAL

Jamel is a 3-year-old boy who loves to play with balls. His mother notes that Jamel enjoys playing by himself. At daycare, he has his own toys so that he does not have to share them. The daycare workers allow Jamel to play in a quiet area outside and he has a corner inside. He becomes upset when he must share things or when there is too much going on.

Jamel has been receiving occupational therapy services in an outpatient setting to prepare him for school. The goal is that Jamel learns to play with others, take turns, and express his needs using his words. The practitioner enjoys their low-key therapy sessions and Jamel has begun to share with the practitioner. Specifically, he will play catch and is starting to accept more noise and activity in the session.

In a conversation with his mother, the practitioner learned that she is concerned that Jamel has difficulty playing with his cousins on Sundays, where the extended family meets after church each week. Furthermore, his parents hear from well-meaning relatives about what they "should do" to make Jamel behave. The stress of his behavior has caused his parents to dread extended family events that they have always enjoyed.

The occupational therapy practitioner listened empathetically to the mother, and they decided to work on this goal. The practitioner asked the mother if she could bring an older cousin into a session so together, they could work on his play skills. After two sessions, his mother reported that the Sunday gatherings had improved. Jamel's older cousin looked after Jamel when they played with the others. Jamel's behavior and play with his cousins improved as he felt comfortable with his older cousin. The extended family members saw Jamel's improvements and remarked on his strengths. As they became more involved with the family's story, they felt connected and empathetic. They began to praise the parents for their patience, and even revealed stories of their own children's behaviors. The parents felt supported once again by their extended family.

### Strengths-Based Approaches

While medical and diagnostic models suggest looking for and then "fixing" or remediating weaknesses, **strengths-based approaches** emphasize a child's strengths and individuality, as everyone has strengths that support their own personal style. Based in positive psychology and disability justice, advocates for strengths-based approaches in the disability community have grown steadily in number and voice (Buntinx, 2013; Niemiec et al., 2017; Russo, 1999), eventually leading to a recent Eleanor Clark Slagle lecture focusing on this topic (Patten, 2022).

Strengths-based approaches owe their origins to White's (1959) focus on competence, but they grew dramatically throughout the 1990s, with the term appearing more than 20 times in one book of the period (Greene & Watkins, 1998). Simple searches of literature from the 1990s document the increasing use of the concept in evaluation and assessment, with an emphasis on empowerment, and giving "voice" to those who are marginalized (Boorman et al., 2009; Corbett, 1998; Cowger, 1994; Dewees, 1999).

Occupational therapists (with input from occupational therapy assistants) evaluate the child and family's strengths as a way to create a rapport and support growth in a child's strengths. They use the child's strengths to work on areas that the child finds challenging. This approach contrasts with the traditional medical model, which focuses intervention on identifying the health or performance problem and resolving that problem (Dunn, 2017). Focusing on a child's performance problems does not always lead to optimal participation and improved quality of life. Because occupational therapy practitioners are concerned with a child's full participation in life activities, focusing solely on impairment narrows the vision of what the child can become and do. Therefore, occupational therapy practitioners working with children and youth empower children and families by focusing on their strengths.

Children and youth with disabilities have unique strengths that, when identified and promoted, can lead to increased participation and confidence. Therefore, occupational therapists evaluate the strengths of a child or youth in addition to trying to understand their difficulties and challenges. Intentionally beginning an evaluation of a child's strengths can build rapport, establish trust, create an atmosphere of positive expectancy, destigmatize treatment, and empower a child

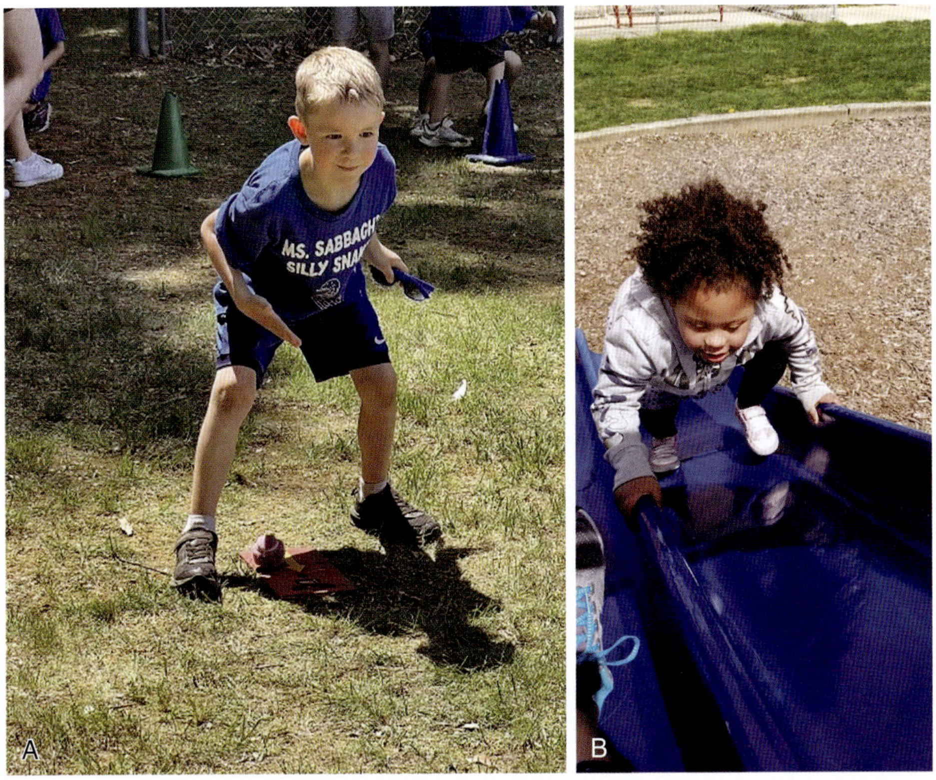


**Fig. 1.7** Occupational therapy supports child engagement in typical school and community activities such as field day (A) and playing in the playground (B).

to begin thinking about their own goals from the very first meeting (O'Brien & Schlechter, 2016). Assessing a child to first determine who they are when they are at their best, and subsequently asking about any barriers or challenges that are preventing them from being their best, engages the child in goal setting. See Fig. 1.8.

Occupational therapy interventions build on a child's strengths. Therefore, occupational therapists identify children's strengths early in the occupational therapy process. By identifying the positive aspects of a child's behavior and areas of greatest competence as well as performance limitations, they can affirm for parents and caregivers that a child's diagnosis does not define them, emphasize ability beyond disability, and instill hope in parents when they are reminded that their child has positive qualities that may only be temporarily shadowed by current challenges (O'Brien & Schlechter, 2016). For example, focusing on the strengths of a child who has autism when communicating with parents has been shown to result in parents displaying more positive affect, making more positive statements about their child, exhibiting greater physical affection toward their child (Steiner, 2011) and increasing leisure participation and self-efficacy (Ullenhag et al., 2020).

In strengths-based approaches, the goal is not that every child does things in the same way or at the same time. Rather, the goal is that children do things in their own way and fulfill their potential. Strengths-based approaches suggest that each child and youth may develop their own abilities to do things in their unique ways. For example, a child with strengths in visual perception and drawing may use these skills to help himself comprehend more difficult academic topics. A child with verbal strengths but difficulty with fine motor skills may engage with schoolwork verbally rather than in written form. The occupational therapy practitioner helps the child capitalize on their strengths in activity choices as well, for example encouraging a child with vocal talent to join with peers in a choir.

The following characteristics determine if an approach is strengths based (Rapp et al., 2008).

- Strengths-based approaches assist people in achieving their goals.
- The individual is encouraged and supported to recognize their own resources and abilities to adapt to or counteract difficulties that they might have.
- The practitioner believes that there is something that the situation or the person has to give or offer that may be useful. It is the practitioner's role to foster that link.
- Strengths-based approaches identify specific methods for determining strengths and using them to achieve goals.
- The relationship between client and practitioner is one of hope.
- Practitioners using strengths-based approaches collaborate with clients and empower client choice and decision-making.

Pediatric occupational therapy practitioners must emphasize a strengths-based approach throughout all aspects of the occupational therapy process to fully embrace the potential of this approach to produce positive changes for families and pediatric clients. As research suggests that the occupational therapy practitioner's documentation is frequently written with a deficit focus (Braun et al., 2017), documentation is a specific aspect of practice to attend to carefully. Case Example 1.3 provides an example of using a strengths-based focus with a child with autism.

## Active Involvement of Child

The pediatric occupational therapy practitioner collaborates with the child to select an activity of interest, make the activity fun and playful, and give the child choices throughout the process (Kuhaneck & Spitzer, 2023). Children are more intrinsically motivated to take on skill challenges that they have designated as

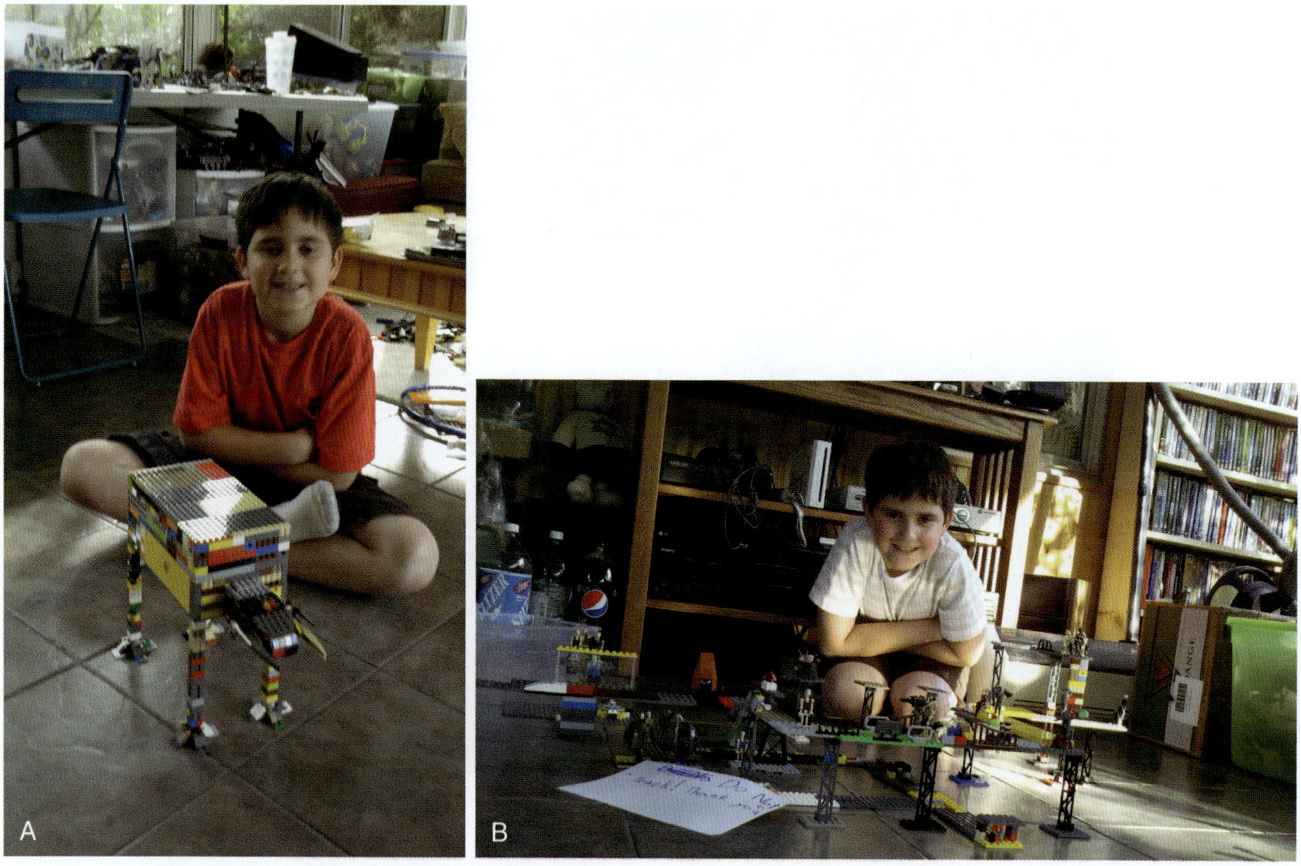

**Fig. 1.8** (A and B) An autistic child with special strengths in visual construction and creativity in design. An important role for occupational therapists is finding out about a child's strengths and preferences during evaluation, so that these can be used in intervention.

important and that the practitioner embeds in preferred activities as shown in Fig. 1.9. The child's engagement in activity is an essential component of a therapy session. This engagement funnels children's energy into the activity, helps them sustain full attention, and implies that they have adopted a goal and purpose that fuels performance in the activity.

When children are provided with support that enables them to focus on and engage fully in a learning activity, they are more likely to persevere and attempt challenging aspects of the activity. Generally, the intrinsic sense of mastery is a stronger reinforcement to the child and youth with greater probability of sustained effects than external rewards, such as verbal praise or other reward systems. When children are motivated to participate and share positive affect and the experience with others involved in an activity, they will more readily sustain engagement with that activity which promotes their learning (Froiland & Oros, 2014; Gopalan et al., 2017; Master et al., 2017).

Activities without social features or those that provide extrinsic motivation may not capture and sustain engagement for as long and may not improve learning outcomes (McKernan et al., 2015; Ronimus et al., 2014). Occupational therapy practitioners working with children and youth seek to actively engage children in activities that are internally motivating for them. Tapping into the child's inner desires promotes engagement and motor, social, and cognitive learning. Engagement is essential because the child's brain responds differently and learns more effectively when they are actively involved in a task rather than merely receiving passive stimulation.

## Just-Right Challenge

A child's active participation and efforts to achieve a task are elicited when therapeutic activities are at just the right level of complexity; that is, where the child not only feels comfortable and nonthreatened but also experiences some challenge that requires effort. An activity that is a child's **just-right challenge** (Ayres, 1972; Burke, 1977; Mack et al., 1982; Yerxa, 1981) has the following elements: the activity (1) matches the child's developmental skills and interests; (2) provides a reasonable challenge to current performance level; (3) engages and motivates the child; and (4) can be mastered with the child's focused effort.

Based on careful analysis of performance and behavior, the occupational therapy practitioner selects an activity that matches the child's strengths and limitations across performance domains. The analysis allows the practitioner to individualize the difficulty, pace, and level of support needed for a child to accomplish a task. The occupational therapy practitioner carefully observes the child's performance to determine whether the activity needs to be "graded," meaning made easier or more challenging, and the precise levels of support that enable the child to succeed. Cognitive, sensory, motor, perceptual, or social aspects of the activity may be made easier or more difficult (see Case Example 1.4). By precisely assessing the adequacy of the child's response, the practitioner finds the just-right challenge. Similarly, they support the child's choice of activity by modifying or adapting it in necessary ways to ensure the child's success.

While the occupational therapy practitioner often presents challenges and asks children to take risks, they also support and facilitate children's performance so that either children succeed, or feel okay when they do not (D'Arrigo et al., 2020). By choosing activities that

### Case Example 1.3 A Strengths-Based Approach

Victor is a 10-year-old autistic boy. He has excellent visual perceptual skills and visual memory. He desperately wants to have a friend to play with. However, he also has difficulty knowing how to interact with his peers on the playground or in unstructured social activities.

Amy, the occupational therapist, uses a strengths-based approach with Victor. To promote Victor's self-determination (ability to make his own choices), she listens to his concern and they focus therapy sessions on his goal of having a friend. Amy works collaboratively with Victor to identify games he is good at, using his visual perceptual and memory skills. She encourages him to consider ways to find friends who might like to play the games he likes to play. He tells Amy about the games he enjoys, such as Lego GearBots and chess. Together they investigate clubs and afterschool activities that involve chess or Lego building. Although they did not find anything appropriate related to Lego, they found a local beginner chess group for people his age.

Together they strategize about how he could engage in that group with new peers. They watch videos of groups of people his age that they find online. They discuss and analyze how the peers interact and they develop specific strategies and scripts for Victor to try, in order to initiate and continue conversations with new people.

Victor practices some of the interactions with her during occupational therapy sessions. They also look for photos online of examples of social interactions (greetings, handshakes, hugs), discuss when each type was appropriate and not appropriate, and together they organize the photos into stories he can use to learn to engage with others socially. They create a visual step-by-step procedure for initiating a social interaction.

After practicing the skills in both occupational therapy sessions and at home Victor felt ready, and he and his family went to the community organization that hosted the chess club. He introduced himself to peers who also liked chess, and as he had rehearsed, Victor had conversations with peers, played chess with new people of his age, and began the process of developing a friendship.

With the strengths-based approach in occupational therapy, Victor learned new skills (e.g., social, planning, problem-solving) while reinforcing his strengths at making choices and carrying out a plan (that might be out of his comfort zone) to meet an important goal for himself. His peers recognized and appreciated his talent, establishing enhanced contexts for social participation.

allow children to feel important and by grading activities to match abilities, occupational therapy practitioners give children the opportunity to achieve mastery and a sense of accomplishment. Practitioners are invested in the children's success, and reinforce the importance of children's efforts. As children experience mastery and success by overcoming challenges, they develop self-confidence and self-efficacy, which promote self-determination and occupational identity.

## Self-Efficacy and Self-Determination

***Self-efficacy*** refers to "beliefs in one's capabilities to organize and execute the courses of action required to produce given attainments" (Bandura, 1997, p. 3). For children, one can think of self-efficacy as children's belief in their ability to do the things they want to do, associated with their perceived confidence. Children who have a positive self-efficacy believe they can achieve in school, have friends, and participate in social activities. They exhibit a positive self-esteem (i.e., I am able to do things well and have a variety of skills).

**Self-determination** is the ability to act in one's life and includes one's perceptions of (1) autonomy (i.e., choice of actions, decisions), (2) competence (i.e., belief that you are effective and have the abilities to act), and (3) relatedness (i.e., sense of belonging) (Deci & Ryan, 2008). Children with positive self-determination can make choices and problem-solve to complete activities, while feeling they are in control of the outcomes and supported in doing the things they want to do. For example, a child who is self-determined is able to decide what to write about during "free writing" time in school. They may feel good about the story and look forward to reading it to classmates. They feel they are a good writer and the story is creative.

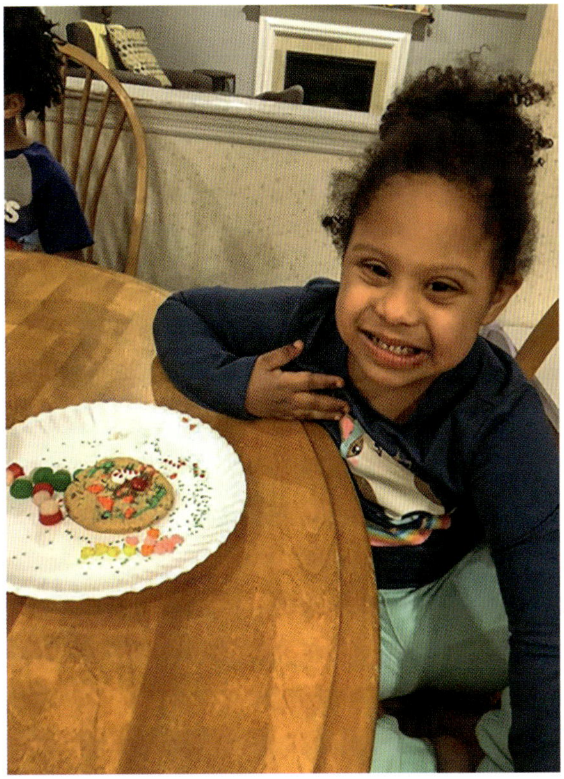

Fig. 1.9 Children are more invested in therapy if the intervention activities are preferred and meaningful, such as decorating cookies for a family party.

Self-efficacy and self-determination are influenced by mindset, skill achievement, success, and mastery. To build confidence and self-efficacy, the activity should not be too easy so the child succeeds every attempt, but rather children benefit from being challenged to problem-solve and "figure things out." The occupational therapy practitioner uses therapeutic reasoning to select tasks that allow the child to experience the excitement that comes with "figuring it out" and problem-solving to complete the task. Occupational therapy practitioners embrace a **growth mindset**, which proposes that skills can be acquired with time as opposed to a fixed mindset, which proposes that skills are innate and fixed (Yeager & Dweck, 2020). Working to accomplish a goal or task that may be considered "out of reach" promotes a growth mindset and feelings of autonomy, mastery, and self-determination, which are important to lifelong learning and confidence in oneself (Ryan & Deci, 2020).

## Occupational Identity

As children and youth realize their strengths and challenges and their ability to make choices, they establish a sense of self within those things that they do, which is referred to as one's **occupational identity** (O'Brien, 2017). A child's occupational identity is reflected in what activities they currently do to make up their day and what they have done in the past. Occupational therapy practitioners engage children

## CASE EXAMPLE 1.4 GRADING ACTIVITIES IN INTERVENTION

Ben is a 6-year-old boy who "hates school." He liked Kindergarten and made friends, but first grade is difficult for him. He does not want to go to school and his teacher says he refuses to participate. The occupational therapist at school was consulted as the teacher noted that Ben has trouble coloring, falls on the playground, and bumps into the desks in the classroom. His mother noted that Ben is slow to follow directions.

The occupational therapy evaluation revealed that Ben likes to please others, but lately he feels he cannot do "anything right." Ben is creative and verbal, and has a sense of humor. He did well on cognitive items where he verbalized answers but scored low on items when he had to copy letters or imitate movements. He showed poor motor planning skills. The therapist hypothesized that Ben's poor motor planning and desire to please others cause him to become very frustrated with himself, leading to low self-efficacy (i.e., belief in his abilities) especially now that in first grade he has to do more writing and activities that require motor planning (such as copying from board, and following more complex instructions for classroom activities).

The occupational therapist conceptualized that Ben's behaviors have arisen since he finds the activities too challenging for his current motor abilities. Since Ben is aware of his challenges, he is handling them by refusing to engage. The therapist worked to grade many of his classroom activities to ensure they were achievable for him. For example, she obtained classroom worksheets ahead of time and, in collaboration with the teacher, reduced the writing demands of the worksheets. Copying from the board was adjusted to copying from another paper at his desk.

The therapist provided Ben with larger rings attached to his zippers to help him grasp and pull the zippers up and also adapted his backpack with a "cool" zipper pull making it easier for him to access. The therapist also consulted with the phys ed teacher to ensure that while Ben plays the same games as his peers, the class is given a variety of options for each activity so that Ben is not singled out, but he can manage the motor demands and succeed. The therapist requires that Ben reflect on his "stars" for the session so that he verbalizes those things he achieved as a way to build his sense of competency. They also discuss classroom "stars" so he begins to see his strengths in the classroom. As Ben begins to feel better about his abilities (and gain more skills), he engages in the learning. The teacher, parent, and therapist all adjust activities so he is successful. They allow Ben to problem-solve, figure things out, and try several times as well so that when he does achieve success, he feels accomplished.

The just-right challenge cannot be too easy or children will not develop that sense of accomplishment. The just-right challenge is also not so hard that it causes children to feel discouraged. Occupational therapy practitioners adjust tasks or activities or the requirements of them to enable children to complete desired occupations while feeling empowered to succeed.

and youth in exploring a variety of activities to experience new occupations or engage in previous occupations in different ways to help them gain new skills, adapt to new challenges, and establish an occupational identity (O'Brien, 2017).

## Generalization of Intervention

The goal of learning is to apply skills and abilities in a variety of situations in flexible ways. Occupational therapy practitioners carefully plan strategies for children to generalize newly learned skills across a variety of environments. Recognizing that transfer of new skills to natural environments does not always automatically follow performance of that skill in an intervention session, occupational therapy practitioners plan multiple ways for children to practice new skills in various ways. To support the generalization of new skills into daily environments, occupational therapy practitioners educate caregivers and teachers to reinforce skills in daily activities. They suggest strategies and opportunities to support the child's practice of skills in a variety of tasks and settings. For example, the child and parent may work on feeding skills at home, daycare, and at a family outing. Each of these settings offers unique challenges and expectations. The practitioner may help the parent adapt or modify the requirements to assure success. They may bring easy-to-eat finger foods to the family outing to avoid carrying around additional feeding equipment. They may provide feeding equipment (such as adapted bowls, cups, and utensils) for daycare. At home, the parent may encourage the child to self-feed without the time constraints of other settings or the expectation that they will always be neat and successful. In this case, the child generalizes skills (e.g., holding feeding equipment to feed self) learned in occupational therapy sessions to home, daycare, and community. Practicing in many environments and engaging in occupations in different ways promotes flexibility and transfer of learning.

## Therapeutic Relationship

The **therapeutic relationship** is critical for the success of pediatric occupational therapy (see Chapter 3). Pediatric occupational therapy practitioners establish therapeutic relationships with the child and family that encourage, support, and motivate (D'Arrigo et al., 2020; Popova et al., 2022). In order to do so, the occupational therapy practitioner first builds rapport to create trust. This trust enables the child and family to feel safe and be willing to take risks. The therapeutic relationship involves acknowledging, validating, and respecting the child's and family's emotions and creating a climate of emotional safety. Occupational therapy practitioners demonstrate a positive effect and seek opportunities for personal connection while conveying positive regard. They show interest in the child and family, make efforts to enjoy their personality, and value the child's and family's contributions to the therapy process.

Occupational therapy practitioners demonstrate mutual respect, positivity, and maintain a nonjudgmental position toward children and families. They cultivate positive relationships with families when they establish open and honest communication and encourage participation of parents and children in occupational therapy sessions. Chapter 22 provides information on empowering families as an essential part of the occupational therapy process.

## Use of Evidence

With extensive availability of research on pediatric practice, competent practitioners read, appraise, and use evidence when making decisions about intervention. Furthermore, to remain current in occupational therapy practice, practitioners must critically analyze research evidence on an ongoing basis. Using knowledge of occupational therapy philosophy and principles, in combination with educational knowledge (such as neurological, social, biological), allows practitioners to make sound decisions regarding assessment and intervention. However, despite wide agreement among professionals regarding the importance of evidence-based practice, the profession continues to have difficulties with the implementation and translation of knowledge to integrate research findings into everyday practice (Juckett et al., 2019; Juckett et al., 2021; Upton et al., 2014). Occupational therapy practitioners often cite limited time to read and consume all the available evidence, and lack of administrative support to develop systems for routinely using evidence in practice.

With the proliferation of published research related to pediatric occupational therapy, organizations, including AOTA, have developed evidence-based practice guidelines. Evidence-based practice guidelines are developed by a group of experts who synthesize the research on a particular intervention or diagnosis to formulate recommendations for practice. These guidelines translate the research evidence to practice by making specific recommendations for evaluations and interventions that prioritize the recommendations using a grading system.

Hospitals and medical systems promote the use of evidence-based practice guidelines to improve the consistency and effectiveness of medical interventions (Kredo et al., 2016). Schools and educational systems have also called for research evidence to be used to guide educational practices and policies (Russo-Campisi, 2017). Clinical guidelines enable efficient consumption of efficacy research; however, implementing the guidelines requires commitment, system and environmental support, and consensus among the agency's or program's team. When evidence-based practice guidelines are implemented within quality improvement processes, they also are embedded in existing processes that include monitoring and examining outcomes.

Following clinical guidelines has the potential of increasing the consistency of practice and its efficacy. The likelihood of positive outcomes is high when occupational therapy practitioners (1) select evidence-based practice guidelines with optimal fit to their clientele and environment; (2) adapt the guidelines to fit their work environment; (3) modify them into user-friendly protocols; (4) examine and resolve barriers to implementation; and (5) establish systems to monitor their outcomes (Carey et al., 2009). Box 1.3 provides the steps of engaging in evidence-based practices. Case Example 1.5 describes using evidence-based practice guidelines in clinical decision-making for a young child with autism spectrum disorder.

**BOX 1.3 Steps in Evidence-Based Practice**

1. Develop an answerable question based on the need for information (e.g., assessments, intervention approaches, evidence for practice)
2. Search the research databases to find the best evidence to answer the research question
3. Critically appraise the evidence for its validity (truthfulness), impact (level of effect), and clinical meaningfulness
4. Critically appraise the evidence for its applicability and usefulness to your practice
5. Apply the information in practice and evaluate the outcomes

## Interprofessional Practice

**Interprofessional practice** involves an "interdependence of professional actions, a focus on user needs, negotiation between professionals, shared decision making, mutual respect and trust among professionals, and acknowledgment of the role and work of the different professional groups" involved in a child's care (Sangaleti et al., 2017, p. 2723). In pediatric practice, occupational therapy practitioners typically work as a member of an interprofessional team with other professions who provide care to children. Health challenges and disability can be broad and complex and demand holistic care that requires the knowledge, expertise, and skills of multiple professions. Additionally, the complexity of the human condition involves interconnected determinants of health including those that are biological, psychological, physical, social, socioeconomic, cultural, and environmental. A team-based approach requires collaboration to effectively organize healthcare services by integrating knowledge and practices from different professions and perspectives. Occupational therapy practitioners who are trained in interprofessional practice help team members understand children and families holistically. They are skilled at synthesizing information from multiple sources to assess how a child's motor, process, and social-emotional strengths and challenges influence their habits, routines, roles and rituals within their specific environment (Johnson, 2017). The occupational therapy practitioner plays a key role in working with a team of professionals to assess and identify environmental and contextual factors that influence a plan of care to best support the goals of a client and family (Johnson, 2017).

**Team Makeup.** Interprofessional teams may be made up of different professionals depending on the context of care, setting, or area of practice. The child and family are always essential members of the interprofessional care team. Other team members may include occupational therapy assistants, speech and language pathologists, physical therapists, social workers, teachers, psychologists, nurses, and doctors among others. See Table 1.1 for an overview of the typical makeup of varied interprofessional care teams.

Occupational therapists and occupational therapy assistants (i.e., occupational therapy practitioners) often collaborate in the care of pediatric clients on the same team. Therefore an understanding of their mutually compatible but varied roles in service delivery is critical. Additionally, fundamental to effective collaborative practice is a deep respect for the knowledge and skills of each. According to AOTA (2020b) "occupational therapy practitioners, after initial certification and relevant state licensure or other governmental requirements, are autonomous practitioners who are able to deliver occupational therapy services independently" (p. 1). Generally, although this is defined at the state level, an occupational therapy assistant is licensed to provide occupational therapy services under the supervision of and in partnership with a licensed occupational therapist. AOTA guidelines (2020b) identify the appropriate levels and types of supervision required but specify that the relationship between the occupational therapist and occupational therapy assistant partners must develop a collaborative plan for supervision that suits their experience levels and their context. Throughout the occupational therapy process for a client, the occupational therapist is directly involved on a regular basis and must decide what portions of the process to delegate to the occupational therapy assistant, once they demonstrate competence to complete the delegated role.

**Competencies.** In 2009, the Interprofessional Education Collaborative (IPEC) began when six national associations of schools of health professions joined together with a goal to prepare future health professionals for enhanced team-based care and improved population health outcomes. IPEC now has membership from 21 national health profession organizations, including the American Occupational Therapy Association. The mission of IPEC is to "ensure that new and current health professionals are proficient in the competencies essential for patient-centered, community- and population-oriented, interprofessional, collaborative practice" (Interprofessional Education Collaborative, 2022, para 4). In 2023, IPEC revised and updated its *Core Competencies for Interprofessional Collaborative Practice.* The current four core competencies include (1) Values and Ethics (Work with team members to maintain a climate of shared values, ethical conduct, and mutual respect.) (2) Roles and Responsibilities (Use the knowledge of one's own role and team members' expertise to address individual and population health outcomes.) (3) Communication (Communicate in a responsive, responsible, respectful, and compassionate manner with team members.) and (4) Teams and Teamwork (Apply values and principles of the science of teamwork to adapt one's own role in a variety of team settings.) (Interprofessional Education Collaborative, 2023)

Working in teams requires a shared identity, a clear role, task, and/or goals, interdependence of team members, integration of teamwork, and a shared responsibility (Reeves et al., 2018). Team members also must engage in collaboration, coordination, and networking, and each

## Case Example 1.5 Using Evidence-Based Practice Guidelines for Food Selectivity and Sensitivity

### Background

Marston is a 4-year-old boy with autism who has a limited diet and is beginning to show signs of poor nutrition. His parents are concerned that his eating behaviors will continue to impede his development. He currently is in the 50th percentile for weight and 60th percentile for height.

Tyrone, an occupational therapist working in an outpatient clinic, often works with children who have eating challenges related to food selectivity and sensitivity. Tyrone evaluated Marston, and his parents reported that he eats five foods (saltines, strawberry jelly sandwich on white bread with no crust, elbow macaroni with white cheese, French fries, yogurt) each day as snacks. He drinks grape-flavored water, water, and milk. He sits at the table with his family for a short time, and takes 3–5 bites of his preferred foods. Tyrone also notes that Marston withdrew when he approached, did not like to manipulate toys with his whole hand, but rather picked things up with the tips of his fingers. His parents reported that Marston does not like getting his hands dirty, washing his face, or playing with Play-Doh. They reported Marston does not like certain clothing and does not like new shoes.

Marston hypothesized that Tyrone exhibits food selectivity and sensitivity issues affecting his eating and feeding. He concluded that the issue may be related to sensory processing deficit resulting in selective behaviors that are reinforced as the child gains control of the foods.

### Research Evidence

Tyrone examines current research, past clinical experiences, with knowledge of Marston's unique strengths and challenges, along with his family situation to create an evidence-based intervention plan. He finds a current systematic review of feeding issues for children with autism (Reinoso et al., 2018) that informs his intervention plan. The reviewers indicate that occupational therapists address both sensory and selectivity issues related to feeding. The Sequential Oral Sensory (SOS) play-based approach addresses both sensory and behavioral challenges (Toomey & Ross, 2011). It is a relatively new approach, with promising results, although no randomized control trials have been conducted to date. Tyrone discusses this with the family and together they decide to cautiously adopt this approach that includes positive social and play reinforcement, grading foods introduced, and introducing the child to new foods.

He also considers the child's sensory processing by providing a calm state for feeding, addressing sensory modulation, and using proprioceptive experiences before introducing new tactile food textures (Reinoso et al., 2018; Suarez, 2015). He will further evaluate Marston's sensory processing as they develop a rapport.

### Professional Reasoning

Tyrone evaluated the research evidence in light of his past clinical experiences and decided that this approach is congruent with his previous work with children with autism. He learned more about the specific SOS approach by reviewing the protocols. As he implemented strategies in practice, Tyrone reflected on the strategies and techniques by revisiting the literature on the topic, discussing concepts with peers, and collaborating with the family. Tyrone used information about Marston to determine the suitability of using this approach in practice. He concluded that the SOS approach includes many practices that have worked with other clients while providing additional ideas and structure to his intervention plan. Tyrone also included the parents in the intervention sessions to promote carryover at home. He carefully monitored Marston's progress throughout the process.

### Summary

Tyrone used research evidence, clinical experience, and information about the client to support collaborative practice decisions. He used professional reasoning to synthesize information for best practice. As he engages Marston in the intervention process, he may revisit the research, discuss with colleagues and the parents, and reflect on the progress to adjust or add strategies to use in practice.

**TABLE 1.1 Examples of Pediatric Interprofessional Care Teams in Varied Settings**

| Setting | Team Members Working With Occupational Therapy (OT, OTA[a]), Child, and Family |
|---|---|
| Hospital | Physical therapist, speech and language pathologist, respiratory therapist, nurse, nurse practitioner, medical doctor, physician associate, pharmacist, social worker, chaplain, psychologist, psychiatrist, play therapist, nutritionist, child life specialist, patient care tech/nursing assistants (PCT/CNA), lactation consultants |
| Birth to three (homecare) | Physical therapist, speech and language pathologist, social worker, teacher, nurse, nutritionist, caregiver, aide |
| School | Regular education teacher, special education teacher, physical therapist, speech and language pathologist, social worker, school psychologist, school nurse, guidance counselor, school principal or assistant principal, special education administrator |
| Outpatient (community, private practice) | Physical therapist, speech and language pathologist, social worker, nurse, aide, nutritionist, physician, caregiver |
| Primary care (pediatrician's office) | Medical doctor, nurse practitioner, physician associate, nurse, lactation consultant, nutritionist, behavioral health provider (social work, counselor, etc.) |

[a]Occupational therapy assistants may be part of any of these teams depending on the state practice acts and licensure laws of individual states.

of these focuses differently on the varied requirements of teamwork (Reeves et al., 2018; Xyrichis et al., 2018). Networking is a different form of "teamwork." In a hospital or acute care setting, the care network for one client can be massive and complex, making face-to-face collaboration almost impossible (Dow et al., 2017). In these types of interprofessional networks the members may communicate via email or online conferencing. Interprofessional networks vary and different professionals enter and leave at varied times, often unpredictably.

**Barriers to Interprofessional Practice.** While there may be an expressed value and commitment to working interprofessionally among practitioners (Bode et al., 2016), they often lack training in it. Without training in teamwork, and when practitioners have a uniprofessional mindset, disciplines tend to provide healthcare services parallel to one another. This may result in excessive contact time with providers for a client and family, as well as interventions or education from individual perspectives without consideration for how interventions or patient education may overlap, complement, or be integrated with other providers from other disciplines (Johnson, 2017). In pediatric practice, for example, an occupational therapy practitioner may have a conversation with a child and caregiver about concerns related to inattention and contributing factors including sensory processing, impulsivity, hyperactivity, developmental stage, behavioral control, or motivating factors. An interprofessional approach involves having one conversation together as a team with multiple providers to discuss the various ways to first assess then treat inattention based on the various frameworks, theories, and principles that inform the practice approaches of different disciplines.

It is important, especially in pediatric practice, that occupational therapy practitioners learn to be competent with the skills that are necessary for interprofessional practice. IPEC core competencies, as well as the many subcompetencies for each, serve as guidelines for practice and professional development for occupational therapy educators, students, and providers. The Accreditation Council for Occupational Therapy Education (ACOTE) includes a standard requiring students to learn how to effectively work in an interprofessional manner (Johnson, 2017).

## SUMMARY

Occupational therapy practitioners working in pediatrics establish therapeutic relationships with children, youth, and their families. The occupational therapy process includes referral, evaluation, creation of an intervention plan, implementation of the plan, and measurement of outcomes. Within this process, practitioners use a strengths-based, child- and family-centered approach to engage children in activities to promote positive self-efficacy, self-determination, and occupational identity. Occupational therapy practitioners work closely with team members. They engage in cultural humility as they commit to life-long learning to understand the family's culture, values, beliefs, roles, and routines. They are committed to identify and address imbalances of power to advocate for children and families. Importantly, practitioners working with children and youth engage in ongoing evidence-based practice and professional reasoning to support children and families.

- Pediatric practice is the provision of occupational therapy services to children and youth from birth to 21 years of age. Occupational therapy practitioners enable children and youth to engage in occupations (e.g., activities of daily living, instrumental activities of daily living, health management, rest and sleep, education, work, play, leisure, and social participation).
- The occupational therapy process includes referral, evaluation, assessment, intervention plan (including goal setting), implementation of the plan, assessment of the outcomes, and discharge planning. The process is not always linear, as therapists may revisit steps along the process.
- Essential concepts in pediatric practice that will be carried throughout this textbook include focus on occupational engagement, cultural humility, and child- and family-centered care; use of strengths-based approaches that involve active involvement of the child, creating the just-right challenge to promote self-efficacy, self-determination, and occupational identity; fostering a therapeutic relationship; using evidence in decision-making; ensuring the generalization of skills gained through intervention; and engagement in interprofessional collaborative practices.

## REFERENCES

Agner, J. (2020). Moving from cultural competence to cultural humility in occupational therapy: A paradigm shift. *American Journal of Occupational Therapy, 74*. :7404347010p1–7404347010p7. https://doi.org/10.5014/ajot.2020.038067.

American Occupational Therapy Association. (2020a). Occupational therapy practice framework: Domain and process—Fourth Edition. *American Journal of Occupational Therapy, 74*(Suppl. 2):7412410010. https://doi.org/10.5014/ajot.2020.74S2001.

American Occupational Therapy Association. (2020b). Guidelines for supervision, roles, and responsibilities during the delivery of occupational therapy services. *American Journal of Occupational Therapy, 74*(Suppl. 3):7413410020. https://doi.org/10.5014/ajot.2020.74S3004.

Ayres, A. J. (1972). *Sensory integration and learning disorders*. Western Psychological Services.

Bandura, A. (1997). *Self-efficacy: The exercise of control*. Freeman.

Baratta-Ziska, F., Oledzka, M., Eannucci, E. F., & Slevin, C. (2021). Patient satisfaction utilizing telehealth for pediatric physical and occupational therapy during COVID-19. *Archives of Physical Medicine and Rehabilitation, 102*, e107. https://doi.org/10.1016/j.apmr.2021.07.503.

Bode, S. F. N., Giesler, M., Heinzmann, A., Krüger, M., & Straub, C. (2016). Self-perceived attitudes toward interprofessional collaboration and interprofessional education among different health care professionals in pediatrics. *GMS Journal for Medical Education, 33*(2), 1–15. https://doi.org/10.3205/zma001016.

Boorman, G., Clarke, G., & Nind, M. (2009). *In their own words: The missing voices of girls with behavioral, social and emotional difficulties*. https://eprints.soton.ac.uk/65965/01/In_Their_Own_Words_v5.doc.

Braun, M. J., Dunn, W., & Tomchek, S. D. (2017). A pilot study on professional documentation: Do we write from a strengths perspective? *American Journal of Speech-Language Pathology, 26*(3), 972–981. https://doi.org/10.1044/2017_AJSLP-16-0117.

Buntinx, W. H. (2013). Understanding disability: A strengths-based approach. *The Oxford Handbook of Positive Psychology and Disability*, 7–18. https://doi.org/10.1093/oxfordhb/9780195398786.013.013.0002.

Burke, J. P. (1977). A clinical perspective on motivation: Pawn versus origin. *American Journal of Occupational Therapy, 31*(4), 254–258.

Cadwgan, J., & Goodwin, J. (2018). Helping parents with the diagnosis of disability. *Paediatrics and Child Health, 28*(8), 357–363. https://doi.org/10.1016/j.paed.2018.06.006.

Cahill, S. M., & Beisbier, S. (2020). Occupational therapy practice guidelines for children and youth ages 5–21 years. *American Journal of Occupational Therapy, 74*(4). https://doi.org/10.5014/ajot.2020.744001.

Camden, C., & Silva, M. (2021). Pediatric telehealth: Opportunities created by the COVID-19 and suggestions to sustain its use to support families of children with disabilities. *Physical and Occupational Therapy in Pediatrics, 41*(1), 1–17. https://doi.org/10.1080/01942638.2020.1825032.

Cano-de-la-Cuerda, R., Molero-Sánchez, A., Carratalá-Tejada, M., Alguacil-Diego, I. M., Molina-Rueda, F., Miangolarra-Page, J. C., & Torricelli, D. (2015). Theories and control models and motor learning: Clinical applications in neurorehabilitation. *Neurologia, 30*(1), 32–41. https://doi.org/10.1016/j.nrl.2011.12.010.

Carey, M., Buchan, H., & Sanson-Fisher, R. (2009). The cycle of change: Implementing best-evidence clinical practice. *International Journal for Quality in Health Care, 21*, 37–43. https://doi.org/10.1093/intqhc/mzn049.

Centers for Medicaid and Medicare Services. (2020). *Children's Health Insurance Program (CHIP Reports and Evaluations)*. https://www.medicaid.gov/chip/reports-evaluations/index.html.

Conijn, J. M., Smits, N., & Hartman, E. E. (2020). Determining at what age children provide sound self-reports: An illustration of the validity-index approach. *Assessment, 27*(7), 1604–1618. https://doi.org/10.1177/1073191119832655.

Corbett, J. (1998). Voice' in emancipatory research: Imaginative listening. In P. Clough, & L. Barto (Eds.), *Articulating with difficulty: Research voices in inclusive education* (pp. 54–63). Paul Chapman.

Cowger, C. D. (1994). Assessing client strengths: Clinical assessment for client empowerment. *Social Work, 39*(3), 262–268.

D'Arrigo, R. G., Copley, J. A., Poulsen, A. A., & Ziviani, J. (2020). Strategies occupational therapists use to engage children and parents in therapy sessions. *Australian Occupational Therapy Journal, 67*(6), 537–549. https://doi.org/10.1111/1440-1630.12670.

Deci, E. L., & Ryan, R. M. (2008). Self-determination theory: A macrotheory of human motivation, development, and health. *Canadian Psychology (Psychologie Canadienne), 49*, 182–185. https://doi.org/10.1037/a0012801.

Dewees, M. (1999). The strengths perspective: A first step in empowerment. *Journal of Baccalaureate Social Work, 4*(2), 95–108.

Dow, A., Zhu, X., Sewell, D., Banas, C., Mishra, V., & Tu, S.-P. (2017). Teamwork on the rocks: Rethinking interprofessional practice as networking. *Journal of Interprofessional Care, 31*, 677–678. https://doi.org/10.1080/13561820.2017.1344048.

Dunn, W. (2017). Strengths-based approaches: What if even the 'bad' things are good things? *British Journal of Occupational Therapy, 80*(7), 395–396. https://doi.org/10.1177/030802261770266.

Froiland, J. M., & Oros, E. (2014). Intrinsic motivation, perceived competence and classroom engagement as longitudinal predictors of adolescent reading achievement. *Educational Psychology, 34*(2), 119–132. https://doi.org/10.1080/01443410.2013.822964.

Gopalan, V., Bakar, J. A. A., Zulkifli, A. N., Alwi, A., & Mat, R. C. (2017). A review of the motivation theories in learning. *AIP Conference Proceedings, 1891*, 020043. https://doi.org/10.1063/1.5005376.

Greene, R. R., & Watkins, M. (1998). *Serving diverse constituencies: An ecological perspective*. Aldine de Gruyter Publishers.

Hemmingsson, H., Ólafsdóttir, L. B., & Egilson, S. T. (2017). Agreements and disagreements between children and their parents in health-related assessments. *Disability and Rehabilitation, 39*(11), 1059–1072. https://doi.org/10.1080/09638288.2016.1189603.

Hoel, V., von Zweck, C., Ledgerd, R., & World Federation of Occupational Therapists. (2021). Was a global pandemic needed to adopt the use of telehealth in occupational therapy? *Work, 68*(1), 13–20. https://doi.org/10.3233/WOR-205268.

Hook, J. N., Davis, D. E., Owen, J., Worthington, E. L., Jr., & Utsey, S. O. (2013). Cultural humility: Measuring openness to culturally diverse clients. *Journal of Counseling Psychology, 60*, 353. https://doi.org/10.1037/a0032595.

Hooper, B., & Wood, W. (2019). The philosophy of occupational therapy: A framework for practice. In B. A. B. Schell, & G. Gillen (Eds.), *Willard and Spackman's occupational therapy* (13th ed.) (pp. 43–55). Lippincott Williams and Wilkins.

Individuals With Disabilities Education Improvement Act of 2004, Pub. L. 108–446, 20 U.S.C. §§ 1400–1482.

Interprofessional Education Collaborative. (2022). *About us*. https://www.ipecollaborative.org/about-us.

Interprofessional Education Collaborative. (2023). *IPEC core competencies for interprofessional collaborative practice: Version 3*. Washington, DC: Interprofessional Education Collaborative. https://ipec.memberclicks.net/assets/core-competencies/IPEC_Core_Competencies_Version_3_2023.pdf. (Accessed 2 August 2024).

Johnson, C. (2017). Understanding interprofessional collaboration: An essential skill for all practitioners. *OT Practice, 22*(11), CE1–CE8. https://www.aota.org/~/media/Corporate/Files/Publications/CE-Articles/CE-Article-June-2017.pdf.

Juckett, L. A., Robinson, M. L., & Wengerd, L. R. (2019). Narrowing the gap: An implementation science research agenda for the occupational therapy profession. *American Journal of Occupational Therapy, 73*(5):7305347010. https://doi.org/10.5014/ajot.2019.033902.

Juckett, L. A., Robinson, M. L., Malloy, J., & Oliver, H. V. (2021). Health Policy Perspectives—Translating knowledge to optimize value-based occupational therapy: Strategies for educators, practitioners, and researchers. *American Journal of Occupational Therapy, 75*. :7506090020. https://doi.org/10.5014/ajot.2021.756003.

Kredo, T. , Bernhardsson, S. , Machingaidze, S., & Young, T. , Louw, Q., Ochodo, E., & Grimmer, K. (2016). Guide to clinical practice guidelines: The current state of play. *International Journal for Quality in Health Care, 28*(1), 122–128. https://doi.org/10.1093/intqhc/mzv115.

Kreider, C. M., Bendixen, R. M., Huang, Y. Y., & Lim, Y. (2014). Review of occupational therapy intervention research in the practice area of children and youth 2009–2013. *American Journal of Occupational Therapy, 68*, e61–e73. https://doi.org/10.5014/ajot.2014.011114.

Kuhaneck, H., & Spitzer, S. (Eds.). (2023). *Making play just right: Unleashing the power of play in occupational therapy* (2nd ed.) Jones and Bartlett Learning.

Lekas, H. M., Pahl, K., & Fuller Lewis, C. (2020). Rethinking cultural competence: Shifting to cultural humility. *Health Services Insights, 13*:1178632920970580.

Little, L. M., Pickett, K. A., & Proffitt, R., & Cason, J. (2021). Keeping PACE with 21st century healthcare: A framework for telehealth research, practice, and program evaluation in occupational therapy. *International Journal of Telerehabilitation, 13*(1), e6379. https://doi.org/10.5195/ijt.2021.6379.

Mack, W., Lindquist, J. E., & Parham, L. D. (1982). A synthesis of occupational behavior and sensory integration concepts in theory and practice, Part 1. Theoretical foundations. *American Journal of Occupational Therapy, 36*, 365–374. https://doi.org/10.5014/ajot.36.6.365.

Master, A., Cheryan, S. , & Meltzoff, A. N. (2017). Brief report: Social group membership increases STEM engagement among preschoolers. *Developmental Psychology, 53*(2), 201–219. https://doi.org/10.1037/dev0000195.

McKernan, B., Martey, R. M., Stromer-Galey, J., Kenski, K., Clegg, B. A., Folkestad, J. E., Rhodes, M. G., Shaw, A., Saulnier, E. T., & Strzalkowski, T. (2015). We don't need no stinkin' badges: The impact of reward features and feeling rewarded in educational games. *Computers in Human Behavior, 45*, 299–306. https://doi.org/10.1016/j.chb.2014.12.028.

NBCOT. (2018). *Practice analysis of the occupational therapist registered*. https://www.nbcot.org/-/media/NBCOT/PDFs/2017-Practice-Analysis-Executive-OTR.ashx?la=en.

Niemiec, R. M., Shogren, K. A., & Wehmeyer, M. L. (2017). Character strengths and intellectual and developmental disability: A strengths-based approach from positive psychology. *Education and Training in Autism and Developmental Disabilities, 52*(1), 13–25. https://www.jstor.org/stable/26420372.

O'Brien, J. (2017). Model of human occupation. In J. Hinojosa, P. Kramer, & C. B. Royeen (Eds.), *Perspectives on human occupation: Theories underlying practice* (2nd ed.) (pp. 93–136). F.A. Davis.

O'Brien, J. (2023). Models of practice and frames of references: Essential concepts for therapeutic reasoning. In J. O'Brien, M. E. Patnaude, & T. G. Reidy (Eds.), *Therapeutic reasoning in occupational therapy: How to develop critical thinking for practice* (pp. 50–66). Elsevier.

O'Brien, K. H., & Schlechter, A. (2016). Is talking about what's wrong necessarily right: A positive perspective on the diagnostic interview. *Journal of the American Academy of Child and Adolescent Psychiatry, 55*(4), 262–264. https://doi.org/10.1016/j.jaac.2015.12.016.

Önal, G., & Güney, G., Gün, F., & Huri, M. (2021). Telehealth in pediatric occupational therapy: A scoping review. *International Journal of Therapy and Rehabilitation, 28*(7), 1–16. https://doi.org/10.12968/ijtr.2020.0070.

Patnaude, M. E. (2023). Student success: Therapeutic reasoning process. In J. O'Brien, M. E. Patnaude, & T. G. Reidy (Eds.), *Therapeutic reasoning in occupational therapy: How to develop critical thinking for practice* (p. 8). Elsevier.

Patten, K. K. (2022). Finding our strengths: Recognizing professional bias and interrogating systems. Eleanor Clarke Slagle Lecture. *American Journal of Occupational Therapy, 76*. :7606150010. https://doi.org/10.5014/ajot.2022.076603.

PBS. (2018). *Talking with kids*. http://www.pbs.org/parents/talkingwithkids/agebyage.html.

Pesch, M. H., Berlin, K. S., Cesaro, R. J., Rybak, T. M., Miller, A. L., Rosenblum, K. L., & Lumeng, J. C. (2018). Maternal discouragement and child intake of a palatable dessert: A multilevel sequential analysis. *Appetite, 129*, 171–177. https://doi.org/10.1016/j.appet.2018.07.013.

Pfeiffer, B., Clark, G. F., & Arbesman, M. (2018). Effectiveness of cognitive and occupation-based interventions for children with challenges in sensory processing and integration: A systematic review. *American Journal of Occupational Therapy, 72*(1):7201190020p1–7201190020p9.

Pinchover, S. (2017). The relation between teachers' and children's playfulness: A pilot study. *Frontiers in Psychology*, *8*, 2214. https://doi-org.une.idm.oclc.org/10.3389/fpsyg.2017.02214.

Popova, E. S., O'Brien, J. C., & Taylor, R. R. (2022). Communicating with intention: Therapist and parent perspectives on family-centered care in early intervention. *American Journal of Occupational Therapy*, *76*. :7605205130. https://doi.org/10.5014/ajot.2022.049131.

Proffitt, R., Cason, J., & Little, L., & Pickett, K. A. (2021). Stimulating research to advance evidence-based applications of telehealth in occupational therapy. *OTJR: Occupation, Participation and Health*, *41*, 153–162. https://doi.org/10.1177/15394492211011433.

Rapp, C. A., Saleebey, D., & Sullivan, W. P. (2008). The future of strengths-based social work practice. In D. Saleebey (Ed.), *The strengths perspective in social work practice* (4th ed.) (pp. 79–90). Pearson Education.

Reeves, S., Xyrichis, A., & Zwarenstein, M. (2018). Teamwork, collaboration, coordination, and networking: Why we need to distinguish between different types of interprofessional practice. *Journal of Interprofessional Care*, *32*, 1–3. https://doi.org/10.1080/13561820.2017.1400150.

Reinoso, G., Carsone, B., Weldon, S., Powers, J., & Bellare, N. (2018). Food selectivity and sensitivity in children with Autism Spectrum Disorder: A systematic review defining the issue and evaluating interventions. *New Zealand Journal of Occupational Therapy*, *65*(1), 36–42.

Rodger, S., & Polatajko, H. (2017). Cognitive orientation for daily occupational performance (CO-OP): An occupation-centred intervention. In S. Rodger, & A. Kennedy-Behr (Eds.), *Occupation-centred practice with children: A practical guide for occupational therapists* (2nd ed.) (pp. 165–188). Wiley Blackwell.

Ronimus, M., Kujala, J., Tolvanen, A., & Lyytinen, H. (2014). Children's engagement during digital game-based learning of reading: The effects of time, rewards, and challenge. *Computers and Education*, *71*, 237–246.

Russo, R. J. (1999). Applying a strengths-based practice approach in working with people with developmental disabilities and their families. *Families in Society*, *80*(1), 25–33. https://doi.org/10.1606/1044-3894.6.

Russo-Campisi, J. (2017). Evidence-based practices in special education: Current assumptions and future considerations. *Child and Youth Care Forum*, *46*, 193–205. https://doi.org/10.1007/s10566-017-9390-5.

Ryan, R. M., & Deci, E. L. (2020). Intrinsic and extrinsic motivation from a self-determination theory perspective: Definitions, theory, practices, and future directions. *Contemporary Educational Psychology*, *61*, 101860. https://doi.org/10.1016/j.cedpsych.2020.101860.

Ryan, R. M., Deci, E. L., & Vansteenkiste, M. (2016). Autonomy and autonomy disturbances in self-development and psychopathology: Research on motivation, attachment, and clinical process. In D. Cicchetti (Ed.), *Developmental psychopathology* (pp. 385–438). John Wiley and Sons Inc.

Sangaleti, C., Schveitzer, M. C., Peduzzi, M., Zoboli, E. L. C. P., & Soares, C. B. (2017). Experiences and shared meaning of teamwork and interprofessional collaboration among health care professionals in primary health care settings: A systematic review. *JBI Database of Systematic Reviews and Implementation Reports*, *15*, 2723–2788. https://doi.org/10.11124/JBISRIR-2016-003016.

Smithsonian. (2018). *Young or old?* https://anthropology.si.edu/writteninbone/young_old.html.

Steiner, A. M. (2011). A strength-based approach to parent education for children with autism. *Journal of Positive Behavior Interventions*, *13*(3), 178–190. https://doi.org/10.1177/1098300710384134.

Suarez, M. A. (2015). Multicomponent treatment for food selectivity in children: Description and case report. *Nutrition in Clinical Practice*, *30*(3), 425–431. https://doi.org/10.1177/0884533614553638.

Tervalon, M., & Murray-Garcia, J. (1998). Cultural humility versus cultural competence: A critical distinction in defining physician training outcomes in multicultural education. *Journal of Health Care for the Poor and Underserved*, *9*(2), 117–125. https://doi.org/10.1353/hpu.2010.0233.

Toomey, K. A., & Ross, E. S. (2011). SOS approach to feeding. *Perspectives on Swallowing and Swallowing Disorders (Dysphagia)*, *20*(3), 82–87. https://doi.org/10.1044/sasd20.3.82.

Traub, S. (2016). *Communicating effectively with children*. University of Missouri. https://extension2.missouri.edu/GH6123.

Ullenhag, A., Granlund, M., Almqvist, L., & Krumlinde-Sundholm, L. (2020). A strength-based intervention to increase participation in leisure activities in children with neuropsychiatric disabilities: A pilot study. *Occupational Therapy International*, *2020*:1358707. https://www.hindawi.com/journals/oti/2020/1358707/.

Upton, D., Stephens, D., Williams, B., & Scurlock-Evans, L. (2014). Occupational therapists' attitudes, knowledge, and implementation of evidence-based practice: A systematic review of published research. *British Journal of Occupational Therapy*, *77*(1), 24–38. https://doi.org/10.4276/030802214X138876853355.

Varni, J. W., Limbers, C. A., & Burwinkle, T. M. (2007). How young can children reliably and validly self-report their health-related quality of life?: An analysis of 8,591 children across age subgroups with the PedsQL 4.0 Generic Core Scales. *Health and Quality of Life Outcomes*, *3*. https://doi.org/10.1186/1477-7525-5-1.

Whalley Hammell, K. (2015). Respecting global wisdom: Enhancing the cultural relevance of occupational therapy's theoretical base. *British Journal of Occupational Therapy*, *78*(11), 718–721. https://doi.org/10.1177/0308022614564.

White, J. G. (1959). The use of learning theory in the psychological treatment of children. *Journal of Clinical Psychology*, *15*(2), 226–229. https://doi.org/10.1002/1097-4679(195904)15:2<227::aid-jclp2270150232>3.0.co;2-e.

Xyrichis, A., Reeves, S., & Zwarenstein, M. (2018). Examining the nature of interprofessional practice: An initial framework validation and creation of the InterProfessional Activity Classification Tool (InterPACT). *Journal of Interprofessional Care*, *32*(4), 416–425. https://doi.org/10.1080/13561820.2017.1408576.

Yeager, D. S., & Dweck, C. S. (2020). What can be learned from growth mindset controversies? *American Psychologist*, *75*(9), 1269. https://doi.org/10.1037/amp0000794.

Yerxa, E. J. (1981). Book review: Children adapt. *Occupational Therapy Journal of Research*, *1*, 99–101. https://doi.org/10.1177/153944928100100111.

Zaidman-Zait, A., Marshall, S. K., Young, R. A., & Hertzman, C. (2014). Beyond compliance: Mother-child joint action during a "do" task. *Journal of Child and Family Studies*, *20*(3), 1034–1049. https://doi.org/10.1007/s10826-013-9760-z.

# 2

# Creativity as a Building Block of Successful Therapeutic Sessions

*Heather Miller Kuhaneck*

## GUIDING QUESTIONS

1. What is creativity?
2. Where does creativity come from? What is required for it to arise?
3. What characteristics do creative people demonstrate?
4. Why is creativity critical for occupational therapists in pediatric practice?
5. How can we support and encourage the development of creativity in ourselves and our clients? How do we develop creativity within therapy sessions?

## KEY TERMS

| | | |
|---|---|---|
| Associative processes | Elaboration | Innovation |
| Creativity | Fluency | Originality |
| Divergent thinking | Flexibility | Serendipity |

## INTRODUCTION

Creativity has been a cornerstone of occupational therapy practice since the beginning. However, it has not been considered a primary tool for the profession until recently (Hansen et al., 2021; Perruzza & Kinsella, 2010; Royeen, 2015; Schmid, 2004; Thompson & Blair, 1998).

Creativity is widely recognized as an important 21st-century skill (e.g., see Batey, 2011; Vivekanandan, 2019; Voogt & Roblin, 2010). A 21st-century skill is one that broadly applies to how people live and work, such as critical thinking, problem-solving, and collaboration (Vivekanandan, 2019). This chapter focuses on the importance of creativity, which many authors have suggested provides a crucial cognitive capacity for success (Pellegrino & Hilton, 2012). It will provide strategies for the occupational therapy practitioner to foster their own creativity and that of the children they treat, through methods and evidence provided from within and outside of occupational therapy.

## CREATIVITY EXPLORED

### Creativity Defined: Clarification of Terminology for This Chapter

Authors have defined creativity in varied ways. Some, perhaps focusing on the arts, science, or everyday activities, have suggested that *creativity* is an ability to produce novel responses (Shamay-Tsoory et al., 2011). Others, perhaps more oriented toward business and industry, have defined it as a process of developing original ideas related to products, services, processes, procedures, or open-ended problems. Creativity has been both linked to and separated from the concept of innovation.

While creativity is proposed as the generation of useful and novel ideas, *innovation* represents the implementation of these ideas (Anderson et al., 2014). Innovation is typically considered to comprise both the creative idea and its implementation. With this distinction, creativity may be considered a first step in innovation (Moirano et al., 2020). The concepts of both creativity and innovation have been explored extensively in design and manufacturing, as well as in art, education, laboratory research, and many other fields. Both terms are used throughout the literature of those fields. These concepts are not as well researched in occupational therapy, although creativity is often considered an implicit value in our profession.

According to the common definitions just discussed, practitioners in occupational therapy pediatric intervention require innovation. Creativity without innovation does not foster successful therapeutic outcomes, as the occupational therapy practitioner must implement the creative idea with the client for it to achieve its aim. For this chapter, however, we shall use the term creativity because, in lay usage, creativity often suggests artistic endeavors, whereas innovation often denotes creation for profit or industry. As therapy is often considered and discussed as an art as well as a science (Wood, 1995), the word creativity resonates best and is the concept now being explored more scientifically in the occupational therapy literature.

Various criteria have been used to measure creativity. In some situations, two criteria are proposed. The first is *originality* (*newness* or *uniqueness*), and the second is effectiveness (*ability to meet task constraints in a meaningful way*) (Plucker et al., 2004; Runco & Jaeger, 2012). Other methods of measuring creativity have focused on four criteria: fluency, originality, flexibility, and elaboration (Guilford, 1967). *Fluency* is the ability to produce many ideas or problem solutions in rapid succession. *Flexibility* is the capacity to consider multiple solutions to a problem at the same time. *Elaboration* is the ability to consider the details of an idea to carry it out. Here, originality is the tendency to produce ideas that differ from those of others. Children may engage in creativity as they develop new ways of building sand sculptures (Fig. 2.1A) and constructing a drinking invention (Fig. 2.1B).

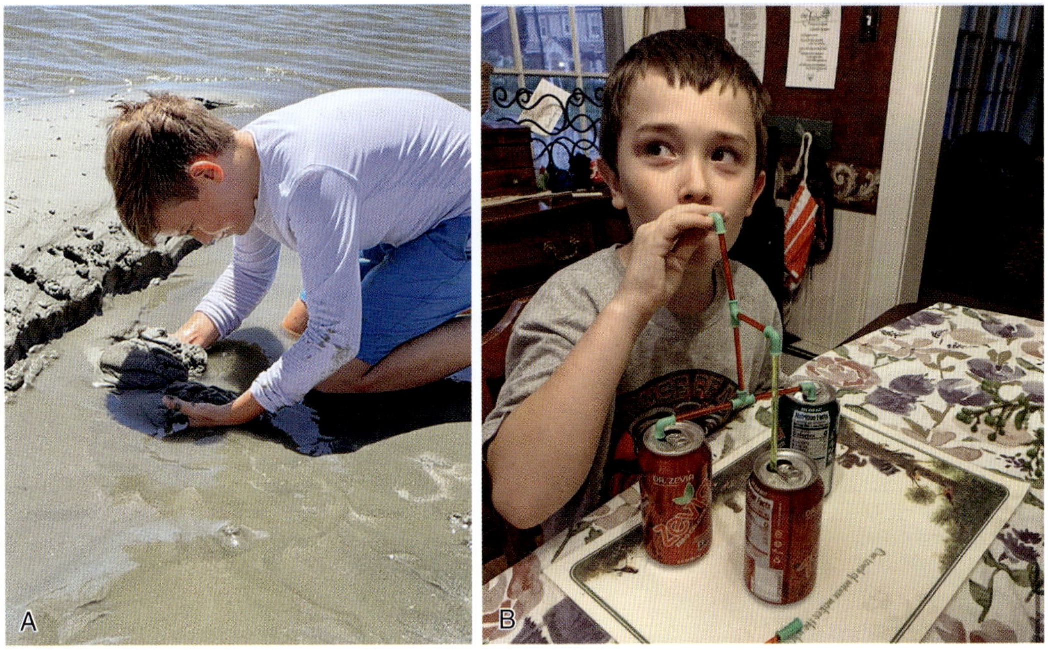


**Fig. 2.1** (A) Child figures out new sand structures to build. (B) Constructing various drinking structures promotes problem-solving, creativity, and divergent thinking. ((A) Courtesy Kirsten Anderson. (B) Courtesy Patricia Schaefer.)

## Related Terminology for this Chapter

Terms commonly associated with creativity are divergent thinking and associative processes. *Divergent thinking* is a process of generating multiple ideas or solutions to problems and it involves aspects of fluency, flexibility, and originality. Research suggests that divergent thinkers are more creative and open and can easily identify problems to solve. They also view problems in various ways, thereby supporting alternative solutions (Dirette, 2017; Said-Metwaly et al., 2022). *Associative processes* are those by which cognitive connections are made between things. These connections (associations) may be formed by specific cues about things, such as similarities or their nearness in time and space. Often measured by tasks that ask about the relationships between words, these abilities have been studied and related to other aspects of creativity such as divergent thinking (Benedek & Neubauer, 2013). The link from these measures to creativity began with Mednick (1962), who defined creative thinking "as the forming of associative elements into new combinations which either meet specified requirements or are in some way useful" (p. 221).

## Types or Levels of Creativity

One popular model of creativity describes four different types or levels labeled mini-C, little-C, Pro-C, and Big-C and is known as the Four C Model (Kaufman & Beghetto, 2009). At the first level, mini-C describes creativity used by people for everyday, personally meaningful activities. This level is the foundation for developing higher levels of creativity. At its highest level, creativity may be life altering—for example, the development of an understanding of human DNA or the creation of the internet. See Table 2.1 for examples of each type of creativity.

Creativity is likely somewhat domain specific at varied levels. For example, Big-C creativity in some domains may require a thorough historical knowledge of the field, whereas in others it may not be necessary.

## Where Does Creativity "Live" in the Brain?

Scientists have studied the neural underpinnings of creativity and have found specific areas of the brain related to various aspects of creativity (Aziz-Zadeh et al., 2013; Gonen-Yaacovi et al., 2013). For example, researchers suggest that the default mode network is implicated in the generation of spontaneous ideas, whereas the frontoparietal control network is involved with divergent thinking and the novel generation of metaphors (verbal creativity) (Gonen-Yaacovi et al., 2013; Lifshitz-Ben-Basat & Mashal, 2021).

Although often considered a right hemisphere function, studies suggest a strong left hemisphere component as well. The left parietal cortex has been linked to originality (Shamay-Tsoory et al., 2011), and in one study, a visual creativity task more strongly activated left hemisphere regions such as the posterior parietal cortex, premotor cortex, dorsolateral prefrontal cortex (PFC) and medial PFC (Aziz-Zadeh et al., 2013). These authors also found that a creative task activated left hemisphere motor areas such as the supplementary motor area, inferior frontal gyrus, and premotor cortex. Motor planning may be a component of improvisation and novel solution development. Other researchers found that providing specific cognitive stimulation (providing subjects with the ideas of others) improved originality with documented activation differences in posterior brain regions such as temporoparietal areas (Fink et al., 2010). The generation of original ideas was associated with activation in the (anterior) supramarginal gyrus and widespread deactivation in the inferior parietal cortex, particularly in the right hemisphere. Interestingly, researchers have recently been able to enhance creativity via transcranial direct current stimulation of areas of the frontoparietal control network (Lifshitz-Ben-Basat & Mashal, 2021). Similarly, evidence that left hemisphere inhibition with right hemisphere facilitation may lead to extraordinary abilities led to a study of transcranial direct current stimulation. Researchers used stimulation to diminish left hemisphere dominance, specifically, cathodal stimulation (decreasing excitability) of the left anterior temporal lobe with anodal stimulation (increasing excitability) of the right anterior temporal lobe increased creativity for problem-solving (Chi & Snyder, 2012).

The intense growth in research on neuroscience and creativity suggests that creative cognition is associated with widespread neural networks that support executive functions, memory, attention, and spontaneous modes of thought (Fink & Benedek, 2019).

**TABLE 2.1 Types of Creativity With Examples**

| Levels | Description | Examples |
|---|---|---|
| Mini-C | The production of something new and meaningful for a single individual within a developmental sequence. | • Learning to do something in a novel way for a child, although the solution may be well known to others<br>• Exploring mixing primary colors of paint to create other colors for an art project<br>• Building with Legos to create novel objects |
| Little-C | Everyday production of novel solutions to minor problems | • Creating a brand-new recipe from ingredients on hand<br>• Creating a new game to play outside with sticks and rocks when there are no toys to use |
| Pro-C | Work by professional practitioners who do valuable novel work but perhaps not historically important contributions | • Designing a living room for a client (interior design)<br>• Sewing a unique outfit for a client (seamstress)<br>• Designing a novel building space for a specific use (architect) |
| Big-C | Productions of importance in scientific, technological, social, or artistic endeavors | • Developing a new theory (Darwin's theory of evolution)<br>• Creating the light bulb or the printing press<br>• Creating the Mona Lisa or designing the first skyscraper |

Adapted from Jones, R. H. (2015). Creativity and discourse analysis. In *The Routledge handbook of language and creativity* (pp. 61–77). Routledge and Beghetto, R. A., & Kaufman, J. C. (2007). Toward a broader conception of creativity: A case for mini-c creativity. *Psychology of Aesthetics, Creativity, and the Arts*, 1, 73–79.

Both divergent and convergent thinking for creative cognition are modulated by metacontrol (Zhang et al., 2020). Divergent thinking may benefit from metacontrol biases toward flexibility. However convergent, analytical thinking appears to benefit from metacontrol biases toward persistence. Both are reflected in specific brain-activation patterns in the left frontal and right temporal/parietal networks.

## Requirements for Creativity

For someone to generate something creative, basic knowledge about the task or situation must first exist. The level of knowledge required is related to the ability to judge what is novel and useful and when to throw out "junk" ideas. Creativity also requires the right environment, enjoyment, and proper motivation. Intrinsic motivation is critical for creativity, and when there is an element of service to others, the link between motivation and creativity increases (Cerasoli et al., 2014; Fischer et al., 2019; Liu et al., 2016).

## The Process of Creativity

Young (1939) suggests a five-step process for creating a new idea (Clear, n.d.; Walsh, 2015). First one must gather new material related to the task along with material gathered because of general fascination with a wide range of concepts. Second, one must mentally "chew" on the material. This includes looking at it from different angles. Additionally, one should experiment with fitting ideas together. Next, it is important to *stop* thinking about new ideas. Often while doing something else an idea will come with a flash of insight. Then, lastly, one develops the idea into practical usefulness. These ideas are similar to the stages discussed related to creativity through flow (Csikszentmihalyi, 1997). These stages have been discussed as well by Taylor (n.d.), who labels them slightly differently. Taylor suggests that the five steps of creativity are preparation, incubation, insight, evaluation, and elaboration.

In terms of occupational therapy practice, practitioners may wish to be creative around new programming for a facility, intervention activities for a child who is struggling to engage in specific tasks, or ideas for an in-service one must perform. An understanding of the process of creativity encourages the practitioner to:

- Read widely from inside and outside the profession so that one has a large "cache" of material to draw from
- Ensure that the practitioner is familiar with a wide range of preferred childhood activities, movies, TV shows, toys, and games
- Think about "thorny" therapeutic issues and try to consider them in new ways!
- Then put those thoughts away and do something else (*go for a walk, run, hike, or engage in self-care activities or household chores*) for a while to see if ideas pop into being

Perry-Smith and Mannucci (2017) discuss a four-step process that chronicles the "journey" of an idea from conception to completion. These four stages are idea generation, elaboration, championing, and execution, as illustrated in Fig. 2.2. These authors discuss creativity as a social process. There is a critical interplay between an individual's idea and the initial efforts to make the idea a reality, the work of a team, the individual's networks, and the organization the individual works for. The individual often must win the support of others before an idea can become reality. Interpersonal skills are critical throughout this process.

In terms of occupational therapy practice, this second depiction of the process of creativity would most likely apply to program development as opposed to the creation of an intervention within a session. For program development, the occupational therapy practitioner becomes familiar with the needs of the community, the range of programs available, and innovative programming from across the globe that could be adapted to the local community. Attending international webinars, engaging online international social networks, and observing the programming in related fields (play therapy for example) may spark creativity for new occupational therapy programming.

Researchers have just begun to operationalize and study the process or trajectory of idea generation, now called ideational pathways (Tanggaard & Beghetto, 2015). An ideational pathway is the trajectory of an idea as it travels through space and time regardless of whether the idea results in a creative outcome. Using diagrams, researchers can document transcripts of interactions between people as a group or team seeks to perform creatively. Studies of ideational pathways may eventually help creativity science better understand the development and growth of creativity in groups and individuals.

## Personality Characteristics of the Creative

Personality is considered a relatively stable set of a person's characteristics that influence that person's performance in varied situations, as well as something that matures and changes over time (Damian et al., 2019). Research supports a variety of associations between specific personality traits and measures of creativity (Baas et al., 2013). For example, in studies with the five-factor model of personality, creativity was

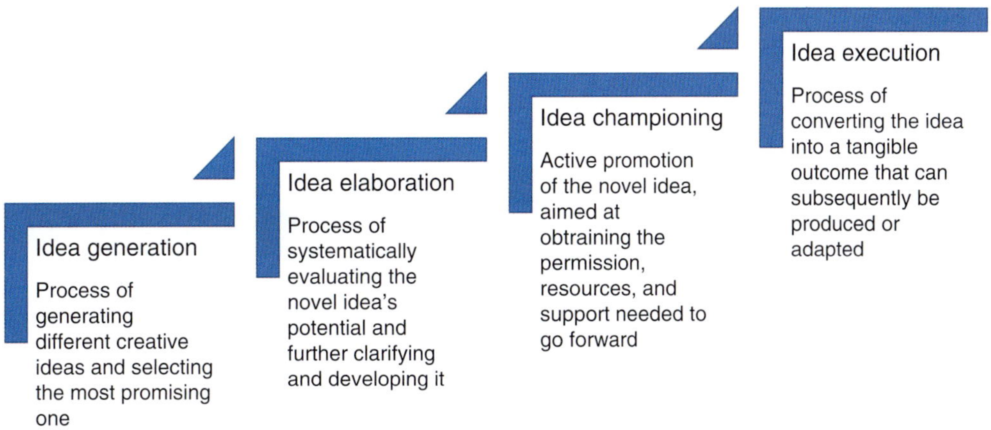


**Fig. 2.2** Journey of an idea, Perry-Smith and Mannucci's (2017) four-step process that chronicles the "journey" of an idea from conception to completion. (Adapted from Perry-Smith, J. E., & Mannucci, P. V. (2017). From creativity to innovation: The social network drivers of the four phases of the idea journey. *The Academy of Management Review*, 42(1), 53–79.)

most related to the characteristic of openness to experience (Conner & Silvia, 2015; Feist, 1998; Ivcevic & Brackett, 2015; van Tilburg et al., 2015). Open people may be more likely to be interested in and even fascinated by ambiguity and new experiences, thus allowing them the capacity to engage in creative activities (Costa & McCrae, 1992). This association between openness to experience and creativity has been documented in multiple studies (Feist, 1998; Grosul & Feist, 2014; Tan et al., 2019; Zhang & Bartol, 2010).

Other personality traits and abilities often linked with creativity include divergent thinking, wonder and curiosity, imaginativeness, originality, willingness to take risks, intrinsic motivation, affinity to collaborate with others, problem-finding/posing/solving, flexibility, perseverance, and playfulness (Csikszentmihalyi & Getzels, 1971; Guilford, 1975; John-Steiner, 2000; Starko, 2013; Sternberg & Lubart, 1999). Creative people have both strong associative abilities and divergent thinking, and these two characteristics are related (Benedek et al., 2012; Benedek & Neubauer, 2013). Creativity is also related to one's level of persistence (Grohman et al., 2017; Nijstad et al., 2010). To understand this chapter, however, it is important to note that while personality traits are related to creativity in many ways, individuals can improve their creativity, and both personality and creativity are formed through developmental processes (Chávez-Eakle et al., 2012).

For occupational therapy practitioners who wish to enhance creativity in practice, investing time in practices that increase openness to new experiences is a good place to start. If one can do so, engaging in travel to new places to learn about new cultures stimulates interests and promotes new ideas (Schwaba et al., 2019; Sparkman et al., 2016). Similarly, trying new foods or new music might help. Trying a new hobby that pushes one outside one's comfort zone may encourage creativity. One study of older adults even suggests that engaging in puzzles and cognitive training supports more open thinking (Jackson et al., 2012). Also, engaging in activities that provide a boost of confidence may foster creativity because confidence may increase one's willingness to try new things.

## CREATIVITY WITHIN OCCUPATIONAL THERAPY

There is a long history in occupational therapy of using creative and expressive arts therapeutically (Perruzza & Kinsella, 2010), and these types of interventions often require creativity on the part of the client for their completion and on the part of the therapist in their selection and modification for success. Early in the profession's historical roots, arts and crafts activities were a mainstay of intervention, particularly in the realm of occupational therapy practice in mental health.

Occupational therapy practitioners often report their belief that creative arts are useful tools, and many practitioners around the globe still value and use them as modalities for intervention and as an outlet for creativity in clients (Bruce, 1933; Vehlow, 1938). A survey of Swedish therapists suggested that 44% used creative activities from once a week to once every 6 months (Müllersdorf & Ivarsson, 2012). Another revealed that one-third of the respondents did not use creative activities at all (Müllersdorf & Ivarsson, 2016). Those who did use them used them most commonly for adult clients and cognitive or mental health challenges. More than 60% reported that they were used for motivation. However, in many practice areas in the United States, creative activities are no longer the norm (Müllersdorf & Ivarsson, 2012; Perruzza & Kinsella, 2010; Thompson & Blair, 1998).

### Importance of Creativity for Occupational Therapy Practitioners

In addition to the use of crafts commonly thought to encourage creativity as a primary intervention, authors have also commented on the creativity required for the profession of problem-solving (Graham, 1983; Lewin & Reed, 1998; Watson, 1970). Creativity in occupational therapy may be critical for client centeredness and has been specifically described as integral knowledge for implementing client-centered approaches in nursing (Merritt & Boogaerts, 2014; Oven & Lobe, 2019).

Occupational therapy practitioners may be considered the "original makers" (Cohen, 2016). The point of the maker movement is for individuals to make something creative, new, and innovative with the tools and materials on hand in a do-it-yourself (DIY) fashion. Many early occupational therapy practitioners did exactly this. They created original and novel solutions to client problems using whatever scraps and materials were available. Occupational therapy practitioners built up handles using dental compound, modified chairs for clients, built a loom that could be used on a bed, and adapted a pen to be held in the mouth; they made cigarette holders and sandwich holders and meal cutting wheels for one-handed clients (Gleave, 1939; Green, 1922; Jackes, 1935; Kaliher, 1967; Langan, 1967; Randall & Schane, 2019; Souza, 1968; Weiss & Weiss, 1976). All these items required practitioners' creativity.

The job of the pediatric occupational therapy practitioner is considered complex, requiring frequent problem-solving employing

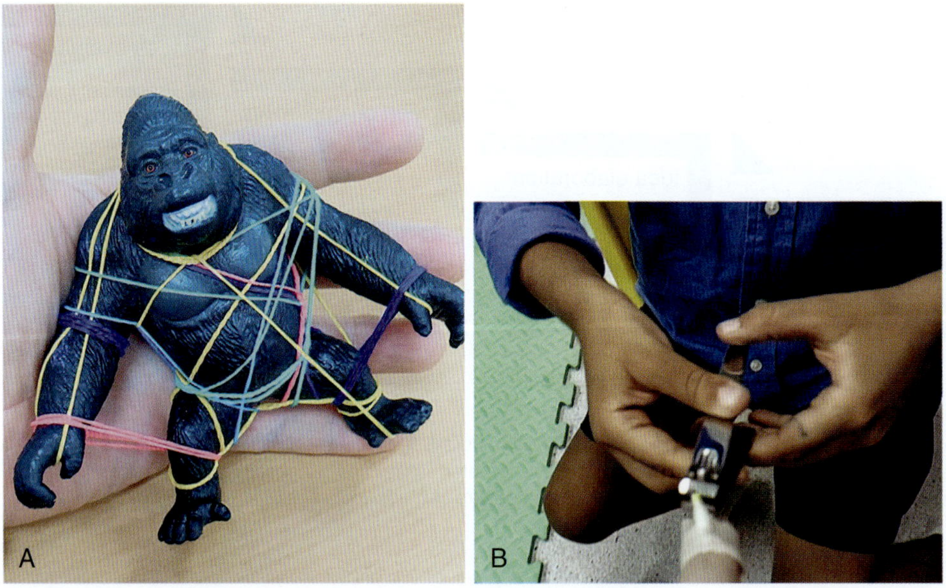


**Fig. 2.3** (A) The occupational therapy practitioner capitalized on the child's interest in the movie King Kong to play "Capture the gorilla" using rubber bands. (B) The practitioner worked on nail cutting by pretending to cut the "witch's nails" using Q-tips taped to the ends of the fingers. (Courtesy Adam Griffin.)

both prior knowledge and experience but also the development of novel solutions to newly arising or never-encountered problems. Practitioners who excel in both areas may experience greater job satisfaction and less likelihood of burnout (Derakhshanrad et al., 2019; Oven & Lobe, 2019). Additionally, creativity is an essential attribute for occupational therapy students and is listed as such by a large majority of fieldwork educators (86.6%) (Campbell et al., 2015). Of fieldwork educators in pediatric settings, 95% listed creativity as essential. Finally, for fluid, playful, child-directed sessions to occur in occupational therapy, practitioners primarily use creative activities. Since each child is unique with individualized preferences and behaviors, the occupational therapy practitioner must be creative to design successful activities (Oven & Lobe, 2019; Spitzer, 2023) (see Fig. 2.3A and B).

## Fostering Creativity in Practice

Although many individuals may feel they are "just not creative," it is important to understand that current science suggests that creativity can be taught or learned and is not an innate trait specific only to certain individuals (Craft, 2005; Kaufman & Sternberg, 2006). Research is converging on many ideas about enhancing one's creativity (Beda et al., 2020). This section provides a variety of suggestions to improve one's creativity, specifically within occupational therapy and pediatric practice.

**Making Time.** Although experienced and established pediatric occupational therapy practitioners typically can quickly implement a creative activity with a child, a newer practitioner or student may need to make some time to think specifically about creative ideas for each upcoming client. Children may refuse some predetermined activities, but when a practitioner is well-stocked with a bucketful of ideas as opposed to just one, the practitioner stands a much better chance of enjoying the fruits of creativity in a successful session. Therefore, it is important to set aside time for creative thinking. This may require quiet periods, without distraction, to consider a specific problem to be addressed with a client and to engage in thought experiments to allow creative ideas to come. See Table 2.2 for thought experiment activities to engage in during this time of creative focus, and see the section on mindsets below as well.

Another aspect of time and creativity is the amount of work time devoted to initiating creative solutions to work-related problems. Pediatric occupational therapy practitioners often face a variety of challenging problems. Some of these may be workplace related, whereas others may be policy related. Work teams may be organized to problem solve solutions.

Because of typical schedules in healthcare, these teams may be able to meet infrequently or weekly over an extended period. This approach can be inefficient and ineffective. An alternative approach sometimes used to foster creativity in business and engineering is the Kaizen or rapid improvement event (Manos, 2007; Van Aken et al., 2010). For these events, teams are structured to address a specific discrete problem within a shortened time frame. The following suggestions can support success with these Kaizen or rapid improvement events: team member authority/autonomy; a well-defined problem; and an action orientation (Glover et al., 2014). When there is a problem in a pediatric worksite, consider scheduling some specific time for group problem-solving following the principles of the Kaizen event.

**Establish a Favorable Environment.** To promote creativity, an important step is to create an environment that is conducive to creativity. This environment can include people to be creative with, the space in which to do creative work, and the "rules" or parameters for creative thinking. For example, an environment that supports creativity likely has "rules" about it being a judgment-free zone for brainstorming. See Box 2.1 for ideas on how to establish a favorable environment and promote creativity in the workplace.

***People.*** Creativity is often social (Marone, 2021). Both the number and type of people one interacts with may influence one's creativity. Creativity has many paradoxes, however (Marone, 2021; Perruzza & Kinsella, 2010). For example, some evidence suggests that working in multidisciplinary groups and with people who have other backgrounds assists a team in generating a greater variety of ideas and novel approaches. However, some research suggests that individuals will generate more ideas or better ideas than groups when asked to

**TABLE 2.2 Thought Experiments to Enhance Creativity**

| Thought Experiment | What to Do |
|---|---|
| The model of excellence | Think about a model person who is excellent at something you are grappling with. Ask yourself ...<br>• Who represents excellence in handling these issues? Is it a famous author? Or is it a historical genius like Einstein? A fictional person? Or a superhero like Wonder Woman?<br>Now imagine you are watching a movie of that person, in your situation<br>• What would be different if this person or character took your place in dealing with your challenges and opportunities? How might things turn out differently?<br>Now imagine the movie again, but with yourself in the place of the model you had selected. How might you address these issues differently? |
| The time machine | Think of something you have accomplished that 5 or 10 years before you did it you would have thought impossible. Now ask yourself, if you could time travel back to your younger self:<br>• How would it change your perspective?<br>• What resources would you give your younger self to help achieve even more?<br>• Consider what you might learn from your future self if your "future you" visited you from 10 or 20 years into the future?<br>• What would you be especially pleased to find out you learned or accomplished? |
| The abstract sculpture | Ask yourself "what would I accomplish if anything was possible, and I could not fail?" then see that result or accomplishment as an abstract art sculpture. What would it look like?<br>Then think about what you value about that accomplishment and focus on the higher level of the value. How would the sculpture change if it represented what you value about the accomplishment versus the accomplishment itself? What new perspective emerges when you return to thinking about the original issue?<br>This can work with different sensory systems (instead of visual with art, try it as auditory—with a piece of instrumental music or taste and touch- with a gourmet meal). |
| The computer simulation | Imagine we are all living in a computer simulation. We are living in a big video game so that nothing you experience is "real" in the sense you thought it was. Ask yourself:<br>• What would you change if you were the programmer?<br>• How would that make things different? |

Adapted from Thought Leadership Studio Podcast Episodes: 3 and 16.

**BOX 2.1 Principles to Adopt to Promote Creativity in Your Eventual Workplace**

- Begin with problem-finding. What problem needs to be solved?
- Focus on the child's interests, desires, and hopes. If they are bored or refusing your activities, consider it your job to do something creative to change the situation.
- Make thoughtful and deliberate choices.
- Create a safe environment for children to take creative chances. Consider it your job to create the environment to nurture exploration and innovation.
- Your role is to model creativity for your pediatric clients, their family members, and even your coworkers.

complete brainstorming tasks (Coursey et al., 2020; Michinov & Jeanson, 2021; Vestal & Mesmer-Magnus, 2020; Yong et al., 2014). This literature, developed in various fields of science, cultural studies, design, and business, suggests that idea generation depends on the type of team diversity present, the level of expertise of the individuals, and their cognitive capacity and skill (Kurtzberg, 2005; Valacich et al., 2006). The team's impact on creativity may also change based on where in the process the team is (idea generation through to implementation) (Perruzza & Kinsella, 2010). Diversity may include functional diversity, which includes differences in knowledge, skills, expertise, or abilities, and demographic diversity (sex, culture, race). Functional diversity may improve group performance (Mello & Rentsch, 2015; Michinov & Jeanson, 2021).

The study of interdisciplinary collaboration and creativity is relatively new, and much remains to be learned about the best ways to create and manage teams to foster this type of creativity (Moirano et al., 2020). Ideally, researchers believe that more diverse and multidisciplinary groups generate the best ideas and select the best ideas from those generated (Baruah & Paulus, 2019; Cirella, 2021; Kuo et al., 2017), as well as that creativity and innovation within teams can be taught and measured. This literature suggests that employment situations where occupational therapy practitioners can work with a diverse team of coworkers promote creativity. This may be one specific benefit of employment in places with a strong interprofessional practice.

In pediatric occupational therapy, the clients themselves may promote creativity as well. Therapists have reported via surveys that their interactions with specific clients often prompted some of their most creative ideas (Oven & Lobe, 2019). Children often make requests that can foster a creative response from a therapist seeking to be child directed and client centered. See Case Example 2.1 of Fiorella for an illustration of one therapist's creative reaction to a child's requests.

***Space and Materials.*** It can be helpful to create a space for daydreaming and thinking if one wishes to foster creativity. In business, these spaces have been called "the lightbulb" (Walsh, 2015). Often the spaces include objects and items to help people be creative, such as musical instruments and Lego bricks (Gauntlett, 2014). A practitioner may make a small space such as this by hanging a blanket over a table and going under the table with the child to their "lightbulb" or "thinking" room as they plan an activity together. Practitioners may include objects in that space to help a child generate ideas.

## CASE EXAMPLE 2.1 FIORELLA: CREATIVITY IN PRACTICE

Fiorella is a 7-year-old girl who loves princesses. She was in therapy because of her difficulties with social play, playground safety, and dressing skills at home. The occupational therapy practitioner incorporated princesses into many of the activities of daily living (ADL), fine motor, and visual perceptual motor activities they engaged in. In the outpatient clinic, the practitioner had a readily available supply of activities and objects to use with the princess theme.

However, during one session, Fiorella mentioned wanting to make a BIG castle. The practitioner could have offered the activity of drawing a big castle, building one with Legos, or other construction toys, or grabbing a prepared castle toy to use. However, the practitioner reasoned that they could use making a big castle as an opportunity to work on upper body strength and endurance needed for playground safety, as well as social play, and specific social skills.

The clinic had multiple rooms, each with four to six large and heavy pillows (16 × 16 in squares). Thinking quickly and creatively, the practitioner suggested they go to each room, and ask the other therapists and children politely if they could have all of the pillows for a few minutes to build a castle. Fiorella loved this idea and readily went along. Fiorella had to knock on each door, then say excuse me, and then ask her questions about the pillows. They subsequently gathered all of the clinic's pillows into the main hallway. Fiorella carried them all one at a time to her clinic space. They built the castle and used it for an additional activity.

The practitioner reflected that they had never played that particular game before and might have never thought of it if Fiorella had not asked to make a big castle. This spark of creativity required the practitioner to be familiar with the materials available, to quickly complete activity analysis to know that the castle building would work on something important for Fiorella and to have the professional attitude of client centeredness to prompt her to want to engage with Fiorella in a way that Fiorella requested.

Makers' spaces have recently cropped up in universities, libraries, camps, and elementary schools (Carey et al., 2014; Schön et al., 2014; Withagen & van der Kamp, 2018). The maker movement is a recent invention brought about by 21st-century developments. Tools such as 3-D printing, electronics, and robotics are combined with more traditional tools and arts and crafts materials in a space to foster creativity (Cal Maritime, 2022). The idea behind the maker movement is to create something new by innovating and developing using these new tools. The movement therefore combines innovation with DIY initiative (Anderson, 2012; Schön et al., 2014). Maker spaces bring people together to engage in the experimental use of materials and technologies to create. A related mindset, called the makerspace mindset, is a view of collaboration that exists and happens across the global community without borders or the restraints of time and space (Culpepper & Gauntlett, 2020).

In pediatric occupational therapy, makers' spaces can also be therapeutic and useful for a variety of cognitive, mental health, and praxis issues. Used as arts and crafts in occupational therapy practice, makers' spaces can be a new, innovative, and current solution to engaging children in therapy.

A related concept to the maker model is the DIY assistive technology model, which is growing in the areas of rehabilitation engineering and assistive technology (Moraiti et al., 2015). This model refers to the movement of engineering to enable individuals to create, modify, or repair items and objects without the need for substantial training. The purpose is to reduce assistive technology abandonment and include users in the development of the technologies. Occupational therapy practitioners who have access to engineers can leverage this interaction and their creativity to generate novel solutions for clients who need them. One specific interaction came out of the Skweezee Lab, where engineers worked specifically with occupational therapists to design tools for their clients (see https://iiw.kuleuven.be/onderzoek/emedia/projects/skweezee).

Years ago, Fazio (1992) described the use of metaphor in occupational therapy practice. A metaphor is a term or description of something in terms of something else (such as "life is a highway"). Fazio encouraged occupational therapy practitioners to use dramatic play, doll play, and puppets as strategies to engage children in the use of metaphors. Acts such as caring for plants in a garden can become metaphors for other actions of caring in life. Games such as blowing up balloons and letting them go can become metaphors for what happens when children "hold on" versus "let go." In therapy, children can draw pictures of their pain and then crumple them up and throw them away. Children can create comic book heroes to engage in symbolic strength and courage in the face of their fears. While Fazio was not specifically promoting creativity per se, her paper opened with the line, "In the crafting of therapeutic intervention, pediatric occupational therapists are challenged to provide therapeutic modalities that are as stimulating and imaginative as the child's world, while offering appropriate and meaningful solutions to the child's problems" (Fazio, 1992, p. 112). What could require more creativity than that?

***Rules.*** To foster creativity, leaders may provide individuals with a variety of rules for time and space to reduce obstacles and barriers that hinder creativity. The following is a set of possible "rules" to initiate in the creative space, such as a pediatric intervention session.

**Be Open to Serendipity.** Occupational therapy practitioners, particularly new practitioners, may approach pediatric sessions with a treatment plan in mind, activities already decided, and an attitude of "I must get XYZ accomplished." However, pediatric sessions may go much better, particularly with certain children, if the practitioner is open to serendipity. Occupational therapy practitioners may enjoy their jobs more if they encounter moments of serendipity or spontaneity, as they may bring with them simple pleasures and happiness (Rubin et al., 2011).

*Serendipity* is an openness to the unexpected (McCay–Peet & Toms, 2015) and is defined as "the interactive outcome of unique and contingent 'mixes' of insight coupled with chance" (Fine & Deegan, 1996, p. 434). One model of serendipity fits well with occupational therapy intervention processes, as it discusses the unexpected event, something that happens often with pediatric clients, and the valuable outcome, something that practitioners would want to see as the destination of the therapeutic session (McCay–Peet & Toms, 2015). See Fig. 2.4 for an illustration of this model. In this model, the trigger is external to the individual and is typically relational. Another person does something or says something that triggers a novel thought or perception about a situation. The trigger initiates some novel connection between disparate ideas or practices. At times, the trigger needs time and self-reflection to "catch," but other times, an instant opportunity is created. These are the magic moments of pediatric therapy sessions; when serendipity strikes, the practitioner sees a new opportunity for intervention, and the child responds with enthusiasm, joy, and engagement, leading to improvement in an important area of function. Serendipity is experienced as positive for both the practitioner and the child, as shown in Fig. 2.5.

**Listen and Watch.** For serendipity to occur, the occupational therapy practitioner must listen and watch for the trigger. This may be something as simple as a child's request, as described in the Fiorella case. Or it can be more subtle, as in Case Example 2.2 of Jordan, whose slight inclination of the head and facial expression prompted the practitioner to change plans during a session.

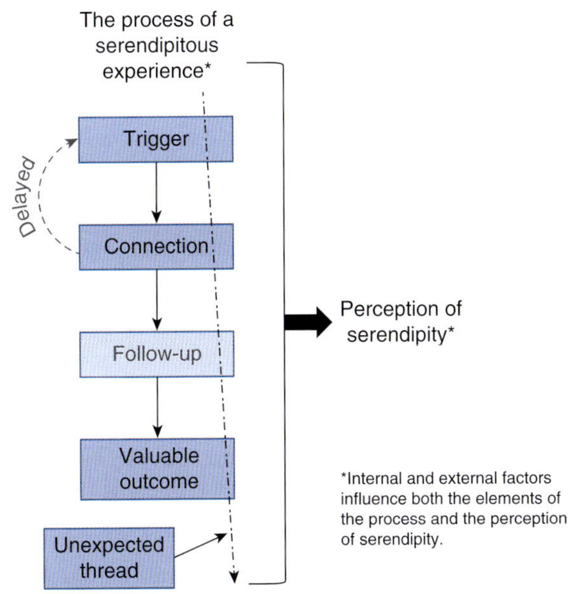


**Fig. 2.4** The process of a serendipitous experience. (From McCay-Peet, L., & Toms, E. G. (2015). Investigating serendipity: How it unfolds and what may influence it. *Journal of the Association for Information Science and Technology*, 66(7), 1463–1476.)

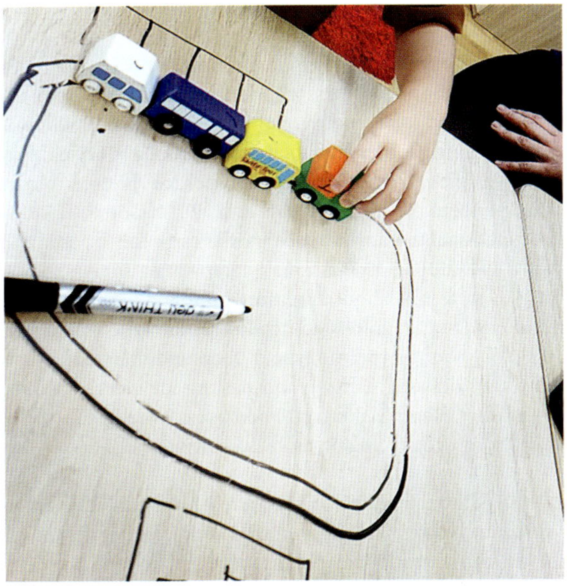

**Fig. 2.5** In a moment of serendipity, the child showed interest in the train and the practitioner quickly drew a track on the table using a whiteboard marker. The child enjoyed "following the road." Serendipity is experienced as positive for both the practitioner and the child.

## CASE EXAMPLE 2.2 JORDAN: SERENDIPITY

An occupational therapist was engaged in an activity with Jordan in a therapy room with more than one practitioner and child present. Jordan had a variety of goals related to ADLs including feeding and oral motor goals. During one session while they were addressing buttoning through a button tic-tac-toe board (Fig. 2.6), Jordan heard another child blowing a whistle and he stopped and turned his head toward the sound, smiling. Serendipity. The subtle change in head position and the smile were a trigger for this therapist to think about using whistles with Jordan. The therapist took this cue as an indication that perhaps he might be ready to try working on lip closure with blowing activities (such as the whistle) that captured Jordan's attention before their self-feeding activity with a spoon.

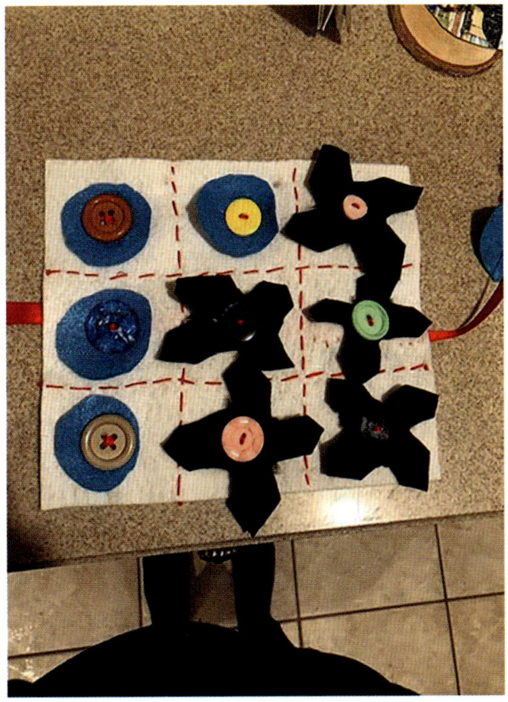

**Fig. 2.6** A large button tic-tac-toe board encourages hand skills. (Courtesy Julia Chiapetta.)

## CASE EXAMPLE 2.3 PETER: PROMOTING IMAGINATION IN PRACTICE

Peter is a 9-year-old boy who receives occupational therapy at school for difficulties with handwriting and expressing what he is learning at school. Often in therapy, the occupational therapy practitioners work on keyboarding, and Peter generally dislikes practicing writing. However, Peter is quite imaginative, and he enjoys science fiction. The occupational therapy assistant discovered that if they worked together discussing odd combinations of items, Peter enjoyed drawing them and labeling them with a made-up word. For example, Peter relayed that he was reading with his mother, "A Wrinkle in Time" which was an old book that his mother loved when she was his age.

The occupational therapy assistant prompted Peter to elaborate on what he loved about the book. He described the dark thing; a cloud that eats stars and the robot that Charles turns into as his favorite parts of the story. The practitioner suggested Peter create a drawing that shows what might happen if the robot and the dark cloud were joined together. Peter laughed and agreed and drew a cloud-shaped body and head with robot arms and legs. Then the practitioner asked Peter what to call it. He named it a Clobot (cloud robot) and eagerly wrote the name on the picture. The practitioner was pleased with Peter's engagement in the session. Peter was excited to bring this work home and show his mother.

**Combine.** Some studies and theories of creativity suggest that the ability to combine elements is an important aspect of creative innovation (Benedek et al., 2012; Benedek & Neubauer, 2013). Mednick (1962) suggested that "any ability or tendency which serves to bring otherwise mutually remote ideas into contiguity will facilitate a creative solution" (p. 222). In therapy, pediatric occupational therapy practitioners can use unusual combinations of items and tools to facilitate novel therapeutic activities. They can also help the child to become more creative by suggesting or questioning using "what if?" and various unusual combinations of items, objects, and activities. Case Example 2.3 illustrates this practice in therapy. Combining old elements in novel ways prompts new ideas. The idea of "combine" is often used in business related to association tools that help the mind

**TABLE 2.3 Association Tools to Help You Think Differently About Something**

| Tool | Description |
|---|---|
| Heroes and Villains | In relation to an issue, ask yourself, What would Batman do in this situation? Or Genghis Khan? |
| Similarities and differences | Think about your issue/item or object and compare it to an item from nature. In what ways is X similar to a storm? A cloud? A tree? A spider? |
| Storytelling | Use the storytelling mountain with your issue to create a fictional story about it. |
| SCAMPER: Substitute, Combine, Adapt, Modify/ Magnify, Purpose, Eliminate/ Minimize and Rearrange/ Reverse | To practice, grab a few objects: a hat, a chair, some craft items, etc. Gather your team in a room (or do this with a child). Throw the objects on the floor and have them start to ask questions below. In this approach, you ask yourself: • What can be replaced? • What can be combined? • What can be added? • What can be modified? • How could you put this thing to another use? • What can be removed or simplified? • What can be swapped or flipped? |

Adapted from Elmansy (2015), Imagine Forest (2022) and Swords and Stationary (2024).

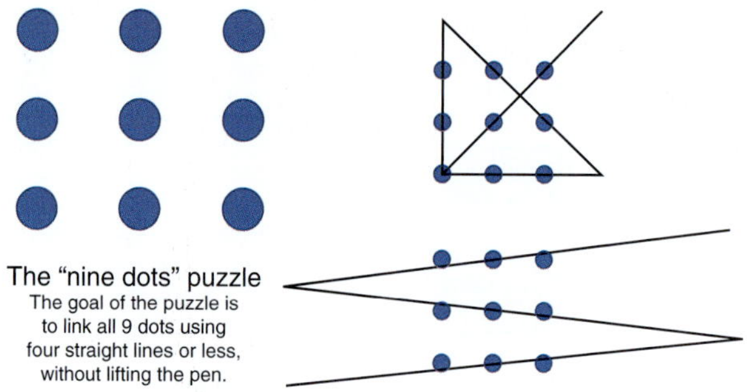


**Fig. 2.7** The nine dots puzzle encourages divergent thinking, perseverance, and creativity (www.artofplay.com/blogs/stories/history-of-the-nine-dot-problem).

think about things in novel ways. Some specific association tools are listed in Table 2.3. Also see the section below on sketching to consider other ways to use "combine."

**Altered Pathways.** Know where you want to end up but that there are many ways to get there. Think about planning a road trip from the east to the west coast of the United States. One would begin knowing the starting and final destinations, but having an openness concerning decisions regarding the pathway or journey to get there can foster opportunities for creativity (and adventure). This type of openness to the journey can be particularly important in pediatric occupational therapy. When a child refuses activities suggested by the practitioner, the practitioner can suggest a creative alternative way to get to the same destination.

**Mindsets.** An important change when trying to foster creativity is to switch one's mindset. Often what hinders creativity is the mindset that "I am not creative." Other mindsets that hinder creativity are linear thinking; benchmarking thinking; simply copying the work of others; the prediction mindset, or trying to predict what will become the next big thing; the mindset that focus is required for creativity when some creativity is inspired by unfocused time; and the naysayer mindset, where ideas are nipped in the bud before being fully explored (Roberto, 2019). Therefore, one of the "rules" to foster creativity is to reject those types of mindsets. Instead, take a "what if?" approach. This is often called "out of the box" thinking, and it is typified by exercises like the nine dots puzzle and Duncker's candle problem (Markov, 2018). See Fig. 2.7 for the nine dots puzzle. Another mindset switch is to take a "devil's advocate" approach and purposely try to shift ideas on their heads. A third is to "time travel" in one's mind and imagine a future where things are radically different from now. Finally, one can purposely change from vertical to lateral thinking. Vertical thinking is logical and sequential. Lateral thinking means to remove preconceived notions and work with ideas that at first seem wrong. Using lateral thinking allows the brain to randomly jump between thoughts to see what emerges. Techniques to foster lateral thinking include using analogies, reversing the order of processes, and trying to connect to random things (Walsh, 2015).

While many of these approaches were designed for teams in business, they can also be used by occupational therapy practitioners who may be stuck on what to do for a particularly difficult client. Similarly, occupational therapy practitioners who work for healthcare organizations and are facing barriers to program initiation/creation may try using some of these techniques to break through those barriers to come up with new and creative solutions.

**Storytelling.** Storytelling fosters imagination and creativity. Stories have been used both to assess children's creativity (Hennessey & Amabile, 1988) and to promote creativity for children (Phillips, 2000). Digital storytelling has benefits similar to traditional storytelling methods, as long as the activities include strategies for children to cocreate, share, and perform the stories (Fields et al., 2014; Göttel, T. 2011).

In occupational therapy practice, stories can easily be used to guide activities. For example, occupational therapy practitioners may cocreate a story with a child about a treasure hunt and pirates while developing and engaging in an obstacle course. Another example might be to read a story about a specific type of food and then make that food either through drawing, cutting and pasting, or using playdough or clay. As another example, a favorite book or codeveloped story can be used to work on sequencing or problem-solving skills.

**Sketching.** Although brainstorming often consists of idea generation using verbal or written language, studies in the field of design, suggest that the use of sketching may prompt idea generation in varied types of activities (van der Lugt, 2005). Three types of sketches are used for these purposes: the thinking sketch, the talking sketch, and the prescriptive sketch. A thinking sketch helps a designer support individual thinking processes during designing. A talking sketch is used to support group discussion. A prescriptive sketch is used to communicate decisions to others who are outside the design process.

In a technique called "brain sketching," individuals sketch their ideas and then share them with others who build upon the original ideas. This process is typically repeated five times (van der Lugt, 2002). Another technique, referred to as "brainsketching with additional context cues," gives participants a context cue card as a source of additional inspiration after the round of individual idea generation. Examples of concrete context cards include things like augmented reality, whereas abstract context cards present things like stressful situations, the weather, or the environment. Adding context cues to a sketching session further assists group creativity (Paay et al., 2023; van der Lugt & van der Graaf, 2002).

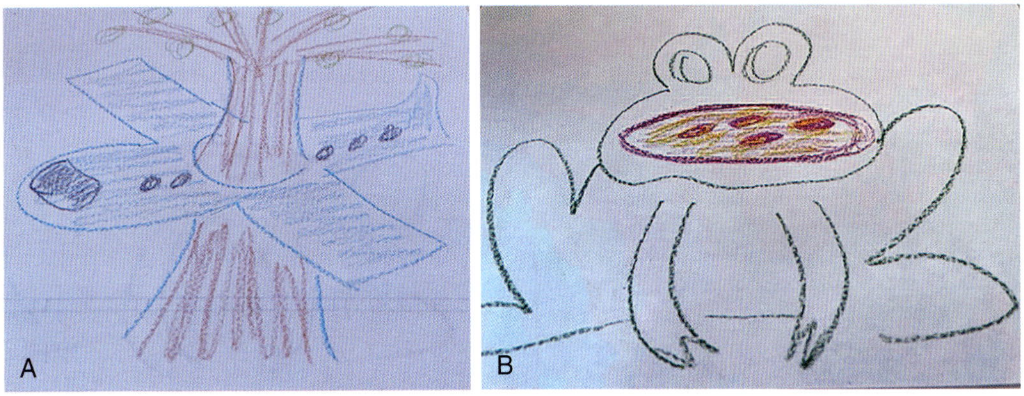

**Fig. 2.8** Combining two things that do not usually go together can lead to creativity. (A) These drawings are a combination of a tree and an airplane and (B) a frog with a pizza. Children can be prompted to draw any two items they prefer and to combine them creatively.

These techniques can be used in occupational therapy with children. The practitioner can work with the child to identify two or more things that do not usually go together but then put them together and try to draw what that might look like. The practitioner and child can take turns adding parts to the drawing so that it becomes increasingly creative but also nonsensical. For example, one could combine two different animals, an animal and a superhero, or an animal and food. Any of these can result in silly and creative pictures that can also engage a child in a variety of fine and visual perceptual motor activities. These types of activities can be readily adapted for home use as well. A child can play these games with peers, siblings, or caregivers. See Fig. 2.8A and B for two examples of this type of activity. Children can also be prompted with unusual contexts for their drawing ideas. For example, what do you think a whale might look like flying over New York City? Or, what would a boat look like in the desert?

**Serious Games and Gamification.** The term "serious game" was initially coined in the 1970s (Abt, 1970; Laamarti et al., 2014). A serious game is not meant for fun or entertainment but instead for learning and skill practice. The beginnings of the gamification movement grew out of military applications where games were used to train soldiers (Laamarti et al., 2014). Often the term serious game refers to methodologies using role play and immersive game situations in industrial and educational settings (Ritterfeld et al., 2009). Some suggest that "serious" comes from the game's role in conveying some message, such as knowledge or skill, to the individual player.

In a serious game, the player is exposed to a game environment that delivers content emanating from some know-how or experience (Laamarti et al., 2014). These games in industry are used to support learning and collaboration. They have been promoted as methods of fostering creativity (AlSaad & Durugbo, 2021; Galetta, 2013; Nivedhitha & Manzoor, 2020) and emerging evidence indicates that serious games can improve creativity (Romero et al., 2015). Some serious games have been developed specifically to enhance creativity by teams and students (Agogué et al., 2015; Hauge et al., 2013) with varying levels of success. However, some research suggests that while serious games may promote knowledge-sharing and collaboration between individuals, they may not support originality on their own (Agogué et al., 2015). Serious games do provide an opportunity to demonstrate learning and change through the analysis of gaming data, which may be helpful in rehabilitation settings (Serrano-Laguna et al., 2018).

Using a combination of manual toolkit-based modeling and serious play may become a way to foster innovation (Schulz et al., 2015).

**BOX 2.2 Prompts to Support Fluency, Originality, Flexibility, and Elaboration**

- Make a list about _____ without stopping for 2 min.
- What are some different ways to _____?
- What ideas from _____ would improve _____?
- What details would improve the idea(s)?
- What is an unusual or another way to _____?
- What could improve _____?
- What would happen if _____?

Adapted from Maloney (n.d.).

Physical models are built and then explained to others through stories. The model or mock-up, built through playful action while incorporating principles of design, then is given meaning through the builder's storytelling. The toolkits to create the models may include pictures, materials for sketching, crafting cardboard, building blocks, or playdough. Lego bricks have also been used in this form of serious game (Barajas et al., 2017; Schulz & Geithner, 2013).

Occupational therapy practitioners who enjoy gaming may try these types of games for themselves to improve creativity and problem-solving. Serious games may also be used with children in therapy. For example, multiple forms of serious games have been used successfully with children with autism (Derks et al., 2022; Mihova et al., 2022; Tsikinas & Xinogalos, 2019), although not yet specifically to improve creativity. The occupational therapy practitioner can also provide children with toolkits for modeling to prompt their creative output.

**Fluency, Originality, Flexibility, and Elaboration.** Fluency, originality, flexibility, and elaboration (FOFE; Mahoney, n.d.) are characteristics that have been used as criteria to measure creativity. They are now specifically used to train students in original thinking. Teachers or practitioners can facilitate FOFE by asking students or children to add more details, continue to add more ideas, or consider ideas from new angles. See Box 2.2 for specific prompts to support creativity with FOFE. Practice and repetition using these strategies promote creativity and thought processes by engaging children to think in novel ways.

**Improvisation.** Engaging in interventions that teach or coach individuals in improvisation may improve children's creativity (Schwenke et al., 2021a, 2021b) and divergent thinking (Hainselin et al., 2018;

Lewis & Lovatt, 2013). Improvisation is the process of spontaneous creation of dialogue, characters, and story for the theater. It works on the assumption of "yes and" which means that the people engaged in this activity together take whatever the improv partner gives them (yes) and then embellish or add to it (and). Those engaged in improv must also work with the assumption that there are no mistakes on stage, merely opportunities. Therefore, actors are taught to take their first inspiration without hesitation and "run with it." To do this, the actors must have the skills to make decisions quickly, take risks, be present in the moment and open to the offers of others, and observe those they are interacting with carefully. Lastly, they must accept each other's ideas in a collaborative way that promotes trust (Schwenke et al., 2021a, 2021b). In many ways, these are the same skills as those of the occupational therapy practitioner, who can play collaboratively and playfully with a child in the moment during an occupational therapy session. This research suggests that training in the skills of improv could promote creativity in pediatric occupational therapy practitioners as well. It may also suggest a method of teaching students to be more creative in pediatric sessions through specific role-play activities (Krusen, 2012). See Case Example 2.4 of Omar and his therapist, who uses the "yes-and" approach in a therapy session to promote Omar's engagement in pretend and play.

### Nonordinary States of Consciousness

Research is beginning to suggest that nonordinary states of consciousness with shifts in thoughts, emotions, and perception can drive creativity. Two mechanisms of obtaining these states are readily available to occupational therapy practitioners, meditation and engaging in flow (a state of total absorption in the present moment). Meditation has been shown to increase creativity in a word fluency test after just 4 days (Zeidan et al., 2010). Flow states can be triggered by having clear goals, intrinsic motivation (curiosity, autonomy, passion, mastery), the "just right challenge," novelty, complexity, unpredictability, insight, risk, and sensory awareness (Kotler et al., 2022). Research supports the link between flow and creativity (Byrne et al., 2003; Csikszentmihalyi, 1997; Schutte & Malouff, 2020; Zubair & Kamal, 2015). Occupational therapy practitioners who wish to improve their creativity may try engaging in meditation or specific occupations that prompt them to find flow. Children may be encouraged to experience "flow" by playing, being engaged in nature activities, dancing, reflecting, or reading.

### CASE EXAMPLE 2.4 OMAR - USING "YES AND" IN THERAPY SESSIONS

Omar is a 6-year-old boy on the autism spectrum who has difficulty with playing, pretending, and being creative. When the occupational therapy practitioner suggests anything even mildly unusual or creative and tries to get him to role-play or pretend himself, he responds, "No, I'm not a _____, I am Omar" or "No, that isn't a _____ it's a _______," or "No that can't happen, that isn't real."

Omar enjoys puppet characters however and the practitioner decides to use this preferred activity, with aspects of improvisation and drama, to work on Omar's ability to pretend and be creative. Omar likes rules and is typically able to follow them. The practitioner has him select his favorite puppet, she selects one as well, and then she describes this new game called "Yes-and." The rules are that Omar cannot say no to anything the puppets say and he has to add to the story. They practice a bit before they begin with the puppets to make sure he understands the rules.

The practitioner tells Omar that they will act out a puppet scene together and have a silly conversation between their two puppets. She lets him choose the topic of their "play" and start the conversation. He chose to play "going to school" which is a familiar routine for him. He starts by saying "I'm going to go get on the bus" as he moves his puppet. She then says, "I am going to school too, but I am going to fly there on my favorite frisbee." He starts to protest that you cannot fly to school on a frisbee but before he can, her puppet says "yes-and" to remind him.

Omar pauses, thinks, and then says, "Yes, that's a good idea, you will get to school very fast, and I will meet you there." The practitioner responds "Yes, I will meet you there and we can have vanilla bananas for breakfast." Again, Omar pauses, makes a face indicating he thinks this is ridiculous, but continues the game, "Yes, and, ummmm, we can make faces on the bananas with M&Ms." The practitioner gives his puppet a high five and they continue with this game for a few more rounds.

The practitioner tries to play the game with Omar using props instead of puppets. They decide to be "firemen." With the practice and props, over time, Omar can begin to role-play and pretend he is a fireman without saying no.

## SUMMARY

Creativity is not a static fixed trait, and it can be learned, enhanced, and facilitated. Creativity is a critical skill for pediatric occupational therapy practitioners but is also a critical "21st-century skill" for children growing up in our current economy and time. This chapter described the importance of creativity, the mechanisms and characteristics of creativity, and provided a variety of strategies for promoting it:

- Creativity is the ability to produce appropriate novelty and useful ideas in responses. It has been linked to and separated from the concept of innovation. Innovation is both the creative idea and the implementation.
- Scientists have studied the neural underpinnings of creativity and found that specific areas of the brain are related to varied aspects of creativity.
- For someone to generate something creative, there must first be a basic level of knowledge about the task or situation. Creativity also requires the right environment, enjoyment, and proper motivation.
- Creative people demonstrate characteristics of openness to ambiguity and new experiences, divergent thinking, wonder and curiosity, imaginativeness, originality, willingness to take risks, intrinsic motivation, flexibility, perseverance, and playfulness. They enjoy collaborating with others and problem-finding, posing, and solving.
- Occupational therapy practitioners working in pediatric settings work with children of all ages, with varied interests, and diverse strengths and challenges. Practitioners use creativity to problem solve novel solutions to newly arising or never-encountered problems. Finally, for fluid, playful, child-directed sessions to occur in occupational therapy, practitioners primarily use creative activities. Since each child is unique with individualized preferences and behaviors, the occupational therapy practitioner must be creative to design successful activities (Oven & Lobe, 2019; Spitzer, 2023).
- There are numerous strategies to foster creativity in occupational therapy practitioners and their clients. Strategies such as making time, establishing a favorable environment, creating "thought" rules, demonstrating openness, listening, and working to find alternative ideas all may prompt creativity. Additional techniques that promote creativity include shifting mindsets, storytelling, brain sketching, serious games and gamification, and improvisation techniques. Prompts based on fluency, originality, flexibility, and elaboration are effective in promoting creativity in children and occupational therapy practitioners.

## REFERENCES


Abt, C. C. (1970). *Serious games*. The Viking Press. 1970.

Agogué, M., Levillain, K., & Hooge, S. (2015). Gamification of creativity: Exploring the usefulness of serious games for ideation. *Creativity and Innovation Management*, *24*(3), 415–429.

AlSaad, F. M., & Durugbo, C. M. (2021). Gamification-as-innovation: A review. *International Journal of Innovation and Technology Management*, *18*(5), 2130002.

Anderson, C. (2012). *Makers: The new industrial revolution*. Crown Business.

Anderson, N., Potoènik, K., & Zhou, J. (2014). Innovation and creativity in organizations. *Journal of Management*, *40*, 1297–1333.

Aziz-Zadeh, L., Liew, S. L., & Dandekar, F. (2013). Exploring the neural correlates of visual creativity. *Social Cognitive and Affective Neuroscience*, *8*(4), 475–480.

Baas, M., Roskes, M., Sligte, D., Nijstad, B. A., & De Dreu, C. K. (2013). Personality and creativity: The dual pathway to creativity model and a research agenda. *Social and Personality Psychology Compass*, *7*(10), 732–748.

Barajas, A. O., Al Osman, H., & Shirmohammadi, S. (2017). A serious game for children with autism spectrum disorder as a tool for play therapy. In *IEEE 5th international conference on Serious Games and Applications for Health (SeGAH)* (pp. 1–7). IEEE.

Baruah, J., & Paulus, P. B. (2019). Collaborative creativity and innovation in education. In *Creativity under duress in education? Resistive Theories, Practices, and Actions* (pp. 155–177). Springer International Publishing.

Batey, M. (2011). Is creativity the number 1 skill for the 21st century? Creativity is the essential skillset for the future. *Psychology Today*. https://www.psychologytoday.com/us/blog/working-creativity/201102/is-creativity-the-number-1-skill-for-the-21st-century.

Beda, Z., Smith, S. M., & Orr, J. (2020). Creativity on demand–Hacking into creative problem solving. *NeuroImage*, *216*, 116867.

Beghetto, R. A., & Kaufman, J. C. (2007). Toward a broader conception of creativity: A case for mini-c creativity. *Psychology of Aesthetics Creativity, and the Arts*, *1*, 73–79.

Benedek, M., Könen, T., & Neubauer, A. C. (2012). Associative abilities underlying creativity. *Psychology of Aesthetics, Creativity, and the Arts*, *6*(3), 273.

Benedek, M., & Neubauer, A. C. (2013). Revisiting Mednick's model on creativity–related differences in associative hierarchies. Evidence for a common path to uncommon thought. *Journal of Creative Behavior*, *47*(4), 273–289.

Bruce, H. A. (1933). An address. *Canadian Journal of Occupational Therapy*, *1*(2), 6–9.

Byrne, C., MacDonald, R., & Carlton, L. (2003). Assessing creativity in musical compositions: Flow as an assessment tool. *British Journal of Music Education*, *20*(3), 277–290.

Cal Maritime. (2022). *Makerspace tool list & guide*. https://www.csum.edu/makerspace/tool-list.html.

Campbell, M. K., Corpus, K., Wussow, T. M., Plummer, T., Gibbs, D., & Hix, S. (2015). Fieldwork educators' perspectives: Professional behavior attributes of level II fieldwork students. *The Open Journal of Occupational Therapy*, *3*(4), 7. https://doi.org/10.15453/2168-6408.1146.

Carey, B., Hernberg, M., Hobbs, T., et al. (2014). *Thinkers and tinkers: The maker movement*. EDEL 545 University of Alberta TLDL Program. https://hernbergm.wixsite.com/maker-movement/background.

Cerasoli, C. P., Nicklin, J. M., & Ford, M. T. (2014). Intrinsic motivation and extrinsic incentives jointly predict performance: A 40-year meta-analysis. *Psychological Bulletin*, *140*(4), 980–1008. https://doi.org/10.1037/a0035661.

Chávez-Eakle, R. A., Eakle, A. J., & Cruz-Fuentes, C. (2012). The multiple relations between creativity and personality. *Creativity Research Journal*, *24*(1), 76–82.

Chi, R. P., & Snyder, A. W. (2012). Brain stimulation enables the solution of an inherently difficult problem. *Neuroscience Letters*, *515*(2), 121–124.

Cirella, S. (2021). Managing collective creativity: Organizational variables to support creative teamwork. *European Management Review*, *18*(4), 404–417.

Clear, J. (n.d.) A technique for producing ideas by James Webb Young. https://jamesclear.com/book-summaries/a-technique-for-producing-ideas.

Cohen, H. (2016). *Accessible fart machines and hand-less video game controllers*. https://www.youtube.com/watch?v=-We84cxubCY&t=1s.

Conner, T. S., & Silvia, P. J. (2015). Creative days: A daily diary study of emotion, personality, and everyday creativity. *Psychology of Aesthetics, Creativity, and the Arts*, *9*(4), 463.

Costa, P. T., Jr., & McCrae, R. R. (1992). Four ways five factors are basic. *Personality and Individual Differences*, *13*(6), 653–665.

Coursey, L. E., Williams, B. C., Kenworthy, J. B., Paulus, P. B., & Doboli, S. (2020). Divergent and convergent group creativity in an asynchronous online environment. *Journal of Creative Behavior*, *54*, 253–266.

Craft, A. (2005). *Creativity in schools: Tensions and dilemmas*. Psychology Press.

Csikszentmihalyi, M. (1997). Flow and creativity. *NAMTA Journal*, *22*(2), 60–97.

Csikszentmihalyi, M., & Getzels, J. W. (1971). Discovery-oriented behavior and the originality of creative products: A study with artists. *Journal of Personality and Social Psychology*, *19*(1), 47.

Culpepper, M. K., & Gauntlett, D. (2020). Making and learning together: Where the makerspace mindset meets platforms for creativity. *Global Studies of Childhood*, *10*(3), 264–274.

Damian, R. I., Spengler, M., Sutu, A., & Roberts, B. W. (2019). Sixteen going on sixty-six: A longitudinal study of personality stability and change across 50 years. *Journal of Personality and Social Psychology*, *117*(3), 674.

Derakhshanrad, S. A., Piven, E., & Zeynalzadeh Ghoochani, B. (2019). The relationships between problem-solving, creativity, and job burnout in Iranian occupational therapists. *Occupational Therapy in Health Care*, *33*(4), 365–380.

Derks, S., Willemen, A. M., & Sterkenburg, P. S. (2022). Improving adaptive and cognitive skills of children with an intellectual disability and/or autism spectrum disorder: Meta-analysis of randomized controlled trials on the effects of serious games. *International Journal of Child-Computer Interaction*, *33*, 100488.

Dirette, D. P. (2017). Cultivating new ideas and solutions in the occupational therapy profession by fostering divergent thinking. *The Open Journal of Occupational Therapy*, *5*(4). https://doi.org/10.15453/2168-6408.1459.

Elmansy, R. (2015). *A guide to the SCAMPER technique for design thinking*. https://www.designorate.com/a-guide-to-the-scamper-technique-for-creative-thinking/.

Fazio, L. S. (1992). Tell me a story: The therapeutic metaphor in the practice of pediatric occupational therapy. *American Journal of Occupational Therapy*, *46*(2), 112–119.

Feist, G. J. (1998). A meta-analysis of personality in scientific and artistic creativity. *Personality and Social Psychology Review*, *2*(4), 290–309.

Fields, D. A., Kafai, Y. B., Strommer, A., Wolf, E., & Seiner, B. (2014). Interactive storytelling for promoting creative expression in media and coding in youth online collaboratives in Scratch. *Proceedings of Constructionism*, 19–23.

Fine, G. A., & Deegan, J. G. (1996). Three principles of Serendip: Insight, chance, and discovery in qualitative research. *International Journal of Qualitative Studies in Education*, *9*(4), 434–447.

Fink, A., & Benedek, M. (2019). The neuroscience of creativity. *Neuroforum*, *25*(4), 231–240.

Fink, A., Grabner, R. H., Gebauer, D., Reishofer, G., Koschutnig, K., & Ebner, F. (2010). Enhancing creativity by means of cognitive stimulation: Evidence from an fMRI study. *NeuroImage*, *52*(4), 1687–1695.

Fischer, C., Malycha, C. P., & Schafmann, E. (2019). The influence of intrinsic motivation and synergistic extrinsic motivators on creativity and innovation. *Frontiers in Psychology*, *10*, 137.

Göttel, T. (2011). Reviewing children's collaboration practices in storytelling environments. In *Proceedings of the 10th international conference on interaction design and children* (pp. 153–156). https://doi.org/10.1145/1999030.1999049.

Galetta, G. (2013). The gamification: Applications and developments for creativity and education. In *Proceedings of the 2013 conference on creativity and innovation in education* (Vol. 10).

Gauntlett, D. (2014). The LEGO System as a tool for thinking, creativity, and changing the world. In *Lego studies: Examining the building blocks of a transmedial phenomenon* (pp. 1–16). Routledge.

Gleave, M. (1939). Prize essay – A new loom for the application of occupational therapy. *Occupational Therapy and Rehabilitation, 18*, 385–389.

Glover, W. J., Farris, J. A., & Van Aken, E. M. (2014). Kaizen events: Assessing the existing literature and convergence of practices. *Engineering Management Journal, 26*(1), 39–61.

Gonen-Yaacovi, G., de Souza, L. C., Levy, R., Urbanski, M., Josse, G., & Volle, E. (2013). Rostral and caudal prefrontal contribution to creativity: A meta-analysis of functional imaging data. *Frontiers in Human Neuroscience, 7*, 465.

Graham, J. (1983). Occupational therapy: Is it the creative problem solving process which the profession claims? *Australian Occupational Therapy Journal, 30*, 89–102.

Green, N. (1922). Occupational therapy for orthopedic patients. *Archives of Occupational Therapy, 1*, 269–278.

Grohman, M. G., Ivcevic, Z., Silvia, P., & Kaufman, S. B. (2017). The role of passion and persistence in creativity. *Psychology of Aesthetics, Creativity, and the Arts, 11*(4), 376.

Grosul, M., & Feist, G. J. (2014). The creative person in science. *Psychology of Aesthetics, Creativity, and the Arts, 8*(1), 30.

Guilford, J. P. (1967). Creativity: Yesterday, today, and tomorrow. *Journal of Creative Behavior, 1*, 3–14.

Guilford, J. P. (1975). Varieties of creative giftedness, their measurement and development. *Gifted Child Quarterly, 19*(2), 107–121.

Hainselin, M., Aubry, A., & Bourdin, B. (2018). Improving teenagers' divergent thinking with improvisational theater. *Frontiers in Psychology, 9*, 1–9.

Hansen, B. W., Erlandsson, L. K., & Leufstadius, C. (2021). A concept analysis of creative activities as intervention in occupational therapy. *Scandinavian Journal of Occupational Therapy, 28*(1), 63–77.

Hauge, J. B., Duin, H., & Thoben, K. D. (2013). The evaluation of serious games supporting creativity through student labs. In *Serious games development and applications: 4th international conference*, SGDA 2013, Trondheim, Norway, September 25-27, 2013: Proceedings (pp. 188–199). Springer.

Hennessey, B. A., & Amabile, T. M. (1988). Story–telling: A method for assessing children's creativity. *Journal of Creative Behavior, 22*(4), 235–246.

Imagine Forest. (2022). *Story mountain explained with examples + free templates*. https://www.imagineforest.com/blog/story-mountain/.

Ivcevic, Z., & Brackett, M. A. (2015). Predicting creativity: Interactive effects of openness to experience and emotion regulation ability. *Psychology of Aesthetics, Creativity, and the Arts, 9*(4), 480.

Jackes, E. (1935). Occupations for recumbent spinal cases. *Canadian Journal of Occupational Therapy, 3*, 12–15.

Jackson, J. J., Hill, P. L., Payne, B. R., Roberts, B. W., & Stine-Morrow, E. A. (2012). Can an old dog learn (and want to experience) new tricks? Cognitive training increases openness to experience in older adults. *Psychology and Aging, 27*(2), 286.

John-Steiner, V. (2000). *Creative collaboration*. Oxford University Press.

Jones, R. H. (2015). *Creativity and discourse analysis. The Routledge handbook of language and creativity* (1st ed., pp. 61-77). Routledge.

Kaliher, M. M. (1967). Picture page: Peeling and cutting board. *American Journal of Occupational Therapy, 21*, 171.

Kaufman, J. C., & Beghetto, R. A. (2009). Beyond big and little: The Four C model of creativity. *Review of General Psychology, 13*(1), 1–12.

Kaufman, J. C., & Sternberg, R. J. (Eds.). (2006). *The international handbook of creativity*. Cambridge University Press.

Kotler, S., Mannino, M., Kelso, S., & Huskey, R. (2022). First few seconds for flow: A comprehensive proposal of the neurobiology and neurodynamics of state onset. *Neuroscience and Biobehavioral Reviews, 143*, 104956.

Krusen, N. E. (2012). Improvisation as an adaptive strategy for occupational therapy practice. *Occupational Therapy in Health Care, 26*, 64–73.

Kuo, H. C., Burnard, P., McLellan, R., Cheng, Y. Y., & Wu, J. J. (2017). The development of indicators for creativity education and a questionnaire to evaluate its delivery and practice. *Thinking Skills and Creativity, 24*, 186–198.

Kurtzberg, T. R. (2005). Feeling creative, being creative: An empirical study of diversity and creativity in teams. *Creativity Research Journal, 17*(1), 51–65.

Laamarti, F., Eid, M., & El Saddik, A. E. (2014). An overview of serious games. *International Journal of Computer Games Technology, 2014* Article 358152.

Langan, T. (1967). Cigarette holder and ashtray. *American Journal of Occupational Therapy, 21*(3), 169.

Lewin, J. E., & Reed, C. A. (1998). *Creative problem solving in occupational therapy: With stories about children*. Lippincott.

Lewis, C., & Lovatt, P. J. (2013). Breaking away from set patterns of thinking: Improvisation and divergent thinking. *Thinking Skills and Creativity, 9*, 46–58.

Lifshitz-Ben-Basat, A., & Mashal, N. (2021). Enhancing creativity by altering the frontoparietal control network functioning using transcranial direct current stimulation. *Experimental Brain Research, 239*(2), 613–626.

Liu, D., Jiang, K., Shalley, C. E., Keem, S., & Zhou, J. (2016). Motivational mechanisms of employee creativity: A meta-analytic examination and theoretical extension of the creativity literature. *Organizational Behavior and Human Decision Processes, 137*, 236–263. https://doi.org/10.1016/j.obhdp.2016.08.001.

Maloney, K. (n.d.). *Fluency, originality, flexibility, & elaboration*. https://sites.google.com/view/kirsten-maloney/critical-and-creative-thinking/9-cct-strategies/fluency-originality-flexibility-elaboration.

Manos, A. (2007). The benefits of Kaizen and Kaizen events. *Quality Progress, 40*(2), 47.

Markov, S. (2018). *The Candle problem by Karl Duncker, 1945*. https://geniusrevive.com/en/the-candle-problem-by-karl-duncker-1945/.

Marone, M. (2021). *Creativity is social*. Dale Carnegie White Paper. https://www.dalecarnegie.com/en/resources/creativity-is-social.

McCay–Peet, L., & Toms, E. G. (2015). Investigating serendipity: How it unfolds and what may influence it. *Journal of the Association for Information Science and Technology, 66*(7), 1463–1476.

Mednick, S. (1962). The associative basis of the creative process. *Psychological Review, 69*(3), 220.

Mello, A. L., & Rentsch, J. R. (2015). Cognitive diversity in teams: A multidisciplinary review. *Small Group Research, 46*, 623–658.

Merritt, A., & Boogaerts, M. (2014). Creativity and power: A qualitative, exploratory study of student learning acquired in a community nursing setting that is applied in future settings. *Contemporary Nurse, 46*, 225–233. https://doi.org/10.5172/conu.2014.46.2.225.

Michinov, N., & Jeanson, S. (2021). Creativity in scientific research: Multidisciplinarity fosters depth of ideas among scientists in electronic "Brainwriting" groups. *Human Factors, 65*(7), 1542–1553.

Mihova, P., Stankova, M., Andonov, F., & Stoyanov, S. (2022). The use of serious games for developing social and communication skills in children with Autism Spectrum Disorders. In *Artificial intelligence and machine learning for healthcare, Vol. 2: Emerging methodologies and trends* (pp. 181–196). Springer International Publishing.

Moirano, R., Sánchez, M. A., & Štěpánek, L. (2020). Creative interdisciplinary collaboration: A systematic literature review. *Thinking Skills and Creativity, 35*, 100626.

Moraiti, A., Vanden Abeele, V., Vanroye, E., & Geurts, L. (2015). Empowering occupational therapists with a DIY-toolkit for smart soft objects. In *Proceedings of the ninth international conference on tangible, embedded, and embodied interaction* (pp. 387–394).

Müllersdorf, M., & Ivarsson, A. B. (2012). Use of creative activities in occupational therapy practice in Sweden. *Occupational Therapy International, 19*, 127–134.

Müllersdorf, M., & Ivarsson, A. B. (2016). What, why, how—creative activities in occupational therapy practice in Sweden. *Occupational Therapy International, 23*(4), 369–378. https://doi.org/10.1002/oti.1438. PMID: 27463409.

Nijstad, B. A., De Dreu, C. K., Rietzschel, E. F., & Baas, M. (2010). The dual pathway to creativity model: Creative ideation as a function of flexibility and persistence. *European Review of Social Psychology, 21*(1), 34–77.

Nivedhitha, K. S., & Manzoor, A. S. (2020). Gamification inducing creative ideation: A parallel mediation model. *Behaviour and Information Technology, 39*(9), 970–994.

Oven, A., & Lobe, B. (2019). Occupational therapists' creativity: Tapping into client centeredness using a novel creativity questionnaire. *American Journal of Occupational Therapy, 73*, 7304205110.

Paay, J., Kjeldskov, J., Bønnerup, M., & Rasenthiran, T. (2023). Sketching and context: Exploring creativity in idea generation groups. *Design Studies, 84*, 101159.

Pellegrino, J. W., & Hilton, M. L. (Eds.). (2012). *Education for life and work: Developing transferable knowledge and skills in the 21st century. National Research Council of the National Academes:* The National Academies Press.

Perruzza, N., & Kinsella, E. A. (2010). Creative arts occupations in therapeutic practice: A review of the literature. *British Journal of Occupational Therapy, 73*(6), 261–268.

Perry-Smith, J. E., & Mannucci, P. V. (2017). From creativity to innovation: The social network drivers of the four phases of the idea journey. *Academy of Management Review, 42*(1), 53–79.

Phillips, L. (2000). Storytelling: The seeds of children's creativity. *Australasian Journal of Early Childhood, 25*(3), 1–5.

Plucker, J., Beghetto, R. A., & Dow, G. (2004). Why isn't creativity more important to educational psychologists? Potential, pitfalls, and future directions in creativity research. *Educational Psychologist, 39*, 83–96.

Randall, K., & Schane, M. (2019). *Adaptive equipment through the ages: A historical review of occupational therapy*. https://digitalservices.scranton.edu/digital/collection/scholarship/id/184/.

Ritterfeld, U., Cody, M., & Vorderer, P. (2009). *Serious games: Mechanisms and effects*. Routledge.

Roberto, M. A. (2019). *Unlocking creativity: How to solve any problem and make the best decisions by shifting creative mindsets*. Wiley.

Romero, M., Usart, M., & Ott, M. (2015). Can serious games contribute to developing and sustaining 21st century skills? *Games and Culture, 10*(2), 148–177.

Royeen, L. (2015). Embracing creativity in occupational therapy. *The Open Journal of Occupational Therapy, 3*(1), 8.

Rubin, V. L., Burkell, J., & Quan-Haase, A. (2011). Facets of serendipity in everyday chance encounters: A grounded theory approach to blog analysis. *Information Research, 16*(3). paper 488 http://www.informationr.net/ir/16-3/paper488.html.

Runco, M. A., & Jaeger, J. (2012). The standard definition of creativity. *Creativity Research Journal, 24*(1), 92–96.

Said-Metwaly, S., Taylor, C. L., Camarda, A., & Barbot, B. (2022). Divergent thinking and creative achievement—How strong is the link? An updated meta-analysis. *Psychology of Aesthetics, Creativity, and the Arts*. https://doi.org/10.1037/aca0000507.

Schön, S., Ebner, M., & Kumar, S. (2014). The Maker Movement. Implications of new digital gadgets, fabrication tools and spaces for creative learning and teaching. *eLearning papers, 39*, 14–25.

Schmid, T. (2004). Meanings of creativity within occupational therapy practice. *Australian Occupational Therapy Journal, 51*(2), 80–88.

Schulz, K. P., & Geithner, S. (2013). Creative tools for collective creativity: The serious play method using Lego bricks. In *Learning and collective creativity* (pp. 191–209). Routledge.

Schulz, K. P., Geithner, S., Woelfel, C., & Krzywinski, J. (2015). Toolkit–based modelling and serious play as means to foster creativity in innovation processes. *Creativity and Innovation Management, 24*(2), 323–340.

Schutte, N. S., & Malouff, J. M. (2020). Connections between curiosity, flow and creativity. *Personality and Individual Differences, 152*, 109555.

Schwaba, T., Robins, R. W., Grijalva, E., & Bleidorn, W. (2019). Does openness to experience matter in love and work? Domain, facet, and developmental evidence from a 24-year longitudinal study. *Journal of Personality, 87*(5), 1074–1092.

Schwenke, D., Dshemuchadse, M., Rasehorn, L., Klarhölter, D., & Scherbaum, S. (2021). Improv to improve: The impact of improvisational theater on creativity, acceptance, and psychological well-being. *Journal of Creativity in Mental Health, 16*(1), 31–48.


Schwenke, D., Dshemuchadse, M., Rasehorn, L., Klarhölter, D., & Scherbaum, S. (2021). Improv to improve: The impact of improvisational theater on creativity, acceptance, and psychological well-being. *Journal of Creativity in Mental Health, 16*(1), 31–48.


Serrano-Laguna, Á., Manero, B., Freire, M., & Fernández-Manjón, B. (2018). A methodology for assessing the effectiveness of serious games and for inferring player learning outcomes. *Multimedia Tools and Applications, 77*, 2849–2871.

Shamay-Tsoory, S. G., Adler, N., Aharon-Peretz, J., Perry, D., & Mayseless, N. (2011). The origins of originality: The neural bases of creative thinking and originality. *Neuropsychologia, 9*(2), 178–185.

Souza, C. M. (1968). Meat cutting wheel for one-handed patients. *American Journal of Occupational Therapy, 22*(3), 211.

Sparkman, D. J., Eidelman, S., & Blanchar, J. C. (2016). Multicultural experiences reduce prejudice through personality shifts in openness to experience. *European Journal of Social Psychology, 46*(7), 840–853.

Spitzer, S. (2023). Being playful: Therapeutic use of self in pediatric occupational therapy. In *Making play just right: Unleashing the power of play in occupational therapy*. Jones & Bartlett Learning.

Starko, A. J. (2013). *Creativity in the classroom: Schools of curious delight*. Routledge.

Sternberg, R. J., & Lubart, T. I. (1999). *The concept of creativity: Prospects and paradigms. Handbook of Creativity* (pp. 3–15. Cambridge University Press.

Swords and Stationary. (2024). https://swordsandstationery.com/learning/story-mountain-awesome-writing-tool/.

Tan, C. S., Lau, X. S., Kung, Y. T., & Kailsan, R. A. (2019). Openness to experience enhances creativity: The mediating role of intrinsic motivation and the creative process engagement. *Journal of Creative Behavior, 53*(1), 109–119.

Tanggaard, L., & Beghetto, R. A. (2015). Ideational pathways: Toward a new approach for studying the life of ideas. *Creativity. Theories–Research-Applications, 2*(2), 129–144.

Taylor, J. (n.d.) The five stages of the creative process. https://www.jamestaylor.me/creative-process-five-stages/.

Thompson, M., & Blair, S. E. E. (1998). Creative arts in occupational therapy: Ancient history or contemporary practice? *Occupational Therapy International, 5*, 48–64.

Thought Leadership Studio. (*Podcast episode 3: The time machine thought experiment*. https://www.thoughtleadershipstudio.com/b/podcast/the-time-machine-thought-experiment.

Thought Leadership Studio. (*Podcast episode 16*. https://www.thoughtleadershipstudio.com/b/podcast/Training-Your-Creativity---The-Abstract-Sculpture-Thought-Experiment.

Tsikinas, S., & Xinogalos, S. (2019). Studying the effects of computer serious games on people with intellectual disabilities or autism spectrum disorder: A systematic literature review. *Journal of Computer Assisted Learning, 35*(1), 61–73.

Valacich, J. S., Jung, J. H., & Looney, C. A. (2006). The effects of individual cognitive ability and idea stimulation on idea- generation performance. *Group Dynamics: Theory, Research, and Practice, 10*, 1–15.

Van Aken, E. M., Farris, J. A., Glover, W. J., & Letens, G. (2010). A framework for designing, managing, and improving Kaizen event programs. *International Journal of Productivity and Performance Management, 59*(7), 641–667.

van Der Lugt, R. (2002). Brainsketching and how it differs from brainstorming. *Creativity and Innovation Management, 11*(1), 43–54.

van der Lugt, R. (2005). How sketching can affect the idea generation process in design group meetings. *Design Studies, 26*, 101–122.

van der Lugt, R., & van der Graaf, A. (2002). Context indicators for determining links between design ideas. In *DS 30: Proceedings of DESIGN 2002, the 7th international design conference*. Dubrovnik.

van Tilburg, W. A., Sedikides, C., & Wildschut, T. (2015). The mnemonic muse: Nostalgia fosters creativity through openness to experience. *Journal of Experimental Social Psychology, 59*, 1–7.

Vehlow, E. L. (1938). The value of occupational therapy. *American Journal of Physical Medicine & Rehabilitation, 17*(1), 41–48.

Vestal, A., & Mesmer-Magnus, J. (2020). Interdisciplinarity and team innovation: The role of team experiential and relational resources. *Small Group Research, 51*, 738–775.

Vivekanandan, R. (2019). *Integrating 21st century skills into education systems: From rhetoric to reality*. https://www.brookings.edu/blot/eduction-plus-development/2019/02/14/integrating-21st-centrury-skills-into-education-systems-from-rhetoric-to-reality/.

Voogt, J., & Roblin, N. P. (2010). *21st century skills*. Discussion Paper Kennisnet, 23. http://opite.pbworks.com/w/file/fetch/61995295/White%20Paper%2021stCS_Final_ENG_def2.pdf.

Walsh, B. (2015). *Releasing creativity*. https://www.burgehugheswalsh.co.uk/Uploaded/1/Documents/CREATIVITY-v8.pdf.

Walsh, S. (2015). *How to transform your problem-solving and creativity*. https://www.smashingmagazine.com/2015/01/transforming-problem-solving-creativity/.

Watson, L. A. (1970). *The nature of creativity in occupational therapy*. Doctoral dissertation University of Pretoria. https://repository.up.ac.za/bitstream/handle/2263/33009/Watson_Nature%20of%20Creativity_1970.pdf;sequence=1.

Weiss, D., & Weiss, L. (1976). The sandwich holder. *American Journal of Occupational Therapy*, *30*(6), 384.

Withagen, R., & van der Kamp, J. (2018). An ecological approach to creativity in making. *New Ideas in Psychology*, *49*, 1–6.

Wood, W. (1995). Weaving the warp and weft of occupational therapy: An art and science for all times. *American Journal of Occupational Therapy*, *49*(1), 44–52.

Yong, K., Sauer, S. J., & Mannix, E. A. (2014). Conflict and creativity in interdisciplinary teams. *Small Group Research*, *45*, 266–289.

Young, J. W. (1939). *A technique for producing ideas*. McGraw-Hill.

Zeidan, F., Johnson, S. K., Diamond, B. J., David, Z., & Goolkasian, P. (2010). Mindfulness meditation improves cognition: Evidence of brief mental training. *Consciousness and Cognition*, *19*(2), 597–605.

Zhang, W., Sjoerds, Z., & Hommel, B. (2020). Metacontrol of human creativity: The neurocognitive mechanisms of convergent and divergent thinking. *NeuroImage*, *210*, 116572.

Zhang, X., & Bartol, K. M. (2010). Linking empowering leadership and employee creativity: The influence of psychological empowerment, intrinsic motivation, and creative process engagement. *Academy of Management Journal*, *53*(1), 107–128. https://doi.org/10.5465/amj.2010.48037118.

Zubair, A., & Kamal, A. (2015). Work related flow, psychological capital, and creativity among employees of software houses. *Psychological Studies*, *60*(3), 321–331.

3

# Intentional Relationships: Working With Children and Families

Evguenia S. Popova, Jane Clifford O'Brien, and Renee Taylor

## GUIDING QUESTIONS

1. What is the therapeutic use of self?
2. How do occupational therapy practitioners develop and maintain therapeutic relationships with children and families?
3. What therapeutic communication modes do occupational therapy practitioners use with children and families?
4. How do the situational and enduring interpersonal characteristics of children and families influence a therapist's use of self?
5. How do inevitable interpersonal events in therapy influence a therapist's use of self?
6. How do occupational therapy practitioners use self therapeutically to respond to strong emotions and challenging interpersonal behaviors?
7. What strategies can occupational therapy practitioners use to develop interpersonal competencies associated with the therapeutic use of self?

## KEY TERMS

Activity focus
Advocating
Collaborating
Empathizing
Encouraging
Enduring interpersonal characteristics
Inevitable interpersonal events
Instructing
Intentional Relationship Model (IRM)
Interpersonal focus
Interpersonal reasoning
Problem-solving
Situational characteristics
Therapeutic relationship

## BUILDING INTENTIONAL RELATIONSHIPS IN PEDIATRICS

Family-centered care is a critical component of occupational therapy practice. Oftentimes, occupational therapy practitioners meet children and families during stressful and unpredictable times in those clients' lives. To ensure family-centered care, occupational therapy practitioners rely on interpersonal skills to empathize and respond to verbal and nonverbal cues as they establish and maintain a ***therapeutic relationship*** with the child and their family. This therapeutic relationship connecting the occupational therapy practitioner, child, and family facilitates trust and open communication. The practitioner can thus ensure a safe and supportive social environment for the whole family when trying something new, challenging, or uncertain (Fig. 3.1). In addition to promoting active participation and engagement, a therapeutic relationship empowers collaborative goal-setting and catalyzes conversations that promote self-efficacy, self-determination, and self-advocacy in children and their families. This chapter discusses strategies for occupational therapy practitioners to develop their interpersonal competencies and explores applying the *Intentional Relationship Model* (IRM; Taylor, 2020) in pediatric occupational therapy practice.

## THERAPEUTIC USE OF SELF

Occupational therapy practitioners develop skills in the therapeutic use of self through practice, supervision, feedback, and reflection. The *Occupational Therapy Practice Framework: Domain and Process—Fourth Edition* (AOTA, 2020b, p. 20) describes therapeutic use of self as "an integral part of the occupational therapy process," which encompasses "professional reasoning, empathy, and a client-centered, collaborative approach to service delivery." Therapeutic use of self supports practitioners in maintaining a balanced approach among an *activity focus* (i.e., an emphasis on "doing" and progressing toward therapeutic goals), and an ***interpersonal focus*** (i.e., emphasis on "feeling" and "relating" with the client) in therapy. Occupational therapy practitioners rely on the therapeutic use of self across all client interactions and draw on their interpersonal characteristics, communication, and therapeutic style to best match client needs.

### Communication

*Verbal and nonverbal communication* is foundational to the therapeutic use of self and family-centered occupational therapy practice (Taylor, 2020). While supporting occupational participation on individual and family levels, occupational therapy practitioners work with families during times of change, uncertainty, and stress. To ensure effective rapport-building and knowledge transfer, occupational therapy practitioners must be cognizant of communicating in a way that is accessible and relevant to the child's and family's immediate needs. While providing family education, practitioners must maintain mindfulness, awareness, and the flexibility to adjust their communication and avoid excessive use of jargon and technical language. For example, while providing parent education and

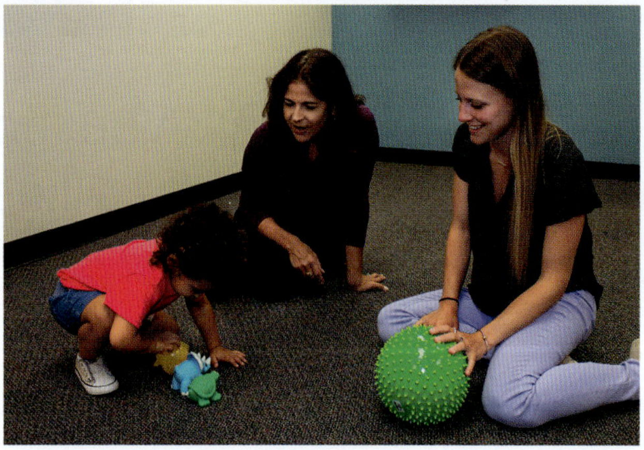

Fig. 3.1 The occupational therapy practitioner creates a safe and welcoming environment to develop a positive therapeutic relationship with the child and parent.

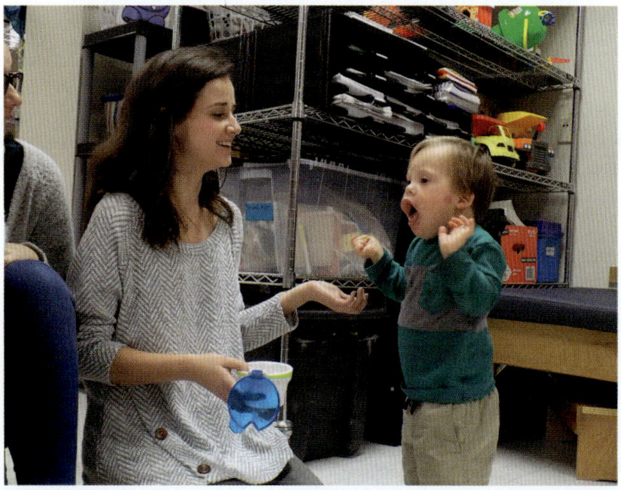

Fig. 3.2 The practitioner uses relaxed body language (by not sitting too close, open hand, smiling facial expression) to support the child while he has a snack break.

instruction, practitioners can apply their interpersonal competencies by using plain language, being mindful of the family's health literacy needs, and ensuring clear and respectful knowledge sharing with children and families. Beyond facilitating family-centered care, the same strategies can be employed to establish a shared understanding and empower interprofessional collaboration across all members of the interdisciplinary team.

In addition to being mindful of their verbal communication, occupational therapy practitioners practice intentionality in their nonverbal communication, including tone of voice, facial expression, and body language. Nonverbal communication is the driving force behind how children and families perceive their relationship with the occupational therapist. For example, the therapist's body language (including posture, movement, and eye contact) can communicate a sense of trust or distrust between the therapist and the client. Fig. 3.2 shows a therapist using welcoming relaxed body language to interact with a child. An occupational therapist can communicate confidence in their clinical practice through eye contact, relaxed body posture, and positioning themselves at the clients' eye level. Alternatively, an occupational therapist who presents themselves by looking away from the client, keeping their hands crossed, and continuously moving away from the client may be perceived as uninterested, nervous, or lacking confidence. Occupational therapy practitioners' interpersonal competencies can also be seen through written communication, including written resources, daily documentation, reports, emails, or text messages. Fig. 3.3A and B illustrate how a practitioner may use therapeutic use of self and therapeutic communication while interacting with a young child.

### Therapeutic Style

***Therapeutic style*** refers to the therapist's interpersonal approach to working with children and families, including preferred modes of communication (Taylor, 2020). Many practitioners may find that their therapeutic style may change depending on contextual demands and the client's interpersonal needs. Understanding the client's unique circumstances, as well as the contextual demands of the clinical setting, helps the occupational therapist adjust their therapeutic style to create a safe and comfortable space for children and families to participate in therapeutic activities. Fig. 3.4 shows practitioners supporting a child as they practice handwriting in a comfortable safe space. For example, an occupational therapist may work in two pediatric settings, seeing families in a neonatal intensive care unit (NICU) and early intervention. When working with families in the NICU, they may recognize the family's increased need for structure, direction, and education. In this instance, the therapist may rely most consistently on structured communication approaches that promote the family's awareness and knowledge of the child's medical condition through instruction and collaborative problem-solving. Yet, when the same therapist sees families through early intervention in a home-based setting, they may rely on more relaxed and flexible communication approaches that promote the family's autonomy through coaching and advocacy.

While occupational therapy practitioners use a wide range of interpersonal approaches when working with clients, the use of humor and playfulness is frequently seen as foundational characteristics of a pediatric occupational therapist Box 3.1 discusses how play and playfulness can support the therapeutic use of self in pediatric occupational therapy practice.

## THE INTENTIONAL RELATIONSHIP MODEL

The IRM (Taylor, 2020) is recognized as the guiding model for the therapeutic use of self in occupational therapy practice (Solman & Clouston, 2016). Consistent with family-centered care, the IRM places the client's experience and needs at the forefront of the therapeutic process. The model stresses that the client is the only person within the therapeutic relationship to determine its success, highlighting the importance of emotional attunement to the child's and family's interpersonal needs in pediatric occupational therapy practice. The IRM views the therapeutic relationship as a process that: (1) supports the client's engagement and (2) provides a space where the client's interpersonal needs can be addressed (Taylor, 2020). As such, the IRM views client- and family-centeredness as an outcome that can indirectly enable the potential for engagement. Box 3.2 shows how occupational therapy practitioners use intentional communication across all aspects of their clinical practice.

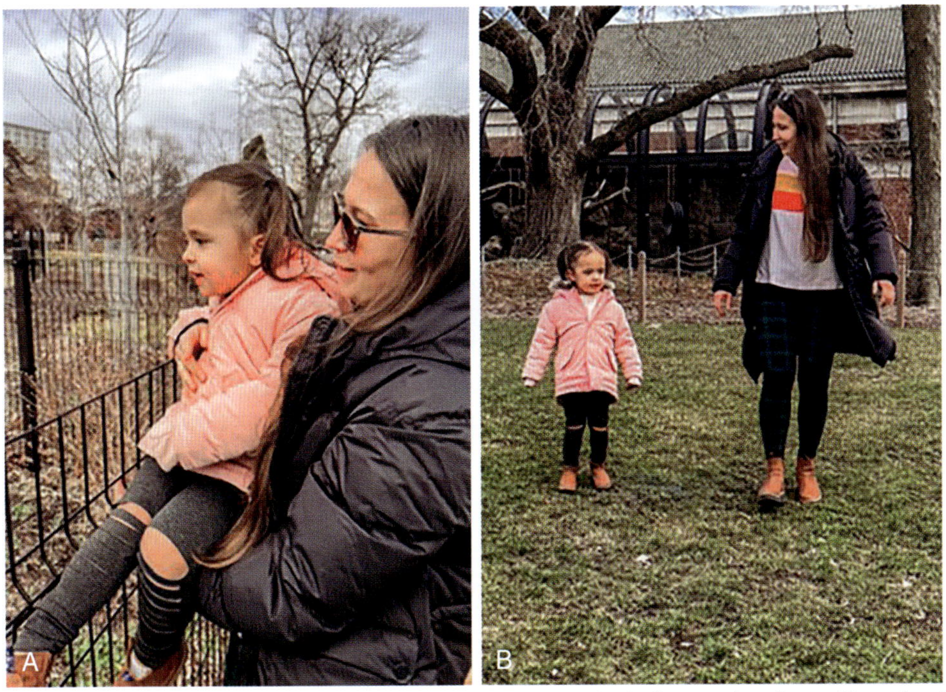


**Fig. 3.3** (A) The occupational therapy practitioner and child share physicality, emotionality, and intentionality as they play "I Spy" at a park. (B) The practitioner uses their therapeutic use of self to mirror the child's body language while playing outside.

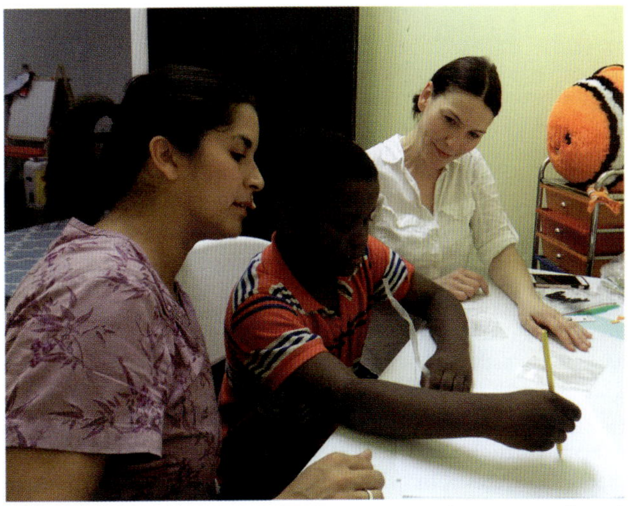

**Fig. 3.4** The practitioners provide a quiet calm safe space to allow the child to practice handwriting. They use their body language to support him, and they observe without providing instruction (since he is engaged in a task which he previously refused).

To promote effective communication and therapeutic use of self, the IRM offers strategies and recommendations that can be used to guide critical self-awareness and interpersonal reasoning throughout the therapeutic process. The IRM defines **interpersonal reasoning** as "a highly individualized, subjective decision-making process grounded in the disciplined application of a set of concepts aimed at meeting the client's interpersonal needs" (Taylor, 2020, pp. 51-52). The IRM model recognizes that a therapeutic relationship emerges from a dynamic interaction between (1) the client's interpersonal characteristics and preferences, (2) the therapist's interpersonal skill base and clinical reasoning, (3) the inevitable (or naturally occurring) interpersonal events, and (4) the client's engagement in occupations

### BOX 3.1 Therapeutic Use of Self and Playfulness in Pediatric Occupational Therapy Practice

Play is an essential building block of child development and lays the foundation for learning, creativity, and problem-solving. Play is used by occupational therapy practitioners across all aspects of pediatric occupational therapy practice and often serves as the driving force behind rapport building and therapeutic use of self as illustrated in Fig. 3.5. Through play, occupational therapy practitioners share and model playfulness and curiosity while inviting children and their families into the therapeutic process. A playful and curious attitude supports the therapeutic use of self by enabling the practitioner to communicate in a flexible manner that follows the interests of the child and their family.

When working with clients who are hesitant or disengaged from the therapeutic process, occupational therapy practitioners can use their playfulness to facilitate trust-building. To build rapport and open communication with the child, practitioners can employ their therapeutic use of self by following the child's lead, joining the child in play, and imitating the child's actions to establish a common understanding. As the child begins to open up and engage with the practitioner, the practitioner can shift their communication to incorporate humor and "conversation temptations" to further build on what the child is doing. For example, while playing with a school bus, a practitioner may invite the child to try something new by singing "Wheels on a Bus" or introducing a new pretend-play idea by having other toys ask to join aboard.

By expanding on the child's ideas, occupational therapy practitioners can capitalize on their playfulness, curiosity, and imagination and create a "just right challenge" to empower the client to try and learn something new. In doing so, the occupational therapy practitioner ensures that the child is challenged and working toward their goal while building a therapeutic relationship and facilitating a foundation for the child's love for learning. Playfulness can also serve as a bridge between the practitioner, the child, and the child's family while communicating via telehealth (Popova, 2022). An open and imaginative approach to communication can strengthen emotional attunement and break down the barrier of physical distance in a virtual setting. For example, the practitioner can create shared moments of understanding and connectedness with the child by giving a "high five" through a camera, sharing a toy, or adding an element of surprise by having toys "come alive" and interact with the child through the camera.

## BOX 3.2 Intentional Communication in all Aspects of Practice

Intentional communication is an essential component of all therapist-client interactions in occupational therapy practice. From the first hello to the last goodbye, occupational therapists practice intentionality and therapeutic use of self to ensure a safe and comfortable space for their clients. Therapists must be mindful of the power of initial impressions and should practice intentionality from the very first interaction with their clients. For example, therapists can use the initial email, phone call, or meeting with the family to communicate their interpersonal style and set the stage for the therapeutic relationship. In the session, therapists practice intentionality as they switch between activity- and interpersonal focus to ensure that they build a strong foundation for relating therapeutically while helping clients work toward their goals. Best practices for maintaining a strong interpersonal focus include dedicating time and space to establish rapport at the start of the session, reflecting and responding to clients' verbal and nonverbal communication throughout the session, and creating closure and reflection on progress in therapy at the end of the session.

Therapists can use various empathic communication strategies to establish rapport at the start of the session, including active listening and observation. Therapists can begin the session by checking in with the client about their week and observing their response. Therapists can pay close attention to verbal and nonverbal communication while considering the client's appearance and immediate context (See Fig. 3.6). Throughout the session, therapists can pause between activities to check in with the client and gather their perspective on the activity. In these times, therapists can ensure that the client is not only actively learning and acquiring information but also feeling comfortable with the therapist's approach. Lastly, at the end of the session, the therapist can document their session while engaging the family in a moment of reflection on their progress.

For example, while working with a family in early intervention, an occupational therapist can take time to ask the family about their week while making a note of any changes in the home environment. A therapist may notice new decorations in the family home and follow up with a question about any upcoming celebrations in the household. Throughout the session, a therapist can pause to ask the family about their perspective on the activities and reflect on their communication to see if it aligns with the family's needs. At the end of the session, the therapist can invite the family to join them in the reflection as they write their notes while using summary statements and enrichment questions to pull the family into the reflecting process.

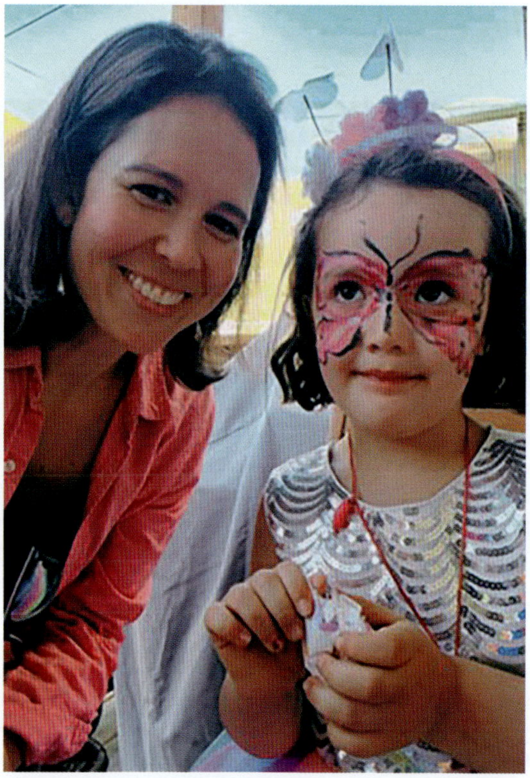

**Fig. 3.5** Being playful in therapy sessions with children helps establish a collaborative relationship and promotes curiosity and engagement.

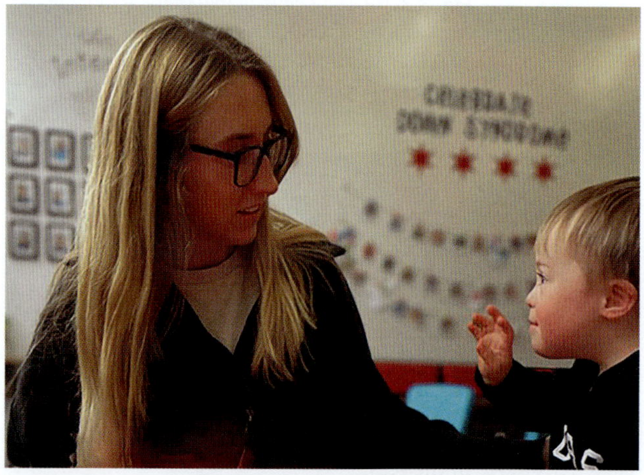

**Fig. 3.6** Practitioners create rapport with children as they listen, communicate honestly (verbally and nonverbally), and build trust.

(or therapeutic activities) (Taylor, 2020). Fig. 3.7 illustrates the IRM model (Taylor, 2020).

The IRM places a strong emphasis on the therapist's responsibility over the positive and the negative ***inevitable interpersonal events*** that occur in therapy, stressing that the therapist should be critically aware of the interpersonal events that occur in therapy, their interpersonal approach, and the client's response (Taylor, 2020). The model proposes that the therapist's ability to adapt their communication to the client's needs can facilitate, or hinder, the client's ability to engage in therapy (Taylor, 2020). Practitioners should have a strong understanding of the client's ***enduring*** (interpersonal tendencies that are typical for the client across a variety of situations) and ***situational characteristics*** (an acute reaction to a situation that is not typical of how the client generally interacts with others), such as communication style, need for control, and ability to receive and provide feedback (Taylor, 2020). To ensure the therapist can work with a wide variety of clients, IRM recommends a lifelong commitment to building interpersonal competency. This competency includes the effective use of interpersonal skills (rapport building, therapeutic communication, strategic questioning) and intentionality in the interpersonal reasoning process. Each of these concepts is discussed in further detail later in this chapter.

The IRM recognizes the importance of social systems and stresses that as the number of people within an interaction increases, the therapist must become more intentional in their communication due to the higher likelihood of an interpersonal event occurring (Taylor, 2020). This concept is especially relevant within pediatric occupational therapy, where practitioners work with children and their families, including parents, siblings, and others. To sustain intentionality within the therapeutic relationship, the therapist must be intimately aware of the unique dynamics within the family. The therapist must recognize that all family members (including the child, parents, siblings, and others) are intimately connected, and a change in one person's emotional state is likely to lead to a change in others. The therapist must be critically aware of the

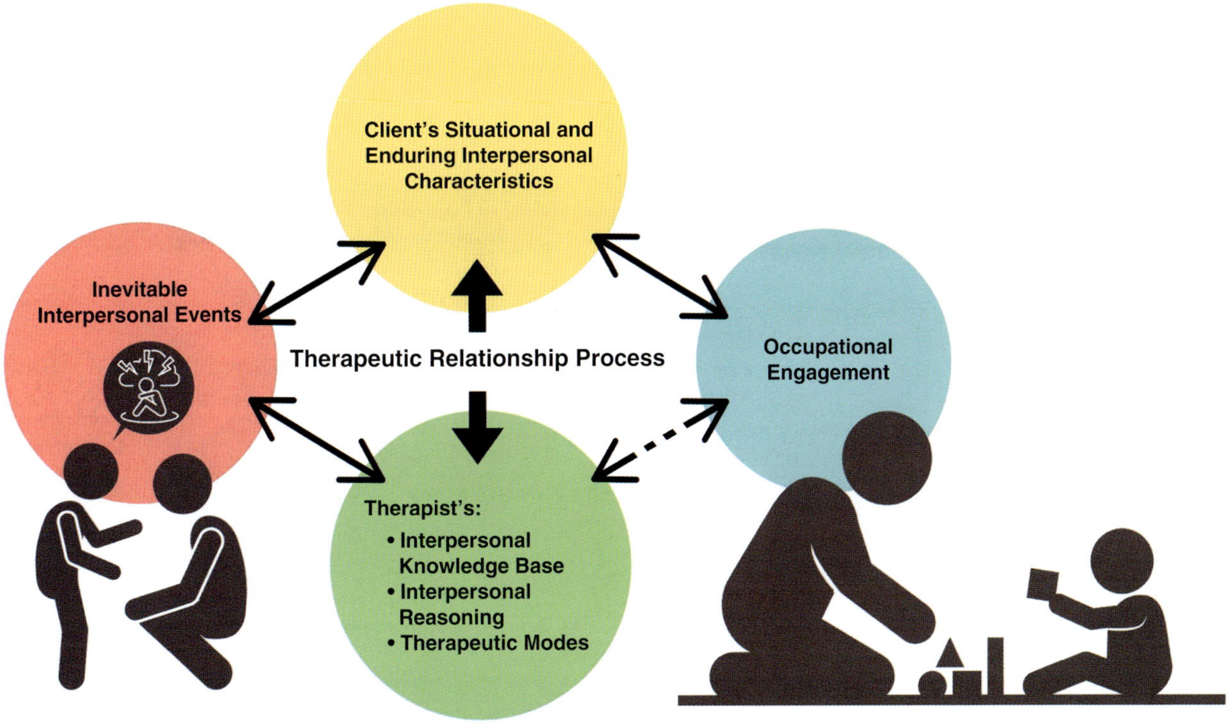


**Fig. 3.7** Illustration of the therapeutic relationship according to the Intentional Relationship Model (Taylor, 2020).

interpersonal dynamics of the client's relationships with others and be able to distinguish between adaptive (trust, collaboration, problem-solving) and maladaptive (dominance, disengagement, manipulation, helplessness, scapegoating) dynamics that may exist within a family (Taylor, 2020). For example, a child showing a high level of excitement in therapy may motivate their parents to be more active in the session. Alternatively, if the child is fearful and hesitant to engage, their parent(s) may become disengaged or reluctant to participate in the session.

## PRINCIPLES OF THE INTENTIONAL RELATIONSHIP MODEL

The IRM is guided by 10 underlying principles.

1. *Critical self-awareness* is key to intentional communication and therapeutic use of self.
2. *Interpersonal self-discipline* is fundamental to effective communication and therapeutic use of self.
3. *Keeping head before heart* supports intentional communication and therapeutic use of self.
4. *Mindful empathy* is required to understand and empathize with the client.
5. Practitioners are responsible for maintaining *professional development* and expanding their interpersonal competencies and knowledge base.
6. A wide range of *therapeutic modes* can be used if the modes are used in flexible, emotionally congruent, and well-matched to the client's interpersonal needs.
7. Clients define a successful therapeutic relationship in practice.
8. An activity focus must be balanced with an interpersonal focus in practice.
9. Therapeutic communication must be informed by professional *values and ethics.*
10. Therapeutic communication must be informed by *cultural sensitivity* (Taylor, 2020, p. 71).

According to the IRM, effective therapeutic use of self is grounded in practitioners' capacity to remain *critically self-aware*. Through reflection on their communication, occupational therapy practitioners can expand their capacity to understand their client's experiences and effectively adjust their communication in response to the client's feedback. Understanding how one is perceived requires a willingness to learn and accept recommendations from others. It also requires that the occupational therapist is aware of how to control their emotions and interpersonal responses. Practitioners can work to build their *interpersonal self-discipline* to ensure that they can "*keep head over heart*" and remain intentional in their communication. This helps the therapist rely on interpersonal reasoning rather than responding to children and families solely based on their initial emotional reaction, which becomes especially important in times of interpersonal stress or uncertainty.

Learning how to remain in the moment or to put one's personal needs aside while working with children and families is essential to family-centered care and promotes *mindful empathy* for children and their families. Practicing mindful empathy requires practitioners to feel and understand another person's underlying emotions and feelings while remaining objective. Since occupational therapy practitioners work with a variety of children and families who may have differing interpersonal needs, they must continuously strive to expand their *professional development* and interpersonal competencies. By expanding their interpersonal competencies and *therapeutic mode* use, occupational therapy practitioners can ensure that their communication is flexible, emotionally congruent, and well-matched to the client's interpersonal needs. Additionally, by empowering the *client to define what a successful therapeutic relationship* looks like, occupational therapy practitioners can work to maintain a *balanced approach between* ***activity focus*** (i.e., an emphasis on "doing" and progress toward achieving therapeutic goals) *and interpersonal focus* (i.e., emphasis on "feeling" and "relating" with the client) in therapy.

Lastly, IRM reminds us that all therapeutic interactions must be grounded in *professional values and ethics* that are core to occupational therapy practice. Staying true to the profession's philosophy

### CASE EXAMPLE 3.1 APPLYING PRINCIPLES OF THE INTENTIONAL RELATIONSHIP MODEL IN OCCUPATIONAL THERAPY PRACTICE

Kai is an inpatient pediatric occupational therapist. One month ago, Kai began working with Heba, a 5-year-old girl that experienced an anoxic brain injury after a near-drowning accident during a family vacation. Kai worked closely with Heba's parents (Karim and Tiye) throughout the rehabilitation stay and established a close and trusting relationship with Heba and her family. While at first Heba was fearful in therapy, her confidence grew with time, and Heba's parents described Heba as "more fearless than ever" as the family prepared to discharge her home.

On the last day of Heba's rehabilitation, Karim and Tiye presented Kai with a basket of fruit and flowers. They thanked Kai for her work with Heba and extended an invitation to Kai to visit their family home and continue working with Heba as a private occupational therapist. While Kai was happy to know that the family saw value in her services and wanted to continue to work with her, she also knew that she would not be able to continue to see them outside of inpatient rehabilitation. She was also critically aware that she needed to be intentional in communicating this information back to the family to ensure that they felt supported, and the therapeutic relationship was not impacted by these limitations in services. She reflected on the cultural importance of gifts to celebrate big life events and professional connections with others and wanted to ensure that she could communicate her gratitude for this gesture and offer to continue working together.

Kai thanked the family for their generosity and shared that the rehabilitation team was so excited about Heba's progress, and Kai was excited to share a gift with the rest of the team. Kai also explained that she was humbled by the invitation to continue working with Heba. However, she would not be able to visit the family or continue working with Heba beyond her current role in the inpatient unit. The family explained that they understood and shared that they included their phone number and email in the thank you card inside the gift basket. After the session, Kai opened the gift basket and placed it in the common break room area. She opened the thank you note to display it for the rest of the team and noticed that in addition to the family's contact information, they included a $100 gift card. Kai knew this gift was beyond an allowable amount at her hospital and was nervous that giving the gift card back to Heba's family would be perceived as insensitive. She remembered, however, that employees were allowed to donate the amount equal to the gift in lieu of returning it. She decided to donate 100 dollars to St. Jude Children's Research Hospital so that the gift would continue supporting children like Heba in the future.

while facilitating occupational performance in children is essential to pediatric occupational therapy practice. Professionalism requires that occupational therapy practitioners follow the American Occupational Therapy Association (AOTA) Code of Ethics (AOTA, 2020a), which includes the principles of beneficence, nonmaleficence, autonomy, justice, veracity, and fidelity. In addition to upholding professional values and ethics, by practicing *cultural sensitivity*, occupational therapy practitioners support their capacity to understand the child's and family's worldviews, beliefs, practices, and traditions and integrate clients' cultures throughout the occupational therapy process. Case Example 3.1 illustrates how these principles may be applied in practice.

## UNDERSTANDING THERAPEUTIC COMMUNICATION MODES

The IRM (Taylor, 2020) describes six therapeutic modes used by occupational therapy practitioners: ***advocating***, ***collaborating***, ***empathizing***, ***encouraging***, ***instructing***, and ***problem-solving*** Fig. 3.8). Each mode is unique in its interpersonal approach and is associated with

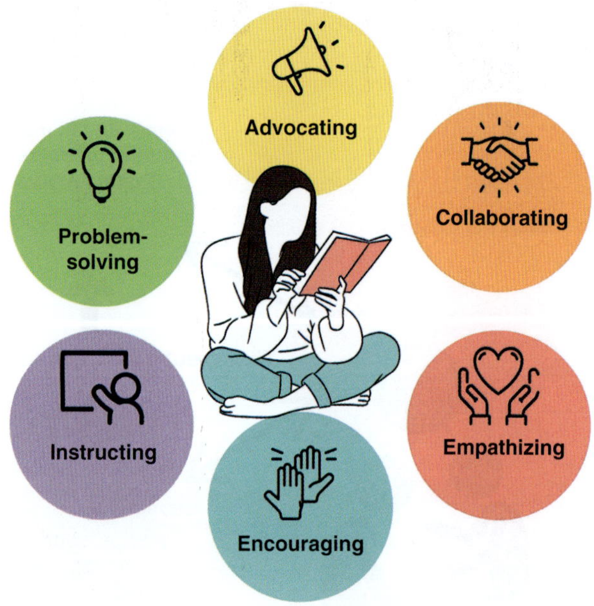


**Fig. 3.8** Therapeutic modes according to the Intentional Relationship Model.

specific communication styles and strategies. The notion of the six therapeutic communication modes proposed by the IRM has been supported by descriptive (Bonsaksen, 2013; Taylor et al., 2011; Yazdani et al., 2017) and psychometric research (Fan & Taylor, 2016). The six modes are also consistent with communication styles reported across pediatric practice settings (Barton & Fettig, 2013; Colyvas et al., 2010; Friedman et al., 2012; Salisbury et al., 2010).

Therapeutic modes can be delivered through verbal or nonverbal means, and the IRM stresses that each mode has the potential to be experienced as therapeutic if it is guided by the needs and preferences of the individual client (rather than being driven by the needs of the therapist) (Taylor, 2020). Different circumstances within a therapeutic interaction may call for mode shifts (an intentional change of modes based on the client's needs in a given situation) (Taylor, 2020). Several roadblocks can prevent therapy practitioners from communicating intentionally and therapeutically, including *mode incongruence* (the mode is perceived as insincere by the client), *mixed mode use* (blending of modes in a way that creates confusion as to what message is being communicated to the client), and *mode mismatch* (the mode is not well matched to the needs of the client) (Taylor, 2020). A therapist who can effectively use a variety of modes is considered to have a *multimodal interpersonal style* by the IRM (Taylor, 2020). A core objective of the IRM is to support the therapist in being able to identify and expand the number of modes that they can comfortably use in practice. Table 3.1 describes an overview of the style and strategies that depict each mode, along with examples from pediatric practice.

Many occupational therapy practitioners can identify modes that are most consistent with their therapeutic style and find that they most consistently rely on those modes in their interactions with clients. Since clients differ in their interpersonal needs, occupational therapy practitioners may also identify professional development opportunities to expand their capacity to communicate multimodally with clients. For example, in early intervention, occupational therapy practitioners are reported to most frequently rely on empathizing, encouraging, and instructing modes in their interactions with children and families (Popova et al., 2022). These findings highlight opportunities to expand the use of collaborating, problem-solving, and advocating modes as a means of ensuring collaborative communication that facilitates the

**TABLE 3.1 Therapeutic Mode Use in Pediatric Practice**

| Therapeutic Mode and Associated Strategies | Examples |
|---|---|
| **Advocating**—working with the client on overcoming physical, social, and environmental barriers that they may encounter, supporting the client's access to resources and services, normalizing the client's experience.<br>• Encouraging client's self-advocacy.<br>• Empowering awareness and knowledge of legal rights.<br>• Promoting access to support and resources.<br>• Connecting clients to others with similar experience.<br>• Making space for the client's feelings about their experiences. | • Talking to an adolescent with an attention-deficit/hyperactivity disorder (ADHD) diagnosis about their educational rights and accommodations available following postsecondary transition.<br>• Talking to parents of a school-aged child who was recently diagnosed with Autism about the Individuals with Disabilities Education Act (IDEA).<br>• Talking to a parent of a neonatal intensive care unit (NICU) graduate about support and services offered through the early intervention system.<br>• Connecting a school-aged child with a down syndrome diagnosis with an online gaming community that was started by an adolescent with a developmental disability.<br>• Validating a parents' perspective on barriers to service access for children with disabilities in the community. |
| **Collaborating**—letting go of control, supporting the client's autonomy and independence in the decision-making process, ensuring that the client has an active role throughout the treatment process.<br>• Empowering autonomous decision-making.<br>• Creating opportunities for clients to take an active lead in therapy.<br>• Soliciting clients' feedback and recommendations.<br>• Making changes based on client's input.<br>• Following-up on client's goals for therapy. | • Supporting an adolescent in establishing their own goals during a postsecondary transition planning.<br>• Asking the child to contribute their ideas to the session agenda.<br>• Asking a parent to provide their feedback on a child's progress in therapy.<br>• Adjusting an intervention activity based on the child's feedback.<br>• Following-up with a teacher on a students' progress toward academic outcomes and asking for their recommendations to help inform future sessions. |
| **Empathizing**—understanding and validating the client's physical, psychological, and emotional experience using active listening strategies.<br>• Striving to understand a client's perspective as accurately as possible through open-ended questions.<br>• Actively listening to the client's verbal and nonverbal communication.<br>• Using active observation to understand the client's experience.<br>• Noticing and responding to the nuances in client's affect and behavior.<br>• Validating of client's emotions through paraphrasing and summary statements. | Asking open-ended questions to understand a child's perspective on their participation at school.<br>• Listening without judgment by paying attention, reflecting, clarifying, and summarizing a parents' perspective.<br>• Paying attention to a toddler's nonverbal communication by watching how they interact with toys and their parents.<br>• Noticing and responding to a change in an adolescent's facial expression by asking an open-ended follow up question on how they are feeling.<br>• Validating a teachers' experience by paraphrasing and summarizing what they shared. |
| **Encouraging**—Fostering hope, encouragement, celebration of the client's successes.<br>• Rewarding the clients' successes using positive reinforcement.<br>• Instilling hope, courage, and the will to explore, participate, or perform a given activity.<br>• Investigating what motivates clients, including their unique interests and goals.<br>• Integrating the client's preferred activities into the session.<br>• Using feedback, humor, cheer and motivational words and gestures. | • Celebrating the child's success in therapy with clapping and praise.<br>• Talking to parents about the child's progress in therapy and positive outcomes resulting from intervention.<br>• Exploring the child's interests and incorporating them into treatment activities.<br>• Developing a session agenda that incorporate the child's highly preferred activities.<br>• Incorporating humor into a child's creative writing assignment. |
| **Instructing**—taking on a role of an expert guide or a teacher, providing structure and feedback, providing clear feedback on the client's performance.<br>• Emphasizing educational aspects of therapy and assuming a teaching stance.<br>• Sharing professional opinions, information and structure therapy process and activities.<br>• Using educational and training approaches, such as the teach-back method and modeling.<br>• Providing constructive feedback.<br>• Setting clear structure and boundaries for therapy. | • Providing a teacher with an infographic on strategies to incorporate mental-health promotion into the classroom routine.<br>• Talking to the parent about the roles and expectations of different interprofessional members on the individualized family service plan (IFSP) team.<br>• Using the teach-back method with an adolescent who is learning how to shave with an adapted razor.<br>• Reminding children about the rules and expectations for the afterschool group.<br>• Providing a child with a visual schedule for the session. |
| **Problem-solving**—utilizing logic, facilitating problem-solving and analytical reasoning, using strategic questioning, outlining the options available to their client as well as any potential outcomes.<br>• Asking strategic questions to guide clients' problem-solving.<br>• Discussing the clients' options, including pros and cons of different decisions.<br>• Using logic to guide client's decisions and analytic reasoning.<br>• Using intentional pauses to provide enough time and space for clients to make their own decisions.<br>• Asking questions to help the client identify alternatives. | • Asking a teacher about different strategies that have supported their students' participation in the classroom.<br>• Brainstorming benefits and challenges of different wheelchair options with an adolescent with a spinal injury.<br>• Outlining postsecondary opportunities with parents of young adult with a developmental disability.<br>• Pausing and "wondering" with a parent about the next steps and possible actions in the potty-training process.<br>• Asking a child a strategic question to help them come up with a solution to a math problem. |

family's capacity to independently problem-solve and advocate for their needs.

Occupational therapy practitioners must be mindful of the unique interpersonal preferences and needs of all clients and recognize that some children and families may respond better to different modes. A change may be required when the mode is not consistent with the child or family's interpersonal needs. For example, if the practitioner uses the instruction mode for a family who prefers collaborating, the family may perceive that the practitioner is not listening to them and become distant, interfering with the therapeutic process. This may lead to reluctance to share pertinent information with a therapist or engage in therapeutic activities during the session. Occupational therapy practitioners may also need to change modes when the timing is not right for the client due to situational demands. For example, a family just learning about a child's diagnosis and prognosis may require an empathizing rather than an encouraging mode.

## Advocating Mode

The ***advocating mode*** encompasses communication strategies that ensure that children and families have access to the resources, materials, and services they need (Taylor, 2020). Practitioners use the advocating mode to ensure that their clients are active advocates for their needs. Occupational therapy practitioners who use the advocating mode have a deep understanding of children's and families' rights, including laws that impact access to resources and services. While using the advocating mode, therapy practitioners work with families and children to raise their awareness of their legal rights and the connections they have to those who share similar experiences.

The advocating mode facilitates discussions that raise clients' awareness and capacity to overcome physical, social, and environmental barriers to occupational participation. These discussions can span a variety of occupational domains, including discussions of occupational and disability justice. The advocating mode is essential for supporting families in understanding their legal rights, advocating for services from service providers and insurance companies, and connecting with others who have had similar experiences. However, practitioners must be cognizant of the family's readiness for change and orientation toward disability advocacy.

## Collaborating Mode

The ***collaborating mode*** encompasses communication strategies that promote clients' autonomy and independence in decision-making. While working with children and families, the occupational therapist may use the collaborating mode to encourage active participation in therapy, collaborative discussion of goals, and self-direction throughout the therapeutic process. The collaborating mode empowers children and families to actively participate in the therapy process and reinforces child and family input, choices, and decision-making.

The collaborating mode is a powerful mechanism behind family-centered care. However, practitioners must also acknowledge that some families may become overwhelmed by being invited as collaborative partners in the intervention process. Families may seek expertise and direction from the occupational therapist or show a strong preference for following suggestions from the therapist without being responsible for creating the plan. This may give families more psychological security and emotional stability in times of uncertainty or stress. Practitioners must also be aware that, when used without intentionality and structure, the collaborating mode may appear as uncertainty or reluctance on the part of the therapist.

## Empathizing Mode

The ***empathizing mode*** encompasses active listening and observation to understand the child's and family's experience. This mode includes open-ended questions to gain a deep understanding of the family's experience. While using the empathizing mode, occupational therapy practitioners notice and respond to the client's emotional, psychosocial, and physical needs. The empathizing mode effectively validates the client's feelings as the therapist uses summary statements to paraphrase the client's experience. The therapist demonstrates understanding the client's point of view.

When using the empathizing mode, practitioners must slow down, listen, and be mindful of the child's and parents' thoughts and feelings. While the empathizing mode is a powerful approach to supporting children and families, if overused, it may not lead to the momentum required for children and families to reach their goals. Excessive use of the empathizing mode can lead to dependence on the therapist and may not challenge the client to engage in occupations outside their comfort zone. Additionally, a therapist who does not practice mindful empathy may risk overidentifying with the client, leading to interpersonal stress and burnout.

## Encouraging

The ***encouraging mode*** encompasses communication strategies that remind the client of their strengths, accomplishments, and progress. Occupational therapy practitioners who use the encouraging mode present as positive, enthusiastic, and hopeful. They may provide frequent reinforcement, praise, and upbeat comments to motivate the client. Fig. 3.9 shows a practitioner using the encouraging mode to promote fine motor and cognitive development. Additionally, the therapist can use the encouraging mode to celebrate small successes and use hopeful language or humor to promote engagement.

Encouragement is an essential component of any therapeutic or mentorship relationship and helps clients persevere through times of change and challenge. The encouraging mode can help children and families through difficult times and promote further efforts toward goals. However, occupational therapy practitioners must be cognizant that clients may become desensitized to positive encouragement if it is overused. Furthermore, excessive use of the encouraging mode may diminish a client's intrinsic motivation; rather, the client may become dependent on external praise to feel good about their abilities. Additionally, some clients may view encouragement as insincere or foolish. Practitioners must practice intentionality and self-awareness to prevent the risk of emotional incongruence.

## Instructing

The ***instructing mode*** emphasizes communication that promotes structure, information-sharing, and client education in therapy. The

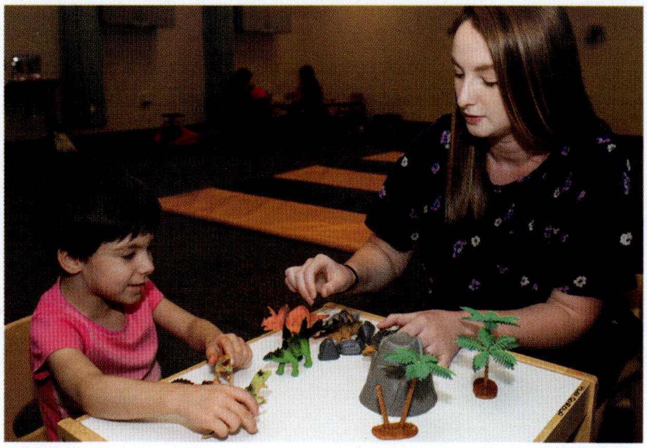

**Fig. 3.9** The practitioner uses encouraging mode to promote cognitive, social interaction, and fine motor skills as they play with the small figurines.

instructing mode assumes that the occupational therapist is knowledgeable and an "expert" in intervention strategies and approaches. Practitioners who use the instructing mode tend to be directive and skilled at teaching others. They develop a plan and review it with the client to ensure follow-through. They may use the "teach-back" approach to review the material and ask the child or a family member to demonstrate the strategy. Case Example 3.2 illustrates how a practitioner might use the teach-back method (Fig. 3.10A and B).

Instruction and information-sharing are core therapy components, and families rely on practitioners to obtain relevant information. However, overusing the instructing mode may distance occupational therapy practitioners from the client and lead to power dilemmas. While using the instructing mode, occupational therapy practitioners may become highly invested in the child's success, leading them to place a stronger emphasis on the activity focus than on the interpersonal focus. Furthermore, overreliance on the instructing mode may lead practitioners to quickly turn to remediation, or "fixing the problem," instead of allowing the child or family the opportunity to problem-solve and determine a solution on their own.

### CASE EXAMPLE 3.2 TEACH-BACK METHOD

Diego is a young adult practicing work-readiness skills through a community-based organization. The practitioner uses an instructing mode to teach Diego how to make a bouquet of flowers in preparation for a Mother's Day Event. While using this mode, the practitioner applies the teach-back method to ensure that Diego is able to understand and remember all parts of the work task. Together, they work on arranging and wrapping flowers (See Fig. 3.10A). The practitioner observes Diego complete the task. Together they develop a plan to ensure follow-through at work. Before beginning the task, Diego reviews the three step-plan and then demonstrates his skills by completing the task. As Diego reflects back on this activity, he is able to confidently explain the 3-step process back to his supervisor Fig. 3.10B.

### Problem-Solving

The ***problem-solving mode*** relies on communication strategies that emphasize logic and reasoning. In their communication, occupational therapy practitioners may use Socratic questioning, a discussion of pros and cons, and an exploration of supports and barriers to families' occupational participation. The problem-solving mode can also empower clients to evaluate their strengths and opportunities to improve their occupational performance through task analysis.

The problem-solving mode may help children and families understand and address how to progress toward their goals logically and systematically. However, overusing problem-solving mode may discount the child's and family's views, resulting in their needs not being adequately addressed. If the problem-solving mode is used too early in the therapeutic process, practitioners may unintentionally introduce jargon and technical terms in ways that families find confusing, leading to frustration and disengagement.

## UNDERSTANDING CHILD AND FAMILY INTERPERSONAL CHARACTERISTICS

In pediatric occupational therapy, the therapeutic relationship encompasses the therapist, the child, and the child's family. While the child is the focal point of the therapeutic relationship, understanding the child's social context and the interpersonal needs of the entire family supports the therapist's effective adjustments in interpersonal style and responses to interpersonal events in therapy. According to IRM, one of the first steps in establishing a therapeutic relationship is gaining a strong understanding of the client's interpersonal style and characteristics (Taylor, 2020). This allows occupational therapy practitioners to effectively anticipate and respond to the child's or parents' responses to various activities and events in therapy. Table 3.2 outlines 14 interpersonal characteristics and provides examples of ways that children and parents may demonstrate each.

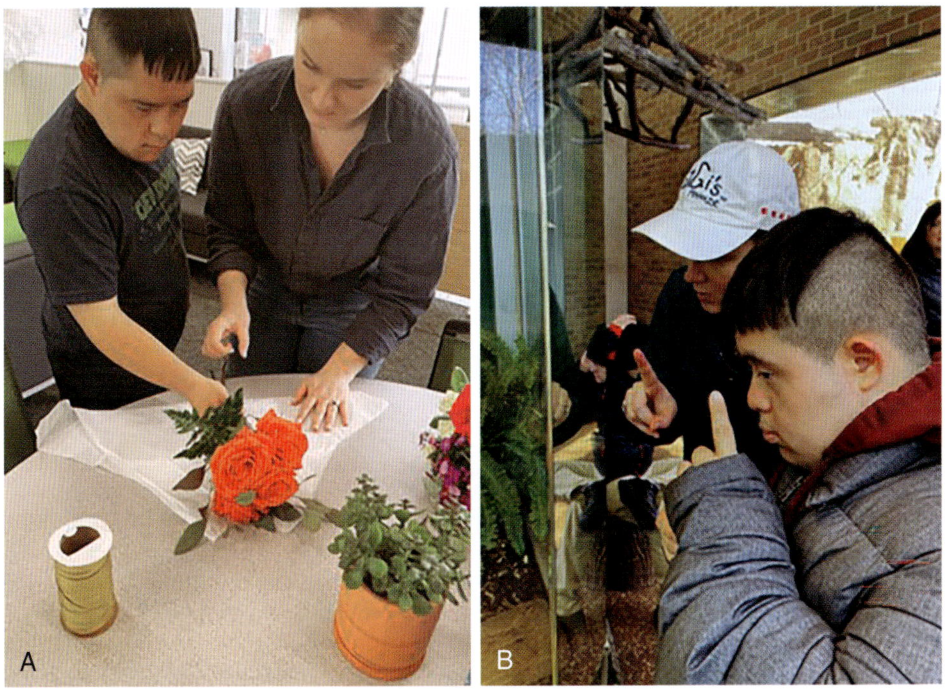


**Fig. 3.10** (A) The therapist uses a 3-step plan to teach Diego how to wrap flowers for work. (B) Diego "teaches back" how he uses the 3-step plan in the workplace to complete work duties.

TABLE 3.2 **Interpersonal Characteristics of Children and Families**

| Interpersonal Characteristic | Examples in Pediatric Practice |
|---|---|
| **Communication style**—Quality, quantity, and pace with which a person expresses themselves verbally or nonverbally | A child closes their eyes and hides behind their parents. The parent responds by saying, "It's ok, I am right here. You are safe." |
| **Tone of voice**—Quality, quantity, and pace with which a person modulates their tone of voice | A child begins to cry and screams out, "homework is too hard!" A parent responds with a lowered voice, "let's try doing this together." |
| **Facial expression**—Quality of nonverbal expression, including affect and facial mannerisms | A child tells a joke and begins to giggle. Another child responds by smiling and laughing. |
| **Body language**—Quality of nonverbal communication, including body position and posture. | An adolescent slouches in the chair and covers their eyes with the hood of their sweatshirt at the start of class. |
| **Interpersonal Reciprocity**—ability to communicate with others in a reciprocal manner | A child looks at a toy and asks, "can I have a turn"? The therapist responds by handing the child the toy. |
| **Orientation toward relating**—Degree to which the person attempts to establish and maintain a relationship with others, including personal and professional relationships | A parent asks the therapist about their plans for the weekend. |
| **Need for control**—degree to which the person attempts to assume and retain control | An adolescent responds with "I do not care" when asked what they want for dinner. |
| **Level of trust**—ability to take confidence in the intentions and actions of others | A child jumps in the pool for the first time while holding onto their parent's hands. |
| **Response to change and challenge**—ability to manage and respond to change and challenge | A child refuses to leave the house and hides their shoes under the couch. |
| **Approach to asserting needs**—ability to communicate wants and needs to others | A parent outlines their weekly responsibilities and shares their preferred days and times for therapy. |
| **Predisposition to giving feedback**—ability to provide feedback to others, including positive and constructive feedback | An adolescent shrugs their shoulders in response to the therapist asking, "How was your day?" |
| **Response to feedback**—ability to receive and respond to feedback from others, including positive and constructive feedback | The therapist says, "Slow down," and the child watches the therapist place the block on top of the other one slowly. The child responds by adding blocks slowly as they build a block tower. |
| **Response to human diversity**—ability to relate to people from diverse backgrounds | A child becomes tearful in the presence of unfamiliar people. |
| **Preference for touch**—preference for physical contact, including physical assistance and cueing | A child sits close to their parents and asks for "squishes" while reading a book. |

The IRM categorizes interpersonal characteristics according to enduring and situational characteristics (Taylor, 2020). ***Enduring interpersonal characteristics*** describe how a client (child or family) most commonly responds to interpersonal aspects of occupational therapy practice and encompass persistent aspects of the client's interpersonal behavior (Taylor, 2020). For example, a child who prefers a consistent routine may react with distrust and an increased need for control when the occupational therapist comes to the classroom earlier and wants the child to skip a regular classroom activity. In this instance, the child may have trouble effectively communicating their needs. Instead, they may throw their book on the floor or attempt to run away from the therapist. The therapist may rely on others who know the client well, and in this example, the therapist may ask the teacher if this behavior is the child's common response to something unexpected or not preferred.

***Situational characteristics*** refer to how a client responds to a specific event or situation and may be inconsistent with the client's typical response. Situational characteristics include interpersonal behaviors that are unexpected or uncharacteristic for a client and may signal to the therapist that the client needs increased support. For example, a generally cooperative child may cry if their parents ask how the school day went. This may signal to the family that something that happened during the school day contributed to the child feeling sad, anxious, or stressed.

Situational characteristics for families may involve responses to changes in the child's or family's life. For example, parents of a young child may not be getting enough sleep, resulting in increased stress and irritability. In therapy, the family may present as distanced and disengaged as a result of this increased stress, which may be taken personally by the therapist when examined without considering contextual factors.

Occupational therapy practitioners working with children and families must seek to understand the situational and enduring characteristics of the whole family and consider how the therapeutic relationship may be impacted by contextual and personal factors. This knowledge can help the therapist best support the family's communication needs and effectively respond in the moment to the child's and family's communication. For example, knowing that the family is under increased stress and may not have the capacity to effectively communicate their needs may prompt the occupational therapist to ask the family if they would prefer to skip or reschedule their session to make more time for self-care and rest. Fig. 3.11A and B show examples of how practitioners may take time to observe and better understand a child's enduring and situational characteristics.

## Understanding Inevitable Interpersonal Events in Therapy

While working with children and their families, occupational therapy practitioners are invited into the family's lives and support them through major life events and transitions. In practice, occupational therapy practitioners may be there for families as they experience the birth of new family members, the loss of loved ones, and life milestones from first birthdays to high school graduations. These times can bring about various ***inevitable interpersonal events***, defined as

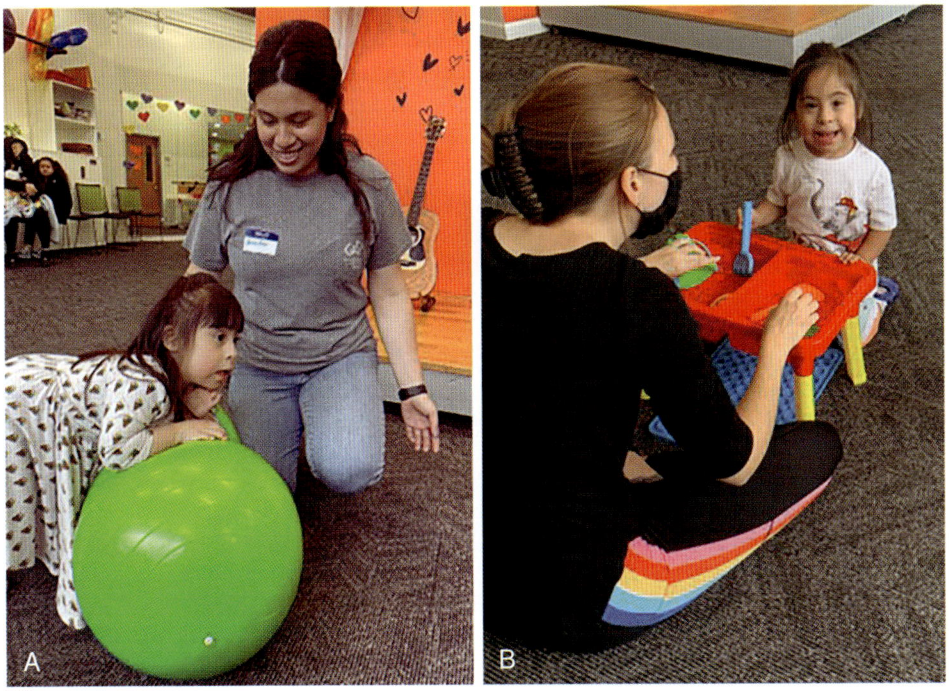


**Fig. 3.11** (A) The practitioner creates space to observe and learn more about the child's interpersonal characteristics, as they witness a child observe others in the therapeutic space. (B) The practitioner mirrors the child's positive affect to empower communication and shared experiences during the session.

emotionally charged or otherwise challenging moments that emerge naturally during the relationship. According to the IRM, inevitable interpersonal events have the power to strengthen or damage the therapeutic relationship depending on how the therapist responds to them (Taylor, 2020).

The occupational therapist must be especially mindful of interpersonal tendencies and communication when responding to inevitable interpersonal events. These moments may produce disappointment, despair, worry, or anger. However, when responded to with intentionality, these events can lead to positive outcomes, clarity, and a strengthened therapeutic relationship. Communicating with intentionality and empathy can help ensure that the child and the family feel supported and understood. Many inevitable events occur during therapy, and while some may be quickly resolved, others may take more time to address. Avoiding inevitable interpersonal events may interfere with the therapeutic process and result in the client feeling ignored, dismissed, or invalidated by the therapist. Table 3.3 outlines 12 categories of inevitable interpersonal events according to the IRM (Taylor, 2020) and provides examples that occur in pediatric occupational therapy.

## Applying the Interpersonal Reasoning Process

Children and families have different priorities, strengths, and challenges. Naturally, some clients may disagree or not connect with the therapist. Additionally, the therapist's communication style may not resonate with the client, and the therapist may be left at the end of the session wondering, *"What happened?"* While these moments may be frustrating, practitioners need to take ownership of the situation and apply their therapeutic use of self to repair the therapeutic relationship. Case Example 3.3 shows how the therapeutic relationship may be impacted by interpersonal events, situational characteristics, and the practitioner's communication.

While working with children and families, occupational therapy practitioners can use interpersonal reasoning to build rapport, establish a common understanding, and set the tone for future interactions. Interpersonal reasoning can also support the occupational therapist's capacity to set an appropriate emotional climate for the session by helping the occupational therapist identify communication strategies that support an optimal tone of communication. For example, while supporting the child or their family through high-emotional-intensity situations (e.g., participation in activities or discussions that result in intense joy, anxiety, or anger), the occupational therapist may rely more on instructing and encouraging modes. In instances of low emotional intensity (e.g., participation in activities or discussions that result in calmness, wonder, or sadness), the occupational therapist may rely more on collaborating, problem-solving, and advocating modes. Alternatively, the occupational therapist may use the empathizing mode to best understand the emotional tone of the activity or the situation to best match the interpersonal needs of the child or their family. Doing so supports occupational therapy practitioners in ensuring that they are appropriately matching their modes to the interpersonal needs of the client while encouraging them to practice mode versatility and mode shifts in a way that promotes a multimodal interpersonal style.

When interpersonal challenges arise, the IRM recommends relying on the interpersonal reasoning process for support in responding therapeutically and intentionally. The IRM outlines a six-step interpersonal reasoning process (Taylor, 2020).

- Anticipate.
- Identify and cope.
- Determine whether a mode shift is required.
- Choose a response mode or mode sequence.
- Draw upon any relevant interpersonal skills associated with the mode(s).
- Gather feedback.

We discuss how these steps can be applied in practice in the sections that follow.

**TABLE 3.3 Inevitable Interpersonal Events in Pediatric Occupational Therapy**

| Inevitable Interpersonal Event | Examples |
|---|---|
| **Expression of strong emotion**—emotional expression that extends beyond what would be normally expected for the interaction, including expression of happiness, sadness, fear, or anger. | A child responds to a joke by laughing loudly and rolling around on the floor. |
| **Intimate self-disclosure**—sharing information that is personal, private, or otherwise sensitive about oneself or others | An adolescent shares that they broke up with their boyfriend. |
| **Power dilemmas**—interpersonal tension because of power issues within a relationship, including circumstances where a person perceives a lack, or a loss, of power within a relationship | A child tells their parents that they want to push the shopping cart all by themselves. |
| **Nonverbal cues**—nonverbal expression of an internal state, including facial expression and body language | A child quickly moves away from the sensory table and puts their hands behind their back. |
| **Verbal Innuendos**—indirect communication that serves as a hint or an insinuation about a person, thing, or situation | An adolescent says "I cannot believe you were actually able to come up with something fun" after seeing the schedule for the day. |
| **Crisis points**—Unanticipated event that results in high stress or pressure in the person's life | A teacher shares that one of their students was hospitalized after being injured in a car accident. |
| **Resistance and reluctance**<br>• ***Resistance***—active or passive refusal to participate in an activity.<br>• ***Reluctance***—active or passive expression of hesitation in response to the activity | A child looks away from the therapist in response to a new activity. They then cross their arms and say, "no, I do not want to play that game." |
| **Boundary Testing**—A request that goes beyond the defined limit within a therapeutic relationship | A child invites the therapist to go with them to a family vacation. |
| **Empathic breaks**—Missed opportunity to notice communication from the client that is perceived as insensitive or hurtful | A therapist does not notice the child attempting to give them a toy. The child responds by fussing and pulling on the therapist's arm. |
| **Emotionally charged therapy tasks and situations**—events that lead to an experience of overwhelm or discomfort | An adolescent is taught a self-catheterization technique after a spinal cord injury. |
| **Limitations of therapy**—Restrictions in available resources and services, including restrictions related to the availability of time, space, and funding | A therapist shares with a parent that insurance will not cover a recommended assistive technology device. |
| **Contextual Inconsistencies**—unexpected change in the interpersonal, occupational, or physical environment | A teacher changes the class schedule after a fire drill. |

## CASE EXAMPLE 3.3 INTERPERSONAL EVENTS, CHARACTERISTICS, AND COMMUNICATION

### Background

Marion, the occupational therapist, prides herself on being a positive, strengths-based, and solution-oriented practitioner. She frequently uses encouraging and problem-solving modes and is confident in their benefit for the clients she sees. Marion is recognized by her clients and co-workers as highly knowledgeable, approachable, and empathic in her communication with others. She enjoys working with children and families and is often approached for advice by other practitioners at her Early Intervention practice.

### Scenario

Marion prepares to evaluate Ty, an 18-month-old boy who was referred to Early Intervention due to his parents' concerns related to global developmental delays. She arrives at Ty's house, only to realize that she is accidently 30 min late for the session. Ty's mother (Ava) invites Marion in and explains that she must leave in 30 min to pick up her older children from school. Marion can see that Ava is stressed out and is having difficulty responding to evaluation questions. Ava frequently looks away, and her answers are short and abrupt. Marion feels embarrassed about being late and frustrated that she is not getting the in-depth answers she needs for the evaluation report. While Ty explores Marion's evaluation toys, he shows little interest in interacting with Marion and does not respond to her attempts to engage. Ava ends the session 15 min into the appointment by abruptly saying "I have to leave so I can pick up my kids from school." Marion apologizes for being late and asks, "what can I do to help?" Ava does not respond, and Marion follows up with "I wonder if I can help Ty with his shoes while you get ready." Ava responds "no, I got this" and begins to help Ty put on his shoes.

Marion leaves the session feeling frustrated. She does not feel that she got a good understanding of Ty's needs for the evaluation report. Although she feels bad for being late, she also feels that Ava was rude and ended the appointment earlier than necessary because she was mad at Marion. She wonders if Ava is not interested in services or seeing Marion again for a full evaluation.

In the hope of repairing the therapeutic relationship, Marion decides to call Ava the next day. At the start of the call, Marion begins the conversation by apologizing for being late and not being able to complete the evaluation. She then pauses and asks Ava how she is doing and if she made it to school to pick-up on time. Ava's voice begins to tremble, and she explains that it was her older child's first day back in school after a long medical leave. She was nervous about his day and wanted to make sure to be at the school early to get a good spot in the pickup line. She shares that she does not have any close family or friends nearby and feels alone. Her husband is trying to help the best he can but has been working two jobs and is almost never home.

### Analysis

Marion generally uses encouraging and problem-solving modes. However, situational characteristics interfered with the session, and she was late for the evaluation. As a therapist who is generally timely, Marion feels upset and embarrassed about the situation. Additionally, Ty's mother is concerned that she will not make it on time to pick up her children from school. The more anxious Ava becomes, the more frustrated she is with Marion's attempts in a positive and encouraging mode. Ty's mother does not feel she is being respected or that her concerns are taken seriously by Marion. Although Marion is trying to help, she does not realize that her attempts at problem-solving mode are adding to Ava's stress at the end of the session. Instead, these attempts further exacerbate Ava's and Marion's frustration with the situation.

**Anticipate.** Inevitable interpersonal events in therapy are natural and expected in the therapeutic process. Occupational therapy practitioners anticipate possible interpersonal events, which may be based on knowledge of one's interpersonal strengths and challenges, feedback from others, and understanding of the clients' enduring and situational characteristics. As practitioners reflect on their communication and anticipate their clients' interpersonal needs, they may ask themselves.

- What are the client's interpersonal characteristics?
- What interpersonal events happened in the past?
- What interpersonal events might happen in the future?

Critical reflection on the client's needs and past experiences can help the therapist best prepare for the client's interpersonal needs in the session. For example, an occupational therapist working with the family of a child with a new diagnosis may anticipate the family needing increased time and space for discussing their experience while asking for increased support and education to feel confident in the next steps. The therapist may reflect on the need to start the session with empathizing and instructing modes to best meet the family where they are.

**Identify and Cope.** In the session, the therapist should apply the empathizing mode to help identify and label interpersonal events that may arise throughout the therapeutic process. Therapists can draw from their knowledge of interpersonal events to identify, cope, and strive for understanding. This process of inquiry and reflection supports objectivity and responds intentionally to help the therapist be:

- *Mindful*—pausing and being present in the moment
- *Self-compassionate*—taking time to empathize with personal experience, feelings, and thoughts
- *Empathic*—taking time to empathize with the client, their experience, feelings, and thoughts

In these moments, the occupational therapy practitioner may take time to observe, ask open-ended questions, or use summary statements to ensure their understanding of the child's and parents' experiences.

After identifying and labeling the event, the occupational therapy practitioner takes time to cope with the situation so that proceeding and responding occur with intentionality. Some strategies that the practitioner might use to cope with feelings of stress, frustration, or unknown include:

- Pausing and taking a deep breath
- Normalizing the event as a natural occurrence in therapy
- Reminding oneself that it is important to validate the client's experience even if no harm was intended
- Reminding oneself that each client is different and may not share the same perspective about the situation
- Reminding oneself that interpersonal events can strengthen the relationship as long as one proceeds with intentionality

Practicing mindful self-awareness helps occupational therapy practitioners realize that the responses are not personal, and can help the practitioner remain mindful, respond with self-compassion, and practice intentionality while responding to the client with empathy. Additionally, taking time to cope and reflect supports the therapy practitioners' capacity to keep head over heart, and avoid responding unintentionally by proceeding with communication that may be easiest or habitual (Taylor, 2020). Fig. 3.12 highlights how an occupational therapy practitioner may dynamically adapt and shift modes during therapy.

**Determine Whether a Mode Shift Is Required.** Once the occupational therapy practitioner has identified that an interpersonal event has occurred, the next step is to determine whether a *mode shift* is required. The occupational therapy practitioner carefully considers how they responded to the situation and the situational factors that may have resulted in the child or family member's interpersonal response. A variety of different interactions may result in a need to mode shift. For example, a *mode mismatch* may occur if the mode selected by the practitioner is not well matched to the needs of the client. The occupational therapy practitioner may decide that the child would benefit from a different style of response. In this case, the occupational therapy practitioner may decide to use another mode. Mode shifts may be necessary if the current mode is not working, and the child's response continues to be problematic and does not allow the therapeutic process to continue (Taylor, 2020).

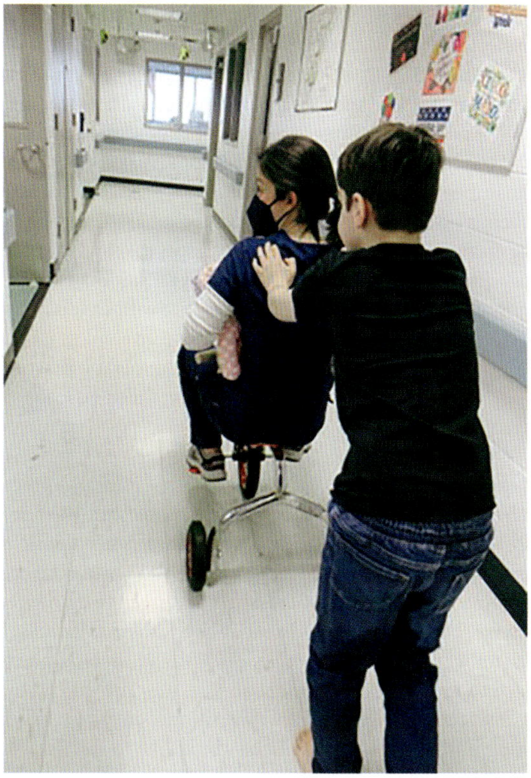

**Fig. 3.12** While working with a student with low vision, a school-based occupational therapist adapts their communication modes to amplify their use of encouraging mode through verbal and nonverbal communication by integrating additional opportunities for play and humor into their session.

Alternatively, the practitioner may decide that the mode was well matched to the needs of the client, however, it was not delivered appropriately. For example, the practitioner may have used a mode in a way that resulted in *mode incongruence*, where the practitioner's verbal and nonverbal communication was not aligned, and the mode may have been perceived as insincere by the client. The practitioner may have also demonstrated *mixed mode use*, which may have resulted in the blending of modes in a way that resulted in a lack of clarity in the message communicated to the client.

**Choose a Response Mode or Mode Sequence.** Practitioners' knowledge of the client's interpersonal characteristics and interpersonal events helps guide their decision and selection of response modes. The practitioner may choose to proceed with a single mode or determine that the situation would be best addressed through a sequence of different modes. For example, while responding to parents' concerns related to the child's academic performance, the practitioner may first begin with an empathizing mode to learn more about the parents' experience before proceeding with the advocating mode to help connect the family to additional support and resources.

***Draw Relevant Interpersonal Skills.*** Choosing a response mode (or mode sequence) requires knowledge of the modes and how they are used in practice. The practitioner must be reflective of opportunities to effectively apply the modes using both verbal and nonverbal communication to ensure that their communication is emotionally congruent and attuned to the client's needs. For example, an occupational therapy practitioner using the encouraging mode with a child engages the child in entertaining behavior with joyful emotions and high energy. They may use humor in the session, and they smile, nod, and are positive with children. Using the encouraging mode with children is typically effective unless it is used too much, and the child perceives the occupational therapy practitioner as being "silly" or insincere. This may frustrate the child and lead to further disengagement in the session.

**Gather Feedback.** Finally, the occupational therapy practitioner gathers feedback to determine whether the mode shift was useful and successful in creating a therapeutic relationship. Since the IRM views successful therapeutic interactions from the child's or caregiver's viewpoint, occupational therapy practitioners are urged to gather feedback from them. This may be as informal as checking in with the child or family member regarding how the occupational therapy practitioner responded to the event. Anonymous surveys may provide useful information. The occupational therapy practitioner may also ask if there is anything unresolved that the client would like to discuss. The IRM (Taylor, 2020) recommends that occupational therapy practitioners work toward a mutual understanding of the event with the child and caregiver. Box 3.3 illustrates how the interpersonal reasoning process can be applied in pediatric occupational therapy practice.

**Responding to Strong Emotions.** It is not uncommon for occupational therapy practitioners to support clients through moments of sadness, anxiety, and anger. The expression of strong emotions is especially prevalent in pediatric practice, and occupational therapy practitioners frequently support clients in their capacity to effectively communicate and regulate emotions in response to change and challenge. Box 3.4 provides an exercise to help readers understand and apply IRM approaches to managing emotional intensity. The IRM (Taylor, 2020) recommends four approaches to managing emotional intensity. They are:

- *Witnessing*—being a silent witness
- *Emotional Resonance*—feeling the same type of emotion as the client and letting your feelings show through verbal or nonverbal means
- *Labeling*—verbally labeling your interpretation of the client's emotional expression
- *Intervening*—acting to change the emotional expression through instruction or problem-solving

***Responding to Sadness.*** When working with clients through moments of sadness, IRM recommends providing clients with enough time to collect themselves and feel their emotions (Taylor, 2020). To do so, occupational therapy practitioners can use witnessing, followed by labeling and emotional resonance once the client is ready to reengage in the interaction. The IRM also recommends that intervening should only take place if sadness becomes maladaptive or chronic or interferes with the client's occupational engagement.

***Responding to Anxiety.*** In instances where the client experiences anxiety, the IRM recommends avoiding prolonged validation of the client's anxiety, as these efforts may only heighten anxiety. Instead, occupational therapy practitioners can intervene through the instructing, collaborating, encouraging, or problem-solving modes. If the occupational therapy practitioner is unclear about the client's emotional state, the therapist can use emotional resonance or labeling to gain a richer understanding of the client's lived experience.

***Responding to Anger.*** Lastly, in situations where the client expressed anger, the IRM recommends that the occupational therapy practitioner evaluates whether the emotional expression was adaptive (i.e., an appropriate emotional response to the situation) or maladaptive (i.e., an inappropriate emotional response that may result in a risk of harm to the client or those around them). According to the IRM, an adaptive expression of anger can activate increased client engagement and should be validated to empower the client and help quell feelings of anger. Furthermore, the IRM recommends that restoring the client's control over the situation helps de-escalate

### BOX 3.3 Applying the Interpersonal Reasoning Process in Pediatric Occupational Therapy Practice

Ari, an occupational therapist, works in a post-secondary college readiness program for young adults with developmental disabilities. Ari works with Parker, who is 19 years old, Autistic, nonbinary, and uses they/them pronouns. Parker was diagnosed with Autism at a young age and is an avid advocate within the Autistic community. Parker's goals are to start a nonprofit for LGBTQ neurodiverse youth, buy their own house, and find a romantic partner.

Ari and Parker have been working together for 6 months, and Parker has been consistently an open communicator who is always ready to jump into action and learn something new. Ari prepares for an upcoming session, and based on previous discussions, anticipates talking to Parker about online dating. Ari opens the topic of dating at the start of the session by beginning to outline different steps and options related to online dating. Parker begins to bite their nails and says, "dating is just a waste of time." This response catches Ari off guard. After taking a deep breath and pausing to reflect on what happened, Ari asks "did you change your mind about starting to date?"

Parker explains that they tried asking out a friend but were rejected without a clear explanation. Ari takes this as a cue to shift from problem-solving mode, and to empathizing mode to help Parker process what happened. Ari draws on strategies of empathic listening and uses summary statements to validate Parker's perspective. At the end of the session, Ari asks Parker how they are feeling, and whether they wish to continue talking about what happened in the following session.

### BOX 3.4 Learning Activity: Responding to Strong Emotions in Pediatric Occupational Therapy Practice

Watch the Pixar animated film Inside Out. Pay attention to the characters during the dinner scene. Apply the IRM recommendations as you reflect on the following questions.

- What interpersonal characteristics do you notice?
- What interpersonal events occurred? Were they responded to in a therapeutic manner?
- What therapeutic modes did you notice? Did you notice any mode incongruence, mismatches, or mixed mode use?

Based on your analysis of this situation, develop a set of IRM-based recommendations that you would give to the characters in the film. Reflecting on the young girls' interpersonal characteristics, and events that took place during the dinner scene, would you have different recommendations for her mother and father? Consider how you could use parent education or coaching to support conflict resolution at that moment.

feelings of anger. On the contrary, a maladaptive expression of anger should be addressed immediately using the instructing mode to ensure the safety of the client and others. This can be done by reinforcing expectations for appropriate behavior and providing instructions to de-escalate the situation. See Learning Activity 3.1 to engage with suggested opportunities to practice with this content.

**Responding to Challenging Interpersonal Behaviors.** While describing the interpersonal aspects of occupational therapy practice, practitioners experience a variety of challenging interpersonal interactions while working with clients across rehabilitation settings and report a wide range of strategies associated with the therapeutic use of self (Taylor et al., 2011; Taylor et al., 2009). The IRM defines *difficult behavior as* recurring, enduring, or high-intensity interpersonal behavior that prompts one (or more) negative emotional reactions in another individual (Taylor, 2020). Most often, challenging behavior is also paired with strong emotion. Occupational therapy practitioners must practice increased mindfulness and intentionality in times of emotionally charged events and strong emotional expression, as these instances may place the relationship at a heightened risk of an empathic break. *Empathic breaks* are a natural consequence of therapy that occur when a practitioner approaches the client in a manner that is perceived as hurtful or insensitive. Unresolved empathic breaks are likely to lead to difficult client behavior and further ruptures in the therapeutic relationship. As such, empathic breaks are best addressed immediately to avoid further escalation and the expression of challenging behaviors. Table 3.4 provides examples of challenging behaviors and suggested modes to support the therapeutic process.

Much like inevitable interpersonal events, depending on how difficult behavior is managed, it can result in negative or positive therapeutic outcomes. Occupational therapy practitioners use the interpersonal reasoning process to select the appropriate mode(s) to understand the client's perspective, support the client's interpersonal needs, and help find an alternative behavior that would be an appropriate expression of the client's experience. As a general rule, the IRM recommends addressing challenging interpersonal behaviors using collaborating, empathizing, instructing, or problem-solving modes. While the practitioner may switch to advocating and encouraging modes once the challenging behavior is resolved, it is not advised to respond initially using those modes, as they run the risk of reinforcing the behavior.

## Strategies to Develop Therapeutic Use of Self

"Developing therapeutic use of self is a lifelong endeavor" (Taylor, 2020, p. 348). The IRM (Taylor, 2020) provides a structure to examine one's therapeutic use of self and explains the process involved when working therapeutically with children and their families. Occupational therapy practitioners can support their professional development and interpersonal competencies by practicing critical self-awareness, recognizing one's strengths and opportunities, creating opportunities to develop new strengths, and being mindful of why one is an occupational therapy practitioner. Additionally, the model provides tools that can give occupational therapy practitioners personal insight into their modes and opportunities for reflecting on the therapeutic use of self.

Hussain et al. (2018) used the IRM to investigate changes in occupational therapy students' short-term self-efficacy for therapeutic mode use, recognizing interpersonal characteristics, and managing

**TABLE 3.4 Challenging Behaviors in Pediatric Occupational Therapy**

| Challenging Behavior & Recommended Modes | Example |
|---|---|
| **Denial**—coping with a painful or uncomfortable event by denying some, or all aspects, of a disability or situation.<br>***Recommended modes:***<br>• Empathizing<br>• Collaborating<br>  • Problem-solving (may be appropriate if the client's safety is at risk) | Despite recommendations to proceed with a medical diagnostic procedure, the parent insists on waiting until the child goes to school. They mention that they have heard that some kids "grow out of it" and believe that this might be the same case for their child.<br>The therapist responds with an empathizing mode by validating the parents' perspective and uses a summary statement "Children change as they get older." they then proceed with a collaborating mode, and ask "would you like to talk through the pros and cons of the medical diagnostic outcomes together?" the parent responds with a yes, and the therapist engages in problem-solving mode. |
| **Difficulty with rapport/trust**<br>• ***Difficulty with rapport***—The client is unfriendly or unresponsive to casual conversation.<br>  • ***Difficulty with trust***—The client expresses skepticism and uneasiness.<br>***Recommended modes:***<br>• Prerequisite: Empathizing<br>• Collaborating<br>• Instructing<br>  • Problem-solving *(not as efficient)* | A therapist transitions to a new case with a client who has been receiving occupational therapy at a different clinic for the past 3 years. At the start of the session, the parent brings up a concern that the child has not been sleeping well at night and seems drowsy during the day. The therapist makes a recommendation to adjust the child's bedtime routine to promote sleep, and the parent responds, "I'm not sure that is a good idea, my other therapist told me our bedtime routine was great."<br>The therapist begins with an empathizing mode by taking time to listen and learn more about the current bedtime routine. They then shift to collaboration by discussing the parent's goals and ideas that could be implemented in the upcoming week. |
| **Emotional disengagement**—A lack of spontaneous and authentic emotional reactions in response to the therapist's attempts to engage.<br>***Recommended modes:***<br>• Empathizing<br>• Problem-solving | An adolescent appears distant and shows minimal social-emotional reciprocity during a therapeutic group. The therapist observes the client slouching in the chair and doodling in their notebook.<br>The therapist approaches the client during the break and asks them how they are feeling. The client shares they are worried about an upcoming test. The therapist responds by saying, "I wonder if it would be helpful for us to do a mindfulness break as a group, what mindfulness strategy do you think would help you feel better in preparation for the test?" |

*Continued*

**TABLE 3.4 Challenging Behaviors in Pediatric Occupational Therapy—cont'd**

| Challenging Behavior & Recommended Modes | Example |
|---|---|
| **Excessive Dependency**—Resistance to the therapist's attempt to promote the client's independent thinking or functioning.<br>***Recommended modes:***<br>• Empathizing (must be accompanied by one or more other modes to be effective)<br>• Collaborating<br>• Instructing<br>• Problem-solving | As the family prepares for discharge from the NICU, the parent shares" this is all just too hard. There is no way that we will be able to do this without your help."<br>The therapist responds with, "this is a difficult time, and there is a lot to do between now and your return home. Remember that I will still see you during your NICU follow-up visits." (i.e., empathizing and collaborating). The therapist pauses, and the parent nods. The therapist follows up with "what are your top three priorities between now and your discharge date that I can help you with?" (i.e., collaborating, and problem-solving). |
| **Hostility**—A multifaceted expression of anger or rage; can be subtle and not always immediately obvious.<br>***Recommended modes:***<br>• Empathizing<br>• Instructing<br>  • Collaborating (*may be used following instructing mode to move toward conflict resolution*) | At the start of an inpatient rehabilitation session, an adolescent says "you clearly know nothing. I don't even know why they have you work with me."<br>The therapist pauses to listen, copes by taking a deep breath, then responds with "I am here to help. Progress takes time, and while I do not know everything, it is important to be respectful of each other." (i.e., empathizing, instructing). |
| **Manipulative behaviors**—Underhanded efforts to maintain control or have one's way when interacting with others.<br>***Recommended modes:***<br>• Empathizing<br>• Collaborating<br>• Instructing<br>  • Problem-solving (requires self-awareness on the part of the client) | A child lays down on the mat, closes their eyes, and says: "I am too sleepy to do anything today. Everything we do is so boring. You never let me do anything fun!"<br>The therapist responds by saying "Let's take a 3-minute rest break, and then make a list of 10 fun things we can do together. Then we can take turns making our schedule for the day." they then proceed by setting a timer to 3 min and getting supplies ready while the child rests. |
| **Resistance**—actively refusing to participate in some aspect of therapy, including withdrawal or avoidance of some aspect of therapy.<br>***Recommended modes:***<br>• Prerequisite: Empathizing<br>• Collaborating<br>• Problem-solving | A child begins to cry and runs to the opposite side of the room during a handwriting activity.<br>The therapist follows the child and takes time to observe what the child is doing. They then ask the child "how can I help you find what you are looking for?" |
| **Symptom focusing**—Spending excessive energy, time, and effort on examining symptoms/impairment, rather than attempting to endure or adjust to symptoms in order to engage in an occupation.<br>***Recommended modes:***<br>• Prerequisite: Empathizing<br>  • Collaborating (should be used following empathizing mode) | After getting a small cut on his foot, a child refuses all activities that require taking off his socks. He insists on having a band-aid on his foot even after the area is fully healed. When the therapist attempts to practice dressing, the child points to his foot and asks for a band-aid.<br>The therapist responds, "sounds like you want a new band-aid. Let's go and get you one from our first Aid Kit." |

interpersonal events of therapy. The authors reported that students improved in all areas and suggested that both classroom and fieldwork experiences influence students' self-efficacy.

Taking time to reflect on one's communication and effectiveness can be a powerful tool in raising self-awareness and developing action steps toward ongoing professional development. Additionally, video-taping sessions and analyzing one's therapeutic modes and the effectiveness of these in practice can prove valuable. In addition to reflecting on their communication, practitioners may benefit from client and peer feedback on their communication. Feedback can be requested in a variety of ways, including informal discussions or structured surveys. Supervisory and mentorship meetings can serve as opportunities for reflection on communication and address therapeutic interactions and client perceptions of the practitioner's therapeutic use of self. Self-reflection and feedback can support practitioners' understanding of their professional strengths and opportunities within each of the six modes. This can also empower ideas of continuing education courses that can help the practitioner strengthen individual mode use. For example, a practitioner may recognize that it can be challenging for them to stay in problem-solving mode when working with families who are reluctant to engage in therapy or indirectly communicate their needs. In this instance, they may consider taking a continuing education course on the use of coaching to further strengthen their skill set and strategies within the problem-solving mode.

The help structure self-reflection and feedback on the therapeutic use of self, three tools have been developed for use in education and clinical practice that can be used to guide self-reflection related to practitioner's communication in practice: the Clinical Assessment of Modes (CAM), the Clinical Assessment of Sub-optimal Interaction, and the Self-Assessment of Modes Questionnaire (SAMQ). The Clinical Assessment of Modes (CAM) (Taylor & Popova, 2018), a measure of therapeutic mode use, and the Clinical Assessment of Sub-optimal Interactions (CASI) (Taylor & Popova, 2018), a measure of nontherapeutic communication that may damage or otherwise hinder the therapeutic relationship, have been developed for evaluating the practitioner's delivery of communication during a clinical interaction. The CAM and the CASI have been shown to be reliable and valid for evaluating practitioners' therapeutic and suboptimal communication in pediatric outpatient settings (Popova & Taylor, 2020; Popova & Taylor, 2019). Additionally, the CAM has been utilized in entry-level occupational therapy education to examine the practitioner and patient perspectives on students' mode use in the classroom (manuscript in preparation). However, findings from these studies have not been published to date.

The SAMQ has been developed as a teaching tool that could be used in a variety of educational and professional development settings to support self-reflection on their preferred mode of use based on individual's responses to clinical vignettes that describe interpersonal situations in occupational therapy (Taylor, 2008, 2020). In addition to the original English version, the Norwegian translation is available (Bonsaksen et al., 2016) and has been utilized in IRM research in Norway. Research examining the mode preferences of students in Norway found that students may be most consistently drawn toward the problem-solving mode (Bonsaksen, 2013; Yazdani et al., 2017).

Provided that the CAM, CASI, and SAMQ are theoretically grounded in the IRM, these assessments can be used to guide critical self-reflection on the use of therapeutic communication. These tools may be particularly effective in instances where the practitioner experiences an interpersonal challenge while attempting to establish a therapeutic relationship with a client. The process of assessment completion can support a systematic approach to evaluating positive and negative aspects of interpersonal communication, and assessment results can shed light on specific areas of professional development.

**Cultivating Interpersonal Mindfulness.** Taylor (2020) advises occupational therapy practitioners remember why they are occupational therapy practitioners and keep the meaningfulness of the work at the forefront of their minds. Mindfulness allows a person to be present in the moment. This may also be referred to as centering and intention setting. Thornton (2007) listed techniques to promote centering before entering a person's room, which includes things such as pausing; setting aside concerns; gently closing your eyes; breathing deeply; repeating, "I am here for the greater good, and I will give my full attention; " direct awareness to your heart; and state, "I am present to the moment." In occupational therapy, this refers to being with the child and their family member and focusing on the session while letting go of work, home, and personal pressures. Being present in the moment with the child and family allows the occupational therapy practitioner to make a difference and enjoy the process (even when it is not going smoothly). It ensures that the interpersonal relationship is a priority and that the child and family receive thoughtful interventions and care. It also allows the occupational therapy practitioner to think through situations and act professionally without the burden of outside pressures.

**Cultivating Critical Self-Awareness.** Being self-aware allows occupational therapy practitioners to continue to develop therapeutic use of self, and therefore, it is a critical skill to master. *Self-awareness* requires that a person first have a sense of who they are, along with their strengths and opportunities for professional development. Being able to critically analyze one's interpersonal relationships with children and families allows the occupational therapy practitioner to learn from the interactions and possibly change modes or behaviors to be more effective. As occupational therapy practitioners try out new ways of interacting, they become more skillful and have more modes and strategies to apply in practice. A pilot program with social care staff explored new ways to explore the therapeutic use of self through a 2-day workshop using case vignettes; they found that participants focused on self-awareness, personal values, self-reflection, empathy, and emotional costs (Kwiatek et al., 2005), suggesting that examining case vignettes may be a successful technique to promote self-awareness and therapeutic use of self.

Understanding one's motivations, personality, style, strengths, limits, and challenges is essential to one's therapeutic use of self. The more self-aware an occupational therapy practitioner becomes, the better they become at examining relationships and making necessary changes. The IRM textbook (Taylor, 2020) provides self-assessment worksheets at the end of each chapter and on the website to help occupational therapy practitioners reflect and develop self-awareness. Discussing one's interpersonal abilities with a trusted colleague may also provide insight. It is important to get feedback from children and their families. This may be done anonymously through a client satisfaction survey or informally as a discussion at the end of a therapy session. Supervisors may provide insight and videotaping sessions may prove useful. Some occupational therapy practitioners benefit from discussion groups that allow members to talk about therapeutic issues informally to develop therapeutic skills.

**Cultivating a Growth Mindset.** Everyone has strengths and opportunities for professional development. Although admitting one's opportunities for growth may be a sensitive subject for many, a growth mindset is a critical characteristic of evidence-based practitioners. Recognizing one's challenges may allow the occupational therapy practitioner to reach out and receive support, education, and feedback for fostering positive therapeutic relationships, understanding things better, or even caring for oneself. Occupational therapy practitioners may even help parents understand that there is always more to learn by admitting that they do not have all the answers but will work with the child and family to figure things out together. This honest discourse allows parents of children with disabilities to realize that all the answers may not be there, and it is a process of understanding the child's development. The occupational therapy practitioner may develop trust by being honest and letting the family know that they will seek out answers to their questions and follow through by the next intervention session.

Occupational therapy practitioners bring their traits, personalities, temperaments, and mannerisms into the therapeutic relationship (Taylor, 2020). Understanding oneself allows the practitioner to use these strengths to connect to children and families. It also allows therapists to seek out resources or continuing education opportunities. For example, many times, caregivers appreciate the honesty of, "I have a colleague who has worked in the school system, and I know she understands the laws in detail. I will ask her to come to the next session, so we are sure to address your child's needs." Knowing when to seek resources shows self-awareness. Occupational therapy practitioners may determine that they work better with certain children and have more difficulty with others and therefore seek out continuing education, observe colleagues, or develop strategies to try to better address the client's needs. It may be that the occupational therapy practitioner seeks out other professionals who are successful with children who exhibit specific symptoms. Gaining new perspectives may provide insight into interpersonal relationships.

Each occupational therapy practitioner will have preferences and limitations. Sometimes, occupational therapy practitioners feel they enjoy working with a certain type of child (e.g., children with a learning disability). It is important to acknowledge one's preferences while working to establish competence in addressing various children's needs. It is also important for occupational therapy practitioners to have a sense of their limits and to identify how to best assist the client despite one's limitations. When practitioners feel that they may not be effective in meeting the child's and family's needs, they may have to refer the child to a different occupational therapist. Occupational therapy practitioners may expand their worldview to provide intervention to various children and families by exploring opportunities for education, experiences, and reflection. Reading about issues that affect persons outside of one's comfort zone may help occupational therapy practitioners gain insights. Visiting children and their families in their community, engaging in events outside of one's community, and speaking with people who have experienced different events help people expand their viewpoints. Importantly, occupational therapy practitioners must be open to experiences and attempt to integrate concepts learned when working with children and their families.

**Recognizing Opportunities for Self-Care.** Taking care of oneself allows an occupational therapy practitioner to be present in therapy and address the needs of children and their families from a fresh perspective. Resting and engaging in self-care allows practitioners to develop new strengths that may bring a new understanding to the therapy process. For example, engaging in a leisurely walk outside on a crisp fall day may lighten an occupational therapy practitioner's mood and allow the therapist to be creative when developing an intervention. In this example, the occupational therapy practitioner picked up some brightly colored leaves and used them in a fall-themed art project to work on hand skills. Taking care of oneself may provide the rest to promote clarity, creativity, and a new outlook on a child's and family's needs.

## SUMMARY

Therapeutic use of self is an essential feature of occupational therapy practice. The IRM (Taylor, 2020) provides a structure to examine one's interpersonal interactions, self-reflection, and understanding of children and their families. The IRM defines various inevitable events that may occur during occupational therapy and provides occupational therapy practitioners with information regarding how to approach the events. The IRM acknowledges people's strengths and suggests that occupational therapy practitioners expand their capabilities (not change who they are). Each occupational therapy practitioner has their own style and life experiences that they bring to practice. This is the beauty of human performance. Instead of trying to change one's style, the IRM embraces each person's uniqueness and provides strategies for expanding one's modes. The IRM allows occupational therapy practitioners to carefully examine their therapeutic use of self so that they can better address the needs of children and their families.

- *Therapeutic use of self* (AOTA, 2020) refers to how the occupational therapy practitioner uses their personality and style to form relationships for the good of the child and family. A therapeutic relationship differs from other relationships in that it is designed to benefit the child and family (not the practitioner). While occupational therapy practitioners gain a sense of accomplishment and achievement when children and families succeed, the therapeutic relationship addresses the child's and family's needs and goals.
- The therapeutic relationship is built on listening, responding, clarifying, and negotiating with children and their families. Occupational therapy practitioners present an open and approachable style that fosters therapeutic interactions with children and families. They use body language (posture, mannerisms, movement, eye contact, and touch) that is warm and open while remaining professional. They communicate clearly and often with children and families and listen and observe responses so they can adjust interventions to meet the needs of a child and family. They are clear and confident and provide a safe environment for parents and children to express themselves, challenge themselves, and try out new things.
- The IRM (Taylor, 2020) identifies six therapeutic modes used by occupational therapy practitioners when interacting with children and families. These six modes are advocating, collaborating, encouraging, empathizing, instructing, and problem-solving. Generally, occupational therapy practitioners have modes they naturally use, and each mode has an associated style and strategy. Since clients differ in their needs, occupational therapy practitioners must develop some underused modes of interaction.
- The IRM categorizes interpersonal characteristics according to enduring and situational characteristics (Taylor, 2020). Enduring interpersonal characteristics describe how a client (child or family) most commonly responds to interpersonal aspects of occupational therapy practice and encompass persistent aspects of the client's interpersonal behavior (Taylor, 2020). Situational characteristics refer to how a client responds to a specific event or situation and may not be consistent with the client's typical response. Practitioners use knowledge of interpersonal characteristics as they determine how to best interact with the child and family to promote the therapeutic process. They may adjust their mode use depending on the situational characteristics influencing the child or family.
- Occupational therapy practitioners respond to clients' inevitable interpersonal events (i.e., emotionally charged or otherwise challenging moments that emerge naturally during the relationship) using the interpersonal reasoning process. The occupational therapy practitioner first anticipates, identifies, and copes with interpersonal events as they present themselves in therapy. The practitioner then proceeds by reflecting on their communication and deciding whether a mode shift is required. They then proceed by drawing upon strategies that are consistent with that mode (or a mode sequence) and gather feedback from the client on the effectiveness of the communication.
- The IRM defines difficult or challenging behavior as recurring, enduring, or high-intensity interpersonal behavior that prompts one (or more) negative emotional reactions in another individual (Taylor, 2020). Occupational therapy practitioners use the interpersonal reasoning process to select the appropriate mode(s) to understand the client's perspective, support the client's interpersonal needs, and help find an alternative behavior that would be an appropriate expression of the client's experience. As a general rule, the IRM recommends addressing challenging interpersonal behaviors using collaborating, empathizing, instructing, or problem-solving modes. While the practitioner may switch to advocating and encouraging modes once the challenging behavior is resolved, it is not advised to respond initially using those modes as they may run the risk of reinforcing the behavior.
- Occupational therapy practitioners develop effective therapeutic use of self by engaging in self-awareness activities, reflecting, discussing one's interpersonal abilities with a colleague or supervisor, receiving and responding to feedback from children and families, attending continuing education, reviewing video clips of oneself, and analyzing one's performance, and attending discussion groups.

## REFERENCES

American Occupational Therapy Association. (2020a). Occupational therapy practice framework: Domain and process-Fourth Edition. *American Journal of Occupational Therapy*, *74*(Suppl. 2). https://doi.org/10.5014/ajot.2020.74S2001.

American Occupational Therapy Association. (2020b). AOTA 2020 occupational therapy code of ethics. *American Journal of Occupational Therapy*, *74*(Suppl. 3). https://doi.org/10.5014/ajot.2020.74S3006.

Barton, E. E., & Fettig, A. (2013). Parent-implemented interventions for young children with disabilities: A review of fidelity features. *Journal of Early Intervention*, *35*(2), 194–219. https://doi.org/10.1177/1053815113504625.

Bonsaksen, T. (2013). Self-reported therapeutic style in occupational therapy students. *British Journal of Occupational Therapy, 76*(11), 496–502. https://doi.org/10.4276/030802213X13833255804595.

Bonsaksen, T., Kvarsnes, H., Eirum, M. N., Torgrimsen, S., & Hussain, R. A. (2016). Development and content validity of the Norwegian self-assessment of modes Questionnaire (N-SAMQ). *Scandinavian Journal of Occupational Therapy, 23*(4), 253–259. https://doi.org/10.3109/11038128.2015.1091896.

Colyvas, J. L., Sawyer, L. B., & Campbell, P. H. (2010). Identifying strategies early intervention occupational therapists use to teach caregivers. *American Journal of Occupational Therapy, 64*, 776–785. https://doi.org/10.5014/ajot.2010.09044.

Fan, C. W., & Taylor, R. R. (2016). Assessing therapeutic communication during rehabilitation: The clinical assessment of modes. *American Journal of Occupational Therapy, 70*(4). https://doi.org/10.5014/ajot.2016.018846.

Friedman, M., Woods, J., & Salisbury, C. (2012). Caregiver coaching strategies for early intervention providers: Moving toward operational definitions. *Infants & Young Children: An Interdisciplinary Journal of Early Childhood Intervention, 25*(1), 62–82. https://doi.org/10.1097/IYC.0b013e31823d8f12.

Hussain, R. A., Carstensen, T., Yazdani, F., Ellingham, B., & Bonsaksen, T. (2018). Short-term changes in occupational therapy students' self-efficacy for therapeutic use of self. *British Journal of Occupational Therapy, 81*(5), 276–284.

Kwiatek, E., McKenize, K., & Loads, D. (2005). Self-awareness and reflection: Exploring the 'therapeutic use of self.' *Learning Disability Practice, 8*(3), 27–31. https://doi.org/10.7748/ldp.8.3.27.s22.

Popova, E. S., & Taylor, R. R. (2020). Evaluating students' use of therapeutic communication in entry-level education: The observer version of the clinical assessment of modes (CAM–Observer). *American Journal of Occupational Therapy, 74*. https://doi.org/10.5014/ajot.2020.039396.

Popova, E. S., O'Brien, J. C., & Taylor, R. R. (2022). Communicating with intention: Therapist and parent perspectives on family-centered care in early intervention. *American Journal of Occupational Therapy, 76*. https://doi.org/10.5014/ajot.2022.049131.

Popova, E. S., Ostrowski, R. K., Wong, S. R., & Taylor, R. R. (2019). Reliability and validity of the pediatric clinical assessment of modes in outpatient pediatric rehabilitation. *British Journal of Occupational Therapy, 83*(8), 514–522. https://doi.org/10.1177/0308022619868091.

Popova, E. S. (2022). Promoting rapport and caregiver engagement in early intervention delivered via telehealth. In L. M. Little, & A. Wallisch (Eds.), *Telehealth and occupational therapy in early intervention*. AOTA Press.

Popova, E. S., & Taylor, R. R. (2019). Reliability and validity of the clinical assessment of sub-optimal interaction in outpatient pediatric rehabilitation. *Occupational Therapy in Mental Health, 36*(2), 176–187. https://doi.org/10.1080/0164212x.2019.1666771.

Salisbury, C. L., Woods, J., & Copeland, C. (2010). Provider perspectives on adopting and using collaborative consultation in natural environments. *Topics in Early Childhood Special Education, 30*(3), 132–147. https://doi-org.une.idm.oclc.org/10.1177/0271121409349769.

Solman, B., & Clouston, T. (2016). Occupational therapy and the therapeutic use of self. *British Journal of Occupational Therapy, 79*(8), 514–516. https://doi.org/10.1177/0308022616638675.

Taylor, R. R., Lee, S.-W., Kielhofner, G., & Ketkar, M. (2009). The therapeutic relationship: A nationwide survey of practitioners' attitudes and experiences. *American Journal of Occupational Therapy, 63*, 198–207.

Taylor, R. R., Lee, S.-W., & Kielhofner, G. (2011). Practitioners use of interpersonal modes within the therapeutic relationship: Results from a nationwide study. *OTJR: Occupation, Participation and Health, 31*, 6–14.

Taylor, R. R. (2020). *The intentional relationship: Occupational therapy and use of self* (2nd ed.). F.A. Davis.

Taylor, R. R., & Popova, E. S. (2018). *Clinical assessment of sub-optimal interaction (CASI), version 1.0. The intentional relationship model clearinghouse, department of occupational therapy. College of applied health sciences.* Chicago, IL: University of Illinois at Chicago. Retrieved from http://irm.ahslabs.uic.edu/assessments/.

Taylor, R. R., & Popova, E. S. (2018). *Clinical assessment of modes (CAM), version 3.0. Intentional relationship model clearinghouse, department of occupational therapy, college of applied health sciences.* Chicago, IL: University of Illinois at Chicago. Retrieved from http://irm.ahslabs.uic.edu/assessments/.

Taylor, R. R. (2008). *The intentional relationship: Occupational therapy and use of self.* Philadelphia: F. A. Davis.

Thornton, L. (2007). Holistic nursing: A way of being, a way of living, a way of practice. *Imprint, 55*(1), 32–39. https://pubmed.ncbi.nlm.nih.gov/18286996/.

Yazdani, F., Carstensen, T., & Bonsaksen, T. (2017). Therapeutic mode preferences and associated factors among Norwegian undergraduate occupational therapy students: A cross-sectional exploratory study. *Scandinavian Journal of Occupational Therapy, 24*(2), 136–142. https://doi.org/10.1080/11038128.2016.1220620.

# 4

# Embracing Diversity and Bridging Differences in Pediatric Occupational Therapy Practice

*Elizabeth W. Stevens-Nafai, Said Nafai, Jane Clifford O'Brien, and Heather Miller Kuhaneck*

## GUIDING QUESTIONS

1. Why is it important for pediatric occupational therapy practitioners to show cultural humility in practice?
2. What steps can occupational -therapy practitioners take to develop cultural humility in practice?
3. What does it mean to bridge differences?
4. How can occupational therapy practitioners bridge differences in their work with others?

## KEY TERMS

Ableism
Bias
Bridging differences
Capabilities approach
Cultural competence
Cultural humility
Cultural sensitivity
Cultural safety
Diversity
Equity
Implicit bias
Inclusion
Occupational justice

## INTRODUCTION

According to the 2020 United States Census, "the chance that two people chosen at random will be from different racial or ethnic groups has increased (to 61.1% in 2020)" (Jensen et al., 2021). Given this rising percentage, this statistical reality makes it imperative for occupational therapy practitioners, students, and educators to be prepared to work and interact with people with backgrounds different from their own. An occupational therapy practitioner will likely work with people, both as clients and coworkers, who are different from themselves throughout their careers. Some parts of the country remain less racially diverse; however, that does not minimize the need to have skills to interact with people different from oneself.

The concept of diversity means considering the many ways in which people differ. Diversity includes ethnicity, race, socioeconomic class, ability (ableness), gender, sexual orientation, age, or religious differences (Froehlich & Thornton-Marsh, 2021). Diversity can encompass even more than these commonly recognized categories; people bring all manner of differences with them to the occupational therapy process, whether as the practitioner or the client. These differences are important to understand as part of client-centered care but also relative to the healthcare and educational systems in which occupational therapy practitioners find themselves. Throughout most of US history, these differences have led to inequity. There is now widespread acceptance that healthcare inequity exists and is often fueled by systemic biases (FitzGerald & Hurst, 2017; Hall et al., 2015; Hamed et al., 2022; Ricks et al., 2022). Research indicates that these same biases exist among healthcare workers (Hall et al., 2015).

This chapter encourages each occupational therapy practitioner to lean into differences, educate themselves, and embrace the experiences that this understanding brings to therapeutic relationships. The authors begin the chapter by defining terms and providing examples to show how the concepts may be observed in occupational therapy practice with children and families. They present ways that practitioners may identify and alter their worldviews to provide services more effectively to children and families. The chapter provides strategies for supporting diversity, equity, and inclusion for children and their families.

## TERMINOLOGY RELATED TO EMBRACING DIVERSITY

As one seeks to educate oneself as an occupational therapy practitioner to embrace children's and families' unique situations, it is important to begin with a shared understanding of terms. The following section briefly defines important terms and provides examples related to occupational therapy practice.

### Diversity, Equity, and Inclusion

Occupational therapy practitioners embrace diversity, equity, and inclusion through child- and family-centered practices (AOTA, 2020a). The definition provided by the American Occupational Therapy Association's (AOTA's) statement of diversity, equity, and inclusion (DEI; AOTA, 2020a), defines **diversity** as unique attributes, values, and beliefs of an individual when compared with a group (Taff & Blash, 2017). The term diversity is meant to describe a characteristic of a group rather than an individual (Kornhaber, 2016). Equity means that everyone can access the same opportunities (World Health Organization [WHO], 2023). **Equity** is not the same thing as equality. Equity suggests that opportunities are not equally accessible and that both advantages and barriers exist to access because of individual differences and social structures. Not everyone is afforded the same opportunities for occupation. Striving for equity means that the occupational therapy practitioner acknowledges unequal starting places for varied clients and strives to correct imbalances. **Inclusion** is a practice of not only recognizing diversity but specifically valuing the

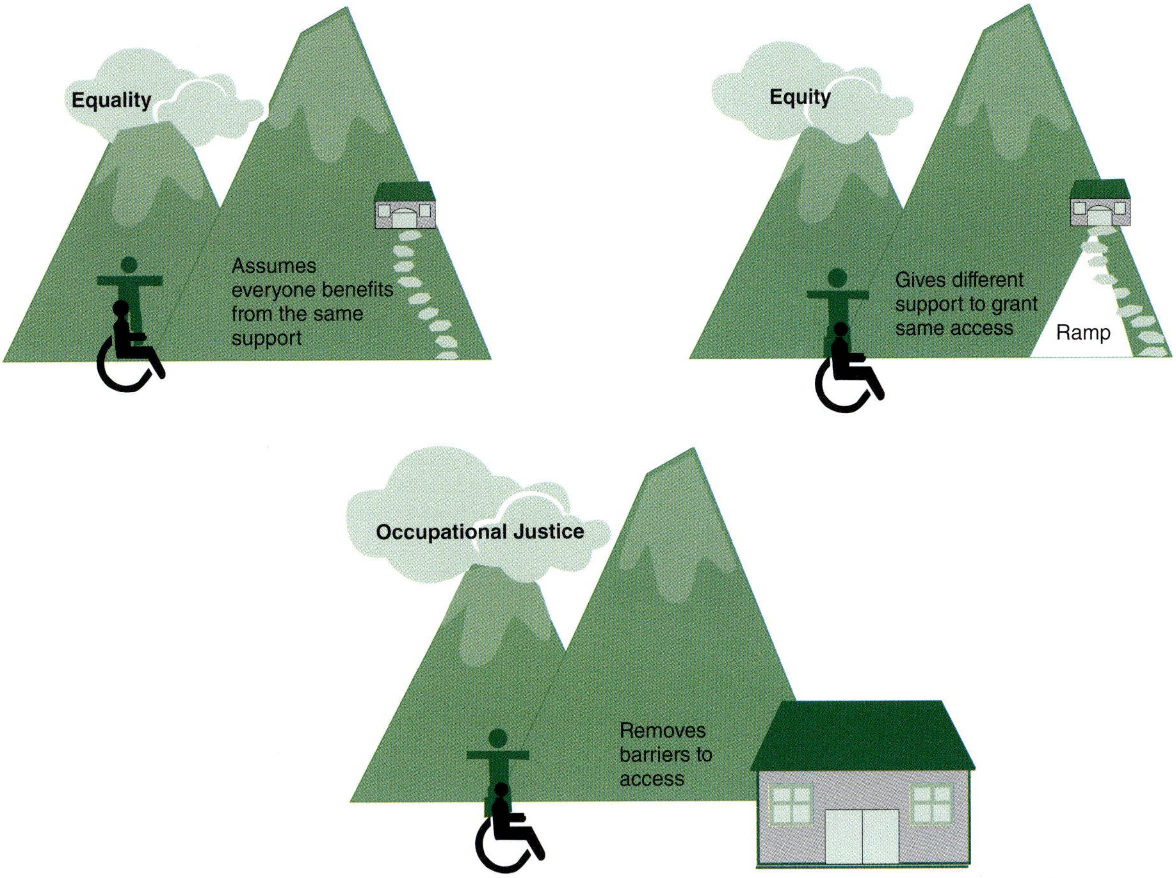


**Fig. 4.1** Equality versus equity. (From O'Brien & Conners. (2024). *Introduction to occupational therapy* (6th ed.), Elsevier. p. 64, Fig. 5.1.)

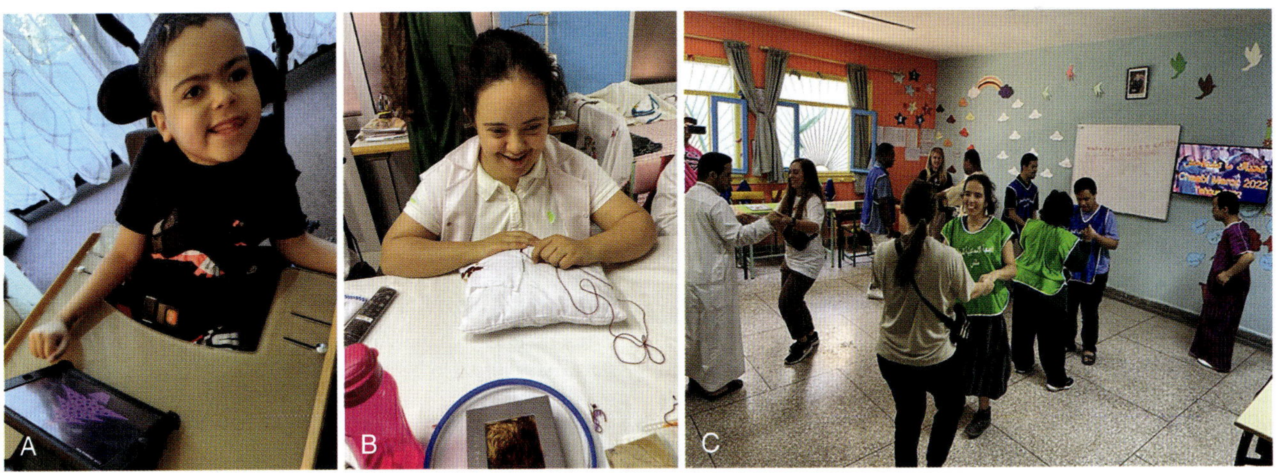


**Fig. 4.2** (A) child uses adaptive equipment to complete his schoolwork. (B) This youth enjoys embroidering a simple pattern as a leisure activity. (C) Children of all abilities are included in this dance class.

uniqueness of beliefs, values, and attributes of others in a way that creates belonging and engagement (Taff & Blash, 2017). Fig. 4.1 illustrates these concepts.

In pediatric occupational therapy, equity may include supporting a child's and family's access to occupations of choice. For example, practitioners work in school settings to enable children to learn with their peers. They may provide children with adapted seating, positioning devices, writing devices, or technology so that they can access their education with their peers. A focus on equity allows children of diverse abilities to participate in occupations (such as school, play, and leisure) as illustrated in Fig. 4.2 A–C. Inclusion refers to providing access to occupations that allow children and families to engage with peers. For example, inclusive dance classes adapt and modify sequencing and physical skills so that all children can participate at their level. All children participate and dance, learn steps, and engage in teamwork. Equitable opportunities require more than access to space, they require options and opportunities for children to engage in space with their peers. For example, inclusive playgrounds include

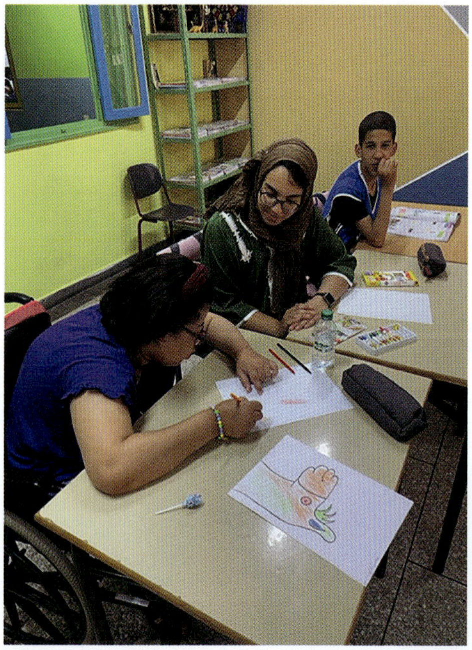

**Fig. 4.3** The occupational therapy practitioner creates a safe social-emotional space, where children who have diverse abilities participate in creative activities, feel they belong, and can express themselves openly without fear.

adapted swings, ramps, or quiet places so that all children can choose activities and engage in play with peers. Occupational therapy practitioners working with children and youth identify opportunities to include them in desired occupations. This also includes supporting safe social-emotional spaces, where children from diverse backgrounds participate in desired occupations, feel they belong, and can express themselves openly without fear. Fig. 4.3.

## Bias

**Bias** refers to "prejudicial attitudes toward and stereotypical beliefs about a particular social group or members therein." (Hagiwara et al., 2020). *Explicit bias* is intentional and purposeful whereas **implicit bias** is based on unconscious beliefs and acts. Implicit bias has been found difficult to change (Vuletich & Payne, 2019), therefore each healthcare practitioner who seeks a more equitable healthcare system must actively engage in methods to understand their own biases and engage in work to foster equity for all clients (Greenwald & Lai, 2020; Mason, 2020). Unconscious or implicit biases may interfere with establishing a therapeutic relationship with children and families.

Occupational therapy practitioners strive to learn about each family's routines, cultures, environments, and expectations so that they can collaborate with families to develop interventions that are meaningful to the child and family. They develop a rapport with parents or caregivers and children by showing interest and curiosity about the family's life and situation. This requires that they do not jump to conclusions, and they seek to understand the entire family's unique situation by asking important questions and listening carefully. They create intervention plans based on information they learn from the family and child, not on stereotypes, or conventions, but rather on the family's expectations and circumstances as they express them. Fig. 4.4 shows a practitioner collaborating with family. This requires that the occupational therapy practitioner listen carefully, ask probing questions, and speak compassionately to families and children who may be experiencing stressful events. As they develop the therapeutic relationship and

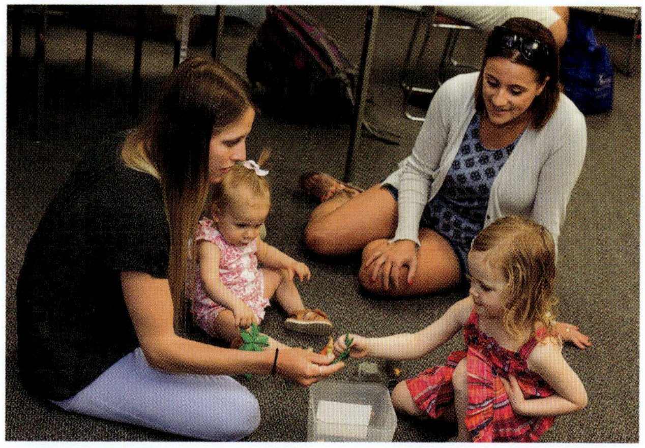

**Fig. 4.4** The occupational therapy practitioner listens carefully, asks probing questions, and speaks compassionately to a young mother during the therapy session.

begin to understand the child and family's unique situation, they may find commonalities in the human experience. They begin to understand and embrace the family and child's strengths and identify areas where the child and family may need support. Occupational therapy practitioners collaborate with families and children to create intervention plans to address their specific goals. Since children and families differ in many ways, goals and intervention plans are unique to each child.

## Cultural Humility

**Cultural humility** is defined as the "ability to maintain an interpersonal stance that is other-oriented (or open to the other) in relation to aspects of cultural identity that are most important to the [person]" (Hook et al., 2013, p. 2). As discussed briefly in Chapter 1, cultural humility requires ongoing reflection, constant learning, acknowledgment of implicit and explicit biases, and a commitment to work toward positive change. The critical actionable steps required of this concept are that the occupational therapy practitioner who engages in cultural humility will be committed to self-evaluation, be open to change, recognize their power in the therapeutic relationship, and use that power through partnering with others to change systems that create bias and inequity (Agner, 2020; McGee-Avila, 2018). See Case Example 4.1 illustrating how an occupational therapy practitioner practices cultural humility.

## Cultural Sensitivity

Often used interchangeably with cultural humility, the term **cultural sensitivity** refers to being aware of others' cultural beliefs and practices as well as one's cultural position relative to others (Agner, 2020; Foronda et al., 2015; Resnicow et al., 1999). It includes the concepts of knowledge, consideration, understanding, respect, and tailoring (Foronda et al., 2015). Knowledge is an understanding of cultural differences and values. Consideration means to include this knowledge in the care provided while avoiding stereotyping. Understanding means comprehending the significance of the client's culture and values and their effects. Respect means appreciating differences, and tailoring refers to altering one's perspective and adapting or modifying approaches based on the needs of the client. Fig. 4.5A and B shows clients engaging in crafts associated with their culture. Culturally sensitive care promotes safe environments for children and families to express themselves and participate in activities. Case Example 4.2 provides an example of how one practitioner showed cultural sensitivity and promoted positive changes.

### CASE EXAMPLE 4.1 PRACTICING CULTURAL HUMILITY

Malcolm is an occupational therapy practitioner who is about to meet a female client who is a recent immigrant from a country and culture he is unfamiliar with. As a practitioner who tries to practice cultural humility, and who seeks to bridge differences, he engages in the following specific steps to prepare:

- He journals and self reflects on any assumptions or biases that come to mind about the culture and country.
- He reflects upon his own ideas about gender and how the female client might view the power differential in having a male therapist. He considers how he can actively attempt to diminish the power differential between them.
- He considers what he might say to indicate his intent for them to be partners in her care, and to show his respect for her worldview.
- He reflects on all the ways in which their worldviews could differ, and on the ways they will likely be similar.
- He attempts to learn more about common power dynamics between the genders in that country and any potential missteps he could make. For example, he thinks he recalls that in some cultures a healthcare provider should not touch a person of the opposite sex. He does some research about this to become more familiar, however he will not assume that the client will act in the way he has read about, but he will make sure to ask.
- When he meets the client, he will ask the client about their identity first, and then he will listen more than he speaks.
- He will listen to the client's narrative for areas where inequity or lack of access exists for this client, and if/when those areas present themselves, he will consider ways to partner with her to address them.

Malcom learns through an interpreter that the woman has diabetes and engages in minimal physical activity. She does understand the need for exercise and a better diet. He later learns that part of the reason for the lack of physical activity is her living situation and lack of a safe space for her to exercise. He will actively work with her to find a solution so that she is able to better manage her disease through an occupation that she chooses that provides physical activity.

## Cultural Safety

Cultural safety has been proposed as more important than cultural humility or competence (Curtis et al., 2019) and as a process that leads to healthcare equity. The term cultural safety suggests that the healthcare practitioner is willing to critique the structures and systems that have been 'taken for granted' and challenge their systems as opposed to trying to be 'competent' in the cultures of others. The primary difference between cultural safety and cultural competence is the understanding of power, the power differential between healthcare providers and their clients, and the structural power differentials in society. The focus of cultural safety is on the culture of the provider rather than the client as an "exotic other." A healthcare practitioner who promotes cultural safety intentionally reflects on these power differentials and attempts to shift or transfer power (Curtis et al., 2019).

### CASE EXAMPLE 4.2 CULTURAL SENSITIVITY

Bijon is an occupational therapist working in a community pediatric setting. To meet productivity standards, evaluations are scheduled for Mondays from 9–5:00 p.m. Therapists working at the clinic work a 40-hour week from 9–5:00 p.m. The clinic, which is in an affluent neighborhood, does very well and has many clients.

Bijon receives a call from a young single mother of three who is unable to bring her child in for an appointment at that designated time since she works and will not get paid if she does not show up for work. Furthermore, she has limited paid time off and has already used that time.

Upon reflection of the power imbalance of this policy, Bijon realizes that the clinic is not addressing the needs of working parents adequately, further promoting inequality in healthcare services. While parents with dual family income or from higher socioeconomic status can meet this time, it is preventing others from much-needed services. Bijon advocates for the team to change this policy and open evening and weekend hours to provide access to services for all families and children. He thanks the parent for expressing her concern when he relays the positive changes to her.

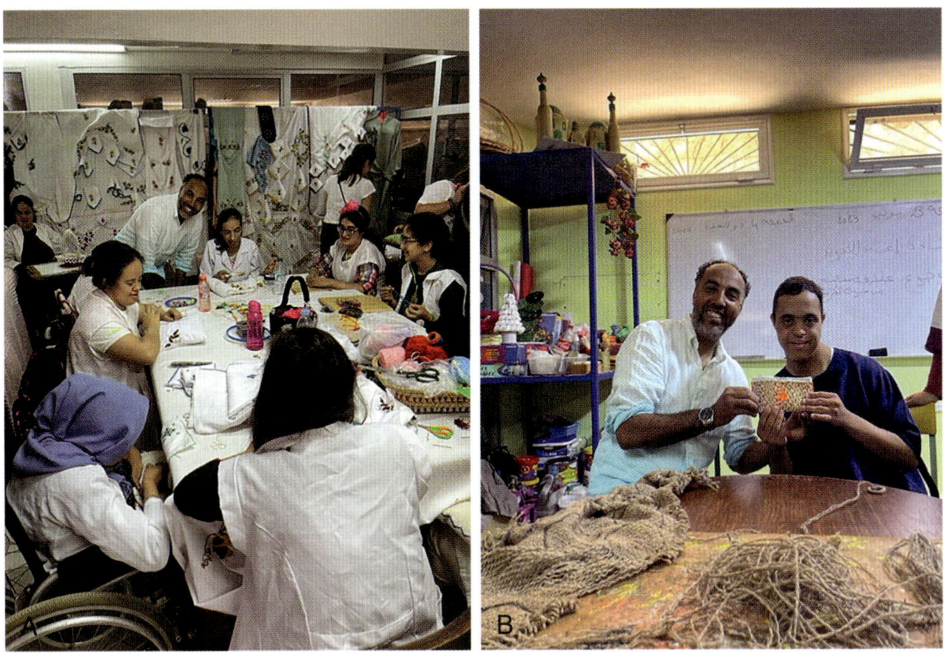


**Fig. 4.5** (A) A group of young girls of varying abilities engage in embroidery activities associated with their culture. (B) A young boy enjoys completing a weaving activity that is valued by his culture.

For an example of methods to promote cultural safety in practice, refer to Case Example 4.3.

## Decolonization

*Decolonization* of healthcare refers to the partnership with and the empowerment of indigenous communities while allowing for engagement and participation in decision-making (Mulumba et al., 2021). Decolonizing involves questioning Western assumptions about knowledge, human beings, and occupation to collaborate with clients to address their occupational needs (Ramugondo, 2018). Occupational therapy began in the United States and the philosophy and concepts associated with the profession are originally based on this culture. To date, much of the research, textbook publications, assessments, techniques, and philosophy of occupational therapy are Western-based. In pediatrics, for example, assessments may be normed on children from North America and not reflect a diversity of cultures. Concepts of occupation, play, and customs of feeding, dressing, and bathing differ among cultures and families. Guidelines may be based on data from one ethnicity, gender, or region and do not represent the diversity of children and their families. Many of the original concepts, writings, and terminology of occupational therapy have been critiqued extensively (See Hammell, 2020a,b; Hammell & Beagan, 2017 for example). Lavalley and Johnson (2020) assert that occupational therapy is largely influenced by the deeply ingrained racist biases and beliefs of society that have been embedded into the United States since its inception.

Occupational therapy practitioners frequently work with children and families outside of Western cultures, requiring that they carefully reflect upon the usefulness of the information, assessment, or strategies created to address children's and families' needs. Furthermore, the major language of research and occupational therapy literature is English, despite there being a statistical minority of English speakers on the planet, which may result in bias (Hammell, 2018). Occupational therapy practitioners are advised to carefully examine the evidence for practice decisions to determine its usefulness to the children and families they are serving. For example, occupational therapy practitioners identify where the research has been conducted and how that may influence the findings specifically related to their clients. Evidence-based practice requires that practitioners use knowledge of the research evidence (including any bias that may exist), clients' expressed desires and choices, and practitioners' experience to make decisions. Box 4.1 provides an example of research to support the decolonization of a health care system.

### CASE 4.3 CULTURAL SAFETY

Shae is an occupational therapist who works in a NICU in a healthcare organization that embarked on a program to hold itself accountable for cultural safety. As part of this initiative, the organization reviewed all its policies and practices, assembled baseline data on healthcare inequities, required and implemented employee training that Shae attended, and reviewed and monitored for outcomes in relation to reduction of inequities at the organizational level. The clients of this organization reported on whether they felt culturally safe. Three specific changes were instituted quickly based on data that surfaced.

1. Indigenous women in the hospital for childbirth documented that they felt unable to engage in their typical cultural practices such as keeping the placenta and holding welcoming ceremonies. These practices are now allowed, and women are informed of this when they arrive.
2. The organization also provided a safe space for prayer and reflection for clients and visitors who did not wish to visit the chapel.
3. Lastly, both halal and kosher alternatives for certain medications are provided.

The occupational therapist reviewed her knowledge of cultural practices to determine how she could better support families. She reflected on how she asked questions and possible "misunderstandings" as a result. She changed some of her questions and added additional questions on the occupational therapy interview to better understand how the family's cultural practices may influence intervention approaches, suggestions, and the family and child's needs. Since the organization implemented new practices, demonstrating their goal to address clients' needs, the occupational therapist was re-energized to review her practices for her clients.

### BOX 4.1 Decolonization of Health Care System

Researchers from Canada (Eni et al., 2021) examined perspectives of the health care system in the Manitoba First Nation. They completed 183 interviews and additional focus groups in eight Manitoba First Nation communities. Four main themes emerged: (1) First Nation control of their healthcare (e.g., desire for less interference from government, systems to protect them, better access) (2) traditional medicine and healing activities (e.g., desire to continue their healing activities without ridicule, revival of traditional medicine, reconnecting with traditional health), (3) full and meaningful community participation (e.g., giving everyone a voice in community matters, creating open dialog, participating in decision-making), and (4) diminishing impacts of colonization (e.g., need for hospitals, resources, consistency in health care, going back to land) (Eni et al., 2021). The findings supported the need for concrete actions towards a decolonizing agenda in this healthcare system. This study illustrates the importance of listening to jointly create solutions within communities. Occupational therapy practitioners may collaborate with communities to enable children and families to engage in desired occupations.

## Occupational Justice

**Occupational justice** refers to occupational rights for all and "is the fulfillment of the right for all people to engage in the occupations they need to survive, define as meaningful, and that contribute positively to their own wellbeing and the wellbeing of their communities." (WFOT, 2019). Occupational therapy practitioners advocate for the right of people to engage in desired occupations. They may create programming, support children and families in finding resources, and address performance challenges that interfere with a child's ability to participate in school, home, or community events. For example, children who receive special education are entitled to accommodations so they may participate in the school day with their peers. They also are entitled access to after-school programs (e.g., sports, dances, field trips, and events). Occupational therapy practitioners may consult with others on the design of adaptive playgrounds so all children can participate in recess activities. These are all forms of occupational justice.

However, there are occupational therapy practitioners who do not like the use of the term occupational justice and the concepts and definitions proposed around its use (See Hammell, 2020a, 2020b; Hammell & Beagan, 2017; Lavalley & Johnson, 2020; for example). For many occupational therapy practitioners outside of the U.S. rather than focusing on occupational justice, they suggest the use of a capabilities approach.

## Capabilities Approach

A capabilities approach grew out of work on poverty and economic development, into a consideration of quality of life and well-being (Gasper, 2002; Nussbaum, 2009; Sen, 1993). A shift in attention from aspects of human welfare focused on basic economics, to areas such as choice and opportunity suggests a model where capability is understood as a way of living that could be attained, highlighting differences between potential and achievement. Essentially, the capability model considers people's opportunities to be healthy (Kellock, 2020; Robeyns, 2005).

The **capabilities approach**, now applied to disability and occupation, focuses on opportunities in addition to abilities. This approach considers not only whether a person *can* engage in valued experiences but also whether their circumstances *allow them to* engage in a valued way. A capabilities approach considers whether a person can use their abilities in chosen ways (Entwistle & Watt, 2013). It recognizes that what individuals choose to do is influenced by what they envision being open to them to do, and what is realistically available to them to do. For occupational therapy practitioners, this type of approach aligns with human rights initiatives (Mousavi et al., 2015) and is a way to refocus the profession on equality of opportunity to "do" (Hammell, 2015, 2023). The Occupation, Capability, and Wellbeing Framework for Occupational Therapy (OCWFOT: Hammell, 2020a,b; Hammell, 2023) has evolved from this work. This global framework promotes a strengths-based approach, focuses on occupations that matter most to people, and highlights the occupational therapy practitioner's role in promoting or advocating for opportunities or access. The framework examines the well-being needs and aspirations of individuals, families, groups, communities, and populations and emphasizes the importance of relating to people as interdependent and embedded within families and communities (Hammell, 2023).

## BARRIERS TO DIVERSITY, EQUITY, AND INCLUSION EFFORTS

Occupational therapy practitioners working with children and their families are committed to providing equitable and inclusive services to all (AOTA, 2020a; 2020b) and therefore must be aware of, seek to understand, and actively work towards removing barriers to equitable healthcare services. As stated earlier, healthcare workers are not immune to the unconscious or implicit biases and the behavioral outcomes they may lead to. Occupational therapy practitioners must become aware of both their own and systemic biases, so they can support children and their families and create safe social-emotional spaces.

### Microaggressions, Microinvalidations, Microinsults and Microassaults

Implicit bias and stereotypes lay at the root of microaggressions. *Microaggressions* are "small acts or remarks that make someone feel insulted or treated badly because of their race, sex, etc., even though the insult or act may not have been intended, and that can combine with other similar acts or remarks over time to cause emotional harm" (Cambridge Dictionary). Microaggressions encompass microinvalidations, microassaults, and microinsults (Sue et al., 2007).

Microinvalidations are the most insidious of microaggressions and are attempts to dismiss or minimize the experiences of members of marginalized groups. They can leave the victim feeling dismissed or invisible. Examples of microinvalidation in pediatric practice can be as innocuous as providing a writing prompt in an elementary fine motor group, "What were you for Halloween?" assuming all the students participate in the practice of dressing up in costumes.

Microinsults are insensitive or rude comments that imply judgment of someone's identity. For example, during a high school presentation on diversity, students were asked to "raise your hand if you're African." Looking around and noting the raised hands, a Black student of Ghanaian descent commented to a light-complexioned girl in the next row, "Why did you raise your hand? You can't be African, you're not Black" dismissing her classmate's North African identity. An example of microinsult based on ability is when a special education teacher says to a student with dyslexia in front of the whole class, "This text is probably too hard for you Felix, just try your best to keep up." Another example of a microinsult is an administrator entering a staff room and asking, "Why is there a parent in here?" referring to a new staff member who was wearing a hijab (Muslim headscarf), implying this person is not appropriate in some way to be a staff member. Microinsults lead to feelings of rejection and exclusion.

Microassaults are intentional and more deliberate. Microassaults are often couched in a joke or involve an action that is explicitly discriminatory. An example would be a veteran staff member orienting a new staff member and stating things they perceive to be helpful but are in fact discriminatory. For example, one might hear "Oh when I go to that neighborhood school I leave my purse in my trunk, I don't want it being stolen if I bring it into that building," or while comparing an inner city to a suburban school, "I make sure to tie my hair up so I don't get lice when I go to that school, but you don't have to worry about that in this school."

Case Example 4.4 describes strategies for handling microaggressions in the workplace.

#### CASE EXAMPLE 4.4 STRATEGIES TO ADDRESS MICROAGGRESSIONS IN THE WORKPLACE

Tamara is an occupational therapy practitioner who traveled to another state for her first job. She was nervous, self-conscious, and excited to begin this new job. She did not know anyone at the site. Tamara is a Black woman who moved to be close to her boyfriend who worked in a tech firm in the same city.

At first, Tamara ignored some of the comments that make her uncomfortable, such as, "Are you the first person in your family to get a master's degree?"; "I have a Black friend," "How did you get into such a great school?" However, the microaggressions continued. In one such example, her supervisor gave her a difficult case, stating, "I am giving you this case because the family is Black and you can relate to them." In the lunchroom, the practitioners called Tamara out as the only Black person by asking, "Tamara, why do Black people always do that?"

Tamara started feeling alienated, stressed at work, and uncomfortable. She did not know where to turn to. She liked her new job and her new home. She did not want to leave. She also did not want to "make trouble."

Knowing what to do when persistent microaggressions happen in the workplace can be a challenge. Calling people out, coworkers, classmates, teachers, and ourselves is potentially uncomfortable. Washington (2022) suggests that people consider (1) the right moment to say something; (2) their relationship to the person who made the comment; and (3) their awareness of the microaggression's subject.

Tamara decided that she would address her supervisor alone, during their "catch up" meeting that is generally relaxed and supportive. Tamara would use the "*I know you intended to* be supportive of me, *but the way I received it was* that I do not belong in the profession, or for some reason Black people are not as qualified." Tamara felt that she had a good relationship with her supervisor, and that generally the occupational therapy practitioners want to be inclusive. She planned to ask her supervisor for advice on how to address the practitioners (during lunch) and the general atmosphere of the setting.

Tamara's supervisor listened carefully, acknowledged, and apologized for the offenses and suggested the department receive some support from Human Resources. The supervisor suggested Tamara also speak to Human Resources and document her concerns. The supervisor scheduled an Inservice training session (with an outside facilitator) to address the topic and establish departmental goals to show a commitment to an inclusive work environment. The team (including Tamara) found the Inservice session helpful, and many practitioners apologized to Tamara.

## EMBRACING DIVERSITY AND BRIDGING DIFFERENCES

Beyond merely valuing the differences that exist between humans in differing situations, occupational therapy practitioners who seek to engage in best practices actively attempt to bridge differences.

### Bridging Differences

**Bridging differences** refers to a person's attempt to connect with another based on a recognition of their shared humanity and with the attitude of valuing the differences each brings to the interaction (Mendoza-Denton & Briscoe-Smith, 2023). The work of bridging differences does not mean that the parties will always agree, always find compromise, or always be friends. It does mean that even in those moments of disagreement, one never sees the other as less than human, less than worthy, or less entitled to the health and happiness that one enjoys, than oneself. Bridging differences is not about persuading another to one's viewpoint but instead trying to understand another's perspective. Coming from a place of modesty and humility, bridging differences means accepting that one does not have a monopoly on the truth (Mendoza-Denton & Briscoe-Smith, 2023). Box 4.2 lists eight skills required for bridging differences.

There are times, however, when it is not appropriate to attempt to bridge differences. This may occur when one feels personally unsafe or threatened by another or when engaging in the work to connect with someone might put others in danger. Occupational therapy practitioners should never feel compelled to try to compromise with someone who is using aggression or threatening violence for example. Bridging differences should also not be attempted when the process is rushed.

Occupational therapy practitioners must learn how and when to skillfully bridge differences. Pediatric occupational therapy practitioners frequently work with families and children who are different from themselves. To provide optimal child- and family-centered care, they learn to listen to families and create trusting and honest therapeutic relationships. Fig. 4.6A and B show practitioners interacting with children during intervention to develop trusting relationships. Occupational therapy practitioners striving to bridge differences to create strong therapeutic relationships, practice the following strategies:

- Intentionally learn about and attempt to neutralize their own unconscious biases;
- Engage in active listening and compassionate speaking;
- Find shared identities and values; and
- Work toward common goals.

Case Example 4.5 describes how an occupational therapy practitioner may use bridging strategies with a child and family.

**BOX 4.2 Eight Essential Skills for Bridging Differences (Mendoza-Denton & Briscoe-Smith, 2023)**

1. Recognize common humanity.
2. Focus on understanding (not persuading) others.
3. Attempt to find common ground.
4. Engage in inner personal work.
5. Demonstrate modesty and humility.
6. Make small shifts in thoughts and actions, consistently.
7. Take risks and accept vulnerability.
8. Recognize times when one should not attempt bridging because of prior trauma.

### Bridging Differences: Relevance to Pediatric Practice

The work of bridging differences can be considered part of an occupational therapy practitioner's adherence to the profession's code of ethics (AOTA, 2020b). It is critical that practitioners are both aware of clients' cultural backgrounds and that they practice in inclusive ways, respecting people's views and opinions regardless of their backgrounds. The AOTA supports and promotes diversity, equity, and inclusion

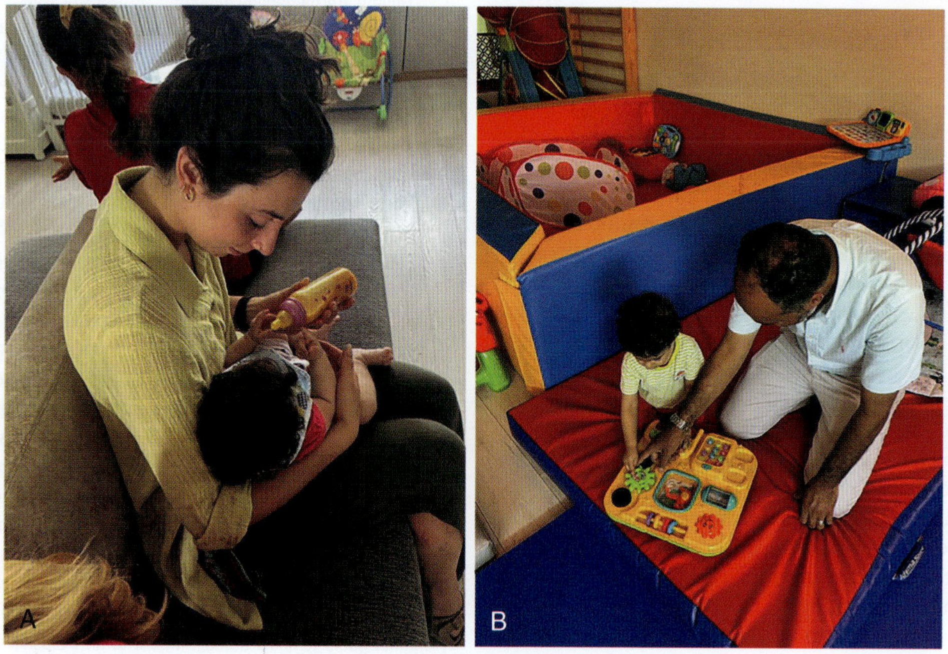


**Fig. 4.6** Occupational therapy practitioners bridge differences through recognizing and working towards common or shared values and goals. (B) Occupational therapy practitioners interact with children during intervention to develop trusting relationships through shared goals.

## CASE EXAMPLE 4.5 BRIDGING THE DIFFERENCES

Mourad is a 15-month-old from Sudan whose mother is concerned that he does not walk or manipulate objects. He was referred to early intervention services by the pediatrician who diagnosed him with right hemiplegia. The family (parents and two children) immigrated to the United States 3 months ago. They are living in temporary housing.

*Intentionally learn about and attempt to neutralize unconscious biases:* The occupational therapy practitioner treating Mourad, has read the news about the Sudanese immigrants, who are struggling with housing, employment, and transportation. The therapist also had a positive experience working in home health with a Sudanese man who worked as an Aide to one of her clients. The man was a physician in Sudan and in the US to earn money so his family can join him.

The occupational therapy practitioner enjoys hearing people's stories and meeting people from other places. The practitioner travels to experience other cultures, reads stories, and reflects on their implicit and explicit biases. To better understand the Sudan culture before meeting Mourad, the practitioner explores the culture. The practitioner also reflects upon any preconceived notions or biases that they may hold regarding people from Sudan.

*Engage in active listening and compassionate speaking:* During the interview the practitioner listens carefully to the mother's concerns regarding Mourad's use of both upper extremities and his gross motor skills. The mother expresses concern over their housing and her difficulty meeting the children's needs. She worries that her oldest son (5 years) will have trouble in public school because he cannot speak English well. The occupational therapy practitioner learns that Mourad's parents want their children to have friends and succeed in school in America. They hope that their children will have opportunities to reach their dreams and that they can provide for their children. The practitioners speaks with the mother compassionately about these fears and concerns.

*Find shared identities and values:* As the mother shares her values, the occupational therapy practitioner notes how universal these parenting goals are, despite their varied backgrounds.

*Work toward common goals:* The practitioner provides the mother with information about the school system, including an open house session to alleviate some of the mother's concerns. The practitioner and mother collaborate to create goals and prioritize intervention sessions.

As intervention continues, the practitioner addresses issues of health equity and follows the state laws to provide services to immigrant children. The practitioner reflects on their communication with the mother, and they frequently stop and define terms more clearly. The practitioner looks at the mother's facial expressions during instruction or the session to make sure the mother is following the practitioner and responding to any signs that things need to be clarified more clearly. The practitioner develops a rapport with the child while engaging him in playful fun activities. As the practitioner works with the child, they highlight the child's strengths, validate the mother's efforts, and celebrate the child's progress. They suggest programs and support groups for parents that may provide additional opportunities for children and parents.

(AOTA, 2020a). The AOTA statement on justice and systemic racism (AOTA, 2021) released after the death of George Floyd states "We acknowledge and condemn the multifaceted aspects of systemic racism and oppression. We stand with occupational therapy practitioners and students in their expressions of pain, anger, and demands for change. The impact of systematic racism spans the history of our country." Recent data suggests that 87.9% of the occupational therapy profession is White and non-Hispanic, and with this comes a specific worldview (US Bureau of Labor Statistics, 2022). Whiteford (2019) asserts that "we act in ways that reinforce and reproduce power relations and the dominance of certain discourses over others." One's unconscious worldview leads to instinctive assumptions that marginalize or exclude others, like instinctive heteronormative or ableist assumptions. **Ableism** refers to "the notion that certain bodies are 'normal', appropriate and desirable, and that upholds as 'natural' the inequitable opportunities and advantages that flow to those with usual bodies" (Hammell, 2023, p. 5). This approach suggests that children and youth who do not meet these standards are somehow flawed, abnormal, or atypical (Hammell, 2023). Occupational therapy practitioners seek to embrace diversity by viewing all abilities and promote a person's engagement in occupations as each person is capable while not requiring that children adhere to what is "normal" or "typical."

Occupational therapy practitioners are trained healthcare providers who have a specific skill set to support and enable children and families to achieve their goals and aspirations. However, the presumption that the occupational therapy practitioner "knows better" than the family or child perpetuates colonial myths and unconsciously feeds into "white coat" or "blind respect of teachers/officials" colonial paradigms.

Effective occupational therapy practice in pediatrics requires practitioners and families both respect each other's knowledge about the child. Occupational therapy practitioners create ways to work with children and their families from diverse backgrounds and create collaborative relationships that benefit the child and family (Popova et al., 2022). The goal of pediatric therapy is to promote a child's skills and abilities, to support families and their children, and to empower parents and caregivers to advocate for their children so that children can engage in personal, family, and community occupations. Occupational therapy practitioners working in the US are exposed to many families from different backgrounds, who have unique circumstances, values, and routines. Therefore, they must be aware of and understand the influence of inequitable systems on the child's and family's health, quality of life, and resources.

Children as young as birth to 3 years, who are non-White, are impacted by significant healthcare discrepancies (Barger et al., 2022; Chaudry & Wimer, 2016; Wexler et al., 2022). In early intervention, where occupational therapy specifically plays a crucial role, children who are non-White receive lower rates of screening, monitoring, and early identification of developmental disabilities (Barger et al., 2022). They also are more likely to live in poverty, which has a potential additional impact on developmental outcomes (Chaudry & Wimer, 2016; Wexler et al., 2022). For children and youth, lack of access, or even delayed access, can lead to lifelong consequences. The lack of access to early identification and intervention services (e.g., occupational, physical, and speech therapy) may lead to altered developmental trajectories affecting the child's cognitive, gross motor, fine motor, self-care, play, language, and social-emotional development) and marginalization (Agorastos et al., 2019; Halfon & Hochstein, 2002; Luyster et al., 2011; Thomas, 2016). See Fig. 4.7 for an illustration of the importance of early intervention for developmental trajectories.

As healthcare providers, occupational therapy practitioners working with children, youth, and their families acknowledge the importance of recognizing how race, ethnicity, and socioeconomic class impact children and their families (Lavizzo-Mourey et al., 2021; Williams & Cooper, 2019). Additionally, occupational therapy practitioners address the mental health needs of children and youth, which requires they consider the impact of biases, policies, and societal views on marginalized populations such as those with disabilities, and those in the LGBTQIIA + communities. Occupational therapy practitioners seek to create positive changes in systems to benefit children and families, advocate for services, and address inequities in care and occupational possibilities.

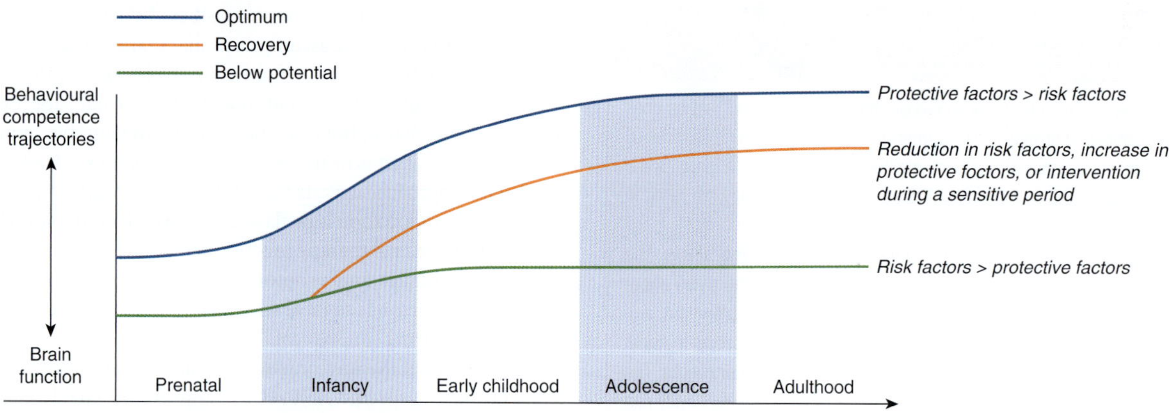


**Fig. 4.7** Importance of early intervention for child development. www.researchgate.net/publication/370818276_PoM_ToM_-Harnessing_the_Power_of_Mind_in_Theory_of_Mind_by_shaping_beneficial_mental_states_in_Preschoolersand_the_ICT%27s_role.

## A Roadmap to Change: Challenging One's Worldview

Hammell (2021) encourages occupational therapy practitioners to expand their views on diversity categories and address the systemic failures of racism and classism in society to rectify healthcare injustices. Occupational therapy, as a global profession, can play a part in changing healthcare systems to become fairer and more equitable. Occupational therapy practitioners can engage in a variety of activities to expand their worldview and foster greater opportunities for family-centered care with cultural humility. Practitioners begin by reflecting on their own biases, communicating, and acting to avoid microaggressions based on these biases, and engaging in the continual work of reflection and learning. Table 4.1 outlines activities that enable practitioners to expand their worldview with examples of how they may engage in those activities. Engaging in activities to expand one's perspective is an essential part of being an occupational therapy practitioner (Perryman-Fox et al., 2022). Broadening one's perspective helps practitioners avoid perpetuating social inequities. Occupational therapy practitioners reflect upon their social context to understand children and families and how social and economic factors influence their lives (Malfitano & Lopes, 2018).

**Self-Reflection.** Occupational therapy practitioners engage in self-reflection to understand the role of implicit bias in their work with others. Implicit biases can be ingrained and accepted without conscious consideration. These biases often come from exposure to media or others (Mendoza-Denton & Briscoe-Smith, 2023). Long-term exposure to negative stereotypes, for example through media use, can lead one to become subconsciously fearful or mistrustful of others or may influence one's expectations of the behavior of others.

When invoked, stereotypes may trigger inaccurate beliefs and assign people negative qualities associated with the stereotype of the group (Blair, 2001). In turn, stereotypes may lead to changes in expectations through subtle changes in behavior. Therefore, stereotypes can have long-term consequences for those who are stereotyped. For example, teachers' expectations impact student performance. A classic study documented that when teachers believed certain students would be "late bloomers" because they were told so, they engaged differently with those students and made the belief into a reality (Rosenthal & Jacobson, 1968). Although the original study has been criticized, recent reviews of the entire body of work on teacher expectancy and self-fulfilling- prophecy suggest that the beliefs of teachers impact student performance over time (Jussim & Harber, 2005; Lorenz, 2021; Wineburg, 1987). Other examples include evidence that negative stereotypes influence judges' decisions for sentencing, decisions by employers for hiring, and decisions police officers make regarding the use of force (Moskowitz et al., 2012), as well as differential access and outcomes in healthcare (Hall et al., 2015; Madeira et al., 2022; Zestcott et al., 2021).

Self-reflection regarding one's own implicit biases or assumptions allows practitioners to examine "blind spots" and investigate belief systems to meet the needs of children and their families (Kinsella & Whiteford, 2008). Self-reflection involves understanding one's own race, class, gender, sexual orientation, religion, age, ethnicity, and (dis)ability status. See online resources for examples of activities for self-reflection and investigation of assumptions and learning activities related to self-reflective practices.

**Expanding One's View Through Education and Networking.** In addition to self-reflection, occupational therapy practitioners engage in ongoing education about diversity, cultural humility, and research on healthcare equity across the globe to better understand systems that affect children and families. They show curiosity for learning and engaging in inclusive practice by joining occupational therapy organizations, such as the World Federation of Occupational Therapists (WFOT) to learn about and from others and expand their knowledge base for practice. They attend national and international conferences and join groups representing diversity within the profession and community (e.g., local groups, the Black OT Caucus). They may participate in international service-learning activities to experience cultural exchanges. Research suggests that international service learning leads to long-term changes in cultural humility and increases occupational therapy students' confidence and comfort in working with diverse people (Chabot et al., 2021; Stevens-Nafai & Nafai, 2019).

Practitioners may learn about others through volunteering. However, volunteerism can also incidentally reinforce the oppressive dynamics of "the white savior complex" (Finnegan, 2022), so practitioners must reflect upon their motivations while volunteering. White savior complex is a term referring to White people "helping" non-White people in a way that promotes the differences and exploits the experience.

Occupational therapy practitioners using media and social media to learn about others must carefully reflect upon the information provided. For example, the media may perpetuate stereotypes and

**TABLE 4.1 Activities to Challenge One's Worldview**

| Activity | Examples |
|---|---|
| Self-reflection | • Take an implicit bias test (https://implicit.harvard.edu/implicit/takeatest.html) and reflect on their findings.<br>• Identify gaps in knowledge about cultures.<br>• Identify explicit biases.<br>• Seek out supervision on your work with families.<br>• Ask feedback from families.<br>• Reflect on interactions with children and families.<br>• Create a personal action plan. |
| Education | • Engage in journal clubs.<br>• Read literature, journal articles, novels, history of cultures.<br>• Take classes or continuing education.<br>• Read OT literature outside of United States to learn different perspectives.<br>• Examine research on disability studies, cultural humility, diversity, equity, and inclusion.<br>• Educate yourself on policies that affect people. |
| Occupational therapy organizations | • Engage in the World Federation of Occupational Therapists, American Occupational Therapy Association (AOTA), and state associations.<br>• Participate in the Coalition of occupational therapy advocates for diversity (COTAD, 2022),<br>• Join AOTA groups that represent diversity. |
| International service learning | • Seek out international service learning or international fieldwork experiences. |
| Group membership | • Join community groups (e.g., local groups for women, support groups, school committees) to learn about the community. |
| Volunteer | • Volunteer for agencies within the community |
| Media and social media | • View, critique, and reflect upon content of documentaries, podcasts, and television shows.<br>• Critique the portrayal of people through media.<br>• Engage in discussions with occupational therapy practitioners and people who are a part of the groups portrayed (e.g., people with disability). |

uninformed views regarding people with disabilities, indigenous people, and immigrants. Material for media sources should be viewed with caution when learning about the community.

## Action Steps

In addition to self-reflection and education, if one truly wants to see change in the world, one must act. There are numerous action steps occupational therapy practitioners can take to practice cultural humility with children and their families so that they receive quality, effective, and equitable occupational therapy services. These steps are not linear, and practitioners revisit them often during practice. They seek out opportunities to understand diversity by engaging in personal (e.g., befriending someone who represents a group or culture), community (e.g., participating in local events that provide exposure to customs, traditions, or practices), or professional events (such as international conferences and networking). The more different groups have opportunities to interact and have positive contact with each other, the more likely the members are to see another's perspective (Hewstone & Greenland, 2000). See Fig. 4.8A and B. Cross-group friendships can be particularly important in improving attitudes toward "others," and may be beneficial for enacting social change (MacInnis & Hodson, 2019; Reimer & Sengupta, 2022).

As it is human nature to categorize others, practitioners actively challenge implicit biases and stereotypes by purposely taking the time to humanize others. To assist in the shift away from seeing another as merely an anonymous member of a group, look for specific features or even quirks that define them as an individual (Mendoza-Denton & Briscoe-Smith, 2023). For example, you might ask about the person's favorite color, or favorite vegetable, or ask if they are a "morning or night" person in their schedule. The idea is to humanize the other person and perhaps find common ground despite differences in group membership. Therefore, avoid questions that may elicit stereotypes in one's mind. For example, discussing musical preferences can invoke group identities of "opera lover" or "country music lover" or "hip-hop fan" and those associations, which is the opposite of the desired outcome of these questions.

**Language.** Occupational therapy practitioners must examine the language of occupational therapy (Mahoney & Kiraly-Alvarez, 2019). For example, there is a difference between the words patient and client that highlights a power differential. In pediatric practice, practitioners use the child's name and refer to parents in a way that fits with their cultural expectations. They avoid the use of professional jargon and clearly explain things. They also ask children and families to show that they understand the directions, techniques, or information to make sure they are communicating clearly. Since occupational therapy terminology and concepts may not translate well in other languages and are not understood by all, practitioners use everyday language with children and families. Additionally, practitioners from non-western cultures find the ambiguity of the English language often difficult to translate (Hammell, 2020a,b; Magalhaes & Galheigo, 2010).

Occupational therapy practitioners need to learn from other languages and cultures for occupational therapy to apply across cultural and language groups (Creek, 2020). For example, the word "occupation" or even "occupational" is a significant trigger to populations who lived through occupation or attack, such as refugees from Palestine or the war in Ukraine.

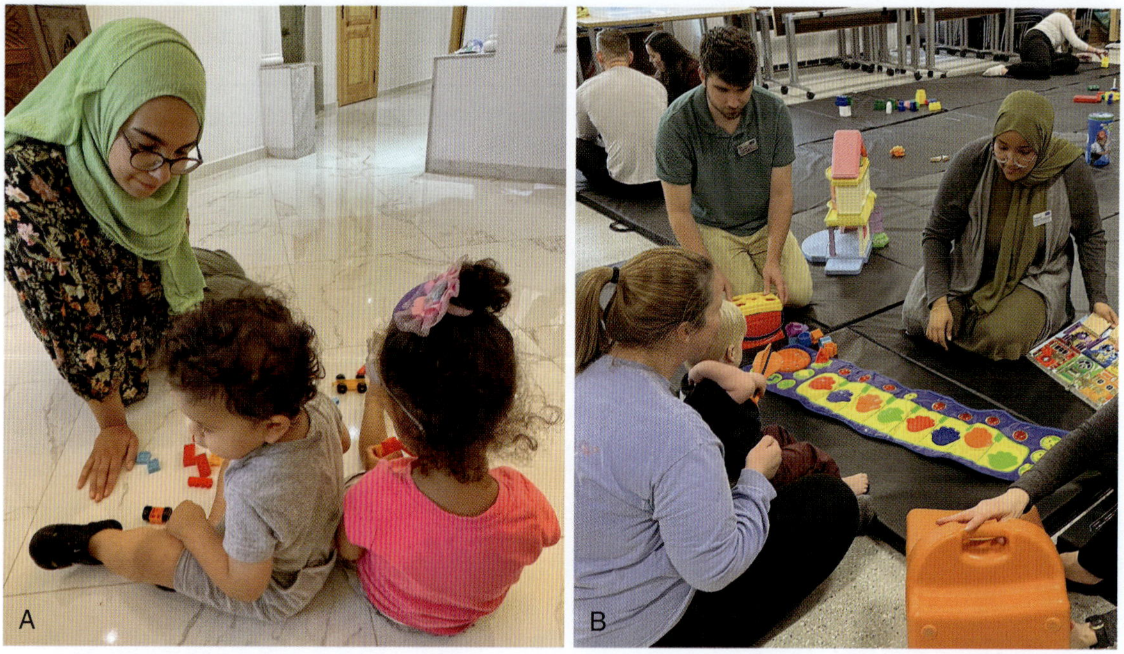

Fig. 4.8 (A) Occupational therapy practitioners gain expertise by learning from parents and children from diverse backgrounds. (B) Occupational therapy practitioners gain expertise by learning from other professionals and working in teams.

**Critically Analyzing.** Occupational therapy practitioners can evaluate, critique, and examine research and clinical practice to enhance and improve health equity and access (Bass & Baker, 2017; Restall et al., 2018) for all clients. They may engage in activities within their clinical practice to advocate for and promote occupational opportunities. For example, securing a grant to provide people who require wheelchairs for mobility access to parks, playgrounds, and water sports (such as adapted kayaking ramps). Broadening occupational therapy's scope of practice to include opportunities to engage in occupations fosters health and quality of life.

**Advocating.** Advocating for occupational opportunities for children and families involves participating in political elections. In the United States, voting in local, state, and national elections is a way to support representatives who may have an inclusive platform for people who would not otherwise have a voice or who are from less-represented groups. Voting can influence everything from a local school committee's budget for special education to federal immigration policies.

**Creating Inclusive Programs.** Occupational therapy practitioners working with children and families may promote occupational engagement by providing creative inclusive programs designed for all children. They may consult with agencies and communities to create inclusive playground spaces, museums, and safe spaces for children who have sensory needs. There are numerous examples of programs supporting children and families. For example, faculty and students created a 'sensory space' at a local ballpark so children could "take breaks" from the game. While the space was created for children with autism so they could enjoy the game with their family, their family and friends also enjoy this annual event. An occupational therapy practitioner created an adaptive dance program for young children with Down syndrome. The program was so successful, in subsequent years, they included the children in the regular lessons by making some adaptations as needed. Faculty and occupational therapy students created an afterschool program to promote physical activity and nutrition at a rural elementary school. Occupational therapy practitioners have secured grants to provide free constraint-induced movement therapy for children using a fun camp-based program. They have involved children and families in adaptive skiing, surfing, and hiking programs.

Creating opportunities with communities and listening to families results in culturally relevant programming addressing the communities' needs. Suarez-Balcazar et al. (2018, 2022) collaborated with Latino immigrant families with youth with disabilities to create programs addressing their needs for food security and programming for healthy lifestyles. Others have engaged parents who have children receiving occupational therapy services in focus groups to better understand their circumstances before creating programs.

Creating culturally relevant programs to include children and families requires that the occupational therapy practitioner listen to the community (such as with focus groups), address their needs, consider practical contexts (such as funding sources, time, setting, and language), and include the community in the design, implementation, and follow-up.

## Communicating With Clients

Communicating effectively with children and family is essential to creating a therapeutic relationship (See Chapter 3). Pediatric occupational therapy practitioners listen to parents and children throughout the process and communicate in a way that is effective for the client. For example, the child may need to communicate using an augmentative communication device that relies on symbols, pictures, or American Sign Language. Children and families who speak a different language may need an interpreter. Working with children and youth who have a specific physical condition or sensory difference may require modifications to the way they are addressed. Box 4.3 provides guidelines to enhance open communication with clients different from oneself, but those who speak the same language. See Fig. 4.9A–C for examples of how this careful communicating can result in trusting relationships, shared goals and relevant interventions. Case Example 4.6 provides an example of the importance of careful communication and bridging differences

Occupational therapy practitioners working with children and families communicate clearly, and in plain language (avoiding the use of professional jargon). The occupational therapy practitioner simplifies language without infantilizing. They speak in clear, short sentences, using everyday wording.

Occupational therapy practitioners examine vocal tone and pitch, energy level, eye contact, and the environment to support effective

## BOX 4.3 Guidelines for Communicating with Children and Families

- Assume good intentions of children and families.
- Approach all families as including individuals who want the best for their children.
- Invite children and families to share knowledge about their hopes, dreams, interests, and struggles.
- Encourage children and families to share information about family culture and traditions often.
- Respect differences in family structures and activities.
- Recognize how children and family members' identity may shape interactions with professionals (such as yourself).
- Bring a sense of openness to all interactions.
- Reflect on how one's own culture, values, and beliefs may influence the interaction.
- View diversity as a strength.
- Use a tone of respect in all communications.
- Ask questions politely, showing interest in the child or family members' response.
- Be honest, truthful, and open when communicating.
- Provide others with the opportunity to ask questions.
- Be comfortable with silence to allow others to process information.

Adapted from Learning for Justice. (2018). Family and community engagement. *Critical practices for anti-bias education.* (p. 14). https://www.learningforjustice.org/sites/default/files/2021-11/LFJ-2111-Critical-Practices-for-Anti-bias-Ed-November-2021-11172021.pdf

## CASE EXAMPLE 4.6 CAREFUL COMMUNICATION WITH CLIENTS AND FAMILIES

Taz is a 14-year-old boy with a learning disability in high school.

The occupational therapy practitioner is part of Taz's team and will work with Taz to provide exploration of potential career options as he moves towards transition out of school. They focus on identifying Taz's aspirations and desired outcomes, exploring opportunities, and creating future visions through collages of possibilities. As they engage in this work, the practitioner addresses Taz's strengths, encourages that he try new things, provides opportunities for him to experience possible options for his future, and seeks to understand the family and community situation he is in.

The occupational therapy practitioner considers family and community characteristics to support Taz's exploration. His family has limited financial resources and his parents struggle to make ends meet. They envision their child working at a local store upon graduation and the family does not value higher education. Taz looks up to his older brother and cousins who work in similar jobs at a store. Taz sees himself doing this when he graduates. The therapist is a practitioner with a higher education degree and a family that strongly values higher education and achievement as part of a profession. The practitioner had to self-reflect and work to understand the potential biases and judgments that could influence their work together. The practitioner had to actively listen to Taz and his family members, and communicate with them clearly and with respect. The practitioner had to do the important work to bridge differences and identify shared values, such as engaging in employment that one enjoys and is good at.

As the practitioner works with Taz and his family, the practitioner's respectful and open communication, use of active listening, and the use of an interpreter when required for conversations with specific family members allows Taz's family members to build a trusting relationship with the practitioner. Taz is able to identify his strengths (e.g., verbal communication, ability to get along with others, creativity, and motivation to become employed) and express his hopes and dreams for employment in a specific local store. Together they learn more about the specific skills required for that job and they work towards building those skills. By understanding Taz's family and community, through careful communication, and identifying and focusing on Taz's hopes and dreams the practitioner was able to engage Taz in intervention that addressed their shared goal of finding meaningful employment, and was relevant to Taz, and his family.

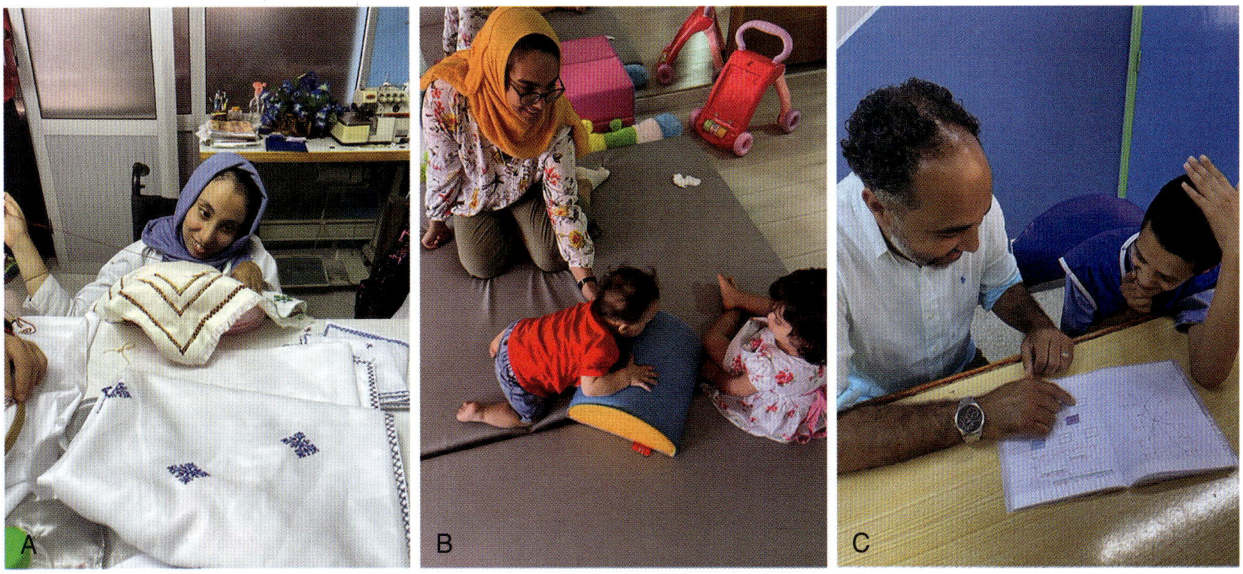


**Fig. 4.9** Engaging in careful communication with families ensures the relevance of occupational therapy interventions. (A) Intervention to improve ability to engage in embroidery resulted from communication regarding an important family tradition. (B) Intervention to promote sibling play resulted from communication regarding the importance of sibling relationships for that family. (C) This therapist makes sure to be on the same level with the client, while engaged in an activity chosen based on the child's communication regarding his hopes and dreams for school.

communication. They are aware of their tone and pitch to communicate in a calm, firm, and respectful manner that is easy for others to hear and process (e.g., not too high, or low). They adjust their energy level relative to the content of the communication and the situation. For example, when discussing a serious intervention issue, the practitioner uses a calmer subdued energy level, whereas if communicating in a playful session with the child, the therapy practitioner opts for a high energy level.

Eye contact can vary by culture. Practitioners ensure a shared understanding of eye contact relative to its use or avoidance. When appropriate, they make eye contact with children before providing instructions, make eye contact with parents (without staring), and nod to indicate they are listening.

When interacting with children, practitioners communicate at the child's level. For example, they position their body so they are at eye level with the child, so the child does not have to crane their neck. They approach children from their height as much as possible. One can half-kneel to have a productive exchange with a kindergartner for example. For clients with a history of trauma, avoid approaching from behind or the side unexpectedly. Similarly, practitioners position their bodies so they are at the same level (for example, both sitting in chairs at the same height).

Lastly, occupational therapy practitioners ensure the environment is conducive to effective communication. For some children, the practitioner may have to reduce noise and visual distractions. Occupational therapy practitioners working with children with specific visual needs, such as cortical visual impairment or traumatic brain injury should wear dark and solid colors. Busy patterns, stripes, or dots can make it difficult for the child to attend to the speaker.

**Interpreters.** Interpreters may be necessary when there is a language barrier. Occupational therapy practitioners working with interpreters follow specific behaviors. They "do not talk to the interpreter instead, speak to the client." If the conversation is happening at a table, such as a caregiver intake interview or at an annual individualized education plan (IEP) meeting, they consider the position of people in the room/at the table. The interpreter may be taking notes and prefer a physical seat at the table. In this case, the interpreter may be seated behind or past the person they are interpreting for. It is important to remember that the interpreter is not a representative of the family or child you are working with.

Occupational therapy terms like "proprioception" can be challenging to explain in English, and even more difficult in a different language. Occupational therapy practitioners are mindful to use straightforward language or briefly explain complex terms in everyday language. Interpreters all have different skill training and occasionally they may forget that their job is to translate verbatim what is being said. If an interpreter seems to be taking too much time or is going back and forth (seemingly answering questions to the family), the practitioner may stop the process and check in. Perhaps the interpreter needs more information, or the caregivers do. For example, at a meeting if the IEP team proposes "curb to curb" special education transportation and an interpreter uses the phrase "door to door" there can be a serious gap in child safety and caregiver expectations.

There are times when caregivers or family members end up interpreting. This can happen when a family rejects the need for interpretation services. While this is the family's right, they may select a member who is not the primary legal decision-maker to interpret or explain. This may also happen when an agency does not have access to a specific language through the interpretation services. This is not ideal and perhaps not considered legal depending on the system. It is always helpful to stop and frequently ask the family if they understand the conversation or have any questions. To ensure accurate communication, occupational therapy practitioners may ask family members to demonstrate techniques, relay suggestions, or summarize content from the session. Providing simple written summaries (transcribed into their language) and pictures may support communication.

**Technology for Interpretation.** Using technology to translate written or spoken information is increasingly an option. A best practice is to document the translated phrases *and* the original language phrases. For example, if communicating in writing with Albanian-speaking caregivers regarding an upcoming visit to the home via email, copy and paste first that caregiver's language, then the English next, to have a record of what you intended, if the translation is somehow inaccurate and so that you can refer to it later if need be.

Sample email to caregiver whose primary language is Albanian, scheduling an Early Intervention OT visit: *"Zonja F, për shkak të stuhisë së borës duhet ta ndryshoj vizitën e sotme me të enjten në orën 15.00. A do të funksionojë kjo për ju? Nëse jo, ju lutem më njoftoni. Faleminderit, OT Mary."*

"Ms. F, due to the snowstorm I need to change today's visit to Thursday at 3:00 p.m. Will this work for you? If not, please let me know. Thanks, OT Mary."

**Assessing with Interpreters.** Using an interpreter to work directly with children varies depending on the child's age. However, regardless of age, it is important to set expectations or ground rules with the interpreter before the child is present. Therapeutic use of self, body positioning and proximity to child, tone, and volume are occupational therapy "tools" used while evaluating or working with children. An interpreter may not understand them and therefore may use multiple and loud cues to attempt to gain a child's attention. They may attempt to physically redirect the child to get them to do what the interpreter "thinks" the occupational therapy practitioner wants. The interpreter may present the child with manipulatives or materials that are unsafe or inappropriate to the child but happen to be in the room at the time, such as scissors or a scooter board. Since the occupational therapist is responsible for the assessment session, they must communicate with the interpreter.

The goal is always to speak directly to the child, not the interpreter. If the therapist asks the interpreter to use extra language to gain the child's attention, such as in a play-based observation of an evaluation of a three-year-old, they must document it. When administering a standardized evaluation an interpreter may repeat directions or suggest corrections to the child during the evaluation that are not part of the intended assessment, which affects the validity of the scores and must be documented. Furthermore, many standardized assessments have not been normed on children who need interpreters. A standardized assessment given in this manner becomes subjective and can only be used to gather data on skills informally. Standardized scores cannot be reported in this case and other forms of assessment need to be used as well.

## MANAGING MISSTEPS

Even with the best of intentions, it is inevitable that mistakes will happen when working with children and families. See Chapter 3 for descriptions of inevitable interpersonal events. Occupational therapy practitioners reflect upon each interaction and communicate with children and families. It is the practitioner's responsibility to address any conflicts, mistakes, or missteps to maintain a therapeutic relationship.

There is a four-step process for correcting mistakes:

1. Acknowledge the error,
2. Apologize sincerely or make amends.
3. Ask how to correct things.
4. Affirm or commit not to make the same mistake again.

Apologize for the *actions*, not for how someone *feels*. First acknowledge the error by reflecting and identifying the error. This means identifying the actual thing that was done or not done, whether intentional or otherwise. Label that action with a verb if possible; *misgendered, mislabeled, mistook, misunderstood*, and *assumed* are all useful action verbs.

Apologize or make amends. A simple, "I'm sorry" or "Pardon my mistake please," works. Do not be defensive in this step, with phrases like, "No one told me." Be clear and succinct to make sure the person understands what you are apologizing for.

Ask how to rectify the error. This gives power and respect to the offended party and takes ownership that the offender has a behavior to change. "How can I fix this?" "What would be a better way to say or do this?"

Lastly, and in some ways, the most important step, affirm or commit to not making this mistake again. This may be difficult. Everyone has natural patterns and ways of going about things that are often automatic; however, this is where the conflict arises. Changing behavior is the truest way to show remorse and acknowledge an error. For example, if inadvertently misgendering a teen client, perhaps based upon their physical appearance or the medical documentation that states their biological sex rather than gender, a teen may respond with, "Hey! I'm not a boy!" The occupational therapy practitioner could respond, "I'm sorry, I didn't mean to misgender you. What pronouns do you prefer?" If the teen were to respond, "I go by Taylor, I use they/them pronouns." The practitioner could then reply, "Thanks for letting me know that. That was my error, I won't do it again."

It is not the child's or family's role to educate occupational therapy practitioners on their customs or culture. However, occupational therapy practitioners incorporate cultural needs into practice and may ask questions to learn how the family may carry out cultural traditions. Families and children may present themselves as defensive or standoffish around certain topics. Do not take this personally. It can be uncomfortable to open up and they may not know they have the right to speak up.

If corrected about a custom, cultural term, or client expectation, avoid a defensive response. Even well-intentioned mistakes are a way to learn. Ironically, one mistake that can happen comes from having had exposure or learned about a specific cultural group and assuming all members of that group have the same beliefs or practices. It can be easy to latch onto superficial bits of knowledge and overgeneralize them. For example, assuming that all Jewish clients will be unable to bring their child to an outpatient occupational therapy clinic on a Saturday because it is their day of worship may not apply to every family.

## TIPS FOR SUCCESS WHILE WORKING WITH CHILDREN AND FAMILIES

Working with people different from you can be rewarding, exciting, and challenging for personally unique reasons. Engaging in self-reflection, education, professional and community organizations, and gaining practical experience communicating with people from different cultures and backgrounds, with different beliefs, customs, and situations, allows occupational therapy practitioners to gain confidence in their abilities. Through self-reflection, practitioners learn to ask questions, seek support from others, and communicate clearly. They develop an understanding of families and children and acknowledge interpersonal events within the therapeutic relationship. Occupational therapy practitioners take ownership of their part in the process and engage children and families in conversations to correct missteps so that children can achieve the full benefits of occupational therapy services.

Seeking support, ideas, and strategies from colleagues, supervisors, and mentors is key to success in working with families. This requires that the practitioner ask questions, seek out others, clarify situations, and show insight into the process and importance of establishing inclusive and equitable relationships for children and families. In work settings, occupational therapy practitioners may collaborate with other professionals on the team to find solutions or understand family reasons, behaviors, and needs. Employer diversity or inclusivity teams and human resource departments are also good places to look for work-related support.

Sometimes just asking the question brings much-needed attention to the topic. Asking questions lets others know that they can also ask questions and can signal to the administration that there is a skill or knowledge deficit. Deficits should be supported through additional professional development or by examining institutional policies and procedures, including systemic bias.

Occupational therapy practitioners work directly with children and families who experience diverse healthcare needs. Consequently, they are in a unique position to be agents of change and advocate for services or policies to support children and families. Seeking support from others who advocate for children and families (such as clinicians, occupational therapy professional groups, state associations, and scholars) may stimulate change and energize practitioners. Many creative ideas originate from practitioners' discussions of problems or needs. For example, a practitioner frustrated with the long wait times and high costs of assistive technology created a free loan program for children in inner-city Chicago and South Carolina (O'Brien, 1990). Being aware of service needs and committing to addressing needs are the first steps in advocating for children and families. Seeking out solutions with children and families as partners ensures that creative programs are culturally responsive to the community's needs.

## SUMMARY

Occupational therapy practitioners have the privilege to work with children and families representing diversity in ethnicity, race, socioeconomic status, ability (ableness), gender, sexual orientation, age, and or religion. Together, with children and families, occupational therapy practitioners synthesize information about the family's beliefs, values, customs, roles, routines, expectations, and environment to create intervention plans that support the child's ability to engage in valued occupations within their community. The intervention takes place within societal, political, and institutional parameters. Additionally, the occupational therapy practitioner holds implicit biases from their own unique background, family structure, and environment that may influence their behaviors. The goal of occupational therapy intervention with children and youth is to enable them to participate in desired occupations. However, some children begin at a disadvantage, not only due to their abilities but also due to their life circumstances. They may not be afforded the same opportunities due to systemic racism and may begin life with health disadvantages caused by generational trauma (lack of healthcare access over time affecting generations).

Occupational therapy practitioners work to advocate for children and families by acknowledging diversity, identifying systems or policies that interfere with children and family health, and establishing therapeutic relationships with children and families who have been underrepresented. They advocate for children and families and seek to provide occupational opportunities (through modifications, adaptations, and skill acquisition) so that children with cognitive, physical, mental, or social disabilities from all communities and groups can participate in a range of meaningful occupations.

1. Occupational therapy practitioners work with children and families from diverse backgrounds. To provide effective occupational therapy intervention, they establish a therapeutic relationship and seek to understand the child and family's situation, beliefs, routines, expectations, goals, and choices. To effectively understand people from various backgrounds, they demonstrate cultural humility (i.e., the ability to maintain an other-oriented stance). Occupational therapy practitioners who engage in cultural humility are committed to self-evaluation, open to change, recognize their power in the therapeutic relationship, and use that power through partnering with others to change systems that create bias and inequity (Agner, 2020). Occupational therapy practitioners who show cultural humility in practice learn from children and families so that they can better address children's challenges and empower families.
2. Cultural humility requires ongoing reflection, constant learning, acknowledgment of implicit and explicit biases, and a commitment to working toward a positive change. Critical actionable steps to develop cultural humility include commitment to self-evaluation, openness to change, recognition of one's power in the therapeutic relationship, and use of that power through partnering with others to change systems that create bias and inequity (Agner, 2020).
3. Bridging differences refers to developing therapeutic relationships by interacting and connecting with those who are different from us or a diverse group (such as ethnicity, race, socioeconomic status, ability, gender, sexual orientation, age, and/or religion). Bridging differences involves understanding one's own biases and engaging in work to foster equity for all clients.
4. Pediatric occupational therapy practitioners can bridge differences by expanding their worldviews, learning to recognize and examine their own biases, and demonstrating specific actions with clients that promote understanding, respect, and family-centered care. They can expand their skills in cultural humility through self-reflection, education, participation in organizations, international service learning, group membership, volunteering, and media. They benefit from supervision, mentorship, and collegial support.

## REFERENCES


Agner, J. (2020). The issue is—moving from cultural competence to cultural humility in occupational therapy: A paradigm shift. *American Journal of Occupational Therapy, 74*, 7404347010. https://doi.org/10.5014/ajot.2020.038067.

Agorastos, A., Pervanidou, P., Chrousos, G. P., & Baker, D. G. (2019). Developmental trajectories of early life stress and trauma: A narrative review on neurobiological aspects beyond stress system dysregulation. *Frontiers in Psychiatry, 118.*

American Occupational Therapy Association. (2020a). Occupational therapy's commitment to diversity, equity, and inclusion. *American Journal of Occupational Therapy, 74*(Suppl. 3), 7413410030. https://doi.org/10.5014/ajot.2020.74S3002.

American Occupational Therapy Association. (2020b). AOTA 2020 occupational therapy code of ethics. *American Journal of Occupational Therapy, 74*(Suppl. 3), 7413410005. https://doi.org/10.5014/ajot.2020.74S3006.

American Occupational Therapy Association. (2021). In *AOTA's statement on justice and systemic racism.* https://www.aota.org/about/diversity-equity-and-inclusion/aota-statement-on-justice-and-systemic-racism.

Barger, B., Benevides, T., Rizk, S., Rice, C., Heiman, H., Salmon, A., & Sanchez-Alvarez, S. (2022). Race/ethnic inequities in conjoint monitoring and screening for U.S. children 3 and under. *Disability and Health Journal, 15*(1), 101179. https://doi.org/10.1016/j.dhjo.2021.101179.

Bass, J. D., & Baker, N. A. (2017). Occupational therapy and public health: Advancing research to improve population health and health equity. *OTJR: Occupation, Participation and Health, 37*(4), 175–177.

Blair, I. (2001). Implicit stereotypes and prejudice. In G. B. Moskowitz (Ed.), *Cognitive social psychology: The Princeton symposium on the legacy and future of social cognition* (pp. 359–374). Lawrence Erlbaum.

Cambridge Dictionary. Microaggression. In Dictionary.Cambridge.org dictionary. Retrieved December 18, 2022, from https://dictionary.cambridge.org/us/dictionary/english/microaggression.

Chabot, M. C., Sanchez, A., Nafai, S., & Stevens-Nafai, E. (2021). All work or all play? The impact of cultural and clinical activities on perceived cultural sensitivity development during an occupational therapy service learning experience. *Journal of Occupational Therapy Education, 5*(3). https://encompass.eku.edu/jote/vol5/iss3/5.

Chaudry, A., & Wimer, C. (2016). Poverty is not just an indicator: The relationship between income, poverty, and child well-being. *Academic Pediatrics, 16*(3), S23–S29.

Creek, J. (2020). More than words can say: Decolonising occupational therapy terminology. In *The occupational therapy hub.* Retrieved from https://www.theothub.com/article/more-than-words-can-say-decolonising-occupational-therapy-terminology.

Curtis, E., Jones, R., Tipene-Leach, D., Walker, C., Loring, B., Paine, S. J., & Reid, P. (2019). Why cultural safety rather than cultural competency is required to achieve health equity: A literature review and recommended definition. *International Journal for Equity in Health, 18*(1), 1–17.

Eni, R., Phillips-Beck, W., Achan, G. K., et al. (2021). Decolonizing health in Canada: A Manitoba first nation perspective. *International Journal for Equity in Health, 20*, 206.

Entwistle, V. A., & Watt, I. S. (2013). Treating patients as persons: A capabilities approach to support delivery of person-centered care. *The American Journal of Bioethics, 13*(8), 29–39.

Finnegan, A. C. (2022). Growing up white saviors. *Journal of Applied Social Science, 16*(3), 617–636.

FitzGerald, C., & Hurst, S. (2017). Implicit bias in healthcare professionals: A systematic review. *BMC Medical Ethics, 18*(1), 1–18.

Foronda, C., Baptiste, D. L., Reinholdt, M. M., & Ousman, K. (2015). Cultural humility. *Journal of Transcultural Nursing, 27*(3), 210–217. https://doi.org/10.1177/1043659615592677.

Froehlich, J., & Thornton-Marsh, J. (2021). *Transforming racial and cultural lines in health and Social Care: Listening, loving, and lifting spirits when you can.* Routledge.

Gasper, D. (2002). Is Sen's capability approach an adequate basis for considering human development? *Review of Political Economy, 14*(4), 435–461.

Greenwald, A. G., & Lai, C. K. (2020). Implicit social cognition. *Annual Review of Psychology, 71*, 419–445.

Hagiwara, N., Kron, F. W., Scerbo, M. W., & Watson, G. S. (2020). A call for grounding implicit bias training in clinical and translational frameworks. *The Lancet, 395*(10234), 1457–1460.

Halfon, N., & Hochstein, M. (2002). Life course health development: An integrated framework for developing health, policy, and research. *The Milbank Quarterly, 80*(3), 433–479.

Hall, W. J., Chapman, M. V., Lee, K. M., Merino, Y. M., Thomas, T. W., Payne, B. K., Eng, E., Day, S. H., & Coyne-Beasley, T. (2015). Implicit racial/ethnic bias among health care professionals and its influence on health care outcomes: A systematic review. *American Journal of Public Health, 105*(12), e60–e76.

Hammell, K. R. W., & Beagan, B. (2017). Occupational injustice: A critique: L'injustice occupationnelle: Une critique. *Canadian Journal of Occupational Therapy, 84*(1), 58–68.

Hammell, K. W. (2020a). Action on the social determinants of health: Advancing occupational equity and occupational rights. *Cadernos Brasileiros de Terapia Ocupacional, 28*, 378–400.

Hammell, K. W. (2018). Building globally relevant occupational therapy from the strength of our diversity. *World Federation of Occupational Therapists Bulletin, 75*(1), 13–26. https://doi.org/10.1080/14473828.2018.1529480.

Hammell, K. W. (2020b). Engagement in living: Critical perspectives on occupation, rights and wellbeing. In *Canadian Occupational Therapy Association*.

Hammell, K. W. (2023). Focusing on "what matters": The occupation, capability and wellbeing framework for occupational therapy. *Cadernos Brasileiros de Terapia Ocupacional, 31*, e3509. https://doi.org/10.1590/2526-8910.ctoAO269035092.

Hamed, S., Bradby, H., Ahlberg, B. M., & Tharpar-Björkert, S. (2022). Racism in healthcare: A scoping review. *BMC Public Health, 22*, 988. https://doi.org/10.1186/s12889-022-13122-y.

Hammell, K. W. (2015). Quality of life, participation and occupational rights: A capabilities perspective. *Australian Occupational Therapy Journal, 62*(2), 78–85.

Hammell, K. W. (2021). Social and structural determinants of Health: Exploring Occupational therapy's structural (in)competence. *Canadian Journal of Occupational Therapy, 88*(4), 365–374. https://doi.org/10.1177/00084174211046797.

Hewstone, M., & Greenland, K. (2000). Intergroup conflict. *International Journal of Psychology, 35*(2), 136–144. https://doi.org/10.1080/002075900399439.

Hook, J. N., Davis, D. E., Owen, J., Worthington, J. ,E. L., & Utsey, S. O. (2013). Cultural humility: Measuring openness to culturally diverse clients. *Journal of Counseling Psychology, 60*(3), 353–366. https://doi-org.une.idm.oclc.org/10.1037/a0032595.

Jensen, E., Jones, N., Rabe, M., Pratt, B., Medina, L., Orozco, K., & Spell, L. (2021). *2020 U.S. Population more racially and ethnically diverse than measured in 2010*. https://www.census.gov/library/stories/2021/08/2020-united-states-population-more-racially-ethnically-diverse-than-2010.html.

Jussim, L., & Harber, K. D. (2005). Teacher expectations and self-fulfilling prophecies: Knowns and unknowns, resolved and unresolved controversies. *Personality and Social Psychology Review, 9*(2), 131–155.

Kellock, A. (2020). Children's well-being in the primary school: A capability approach and community psychology perspective. *Childhood, 27*(2), 220–237. https://doi.org/10.1177/0907568220902516.

Kinsella, A., & Whiteford, G. (2008). Knowledge generation and utilization in occupational therapy: Towards an epistemic reflexivity. *Australian Occupational Therapy Journal, 56*(4), 249–258. https://doi.org/10.1111/j.1440-1630.2007.00726.x.

Kornhaber, S. (2016). A person can't be diverse. In *The Atlantic*. https://www.theatlantic.com/entertainment/archive/2016/01/ava-duvernay-oscars-so-white-diversity-academy-awards-language/429225/.

Lavalley, R., & Johnson, K. R. (2020). Occupation, injustice, and anti-black racism in the United States of America. *Journal of Occupational Science, 29*(4), 487–499. https://doi.org/10.1080/14427591.2020.1810111.

Lavizzo-Mourey, R. J., Besser, R. E., & Williams, D. R. (2021). Understanding and mitigating health inequities—past, current, and future directions. *New England Journal of Medicine, 384*(18), 1681–1684.

Learning for Justice. (2018). Family and community engagement. In *Critical practices for anti-bias education* (pp. 14–18). https://www.learningforjustice.org/sites/default/files/2021-11/LFJ-2111-Critical-Practices-for-Anti-bias-Ed-November-2021-11172021.pdf.

Lorenz, G. (2021). Subtle discrimination: Do stereotypes among teachers trigger bias in their expectations and widen ethnic achievement gaps? *Social Psychology of Education, 24*(2), 537–571.

Luyster, R. J., Seery, A., Talbott, M. R., & Tager–Flusberg, H. (2011). Identifying early–risk markers and developmental trajectories for language impairment in neurodevelopmental disorders. *Developmental Disabilities Research Reviews, 17*(2), 151–159.

MacInnis, C. C., & Hodson, G. (2019). Extending the benefits of intergroup contact beyond attitudes: When does intergroup contact predict greater collective action support? *Journal of Theoretical Social Psychology, 3*(1), 11–22. https://doi.org/10.1002/jts5.23.

Madeira, F., Costa-Lopes, R., Do Bú, E. A., & Tato Marinho, R. (2022). The role of stereotypical information on medical judgements for black and white patients. *PLoS One, 17*(6):e0268888.

Magalhaes, L., & Galheigo, S. M. (2010). Enabling international communication among Brazilian occupational therapists: Seeking consensus on occupational terminology. *Occupational Therapy International, 17*(3), 113–124.

Mahoney, W. J., & Kiraly-Alvarez, A. F. (2019). Challenging the Status Quo: Infusing non-western ideas into occupational therapy education and practice. *The Open Journal of Occupational Therapy, 7*(3), 1–10.

Malfitano, A. P. S., & Lopes, R. E. (2018). Social occupational therapy: Committing to social change. *New Zealand Journal of Occupational Therapy, 65*(1), 20–26. https://search.informit.org/doi/10.3316/informit.779763971754213.

Mason, B. (2020). *Curbing implicit bias: What works and what doesn't*. https://knowablemagazine.org/article/mind/2020/how-to-curb-implicit-bias.

McGee-Avila, J. (June 21, 2018). *Moving beyond cultural competency to cultural humility acknowledges patients' authority over their lived experience*. Robert Wood Johnson Foundation. https://www.rwjf.org/en/insights/blog/2018/06/practicing-cultural-humility-to-transform-healthcare.html#:~:text=While%20we%20often%20view%20our,dominant%20voice%20in%20the%20conversation.

Mendoza-Denton, R., & Briscoe-Smith, A. (2023). *Bridging differences*. University of California, Berkely. https://ggsc.berkeley.edu/what_we_do/event/bridging_differences_online_course.

Moskowitz, G. B., Stone, J., & Childs, A. (2012). Implicit stereotyping and medical decisions: Unconscious stereotype activation in practitioners' thoughts about African Americans. *American Journal of Public Health, 102*(5), 996–1001.

Mousavi, T., Forwell, S., Dharamsi, S., & Dean, E. (2015). The historical shift towards human rights in occupational therapy with special reference to the Capabilities Approach and its implications. *World Federation of Occupational Therapists Bulletin, 71*(2), 81–87.

Mulumba, M., Ruano, A. L., Perehudoff, K., & Ooms, G. (2021). Decolonizing health governance: A Uganda case study on the influence of political history on community participation. *Health and Human Rights, 23*(1), 259–271.

Nussbaum, M. C. (2009). Creating capabilities: The human development approach and its implementation. *Hypatia, 24*(3), 211–215.

O'Brien, J. (1990). Project ARCH (adapted resources for children) grant. Ronald McDonald's Children's Charities.

Perryman-Fox, M., Cox, D., Morris, K., & Stoffel, V. (2022). *The occupation of the occupational therapy practitioner: Channeling cultural humility through reflection and reflexive practices.*

Popova, E. S., O'Brien, J. C., & Taylor, R. R. (2022). Communicating with intention: Therapist and parent perspectives on family-centered care in early intervention. *American Journal of Occupational Therapy, 76*(5), 1–9. https://doi.org/10.5014/ajot.2022.049131.

Ramugondo, E. (2018). WFOT congress keynote – healing work: Intersections for decoloniality. *World Federation of Occupational Therapists Bulletin, 74*(2), 83–91. https://doi.org/10.1080/14473828.2018.1523981.

Reimer, N. K., & Sengupta, N. K. (2022). Meta-analysis of the "ironic" effects of intergroup contact. *Journal of Personality and Social Psychology, 124*(2). https://doi.org/10.1037/pspi0000404.

Resnicow, K., Baranowski, T., Ahluwalia, J. S., & Braithwaite, R. L. (1999). Cultural sensitivity in public health: Defined and demystified. *Ethnicity & Disease, 9*(1), 10–21.

Restall, G. J., MacLeod Schroeder, N. J., & Dubé, C. D. (2018). The equity lens for occupational therapy: A program development and evaluation tool. *Canadian Journal of Occupational Therapy, 85*(3), 185–195.

Ricks, T. N., Abbyad, C., & Polinard, E. (2022). Undoing racism and mitigating bias among healthcare professionals: Lessons learned during a systematic review. *Journal of Racial and Ethnic Health Disparities*, *9*(5), 1990–2000.

Robeyns, I. (2005). The capability approach: A theoretical survey. *Journal of Human Development*, *6*(1), 61–92.

Rosenthal, R., & Jacobson, L. (1968). Pygmalion in the classroom. *The Urban Review*, *3*(1), 16–20.

Sen, A. (1993). Capability and well-Being. In S. Nussbaum (Ed.), *The quality of life*. Clarendon Press.

Stevens-Nafai, E. W., & Nafai, S. (2019). Global perspectives on occupational therapy practice. In K. Jacobs, & G. McCormack (Eds.), *Occupational therapy manager* (6th ed.) (pp. 55–64). AOTA Press.

Suarez-Balcazar, Y., Early, A., Maldonado, A., Garcia, C. P., Arias, D., Zeidman, A., & Agudelo-Orozco, A. (2018). Community-based participatory research to promote healthy lifestyles among Latino immigrant families with youth with disabilities. *Scandinavian Journal of Occupational Therapy*, *25*(5), 396–406. https://doi.org/10.1080/11038128.2018.1502348.

Suarez-Balcazar, Y., Balcazar, F., Miranda, D. E., Velazquez, T., Arcidiacono, C., & Garcia, R. M. (2022). Promoting justice through community–based research: International case studies. *American Journal of Community Psychology*, *69*(3/4), 318–330. https://doi.org/10.1002/ajcp.12584.

Sue, D. W., Capodilupo, C. M., Torino, G. C., Bucceri, J. M., Holder, A. M., Nadal, K. L., & Esquilin, M. (2007). Racial microaggressions in everyday life: Implications for clinical practice. *American Psychologist*, *62*(4), 271–286. https://doi.org/10.1037/0003-066x.62.4.271.

Taff, S. D., & Blash, D. (2017). Diversity and inclusion in occupational therapy: Where we are, where we must go. *Occupational Therapy in Health Care*, *31*(1), 72–83. https://doi.org/10.1080/07380577.2016.1270479.

Thomas, M. S. (2016). Understanding delay in developmental disorders. *Child Development Perspectives*, *10*(2), 73–80.

U.S. Bureau of Labor Statistics. (2022). *Employed persons by detailed occupation, sex, race, and Hispanic or Latino ethnicity*. U.S. Bureau of Labor Statistics. https://www.bls.gov/cps/cpsaat11.htm.

Vuletich, H. A., & Payne, B. K. (June 2019). Stability and change in implicit bias. *Psychological Science*, *30*(6), 854–862.

Washington, E. (May 10, 2022). Recognizing and responding to microaggressions at work. In *Harvard business review*. https://hbr.org/2022/05/recognizing-and-responding-to-microaggressions-at-work.

Wexler, M. G., McGean, M., Tripodis, Y., Tolliver, D., Messmer, E., Brochier, A., & Garg, A. (2022). The association between racial discrimination, race, and social class with health among US children: Discrimination, race and social class with child health. In *Academic Pediatrics*.

Whiteford, G. E. (2019). Sylvia Docker Memorial Lecture: Together we go further-service co-design, knowledge co-production and radical solidarity. *Australian Occupational Therapy Journal*, *66*(6), 682–689. https://doi.org/10.1111/1440-1630.12628.

Williams, D. R., & Cooper, L. A. (2019). Reducing racial inequities in health: Using what we already know to take action. *International Journal of Environmental Research and Public Health*, *16*(4), 606.

Wineburg, S. S. (1987). The self-fulfillment of the self-fulfilling prophecy. *Educational Researcher*, *16*(9), 28–37.

World Federation of Occupational Therapists. (2019). In *Position statement: Occupational therapy and human rights (Revised 2019)*. https://www.wfot.org/resources/occupational-therapy-and-human-rights.

World Health Organization. (2023). In *Health equity*. https://www.who.int/health-topics/health-equity#tab=tab_1.

Zestcott, C. A., Spece, L., McDermott, D., & Stone, J. (2021). Health care providers' negative implicit attitudes and stereotypes of American Indians. *Journal of Racial and Ethnic Health Disparities*, *8*(1), 230–236.

5

# Pediatric Conditions

*Patricia Bowyer, and Jarrett Wolske*

With contributions from Patty Coker-Bolt, Patricia Fingerhut, Heather Miller Kuhaneck, Erin Naber, Jane Clifford O'Brien, Karen Ratcliff, Teressa Garcia Reidy, Patricia Sharp, Amber Sheehan, Elizabeth Warnken.

## GUIDING QUESTIONS

1. What causes, characteristics and symptoms, and occupational challenges are associated with common childhood conditions?
2. How do occupational therapy practitioners use knowledge of conditions to inform practice?

## KEY TERMS

Adverse Childhood Experiences (ACE)
Ataxia
Athetoid
Dyskinetic
International Classification of Diseases (ICD)
Incidence
Prevalence
Scientific reasoning
Spasticity

## INTRODUCTION

One of the hallmarks of an exemplary occupational therapy practitioner is the ability to clinically reason using multiple methods to help clients achieve their occupational goals. **Scientific reasoning**, one type of clinical reasoning, refers to using knowledge of a client's diagnosis, health impairment, or condition and its potential impact on occupational participation to guide the practitioner's thinking and decision-making (Boyt-Schell, 2019; Patnaude, 2023). Occupational therapy practitioners engage in scientific reasoning when they seek to understand a child's condition and its influence on the child's occupational performance. However, occupational therapy practitioners do not only consider a client's diagnosis or health condition when creating intervention plans. They consider a variety of factors, including the child's strengths and challenges, motivation, occupational interests, unique circumstances, resources, routines, and culture. They use knowledge of the child's diagnoses and health conditions as part of the child's overall story to make decisions regarding a comprehensive evaluation plan, specific assessments, as well as interventions and potential outcomes. The chapter reviews the causes, symptoms, and occupational challenges associated with common conditions that occupational therapy practitioners working with children and youth encounter in practice and illustrates how occupational therapy practitioners use scientific knowledge of the child's diagnosis to understand its potential impact on occupational performance.

## CATEGORIZATION OF CONDITIONS

Diseases, disorders, and diagnoses can be organized or classified according to a variety of dimensions. For example, depending on one's purpose or need for the information, conditions can be organized by patterns of symptoms, parts of the body, the etiology or explanatory mechanism, the developmental course of the disorder, the age of onset, relationship to genetic or environmental factors, and more. There are also classification guidelines and coding schemes provided for medical professionals to standardize diagnosis and communication. One common diagnostic structure for mental health disorders is the DSM-TR (APA, 2022). Another is **The International Classification of Diseases (ICD)**, which is a global standard for recording health information and causes of death that is developed and updated by the World Health Organization. The current version is the ICD-11 (WHO, 2022). Table 5.1 provides the ICD-11 categories for many of the conditions that children who are referred to and treated by occupational therapy practitioners have. The ICD categories were used for the primary headings in this chapter, and a representative but not comprehensive selection of conditions within those sections is described below. It is beyond the scope of this chapter to cover every condition, and there are entire textbooks devoted to this content. Box 5.1 provides ideas about how to approach the situation if one is given a referral for a client with an unknown condition.

Another way to consider and group conditions for this chapter is by how common it is for an occupational therapy practitioner to work with a child with the condition. It is difficult to find evidence regarding the most common pediatric conditions seen by occupational therapy in the United States as recent surveys of occupational therapy practices have focused on adult populations. An annual IDEA report using figures from 2020 suggests that the most common disability categories served (not necessarily by occupational therapy) were developmental delay, speech-language impairment, and then autism (IDEA, 2022). A recent review of occupational therapy interventions with children with disabilities included the

TABLE 5.1 **ICD-11 Categories with selected Conditions and Corresponding Diagnostic Codes**

| Category | Condition and (ICD-11 Code) |
|---|---|
| **Mental, behavioral, or neurodevelopmental disorders (06)**<br>"Mental, behavioral, and neurodevelopmental disorders are syndromes characterized by clinically significant disturbance in an individual's cognition, emotional regulation, or behavior that reflects a dysfunction in the psychological, biological, or developmental processes that underlie mental and behavioral functioning. These disturbances are usually associated with distress or impairment in personal, family, social, educational, occupational, or other important areas of functioning." ICD-11 | Autism spectrum disorder (6A02)<br>Developmental motor coordination disorder (6A04)<br>Attention deficit hyperactivity disorder (6A05)<br>Depressive disorders (6A70-3)<br>Anxiety (6B00-06)<br>Feeding and eating disorders (6B80-85) |
| **Diseases of the nervous system (08)**<br>"This is a group of conditions characterized as being in or associated with the nervous system." ICD-11 | Intracranial hemorrhage (8B20-26)<br>Spinal muscle atrophy (8B61)<br>Brachial plexus (8B91)<br>Muscular dystrophy (8C70)<br>Cerebral palsy (8D20-3)<br>Intracranial injuries (concussion, TBI) (NA07.0-0.7) |
| **Injury, poisoning, or certain other consequences of external causes (22)**<br>"In the ICD, injury means physical or physiological bodily harm resulting from the interaction of the body with energy (mechanical, thermal, electrical, chemical or radiant, or due to extreme pressure) in an amount, or at a rate of transfer, that exceeds physical or physiological tolerance. Injury can also result from a lack of vital elements, such as oxygen. ... Injury usually has a rapid onset in response to a well-defined event (e.g., a car crash, striking the ground after falling) .... These events are often referred to as external causes of injury. The injurious energy can, however, originate from the injured person and/or from his or her immediate environment (e.g., a person running on a hot day sustains heat exhaustion), and injury can be caused by the injured person (i.e., intentional self-harm)." ICD-11 | Spinal cord injury (ND51.2) |
| **Developmental anomalies (20)**<br>"Includes conditions caused by failure of a particular body site or body system to develop correctly during the antenatal period." ICD-11 | Down syndrome (LD40)<br>Spina bifida (LA02) |
| **Neoplasms (cancer) (02)**<br>"An abnormal or uncontrolled cellular proliferation which is not coordinated with an organism's requirements for normal tissue growth, replacement or repair." ICD-11 | There are a multitude of specific cancers named depending on their type and location of the disease. (2A00-2F97) |

ICD-11 codes can be found https://icd.who.int/browse11/l-m/en#/http://id.who.int/icd/entity/2065413738

BOX 5.1 **Exploring Childhood Conditions**

There are a variety of ways to obtain information about childhood conditions that you are not familiar with, including:

- Look up the diagnosis on the internet, finding reputable sources such as peer-reviewed journals or national association websites.
- If possible, find multiple sources for the information, including information on intervention strategies from professionals (within and outside of occupational therapy).
- Look in your textbooks for information on the condition (start with the table of contents and index to quickly determine if the condition is covered in the book).
- Look for online books about the condition.
- Review a medical text such as the Merck Manual, which is now provided online (https://www.merckmanuals.com/professional).
- Find online case examples written by medical professionals.
- Find blogs written by people experiencing the diagnosis to try to understand personal perspectives of having the condition.
- Ask a mentor, supervisor, or more experienced clinician if they have experience working with children who have the condition.
- Synthesize material from multiple sources (publications, professionals, and parents/caregivers) with your professional knowledge and previous experience to understand the child's condition.

following conditions in alphabetical order arthrogryposis, attention deficit hyperactivity disorder (ADHD), autism spectrum disorder (ASD), behavior disorders, brachial plexus, brain injury, burns, cerebral palsy, cancer, chronic pain, developmental coordination disorder (DCD), developmental disability, down syndrome, fetal alcohol spectrum disorder, learning disability, mental health, muscle diseases; intellectual disability, obesity, preterm infants, physical disability, rheumatoid arthritis, spina bifida (Novak & Honan, 2019). These authors found that most research existed on ASD, ADHD, cerebral palsy, and DCD. A simple search of web resources for large rehabilitation facilities that provide occupational therapy lists a variety of diagnoses that may be seen by occupational therapists (see Table 5.2).

The frequency with which any practitioner may work with children and youth with these conditions varies by work setting and the actual **prevalence** and **incidence** of the condition itself.

The prevalence of a condition is the proportion of a population who have a specific disorder during a given time, such as a year, regardless of when they were diagnosed. Incidence is the number of new cases diagnosed in a period. There are generally strong studies of prevalence in the United States and abroad, so we have chosen to order the conditions in this chapter within the ICD-11 primary headings, by prevalence based on United States data. As many of the conditions have similar symptoms and occupational performance challenges, however, not every condition listed in Table 5.2 will be specifically discussed.

## MENTAL, BEHAVIORAL, OR NEURODEVELOPMENTAL DISORDERS

Eight percent of American children have a diagnosed disability of mental, behavioral, or neurodevelopmental disorder (e.g., autism spectrum, developmental motor coordination, attention-deficit hyperactivity, depressive, and anxiety) (CDC, 2022). According to the

**TABLE 5.2 Commonly Listed Diagnoses and Conditions**

| Physical/Orthopedic/Motor | Mental Health/Behavioral and Cognitive/Intellectual |
|---|---|
| Arthrogryposis | ADD |
| Brachial plexus | ADHD |
| Burns | Asperger's syndrome |
| Cancer | Auditory processing disorder |
| Cerebral palsy | Autism spectrum disorders |
| Childhood stroke | Cognitive disorders |
| Developmental coordination disorder | Concussion |
| Developmental delays | Down syndrome |
| Epilepsy/Seizure disorders | Dyslexia |
| Failure to thrive | Fetal alcohol syndrome |
| Feeding difficulties | Learning disabilities |
| Generalized weakness | Oppositional defiant disorder |
| Hemiparesis | Posttraumatic stress disorder (PTSD) |
| High or low Muscle tone | Reading disorders |
| Juvenile rheumatoid arthritis | Sensory processing disorders (SPD) |
| Muscular dystrophy | Specific learning impairments (SLIs) |
| Oral Motor weakness | |
| Prematurity | |
| Spina bifida | |
| Spinal cord injury | |
| Spinal Muscle atrophy | |
| Sports injuries | |
| Torticollis | |
| Traumatic brain injury (TBI) | |
| Upper extremity deformities | |

Created from https://www.nationwidechildrens.org/specialties/occupational-therapyhttps://www.rwjbh.org/treatment-care/pediatrics/conditions-treatments/pediatric-occupational-therapy/https://nyulangone.org/locations/pediatric-rehabilitation-serviceshttps://www.chla.org/rehabilitation-services/occupational-therapy

Centers for Disease Control and Prevention (CDC), the most diagnosed mental disorders in children are ADHD, anxiety, behavior problems, and depression. In 2017, the reported prevalence for ADHD was 9.5%, and for ASD, 2.5% (Zablotsky et al., 2019). The prevalence of ASD reported in 2018 using data from 2014 was 1 in 59 children (Baio et al., 2018); however, the most recent CDC figures suggest 1 in 36. The CDC reports that of children 3–17 years, 9% have anxiety and 4% have depression. DCD affects about 5% of school-aged children (American Psychiatric Association, 2022; Harrowell et al., 2018) and is the most common movement disorder in childhood (Smits-Engleslman et al., 2018). Fewer than 1% of children have feeding and eating disorders (Lindvall Dahlgren et al., 2017). Based on these prevalence rates within the ICD-11 category, we include ADHD, anxiety, DCD, depression, ASD, and feeding and eating disorders, in that order.

## Attention Deficit Hyperactivity Disorder

ADHD is a neurodevelopmental disorder where symptoms present as inattentive, hyperactive-impulsive, or both and lead to difficulties with daily life (Faraone et al., 2021; Krauss & Schellenberg, 2022). A diagnosis of ADHD is made by a licensed clinician and is characterized as the presence of developmentally inappropriate levels of hyperactivity-impulsivity and/or inattentive symptoms occurring for at least 6 months, present across different environmental settings, with symptoms impairing participation in major life domains (Faraone et al., 2021).

**BOX 5.2 Characteristics of Attention Deficit Hyperactivity Disorder**

**Inattention**

✓Carelessness in daily tasks
✓Distracted easily
✓Forgetful of daily activities
✓Poor organization
✓Avoiding tasks
✓Appearing to not listen

**Hyperactivity-Impulsivity**

✓Excessive talking
✓Fidgeting
✓Interrupting others
✓Unable to take turns
✓Difficulty in quiet play

**Causes.** The causes of ADHD are not known but may include a combination of genetic and environmental factors (Faraone et al., 2021). Risk factors can include a familial history of ADHD, and neonatal conditions such as viral infections, nutritional deficiency, and maternal smoking during pregnancy.

**Characteristics and Symptoms.** Children with ADHD can present as primarily inattentive, primarily hyperactive-impulsive, or combined (American Psychiatric Association, 2022; Faraone et al., 2021). The characteristics for each type are listed in Box 5.2. ADHD has a comorbidity with obesity and sleep disorders (Chen et al., 2019; Craig et al., 2020; Faraone et al., 2021).

**Challenges in Occupational Participation.** Children and youth with ADHD experience challenges related to executive functioning. These core executive functioning weaknesses, specifically with skills such as planning, task initiation, emotional regulation, and attention, affect the child's participation across all occupations, as outlined in Box 5.3 (Hahn-Markowitz et al., 2020). For example, in school, a child may struggle to complete assignments, turn in assignments on time, take effective notes, and participate in lectures or class discussions. A youth with ADHD may struggle to attend work on time, resulting in concerns about tardiness and attendance. They may exhibit social skills challenges as they miss cues or subtleties in conversations (Fox et al., 2020). They may struggle to complete various work tasks efficiently or have difficulty prioritizing tasks (Fuermaier et al., 2021).

**Implications for Occupational Therapy.** Occupational therapy practitioners may help children identify strategies to support their performance in school, at home, and in the community (Ianni et al., 2021). Children may benefit from learning cognitive behavioral techniques, self-regulation strategies, or organizational strategies. They may benefit from role-playing situations, learning to "chunk" work into smaller parts, and establishing strategies to listen. Children with ADHD may benefit from sensory strategies, breathing techniques, and support from adults. Many children with ADHD enjoy creative projects where they can show their skills. Occupational therapy practitioners seek to promote children's self-efficacy (belief in their abilities) and self-determination (making choices and acting upon them). They may help children identify their strengths and challenges so that they can develop lifelong skills.

**BOX 5.3 Occupations of Childhood (American Occupational Therapy Association, 2020)**

**Activities of Daily Living (ADLs)**
- Bathing or showering
- Dressing
- Eating and feeding
- Functional mobility
- Personal hygiene and grooming
- Sexual activity
- Toileting and toilet hygiene

**Instrumental Activities of Daily Living (IADLs)**
- Care of pets and animals
- Communication management
- Driving and community mobility
- Financial management
- Meal preparation and clean up
- Safety and emrgency maintenance
- Shopping

**Health Management**
- Medication management
- Nutrition Management
- Personal care device management
- Physical activity
- Social and emotional health promotion and maintenance
- Symptom and condition management

**Rest and Sleep**
- Rest
- Sleep participation
- Sleep preparation

**Play and Leisure**
- Play and leisure exploration
- Play and leisure participation

**Education**
- Formal education participation
  - Reading, writing
  - Listening to teacher
  - Responding to questions
  - Engaging in school routine
- Informal education participation

**Work**
- Employment interests and pursuits
- Employment seeking and acquisition
- Job performance and maintenance
- Volunteer exploration and participation

**Social Participation**
- Community participation
- Family participation
- Friendships
- Peer group participation

Adapted from: AOTA (2020).

Children and youth with ADHD benefit from occupational therapy focusing on social skill interventions incorporating peers. Fox et al. (2020) conducted a systematic review of social skills intervention for children with ADHD. They reported that interventions incorporating peers were effective at increasing skills, reducing undesirable social behaviors, and improving communication and social participation (Fox et al., 2020). Furthermore, the changes remain over time. Occupational therapy practitioners working with children who have ADHD may effectively address play skills at school, at home, and within the community.

## Anxiety

Anxiety disorders are quite common and are noted by extreme concern about the future and intrusive thoughts (American Psychiatric Association, 2022; Szuhany & Simon, 2022; American Psychological Association, 2023c). Children may avoid certain situations because of worry. Feelings of panic and anxiety affect their ability to engage in daily activities, and children cannot control their feelings, which are not in line with actual danger. These feelings can begin during childhood or teen years and continue into adulthood. Anxiety disorders include several types such as generalized anxiety disorder, social anxiety disorder (social phobia), specific phobias, and separation anxiety disorder. Children and youth can have more than one anxiety disorder. Anxiety can also result from a medical condition that needs treatment.

**Causes.** Adverse childhood experiences (ACEs) such as abuse, neglect, trauma, and living in a dysfunctional household before the age of 18 years may cause anxiety in children and youth (Elmore & Crouch, 2020, 2023). Inherited traits also can be a factor.

**Characteristics and Symptoms.** Common anxiety signs and symptoms include:
- Feeling nervous, restless, or tense
- Having a sense of impending danger, panic, or doom
- Having an increased heart rate
- Breathing rapidly (hyperventilation)
- Sweating
- Trembling
- Feeling weak or tired
- Trouble concentrating or thinking about anything other than the present worry
- Having trouble sleeping
- Experiencing gastrointestinal problems
- Having difficulty controlling worry
- Having the urge to avoid things that trigger anxiety

**Challenges in Occupational Participation.** Occupational participation deficits in children and youth with anxiety disorder can occur in any occupation. Children and youth with anxiety disorder experience feelings of anxiety so extreme that they are unable to complete daily activities. For example, children may experience hyperventilation, increased heart rate, sweating, and trembling when going to school. They may have difficulty concentrating and feel a sense of "doom" preventing them from engaging in activity. Children and youth may have trouble sleeping leading to being tired during the day resulting in difficulty engaging in desired occupations. Children may avoid novel situations and activities interfering with their home, school, and community participation. They may self-medicate (e.g., drugs or alcohol) to avoid feelings.

**Implications for Occupational Therapy.** Occupational therapy practitioners address the occupational disruptions that occur because of a child's extreme anxiety. They may engage children in cognitive-behavioral strategies, which may include role-playing, social stories, skill training, and engagement in a variety of activities. Occupational therapy practitioners provide support while children engage in activities scaffolded to be successful.

Practitioners may engage children in occupation-based activities to develop skills to address their anxiety in a safe environment (Cahill et al., 2020). As children engage in activities (the doing of occupation), they develop coping strategies (such as breathing techniques, relaxation, self-mantras, and support people) that allow them to self-soothe and feel success and achievement. For example, sometimes a child can tap their wrist band or take a deep breath, close their eyes, and visualize being outdoors when they begin to feel nervous. Occupational therapy practitioners practice techniques with children and youth and allow them to reflect on strategies that are useful to them. Practitioners may suggest journaling, drawing, yoga, listening to music, or other activities to encourage reflection. Children and youth may benefit from sensory strategies to provide calming sensations.

Children who experience anxiety disorders have difficulty performing school tasks as shown in Fig. 5.1. They benefit from a multi-disciplinary intervention approach to address their feelings in a variety of situations. The team creates an intervention plan to support the child throughout the day. This may include frequent breaks, time in a sensory room, and breaking up or scaffolding work to assure success. The child may benefit from counseling to anticipate challenges. Case Example 5.1 illustrates how anxiety disorder may affect a student.

## Developmental Motor Coordination Disorder

Developmental motor coordination disorder (also called developmental coordination disorder or DCD) affects fine and gross motor coordination. The deficits in motor coordination cannot be explained by some other category such as age, intelligence, or another disability (van Hoorn et al., 2021).

**Causes.** DCD has an unknown etiology, with the only risk factor including preterm birth. DCD has a higher prevalence in males (van Hoorn et al., 2021).

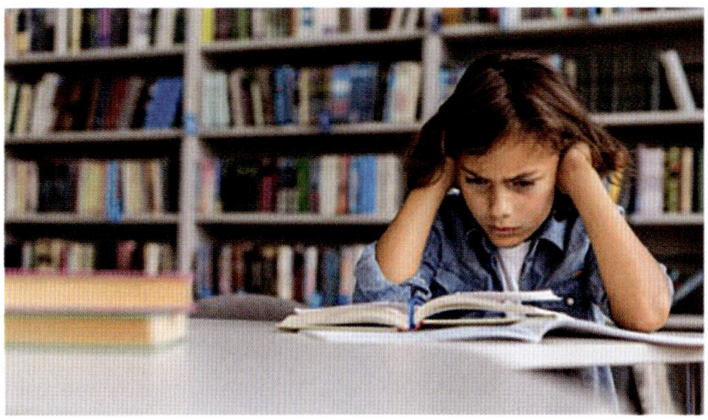

**Fig. 5.1** Children who experience anxiety disorders have difficulty performing school tasks and may benefit from a multi-disciplinary intervention approach to address their feelings in many situations. (Source: https://www.freepik.com/free-photo/front-view-boy-thinking-hard-about-how-solve-his-homework-with-copy-space_10354103.htm#page=8&query=anxious%20kids&position=2&from_view=search&track=ais)

**Characteristics and Symptoms.** Children with DCD exhibit motor challenges. They typically have average intelligence and therefore, they are often aware of their challenges, which may result in frustration and feelings of incompetence. Symptoms include motor difficulties such as balance, coordination, visual motor skills, and manual dexterity (Tamplain & Miller, 2021). Children with DCD experience challenges with timing, sequencing, motor planning, and coordination for both gross and fine motor coordination. They exhibit slow, variable, and less accurate motor performance and difficulty with motor learning (Zwicker et al., 2012). They may have variable balance responses, resulting in poorly coordinated movements. DCD can co-occur with communication difficulties, hyperactivity, and specific learning disabilities. Motor difficulties then lead to difficulties with academic achievement and participation (Harrowell et al., 2018). Children with DCD can later develop psychosocial challenges and internalizing disorders such as anxiety and depression due to motor difficulties resulting in poor school performance leading to poor self-efficacy (Harrowell et al., 2018).

**Challenges in Occupational Participation.** Activities of daily living, education, and social participation are frequently impacted (Smits-Englesman et al., 2018) although any occupation (see Box 5.3) that requires a degree of motor coordination may be impaired. For example, they may lack bilateral coordination skills to complete fasteners such as buttons, or the coordination to put on a shirt, coat, or pants. They may struggle with integrating fine motor, visual motor, and balance skills, resulting in difficulty with a variety of daily activities such as tying shoes, playing sports, or handwriting. They may run with a wide-based gait, fall at times, and have difficulty moving around obstacles effectively. Children with DCD experience difficulties completing activities that require precision, such as tying a knot, cutting with scissors, handwriting, typing, or zipping. Children with DCD may have difficulty completing creative activities in art or eye-foot games in gym classes. They may also struggle to play at recess, which can contribute to challenges in social interaction and peer-engagement. Children with DCD need more time to learn new motor skills. They may experience feelings of inadequacy that may lead to psychosocial concerns (Harrowell et al., 2018).

**Implications for Occupational Therapy.** Occupational therapy practitioners addressing occupational performance challenges with children who have DCD focus on promoting problem-solving, addressing goals that are unique and meaningful to the child, and allowing the child to reflect upon their performance. The practitioner seeks to empower children to understand their strengths and find activities in which they are successful. Children with DCD benefit from practice on self-selected goals, cognitive strategies, and problem-solving with reflection. The Cognitive Orientation to daily Occupational Performance provides a structured program that is effective at "improving self-perceived motor performance and satisfaction in child-chosen motor goals and quality of motor performance" (Izadi-Najafabadi et al., 2022, p. 784). However, children's underlying motor skills did not show a significant improvement. This suggests that practitioners focus intervention on child-chosen goals and create strategies as opposed to targeting underlying motor skills. See Chapter 26 for specifics of this approach.

Other approaches that may support children with DCD include contemporary motor control and motor learning (See Chapter 29), especially the use of motor learning strategies to teach movement when coaching children. Children with DCD benefit from simple direct verbal instructions focusing on the key components of the movements. Motor learning strategies (such as engaging in meaningful activities,

## Case Example 5.1 Annaliesa's High School Experiences

"I don't know" Annaliesa responds timidly as she speaks with Victor (her school-based occupational therapist). Victor continues, "Well, what would be the next step if you are unsure?" Annaliesa shrugs her shoulders. "Perhaps you could email your teacher for a copy of the class notes. You have that right because it is a part of the accommodations that you receive" Victor adds.

Annaliesa is a 17-year-old female recently diagnosed by a private clinician with social anxiety disorder and attention deficit hyperactivity disorder (ADHD). Annaliesa, her parents, and the high school team collaborated to determine and implement her Individualized Education Plan (IEP). Due to the severity of her social anxiety and ADHD, Annaliesa attends school remotely. She receives 60 monthly minutes of direct occupational therapy services, which is rare for a high school student. She receives classroom accommodation, including extended test time, flexibility with due dates, and access to course materials in advance. Annaliesa struggles with self-advocacy and communicating with her instructors regarding her needs and accommodations.

Victor first met with Annaliesa through Zoom several weeks prior to completing Annaliesa's initial evaluation. Annaliesa refused to be on camera, so Victor relied heavily on subjective reporting from her mother (Mary Ellen), and the high school instructors. Mary Ellen explained, "Annaliesa was always fidgeting and bopping around as a child, so her main outlet was sports like running, hiking, track and field." Mary Ellen continued that while Annaliesa received counseling and services in elementary school, she appeared to manage her symptoms and find appropriate outlets so that she could be successful.

After the start of the COVID-19 pandemic, when Annaliesa was in her first year of high school, she became more withdrawn. Mary Ellen stated that Annaliesa demonstrated poor executive functioning skills like time management, organization, and self-monitoring. "My husband and I always had to hound her to do her work," Mary Ellen quipped. Victor heard Annaliesa grow upset by Mary Ellen's comment.

Victor wanted to hear more from Annaliesa and asked her if she still participated in those sports-based activities. Annaliesa said, "No." Victor asked Annaliesa what activities she currently did, but she responded with silence. Mary Ellen chimed in, "She's more reclusive now and afraid of the pandemic. She doesn't want to be around people." Mary Ellen reported that when school returned to in-person instruction during Annaliesa's sophomore year, more problems occurred, including panic attacks, refusing to attend school for fear of the lunchroom and gym class, failing to complete assignments, not paying attention during class, and failing to respond to emails. Due to these concerns voiced by her teachers, the IEP process was initiated, and Annaliesa sought neuropsychiatric testing.

### Role of the Occupational Therapy Practitioner

The occupational therapy practitioner working in the school system completed an evaluation examining Annaliesa's current level of occupational performance. The therapist considered her motor, sensory, cognitive, and social-emotional factors and specifically identified her unique situation, resources, and goals. The practitioner worked with the team to support Annaliesa's academic work, future goals, and social participation. They created organizational strategies tailored to her style. The practitioner allowed her to make choices, at first offering her to select between two options. As time progressed, Victor provided more options. Therapy sessions were designed to empower Annaliesa to complete academic work, show her creativity, and engage with peers. Victor created a small weekly discussion group of peers called "Speak up". The group discusses a topic for 30 minutes with rules that everyone says something. Each week they select a topic, and one member leads the session.

The practitioner also included physical activity sessions, such as yoga, kick-boxing, jump roping games, and walking outside twice a week. Together, they completed the activities (sometimes with peers) and reflected upon the benefits and challenges of physical activity. Together, they developed strategies that may support Annaliesa's success.

using imagery, and providing knowledge of performance) can be integrated into an occupational therapy session to promote motor skills for children with DCD.

Some children with DCD may benefit from Ayres' sensory integration therapy (See Chapter 27). The practitioner evaluates the child's skills and abilities to determine if the child has a sensory-based dysfunction. If the child has sensory integration dysfunction, the practitioner creates an intervention session with the "just right challenge" that will lead to an adaptive response and improved performance in important occupations over time.

## Depressive Disorders

Depression is the most common cause of disability in adolescence (American Psychiatric Association, 2023a). The signs of depression include feeling sadness and loss of interest in activities that children and youth used to enjoy over an extended period. Depression is different from grief or temporary sad feelings (APA, 2022).

**Causes.** Biochemical imbalance, genetics, personality, or environmental factors contribute to depression. Biochemical imbalance refers to the effects of chemicals in the brain. Depression is common among family members, suggesting a genetic cause. People who have low self-esteem, a tendency toward pessimism, or who become easily overwhelmed by stress are prone to depression. Environmental factors such as continuous exposure to abuse, violence, neglect, or poverty are linked to depression in children and youth (American Psychiatric Association, 2023a).

**Characteristics and Symptoms.** Depression can occur at any time but often appears for the first time in a person's late teens to mid-twenties. In young children, depression is linked to social anxiety (Epkins & Seegan, 2015). The symptoms must last longer than 2 weeks and be different from previous levels of functioning. Symptoms of depression range from mild to severe and include (APA, 2022):

- Feeling sad or having a depressed mood
- Loss of interest or pleasure in activities once enjoyed
- Changes in appetite—weight loss or gain unrelated to dieting
- Trouble sleeping or sleeping too much
- Loss of energy or increased fatigue
- Increase in purposeless physical activity (e.g., inability to sit still, pacing, hand-wringing) or slowed movements or speech (these actions must be severe enough to be observable by others)
- Feeling worthless or guilty
- Difficulty thinking, concentrating, or making decisions
- Thoughts of death or suicide

**Challenges in Occupational Participation.** Children and youth with depression may experience deficits in any of their occupations (listed in Box 5.3). They may withdraw from activities, have difficulty initiating activities, and avoid social situations. They may struggle in everyday activities, such as school, play, and community events. They may express negative feelings (or conversely cover up and "pretend" everything is fine). Children who experience severe depression may spend time alone and sleep for long periods.

**Implications for Occupational Therapy.** There is evidence to support the use of activity and occupation-based intervention to address the mental health, behavioral, and social participation concerns for children and youth (Cahill et al., 2020). Interventions include life skills training, vocational skills training, and graded occupational engagement. Occupational therapy practitioners may also address behavior, conflict resolution behaviors, perseverance, school performance, social participation, communication, and cooperative behaviors.

They may work in mental health settings as part of a team of professionals working with children who have depression. In this setting, the practitioner engages the child in activities to learn new effective skills and engage in desired roles in a supportive environment. Practitioners provide safe spaces within the therapy session for children to discuss, display, and process their emotions while engaging in meaningful activities. For example, a practitioner may engage a child in a project to make a colorful creative calendar for the next month. Engaging in activity provides the child with time to reflect on future goals, positive activities, and plans. As the child shares their product, the practitioner can reinforce their work, and strengths (e.g., creativity, thought process, attention, decision-making). This helps the child develop a sense that they have capabilities and support.

Occupational therapy practitioners may address mental health skills (such as attention, decision-making, executive function, memory, and orientation). Practitioners employ the therapeutic use of self (See Chapter 3) to establish a relationship and support children and youth through the process. They begin by understanding the child's unique situation and resources using an occupation-centered model of practice (such as the Model of Human Occupation or Person-Environment-Occupation-Performance), which leads to an assessment of skills that may be interfering with the child's occupational performance. For example, Kielhofner's Model of Human Occupation (Taylor et al., 2024) proposes that children engage in those things that are meaningful to them, interesting, and provide them with a sense of competency. Once practitioners identify areas to address in practice, they create interventions using graded activities to ensure the child is successful (but still challenged) and engage the child in activities or discussions to promote reflection. Evidence suggests that activity-based interventions are successful at addressing mental health concerns in children and youth (Cahill et al., 2020; Read et al., 2018).

Occupational therapy practitioners may use a variety of cognitive approaches to promote occupational engagement for children with depression. Cognitive behavioral therapy (CBT; Brent et al., 2015; Stice et al., 2008) promotes occupational functioning. Occupational therapy practitioners use cognitive behavioral therapy as a child is engaged in an activity. They address negative thought patterns as they occur within the activity. For example, the practitioner intervenes when a child says, "I can't do this, I'm horrible at this." The practitioner may ask the child to explain further and identify just one part of the activity that went well. Together, they discuss that. The practitioner supports the child in continuing the activity and ends the session reflecting upon the child's progress. For some children, acknowledging that the activity was difficult and that they did their best for that moment, which is okay, may be therapeutic. Helping children and youth recognize their strengths and challenges supports mental health. Occupational therapy practitioners provide tools to allow children to continue to engage in life's roles, seek out support systems, as they begin to move out of depression (which may be assisted with medications).

## Autism Spectrum Disorder

ASD is characterized as a neurodevelopmental disorder with symptoms usually appearing in the first 2 years of life (Dominguez-Lucio et al., 2023). Since ASD is a spectrum disorder, the presentation and symptoms vary greatly. Children may be diagnosed with ASD after a general developmental screening and neuropsychological evaluation often before 3 years of age (Zablotsky et al., 2019). However, the age of initial diagnosis is highly variable, ranging from 38 to 120 months (Daniels & Mandell, 2014), and depends on socioeconomic status, race, parental education, gender, and geography (Dallman et al., 2021).

In the population of those diagnosed with autism, there is a conversation occurring regarding identity first or person first language, that occupational therapy practitioners should be aware of. In this chapter, the authors have elected to use the identity-first term autistic rather than person-first language as this is the reported preference of the majority of autistic individuals (Botha et al., 2023; Bury et al., 2023).

**Causes.** There is no known cause for ASD, but the condition is influenced by an interplay of genetics and the environment. Risk factors for ASD include having a sibling or family member with ASD, certain genetic conditions, and low birth weight (American Psychiatric Association, 2022)

**Characteristics and Symptoms.** ASD is a lifelong condition that affects communication and behavior. The characteristics and symptoms of ASD therefore frequently include challenges related to social communication and interaction skills and behaviors. For example, autistic children and youth may have inconsistent eye contact, respond slowly to their names, have difficulty initiating and maintaining conversations, or speak using an unusual tone of voice. Others may have difficulty with perspective-taking or talking at length about a specific topic while unaware of another's interest (American Psychiatric Association, 2022; Peña et al., 2021).

Autistic youth present with specific and repetitive behaviors and interests (American Psychiatric Association, 2022) and may engage in repetitive behaviors including echolalia (i.e., repetition of words or phrases), repetitive motor movements, specific interests, sensitivity to sensory input, and negative behavioral responses to changes in routine (American Psychiatric Association, 2022; Peña et al., 2021). However, many autistic individuals present with great strengths as well as illustrated in (Fig. 5.2A and B). Each child's symptoms and presentation vary.

**Challenges in Occupational Participation.** Typically, a lack of social engagement and play in the first years of a child's life is one of the leading indicators of ASD (American Psychiatric Association, 2022). As a result, play is one of the major occupations impacted by ASD. Autistic children play, but the quality and duration of their play differ, and they may not be as creative as their peers (Kuhaneck et al., 2020). Social difficulties continue to impact occupational participation as the child grows and seeks to develop and maintain interaction with peers (Dominguez-Lucio et al., 2023). The characteristic difficulties with social communication, interaction, and behaviors affect social and educational participation. Autistic children and youth may have trouble eating and feeding and may exhibit fixed routines around mealtime, or rigidity in food preferences. Young autistic children may have difficulty engaging in toilet training and washing their hands to complete the toileting routine. Sleep problems are very common (Cortese et al., 2020; Posar & Visconti, 2020).

Autistic children can demonstrate challenges in multiple skill areas and with many client factors. Of interest to occupational therapy practitioners are the common sensory-motor concerns. Current research suggests that the majority of autistic individuals, perhaps over 70%, exhibit sensory processing difficulties (Kirby et al., 2022). Sensory challenges can interfere with daily activities such as grooming tasks,

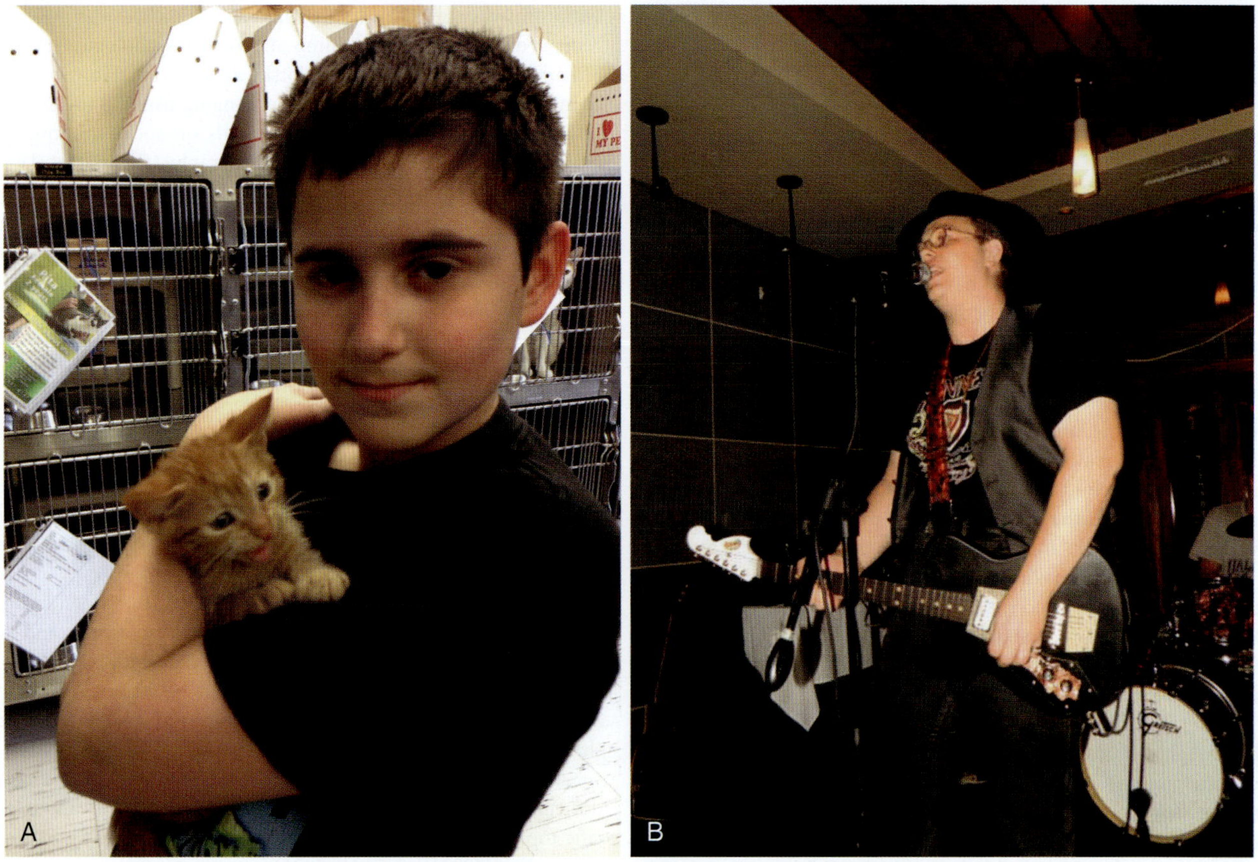


**Fig. 5.2** Children have a variety of strengths unique to them. (A) This child is good at caring for animals and volunteers at an animal shelter. (B) This young adult sings and plays lead guitar at local clubs.

oral healthcare, hair brushing, and nail trimming and also lead to challenging behaviors. Autistic children exhibit variable sensory preferences and also engage in restricted and repetitive behaviors that may relate to these preferences or may serve to reduce discomfort with sensation (Glod et al., 2019; Williams et al., 2021).

Autistic children also demonstrate a variety of motor skill deficits (Zampella et al., 2021). Research suggests that more than 35% of autistic individuals may have challenges with motor skills; however, these are underdiagnosed and underreported (Licari et al., 2020). The range of these difficulties includes gait, balance, postural control, imitation, and motor learning.

**Implications for Occupational Therapy.** Occupational therapy practitioners address an autistic child's participation in feeding and eating and other activities of daily living, educational performance, play, social participation, and instrumental activities of daily living. Practitioners may support children in completing schoolwork, establishing routines, and developing effective strategies for learning (Grandisson et al., 2020). They work to remove the impact of repetitive behaviors on occupational performance (Patriquin et al., 2020). They collaborate with others to manage symptoms and improve performance in intense sensory environments such as the dental office (Como et al., 2021) or the school classroom (Dynia et al., 2023). They help families to improve their child's sleep, or may assist in engaging children in the care of pets as shown in Fig. 5.3. There are a variety of strategies and approaches that may help when working with an autistic

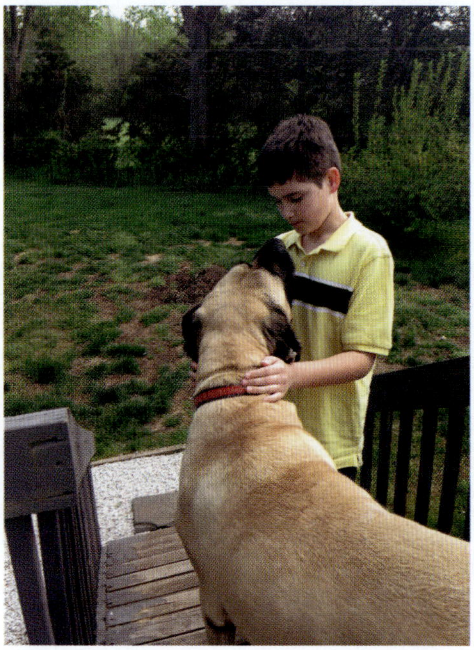

**Fig. 5.3** Children with ASD can become quite bonded to their pets, and research indicates that interaction with animals may improve social skills.

**TABLE 5.3 Interventions for Children With Autism Spectrum Disorder**

| Intervention Name | How Used in Occupational Therapy |
|---|---|
| Reciprocal Imitation Training (RIT) (http://www.ncbi.nlm.nih.gov/pmc/articles/PMC3686149/) | Occupational therapists can use imitation to increase engagement and interaction with a child with ASD. This is particularly useful when a child is avoiding the therapist or disengaged. The occupational therapist imitates the child until the child makes some indication of connection or interaction (a look, touch, smile). For evidence of the efficacy of this type of approach, see https://psychology.msu.edu/news-events/news/msu-autism-lab-study-examines-the-power-of-play.html. The evidence for imitation models is considered to be emerging. |
| Relationship Development Intervention (RDI) (http://www.rdiconnect.com/about-rdi/) | Focuses on coping with change, being more flexible, and integrating information from multiple sources. There is currently minimal evidence of efficacy, but research is occurring. The evidence for relationship-based models is considered to be emerging. |
| Treatment and Education of Autistic and Related Communication Handicapped Children (TEACCH) (http://www.teacch.com/) | Occupational therapists can incorporate many of the visual support strategies into their sessions. Efficacy is unclear at this time but one review suggests it was beneficial for improving motor skill and cognition. TEACCH is considered an emerging approach. |
| Early Start Denver Model (http://www.autismspeaks.org/what-autism/treatment/early-start-denver-model-esdm) | Occupational therapists can use strategies from this model that focus on joint attention and shared interaction using a naturalistic applied behavioral approach. Well-designed studies of the early start model have documented effectiveness in improving IQ, language, and autism symptoms. Also see http://www.effectivehealthcare.ahrq.gov/ehc/products/106/656/CER26_Autism_Report_04-14-2011.pdf. This model is considered established. |
| Miller Method (http://millermethod.org/) | Occupational therapists can use many of the strategies to increase attention (i.e., carefully adding to the number of steps needed to achieve a desired goal or using raised surfaces to enhance attention to mobility). There is minimal evidence regarding the efficacy of the program in its entirety. |
| The Son-Rise Program (http://www.autismtreatmentcenter.org/) | Focuses on using the child's inherent motivations to engage and interact and on helping parents be optimistic and hopeful while helping their child learn and achieve. Very playful approach and open to including sensory-based therapy. There is currently no published evidence of efficacy for this program. See http://www.autismtreatmentcenter.org/contents/reviews_and_articles/research_project.php. |
| Social Communication, Emotional Regulation and Transactional Support (SCERTS) (http://scerts.com/index.php?option=com_content&view=article&id=2&Itemid=2) | SCERTS is a comprehensive model to be used with a team. Occupational therapists are part of this team and are involved in the emotional regulation portion of the intervention. SCERTS can be readily combined with many other of the interventions, although it is considered to be most different from ABA. Evaluation of the SCERTS model is ongoing. See https://scerts.com/ and http://ies.ed.gov/funding/grantsearch/details.asp?ID=978. |
| Pivotal Response Training (PRT) (http://www.koegelautism.com/) | Occupational therapists can use specific strategies such as providing choice, using task variation, rewarding attempts, and using natural reinforcers in play-based sessions. PRT specifically teaches responsivity to multiple cues and the occupational therapist can incorporate this into activities such as visual-perceptual-motor tasks (i.e., "Can you find the big, round, one? Can you find the smooth, red one?"). PRT is a well-studied approach to treatment for ASD and is considered an established approach |
| Animal Assisted Therapy (AAT) (Pet Partners [formerly the Delta society] (http://www.petpartners.org/) | Animals may be calming for individuals with ASD and may help increase language and social interaction. They can be used in occupational therapist sessions if the occupational therapist is trained in this approach (see (Nimer & Lundahl, 2007; O'Haire, 2017; O'Haire et al., 2013)). |

child (see Table 5.3 describing intervention approaches and Box 5.4 providing specific stategies that may be used in occupational therapy sessions Box 5.4).

Autistic children may benefit from sensory integration intervention to improve engagement in daily activities (Schaaf et al., 2018). Ayres sensory integration (ASI) intervention improves motor skills for those with autism (Andelin et al., 2021) and may also influence play outcomes (Kuhaneck et al., 2023; Waldman-Levi & Kuhaneck, 2023).

Occupational therapy practitioners who work with this population need to be well versed in the recent discussions regarding the use of behavioral approaches. In light of the neurodiversity movement (Chapman & Botha, 2023; Dallman et al., 2022; Graber & Graber, 2023) as well as the professional shift to strengths-based focus in all areas of intervention, but specifically for autistic and neurodiverse individuals (Patten, 2022), practitioners must consider the ethical issues surrounding the intentional changing of another's behavior without their consent or desire. Proponents of the neurodiversity movement have conceptualized differences in those with conditions such as autism as a part of biodiversity. As such, proponents suggest society needs to develop support and make space for differences as opposed to trying to eliminate diversity through 'treating' or 'curing' autistic individuals.

## Feeding or Eating Disorders

Eating disorders can range in severity and affect physical, psychological, and social functions. Persistent disturbance in eating behaviors in combination with distressing thoughts and emotions are a hallmark

## BOX 5.4 Specific Strategies for Occupational Therapy Sessions

**Improve Engagement and Interaction, Reduce Fear or Anxiety**

- Imitate the child and wait for the child to initiate interaction via eye contact, touch, or moving into closer physical proximity.
- Alter the therapist's proximity to the child.
- Reduce the use of direct eye contact.
- Alter the therapist's pace both motorically and verbally.
- Alter the therapist's voice volume or intonation.
- Use musical or sing-song vocalizations or word pronunciation that the child finds humorous.
- Use preferred objects, colors, or movements within therapy tasks. For example, hide a favorite object within Theraputty or place it on top of something to encourage climbing, under something to encourage digging, or inside something to encourage fine motor skills like opening or unbuttoning. Be sure the child sees where the object went and, if necessary, make sure that he or she will be able to get it back quickly to avoid distress and difficult behaviors. This should be a fun game.
- Interact playfully make work into play.
- Create fun problems to be solved. For example, "Oh no, the pig (stuffed toy) is trapped in the mud, you have to help him get out. How can we save him?"
- Sing familiar songs and leave out the last word, to encourage the child to vocalize to fill in where you have omitted the word.

**Improve Behavior and Task Completion, Reduce Fear or Anxiety**

a. Use objects, visual cues, or schedules to help the child predict what will come next or what will happen. Provide a visual schedule that indicates how many times a particular action or behavior is expected. For example, place five magnetic coins on the table to be placed in the container. When the five are done, this activity is done.
b. Use the prompts that are familiar to the child.
c. Know and use the child's preferred reinforcers throughout occupational therapy "work"
d. Provide clear boundaries regarding areas of the intervention space so that it is clear which type of activity occurs in each area.
e. Provide choices or choice boards, visual schedules, or other visual materials to aid in understanding what is to be done.
f. Provide written instructions for a child who can read.

**Improve Comfort, Reduce Fear and Anxiety**

- Carefully grade the introduction of novelty into a session.
- Attend to the sensory environment and the child's response (including facial expression, and nonverbal responses) to the sensory environment.
- Alter lighting, noise, and smells.
- Provide opportunities for deep pressure and proprioception through active play.

**Improve Motor Skills/Praxis**

a. Create fun obstacles or challenges that encourage the movements that are therapeutically desired (e.g., require motor planning, bilateral coordination, and sequencing, relate to functional goals) while engaging the child in a preferred activity of his or her choice.
b. Climb, walk, or crawl on raised surfaces to increase attention to motion. For example, climb across a wide balance beam or a horizontal ladder at 2–3 ft off the ground (with mats and pillows for safety and hand-holding if needed).
c. Gradually increase motoric sequences that are completed before a desired event or object is provided. For example, place a favorite toy (or a puzzle piece) in a zip lock bag to be opened. Then wrap it in a wad of tin foil inside a zip lock bag to be opened. Then put it in a closed Tupperware, wrapped in tin foil, and inside a zip lock bag. Then in a closed Tupperware, wrapped in tin foil, inside a zip lock bag placed up a ramp, up a ladder, or through a tunnel.
d. Alternate preferred sensory activities with more challenging motor tasks.
e. Sing about the motor activity you are doing using a familiar tune. For example, using the tune of "Mary Had a Little Lamb," or "Row, Row, Row Your Boat," you can sing about Johnny's going to climb that ramp, or push, push, push that cart gently down the hall.

**Improve Play and Ideational Praxis**

- Use realistic props to begin to introduce role play (fireman's hats, dress-up clothing that is realistic).
- Use movie characters and stories to begin to introduce pretend play.
- Promote imagination in your sessions (What would an animal look like if it were part zebra and part frog?).
- Have the child help you create a game out of unusual materials ("What could we play with this cup, this small ball, and this stuffed animal?").
- Have the child help you build an obstacle course or sensorimotor activity.
- Discuss the ways you can use certain objects based on their properties (affordances) ("Look, this is round. It can roll. These are all square shaped and they can stack. What could we do with this object?").
- Try to add to current ideas with prompting ("Can you think of another way to do that? How many different ways can you do that?").
- Take turns between imitating the child and having the child attempt to imitate you. Use silly motions, vocalizations, and sequences to be playful.

of eating disorders. Eating and feeding disorders result in malnutrition affecting the child or youth's ability to engage in daily living. As children become malnourished, they lose physical strength and endurance, experience cognitive changes (e.g., confusion, disorganization, difficulty problem-solving), and distance themselves from friends and family (who may express concern). As the condition progresses, the child or youth seeks to maintain control of their feeding and eating, which further reinforces the dysfunctional behaviors.

**Types of Feeding and Eating Disorders.** Several types of eating disorders exist, including anorexia nervosa, bulimia nervosa, binge eating disorder, avoidant restrictive food intake disorder, other specified feeding and eating disorders, pica, and rumination disorder (APA, 2022). Although the causes of eating and feeding disorders are similar, each type of disorder presents differently.

**Causes.** Feeding and eating disorders are caused by a complex interplay of factors, including sociocultural influences such as media exposure, personality characteristics such as perfectionism, and even co-morbidities such as autism (Culbert et al., 2015; Gupta, 2021). Exposure to trauma and adverse childhood experiences contribute to eating disorders. As children experience these negative events, they seek to gain control over things within their control, which may be feeding and eating. Three forms of abuse are most linked to eating disorders sexual abuse, physical abuse, and emotional abuse (Trottier & MacDonald, 2023).

**Characteristics and Symptoms.** All eating disorders result in a lack of nutrition and health concerns. The characteristics and symptoms differ based on the type of eating disorder as described below.

***Anorexia Nervosa.*** Anorexia nervosa is diagnosed when a child or youth significantly restricts their caloric intake. They may claim they are trying to gain weight while restricting calories and exercising excessively. The two types of anorexia nervosa include (1) the restricting type, in which children and youth lose weight by dieting, fasting, or excessively exercising, and (2) binge eating and purging, in which children and youth intermittently binge eat and then purge what they have eaten (American Psychiatric Association, 2023b). Anorexia nervosa is characterized by the following signs and symptoms:

- Menstrual periods cease
- Dizziness or fainting from dehydration
- Brittle hair/nails
- Cold intolerance
- muscle weakness and wasting
- Heartburn and reflux (in those who vomit)
- Severe constipation, bloating, and fullness after meals
- Stress fractures from compulsive exercise as well as bone loss resulting in osteopenia or osteoporosis (thinning of the bones)
- Depression, irritability, anxiety, poor concentration, and fatigue (APA, 2022; American Psychiatric Association, 2023b)

***Bulimia Nervosa.*** Children and youth with bulimia nervosa alternate eating low-calorie foods and dieting with binge eating high-calorie foods. Children and youth who have bulimia nervosa rapidly eat resulting in fullness that is uncomfortable and causes nausea. They often eat in secret and experience feelings of shame or embarrassment. The bingeing occurs weekly, followed by a period of corrective actions to keep from gaining weight, such as fasting, laxative misuse, vomiting, or excessive exercise. Children and youth with bulimia nervosa obsessively think about food, weight, and their body, which affects their self-esteem (American Psychiatric Association, 2022, American Psychiatric Association, 2023b). The signs and symptoms of bulimia nervosa include:

- Frequent trips to the bathroom right after meals
- Substantial amounts of food disappearing or unexplained empty wrappers and food containers
- Chronic sore throat
- Swelling of the salivary glands in the cheeks
- Dental decay resulting from erosion of tooth enamel by stomach acid
- Heartburn and gastroesophageal reflux
- Laxative or diet pill misuse
- Recurrent unexplained diarrhea
- Misuse of diuretics (water pills)
- Feeling dizzy or fainting from excessive purging behaviors resulting in dehydration (American Psychiatric Association, 2022, American Psychiatric Association, 2023b)

***Avoidant Restrictive Food and Intake Disorder.*** Avoidant Restrictive Food and Intake Disorder (ARFID) occurs when children and youth, who may be considered 'picky eaters' have food avoidance or a limited number/types of food they will eat, and they fail to meet nutrition and/or energy needs. Children and youth with ARFID may demonstrate the following behaviors (APA, 2022; American Psychiatric Association, 2023b):

- Low appetite and lack of interest in eating or food.
- Extreme food avoidance based on sensory characteristics of foods (e.g., texture, appearance, color, or smell).
- Anxiety or concern about consequences of eating, such as fear of choking, nausea, vomiting, constipation, or an allergic reaction. The disorder may develop in response to a significant negative event such as an episode of choking or food poisoning followed by the avoidance of an increasing variety of foods.

***Pica and Rumination Disorder.*** Pica occurs when children and youth eat inanimate objects. Pica is not diagnosed under the age of 2 because part of normal development is when toddlers put objects in their mouths (APA, 2022; American Psychiatric Association, 2023b). Children and youth may develop pica because of their sensory needs (Bryant-Waugh, 2019). Rumination disorder occurs when children repeatedly voluntarily regurgitate and rechew food. They rechew, reswallow, or spit out the food (APA, 2022; American Psychiatric Association, 2023b). Rumination disorder occurs in infancy, childhood, and adolescence.

**Challenges in Occupational Participation.** Occupational participation deficits in children and youth with eating disorders can occur in any occupation (see Box 5.3) due to the decline in physical strength, health, and nutrition and the child's fixation with eating. Children and youth with eating disorders experience challenges with the routines, habits, and tasks related to eating, swallowing, feeding, and meal preparation. These disruptions in routine affect other areas of their daily activity, such as social participation, academics, and instrumental activities of daily living. They experience mental health challenges as they seek to control their behaviors, often in secret, and equate their self-esteem and efficacy with their control over food. As the disorder progresses, their impaired nutrition interferes with health management, sleep and rest, and physical activity. They may experience confusion affecting formal education. Along with physical challenges, they exhibit social and emotional challenges that interfere with all aspects of daily life, including activities of daily living, health management, rest and sleep, education, play, leisure, work, and social participation.

**Implications for Occupational Therapy.** Occupational therapy practitioners collaborate with a team of professionals (e.g., physician, nurse, physical therapist, psychologist, psychiatrist, recreational specialist, nutritionist, dietician) within an inpatient hospitalization or day treatment program to address the challenges associated with eating disorders (Sharp et al., 2017). As part of the team, occupational therapy practitioners use a holistic approach by completing a comprehensive evaluation (based on an occupation-centered model of practice) to understand the child's situation, strengths, challenges, and resources. They create intervention plans using a variety of approaches including positive reinforcement, extinction by ignoring unwanted behaviors, stimulus shaping and fading, and caregiver involvement and education (Gosa et al., 2017; Gronski, 2021; Gronski & Doherty, 2020; Huston et al., 2019).

Cognitive behavioral interventions (CBT) focus on the interactions between emotions, behaviors, and thoughts. Practitioners using CBT target physical sensations (e.g., deep breathing, guided imagery, progressive muscle relaxation), cognition (e.g., thoughts, problem-solving, planning), and behavior (e.g., actions and performance) (Huston et al., 2019). They help children identify and modify their negative thoughts and replace those thoughts with positive self-statements. Occupational therapy practitioners teach children the techniques within a safe setting where the child can practice with repeated gradual exposure to feared stimuli (Huston et al., 2019). They may address anxiety associated with feeding challenges, self-efficacy (child's belief in their abilities), self-esteem, and self-determination. As children experience repeated successes in a supportive environment, they begin to make needed changes and use the strategies at home. Severe feeding difficulties also cause parental stress, anxiety, and depression (Garro et al., 2005). Practitioners often include family training to support the recovery process and transition.

## DISEASES OF THE NERVOUS SYSTEM

Neurological conditions may affect motor, sensory, and cognitive functioning. Cerebral palsy is the most common chronic childhood disability (CDC, 2022) occurring in 3 of 1000 children in the United States (CDC, 2022), or 1 in 345. According to the NIH, other diagnoses in this category are much rarer, including brachial plexus injuries (1.5 in 1000), spina bifida (2–4 per 10,000), muscular dystrophy (5 cases per 100,000), spinal muscle atrophy (1–2 cases in 100,000) and intracranial hemorrhage (10–20 per million). Regardless, children with these conditions are often referred for occupational therapy evaluation and intervention services.

### Cerebral Palsy

Cerebral palsy is a broad term that indicates a group of motor problems that begin early in life. These motor problems can begin before birth (prenatal), or immediately before or after birth (perinatal) (Pashmdarfard et al., 2021; Sadowska et al., 2020). Cerebral palsy affects motor systems and influences posture, motor control and motor production, sensation, communication, behavior, and cognition. Cerebral palsy results in abnormal muscle tone that may present as spastic or dyskinetic (Brunstrom-Hernadez, Shah, & Tlton, 2022; Garcia Reidy et al., 2021). The condition is typically classified as congenital or acquired and as spastic and dyskinetic types based on motor presentation (Sadowska et al., 2020). Children with cerebral palsy experience challenges with movement which are considered primary, and these in turn may lead to secondary impairments. Box 5.5 describes primary and secondary impairments associated with cerebral palsy.

**Causes.** The typical causes of cerebral palsy are an injury or insult to a developing brain. Risk factors for cerebral palsy can include low birth weight, prematurity, genetic, and metabolic factors. Box 5.6 provides a description of other risk factors associated with cerebral palsy. The diagnosis of cerebral palsy is based on motor presentation, symptoms, clinical interview, and observation (Sadowska et al., 2020).

**BOX 5.5 Examples of Primary and Secondary Impairments in Children Diagnosed With Cerebral Palsy**

| Primary Impairments | Secondary Impairments |
|---|---|
| Muscle weakness or hypotonicity | Contracture in a joint (e.g., elbow, wrist, hip, knee, ankle) |
| Muscle tightness or hypertonicity | Poor or unsteady gait or mobility |
| Spasticity | Impairment of visual processing, hearing, or speech |
| Involuntary movement | Difficulty with bladder and bowel control |
| Weakness of eye muscles | Intellectual disability, learning disabilities |
| Abnormal muscle tone in facial musculature | Problems with breathing because of postural difficulties and weakness in trunk muscles |
| Impaired sensation in affected limbs | Skin integrity: increased risk of pressure sores |
| Possible seizure disorder | Difficulty in feeding, eating, and swallowing |

**Characteristics and Symptoms.** Spastic types of cerebral palsy present as increased muscle tone. Spasticity is often resistant to range of motion and stretching (Garcia Reidy et al., 2021). Spastic types of cerebral palsy are categorized according to the distribution and include hemiplegia (one-sided), diplegia (both lower extremities), and quadriplegia (all extremities).

Dyskinetic cerebral palsy involves abnormal, involuntary, and uncontrolled movements that are observed when a child or youth attempts to initiate movements (Garcia Reidy et al., 2021). Dyskinetic movements are slow, writhing, and involuntary. The movements increase with emotional tension and are not present while asleep. **Atheoid** movement to a fluctuation of muscle tone that presents as writhing extreme movements with inaccurate timing and coordination (Garcia Reidy et al., 2021). Ataxia presents as unsteadiness that leads to poor balance, specifically when ambulating.

Children and youth with cerebral palsy may also exhibit atypical posture, visual difficulties or disorders, cognitive impairments, communicative delays, and motor impairments (Brunstrom-Hernandez et al., 2022). The movement challenges vary in severity from mild to severe. Children with mild motor impairments may experience coordination, timing, and balance difficulties, whereas severe motor challenges may result in children requiring a wheelchair for mobility.

**Challenges in Occupational Participation.** A child or youth with cerebral palsy may experience deficits in occupational participation based on their symptoms and presentation. Their challenges occur across many domains of occupation. For example, a child with

**BOX 5.6 Risk Factors Associated with the Development of Cerebral Palsy**

**Prenatal**

- Genetic disorders
- Gestational hypertension
- Lack of growth factors affecting fetal growth in utero (e.g., hormones, insulin, proteins)
- Maternal health factors (e.g., chronic stress, malnutrition)
- Placental disruption (inability of the placenta to provide the developing fetus with oxygen and nutrients)
- RH blood type incompatibility between mother and infant
- Teratogenic agents (e.g., drugs, chemical exposure, radiation)

**Perinatal**

- Emergency cesarean section
- Low birth weight
- Medical problems associated with prematurity (e.g., compromised respiratory and cardiovascular systems, intraventricular hemorrhage [IVH], periventricular leukomalacia [PVL])
- Multiple births
- Prenatal conditions (e.g., toxemia secondary to maternal diabetes)

**Postnatal**

- Alcohol or drug intoxication transferred during breastfeeding
- Hypoxic ischemic encephalopathy: prolonged loss of oxygen during the birthing process
- Infections (e.g., meningitis, encephalitis, chorioamnionitis)
- Severe and untreated jaundice shortly after birth
- Trauma during birth or shortly after

Adapted from: (Bax et al., 2005; Chen et al., 2019; Johnson et al., 2019).

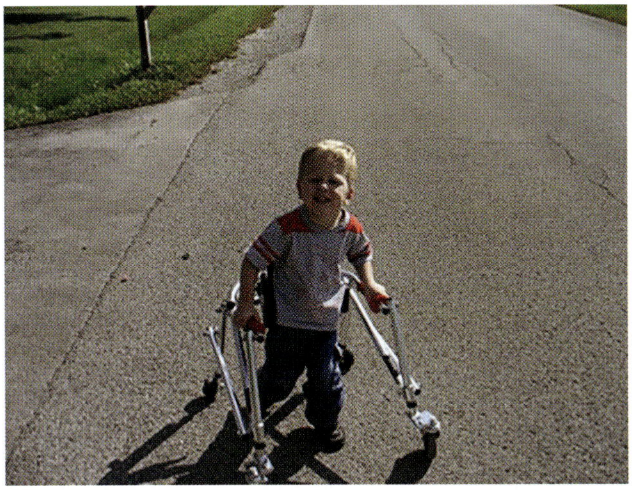

**Fig. 5.4** A walker provides additional support to allow the young boy to move around on his own. (Source: https://openverse.org/image/0be20977-bd21-470a-86f1-1f9937cc7abf?q=child%20with%20cerebral%20palsy Credit: "Ethan" by PaulEisenberg is licensed under CC BY 2.0. To view a copy of this license, visit https://creativecommons.org/licenses/by/2.0/?ref=openverse)

cerebral palsy who experiences spasticity may not have the range of motion to bring food to their mouth. They may have mobility challenges and difficulty with fine motor and oral motor skills. Children may have challenges with grooming, bathing, dressing, and toileting. Fig. 5.4 shows a child who requires a walker for ambulation. Children and youth with cerebral palsy may also exhibit communication challenges related to abnormal oral motor muscle tone which can affect their ability to play and socially engage with their family and friends. Children and youth with mild symptoms may be independent in daily living skills, school, play, and social participation. Cerebral palsy is not a progressive disorder, but as children grow, they may notice challenges in engaging in occupations (such as driving, social participation, and work).

**Implications for Occupational Therapy.** Occupational therapy practitioners working with children who have cerebral address gross and fine motor functioning (Pashmdarfard et al., 2021). Research suggests that engaging children in play and functional activities is effective in improving fine motor skills and participation (Senapati, 2017; Tanner et al., 2020). However, Senapati (2017) found that play activities produced a stronger therapeutic value on fine motor skills as compared to functional activities in children who had spastic diplegia.

Constraint-induced movement therapy (CIMT) is effective in improving upper extremity control in infants and children who have hemiplegic cerebral palsy (Dionsio & Terrill, 2022). This approach requires children to engage in activities with their affected arm and hand while their unaffected arm/hand is restrained (in a cast or mitt). Occupational therapy practitioners grade activities to promote the use of the affected arm and hand in a fun and playful way. Figs. 5.5 and 5.6 illustrate ways of grading activities to promote arm and hand use for children.

Children with cerebral palsy may have oral motor challenges interfering with feeding and eating. Practitioners create interventions with families to address feeding, swallowing, mealtime behaviors, and self-feeding. Practitioners also promote accessibility through mobility devices (such as scooters, walkers, and wheelchairs) (See Chapter 32)

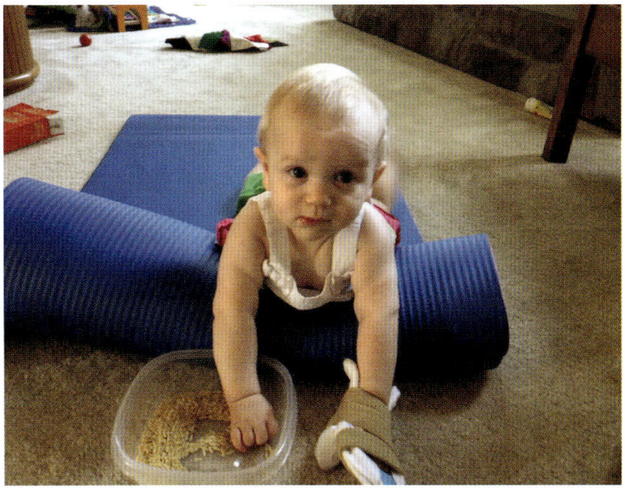

**Fig. 5.5** Children engage in playful activities while engaging in constraint-induced movement therapy.

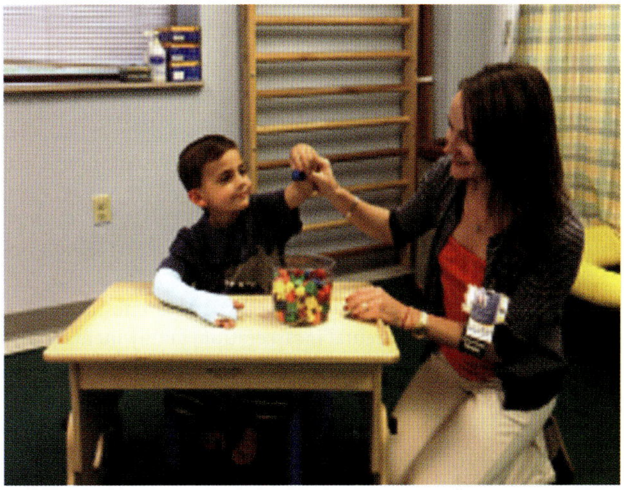

**Fig. 5.6** Constraint-induced movement therapy involves limiting the use of the more functional upper extremity to promote increased strength and function of the impaired side. It is widely supported and can be used following traumatic brain injury (TBI) or any condition that results in hemiplegia.

and advocate for environmental modifications so children can participate in desired occupations. They may provide children with assistive technology to support their participation in home, school, and community (See Chapter 34). They may facilitate external stability at the trunk by providing positioning equipment (such as adapted chairs) so that children may use their hands for feeding, play, and academics. Children with cerebral palsy may require adaptations for driving (See Chapter 20).

## Traumatic Brain Injury

A traumatic brain injury (TBI) is a head injury or concussion that results in loss of consciousness for a minimum of 5 minutes or an overnight hospital stay of at least one night. TBI occurs more frequently among males than females and most males have their first or only TBI between grades five to eight. Forty-one percent of TBIs are sports-related (Boisgontier et al., 2020; Illie et al., 2020). Fifteen- to nineteen-year-olds have the highest hospitalizations, emergency

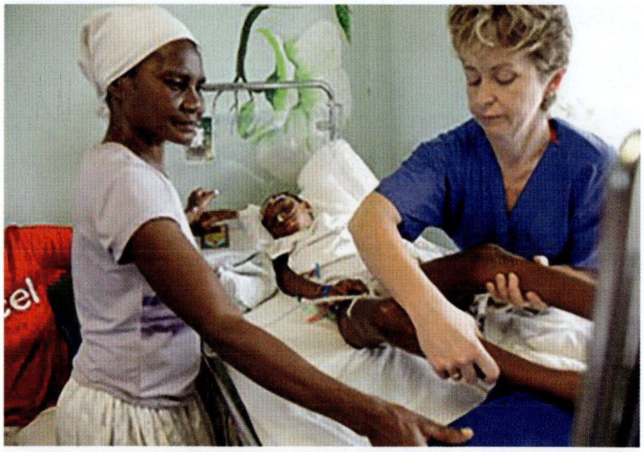

**Fig. 5.7** Children who experience trauma (such as this child who was in an earthquake) may sustain a traumatic brain injury. (Credit: "Haiti Earthquake 2010" by Direct_Relief is licensed under CC BY-NC-ND 2.0. To view a copy of this license, visit https://creativecommons.org/licenses/by-nc-nd/2.0/?ref=openverse. Source: https://openverse.org/image/1a9a4db6-f229-471e-826c-44017f829bf9?q=pediatric%20brain%20injuryhttps://www.flickr.com/photos/43649101@N07/)

department visits, and deaths related to TBIs when compared to other age groups. Approximately 22% of adolescents sustain a TBI (Illie et al., 2020).

**Causes.** Many concussions are sports-related. Hockey-related injuries are more frequent than soccer-related TBIs (Illie et al., 2020). There is also a correlation between ACEs (i.e., domestic violence, neighborhood violence, parental incarceration, family mental illness, and material hardship) and TBIs (Jackson et al., 2022). TBIs can be caused by traumatic events, such as motor vehicle accidents, and natural disasters. Fig. 5.7 shows a child who sustained a TBI during an earthquake.

**Characteristics and Symptoms.** TBI can cause sleep disturbances, somatic issues (headaches or dizziness), emotional (moody, depressed), physical (balance and visual-ocular motor dysfunction), and cognitive (memory, inattention, forgetfulness, executive function) (Boisgontier et al., 2020; Yeo et al., 2021). TBI in children has been associated with other childhood conditions such as ADHD, seizures, behavior problems, mental disorders, and learning and hearing problems (Haarbauer-Krupa, 2018). Recovery from a TBI usually follows a typical progression as indicated by the Rancho Levels of Cognitive Functioning (see Table 5.4).

**Challenges in Occupational Participation.** Occupational participation deficits in children and youth with TBIs can occur in all occupations as outlined in Box 5.3. Children who experience TBI may have corresponding motor difficulties that affect their ability to engage in their occupations. For example, they may experience poor balance making it difficult to sit up and eat, go to the bathroom, or walk around the house. They may lose the use of their hands or arms. They may have cognitive issues such as poor memory, forgetfulness, or problem-solving which interferes with their ability to figure out how to dress, make a sandwich, or do schoolwork. They may tire easily, have difficulty establishing a routine, and sleep throughout the day. Children with TBI present differently depending on the severity of the injury. They may have difficulty paying attention, lose focus quickly, and show erratic behaviors (such as being moody, tearful, or silly).

**Implications for Occupational Therapy.** Occupational therapy practitioners working with a child with a TBI create interventions to address the child's unique situation, challenges, and abilities. Initially, while the TBI is in an acute phase, they may work with the child in the intensive care unit (ICU). Box 5.7 provides examples of occupational therapy intervention for children in the Intensive Care Unit, while Box 5.8 describes intervention in the acute care setting. Later in the course of intervention, they may provide adaptations (such as assistive technology) or compensatory ways of doing things as the child progresses. They may address the child's motor challenges using frames of reference such as biomechanical contemporary motor control and motor learning (See Chapter 29), or developmental approach (See Chapter 8). These approaches help the child regain motor control by engaging them in meaningful repetitive occupation-based activities designed specifically for the child's level of functioning. Laverdure and Beisbier (2021) conducted a systematic review to examine occupational therapy interventions for children and youth ages five to 21. They reported strong evidence for interventions that involve children engaging in occupations and activities in multiple environments along with coaching and feedback to improve participation and performance in ADLs and functional mobility (Laverdure & Beisbier, 2021).

The practitioner may provide strategies to support the child at home or school. For example, the child may need frequent breaks, clear instructions, and sensory considerations (such as lighting, or environmental distractions). Children may need to relearn handwriting. Evidence suggests that this is best accomplished by teaching and practicing handwriting in the context of school (Grajo et al., 2020; Hoy et al., 2011; Tichener et al., 2018). Children may have trouble with cognitive tasks and require strategies to work through the material and show one's knowledge. It may be necessary to educate the child and the team on what to expect and how to provide the child with the best educational experience that allows their brain to heal. As the child progresses, the occupational therapy practitioner adjusts the occupations to support performance. Case Example 5.2 describes the progression of occupational therapy intervention from the intensive care unit to rehabilitation for a child who sustained a SCI. They may increase motor responses, problem-solving, or complexity of the performance as the child makes progress.

Children with TBI experience impairments that affect their social functions. They may not be able to participate in activities that give them meaning and provide them with a sense of belonging. Occupational therapy practitioners may design interventions to address social participation but modify them to support the child with TBI. For example, Jacobs-Nzuzi Khuabi et al. (2022) created a model to facilitate resilience so adolescents with TBI could meet the occupational challenges of school.

## INJURIES TO UNSPECIFIED PART OF TRUNK, LIMB, OR BODY REGION

Children and youth may experience injuries to the trunk, limb, or body region, such as those that result in spinal cord injuries (SCI).

### Spinal Cord Injury

Spinal cord injury is an injury to the spinal cord anywhere from the foramen magnum to the cauda equina resulting from compulsion, incision, or contusion of the spinal cord (Nas et al., 2015). They result

**TABLE 5.4 The Rancho Levels of Cognitive Functioning and Behaviors**

| Rancho Level of Cognitive Functioning | Description of Behaviors |
|---|---|
| Level I: No response | • Demonstrates no response to external stimuli |
| Level II: Generalized response | • Responds inconsistently and non-purposefully to external stimuli<br>• Responses are often the same regardless of stimuli |
| Level III: Localized response | • Demonstrates localized responses to external stimuli<br>• Responds more to familiar people versus strangers<br>• May follow some basic commands |
| Level IV: Confused, agitated | • Demonstrates confusion and agitation (e.g., internal confusion, hyperactive state with bizarre and non-purposeful behavior)<br>• Absent short-term memory<br>• Begins to participate in more basic activities of daily living with maximal assistance |
| Level V: Confused, inappropriate (not agitated) | • Can follow simple step-by-step instructions for completion of self-care skills<br>• Able to complete simple tasks after demonstration<br>• Responses are non-purposeful and random to complex commands<br>• Memory is severely impaired and learning new information is difficult<br>• Behavior and verbalization is often inappropriate<br>• Can show agitation to unpleasant external stimuli |
| Level VI: Confused, appropriate | • Demonstrates confusion due to memory deficits<br>• Follows simple commands consistently<br>• Able to complete familiar routines and task (such as daily self-care)<br>• Exhibits improved attention to functional tasks<br>• Easily distracted by environmental stimuli<br>• Emerging insight into physical deficits<br>• Impulsive with actions and speech<br>• Unaware of safety concerns |
| Level VII: Automatic, appropriate | • Oriented in familiar settings<br>• Emerging independence with routine tasks, functional activities<br>• Demonstrate carry over for new tasks and learning<br>• Poor insight into true physical and cognitive capabilities<br>• Limited safety awareness<br>• Demonstrates inflexibility with though processes and actions<br>• Beginning to show interest in social and recreational activities in structured settings |
| Level VIII: Purposeful, appropriate (stand by assistance) | • Consistently oriented to person, place, and time<br>• Beginning to show awareness of physical and cognitive impairments<br>• Compensates for deficits to independently compete daily tasks<br>• Demonstrates more appropriate problem-solving skills<br>• Illustrates improved memory and learning abilities<br>• Often depressed, irritable and frustrated easily |
| Level IX: Purposeful, appropriate (stand by assistance on request) | • Able to shift between different tasks and complete them independently<br>• Acknowledge their impairments<br>• Use compensatory strategies to cope<br>• With assistance, nticipate obstacles that may arise due to impairments<br>• Able to consider consequences of actions<br>• Continue to demonstrate depression and low frustration |
| Level X: Purposeful, appropriate (modified independent) | • Multi-task in many different environments with extra time or devices<br>• Able to create strategies for memory retention<br>• Independently anticipate obstacles due to impairments<br>• Interact appropriately with others in social situations<br>• May experiences periods of depression and low frustration when under stress |

Adapted from: Hagen et al. (1972); Lin and Wroten (2024)

### BOX 5.7 Occupational therapy Intervention for Children With Traumatic Brain Injury in the Intensive Care Unit

**Preparatory methods:**

- Although the physician manages pharmacologic interventions to address autonomic storming, the occupational therapist may communicate to the medical team whether interventions support improved tolerance of therapy interventions (Lemke, 2007).
- A low-stimulation environment may promote brain healing (Anderson et al., 2006). After brain injury, loud noises, bright lights, and tactile input may overstimulate the child and lead to increased agitation and blood pressure. Increased blood pressure is dangerous to healing brain tissues because the child is already experiencing increased intracranial pressure resulting from swelling (Johnson et al., 2009; Lemke, 2007).

**Purposeful activities and occupation-based interventions:**

- Depending on the child's level of consciousness, the occupational therapist may introduce appropriate sensory stimulation in a controlled manner to evoke a localized, volitional response to the environment (Anderson et al., 2006). Monitoring the autonomic nervous system's response to sensory stimulation can provide information on the client's potential return to consciousness (Wijnen et al., 2006).

**Education:**

- Caregivers may benefit from general education on brain injury including how arousal, acceptance of stimulation, and body movements impact their child. The Rancho levels (Hagen et al., 1972; Lin & Wroten, 2024) may facilitate understanding of the phases of recovery post brain injury and projected outcome.

in paraplegia or complete injuries. Spinal cord injuries are either complete or incomplete, denoted by the level of the injury within the spinal cord, and measured using the American Spinal Injury Association (ASIA) scale for spinal cord injury (See Fig. 5.8) ((Benmelouka et al., 2020; Rupp et al., 2021; van Den Hauwe et al., 2020) Spinal cord injuries are uncommon in children under 5 years of age. Although relatively rare (prevalence about 2%), cervical injuries are the most common spinal cord injury in children under 12 (Shin et al., 2016).

**Causes.** Pediatric SCI typically has different causes than adult SCI. Whereas in adults, the most common cause of SCI is traumatic injury, for children, it is more common to have nontraumatic causes such as congenital anomalies, spinal cord tumors, infections, or vascular malformations. However, when there is a traumatic cause for a pediatric SCI, it is typically due to a motor vehicle accident, or a sports injury. Other traumatic causes include falls, and child abuse (Benmelouka et al., 2020; Cunha et al., 2023; Shin et al., 2016).

**Characteristics and Symptoms.** A spinal cord injury causes impaired mobility and secondary health conditions (Hwang et al., 2020). The secondary health conditions are neurogenic bladder and bowel dysfunction, pressure injuries, spasticity, pain, and autonomic dysfunction (Hwang et al., 2020).

### BOX 5.8 Occupational Therapy Intervention for Children with Traumatic Brain Injury in Acute Care

**Preparatory methods:**

- Muscle hypertonia may become more evident at this stage of recovery, in which case interventions to maximize range of motion are initiated (Mass et al., 2022; Ylvisaker et al., 2005).
- Collaboration with physicians on pharmacologic management of muscle tone, agitation, and/or arousal in addition to pain may support improved participation in therapy and response to interventions (Mass et al., 2022; Ylvisaker et al., 2005).
- Ongoing assessment of the child's ability to perceive or interact with the environment is essential (Anderson et al., 2006). Examples include the ability to localize touch, blink to threat, visually track, startle to sound, localize to sound or react to smells or tastes.
- Sensory stimulation may be used to increase or decrease alertness as appropriate to facilitate participation in functional tasks (Anderson et al., 2006).
- Physical restlessness typically increases in this stage owing to decreased pharmacologic sedation (Anderson et al., 2006). The need for safety measures, such as padding to prevent skin shearing, is continuously assessed.

**Purposeful activities and occupation-based interventions:**

- Once the child is able to perceive environmental stimuli, facilitation of the child's ability to interact with the environment progresses from basic functioning to more complex (Anderson et al., 2006). For example, if a child is demonstrating the ability to visually track and is initiating basic upper extremity movement, facilitating reach for a preferred object in a gravity-lessened, side-lying position may be an appropriate next step for intervention. From this position, the task can be graded in complexity in a variety of ways, including requiring the child to reach against gravity and increasing the distance of the object from the child to incorporate the practice of trunk control.
- Neuromuscular reeducation, including active assist of arm and hand movement and sensorimotor therapeutic interventions, supports the restoration of motor functions.

**Education:**

- Caregivers may benefit from education on how environmental stimuli and the child's level of alertness may affect the child's ability to participate in functional tasks. The occupational therapist may then model how the caregiver can facilitate purposeful interactions.
- Caregivers may benefit from education on how the repetition of motor tasks reinforces motor learning and subsequent function.

## Case Example 5.2 Sam

### History

Sam is an 8-year-old boy who was riding his bicycle in a wind storm and was hit in the head by a large tree branch. He sustained a brain injury, including a large left frontal lobe laceration with an extensive shear injury, multiple subdural hematomas, and many regions of diffuse damage. His skull was fractured in multiple locations, along with fractures of the C7 spinous process and T1–T3 compression fractures. On admission, he underwent emergency bilateral craniectomy surgeries to relieve the intracranial pressure and address the significant subdural hemorrhaging. He spent 1 month in the ICU and was transferred to the inpatient pediatric rehabilitation unit.

### Intensive Care Unit

During his hospital stay, Sam experienced significant muscle spasticity managed by medication, serial casting, and orthosis fabrication. His body's ability to regulate itself was inadequate, causing autonomic storming episodes with a consistent decorticate posturing pattern (tonal pattern involving intense spasticity with shoulders adducted and internally rotated, elbows flexed, forearms pronated, wrists flexed, and digits in composite flexion). Sam always wore a back brace to address his spinal stability needs and a helmet was placed on his head when out of bed. He demonstrated a right-sided hemiplegic presentation due to the nature of his injury.

Occupational therapy assessment: what is interfering with his function?

a. Significant spasticity of extremities
b. Decreased positioning options for comfort
c. Decreased purposeful responses to stimuli
d. At risk for pressure sore development and joint contracture

#### *Goals Areas*

- Development of a positioning plan for skin integrity assurance
- Physiologic tolerance and endurance for upright positioning
- Passive range of motion (PROM) of B UE achieved via tone management techniques (in partnership with medical management)
- Purposeful responses to elicited stimulation
- Caregiver education regarding plan of care and strategies for positioning
- Increased scar integrity

#### Plan

- Working with nursing and support staff regarding positioning alternatives based on Sam's tolerance/responses
- Daily passive range of motion to B UE
- Custom orthoses/serial cast fabrication or positioning of joints with loss of ROM
- Instruct family in care as appropriate
- Provision of various sensory stimuli (auditory, visual, tactile, etc.) to observe consistent responses, quality of responses, etc.
- Exposing Sam to upright/edge of bed/recliner, etc. positioning while closely monitoring Sam's vital signs, etc.
- Working to increase Sam's endurance for upright activity/exposure
- Application of scar massage techniques and education of caregivers in the method

### Inpatient Rehabilitation

Once medically stable, Sam was transferred directly to the inpatient rehabilitation unit. His storming episodes continued, and his purposeful engagement/responsiveness was not yet surfacing consistently. Sam's occupational therapist continued to focus on facilitating consistent, localized responses to stimulation; decreasing his agitation via environmental adjustments and positioning methods; spasticity management via positioning and use of orthoses during times of decreased agitation; facilitating upright and out-of-bed positioning in his wheelchair and in therapy gyms within tolerance; caregiver education regarding necessary adaptive equipment (fully supportive shower chair, tilt-in-space wheelchair with full support); transfers; and handling methods used to facilitate purposeful responses; ongoing scar management using scar massage and monitoring for the need for pressure therapy. Due to his slow functional progress while inpatient, the main difference in his plan of care related to caregiver preparedness/empowerment before discharge to ensure greater competence in caring for Sam.

Occupational therapy assessment: what is interfering with his functioning?

- Ongoing limited responses to sensory stimulation techniques
- Increased spasticity in his affected upper extremity (UE)
- Need for equipment/full support during transfers and mobility
- Caregiver comfort with his status and managing his care

#### *Goals Areas*

- Purposeful responses to elicited stimulation
- Active engagement in activity
- Skin and scar integrity
- Caregiver education regarding plan of care, methods for assistance/facilitating functional responses, etc.
- Within functional limits UE PROM/AROM of affected UE for self-care

#### Plan

- PROM and trials of AAROM to determine if Sam will engage in a portion of the movement actively
- Custom orthoses/serial cast fabrication or positioning of joints with loss of ROM
- Provision of various sensory stimuli (auditory, visual, tactile) to observe consistent responses, quality of responses, etc.
- Exposing Sam to an upright/wheelchair/sitting on the edge of the mat
- Working to increase Sam's endurance for upright activity/exposure
- Application of scar massage techniques and education of caregivers in methods
- Caregiver education regarding managing equipment, activities of daily living (ADLs), transfers, home accessibility, etc.

### Outpatient Rehabilitation

After 3 months of hospitalization, Sam was discharged home. His recovery had stabilized and had not progressed significantly; he was fully dependent on all self-care and communication needs. Sam continued to have decreased periods of autonomic storming, hypertonicity, and agitation and was beginning to visually track for brief periods. He was assigned a home nurse who was trained to manage his care during the day while his parents worked. It was decided that he would participate in intensive occupational, physical, and speech pathology treatments on an outpatient basis.

Sam's parents and home health nurse attended the outpatient occupational therapy evaluation. His parents reported feeling overwhelmed with Sam's care and wanting to know how the recovery process for their son would proceed. Sam was agitated and storming during the initial evaluation, making it difficult to fully assess his passive upper extremity range of motion. He postured in a modified decorticate pattern with his trunk in right rotation and pelvis in left rotation, particularly when placed in a supine position on the mat table. His parents reported that the periods when this posturing occurred were becoming less frequent. The occupational therapist noted that his tonal pattern decreased when he was placed in a right-side-lying position, allowing his shoulders to depress and protract. The occupational therapist placed Sam in various supported positions on the mat to observe his tolerance to transitional movements, spasticity patterns, and head and trunk muscle facilitation. He did not demonstrate the ability to visually track during the evaluation; however, his parents reported that he would, at times, demonstrate purposeful visual attention in the home environment (i.e., with the television). During times of increased alertness, Sam's parents reported that he appropriately smiled to auditory input. The occupational therapist explored the family's current adaptive equipment, discussed the parents' and nurse's comfort with using the equipment, observed Sam in his wheelchair, and discussed the home set-up. Additionally, she asked the family questions about Sam's premorbid recreational interests, which included baseball, playing with his friends, karate, telling jokes, and spending time with his older brother.

As outpatient therapies were initiated and his doctors refined his medications, Sam's autonomic storming episodes decreased. As this happened, bilateral upper extremity hypertonicity decreased, and he presented in a right hemiplegic manner. Sam began to demonstrate purposeful use of his left upper extremity, and his right presented as flaccid proximally with simultaneous distal tightness of his long finger flexors and wrist flexors. He continued to hold his left elbow at approximately 90 degrees of flexion with internal rotation and adduction of the shoulder.

The first stage of his outpatient occupational therapy intervention facilitated his emerging purposeful left upper extremity movement. Sam was placed in a right-side-lying position on the mat table to eliminate gravity to promote left upper

*Continued*

## Case Example 5.2 Sam—cont'd

extremity reach. For example, Sam demonstrated early motivation when exposed to a water toy. A basic button switch was connected to the water toy that poured water into a spout with activation. Initially, the occupational therapist used a hand-over-hand strategy to elicit reach in this position. From there, Sam began to visually attend to this toy and engaged in purposeful reach for the switch. The occupational therapist talked with Sam and his parents conversationally, making an effort to discuss with Sam professional baseball scores and tell him silly jokes. During these interactions, Sam demonstrated appropriate smiling and laughing and visually attended to the occupational therapist when she spoke.

Early outpatient sessions also included supported sitting on the edge of the mat table with a mirror in front of Sam for visual feedback to address basic head control, visual attention, and tracking. After a few weeks, he demonstrated independent head control, and trunk control became a more significant focus of intervention. Functional activity was incorporated throughout each stage, engaging Sam's interests while maximizing his ability to move his left upper extremity against gravity. He reached for a baseball while seated, placed a small plastic basketball into a hoop, and participated in self-care. His parents were involved in one session per week on a common day off of work, learning how to work with Sam at home. The occupational therapist developed an orthosis use protocol for his right upper extremity at night and a functional electrical stimulation program. After a few months, Sam began to demonstrate basic reach and grasp with his more affected right side.

Sam's outpatient rehabilitation then incorporated aquatic therapy and weekly exercises for upper extremity and trunk strength. His ataxia and right upper extremity mobility continued to improve, allowing him to focus on bimanual skills. The occupational therapist balanced the use of compensation and restoration techniques as his progress continued. Continued outpatient sessions focused on any barriers to functioning fully in the home, school, and community environments.

The occupational therapist participated in ongoing, consistent communication with other care team members regarding Sam's progress. As Sam's agitation diminished, his occupational performance increased with left-sided functional use and engagement in purposeful activity. He began attending school 2 days per week. Sam's large, tilt-in-space manual wheelchair was becoming a barrier to his function owing to components no longer being needed. In therapy he trialed power wheelchairs with an equipment vendor on multiple occasions and, after educating the family and understanding his capabilities, he was deemed appropriate to use a power wheelchair. He received a new wheelchair and additional training on its use; within a few short weeks, he was able to navigate his school, home, and community environments with supervision. Sam's mindset greatly improved with his newfound independence.

What is interfering with his functioning?

a. Ongoing storming/posturing episodes
b. Inconsistent responses to stimuli
c. Decreased UE mobility/right-sided weakness
d. Decreased head/trunk control
e. Caregiver fatigue/uncertainty/feelings of being overwhelmed

### *Goal Areas*

- Consistency with purposeful responses to stimuli
- Ongoing tone management strategies for increased participation in functional activities
- Facilitation of purposeful UE, trunk, and cervical mobility for ADL participation
- Facilitation of development of fine motor skills for functional application
- Improved cognition for functional problem-solving participation
- Focus on visual processing and hand/eye coordination tasks for functional performance
- Ongoing motor planning of bilateral UE, particularly affected right UE
- Increased participation in self-care participation
- Increased competence with stand pivot transfers
- Engagement in school-related activities as appropriate
- Increased caregiver engagement/comfort in Sam's care
- Increased independence with mobility for home, school, and community environments

### *Plan*

a. Facilitating B UE mobility via NMES, hand-over-hand strategies, positioning, etc.
b. Use of splinting and positioning methods for tone management
c. Participation in B UE, trunk, and cervical strengthening tasks (on land and in an aquatic environment) for increased engagement in occupational performance
d. Engagement in graded ADL and other activities for eliciting ongoing purposeful responses/mobility
e. Use of basic identification of objects via visual regard, with the ongoing increased complexity of task and movement requirements for increased cognitive and motor demands
f. Involvement of caregivers in sessions and ongoing goal development discussions/strategies based on caregiver-reported readiness/comfort
g. Collaboration with Sam's school occupational therapist regarding strategy use in an outpatient setting for carryover in the school environment when appropriate (and vice versa)
h. Facilitation of transfers during functional tasks with ongoing caregiver participation
i. Implementation of various visual strategies for increased understanding of Sam's visual skills, including tracking, convergence, saccades, smooth pursuits, etc. during functional tasks
j. Wheelchair evaluation for modification of equipment based on increased functional skills

### *Outcomes*

- ADLs: during the first year of Sam's outpatient rehabilitation course, he made significant gains in his occupational performance in general. He progressed from inconsistent visual regard and responses to stimulation to purposeful engagement. He was performing UE dressing with moderate assistance, lower extremity (LE) dressing with maximum assistance, toileting with maximum assistance, toothbrushing with moderate assistance, and self-feeding finger foods with minimum assistance.
- Range of motion: Sam's left UE AROM increased to within functional limits. His right UE, the affected UE, continued to demonstrate increased tone distally, with increased purposeful movements throughout. By the end of the first year of outpatient rehabilitation, Sam was using his affected UE as a stabilizer during functional tasks.
- Functional mobility: Sam required supervision of his functional mobility while using his power wheelchair in his various contexts.
- Leisure skills: Sam began to engage in leisure activities such as participation in social outings with friends to the movies, baseball games, etc. Additionally, he began to use modified computer control skills for engagement in video games; he participated in basic ball play, swimming, playing with his pets, tabletop tasks with minimum to maximum assistance, as well as various additional modified activities.
- School participation: Sam attended school 5 days per week and was engaging with peers and in educational activities on a modified basis. He used a one-handed keyboard for writing and assignment participation, as writing continued to be an ongoing challenge and frustrating task for him.
- Caregiver education: his parents were educated on an ongoing basis about ways to support Sam's functional status with ADLs, transfers, engagement in leisure tasks, etc. and to continue to facilitate his function at home and in the community. They received ongoing education regarding the role of occupational therapy and the development of his care plan. Their comfort with his care improved yet they continued to struggle with the emotional experience of seeing their child go through such a traumatic experience and continued to hope and assume that, at some point, he would walk again and be significantly closer to how he was functioning before his accident, despite the severity of his injury and ongoing education from the care team.

**Challenges in Occupational Participation.** Occupational participation deficits in children and youth with SCI can occur in any of the occupations listed in Box 5.3. The motor deficits vary depending on the level and type of injury (complete or incomplete). Complete injury to the spinal cord level refers to a loss of both motor and sensory functions at the level below the injury. Incomplete injuries to the spinal cord refer to instances where partial sensory and motor functions below the level are present (Nas et al., 2015).

Children with spinal cord injuries may have challenges with mobility and require assistive devices (such as walkers and wheelchairs). They may have upper extremity challenges requiring assistive technology (such as a tenodesis splint), or requiring adaptations to keyboards to communicate. Children may have challenges breathing, eating, and communicating. Technology may allow them to use suck-swallow-breathe to operate an electronic wheelchair.

**Implications for Occupational Therapy.** Occupational therapy practitioners use knowledge of the level of the injury and type of injury when creating intervention plans to address the child's daily activities. They also vary their interventions based on the timing of the injury and the setting. Boxes 5.9 and 5.10 describe intervention for children with SCI in intensive care and acute care settings. They may use strategies from motor control motor learning, biomechanical, and developmental approaches to promootor functioning. They provide assistive technology and mobility equipment and consult on home modifications to support children in engaging in daily activities. For example, they may be a part of the team to consult on home and school modifications that allow the child to reach objects in the kitchen, use the bathroom, and move throughout the house using a wheelchair, walker, or scooter Chapter 32 They may suggest leisure opportunities and equipment modifications to allow children and youth to engage in adapted basketball, sailing, kayaking, or hiking. Fig. 5.9 shows a child using a specially designed wheelchair that allows them to turn and move quickly to participate in a sports team. Children and youth may also require training and adaptations for driving (See Chapter 20). See Case Example 5.3 for an example of intervention for a child with SCI progressing through varied treatment settings.

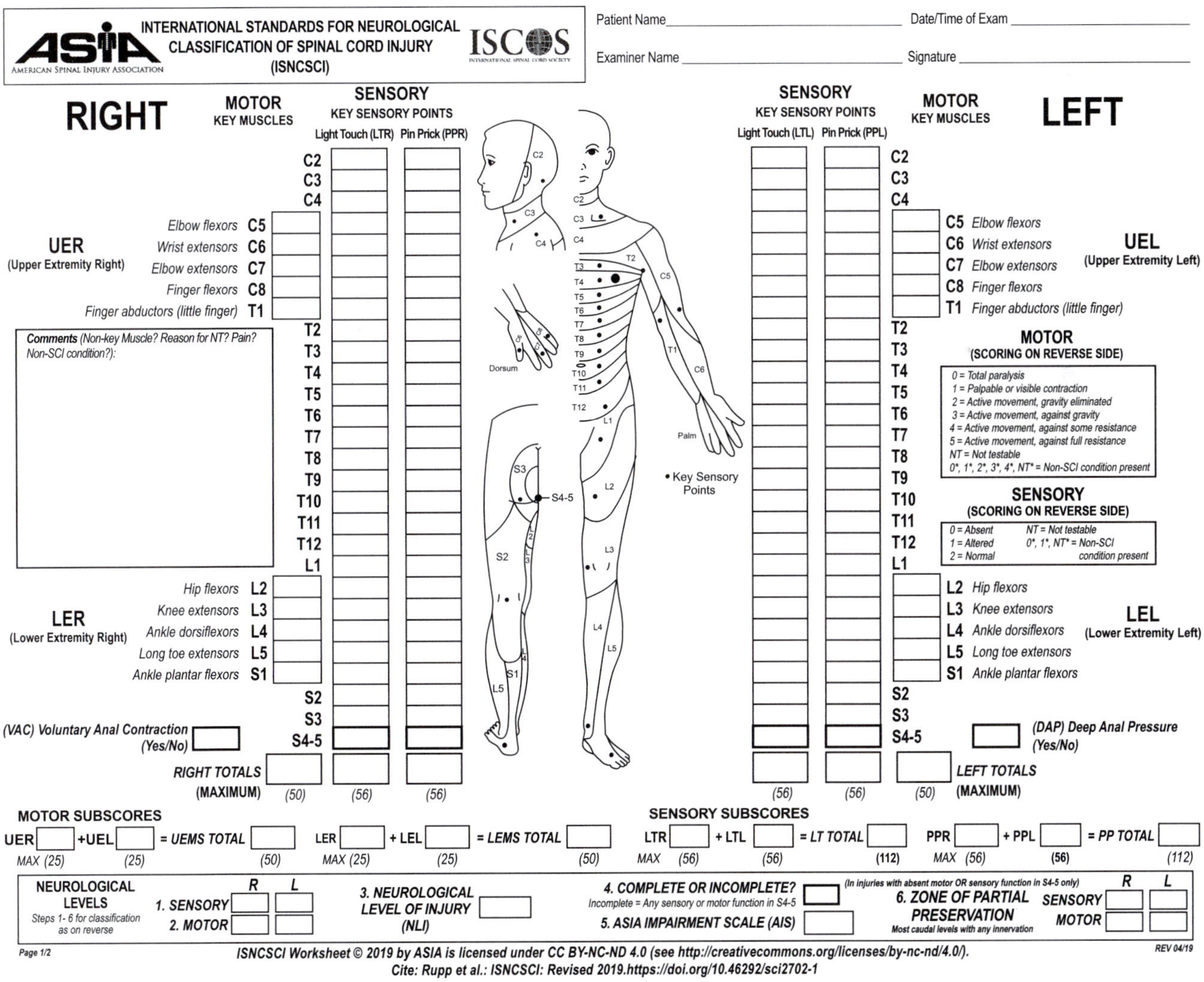


**Fig. 5.8** International Standards for Neurological Classification of SCI (ISNCSCI) Worksheet ©2019 by Rupp et al., (2021).

*Continued*

### Muscle Function Grading

**0** = Total paralysis

**1** = Palpable or visible contraction

**2** = Active movement, full range of motion (ROM) with gravity eliminated

**3** = Active movement, full ROM against gravity

**4** = Active movement, full ROM against gravity and moderate resistance in a muscle specific position

**5** = (Normal) active movement, full ROM against gravity and full resistance in a functional muscle position expected from an otherwise unimpaired person

**NT** = Not testable (i.e. due to immobilization, severe pain such that the patient cannot be graded, amputation of limb, or contracture of > 50% of the normal ROM)

**0*, 1*, 2*, 3*, 4*, NT*** = Non-SCI condition present [a]

### Sensory Grading

**0** = Absent **1** = Altered, either decreased/impaired sensation or hypersensitivity

**2** = Normal **NT** = Not testable

**0*, 1*, NT*** = Non-SCI condition present [a]

[a] Note: Abnormal motor and sensory scores should be tagged with a '*' to indicate an impairment due to a non-SCI condition. The non-SCI condition should be explained in the comments box together with information about how the score is rated for classification purposes (at least normal / not normal for classification).

### When to Test Non-Key Muscles:

In a patient with an apparent AIS B classification, non-key muscle functions more than 3 levels below the motor level on each side should be tested to most accurately classify the injury (differentiate between AIS B and C).

| Movement | Root level |
|---|---|
| **Shoulder:** Flexion, extension, adbuction, adduction, internal and external rotation<br>**Elbow:** Supination | C5 |
| **Elbow:** Pronation<br>**Wrist:** Flexion | C6 |
| **Finger:** Flexion at proximal joint, extension<br>**Thumb:** Flexion, extension and abduction in plane of thumb | C7 |
| **Finger:** Flexion at MCP joint<br>**Thumb:** Opposition, adduction and abduction perpendicular to palm | C8 |
| **Finger:** Abduction of the index finger | T1 |
| **Hip:** Adduction | L2 |
| **Hip:** External rotation | L3 |
| **Hip:** Extension, abduction, internal rotation<br>**Knee:** Flexion<br>**Ankle:** Inversion and eversion<br>**Toe:** MP and IP extension | L4 |
| **Hallux and Toe:** DIP and PIP flexion and abduction | L5 |
| **Hallux:** Adduction | S1 |

### ASIA Impairment Scale (AIS)

**A = Complete.** No sensory or motor function is preserved in the sacral segments S4-5.

**B = Sensory Incomplete.** Sensory but not motor function is preserved below the neurological level and includes the sacral segments S4-5 (light touch or pin prick at S4-5 or deep anal pressure) AND no motor function is preserved more than three levels below the motor level on either side of the body.

**C = Motor Incomplete.** Motor function is preserved at the most caudal sacral segments for voluntary anal contraction (VAC) OR the patient meets the criteria for sensory incomplete status (sensory function preserved at the most caudal sacral segments S4-5 by LT, PP or DAP), and has some sparing of motor function more than three levels below the ipsilateral motor level on either side of the body. (This includes key or non-key muscle functions to determine motor incomplete status.) For AIS C – less than half of key muscle functions below the single NLI have a muscle grade ≥ 3.

**D = Motor Incomplete.** Motor incomplete status as defined above, with at least half (half or more) of key muscle functions below the single NLI having a muscle grade ≥ 3.

**E = Normal.** If sensation and motor function as tested with the ISNCSCI are graded as normal in all segments, and the patient had prior deficits, then the AIS grade is E. Someone without an initial SCI does not receive an AIS grade.

**Using ND:** To document the sensory, motor and NLI levels, the ASIA Impairment Scale grade, and/or the zone of partial preservation (ZPP) when they are unable to be determined based on the examination results.

ASIA
AMERICAN SPINAL INJURY ASSOCIATION

**INTERNATIONAL STANDARDS FOR NEUROLOGICAL CLASSIFICATION OF SPINAL CORD INJURY**

ISCOS
INTERNATIONAL SPINAL CORD SOCIETY

Page 2/2

### Steps in Classification

The following order is recommended for determining the classification of individuals with SCI.

**1. Determine sensory levels for right and left sides.**
*The sensory level is the most caudal, intact dermatome for both pin prick and light touch sensation.*

**2. Determine motor levels for right and left sides.**
*Defined by the lowest key muscle function that has a grade of at least 3 (on supine testing), providing the key muscle functions represented by segments above that level are judged to be intact (graded as a 5).*
*Note: in regions where there is no myotome to test, the motor level is presumed to be the same as the sensory level, if testable motor function above that level is also normal.*

**3. Determine the neurological level of injury (NLI).**
*This refers to the most caudal segment of the cord with intact sensation and antigravity (3 or more) muscle function strength, provided that there is normal (intact) sensory and motor function rostrally respectively.*
*The NLI is the most cephalad of the sensory and motor levels determined in steps 1 and 2.*

**4. Determine whether the injury is Complete or Incomplete.**
*(i.e. absence or presence of sacral sparing)*
*If voluntary anal contraction = **No** AND all S4-5 sensory scores = **0** AND deep anal pressure = **No**, then injury is **Complete**.*
*Otherwise, injury is **Incomplete**.*

**5. Determine ASIA Impairment Scale (AIS) Grade.**
**Is injury Complete? If YES, AIS=A**

**NO ↓**

**Is injury Motor Complete? If YES, AIS=B**

**NO ↓** (No=voluntary anal contraction OR motor function more than three levels below the motor level on a given side, if the patient has sensory incomplete classification)

**Are at least half (half or more) of the key muscles below the neurological level of injury graded 3 or better?**

**NO ↓** → **AIS=C**

**YES ↓** → **AIS=D**

**If sensation and motor function is normal in all segments, AIS=E**
*Note: AIS E is used in follow-up testing when an individual with a documented SCI has recovered normal function. If at initial testing no deficits are found, the individual is neurologically intact and the ASIA Impairment Scale does not apply.*

**6. Determine the zone of partial preservation (ZPP).**
*The ZPP is used only in injuries with absent motor (no VAC) OR sensory function (no DAP, no LT and no PP sensation) in the lowest sacral segments S4-5, and refers to those dermatomes and myotomes caudal to the sensory and motor levels that remain partially innervated. With sacral sparing of sensory function, the sensory ZPP is not applicable and therefore "NA" is recorded in the block of the worksheet. Accordingly, if VAC is present, the motor ZPP is not applicable and is noted as "NA".*

**Fig. 5.8, cont'd**

## CHROMOSOMAL ANOMALIES, EXCLUDING GENE MUTATIONS

Children may be born with chromosomal anomalies, which may affect their motor, neurological, and other bodily systems (such as cardiac, immunological, and gastrointestinal). Each syndrome presents differently. Down syndrome is the most common chromosomal syndrome in the United States, with a birth prevalence of 1 in 700 births (CDC, 2023). Children with Down syndrome are living longer and experiencing improved quality of life due to improved medical care and reduced institutionalism (Presson et al., 2013).

### Down Syndrome

Down syndrome or Trisomy 21, is a congenital, genetic disorder that affects intellectual ability (Antonarakis et al., 2020). The level of intellectual ability varies among children. Down syndrome occurs in approximately one of 800 births worldwide and about 5000 live births annually In the United States. Social behaviors are often more skilled relative to the individual's cognitive impairment. Cardiac and respiratory complications are common but are managed medically. One important precaution with this disorder is the presence of atlantoaxial instability, which is particularly dangerous as it can lead to spinal cord compression.

**Causes.** Down syndrome is caused by an extra 21st chromosome. While a major risk factor for Down syndrome is advanced maternal age, it is difficult to ascertain the environmental impact and influences that contribute to it (Antonarakis et al., 2020; CDC, 2023; Miller, 2021). Down syndrome is not related to race, nationality, socioeconomic status, religion, or anything the mother and father did during pregnancy (Global Down Syndrome Foundation, 2018). Some children are born with mosaic translocation Down syndrome, which means only some cells have an extra copy of the 21st chromosome.

**Characteristics and Symptoms.** Down syndrome can result in intellectual disability, sleep apnea, epilepsy, expressive language difficulties, and hearing and vision difficulties (Antonarakis et al., 2020). Down syndrome also includes observable features such as low muscle tone throughout, a shorter stature, and a round face with almond-shaped and up-slanting eyes (CDC, 2023).

### BOX 5.9 Occupational Therapy Intervention for Children With Spinal Cord Injury (SCI) in Intensive Care

| | |
|---|---|
| **Preparatory methods:** | • Pain may limit a child's participation, making collaboration with physicians on pain management especially important. |
| **Purposeful activities and occupation-based interventions:** | • If the child is conscious, the occupational therapist can prevent the child's anxiety about mobility limitations by providing adapted call lights and other modified accessibility strategies for increased independence.<br>• Adaptive equipment can also be trialed incorporated as tolerated for completion of self-care activities in bed like feeding or bed baths. |
| **Education:** | • Caregivers and patients may benefit from general education on their child's SCI.<br>• Education also includes autonomic dysreflexia. Symptoms of autonomic dysreflexia may be managed conservatively (e.g., using removal of precipitating stimulus or positioning) and/or pharmacologically (Krassioukov et al., 2009). |

**Challenges in Occupational Participation.** Children with Down syndrome achieve motor milestones later than neurotypical peers and experience low muscle tone and cognitive challenges that interfere with play, activities of daily living, instrumental activities of daily living, educational participation, social interaction, and work and vocational skills. They generally achieve developmental milestones at a later age than their peers. They may experience mild to moderate cognitive impairment and varied abilities. Children with Down syndrome may require additional training for work and educational pursuits and assistance living in the community.

**Implications for Occupational Therapy.** Children with Down syndrome benefit from early intervention services where the occupational therapy practitioner provides intervention in collaboration with the caregiver. Occupational therapy practitioners address challenges in feeding, dressing, bathing, playing, and academics. They encourage motor and sensory development through meaningful repetitive activities during play and use developmental approaches to promote engagement in daily activities. Practitioners engage children in play activities to stimulate movement, including fine motor, gross motor, and oral motor skills. As children develop these skills and repeat them during play, mealtimes, or social interactions with caregivers, they become foundational skills. Occupational therapy practitioners scaffold activities to challenge children while ensuring success. Practitioners address all areas of occupation, prioritizing the parents' goals at first. As children begin to indicate their wants and desires, practitioners can involve them in the goal-setting process.

Children with Down syndrome may require support for feeding due to low oral motor muscle tone. They may require adapted seating to provide support during mealtimes. Practitioners may provide jaw control techniques and intervention to encourage tongue lateralization (to prevent tongue thrusting) (See Chapter 11).

Children with Down syndrome are entitled to a free and appropriate education and many people with Down syndrome complete high school and some attend post-secondary education. Colleges and universities may

### BOX 5.10 Occupational therapy Intervention for Children With Spinal Cord Injury (SCI) in Acute Care

| | |
|---|---|
| **Preparatory methods:** | • Muscle hypertonia may become more evident at this stage of recovery, in which case interventions (such as orthotics) to maximize range of motion are initiated.<br>• Collaboration with physicians on pharmacological management of spasticity (Taricco et al., 2000) in addition to pain may support improved participation in therapy and response to interventions.<br>• Orthostatic hypotension may be managed conservatively (e.g., using functional electrical stimulation) and/or pharmacologically following SCI (Krassioukov et al., 2009).<br>• Vital sign instability may be caused by autonomic dysreflexia. |
| **Purposeful activities and occupation-based interventions:** | • Resumption of motor functions must remain within restrictions of spinal orthopedic equipment such as a neck or back brace. Unfortunately, this equipment may limit independent function (Chafetz et al., 2007).<br>• Neuromuscular reeducation, including hand-over-hand and sensorimotor therapeutic interventions, supports restoration of motor functions. For example, when children are beginning to reinitiate purposeful movements, they often have difficulty with precision and control. The occupational therapist can use his or her own hands, by placing them over the child's hands, as an assist to the child's action. The occupational therapist's assistance provides the child with kinesthetic input for the movement pattern. Additionally, the occupational therapist may use vibration or muscle and tendon tapping techniques to elicit active movement in the context of a functional task and to provide the child with the sensorimotor input of how a particular action of the body should feel.<br>• Adaptive equipment and assistive technology should be introduced to maximize the child's function amidst new motor deficits. This may include the provision of alternative call light and bed controls, abdominal binders, compression stockings, and loaner durable medical equipment, for example, a wheelchair, air mattress, and commode chair. A wheelchair evaluation will determine which model and features are best for each child; optimal fit is important to maximize the child's safety and function. |
| **Education:** | • Occupational therapists may model how to support children's ability to direct their care as appropriate. When children may have long-term movement limitations, it is important to empower them to instruct those who assist them. For example, children can increase their sense of control over their bodies by communicating how they prefer to be transferred or how to position a piece of equipment most effectively for them. |

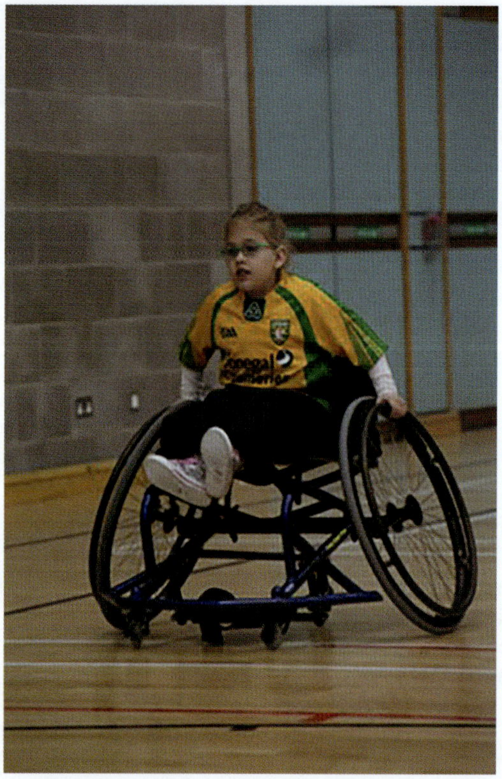

**Fig. 5.9** Children who have spinal cord injuries may require mobility devices, such as this wheelchair designed to turn and move quickly so the child can participate in sports. (Source: https://www.istockphoto.com/photo/basketball-players-using-wheelchairs-gm1083492198-290670783?utm_campaign=srp_photos_top&utm_content=https%3A%2F%2Funsplash.com%2Fs%2Fphotos%2F-child-in---a-wheelchair-playing-basketball&utm_medium=affiliate&utm_source=unsplash&utm_term=child+in+++a+wheelchair+playing+basketball%3A%3Aaffiliate-collections%3Acontrol Credit: Photo by Danny Nee on UnsplashLetterkenny, Donegal, Ireland. Published on September 11, 2020Canon, EOS-1D X. Free to use under the Unsplash License)

have programs to support them (Global Down Syndrome Foundation, 2018). Occupational therapy practitioners working in school settings may support children with Down syndrome by providing organizational strategies, scaffolding assignments as needed, and creating strategies for children to complete academic work, play with peers, and set future goals. See Chapter 15 on the progression from school to transitions and Chapter 21 on work skills and employment.

Intervention may address social participation by engaging children in peer play to take turns, communicate needs, respond to others' cues, and provide cues that one is playing. They benefit from participation in social activities and may enjoy athletic games adapted to support their abilities (such as Special Olympics, adapted baseball, and dance classes). Children with Down syndrome benefit from exploratory play (as shown in Fig. 5.10) and opportunities to engage in daily activities. They engage in fine motor activities to further develop hand arches and in-hand manipulation. Children with Down syndrome may benefit from pencil grips to support grip strength. They may benefit from activities to increase their physical endurance for play.

## NEOPLASMS

Cancer, sometimes referred to as a malignant tumor or a neoplasm, is a group of conditions that indicate the development of abnormal cells (Nurmik et al., 2020; Siegel et al., 2021). While pediatric cancer is rare, it is also one of the leading causes of death among children (Siegel et al., 2021). Two categories of cancer are largely seen in the pediatric population: Leukemia and brain neoplasms (tumors) (Siegel et al., 2021).

### Leukemia and Brain Neoplasms

The two most common types of Leukemia are acute myelogenous leukemia and acute lymphoblastic leukemia, which impact bone marrow and are indicated by a rise in white blood cells (Miller, 2021). Leukemia can be acute or chronic, depending on the percentage of malignant cells, and myeloid or lymphoid based on the size of the malignant cells (Miller, 2021). Brian neoplasm, or a tumor in the central nervous system, is the second largest category of cancer within the pediatric population, with symptoms dependent on the location of the neoplasms (Fischer et al., 2016).

**Causes.** Many genetic and environmental risk factors can lead to the development of cancer. These risk factors can include tobacco use or exposure, maternal age, immunosuppressive medication, and genetics. Disparities in relation to race and ethnicity also exist relative to cancer diagnosis and treatment (Beltrami et al., 2022).

**Characteristics and Symptoms.** The characteristics and symptoms of cancer depend on the type of its type of cancer, the number of tumors, and their locations. Children and youth with Leukemia may experience symptoms such as fatigue, infections, and bruising (Miller, 2021). Children with brain tumors present with motor or sensory difficulties and impairments depending on the tumor(s)' location (Miller, 2021).

**Challenges in Occupational Participation.** Cancer can affect energy, strength, and endurance, which can lead to deficits across all domains of occupation (Box 5.3). Deficits in occupational participation may also depend on the therapies or medication used to treat the child or youth, which can fluctuate. For example, children and youth may feel less engaged with their peers and have limited endurance or stamina to socialize, play, and engage in group activities. Children and youth may experience the same challenges affecting their ability to engage in co-occupations or experiences with families, such as leisure pursuits, and instrumental activities of daily living (e.g., cooking, and cleaning). Due to the influence of the decreased energy, strength, and endurance that cancer and treatment create, many children and youth experience psychosocial challenges. Depending on treatment, a child or youth may miss several weeks, to months, of educational participation.

**Implications for Occupational Therapy.** Occupational therapy practitioners working with children who have cancer may be part of the acute care team, working in the hospital as the child undergoes therapy. They may address pain, provide positioning assistance, and engage children in activity. Children may struggle to complete activities of daily living and benefit from energy conservation techniques or adaptive equipment. As children recover from cancer, they may experience motor challenges that interfere with their daily activities. Occupational therapy practitioners may suggest assistive technology to enable children to fully engage. They may teach compensatory techniques. They may address challenges through rehabilitation approaches, such as contemporary motor control, biomechanical, and repetitive practice of meaningful activities. They may provide strategies for schedules, memory, and organization. They may identify learning strategies (such as chunking material or having material read to the student).

## Case Example 5.3 Keegan

### History

Keegan is a 3-year-old boy admitted to the ICU following a car accident. He was restrained by a lap belt without a booster seat in the back seat when his mother lost control of her car, which sustained a front-end impact and caught on fire. He was transported to the emergency room by ambulance where his immediate injuries were treated and later transitioned to the ICU. Before the injury, Keegan was a typically developing boy who lived with his parents and older brother. He attended a half-day preschool after which his grandmother cared for him. Keegan was outgoing and loved to explore the outdoors and wrestle with his brother.

Keegan sustained a T-12 ASIA B spinal cord injury and 30% total body surface area, full-thickness burns to the neck, right shoulder, and upper extremity proximal to the elbow; he had a nasogastric feeding tube, back brace, and indwelling Foley catheter, was intubated, and was in a pharmacologically induced coma. Therapy was initiated to prevent secondary complications. Burn wound assessment revealed that full-thickness burns crossed joints including the neck and anterior axilla. Passive range of motion was measured to be normal at these joints at this point in care.

### Intervention Progression

#### Intensive Care Unit

The occupational therapist coordinated a positioning schedule with nursing staff to ensure Keegan was turned in bed at least every 2 hours to prevent skin breakdown and prevent deformity caused by wound contracture; he was also issued multipodus boots to avoid direct pressure to his heels while positioning the ankles for future weight-bearing. The occupational therapist educated Keegan's parents on his positioning schedule, posted in his hospital room, and on how they could help nursing staff keep track of his schedule. Following instruction, she asked that each parent demonstrate how to safely assist in transitioning Keegan's position. The occupational therapist completed a passive range of motion (PROM) daily to the neck and shoulder, increasing stretch as tolerated, and fabricated custom orthoses with any loss in the range of motion (ROM). The surgeons performed split-thickness autografting of the burned areas following wound demarcation, and 5 days after surgery, the therapists initiated twice-daily PROM. Keegan began to demonstrate decreased shoulder and neck ROM, so the occupational therapist began positioning the shoulder into abduction using a thermoplastic orthosis and neck extension over a rolled towel when in bed. At that time, Keegan demonstrated improved medical stability; his physician ordered weaning from the coma-inducing medications and transitioned Keegan to acute care.

OT Assessment: what is interfering with his functioning?

1. Limited consciousness, minimal to no purposeful active movement
2. Fear, confusion
3. At risk for joint contracture and pressure area development
4. Goals:
5. Keegan will communicate needs as able.
6. Keegan will participate in his care as able.
7. Keegan will demonstrate maintained PROM at all joints.
8. Keegan will demonstrate good skin integrity in areas at risk for pressure sore development.
9. Caregivers will participate in Keegan's care.

#### *Plan*

- Bedside stimulation and age-appropriate conversation
- Communicate plans of care ("We're going to stretch your arms now.") and facilitate engagement as able ("Help me lift your arm up. Good job!")
- Instruct family in care as appropriate
- Daily passive range to affected joints, increase to twice a day if PROM becomes limited
- Custom orthosis fabrication or positioning for joints with loss of ROM
- Pressure area monitoring and prevention (air mattress, heel lifts)

#### *Acute Care*

As Keegan's level of consciousness increased, he demonstrated significant difficulty tolerating therapy owing to both pain from his burn injury and neuropathic pain in his lower extremities. The occupational therapist provided his physician with input regarding potential pharmacologic pain management in hopes of balancing Keegan's tolerance for therapy with a level of alertness that allowed him to begin participating during sessions. Keegan's mother brought music from his favorite television show and the therapist began to play it during each session. When Keegan was able to follow simple commands, the occupational therapist let him know that it would hurt and assessed his active shoulder and cervical range by asking him to reach for and turn to look at different toys from home. The occupational therapist asked Keegan's brother to hold his tablet computer in a position, so Keegan could only see it if he was upright; she slowly helped Keegan transition to sitting at the edge of the bed and assessed his postural control while he was watching a video clip. He cried and told the occupational therapist not to let go, and she responded by reassuring and engaging Keegan. The occupational therapist instructed his parents on safe transfers so he could sit in a chair with supportive pillows for periods during the day as part of his updated positioning plan. During sessions, the occupational therapist encouraged Keegan to perform active range as much as possible throughout stretches and let him know when she needed to passively range his joints further. She discussed goals and ideas that were meaningful to Keegan in a "guided imagery" format during painful stretching and worked with nursing to complete ROM shortly after receiving scheduled pain medication. He then transitioned to inpatient rehabilitation.

Occupational therapy assessment: what is interfering with his functioning?

- Anxiety, fear, lack of knowledge of the condition
- Upper body procedural pain, lower body neuropathic pain
- Weakness and deconditioning
- No controlled active movement of bilateral lower extremities (BLEs)

#### *Goals*

1. Keegan will communicate his needs and concerns consistently.
2. Keegan will demonstrate the successful use of three nonpharmaceutical pain relief techniques.
3. Keegan will demonstrate functional active and passive range at the neck, trunk, and bilateral upper extremities.
4. Keegan will be independent in completing scar management.
5. Keegan will transfer from bed to chair and reverse with minimum assistance from caregivers.
6. Keegan will participate in self-dressing and hygiene with minimum to moderate assistance and adaptive techniques as needed.
7. Keegan will use both hands to hold and manipulate his tablet as desired.

#### *Plan*

- Educate Keegan on burns and spinal cord injury (SCI) at an age-appropriate level and with small amounts of information at a time. Ensure understanding by having him teach back.
- Instruct and rehearse nonpharmaceutical pain relief techniques; guided imagery, deep breathing, imagination, and distraction with music and TV.
- PROM to neck, trunk, BUEs twice a day to full range with scar massage as indicated.
- Fabrication of orthoses for joints lacking full ROM.
- Measurement for custom pressure garments, use of temporary pressure therapy with elastic bandages (Fig. 31.8).
- Transfer education and rehearsal.
- Strategies for dressing and hygiene, rehearsal with fun clothes, and other simulated hygiene objects (blowing bubbles vs. brushing teeth).
- Play activities with BUEs, sitting or in bed; ball, crafts, games, video games, tablet play.
- Educate and engage parents on all interventions.

*Continued*

## Case Example 5.3 Keegan—cont'd

***Outcomes***

- Functional communication: Keegan learned to use words instead of screams to communicate his needs. It took time for him to gain trust that he would be listened to. He began to participate in strategies to control his pain instead of simply resisting.
- Range of motion: Despite passive stretch and scar massage twice a day, Keegan's scars were quite active and he demonstrated tightness at the end range for neck extension and shoulder abduction. He continued to be positioned in neck extension over a towel roll under his upper back, and in bilateral shoulder abduction using thermoplastic orthoses at night. This kept his actively contracting tissues on a low-load stretch overnight, and caregivers continued daily aggressive stretch. In addition, Keegan's increased participation in games involving BUEs (ball tossing) helped provide some motivation to keep stretching as well as decreased reports of pain.
- Skin integrity: multipodus boots have prevented pressure ulcer development at the heels. Grafts have adhered but are actively scarring. Scar massage and pressure garments assisted with adequate scar management.
- Functional mobility: Keegan could roll in bed independently, come from supine to sit with assistance from the bed rail, and transfer from bed to chair and reverse with minimum assistance from parent. His confidence increased significantly with a little bit of increased movement.
- Self-care skills: Keegan began donning open button-down shirts over his pressure wraps independently. He continued to require maximum assistance for lower body dressing but started showing some increased confidence and a bit of personality in his shirt choices. He started participating in toothbrushing and began initiating more fine motor activities, including crafts, picture books, and puzzles as a result.
- Leisure skills: as Keegan began to use his arms and hands more, he engaged in more games and activities with therapists and caregivers. He enjoyed tossing balls, playing video games, throwing darts, playing with bubbles, and doing crafts. He began to relax and the range of motion in his arms and hands became easier as he participated more.
- Caregiver education: Parents were involved at all stages. They were tearful and hesitant at first but were willing to learn and participate. By the time of transfer, they were able to help Keegan dress himself, transfer him from bed to chair, perform scar massage and gentle range of motion (not yet a full aggressive session), and facilitate any play Keegan enjoyed. They verbalized understanding of the expected course of care and were beginning to make plans for discharge to home.
- Disposition: transfer to a rehabilitation unit.

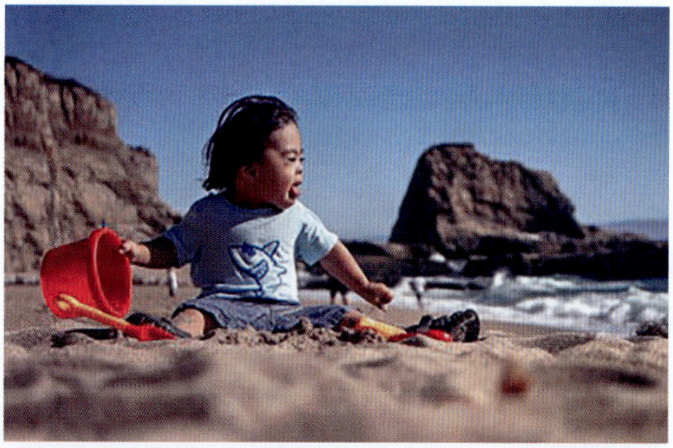

**Fig. 5.10** Children with Down syndrome benefit from exploratory play and opportunities to engage in daily activities. (Source: https://www.flickr.com/photos/98786299@N00/36909177936 https://openverse.org/image/f434fcf9-435e-474c-ab67-6d973e5fbb1d?q=child%20with%20down%20syndrome Credit: "Absorbed in playing with sand" by PeterThoeny is licensed under CC BY-NC-SA 2.0. To view a copy of this license, visit https://creativecommons.org/licenses/by-nc-sa/2.0/?ref=openverse.© Peter Thoeny, CC BY-NC-SA 4.0, HDR, 1 RAW exposure, NEX-6, _DSC7614a_hdr1bal1b.jp)

Importantly, occupational therapy practitioners address mental health challenges by engaging children in self-reflection activities and facilitating discussions, empowering children to make decisions, and involving family and friends. They create opportunities for children to socialize with others. They explore resources (such as camps and programming) to support children and their families.

## TRAUMA/ADVERSE CHILDHOOD EXPERIENCES

Trauma and **adverse childhood experiences (ACEs)** are potentially traumatic events that can have negative lasting effects on health and well-being and occur in individuals under the age of 18 years (Elmore & Crouch, 2020). One in six individuals in the United States experiences four or more ACEs (CDC, 2019). These experiences expose children to situations or events that surpass their ability to cope (such as abuse, neglect, and household dysfunction). The trauma may occur once, as a series of events, or be continuous (National Center on Early Childhood Health and Wellness, 2023). Toxic stress or repeated adverse experiences can cause permanent damage to the developing brain and immune and endocrine systems, predisposing them to considerable risk of chronic diseases and early death (Boullier & Blair, 2018). The specific diagnosis of ACEs does not currently exist in the ICD-11.

**Causes.** ACEs include (National Center on Early Childhood Health and Wellness, 2023):

- Physical abuse
- Sexual abuse
- Emotional abuse
- Emotional neglect
- Physical neglect
- Mentally ill, depressed, or suicidal person in the home
- Drug addict in home
- Alcoholic in home
- Witnessing domestic violence against the mother

**Characteristics and Symptoms.** Children and youth who have experienced ACEs or trauma exhibit psychosocial challenges, such as:

- Extreme fear
- Guilt
- Helplessness
- Shame
- Dissociation from body and surroundings
- Numb to physical and feelings
- Feels like floating outside of the body
- No memories of the event (National Center on Early Childhood Health and Wellness, 2023).

Children who experience a greater number of ACEs and those who experience ACEs for an extended time are prone to challenges disrupting their ability to engage in everyday activities. They may experience behavioral problems, difficulties with concentration, memory, and learning, and poor executive functioning. They may experience cardiovascular disease because of chronic stress. They are more likely to engage in behaviors that are harmful to their health (e.g., smoking, drinking alcohol, antisocial behaviors) leading to poor adult health (Boullier & Blair, 2018). Children as young as 6 years of age who are exposed to one ACE are twice as likely to exhibit poor physical health (Boullier & Blair, 2018).

**Challenges in Occupational Participation.** Occupational participation deficits in children and youth with Trauma/ACE can occur in any occupation (see Box 5.3). Children may be unable to participate in activities because they experience fear, shame, and guilt. They may withdraw, become angry, or be defiant when triggered (i.e., reminded of events). They may cope for some time and then experience an emotional change (which may be triggered by a memory, event, or situation). They may become resistant and afraid of familiar people. For example, a child may refuse to participate in school, recess, or a project.

Children and youth who have experienced ACEs have difficulty participating in school, home, and the community. The adverse experiences (which may be ongoing) interfere with their ability to develop a positive sense of self, develop positive coping methods, and enjoy childhood. They may be afraid for their safety and not able to seek out help. They may withdraw from social activities and find comfort in drugs or unhealthy behaviors. They may have difficulty establishing trusting relationships with adults and others. The uncertainty and fear may interfere with their habits and routines, affecting their academic work.

**Implications for Occupational Therapy.** Occupational therapy practitioners meet children and youth "where they are at" (i.e., emotionally) at that moment in time and use therapeutic use of self to establish a rapport and understand the child's needs. Through an activity-based nonthreatening approach whereby the practitioner grades the activity and provides needed cues, the child engages in the activity. By engaging in the everyday things that are meaningful to the child (such as completing a simple craft project), children develop a sense of competence and efficacy, which leads to a sense of control and self-determination that may not develop in children with a history of ACEs. The occupational therapy practitioner skillfully enables the child to complete daily occupations, such as school, play, and self-care. Together, they create strategies to support performance over time, such as a visual schedule showing breaks. Occupational therapy practitioners may teach children sensory calming strategies, cognitive behavioral therapy techniques, and coping skills to use over time. They engage children in playful, creative, and novel activities that support problem-solving and allow children to develop positive interests and a sense of occupational identity. The practitioner reinforces to the child that they have trusting adults, resources, and friends to support them. The process takes time and children benefit from finding support with counselors as well.

Occupational therapy practitioners can facilitate resilience in youths by creating positive programming to engage children and youth in creating social connections, confidence, character, competence, and contributions (Wilburn et al., 2022). They may engage children in play and leisure activities to empower children and youth to experience positive connections and enjoy feelings of satisfaction and well-being (Wilburn et al., 2022). Occupational therapy practitioners support children and families by providing community-based interventions within their community.

## SUMMARY

This chapter aimed to provide an overview of the causes, characteristics, and symptoms of some health impairments and conditions that children and youth receiving occupational therapy may experience. For each condition, the authors described challenges in occupational participation children and youth may experience and the implications for occupational therapy intervention. Occupational therapy practitioners can use this information to guide professional reasoning.

1. The causes, characteristics, symptoms, and associated occupational challenges vary according to the specific condition.
2. Occupational therapy practitioners use knowledge of conditions as part of scientific reasoning to explore factors that are unique to the condition. Understanding the condition provides initial information that can direct the assessment process. Practitioners evaluate the child's occupational performance, motivations, routines, habits, and interests, along with their cultural expectations, resources, and environment, to gain a thorough understanding of how the child's condition affects occupational performance. Occupational therapy practitioners do not treat conditions but rather treat children.

## REFERENCES


American Occupational Therapy Association. (2020). Occupational therapy practice framework: Domain & process (4th ed.). *American Journal of Occupational Therapy*, *74*(Suppl. 2). https://doi.org/10.5014/ajot.2020.74S2001.

American Psychiatric Association. (2022). In *Diagnostic and statistical manual of mental disorders* (5th ed.). American Psychiatric Association. https://doi.org/10.1176/appi.books.970890425787. (text rev.).

American Psychiatric Association. (2023a). *Depression*. https://www.psychiatry.org/patients-families/depression/what-is-depression.

American Psychiatric Association. (2023b). *Eating disorders*. https://www.psychiatry.org/patients-families/eating-disorders/what-are-eating-disorders.

American Psychological Association. (2023c). *Anxiety disorders*. https://www.apa.org/topics/anxiety#:~:text=People%20with%20anxiety%20disorders%20usually,they%20are%20often%20used%20interchangeably.

Andelin, L., Reynolds, S., & Schoen, S. (2021). Effectiveness of occupational therapy using a sensory integration approach: A multiple-baseline design study. *American Journal of Occupational Therapy*, *75*(6),7506205030.

Anderson, V. A, Catroppa, C., Dudgeon, P., Morse, S. A., Haritou, F., & Rosenfield, J. V. (2006). Understanding predictors of functional recovery and outcome 30 months following early childhood head injury. *Neuropsychology*, *20*(1), 42–57.

Antonarakis, S. E., Skotko, B. G., Rafii, M. S., Strydom, A., Pape, S. E., Bianchi, D. W., Sherman, S., & Reeves, R. H. (2020). Down syndrome. *Nature Reviews Disease Primers*, *6*(1), 9.

Baio, J., Wiggins, L., Christensen, D. L., Maenner, M. J., Daniels, J., Warren, Z., Kurzius-Spencer, M., Zahorodny, W., Robinson Rosenberg, C., White, T., Durkin, M. S., Imm, P., Nikolaou, L., Yeargin-Allsopp, M., Lee, L. C., Harrington, R., Lopez, M., Fitzgerald, R. T., Hewitt, A., Pettygrove, S., … Dowling, N. F. (2018). Prevalence of autism spectrum disorder among children aged 8 years - autism and developmental disabilities monitoring network, 11 Sites, United States, 2014. *Morbidity and Mortality Weekly Report*, *67*(6), 1–23.

Bax, M., Goldstein, M., Rosenbaum, P., Leviton, A., Paneth, N., Dan, B., Jacobsson, B., Damiano, D., & Executive Committee for the Definition of Cerebral Palsy. (2005). Proposed definition and classfication of cerebral palsy. *Developmental Medicine and Child Neurology*, *47*(8), 571–576 10.1017/s001216220500112x.

Beltrami, A., Hilliard, A., & Green, A. L. (2022). Demographic and socioeconomic disparities in pediatric cancer in the United States: Current knowledge, deepening understanding, and expanding intervention. *Cancer Epidemiology*, *76*(102082).

Benmelouka, A., Shamseldin, L. S., Nourelden, A. Z., & Negida, A. (2020). A review on the etiology and management of pediatric traumatic spinal cord injuries. *Advanced Journal of Emergency Medicine*, *4*(2).

Boisgontier, M. P., Cheval, B., & Schmidt, J. (2020). Daily life physical activity and concussion symptoms in adolescents. *Canadian Journal of Occupational Therapy*, *87*(5), 364–371.

Botha, M., Hanlon, J., & Williams, G. L. (2023). Does language matter? Identity-first versus person-first language use in autism research: A response to Vivanti. *Journal Autism and Development Disorders*, *53*(2), 870–878. https://doi.org/10.1007/s10803-020-04858-w.

Boullier, M., & Blair, M. (2018). Adverse childhood experiences. *Pediatrics and Child Health*, *28*(3), 133–137.

Boyt-Schell, B. A. (2019). Professional reasoning in practice. In B. A. B. Schell, & G. Gillen (Eds.), *Willard and Spackman's' occupational therapy* (13th ed.) (pp. 482–497). Wolters Kluwer.

Brent, D. A., Brunwaser, S. M., Hollon, S. D., Weersing, V. R., Clarke, G. N., Dickerson, J. F., & Garber, J. (2015). Effect of a cognitive-behavioral prevention program on depression 6 years after implementation among at-risk adolescents: A randomized clinical trial. *JAMA Psychiatric*, *72*, 1110–1118.

Brunstrom-Hernandez, J., Shah, M., & Tilton, A. (2022). Clinical features and management of cerebral palsy. In H. R. Winn (Ed.), *Youmans and Winn Neurological surgery* (8th ed.) (pp. 2047–2054). Elsevier.

Bryant-Waugh, R. (2019). Feeding and eating disorders in children. *Psychiatric Clinics of North America*, *42*, 157–167.

Bury, S. M., Jellett, R., Spoor, J. R., & Hedley, D. (2023). "It defines who I am" or "It's something I have": What language do [Autistic] Australian adults [on the Austim spectrum] prefer? *Journal of Autism and Developmental Disorders*, *53*(2), 677–687. https://doi.org/10.1007/s10803-020-04425-3.

Cahill, S. M., Egan, B. E., & Seber, J. (2020). Activity- and occupation-based interventions to support mental health, positive behavior, and social participation for children and youth: A systematic review. *American Journal of Occupational Therapy*, *74*,7402180020.

Center for Disease Control and Prevention (CDC; 2023). *Birth defects: Facts about Down syndrome.* https://www.cdc.gov/ncbddd/birthdefects/downsyndrome.html#print.

Center for Disease Control and Prevention (CDC; 2019). *CDC vital signs: Adverse childhood experiences (ACEs).* https://www.cdc.gov/vitalsigns/aces/pdf/vs-1105-aces-H.pdf.

Center for Disease Control and Prevention (CDC; 2022). *Increase in developmental disabilities among children in the United States.* https://www.cdc.gov/ncbddd/developmentaldisabilities/features/increase-in-developmental-disabilities.html.

Chafetz, R. S., Mulcahey, M. J., Betz, R. R., Anderson, C., Vogel, L. C., Gaughan, J. P., Odel, M. A., Flanagan, A., & McDonald, C. M. (2007). Impact of prophylactic thoracolumbosacral orthosis bracing on functional activities and activities of daily living in the pediatric spinal cord injury population. *Journal of Spinal Cord Medicine*, *30*(Suppl.1), 178–183. https://doi.org/10.1080/10790268.2007.1154598.

Chapman, R., & Botha, M. (2023). Neurodivergence–informed therapy. *Developmental Medicine and Child Neurology*, *65*(3), 310–317.

Chen, Q., Hartman, C. A., Kuja-Halkola, R., Faraone, S. V., Almqvist, C., & Larsson, H. (2019). Attention-deficit/hyperactivity disorder and clinically diagnosed obesity in adolescence and young adulthood: A register-based study in Sweden. *Psychological Medicine*, *49*(11), 1841–1849.

Chen, D., Huang, M., Yin, Y., Gui, D., Gu, Y., Zhuang, T., Chen, C., & Huo, K. (2022). Risk factors of cerebral palsy in children: A systematic review and meta-analysis. *Translational Pediatrics*, *11*(4), 22–78. https://doi.org/10.21037/tp-22-78.

Como, D. H., Stein Duker, L. I., Polido, J. C., & Cermak, S. A. (2021). Oral health and Autism Spectrum Disorders: A unique collaboration between dentistry and occupational therapy. *International Journal of Environmental Research and Public Health*, *18*(1), 135.

Cortese, S., Wang, F., Angriman, M., Masi, G., & Bruni, O. (2020). Sleep disorders in children and adolescents with autism spectrum disorder: Diagnosis, epidemiology, and management. *CNS Drugs*, *34*, 415–423.

Craig, S. G., Weiss, M. D., Hudec, K. L., & Gibbins, C. (2020). The functional impact of sleep disorders in children with ADHD. *Journal of Attention Disorders*, *24*(3), 499–508.

Culbert, K. M., Racine, S. E., & Klump, K. L. (2015). Research Review: What we have learned about the causes of eating disorders–a synthesis of sociocultural, psychological, and biological research. *Journal of Child Psychology and Psychiatry*, *56*(11), 1141–1164.

Cunha, N. S., Malvea, A., Sadat, S., Fehlings, M. G., & Ibrahim, G. (2023). Pediatric spinal cord injury: A review. https://www.preprints.org/manuscript/202306.1924/download/final_file.

Dallman, A. R., Artis, J., Watson, L., & Wright, S. (2021). Systematic review of disparities and differences in the access and use of allied health services amongst children with autism spectrum disorders. *Journal of Autism and Developmental Disorders*, *51*, 1316–1330.

Dallman, A. R., Williams, K. L., & Villa, L. (2022). Neurodiversity-affirming practices are a moral imperative for occupational therapy. *The Open Journal of Occupational Therapy*, *10*(2), 1–9.

Daniels, A. M., & Mandell, D. S. (2014). Explaining differences in age at autism spectrum disorder diagnosis: A critical review. *Autism*, *18*(5), 583–597.

Dionsio, M. C., & Terrill, A. L. (2022). Constraint-induced movement therapy for infants with or at risk for cerebral palsy: A scoping review. *American Journal of Occupational Therapy*, *76*,7602205120.

Dominguez-Lucio, S., Compan-Gabucio, L. M., Torres-Collado, L., & de la Hera, M. G. (2023). Occupational therapy interventions using new technologies in children and adolescents with Autism Spectrum Disorder: A scoping review. *Journal of Autism and Developmental Disorders*, *53*(1), 332–358. https://doi.org/10.1007/s10803-022-05431-3.

Dynia, J. M., Walton, K. M., Sagester, G. M., Schmidt, E. K., & Tanner, K. J. (2023). Addressing sensory needs for children with Autism Spectrum Disorder in the classroom. *Intervention in School and Clinic*, *58*(4), 257–263.

Elmore, A. L., & Crouch, E. (2023). Anxiety, depression, and adverse childhood experiences: An update on risks and protective factors among children and youth. *Academic Pediatrics*, *23*(4), 720–721.

Elmore, A. L., & Crouch, E. (2020). The association of adverse childhood experiences with anxiety and depression for children and youth, 8 to 17 years of age. *Academic Pediatrics*, *20*(5), 600–608.

Epkins, C. C., & Seegan, P. L. (2015). Mother-reported and children's perceived social and academic competence in clinic referred youth: Unique relations to depression and/or social anxiety and the role of self-perceptions. *Child Psychiatry and Human Development*, *46*, 656–670.

Faraone, S. V., Banaschewski, T., Coghill, D., Zheng, Y., Biederman, J., Bellgrove, M. A., & Wang, Y. (2021). The world federation of ADHD international consensus statement: 208 evidence-based conclusions about the disorder. *Neuroscience & Biobehavioral Reviews*, *128*, 789–818.

Fischer, C., Petriccione, M., Donzelli, M., & Pottenger, E. (2016). Improving care in pediatric neuro-oncology patients: An overview of the unique needs of children with brain tumors. *Journal of Child Neurology*, *31*(4), 488–505.

Fox, A., Dishman, S., Valicek, M., Ratcliff, K., & Hilton, C. (2020). Effectiveness of social skills interventions incorporating peer interactions for children with attention deficit hyperactivity disorder: A systematic review. *American Journal of Occupational Therapy*, *74*,7402180070.

Fuermaier, A. B., Tucha, L., Butzbach, M., Weisbrod, M., Aschenbrenner, S., & Tucha, O. (2021). ADHD at the workplace: ADHD symptoms, diagnostic status, and work-related functioning. *Journal of Neural Transmission*, *128*, 1021–1031.

Garcia Reidy, T., Cocker-Bolt, P., & Naber, E. (2021). Cerebral palsy. In J. Solomon, & J. C. O'Brien (Eds.), *Pediatric skills for occupational therapy assistants* (5th ed.) (pp. 350–373). Elsevier.

Garro, A., Thomas, S. K., Kerwin, M. E., & Ducett, J. P. (2005). Parent/caregiver stress during pediatric hospitalization for chronic feeding problems. *Journal of Pediatric Nursing, 20*, 268–275.

Global Down Sydrome Foundation. (2018). *FAQ and Facts about Down syndrome.* https://www.globaldownsyndrome.org/about-down-syndrome/facts-about-down-syndrome/?gclid=CjwKCAjwqZSlBhBwEiwAfoZUIN9J3LIBCpoOOZucnp0b9GYghq5MBHbTb-F6T8B2EPgDE4B-LyVFGxoCEnAQAvD_BwE.

Glod, M., Riby, D. M., & Rodgers, J. (2019). Relationships between sensory processing, repetitive behaviors, anxiety, and intolerance of uncertainty in autism spectrum disorder and Williams syndrome. *Autism Research, 12*(5), 759–765.

Gosa, M., Carden, H. T., Jackes, C. C., Threadgill, A. Y., & Sidlowvsky, T. C. (2017). Evidence to support treatment options for children with swallowing and feeding disorders: A systematic review. *Journal of Pediatric Rehabilitation Medicine: An Interdisciplinary Approach, 10*, 107–136.

Graber, A., & Graber, J. (2023). Applied behavior analysis and the abolitionist neurodiversity critique: An ethical analysis. *Behavior Analysis in Practice, 16*(4), 1–17.

Grajo, L., Candler, C., & Sarafian, A. (2020). Interventions within the scope of occupational therapy to improve children's academic participation: A systematic review. *American Journal of Occupational Therapy, 74*,7402180030.

Grandisson, M., Rajotte, É., Godin, J., Chretien-Vincent, M., Milot, É., & Desmarais, C. (2020). Autism spectrum disorder: How can occupational therapists support schools? *Canadian Journal of Occupational Therapy, 87*(1), 30–41.

Gronski, M., & Doherty, M. (2020). Interventions within the scope of occupational therapy practice to improve activities of daily living, rest, and sleep for children ages 0 – 5 years and their families: A systematic review. *American Journal of Occupational Therapy, 74*,7402180010.

Gronski, M. P. (2021). Evidence connection – occupational therapy interventions to support feeding and toileting in children from birth to age 5 years. *American Journal of Occupational Therapy, 75*,7505390010. .

Gupta, R. (2021). Avoidant Restrictive Food Intake Disorder (ARFID)–What is it and what to do with them. *Journal of Medical & Clinical Nursing, 110*(2), 3.

Haarbauer-Krupa, J., Lee, A. H., Bitsko, R. H., Zhang, X., & Kresnow-Sedaca, M. (2018). Prevalence of parent-reported traumatic brain injury in children and associated health conditions. *JAMA Pediatrics, 172*(11), 1078–1086.

Hagen, C., Malkmus, D., & Durham, P. (1972). *Levels of cognitive functioning.* Downey, CA: Rancho Los Amigos Hospital.

Hahn-Markowitz, J., Berger, I., Manor, I., & Maeir, A. (2020). Efficacy of Cognitive-Functional (Cog-Fun) occupational therapy intervention among children with ADHD: A randomized controlled trial. *Journal of Attention Disorders, 24*(5), 655–666.

Harrowell, I., Hollén, L., Lingam, R., & Emond, A. (2018). The impact of developmental coordination disorder on educational achievement in secondary school. *Research in Developmental Disabilities, 72*, 13–22.

Hoy, M. M. P., Egan, M. Y., & Feder, K. P. (2011). A systematic review of interventions to improve handwriting. *Canadian Journal of Occupational Therapy, 78*, 13–25.

Huston, P. L., Dempster, R., & Garbacz, L. (2019). Cognitive and behavioral strategies for the treatment of feeding disorders in adolescents. *Perspectives of the ASHA Special Interests Groups, 4*, 1498–1506.

Hwang, M., Zebracki, K., Vogel, L. C., Mulcahey, M. J., & Varni, J. W. (2020). Development of the pediatric quality life inventory spinal cord injury (pedsql) module: Qualitative methods. *Spinal Cord, 58*, 1134–1142.

Ianni, L., Mazer, B., Thomas, A., & Snider, L. (2021). The role of occupational therapy with children with attention deficit hyperactivity disorder (ADHD): A Canadian national survey. *Journal of Occupational Therapy, Schools, & Early Intervention, 14*(2), 162–183.

IDEA. (2022). 2022 Annual Report to Congress on the Individuals With Disabilities Education Act (IDEA). https://sites.ed.gov/idea/2022-individuals-with-disabilities-education-act-annual-report-to-congress/.

Illie, G., Trenholm, M., Boak, A., Mann, R. E., Adlaf, E. M., Asbridge, M., Hamilton, H., Rehm, J., Rutledge, R., & Cusiman, M. D. (2020). Adolescent traumatic brain injuries: Onset, mechanism and links with current academic performance and physical injuries. *PLoS One, 15*(3). https://doi.org/10.1371/journal.pone.0229489.

Izadi-Najafabadi, S., Gunton, C., Dureno, Z., & Zwicker, J. G. (2022). Effectiveness of Cognitive Orientation to Occupational Performance intervention in improving motor skills of children with developmental coordination disorder: A randomized waitlist-control trial. *Clinical Rehabilitation, 36*(6), 776–788.

Jackson, D. B., Posick, C., Vaughn, M. G., & Testa, A. (2022). Adverse childhood experiences and traumatic brain injury among adolescents: Findings from the 2016-2018 national survey of children's health. *European Child & Adolescent Psychiatry, 31*, 289–297.

Jacobs-Nzuzi Khuabi, L. J., Swart, E., & Soeker, M. S. (2022). Towards occupational resilience: A model to facilitate high school participation post traumatic brain injury. *Work, 72*, 463–482.

Johnson, T. L., Chin, E. M., & Hoon, A. H. (2019). Cerebral palsy. In Batshaw M.L., Roizen N.J., & Pellegrino L. (Eds.), *Children with Disabilities* (8th) (p. 426). Paul H. Brookes Publishing Co.

Johnson, A. R, DeMatt, E., & Salorio, C. F (2009). Predictors of outcome followig acquired brain injury in children. *Developmental Disabilities Research Reviews, 15*(2), 124–132.

Kirby, A. V., Bilder, D. A., Wiggins, L. D., Hughes, M. M., Davis, J., Hall-Lande, J. A., Lee, L. C., McMahon, W. M., & Bakian, A. V. (2022). Sensory features in autism: Findings from a large population-based surveillance system. *Autism Research: Official Journal of the International Society for Autism Research, 15*(4), 751–760.

Krassioukov, A., Warburton, D. E., Teasell, R., & Eng, J. J. (2009). A systematic review of the management of autonomic dyreflexia after spinal cord injury. *Archives of Physical Medicine and Rehabilitation, 90*(4), 682–695. https://doi.org/10.1016/j.apmr.2008.10.017.

Krauss, A., & Schellenberg, C. (2022). ADHD symptoms and health-related quality of life of adolescents and young adults. *European Journal of Health Psychology*, 1–10.

Kuhaneck, H. M., Watling, R., & Glennon, T. J. (2023). Ayres sensory Integration® for addressing play in autistic children: A multiple-baseline examination. *American Journal of Occupational Therapy, 77*(2),7702205080.

Kuhaneck, H., Spitzer, S. L., & Bodison, S. C. (2020). A systematic review of intervention to improve the occupation of play in children with autism. *OTJR: Occupation, Participation and Health, 40*(2), 83–98.

Laverdure, P., & Beisbier, S. (2021). Occupation- and activity-based interventions to improve performance of activities of daily living, play, and leisure for children and youth ages 5 to 21: A systematic review. *American Journal of Occupational Therapy, 75*,7501205050.

Lemke, D. M. (2007). Sympathetic storming after severe traumatic brain injury. *Critical Care Nurse, 27*(1), 30–37.

Licari, M. K., Alvares, G. A., Varcin, K., Evans, K. L., Cleary, D., Reid, S. L., & Whitehouse, A. J. (2020). Prevalence of motor difficulties in autism spectrum disorder: Analysis of a population–based cohort. *Autism Research, 13*(2), 298–306.

Lin, K., & Wroten, M. (2024). *Ranchos Los Amigos Scale. NCBI Bookshelf.* StatPearl Publishing LLC.

Lindvall Dahlgren, C., Wisting, L., & Rø, Ø. (2017). Feeding and eating disorders in the DSM-5 era: A systematic review of prevalence rates in non-clinical male and female samples. *Journal of eating disorders, 5*, 56.

Mass, A., Fitzgerald, M., Gao, G., Gupta, D., Hutchinson, P., Manley, G. T., & Menon, D. K. (2022). Traumatic brain injury over the past 20 years: Research and clinical progress. *The Lancet Neurology, 21*(9), 768–770. https://doi.org/10.1016/S1474-4422(22)00307-6.

Miller, M. (2021). Pediatric health conditions. In J. Solomon, & J. C. O'Brien (Eds.), *Pediatric skills for occupational therapy assistants* (5th ed.) (pp. 214–262). Elsevier.

Nas, K., Yazmalar, L., Sah, V., Aydin, A., & Oneg, K. (2015). Rehabilitation of spinal cord injuries. *World Journal of Orthopedics, 6*(1), 8–16.

National Center on Early Childhood Health and Wellness. (2023). *Trauma and Adverse Childhood Experiences (ACEs).* https://eclkc.ohs.acf.hhs.gov/publication/trauma-adverse-childhood-experiences-aces.

Nimer, J., & Lundahl, B. (2007). Animal-assisted therapy: A meta analysis. *Arthrozoos, 20*(3), 225–238. https://doi.org/10.2752/089279307X224773.

Novak, I., & Honan, I. (2019). Effectiveness of paediatric occupational therapy for children with disabilities: A systematic review. *Australian Occupational Therapy Journal, 66*(3), 258–273.

Nurmik, M., Ullmann, P., Rodriguez, F., Haan, S., & Letellier, E. (2020). In search of definitions: Cancer–associated fibroblasts and their markers. *International Journal of Cancer, 146*(4), 895–905.

O'Haire, M. E. (2017). Research on animal-assisted intervention and autism spectrum disorder. *Applied Developmental Science, 21*(3), 200–216. https://doi.org/10.1080/10888691.2016.1243988.

O'Haire, M. E., McKenzie, S. J., Beck, A. M., & Slaughter, V. (2013). Social behaviors increase in children with autim in the presence of animals compared to toys. *PLoS One, 8*(2):e57010. https://doi.org/10.1371/journal.pone.0057010.

Pashmdarfard, M., Richards, L. G., & Amini, M. (2021). Factors affecting participation of children with cerebral palsy in meaningful activities: Systematic review. *Occupational Therapy in Health Care, 35*(4), 442–479.

Patnaude, M. E. (2023). Student success: Therapeutic reasoning process. In J. O'Brien, M. E. Patnaude, & T. G. Reidy (Eds.), *Therapeutic reasoning in occupational therapy: How to develop critical thinking for practice* (pp. 1–14). Elsevier.

Patriquin, M., MacKenzie, D., & Versnel, J. (2020). Occupational therapy interventions for restricted and repetitive behaviors in children with autism spectrum disorder. *Occupational Therapy in Mental Health, 36*(1), 85–104.

Patten, K. K. (2022). Eleanor Clarke Slagle Lecture - finding our strengths: Recognizing professional bias and interrogating systems. *American Journal of Occupational Therapy, 76*,7606150010.

Peña, M., Ng, Y., Ripat, J., & Anagnostou, E. (2021). Brief report: Parent perspectives on sensory-based interventions for children with autism spectrum disorder. *Journal of Autism and Developmental Disorders, 51*, 2109–2114.

Posar, A., & Visconti, P. (2020). Sleep problems in children with autism spectrum disorder. *Pediatric Annals, 49*(6), e278–e282.

Presson, A. P., Paryka, G., Jensen, K. M., Devine, O. J., Rasmussen, S. A., McCabe, L. L., & McCabe, E. R. B. (2013). Current estimate of Down syndrome population prevalence in the United States. *The Journal of Pediatrics, 163*, 1163–1168.

Read, H., Roush, S., & Downing, D. (2018). Early intervention in mental health of adolescents and young adults: A systematic review. *American Journal of Occupational Therapy, 72*,7205190040.

Rupp, R., Biering-Sorensen, F., Burns, S. P., Graves, D. E., Guest, J., Jones, L., Schmidt Read, M., Rodriguez, G. M., Schuld, C., Tansey, K. E., Walden, K., & Kirshblum, S. (2021). International standards for neurological classification of spinal cord injury: Revised 2019. *Topics in Spinal Cord Injury Rehabilitation, 27*(2), 1–22. https://doi.org/10.46292/sci2702-1.

Sadowska, M., Sarecka-Hujar, B., & Kopyta, I. (2020). Cerebral palsy: Current opinions on definition, epidemiology, risk factors, classification and treatment options. *Neuropsychiatric Disease and Treatment*, 1505–1518.

Schaaf, R. C., Dumont, R. L., Arbesman, M., & May-Benson, T. A. (2018). Efficacy of occupational therapy using Ayres Sensory Integration®: A systematic review. *American Journal of Occupational Therapy, 72*(1),7201190010p1–7201190010p10.

Senapati, B. (2017). The effectiveness of play activities and functional activities on fine motor skills in children with spastic diplegic cerebral palsy. *Indian Journal of Physiotherapy & Occupational Therapy, 11*(1), 85–89.

Sharp, W. F., Volkert, V. M., Scahill, L., McCracken, C. E., & McElhanon, B. (2017). A systematic review and meta-analysis of intensive multidisciplinary intervention for pediatric feeding disorders: How standard is the standard of care? *The Journal of Pediatrics, 181*, 116–124.

Shin, J. I., Lee, N. J., & Cho, S. K. (2016). Pediatric cervical spine and spinal cord injury: A national database study. *Spine, 41*(4), 283–292.

Siegel, R. L., Miller, K. D., Fuchs, H. E., & Jemal, A. (2021). Cancer statistics, 2021. *CA: A Cancer Journal for Clinicians, 71*(1), 7–33.

Smits-Engelsman, B., Vincon, S., Blank, R., Quadrado, V. H., Polatajko, H., & Wilson, P. H. (2018). Evaluating the evidence for motor-based interventions in developmental coordination disorder: A systematic review and meta-analysis. *Research in Developmental Disabilities, 74*, 72–102.

Stice, E., Rhode, P., Seeley, J. R., & Gau, J. M. (2008). Brief cognitive-behavioral depression prevention program for high-risk adolescents outperforms two alternative interventions: A randomized efficacy trial. *Journal of Counseling and Clinical Psychology, 76*, 595–606.

Szuhany, K. L., & Simon, N. M. (2022). Anxiety disorders: A review. *JAMA, 328*(24), 2431–2445.

Tamplain, P., & Miller, H. L. (2021). What can we do to promote mental health among individuals with developmental coordination disorder? *Current Developmental Disorders Reports, 8*, 24–31.

Tanner, K., Schmidt, E., Martin, K., & Bassi, M. (2020). Interventions within the scope of occupational therapy practice to improve motor performance for children ages 0 – 5 years: A systematic review. *American Journal of Occupational Therapy, 74*,7402180060.

Taricco, M., Apolone, G., Colombo, C., Filardo, G., Telaro, E., & Liberati, A. (2000). Functional status in patients with spinal cord injury: A new standardized measurement scale. *Archives of Physical Medicine and Rehabilitation, 81*(9), 1173–1180.

Taylor, R. R., Bowyer, P., & Fisher, G. (Eds.). (2024). *Kielhofner's model of human occupation* (6th ed.). Wolters Kluwer.

Tichener, A., Dunford, C., & Wales, L. (2018). A reflective case review: Relearning handwriting after a traumatic brain injury. *British Journal of Occupational Therapy, 81*(5), 290–293.

Trottier, K., & MacDonald, D. E. (2023). Update on psychological trauma, other adverse experiences and eating disorders: State of the research and future research directions. *Current Psychiatry Reports, 19*(45).

van Den Hauwe, L., Sundgren, P. C., & Flanders, A. E. (2020). Spinal trauma and spinal cord injury (SCI). In J. Hodler, R. A. Kubik-Huch, & G. K. von Schulthess (Eds.), *Diseases of the brain, head and neck, spine 2020-2023: Diagnostic imaging [Internet]*. Springer. https://www.ncbi.nim.nih.gov/books/NBK554330.

van Hoorn, J. F., Schoemaker, M. M., Stuive, I., Dijkstra, P. U., Rodrigues Trigo Pereira, F., Van der Sluis, C. K., & Hadders–Algra, M. (2021). Risk factors in early life for developmental coordination disorder: A scoping review. *Developmental Medicine and Child Neurology, 63*(5), 511–519.

Waldman-Levi, A., & Kuhaneck, H. (2023). Father-child playfulness: A secondary analysis of a multiple-baseline single-subject study of three children with autism spectrum disorder. *American Journal of Occupational Therapy, 77*(2),7702205020.

Wijnen, V. J., Heutink, M., van Boxtel, G. J., Eilander, H. J., & de Gelder, B. (2006). Autonomic reactivty to brain injury. *Clinical Neurolphysiology, 117*(8), 1794–1807.

Wilburn, V. G., Huber, M., Senter, D., & Stoll, H. B. (2022). Considerations for occupational therapists in developing community-level interventions for youth with high adverse childhood experiences (ACEs). *The Open Journal of Occupational Therapy, 10*(1), 13.

Williams, K. L., Campi, E., & Baranek, G. T. (2021). Associations among sensory hyperresponsiveness, restricted and repetitive behaviors, and anxiety in autism: An integrated systematic review. *Research in Autism Spectrum Disorders, 83*,101763.

World Health Organization. (2022). ICD-11: International classification of diseases (11th revision). https://icd.who.int/.

Yeo, V., Phillips, N. L., Bogdanov, S., Brookes, N., Epps, A., Teng, A., Naismith, S. L., & Lah, S. (2021). The persistence of sleep disturbance and its correlates in children with moderate to severe traumatic brain injury: A longitudinal study. *Sleep Medicine*, 387–393.

Ylvisaker, M, Adelson, D. P., Braga, L. W., Burnett, S. W., Glang, A., Feeney, T., Moore, W., Rumney, P., & Todis, B. (2005). Rehabilitation and ongoing support after pediatric TBI: Twenty years of progress. *Journal of Head Trauma Rehabilitation, 20*(1), 95–109.

Zablotsky, B., Black, L. I., Maenner, M. J., Schieve, L. A., Danielson, M. L., Bitsko, R. H., Blumberg, S. J., Kogan, M. D., & Boyle, C. A. (2019). Prevalence and trends of developmental disabilities among children in the US: 2009 – 2017. *Pediatrics, 144*(4),e2019080811.

Zampella, C. J., Wang, L. A., Haley, M., Hutchinson, A. G., & de Marchena, A. (2021). Motor skill differences in autism spectrum disorder: A clinically focused review. *Current Psychiatry Reports, 23*(10), 64.

Zwicker, J. G., Missiuna, C., Harris, S. R., et al. (2012). Developmental coordination disorder: A review and update. *European Journal Pediatric Neurology, 16*, 573–581.

6

# Pediatric Settings

Leslie Jackson

## GUIDING QUESTIONS

1. What types of settings serve children and youth?
2. What laws support occupational therapy services for children and youth in each of the varied settings?
3. What are the similarities and differences in the role of occupational therapy practitioners across settings?

## KEY TERMS

Acute care
Children's hospital
Compensatory techniques
Early intervention
General hospital
Head Start and Early Head Start
Individualized Education Program
Individualized Family Service Plan
Inpatient rehabilitation
Intensive care unit (pediatric and neonatal)
Intraventricular hemorrhage
Least restrictive environment
Retinopathy of prematurity
Trauma center

## INTRODUCTION

Occupational therapy practitioners work with children in a variety of settings. Children may receive occupational therapy services in one setting or across a continuum of care depending on their needs. In each setting, the occupational therapy practitioner works with a variety of people, professionals, and staff who also have roles in caring for children. The team works together to provide coordinated and seamless care (Cahill, 2024; Casimir, 2019; Kovanis & Shivers, 2022). Occupational therapy practitioners must also understand the varied roles of the team members in different settings.

Regardless of the setting in which services are delivered, the occupational therapy practitioner focuses on enhancing occupational engagement to support the child's participation across contexts and forms collaborative partnerships with families and others involved in the care of the child (AOTA, 2020a). These collaborative partnerships with families afford opportunities for salient moments in home and family life that can influence what happens in therapy sessions and how it matters in people's lives (Lawlor & Mattingly, 2019).

Each setting has its requirements and differently determines the type of services provided and how and when a child is eligible for services. Many of these setting-specific requirements are governed by federal or state policy. Therefore, it is important for the pediatric practitioner to understand the variations across settings and the requirements and policies that may impact occupational therapy practice.

## TYPES OF PEDIATRIC HEALTH CARE

Occupational therapy practitioners working with children and families provide services in settings that can be viewed along a continuum from those most closely aligned to the medical model (i.e., hospital) to those least like the medical model (i.e., community, school, or social service agency). Children may enter the healthcare system at any point on the continuum and do not necessarily follow a direct progression through the various settings. See Fig. 6.1 for a depiction of this continuum. The continuum of pediatric settings may include:

- Hospital
- Outpatient therapy center/clinic
- Home health and community-based settings
- Early intervention (EI)
- School system
- Community/social service agency (Robinson & Fisher, 2022).

Decisions about where care is provided have to do with the severity of medical concerns, the ability of the child to leave the home safely, and the specific laws and reimbursement patterns that guide healthcare systems in the United States (US). Each organization has a different mission, method of operation, and internal organizational culture (e.g., values, practices, explicit and implicit ways of working) which affect how occupational therapy services are provided in that setting (Braveman, 2022; Robinson & Fisher, 2022). The role of the occupational therapy practitioner in each of the settings is compared in Table 6.1. Case Example 6.1 illustrates the variety of settings where children may receive services.

### Hospital Settings

Hospitals are often referred to as "medical model" settings because much of the intervention focuses on the remediation of underlying physical impairments to restore health and function (Braveman, 2022). Hospitals provide different levels of care depending on the child's needs, including acute care, intensive care, inpatient rehabilitation, and hospital-based outpatient clinics. Children receive care at a hospital for a wide variety of health, diagnostic, and intervention reasons. Nearly one of every six discharges from US hospitals in 2019 were children aged 17 years and younger, the majority of whom were

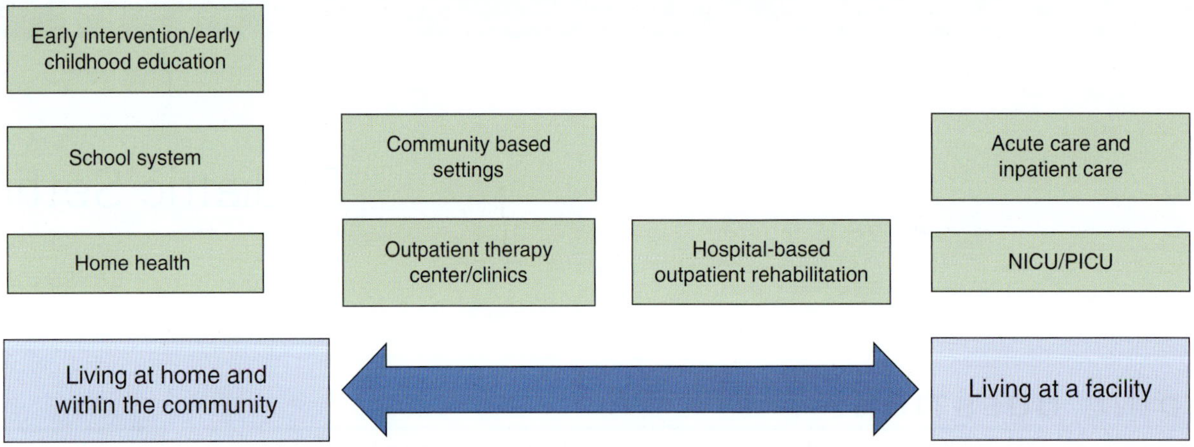


**Fig. 6.1** The continuum of care for children and youth.

**TABLE 6.1 The Role of the Occupational Therapy Practitioner in Each Setting[a]**

| Setting | Occupational Therapy's Role | Special Considerations |
|---|---|---|
| Acute care | • Conduct efficient evaluation and intervention due to short hospital stays.<br>• Support occupational performance within the limits created by the medical event.<br>• Review findings from diagnostic tests.<br>• Be aware of precautions associated with the child's status, lab values, and vital signs.<br>• Be aware of medications and common side effects.<br>• Report changes in status or behavior to the doctor or nurse.<br>• Consider the child's behavioral and mental health and the family's stress level during this time. | Practitioners work as part of a large medical team in a fast-paced environment, with children who have medical concerns. Intervention is often conducted in the child's hospital room, and coordinated around medical procedures, laboratory work, or medication schedules. |
| NICU | • Evaluate infant needs including feeding and positioning.<br>• Support caregivers in creating caregiver-infant bond.<br>• Support caregivers by identifying and helping them recognize the infant's behavioral communication.<br>• Promote infant's development and regulation.<br>• Modify environments to reduce stimulation when necessary.<br>• Consider the parent's mental health and significant stressors that are associated with having an infant in the NICU. | This is a specialized environment requiring advanced training and mentoring. |
| Inpatient rehabilitation | • Focus on resuming the roles and occupations deemed important to the child and family's life.<br>• Address cognitive, neuromuscular and musculoskeletal complications that affect occupational performance.<br>• Target restoration of lost skills and function using biomechanical, sensorimotor, perceptual-cognitive, and rehabilitative approaches.<br>• Fabricate or fit orthoses to maintain positions (e.g., resting hand orthotic), increase range of motion (e.g., dropout orthoses, dynamic orthoses with spring tension forces, or serial casting), or promote function (e.g., wrist cock-up orthosis, tenodesis orthosis).<br>• Recommend **compensatory techniques**.<br>• Teach clients adapted routines, assistive devices, and environmental modifications and/or strategies of energy conservation, joint protection, and work simplification. (See Box 6.2 for information about energy conservation techniques adapted for children.)<br>• Teach or train others to take over specific strategies or methods.<br>• Develop a transition and discharge plan, which may include a home visit.<br>• Consider the child's behavioral and mental health during the rehabilitation process. | Depending on the child's age, the team should be focusing on assisting the child's return to school and other prior activities. Although the focus may be on performance and skills, the practitioner cannot overlook the potential mental health concerns that will arise for the client and family, based on the potential lengthy course of rehabilitation, the major changes to the families' daily life, and the contemplation of long term needs that may accompany a severe illness or injury. |

TABLE 6.1 The Role of the Occupational Therapy Practitioner in Each Setting[a]—cont'd

| Setting | Occupational Therapy's Role | Special Considerations |
|---|---|---|
| Inpatient psychiatric unit | • Assist children to "develop and maintain positive mental health, prevent mental ill health, and recover from mental health challenges in order to live full and productive lives" (AOTA, 2016a).<br>• Promote self-efficacy, self-determination, responsibility, feelings of connectedness, and socialization.<br>• Engage in group intervention to foster skills such as coping, frustration tolerance, problem-solving, and goal setting. | Many units have strict protocols in place regarding client access to certain objects or materials for their safety. Clients may or may not be allowed off the unit or outside to play. These protocols may impact occupational therapy interventions. |
| Palliative care | • Facilitate quality of life.<br>• Engage clients and their caregivers in important occupations that support the families' adaptation and assist them in finding peace and preparing for death.<br>• Modify important occupations to allow their completion for someone with pain, reduced energy, emotional distress, or physical limitations from the illness. | Less a setting than a philosophy, palliative care can be provided in the home or a facility.<br>An important consideration for the practitioner working in palliative care is the necessary support caregivers will need for their roles and their mental health. |
| Outpatient setting | • Evaluate and treat a variety of possible areas of occupation.<br>• Function as a consultant and coordinate care with other settings (schools, for example).<br>• Provide recommendations for, or assist in obtaining needed adaptive equipment, orthotics, or home modifications. | May have to manage multiple insurance plans and requirements for documentation |
| Home health care | • Evaluate and intervene in a variety of occupational performance areas.<br>• Provide parent education.<br>• Advocate for needed community services.<br>• Provide recommendations for environmental adaptations.<br>• Collaborate with the family regarding physical changes to the home.<br>• Consult with others in the client's care.<br>• Case management.<br>• Seek out community-based resources.<br>• Assist the family in obtaining respite care.<br>• Supervise volunteers or run special events.<br>• Consider the child's behavioral and mental health needs. | The practitioner is a guest in the child's home and is subject to certain social rules associated with guests. Appointments should support the family's routines and not interfere with daily schedules. Families may benefit from respite care, which temporarily provides an alternative caregiver for a few hours and up to several days. Healthcare workers in the home occasionally encounter ethical dilemmas, typically involving safety, such as fire and health hazards. They must address these issues with the family openly and honestly. |
| Early intervention | • Services may be provided directly or as a consultative, transdisciplinary model. | In a primary service provider team approach, each child and family have full team support and availability to them, but one discipline or provider functions as the primary support for the family receiving consultation from the other team members. |
| Schools | • Support education and learning for all children and youth including participation in academic, non-academic, and extramural activities.<br>• Provide direct support and consultation with teachers and school staff.<br>• Adapt classroom environments to support attention and behavior.<br>• Teach cognitive strategies.<br>• Promote social-emotional competence and learning.<br>• Support children's social and emotional skill development to promote self-regulation. | A large percentage of occupational therapy practitioners (15.4% of OTAs and 18.8% of OTs) work in school settings (AOTA, 2023).<br>Occupational therapy services in schools are guided by the educational model, where all goals, related services, and supports are focused on the child's participation, performance, and function in the student role. The occupation of education includes academic (e.g., math, reading, writing), nonacademic (e.g., sports, band, cheerleading, club), and prevocational and vocational activities. |

[a]Practitioners must be mindful of the relationship between the occupational therapist and occupational therapy assistant when working in a setting that utilizes both levels. Each practitioner has a role in providing evaluation, treatment, documentation, and discharge planning (American Occupational Therapy Association AOTA, 2016; AOTA, 2016b, 2020a; Nicolson & Salinas, 2022). State practice act requirements provide details on the relationship in each state.

Table created from the following sources: (AOTA, 2013; Boucher, Downing, & Shemilt, 2014; Connecticut Birth to Three, 2016; Dudgeon, 2020; Essential Yeh, & McColl, 2019; Matthies & Smith- Gabai, 2017; Meyers & Cason, 2020; Roberts & Evenson, 2019; Shotwell & Johnson, 2017; Smith-Gabai, 2017; Stoops, 2017; Wilburn, et al., 2021; Zero to Three, 2010).

infants, including newborns (Weiss et al., 2022). Although respiratory and gastrointestinal problems are the most common reasons for hospital care for children (Pelletier et al., 2021), rehabilitation services, including occupational therapy, are provided to children with medical, neurological, musculoskeletal, and mental health disorders.

**Types of Hospitals.** Hospitals in which pediatric patients are served generally fall into three categories: general hospitals, trauma centers, and children's hospitals. **General hospitals** strive to serve the needs of the community in which they are located. Some general hospitals may also have special units dedicated to serving the needs of pediatric

## CASE EXAMPLE 6.1 EZRA'S STORY

Ezra is a happy, chubby-cheeked 15-month-old boy who was born with tetralogy of Fallot and an omphalocele. According to his mother, they found out at her 20-week ultrasound scan that something was wrong with his stomach (Fig. 6.2A). The doctor came in and talked to the parents about what was on the scan and that Ezra might have some deformities and they were unsure of how many or if anything else would come up. The parents later found out that Ezra also had a heart defect after being referred to a pediatric cardiologist (the defect was seen on the 20 week-scan and was confirmed by the cardiologist the following week). At the next doctor's appointment, the parents were asked if they wanted to terminate the pregnancy; they were told they had to decide by a certain date or else it would be too late. The parents chose to continue with the pregnancy and decided to have an amniocentesis done to see if there were any other genetic defects. Due to the nature of Ezra's diagnoses, his parents continued to have scans up until his birth to monitor his condition and make sure nothing had changed.

Ezra was born at 38 weeks gestation via C-section. He was intubated but ended up not needing anything else (Fig. 6.2B). He was in the PICU for about a week and then transferred to the NICU, where he stayed for about 4 days (Fig. 6.2C). The day before Ezra was scheduled to be discharged, the parents started to notice he would turn blue when he was crying, and it seemed like he could not catch his breath. They were so worried that they asked the doctor to take a look. It was then that Ezra's parents learned he was having a tet spell, which can be caused by activities that change the baby's heart pressure and increase the flow of oxygen-poor blood to their body. Ezra had to have surgery to place a stent in his pulmonary valve because it was so narrow. Ezra was transferred back to the PICU and had surgery. He was in the hospital another week before being discharged.

The doctors decided to wait to do a full repair until Ezra was bigger/older. Ezra had open heart surgery at 6 months and was in the hospital for a week and a half (Fig. 6.2D and E)). During this time, he received occupational therapy and physical therapy. After discharge, therapy continued at home. At 11 months Ezra had his omphalocele repaired. He was discharged on the third day and continued therapy at home. He has been receiving therapy at home for a year now, and his sitting balance and mobility have greatly improved since having his stomach repaired (Fig. 6.2F).

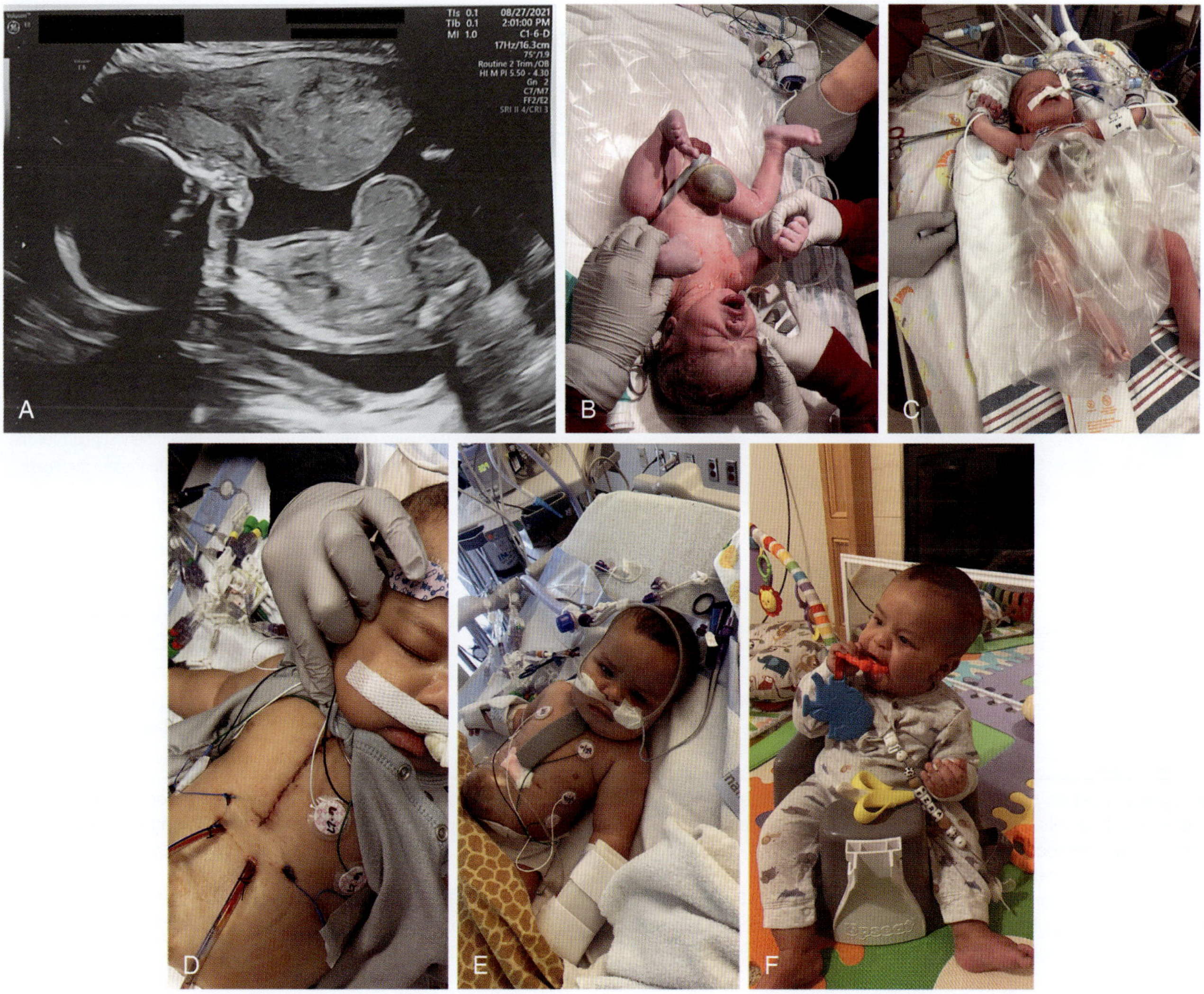


**Fig. 6.2** (A–F) Case Example 6.1 Erzra's Story. (A) Ezra's 20-week ultrasound scan shows an omphalocele. (B) Ezra (at birth) with omphalocele evident. (C) Ezra in NICU with tubes and plastic covering supporting his medical needs. (D) Ezra's at 6 months after heart surgery. (E) Ezra at 6 months after heart surgery. (F) Ezra working on sitting balance at home.

populations; however, children with more complex needs are often referred to a children's hospital.

**Trauma centers** often have burn units and other special units or programs organized to handle evaluations and treatments (e.g., splinting, positioning, and evaluating oral motor skills for feeding) that initially focus on lifesaving and sustaining procedures and preventing unnecessary complications. As a child becomes more stable, intervention may focus on activities of daily living, play, social participation, or education. Once patients are stabilized and intervention has been established, they may receive ongoing care in that hospital, or they may be transferred to a children's hospital or a general hospital closer to their own community.

**Children's hospitals** are designed to provide optimal care to infants, children, and adolescents in an environment that caters to children's needs (Casimir, 2019). Children's hospitals have missions that include advocating for children's health, conducting leading-edge pediatric research to improve clinical outcomes, and creating and implementing models for family-centered and community-based care. Because children's hospitals tend to serve a broader geographic region than general hospitals, children may be hospitalized far from home, increasing the sense of separation from family, peers, and familiar environments. The distance between the home and the hospital may affect the family's ability to visit the child and remain in contact with the health personnel caring for the child. Frequently only one family member may be available to remain with the child. This can pose psychological, social, emotional, and financial stress for families.

**Acute Care Services.** **Acute care** services include those ordered directly from a medical service or unit (e.g., intensive care neurology, neurosurgery, oncology, general surgery, orthopedics, cardiac and pulmonary services). Children are generally referred to acute care services for evaluation and intervention of their immediate needs, and assistance in planning transition to other service settings or discharge to home. Medical intervention in acute care settings is directed toward promoting medical stability and providing for safe, expedient discharge. See Table 6.1 for the practitioner's role in acute care and Table 6.2 for a description of important tests children may receive in the acute care setting.

**Intensive Care Services.** Children requiring medical care for a critical illness may be seen in an **intensive care unit** (ICU) within the hospital. Medical care in the ICU is the most complex level of care that includes spaces for medical procedures and care, family involvement, and consultation (Bigsby, 2020). The ***pediatric intensive care unit*** **(PICU)** is a critical care unit that provides medical care for children up to 18 years of age with life-threatening injuries or illnesses (MedlinePlus, 2020). ***Neonatal intensive care units*** **(NICUs)** provide intensive care to medically fragile infants including those born too early (before 37 weeks gestation) or infants of low birth weight (less than 2500 g or 5.5 lb) (AAP, 2022c). Medical care in the ICU (consisting of mechanical ventilation, neonatal surgery, and special care) is provided 24 hours a day by a team of specially trained providers, which may include occupational therapists.

***Pediatric Intensive Care Unit.*** Children receiving services in the PICU are seriously ill and have intense medical needs that cannot be met on the hospital's main medical floors. For example, children may have severe respiratory conditions, serious infections, complications of diabetes, or have been involved in a serious accident or near-drowning (Torres, 2021). They experience an illness or trauma that requires intense medical interventions from a specialized team. Fig. 6.3 A and B shows a child receiving care in the PICU.

**TABLE 6.2 Common Diagnostic Tests by Category**

| Tests | Description |
|---|---|
| Blood studies | Examine specific functions of blood cells, such as blood counts, electrolyte levels, oxygen, and the presence of markers for certain diseases. |
| Electrodiagnostic | Evaluate the body's electrical activity or performance of electronic medical devices. Examples include evoked potential studies, electrocardiogram, and electroencephalography. |
| Endoscopic studies | Examine internal body structures using an endoscope, such as arthroscopy, colonoscopy, and bronchoscopy. |
| Fluid analysis | Examine the accumulation of fluids in the body, such as lumbar puncture, arthrocentesis, and pericardiocentesis. |
| Microscopic studies | Examine samples of tissue or specimens for the presence of disease and infection. Examples include biopsy and cultures. |
| Nuclear scanning | Involve the use of a radioscope administered to the patient. Often used to stage cancers and includes bone and brain scans, PET, and thyroid scans. |
| Radiographic studies | Penetrate body structures to provide an image based on the density of the structure. Examples include barium swallow tests, cardiac catheterization, chest X-rays, and CT scans. |
| Stool tests | Detect the presence of infections, inflammation, malabsorption conditions, and intestinal bleeding. |
| Ultrasound tests | A noninvasive approach using high-frequency sound waves to create an image of the area being examined and includes Doppler ultrasounds. |
| Urine studies | Detect the presence of infection, kidney, or urinary tract diseases, or metabolic or systemic disease. |
| Misc. | Studies that do not fit into one of the other categories, such as pulmonary function tests and MRI. |

Source: Smith-Gabai, 2017

PICU levels of care from least to most intensive include community-based, tertiary, and quaternary (or specialized) as summarized in Table 6.3. Regardless of the level of PICU care, the American College of Critical Care Medicine recommends that they be cared for in child- and family-centered environments by a multidisciplinary pediatric critical care team, which often includes the occupational therapist (Frankel et al., 2019; Hsu et al., 2019. See Box 6.1 for a summary of occupational therapy practitioners' roles in the PICU and NICU.

***The Neonatal Intensive Care Unit.*** The NICU is also designated by "level" on a continuum of care (AAP, 2012; Atrium Health Floyd, 2021). See Table 6.4. Preterm infants are the largest group represented in the NICU setting. An infant's course in the NICU varies by medical severity, which also can be influenced by maternal health conditions, gestational age at birth (GA), birthweight (BW), and fetal growth in the womb (Bigsby, 2020). See Tables 6.5 and 6.6 regarding birth weight classifications. The team also categorizes birth weight as related to gestational age using standardized growth charts. See Fig. 6.4 of a typical NICU environment.

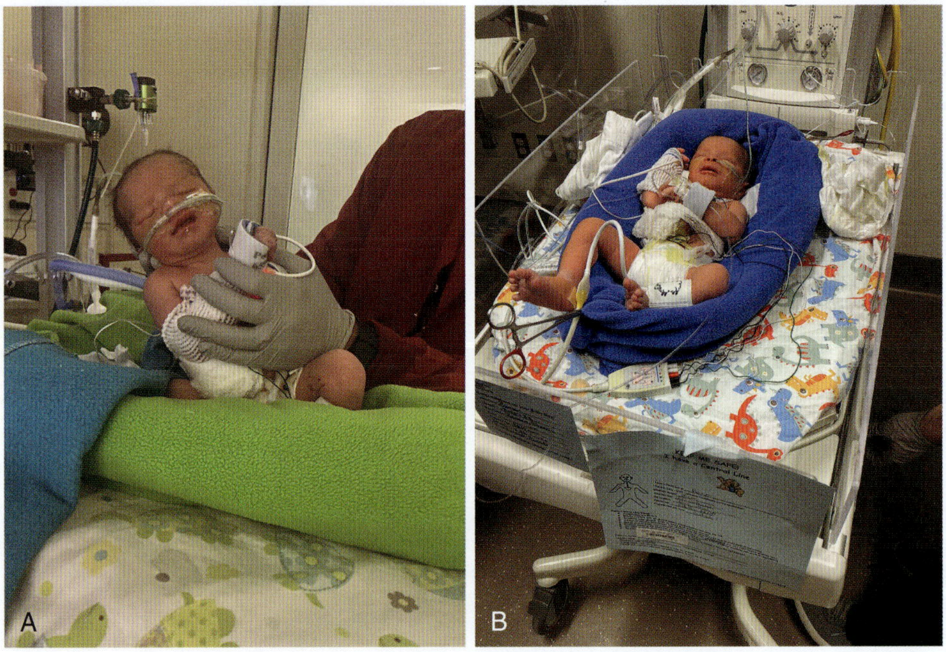

**Fig. 6.3** (A and B) Show an infant receiving care in the PICU.

**TABLE 6.3 Pediatric Intensive Care Unit Levels**

| Level | Services | Institutional Requirements |
|---|---|---|
| Community-based | Broad range of services and resources that may differ depending on the institution, hospital size, and referral base. | Predominantly in general medical-surgical institutions with the capability of treating pediatric patients. |
| Tertiary | Advanced care for medical and surgical illnesses in infants and children, including advanced ventilatory support such as high-frequency oscillatory ventilation and inotropic management (but not extracorporeal membrane oxygenation support). | Ready access to most pediatric medical subspecialties but there may not be in-house coverage. |
| Quaternary (specialized PICU) | Comprehensive care to all complex patients within a regional catchment area that serves large populations. | Provides diagnosis-specific care for select patient populations and has readily available resources to support an American College of Surgeons (ACS) verified level I or level II Children's surgical center or level I or level II pediatric trauma center. |

Adapted from Frankel et al., 2019; Hsu et al., 2019.

Premature infants are at significant risk for neurologic involvement such as **intraventricular hemorrhage** (IVH: bleeding into the ventricles, and potentially into the brain), particularly during the first 48 hours of their NICU stay (Bigsby, 2020). Intraventricular hemorrhage increases the likelihood of an ischemic condition or cystic periventricular leukomalacia, and both conditions disrupt the development of neuronal pathways (white-matter tracts) and increase the likelihood that the infant could present with a significant developmental delay and motor impairments, including cerebral palsy.

Prematurity presents significant challenges to the infant's physiologic and neurobehavioral functioning (Fig. 6.5). Additionally, preterm infants as a group are at increased risk of learning difficulties, language and cognitive delays, problems with executive function, and behavioral problems, such as attention deficit disorder (Bigsby, 2020). Immature organ and central nervous system function influences autonomic, sensory, motor, and behavioral responses.

Although necessary to sustain the infant's life, the preterm infant's prolonged need for supplemental oxygen has the potential to disrupt the maturation of the retinas of the eyes and result in **retinopathy of prematurity**, which may result in visual impairments. Infants may have trouble suckling, swallowing, and breathing, resulting in an inability to suck a bottle or breast for nutrients. They may experience gastrointestinal or sensory (such as difficulty calming) challenges.

**Hospital Inpatient Rehabilitation or Rehabilitation Hospital.** To be eligible for **inpatient rehabilitation** a child must be medically stable and able to engage in a minimum of 3 hours of intensive therapy a day, requiring at least physical therapy and occupational therapy. The typical length of stay in rehabilitation settings ranges from 2 to 3 weeks but varies according to the child's needs. A doctor who specializes in rehabilitative medicine (*physiatrist*) oversees the rehabilitation team.

Children and adolescents who sustain a sudden illness or injury (e.g., traumatic brain injury, spinal cord injury, environmental hazard, accidents, burns, near drowning, infections, neurological disorders, or cancer) may be admitted to a rehabilitation hospital. All these disorders are characterized by typical development until an acute health crisis causes loss of function, a likelihood of prolonged recovery with residual disability, and potential chronic health complications

## BOX 6.1 Occupational Therapy's Role in Pediatric Intensive Care and Neonatal Intensive Care

Due to the acute nature of patients' conditions, occupational therapists should be properly oriented to and trained for the PICU and NICU environment to maintain patient safety during interventions and reach occupational performance goals (Clark, 2017). They should develop competency with specialized equipment, medications, and medical issues. The therapist manages the many lines, tubes, drains, and monitors while also providing effective intervention. They consult and collaborate with members of the care team (i.e., respiratory therapist, nurse) to provide safe interventions for patients who are medically unstable.

The medical status of children in the PICU and NICU can change quickly and frequently, so the occupational therapist must be familiar with the medical factors that might arise, as well as with all types of medical equipment (e.g., ventilator, nasal cannula, feeding tube). The occupational therapist uses knowledge of human development, neurobehavioral organization, the musculoskeletal system, family attachment and bonding, infant and parent or caregiver mental health, stress management, and advanced feeding practices and techniques to implement intervention to address the child's and family's needs (AOTA, 2018).

The OT process in the PICU and NICU includes evaluation, goal setting and treatment planning, intervention, and discharge planning. Each step in the process is affected by the child's medical stability, cognitive ability, and any restrictions based on vital sign parameters, activity orders, attached lines, tubes, or drains (Clark, 2017). Intervention sessions are coordinated with other professionals to optimize the child's involvement. Occupational therapists provide services to prevent such secondary problems (such as decreased endurance) by using graded activities and soliciting the child's participation to maintain strength and to enhance functional capacities. Establishing a routine, including regular therapy times within the intensive care unit, facilitates the child's participation.

Children seen in intensive care settings present with a multitude of medical conditions (e.g., genetic, orthopedic, cardiac, neurological, physical, immunological), ranging in severity. The occupational therapist provides direct patient care, collaborates with families, the medical team, and staff, provides family support and education, facilitates system changes in the ICU environment, and employs caregiving practices that are neuroprotective to the child and supportive of the family as partners in care.

To protect vulnerable infants and children and their families and optimize their outcomes, the pediatric ICU requires continuous assessment and a dynamic approach to intervention planning. Providing optimal care requires experienced therapists who perform at an advanced level of practice, possess excellent critical thinking skills and a high degree of situational awareness, and the ability to participate on an interprofessional team that includes the family (AOTA, 2018; Bigsby, 2020). As such, occupational therapy practice in this area is appropriate only for occupational therapists with advanced knowledge and skills; it is not a recommended area of practice for entry-level therapists (Bigsby, 2020) or occupational therapy assistants because such knowledge and skills are beyond the scope of their practice (AOTA, 2018).

associated with disability. The purpose of rehabilitation is to optimize the child's ability to engage in family and community life. The child may continue to receive services or follow-up at an outpatient therapy clinic (described later in this chapter).

**Inpatient Psychiatric Units.** Children who experience behavioral and mental health challenges interfering with their safety or that of others may be referred to in-patient psychiatric units. Children and adolescents admitted to inpatient units require 24-hour care for short or extended care (Roberts & Evenson, 2019). The focus of in-patient

## TABLE 6.4 NICU Levels of Care

| Level | Brief Description of Services |
|---|---|
| Level 1 NICU well baby nursery | • Provide neonatal resuscitation at every delivery.<br>• Evaluate and provide postnatal care to healthy newborn infants.<br>• Stabilize and provide care for infants born at 35–37 weeks gestation who remain physiologically stable.<br>• Stabilize newborn infants who are ill and those born less than 35 weeks gestation until transfer to a facility that can provide the appropriate level of neonatal care (AAP, 2012). |
| Level II special care nursery | • Provides close observation with continuous monitoring of heart rate, respiration, and oxygen saturation levels (02 saturation), intravenous medications, and basic respiratory support for a brief duration or continuous positive airway pressure (AAP, 2012), for infants born at 32 weeks gestation or older and weighing at least 1500 g who have physiologic immaturity or who are moderately ill with problems that are expected to resolve rapidly and are not anticipated to need subspecialty services on an urgent basis.<br>• Provide care for infants who are feeding and growing stronger or recovering after intensive care.<br>• Stabilize infants born before 32 weeks gestation and weighing less than 1500 g until transfer to higher level NICU (Atrium Health Floyd, 2021). |
| Level III NICU | • Provides more intensive services aimed at sustaining the life of the infant, including higher levels of respiratory support:<br>• Provides critical respiratory support, as well as administration of medications via venous or arterial catheters and percutaneous intravenous central catheters, as well as parenteral feeding.<br>• Surgical interventions varying in complexity, including patent ductus arteriosus ligation, gastrointestinal surgeries, and diaphragmatic hernia repair. |
| Level IV NICU | • Provides the highest level of care that includes highly complex, life-saving interventions, such as extracorporeal membrane oxygenation (i.e., heart-lung bypass) and/or complex cardiopulmonary surgeries. |

## TABLE 6.5 Birth Weight Classifications

| Term | Weight Range |
|---|---|
| Full term | 2500 g–5 kg (5.5–11 lb) |
| Low Birth Weight (LBW) | 1500–2500 g |
| Very Low Birth Weight (VLBW) | 1000–1500 g |
| Extremely Low Birth Weight (ELBW) | Less than 1000g |
| Incredibly Low Birth Weight (ILBW) | Less than 750 g |

**TABLE 6.6 Birth Weight Categories Based on Gestational Age**

| Classification | Percentile |
|---|---|
| Appropriate for gestational age (AGA) | 10th to 90th percentile |
| Small for gestational age (SGA) | Below 10th percentile |
| Large for gestational age (LGA) | Above 90th percentile |

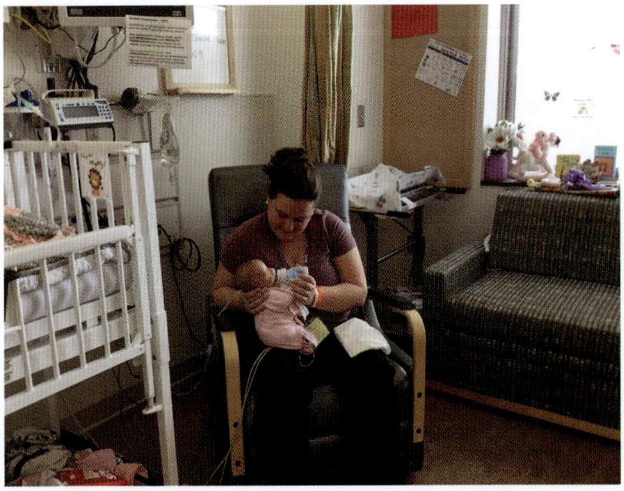

**Fig. 6.4** This former 24-week-old infant has been cared for in a single-family room throughout her NICU stay. Her parents have brought items from home to personalize her room. (Courtesy NICU, Women & Infants Hospital, Providence, RI.)

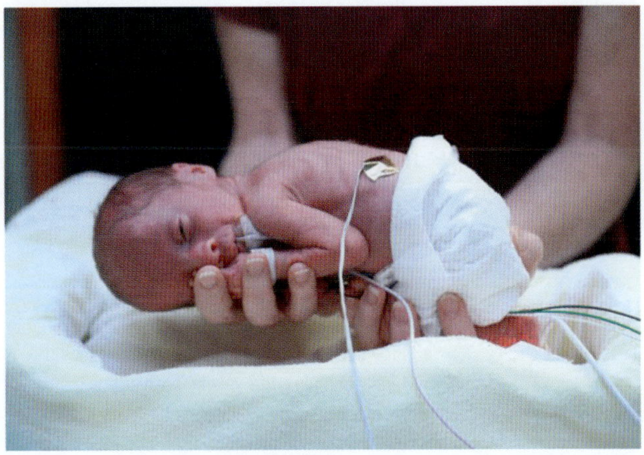

**Fig. 6.5** Infants in the NICU require careful handling. Lifting an infant in a prone position allows gravity to assist with keeping arms and legs tucked for comfort. (Courtesy NICU, Memorial Hermann Hospital Southwest, Houston, TX. Photograph by Beverly Edwards.)

psychiatric hospitalization is to stabilize the patient, which includes addressing basic self-care.

**Palliative Care Units.** Palliative care programs within hospitals have grown substantially in number in the last 20 years, with core team members typically including a doctor, nurse, chaplain, and social worker (Rogers et al., 2021). Although not yet a common setting for pediatric occupational therapy practice (Chow & Pickens, 2020), a variety of pediatric palliative care programs, hospice settings, and facilities are now available for children with life-threatening and life-shortening diseases. Palliative care, in relation to children, is "the active total care of the child's body, mind and spirit, (which) also involves giving support to the family. It begins when illness is diagnosed and continues regardless of whether a child receives treatment directed at the disease. Health providers must evaluate and alleviate a child's physical, psychological, and social distress" (World Health Organization, 2018). Palliative care is a philosophy as opposed to a specific intervention technique.

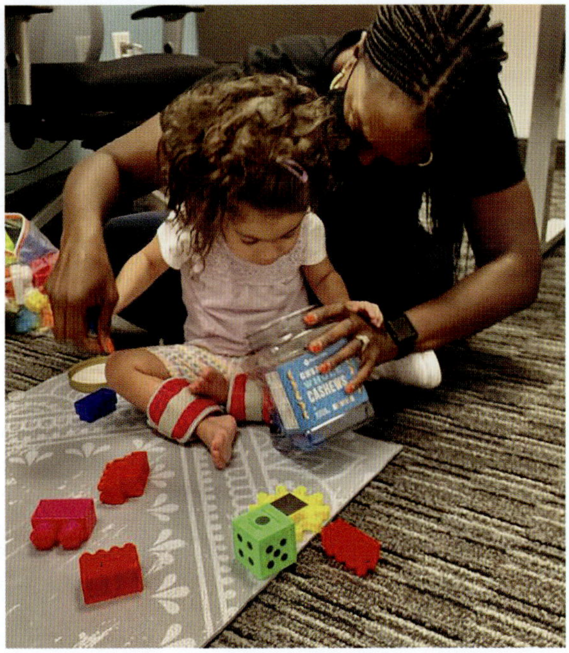

**Fig. 6.6** Young children receive occupational therapy intervention in an outpatient clinic. The practitioner facilitates movement and hand skills for play.

## Outpatient Therapy Clinic or Center

*Outpatient care* is often referred to as "ambulatory care" because the client can "walk in and out" on their own (Askin & Moore, 2014). To be considered for *outpatient rehabilitation,* the child must have a medical or surgical diagnosis with functional limitations that interfere with their ability to participate in daily life activities (Roberts & Evenson, 2019). The typical length of stay in outpatient rehabilitation settings is 3 months. Outpatient services may also include both regularly scheduled hospital-based specialty clinics that address children and families' ongoing needs and individual child services in community-based clinics. Children receiving services in this setting have functional limitations that interfere with their ability to participate in desired activities and roles (Roberts & Evenson, 2019). The child is medically stable and able to engage in a few hours of therapy and travel to an outpatient clinic. Fig. 6.6 shows a child receiving therapy in an outpatient setting.

Children and youth may be referred to an outpatient clinic for ongoing intervention, equipment-related issues, consultation, or reevaluation. The frequency of services varies based on the child's needs. For example, a child may attend therapy weekly to reach their goals after experiencing a traumatic injury. They may attend the clinic monthly to reevaluate the fit of their positioning devices. A child may attend an outpatient clinic for monitoring, such as a clinic for children who were born prematurely that monitors the child's developmental progression.

## Community Health

Community health settings allow practitioners access to the child's natural physical, social, and cultural environments. *Community-based* organizations can be small organizations focused on the delivery of a single type of service to a very specific population, or they can be large and serve a wide range of needs experienced by the community they serve (Braveman, 2022). Communities may offer resources for children and their families such as after-school programming, field trips, inclusive camp experiences, or adapted sports programs. Community-based settings may offer specialized services such as resources for driving or equipment loan programs. Community settings may also include day programs, which are more intensive than outpatient care but less intensive than hospitalization. See Fig. 6.7A and B showing children engaged in their communities.

**Day Treatment Programs.** Day treatment programs provide behavioral and mental health intervention in the community for children who do not need to be hospitalized but continue to need intervention and structure. Children and youth attending day treatment typically live at home but require support and assistance to participate in daily routines and roles. Professionals from multiple disciplines are engaged cooperatively, sharing their expertise to address the child's goals. Children may receive services in this setting to further recover functional skills following an acute injury or illness, a progressively deteriorating disorder, or a mental health diagnosis. The goal is to foster continued participation in occupations, including community reentry and participation, independent living, education, and work activities (Roberts & Evenson, 2019). Fig. 6.8 shows an occupational therapist leading a group in the community.

### Home Health

*Home health* agencies provide care in the home which affords the most natural context for intervention. Home health in pediatrics is often meant to be a transitional service as a child is either returned to school or transitioned to other long-term care services. However, for a child with a severe or chronic condition, home health services allow the family to return home while still

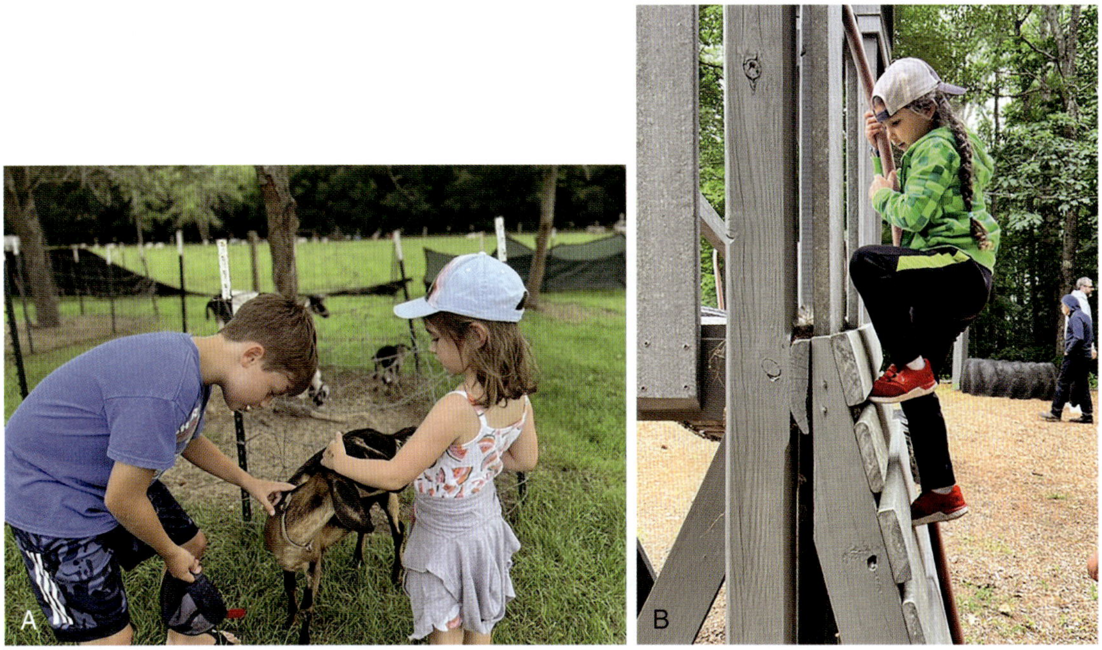


**Fig. 6.7** Children engage in community activities. (A) The children enjoy the petting zoo together. (B) Climbing on the playground equipment is challenging.

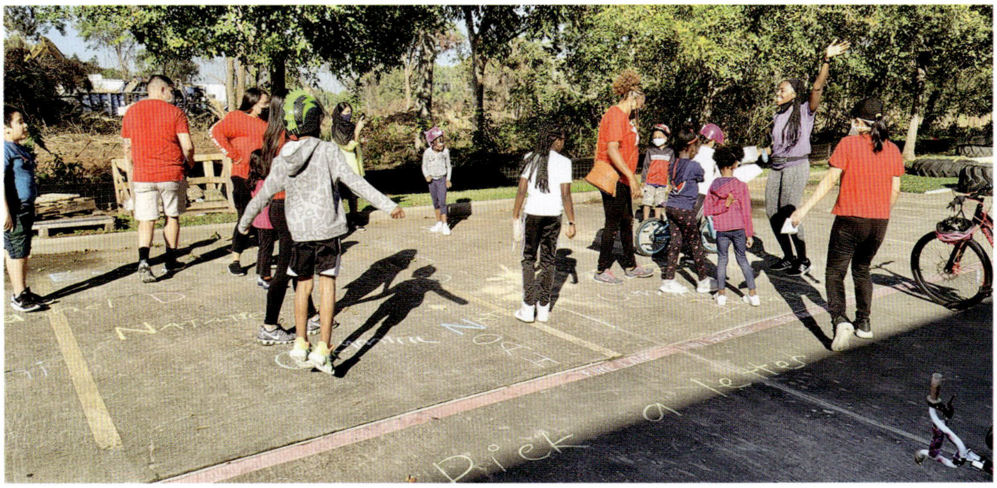

**Fig. 6.8** The occupational therapist leads a group intervention session in the community.

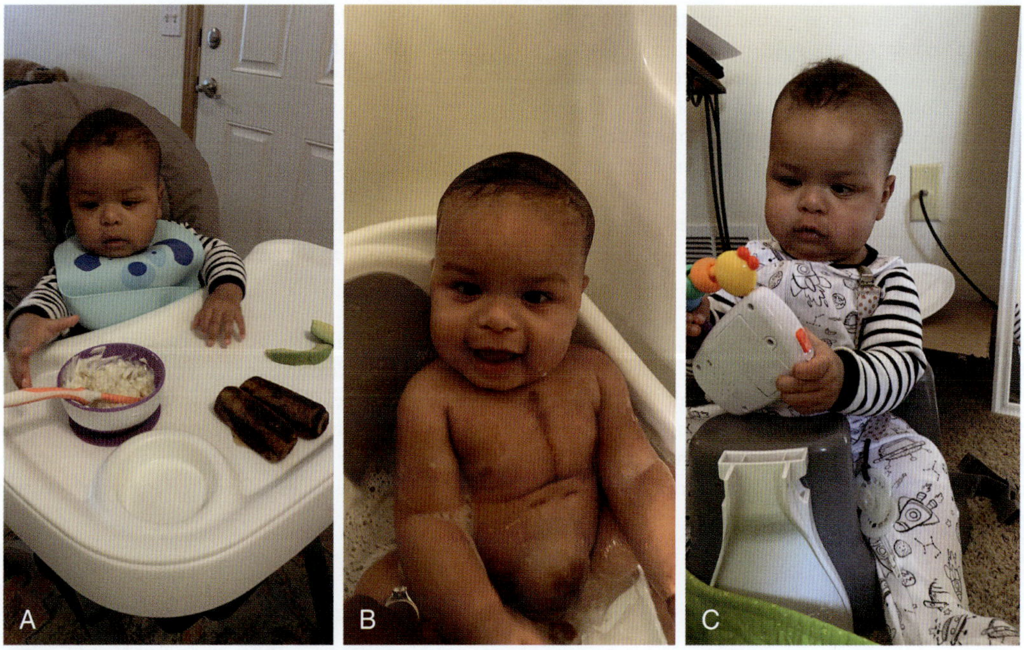


**Fig. 6.9** Occupational therapy practitioners working in early intervention settings address everyday occupations in the home, such as (A) Feeding; (B) Bathing, and (C) Play.

managing a child's intensive and perhaps lengthy medical needs. Fig. 6.9 shows young children receiving occupational therapy for feeding (Fig. 6.9A), bathing (Fig. 6.9B), and play (Fig. 6.9C) in the home. Children receiving home health care can be provided with a variety of medical and nonmedical services such as nursing care, personal care, respiratory support, medication management, wound care, and management of chronic pain. Rehabilitative care, including all therapies, can also be part of the home health package.

## Early Intervention

The early years of a child's life are critical to their health and development. Experiences and opportunities offered in the first 8 years of life lay the foundation for how children grow, learn, build relationships, and prepare for school (AAP, 2022a). Occupational therapy services for young children may be provided in **early intervention** programs, typical early childcare settings (also known as *Early Education and Care*), *Head Start,* and *Early Head Start* programs. See Chapter 15 for more information on the provision of occupational therapy in early intervention.

**Early Intervention Programs.** The EI Program for Infants and Toddlers with Disabilities, or Part C, of the Individuals with Disabilities Education Improvement Act (IDEIA), is a federal grant program that assists states in operating a comprehensive statewide program of services and supports for children birth to 3 years old with developmental delays, including (at state option) children who are "at risk" of developing a delay or special need that may affect their development or impede their education (§1435(a)). The primary goal of the Part C EI program is to enhance the capacity of families to meet the needs of their infants and toddlers.

States that participate in Part C of IDEIA are required to maintain and implement comprehensive, coordinated, multidisciplinary, interagency systems of EI services for infants and toddlers with disabilities and their families, which includes defining developmental delay and setting eligibility requirements. Infants and toddlers are eligible for EI services if they:

- experience a developmental delay in cognitive, physical, communication, social or emotional, and or adaptive development; or
- have a diagnosed physical or medical condition that may result in developmental delay (IDEIA, §1432(5) (A)).

States may also choose to include children under 3 years of age who are at risk of developing substantial delays if EI services are not provided (IDEIA, §1432(5) (B)). See Chapter 15, describing EI services.

**Early Education and Care.** Early care and education (ECE) settings are those in which children are cared for by someone other than their parents and include childcare, preschool, Head Start, prekindergarten, and nonparental home-based arrangements (i.e., babysitting) (Health Affairs, 2019). Many children in the US spend a significant amount of time in early child and education settings. According to Health Affairs (2019), 75% of preschool-age children and 46% of children younger than 1 year attended one or more nonparental arrangements; 4-year-olds were more likely to be in center-based care than 3-year-olds; children with employed mothers and those in higher-income families were more likely to be in center-based settings, while Latino children were less likely to be in such care; and half of the children living below the federal poverty level attended center-based care compared with 57% of children living at or above the poverty level. Forty-three states have some sort of publicly funded preschool program (Health Affairs, 2019), which are typically part-day, school-year programs intended for children during the year before kindergarten (usually 4-year-olds). Most programs are designed to provide care while parents work or promote children's readiness to enter kindergarten by supporting cognitive, social-emotional, and behavioral development (Health Affairs, 2019).

**Head Start/Early Head Start.** **Head Start** (children 3–5 years) and **Early Head Start** (children 0–3 years) services are available at no cost to children in eligible families. Head Start is the largest public investment in early care and education in the US, serving around 40% of 3- and

4-year-olds living in poverty (Health Affairs, 2019). It supports children's growth from birth to age five through services that support early learning and development, health, and family well-being. Head Start staff actively engage parents, recognizing family participation throughout the program as key to strong child outcomes (US Department of Health and Human Services [HHS], 2022). The goal of Head Start is to help children succeed in school and in life through learning experiences tailored to their changing needs and abilities by supporting early learning and development; health and wellness; family well-being, and family engagement (HHS, 2022). Programs deliver child development services in center-based, home-based, or family childcare settings, designed to foster strong relationships between program staff, families, and children (HHS, 2022). See Fig. 6.10 showing a child engaging in center-based learning.

Children enrolled in Early Head Start programs have significantly fewer child welfare encounters related to sexual or physical abuse between the ages of five and nine than those who do not attend (HHS, 2022). Children enrolled in Head Start programs are more likely to graduate from high school and attend college, have improved social, emotional, and behavioral development, and are better prepared to be parents themselves than similar children who did not attend the program (HHS, 2022). Children who participate in Head Start also have improved skills and better long term outcomes (Johnson & Jackson, 2019; Zhang & Dobbs-Oates, 2019).

Head Start and Early Head Start programs provide services for children with disabilities who are IDEIA-eligible (HHS, 2022). Occupational therapy and other Part C services or school services under Part B of IDEIA can be provided in these Head Start settings in accordance with the child's Individualized Family Service Plan or **Individualized Education Program (IEP)**.

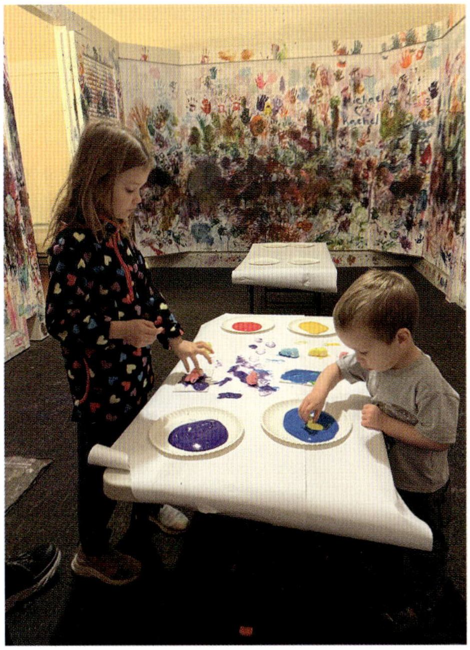

Fig. 6.10 Children engage in center-based learning in a Head Start program.

### School Settings

Each state is required to educate all elementary and high school-aged students who live within its geographic boundaries (Rioux & Chandler, 2019), including students who have disabilities. Children develop a sense of achievement as they assume school responsibilities such as getting dressed, taking the bus to school, and engaging in the school day (See Fig. 6.11). State-specific efforts are supplemented by federal programs and resources targeted to particular populations (i.e., students who are academically disadvantaged and/or have disabilities) to ensure fair and equitable educational opportunities.

Since the start of the COVID-19 pandemic, school officials have reported an increase in the number of students seeking mental health services (National Center on Education Statistics [NCES], 2022) with a concomitant increase in the percentage of staff voicing concerns about their student's mental health. Ninety-six percent of all schools in the United States reported providing mental health services for their students in the 2021–2022 school year; however, 88% did not strongly agree they could effectively meet these needs (NCES, 2022). One of the reasons noted was an inadequate number of mental health professionals.

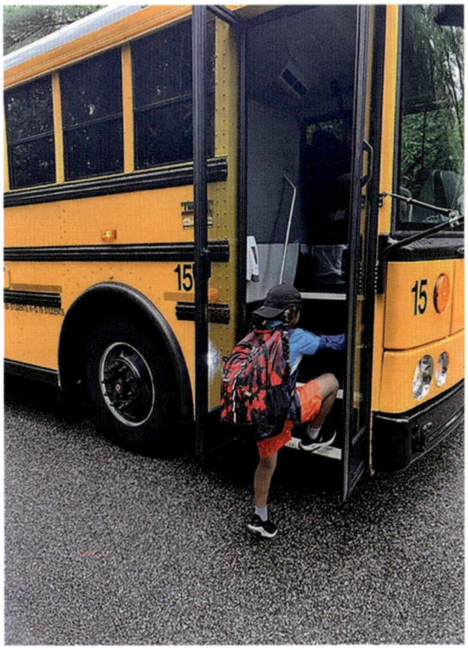

Fig. 6.11 Children enjoy taking the bus to school as part of their daily routines.

## LAWS IMPACTING OCCUPATIONAL THERAPY SERVICES

There are a variety of laws that influence occupational therapy practice in pediatrics. Many of these laws are specific to practice in the schools, but occupational therapy practice is also influenced by each state's Occupational Therapy Practice Act, the Family Educational Rights and Privacy Act of 1974 (FERPA) and related Protection of Pupil Rights Amendment (PPRA), and the Health Insurance Portability and Accountability Act of 1996 (HIPAA). Table 6.7 provides more information about these laws and their scope in relation to occupational therapy.

### Laws That Apply to Practice in the Schools

Occupational therapy practitioners working in schools must be familiar with the laws and regulations that influence service delivery, including who is eligible to receive services, when, and how. Educational systems prepare students for adult roles associated with work and community life (Cahill & Bazyk, 2020). The focus in schools is the occupation of education and the role of the student, and occupational therapy practitioners must remain current on the laws governing practice.

TABLE 6.7 **Laws Influencing Service Delivery in School Settings**

| Law | Description | Role of Occupational Therapy |
|---|---|---|
| Pub. L. 108–446<br>Individuals with Disabilities Education Improvement Act (IDEIA) | Defines special education requirements for children and youth ages 3–21. Provides children with special needs a free and appropriate public education. | Occupational therapy is considered a related service, defined as developmental, corrective, and required to assist the child with a disability to benefit from special education (§1401(26) (A)). |
| Pub. L. 93–112. Rehabilitation Act Amendments of 2004, 29 U.S.C. §794<br>Section 504 of the Rehabilitation Act of 1973 | Provides services for students who have disabilities but are not eligible for special education under IDEIA. | The focus of Section 504 is access to education (Jackson, 2019). Services may include modifications to the general education program (e.g., adjustments in test-taking procedures, or attendance policies) occupational therapy services provided under Section 504 support student engagement in learning, skill development and participation in school activities (Jackson, 2019). |
| Pub. L. 110–325<br>Americans with Disabilities Act (ADA) | ADA requires public places to provide accessibility accommodations so that people with disabilities have equal access to participate in school and community. | Services address accessibility for students with disabilities to education, such as providing ramps, adapted playgrounds, transportation to school events, and tables and chairs that allow children to participate. |
| Pub. L. 114–195<br>Every Student Succeeds Act (ESSA)<br>Previously known as *No Child Left Behind* (NCLB; Pub. L. 107–110) | The purpose of ESSA is to provide full educational opportunity to all children in America's schools, particularly to districts serving low-income students (DOE, n.d.). | Occupational therapists are considered "specialized instructional support personnel" and work to support education, health promotion and prevention, socio-emotional learning, and mental health of children. |
| *OT Practice Act*<br>Official occupational therapy scope of practice codified in state law and regulation. | Provide stipulations for occupational therapy service delivery, including evaluation, intervention, documentation, and supervision of occupational therapy assistants. Ethical and behavioral expectations for professional conduct are often included. | Each state provides stipulations regarding occupational therapy practice. Occupational therapists follow the guidelines listed in the State Practice Act (e.g., licensure law), which includes information on the role of occupational therapy within the state. |
| *FERPA* (20 U.S.C. 1232g)/*PPRA* (20 U.S.C. § 1232h) | Federal law that protects the privacy of student education records in education settings. Also applies to EI programs and other programs funded by the US Department of Education. | Occupational therapists protect the privacy of their records according to FERPA guidelines, which includes not sharing information with people who are not directly part of the team. |
| *HIPAA* | Service providers, school districts, and educational agencies billing Medicaid are also subject to HIPAA rules under protected health information provisions | Occupational therapy records include protected health information. Therapists follow HIPAA guidelines to protect children and families' information. |

Adapted from AOTA, 2017; US DOE, 2022a.

**Individuals With Disabilities Education Improvement Act.** Initially known as the Education for All Handicapped Children Act of 1975 (EHA; Pub. L. 94–142), the law is based on the constitutional principle of equal protection based on the 14th amendment (Rioux & Chandler, 2019) and has undergone multiple revisions and updates since 1975. The current version was last updated in 2004 as the Individuals with Disabilities Education Improvement Act of 2004 (IDEIA; Pub. L. 108–446).

The IDEIA requires states to provide each eligible child or youth with a disability a *free appropriate public education*, which consists of special education and related services in the least restrictive environment that allows students to fully participate and succeed in the range of school activities and prepares them for further education, employment, and independent living (§1400(d)(1)(A)). The IDEIA also guarantees parents and children with special needs certain rights and procedural safeguards (i.e., policies and procedures) that educational teams need to follow to comply with the law (Cahill & Bazyk, 2020).

A free and appropriate public education means that special education and related services meet State education standards and include an appropriate education at all levels (preschool, elementary, and secondary levels). It does not, however, guarantee that children will receive the most advanced or innovative educational methods or have access to state-of-the-art technology and materials to meet their needs.

Eligibility for IDEIA is based on whether a student meets one or more of the 10 disability categories (See Box 6.2 for a list of disability categories) and needs special education and related services (§1401(3)(A)). This means eligibility for occupational therapy and other related services is automatic if the team determines the student needs special education (specially designed instruction). It is up to the team to determine which related services are necessary to help the student benefit from special education, its frequency, duration, and location (§1414(d)) based on the results of the multidisciplinary evaluation (§1414(a)(1)(A); (§1414(b)(2); §1414(3); §1414(4); §1414(c)(1)). The child's special education and related services are described in their IEP, which is tailored to their specific needs (§1414(d)).

Occupational therapy services can be provided directly to the student, on their behalf, and/or as program supports to the teachers and other staff who work with the student (§1414(d)(A)(i)(IV)). Furthermore, occupational therapy may be identified as a supplementary aid and support (§1414(d)(A)(i)(IV)) provided in the general education classroom or other education-related settings to enable children with disabilities to be educated with nondisabled children to the maximum extent appropriate (§1401(33)). All these options present a tremendous opportunity to demonstrate the value of the full breadth of occupational therapy services in helping teachers in their role as educators in promoting student progress.

**BOX 6.2 Disability Categories According to the Individuals With Disabilities Education Improvement Act (IDEIA)**

Intellectual disabilities
Hearing impairments (including deafness)
Speech or language impairments
Visual impairments (including blindness)
Serious emotional disturbance
Orthopedic impairments
Autism
Traumatic brain injury
Other health impairments
Specific learning disabilities

**Additional Option for Children Aged 3-9**

Developmental delays in one or more of the following developmental areas:

- physical
- cognitive
- communication
- social or emotional
- adaptive

IDEIA requires teams to consider the least restrictive environment where the student will receive their educational program, including all their academic and related services. General education should be the first setting considered as potentially meeting the student's needs, before a more restrictive setting is considered. The IEP team considers a more restrictive setting "only when the nature or severity of the disability of a child is such that education in regular classes with the use of supplementary aids and services cannot be achieved satisfactorily" (§1412(5)(A)). All decisions regarding placement must be made on an individual basis, based on the child's unique educational needs, documented in the IEP, and reviewed annually. Placement decisions should not be based on the availability of space or resources.

Another area for occupational therapy support in school is that of transition (§1401(34)), which is defined as a coordinated set of activities to facilitate students' movement from school to postschool activities, including postsecondary education, employment, continuing and adult education, adult services, independent living, or community participation. See Chapters 15 and 21 on transitions.

**Section 504 and the Americans With Disabilities Act.** Section 504, as it is often called, is a civil rights law that prohibits any organization that receives federal funding from discriminating against people with disabilities (Jackson, 2019). Section 504 works in tandem with the IDEIA to ensure that school districts do not discriminate against students with disabilities while also ensuring each student's rights to special education services.

Disability is defined more broadly under Section 504 and the Americans with Disabilities Act (ADA). A student is deemed to have a disability if they (1) have a physical or mental impairment that substantially limits one or more major life activities; (2) have a record of such an impairment; or (3) are regarded as having such an impairment (34 CFR §104.3(j) (2) (i)). School districts are advised to interpret this definition in a way that allows for broad coverage (US DOE, 2022b). Major life activities include caring for oneself, education, learning, performing manual tasks, speaking, and working.

If a student's impairment significantly impacts their school performance, the school district must develop an individualized plan for accommodations and services so the student can access the same education provided to students without disabilities (Jackson, 2019). Even when a student does not need accommodations, they are entitled to other protections, including the right to be free from actions that discriminate on the basis of the student's disability (Jackson, 2019). Under Section 504 and the ADA, school districts must ensure students with disabilities have equal access to all education programs and activities that are provided to students without disabilities (DOE, 2020).

**Every Student Succeeds Act.** The purpose of the Every Student Succeeds Act (ESSA) is to increase accountability and action to effect positive change in the lowest-performing schools, where groups of students are not making progress (i.e., children most at risk of poor performance), and where graduation rates are low over extended periods (Schneider & Chandler, 2019; US DOE, n.d.). A previous version of the law, known as No Child Left Behind (Pub. L. 107-110), stressed the use of high stakes testing and punitive measures in an effort to incentivize schools to improve student performance and progress (National Alliance of Specialized Instructional Support Personnel [NASISP], 2022). As a result, ESSA shifts a great deal of oversight and discretion to the State and local education agencies to establish their own accountability goals and monitoring systems, which may be less reliant on standardized assessments as a single measure of performance or improvement (Cahill & Bazyk, 2020), while retaining the an expectation that there will be appropriate action to effect positive change in the lowest-performing schools (DOE, n.d.; Schneider & Chandler, 2019).

Occupational therapy practitioners are considered "specialized instructional support personnel" in Title II of the law. They work with teachers, administrators, and parents to ensure that all students are successful in school. In this role, practitioners consult with other personnel to support the academic achievement of students, participate in school-wide systems of support (i.e., multitiered systems of support to address learning and mental health needs), and provide professional development training designed to give teachers and instructional staff, "the knowledge and skills to provide instruction and academic support services, to those children, including positive behavioral interventions and supports, multi-tier system of supports, and use of accommodations" (ESSA, §1115(b)(2)(D)). General and special education practices have increasingly aligned providing school personnel, including occupational therapy practitioners, with increasing opportunities to expand their role in schools, particularly in the area of health promotion and prevention (Cahill & Bazyk, 2020).

## Reimbursement for Occupational Therapy Services

Occupational therapy practitioners must be knowledgeable about various payment sources and methods for occupational therapy reimbursement in a constantly changing healthcare system (Robinson & Fisher, 2022). Private insurance policies typically contain information about what they will pay for, what documentation is required, and the maximum number of therapy sessions that are covered by the policy. For governmental payment sources (i.e., Medicaid), official documents detail the rules about what is covered and what is excluded (Robinson & Fisher, 2022). Many payers have a fee schedule that determines the amount they will pay, regardless of what is billed. Payment rates are influenced by many factors, including legislative and regulatory decision-making, fluctuations in the costs of providing care, and the state of the economy (Robinson & Fisher, 2022). Payment for occupational therapy may also be influenced by payment incentives created for other professions, such as the Medicare Physician Fee Schedule, which was created for physicians to increase efficiency and value and led to performance measures that also apply to practitioners (Robinson & Fisher, 2022).

Despite the many private and public insurance options available, many people are uninsured (Robinson & Fisher, 2022). Uninsured families typically have to pay out of pocket for their child's therapy, perhaps at a negotiated or reduced rate. They may have to opt for less frequent therapy sessions and less extensive home programs. It is important that practitioners working in pediatric settings, such as hospitals, establish relationships with community organizations to address limited access to healthcare services, a critical social determinant of health (Robinson & Fisher, 2022).

Higher severity and longer hospital stays also come with increased costs and lower reimbursement. Children with more severe illness tend to be on Medicaid, according to the Children's Hospital Association (CHA, 2022), which reimburses at lower rates than private payers, and these children require specialized resources that may be more costly due to current supply chain shortages. Historically, behavioral health cases receive lower reimbursement (CHA, 2022). See Box 6.3 for more information on limited access to care.

Managed care organizations and episode-of-care payment models may facilitate the use of a clinical or critical pathway as a quality assurance measure in medical settings. These pathways are typically established by the facility. Occupational therapy practitioners need to be involved when these pathways are formulated, to ensure that their role is recognized and integrated within the care plan (Robinson & Fisher, 2022).

For more information on methods of reimbursement and their influence on practice please also see Chapter 7 on documentation and billing.

### BOX 6.3

Many children do not have equal access to healthcare in the United States. Ten to 20 million children and adolescents in the United States (40% of school-aged children) have some form of chronic illness or disability, such as asthma, cystic fibrosis, diabetes, epilepsy, and developmental disabilities, which can last from 3 months to a lifetime (AAP, 2022b; Centers for Disease Control and Prevention [CDC], 2021). Children with chronic illness or disability tend to see more specialists than the rest of the population (Children's Hospital Association, 2022). Chronic illnesses disproportionately affect minoritized children and adolescents, who are 1.5–2 times more likely to be diagnosed with a chronic illness than their white counterparts (Isaac et al., 2020). Minoritized children and adolescents with chronic illness not only experience disparities in health status and outcomes, such as differences in disease burden, injury, or mortality, but also experience significant healthcare disparities, including differences in healthcare coverage, access to care and quality of care, which subsequently impacts upon their health outcomes (Isaac et al., 2020). Occupational therapy practitioners provide services for all children and families fairly and impartially in a way that is free of bias (AOTA, 2020b). They therefore may need to advocate for additional services for children and their families.

## SUMMARY

Occupational therapy practitioners work in a variety of pediatric settings to enable children to participate in daily activities in their own families and communities. While the occupational therapy process is the same in all settings, intervention may emphasize specific factors, depending upon the setting.

1. Occupational therapy practitioners working in pediatrics provide services in hospitals, outpatient therapy centers, home health, EI, school systems, and community-based settings.
2. A variety of federal and state laws impact occupational therapy services for children and youth in each of the varied settings. IDEIA, Section 504 of the Rehabilitation Act, the ADA, and ESSA are just some of the laws that specific aspects of occupational therapy practice in the schools. State OT Practice Acts, FERPA, and HIPAA provide additional guidelines for practice with children and youth.
3. In each setting, the occupational therapy practitioner engages in the process described by the OT Practice Framework. Across settings, occupational therapy practitioners develop therapeutic relationships, evaluate, create intervention plans, implement plans, assess outcomes, and make discharge plans. Throughout the process, practitioners communicate and collaborate with other professionals. While occupational therapy practitioners consider the child's physical, social-emotional, behavioral, and cognition when designing intervention, the focus of the occupational therapy process is influenced by the mission of the setting.

## REFERENCES

American Academy of Pediatrics (AAP). (2022b). *Chronic conditions.* https://www.healthychildren.org/English/health-issues/conditions/chronic/Pages/default.aspx.

American Academy of Pediatrics (AAP). (2022a). *Early childhood.* https://www.aap.org/en/patient-care/early-childhood/.

American Academy of Pediatrics (AAP). (2012). Levels of neonatal care. *Pediatrics, 130*(3), 587–597.

American Academy of Pediatrics (AAP). (2022c). *Preemie.* https://healthychildren.org/English/ages-stages/baby/preemie/Pages/default.aspx.

American Occupational Therapy Association (AOTA). (2013). *Occupational therapy's role in mental health promotion, prevention, & intervention with children & youth: Social and emotional learning (SEL).* https://www.aota.org/practice/clinical-topics/-/media/f282d9a923cc4e1b9e133cb438649f99.ashx.

American Occupational Therapy Association (AOTA). (2016a). Mental health promotion, prevention, and intervention across the lifespan. https://www.aota.org/-/media/corporate/files/practice/mentalhealth/distinct-value-mental-health.pdf.

American Occupational Therapy Association (AOTA). (2016b). The role of occupational therapy in end-of-life care. *American Journal of Occupational Therapy, 70*(Suppl. 2):7012410075.

American Occupational Therapy Association (AOTA). (2017). Guidelines for occupational therapy services in early intervention and schools. *American Journal of Occupational Therapy, 71*(Suppl. 2), 7112410010. https://doi.org/10.5014/ajot.2017.716S01.

American Occupational Therapy Association (AOTA). (2018). Occupational therapy's role in the neonatal intensive care unit. *American Journal of Occupational Therapy, 72*(Suppl. 2):7212410020.

American Occupational Therapy Association. (2020). *Occupational therapy practice framework: Domain and process* (4th ed.). AOTA Press.

American Occupational Therapy Association (AOTA). (2020b). AOTA 2020 occupational therapy code of ethics. *American Journal of Occupational Therapy, 74*(Suppl. 3):7413410005.

American Occupational Therapy Association (AOTA). (2023). *2023 compensation & workforce survey.* Bethesda, MD: AOTA Press.

Americans with Disabilities Act Amendments of 2008, Pub. L. 110–325. 122 STAT. 3553.

Askin, E., & Moore, N. (2014). *The healthcare handbook. A clear and concise guide to the United States Health Care System* (2nd ed.). Washington University.

Atrium Health Floyd. (2021). Levels of neonatal care. https://www.floyd.org/medical-services/maternity/NICU/Pages/Levels-of-Neonatal-Care.aspx.

Bigsby, R. (2020). Neonatal intensive care unit. In J. C. O'Brien, & H. Kuhaneck (Eds.), *Case-Smith's occupational therapy for children and adolescents* (8th ed.) (pp. 565–600). Elsevier.

Boucher, S., Downing, J., & Shemilt, R. (2014). The role of play in children's palliative care. *Children, 1*(3), 302–317.

Braveman, B. (2022). Understanding and working within organizations. In B. Braveman (Ed.), *Leading and managing occupational therapy services: An evidence-based approach* (3rd ed.) (pp. 119–151). F.A. Davis.

Cahill, S. (2024). Education in the United States. In G. Gillen, & C. Brown (Eds.), *Willard and spackman's occupational therapy* (14th) (pp. 744–765). Philadelphia, PA: Wolters Kluwer.

Cahill, S., & Bazyk, S. (2020). School-based occupational therapy. In J. C. O'Brien, & H. Kuhaneck (Eds.), *Case-Smith's occupational therapy for children and adolescents* (8th ed.) (pp. 627–658). Elsevier.

Casimir, G. (2019). Why children's hospitals are unique and so essential. *Frontiers in Pediatrics, 23*(7), 305.

Centers for Disease Control and Prevention CDC. (2021). *Managing chronic conditions.* https://www.cdc.gov/healthyschools/chronicconditions.htm.

Children's Hospital Association (CHA). (2022). *4 trends in pediatric hospital utilization.* https://www.childrenshospitals.org/content/analytics/summary/4-trends-in-pediatric-hospital-utilization.

Chow, J. K., & Pickens, N. D. (2020). Measuring the efficacy of occupational therapy in end-of-life care: A scoping review. *American Journal of Occupational Therapy, 74*(1):7401205020p1-7401205020p14.

Clark, K. (2017). Intensive care unit. In H. Smith-Gabai, & S. E. Holm's (Eds.), *Occupational therapy in acute care* (pp. 115–135). AOTA Press.

Connecticut Birth to Three. (2016). Primary service provider approach to teaming: Connecticut birth to three services & supports. https://www.birth23.org/about-us/psp/.

Dudgeon, D. J. (2020). Hospital and pediatric rehabilitation services. In J. C. O'Brien, & H. Kuhaneck (Eds.), *Case-Smith's occupational therapy for children and adolescents* (8th ed.) (pp. 680–701). Elsevier.

Essential Yeh, H. H., & McColl, M. A. (2019). A model for occupation-based palliative care. *Occupational Therapy in Health Care, 33*(1), 108–123.

Student Succeeds Act of 2015, Pub. L. 114–195, 114 Stat. 1177.

Frankel, L. R., Hsu, B. S., Yeh, T. S., Simone, S. A., Arca, M. J., Coss-Bu, J. A., Fallat, M. E., Foland, J., Gadepalli, S., Gayle, M. O., Harmon, L. A., Hill, V., Joseph, C. A., Kessel, A. D., Kissoon, N., Moss, M., Mysore, M. R., Papo, M. E., Rajzer-Wakeham, K. L., … Conway, E. E. (2019). Criteria for critical care infants and children: PICU admission, discharge, and triage practice statement and levels of care guidance. *Pediatric Critical Care Medicine, 20*(9), 847–887.

Health Affairs. (2019). The effects of early care and education on children's health. *Health Affairs Health Policy Brief.* https://doi.org/10.1377/hpb20190325.519221.

Hsu, B. S., Hill, V., Frankel, L. R., Yeh, T. S., Simone, S., Arca, M. J., Coss-Bu, J. A., Fallat, M. E., Foland, J., Gadepalli, S., Gayle, M. O., Harmon, L. A., Joseph, C. A., Kessel, A. D., Kissoon, N., Moss, M., Mysore, M. R., Papo, M. C., Kari, L., … Agus, M. S. D. (2019). Executive summary: Criteria for critical care of infants and children: PICU admission, discharge, and triage practice statement and levels of care guidance. *Pediatrics, 144*(4):e20192433.

Individuals With Disabilities Education Improvement Act of 2004, Pub. L. 108–446, 20 U.S.C. § 1400 et seq.

Isaac, E. I., Meisman, A. R., Drucker, K., Violante, S., Behrhorst, K. L., Floyd, A., & Rohan, J. M. (2020). The relationship between health disparities, psychosocial functioning and health outcomes in pediatric hematology-oncology and stem cell transplant populations: Recommendations for clinical care. *International Journal of Environmental Research and Public Health, 17*(7), 2218.

Jackson, L. (2019). Best practices in supporting students with a 504 plan. In G. F. Clark, J. E. Rioux, & B. E. Chandler (Eds.), *Best practices for occupational therapy in schools* (2nd ed.) (pp. 219–226). AOTA Press.

Johnson, R. C., & Jackson, C. K. (2019). Reducing inequality through dynamic complementarity: Evidence from head start and public school spending. *American Economic Journal: Economic Policy, 11*(4), 310–349.

Kovanis, C. A., & Shivers, E. (2022). Acute care services and disciplines. In H. Smith-Gabai, & S. E. Holm (Eds.), *Occupational therapy in acute care* (pp. 99–105). AOTA Press.

Lawlor, M. C., & Mattingly, C. (2019). Family perspectives on occupation, health, and disability. In B. A. Boyt Schell, & G. Gillen (Eds.), *Willard & Spackman's occupational therapy* (13th ed.) (pp. 196–211). Wolters Kluwer.

Matthies, J., & Smith-Gabai, H. (2017). Laboratory values. In H. Smith-Gabai, & S. E. Holm (Eds.), *Occupational therapy in acute care* (pp. 149–174). AOTA Press.

MedlinePlus [Internet]. Bethesda (MD): National Library of Medicine (US). [updated August 20, 2020]. Critical care. https://medlineplus.gov/criticalcare.html.

National Alliance of Specialized Instructional Support Personnel. (2022). *ESEA/ESSA.* http://nasisp.org/issues-advocacy/esea/.

National Center on Education Statistics NCES. (2022). Roughly half of public schools report that they can effectively provide mental health services to all students in need. https://nces.ed.gov/whatsnew/press_releases/05_31_2022_2.asp.

Nicolson, J., & Salinas, J. (2022). Occupational therapist/occupational therapy assistant partnership: Supervision and collaboration. In B. Braveman (Ed.), *Leading and managing occupational therapy services: An evidence-based approach* (3rd ed.) (pp. 249–267). F.A. Davis.

Pelletier, J. H., Rakkar, J., Au, A. K., Fuhrman, D., Clark, R. S. B., & Horvat, C. M. (2021). Trends in US pediatric hospital admissions in 2020 compared with the decade before the COVID-19 Pandemic. *JAMA Network Open, 4*(2):e2037227.

Rioux, J. E., & Chandler, B. E. (2019). History of occupational therapy in schools. In G. F. Clark, J. E. Rioux, & B. E. Chandler (Eds.), *Best practices for occupational therapy in schools* (2nd ed.) (pp. 3–9). AOTA Press.

Roberts, P. S., & Evenson, M. (2019). Continuum of care. In B. A. Boyt Schell, & G. Gillen (Eds.), *Willard & Spackman's occupational therapy* (13th ed.) (pp. 994–1010). Wolters Kluwer.

Robinson, M., & Fisher, G. (2022). Understanding healthcare systems and practice contexts. In B. Braveman (Ed.), *Leading and managing occupational therapy services: An evidence-based approach* (3rd ed.) (pp. 73–118). F.A. Davis.

Rogers, M. M., Friebert, S., Williams, C. S., Humphrey, L., Thienprayoon, R., & Klick, J. C. (2021). Pediatric palliative care programs in US hospitals. *Pediatrics, 148*(1).

Schneider, E., & Chandler, B. E. (2019). Laws that affect occupational therapy in schools. In G. F. Clark, J. E. Rioux, & B. E. Chandler (Eds.), *Best practices for occupational therapy in schools* (2nd ed.) (pp. 19–26). AOTA Press.

Shotwell, M. P., & Johnson, K. R. (2017). Evaluation of acute care patients. In H. Smith-Gabai, & S. E. Holm (Eds.), *Occupational therapy in acute care* (pp. 37–61). AOTA Press.

Smith-Gabai, H. (2017). Common diagnostic tests. In H. Smith-Gabai, & S. E. Holm (Eds.), *Occupational therapy in acute care* (pp. 137–147). AOTA Press.

Stoops, K. (2017). Fundamentals of pharmacology for occupational therapy. In H. Smith-Gabai, & S. E. Holm (Eds.), *Occupational therapy in acute care* (pp. 175–182). AOTA Press.

Torres, A. (2021). Nemours KidsHealth: When your child's in the pediatric intensive care unit. https://kidshealth.org/en/parents/picu.html.

U.S. Department of Education. (2022a). 2021 Annual report to Congress on the individuals with disabilities education act (IDEA). https://sites.ed.gov/idea/2021-individuals-with-disabilities-education-act-annual-report-to-congress/.

U.S. Department of Education. (2022b). A history of the individuals with disabilities education act. https://sites.ed.gov/idea/IDEA-History#2000s-10s.

U.S. Department of Education (n.d.). Every Child Succeeds Act. https://www.ed.gov/essa?src=rn.

U.S. Department of Education. (2020). Protecting students with disabilities. https://www2.ed.gov/about/offices/list/ocr/504faq.html. [Accessed 1 December 2022].

U.S. Department of Health and Human Services, Office of Head Start. (2022). *Head Start Services.* https://www.acf.hhs.gov/ohs/about/head-start.

Weiss, A. J., Liang, L., & Martin, K. (2022). Overview of Hospital Stays Among Children and Adolescents, 2019. Statistical Brief #299. https://www.hcup-us.ahrq.gov/reports/statbriefs/sb299-Hospital-Stays-Children-2019.jsp.

Wilburn, V. G., Hoss, A., Pudeler, M., Beukema, E., Rothenbuhler, C., & Stoll, H. B. (2021). Health policy perspectives—Receiving recognition: A case for occupational therapy practitioners as mental and behavioral health providers. *American Journal of Occupational Therapy, 75*:7505090010.

World Health Organization WHO. (2018). *Integrating palliative care and symptom relief into paediatrics: A WHO guide for health care planners, implementers, and managers.* https://www.who.int/publications/i/item/integrating-palliative-care-and-symptom-relief-into-paediatrics.

Zero to Three. (2010). *Making hope a reality: Early intervention for infants and toddlers with disabilities.* https://www.zerotothree.org/resource/making-hope-a-reality-early-intervention-for-infants-and-toddlers-with-disabilities/.

Zhang, C., & Dobbs-Oates, J. (2019). The relations between American children's head start experience and pre-academic skills: A comparison with children from a community group. *Journal of Research in Childhood Education, 33*(4), 623–636.

7

# Documentation and Billing in Pediatric Practice

*Tara J. Glennon*

## GUIDING QUESTIONS

1. What are the legal and ethical considerations for documentation of occupational therapy services?
2. How are ICD-11 and CPT codes utilized to document the need for and provision of occupational therapy services?
3. What rules, regulations, and parameters guide documentation and coding of occupational therapy services within medically-based occupational therapy practice, such as provided to commercial insurance and Medicaid?
4. What are the pragmatic considerations in documenting the occupational therapy process in medically-based contexts, including referral, diagnosis, evaluation, plan of care, treatment session notes, progress notes, denial appeals, letters of medical necessity, and discharge plans?
5. What are the best practices for documenting educationally-based and early intervention occupational therapy services under Parts B and C of the Individuals with Disabilities Education Act (IDEA)?

## KEY TERMS

Coding
Billing
Documentation
Electronic medical record (EMR)
Electronic health record (EHR)
Federal programs
Funding
Insurance
Letter of medical necessity (LOMN)
Medicaid
Plan of care
Prior authorization
Reimbursement
SOAP note

## INTRODUCTION

Documentation within occupational therapy practice serves a variety of purposes, including meeting legal requirements, assuring the ethical provision of services, accurately representing professional processes, clearly articulating the need for services through a client-centered intervention plan, advocating for the skilled therapeutic services occupational therapy practitioners provide, and supporting payment for services from the designated payer source. Documentation is required when professional services are provided to clients, whether an individual, a group, or a population (American Occupational Therapy Association [AOTA], 2018, 2020a).

Pediatric occupational therapy practitioners provide services in a wide variety of settings, each with their own philosophy and regulations for service provision, as well as guidelines, parameters, and requirements for documentation format and frequency. They abide by "time frames, formats, and standards established by practice settings, federal and state laws, other regulatory and payer requirements, external accreditation programs, and AOTA official documents" (AOTA, 2021a, p. 4). Occupational therapy practitioners follow organizational standards for documentation and accurately bill the funding source for the services provided to clients in a variety of pediatric settings (See Chapter 6 for more information on specific pediatric settings).

This chapter focuses on documentation required to substantiate and bill for the person as a client, with some discussion of group and population-based documentation when working in a community-based model. The author reviews common documentation principles with a focus on documentation required by various funding sources that represent the occupational therapy profession when providing services for children and youth. The author describes the nuances of and best practices in documentation for various pediatric funding sources, such as commercial insurance, Medicaid, and federal programs, as well as the core values the public can expect when receiving occupational therapy services (AOTA, 2020b), including professional standards (AOTA, 2021a), as described in the *Occupational Therapy Practice Framework* (OTPF-4).

## CONSIDERATIONS FOR DOCUMENTATION AND REIMBURSEMENT ACROSS SETTINGS

Several factors are considered when documenting the provision of occupational therapy services, remembering that the occupational therapy practitioner represents the profession and the value of services by facilitating functional participation and engagement in occupations for children and youth. Occupational therapy practitioners maintain "current knowledge of legislative, political, social, cultural, societal, and reimbursement issues that affect clients and the practice of occupational therapy" (AOTA, 2021a, p. 3). Legal and ethical principles overarch all documentation and require that occupational therapy practitioners maintain timely, accurate, and complete client records for all client encounters (AOTA, 2020b) and secure and prevent the unauthorized disclosure of information related to their clients.

### Legislation and Privacy

Within pediatric practice, two congressionally authorized pieces of federal legislation are pertinent: the Health Insurance Portability and Accountability Act (HIPPA; Pub. L. No. 104–191), with subsequent Privacy and Security rules, 2000 and 2003, respectively (United States Department of Health and Human Services, 2021) and Family Educational Rights and Privacy Act (FERPA; 20 U.S.C. §1232g; 34 CFR Part 99). HIPPA established federal standards focused on how a client's protected health information (PHI) can be utilized, shared (verbal, written, or electronic communications), stored, and secured; and emphasized that clients should be aware of their rights to know how their PHI is being protected. FERPA provides access to a student's educational record by the parent and an eligible student who is 18 years old; and protects student record information with access to only those people who have a legitimate educational interest in viewing the information (United States Department of Education, 2021).

Although the medical provider (HIPPA) or school system (FERPA) implements and manages required authorizations and consent forms, occupational therapy practitioners have a responsibility to actively protect client information. An occupational therapy practitioner should not discuss client PHI with anyone who does not need to know the information, and unattended files stored in cabinets or on electronic devices should be locked.

Furthermore, occupational therapy practitioners are expected to routinely practice privacy and confidentiality measures, including:

- Assuring that verbal communications with other team members take place in areas where information cannot be overheard
- Refraining from discussing information outside of the team
- Closing files or computer screens when not in use
- Leaving files secured at work settings (not at home or in personal vehicles)
- Using secured wireless access when logging into electronic documentation systems
- Logging off digital platforms when finished documenting or billing
- Refraining from taking or storing pictures on your phone or posting anything about clients on social media

## Electronic Medical Records for Documentation

An **electronic medical record (EMR)** is information typically found in a paper chart but allows electronic (digital) access for multiple departments within an organization for convenience and efficiency. EMR information includes insurance and demographic information, precautions and contraindications, evaluation reports, treatment notes, progress summaries, discharge plans, and communications with external medical professionals. For ease and synchrony of the organization's workflow, EMRs often interface patient data with calendars to schedule patients and record arrivals, session notes for every arrival, and the corresponding invoicing for the therapy provided. Thereafter, an electronic invoice is generated in one of two formats, an insurance claim form or a superbill. Direct billing for commercial and government insurance providers, such as Medicaid or the Children's Health Insurance Program (CHIP) for children and youth considered in low- and lower-income families, utilizes CMS Form 1500—*Health Insurance Claim Form* (United States Department of Health and Human Services [HHS], Centers for Medicare and Medicaid Services [CMS], Office of Management and Budget, 2012). A superbill is provided to the caregiver if the child's services are not covered under an insurance plan (e.g., not eligible per the diagnosis, therapy considered experimental and not approved), the therapist is not contracted to provide services with the patient's insurance plan (e.g., is "out of network"), the family is requesting payment for services from another funding source (e.g., flexible spending account), or the services are considered "out of pocket" or "private pay" for the family/caregiver.

Limitations of an EMR include information sharing across different medical practices and health systems where paper copies might need to be printed and shared with other external providers, such as sending a progress note to the pediatrician from the occupational therapy practitioner providing therapy at an outpatient therapy clinic. Under certain payer requirements, an **electronic health record (EHR)** system is necessary to:

- Share information across and between different health care provider organizations to improve patient care
- Track medical conditions, tests, and procedures
- Afford patients access to their medical information

Larger health care or hospital systems generally have an EHR system, while independent therapy outpatient clinics use an EMR system.

Securing patient information is paramount and HHS issued a report on how to secure and safeguard electronic patient records in EMR and EHR systems (United States Department of Health and Human Services, Health Sector Cybersecurity Coordination Center, 2022). Two cautions when using an EMR or EHR platform are that practitioners must not share usernames or passwords, and the practitioner only logs into the system with their own credentials to prevent fraudulently documenting, billing, or signing/authorizing for another practitioner.

Several companies provide EMR systems designed to support pediatric practice needs. These platforms often include templates for evaluation reports, including common pediatric assessment information and formatting, as well as goal banks for ease of designing and tracking plans of care over the course of intervention. It is also important for the EMR system to allow the occupational therapy practitioner to document each child's affordances and barriers to functional participation clearly and distinctly, rather than all reports looking the same. Ongoing communication with the EMR company may be required to modify the features of the EMR to achieve this outcome. See Fig. 7.1 Electronic Medical Record for an example of how an EMR platform allows the practitioner to choose a template that prepopulates all the required content areas to be completed for a specific age or diagnostic category.

## Professional Writing and Importance of "Audience"

Professional writing reflects on the profession, provides an illustration of an occupational therapy practitioner's professional reasoning skills, and represents the ability to communicate effectively and efficiently before, during, and after the provision of occupational therapy services. All documentation needs to be clear, concise, accurate, timely, objective, grammatically correct, and professionally presented (AOTA, 2018). Carefully chosen words and judicious use of professional terminology commensurate with the intended audience are also important. For example, documentation within a school-based model to foster team collaboration might sound very different from documentation aimed at justifying the need for skilled, medically-based intervention for reimbursement by a commercial insurance carrier. The occupational therapy practitioner documents based on the audience, and each audience reads documentation through a different lens (Sames, 2019).

The various audiences for occupational therapy documentation include payer sources, accreditation agencies, medical professionals, educational staff, parents/caregivers, and the general community (e.g., when working in a community-based model). In a school setting the occupational therapy practitioner uses less jargon and more descriptors that illustrate the child's story and functional engagement in educationally-based activities. In a medical setting, medical terminology is expected by the insurance reviewer per their funding specifications. A progress note for the pediatrician might include professional jargon, whereas classroom suggestions for the paraprofessional use layman's terms to describe how, when, and where to implement each strategy.

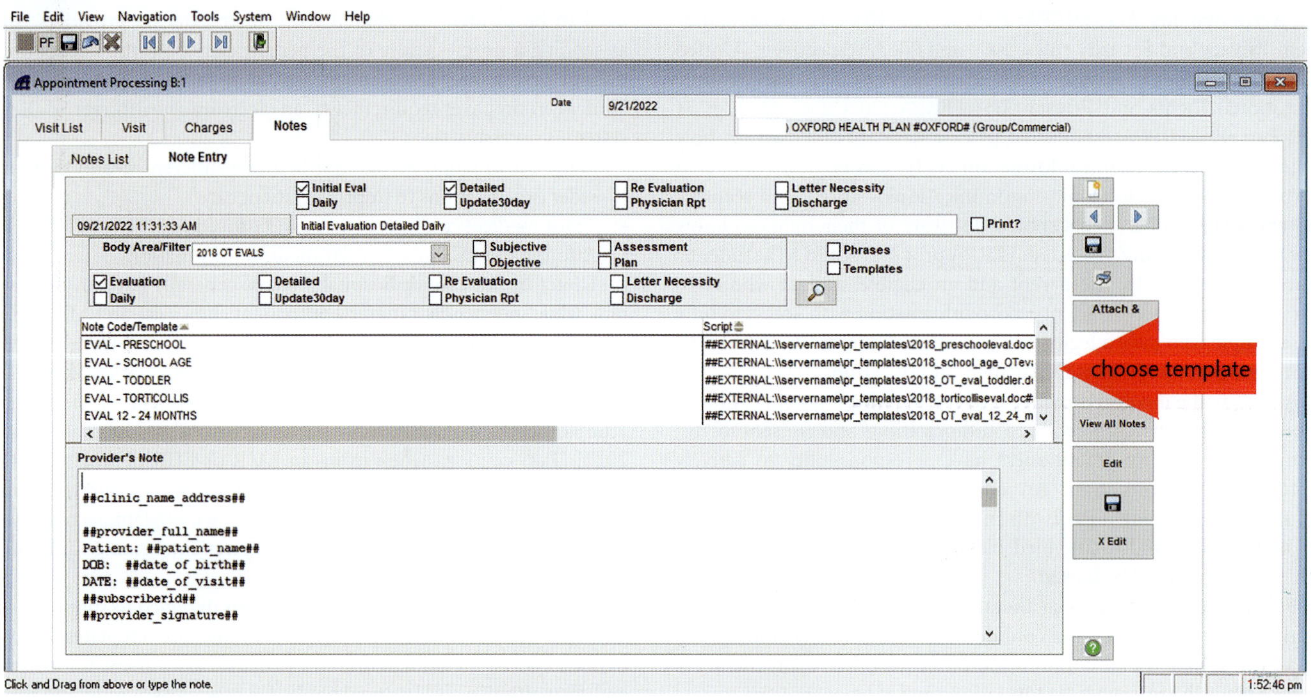


**Fig. 7.1** Electronic medical record.

## BOX 7.1 Words to Avoid in Documentation

- Aggressive
- Angry
- Annoying
- Bossy
- Belligerent
- Bratty
- Careless
- Clingy
- Concerning
- Confrontational
- Controlling
- Cranky
- Cruel
- Defiant
- Destructive
- Finicky
- Hostile
- Incapable
- Inconsiderate
- Lazy
- Manipulative
- Moody
- Naughty
- Obnoxious
- Rebellious
- Sneaky
- Spiteful
- Spoiled
- Stubborn
- Unpredictable
- Unruly
- Volatile
- Worst

## CASE EXAMPLE 7.1

Woman Charged with Larceny and Health Insurance Fraud
State of Connecticut (2019)
Connecticut State—Division of Criminal Justice Press Release (March 9, 2021)

*"According to the arrest warrant affidavit, between February 2016 and August 2019, (Therapist X) instructed her staff to bill for 10 units of service for each patient visit, a unit representing 15 minutes of billable time, regardless of actual time staff spent with the patient. (Therapist X) submitted thousands of claims for reimbursements to the Medicaid program for more time than her therapists spent with the patients. (Therapist X), through (Business Name) billed for two and half hours of occupational therapy and physical therapy services, when patient sessions lasted, on average, less than 45 minutes. (Therapist X) also billed for treatment allegedly provided to patients using employee's provider numbers on dates after those employees resigned, and without their permission."*

Documentation serves as a legal record of what occurred in the occupational therapy process for future reference. Words have connotations, emotions that one perceives from words. Therefore, occupational therapy practitioners document objective data free from harsh or judgmental language that provides a professional view of the child and is non-offensive. For example, "child is noncompliant" can evoke a negative feeling; and "family is noncompliant with home program carryover" indicates that the occupational therapy practitioner has not yet been successful in providing client-centered home suggestions. Box 7.1 provides a list of words (not exhaustive) that have negative connotations in the English language and may offend a family/caregiver or negatively influence a payer.

## Documentation for Billing

The AOTA Code of Ethics (AOTA, 2020b) mandates that occupational therapy practitioners provide honest documentation, and it is against the Code of Ethics to fabricate or falsify documentation or provide inaccurate billing. "Documentation for reimbursement purposes is done in accordance with applicable laws, guidelines, and regulations" (p. 6). The occupational therapy practitioner abides by the "standards established by practice settings, federal and state laws, other regulatory and payer requirements, external accreditation programs, and AOTA official documents" (AOTA, 2021a, p. 4). In addition to narrative session notes and formalized reports recording the outcomes of patient contacts, the codes used for billing a specific therapy service are also a form of documentation and legally verify the service delivered. Therefore, accurate billing for occupational therapy services is important. Improper coding/billing as a form of documentation of occupational therapy services is considered fraud and has legal implications. See Case Example 7.1 for an example of improper billing and the resultant implications.

Administrators of a provider organization offering occupational therapy services outline how occupational therapy practitioners bill various payer sources for occupational therapy staff. These instructions relate to the provider organization's contractual arrangements with various payer sources, including commercial insurance carriers, governmental agencies, local municipalities responsible for educationally-based therapy services, and community programs requesting occupational therapy services. However, invoicing for occupational therapy services is linked to each occupational therapy practitioner's license and credentials, and, in essence, legal assurance for accuracy. The practitioner is obligated to trust but verify the parameters set forth by the supervisor/administrator to ensure legal and ethical billing of the services provided under their credentials. See Table 7.1 for considerations related to invoicing payer sources for occupational therapy services.

## DOCUMENTATION AND REIMBURSEMENT FOR SPECIFIC SETTINGS AND SITUATIONS

Understanding the contexts within which services are provided, best practices in service delivery within those contexts, and funding source requirements supporting practice within those contexts guides the approach to documentation to ensure full and correct reimbursement for services rendered. As mentioned earlier, although there are general considerations for documentation and billing that are carried across all settings, there are also specific issues within varied settings. Pediatric occupational therapy practitioners work in a variety of settings (see Chapter 6), although the majority work in public schools.

### School-Based Practice

Children ages 3–21 years receive special education and related services under Part B of IDEA (Pub L. 108–446). The documentation systems and parameters for all personnel tasked with meeting federal/state laws and requirements are outlined by each state's department of education and implemented by local boards of education. See Chapter 15 for more on school system practice. Documentation of occupational therapy services within special education law adheres to IDEA requirements, with the individualized education program (IEP) serving as the written legal document. Although the layout of IEP forms might vary from state to state, including many states that have moved to an online IEP platform, each format meets federal requirements. Resource materials on completing the federally mandated IEP document are provided via training webinars or video tutorials through each state's department of education. Sections of the IEP that are particularly important for the occupational therapy practitioner's input include (1) present level of academic achievement and functional performance, specifically how the child's disability affects progress or participation in general education; annual goals and objectives; (2) a description of the related services; and (3) accommodations and modifications to assist the child advance or attain annual goals, be involved in and make progress in the general education curriculum, and/or participate in extracurricular and nonacademic activities, including supplemental materials, equipment, or adaptive devices.

The occupational therapy practitioner also adheres to professional standards related to the "development, documentation, and implementation of the occupational therapy intervention plan based on the evaluation, client goals, best available evidence, and professional and clinical reasoning" (AOTA, 2021a, p. 5). It is the occupational therapy department's responsibility to create and implement forms and documentation procedures essential to supporting the occupational therapy process. These documents are not a part of the official educational file, either in a paper record or in an online platform database. Forms to support school-based occupational therapy services include templates for evaluation reports, assessment tool descriptions and score reporting charts, clinical reasoning pathways for intervention planning, attendance tracking, collaboration documents, data collection charts, and group activity schedules. If the local school district does not require a specific paper or electronic record format for recording student contact, the occupational therapy staff needs to create a form or system to log and classify occupational therapy service contacts for each student. See Box 7.2 for various types of service contacts requiring documentation within a school-based model. This section will overview important documentation concepts and requirements related to school-based occupational therapy practice to meet educational documentation requirements under federal programs.

**Screening.** Occupational therapy screenings are not a covered expense under most medical funding sources, but they are common practice within school-based occupational therapy. The intent of a screening (AOTA, 2020a, 2021b) is to identify a child's potential strengths and weaknesses and determine the need for further evaluation and

**TABLE 7.1 Considerations When Invoicing Payer Sources for Occupational Therapy Services**

| Situation or Scenario | Occupational Therapy Practitioner's Responsibility |
|---|---|
| Occupational therapy practitioner submits their documentation and billing for services rendered but the information then goes to another department for actual submission to the payer source | Verifying that the record of services documented is not changed, altered, or "fixed" by other departments within the organization before submission to the payer source. |
| The billing department thinks there is an error in what the practitioner billed and changes it without discussion. | Ensuring that the billing department contacts the occupational therapy practitioner directly if they feel there is an error in the records submitted. This assurance may be added to the therapist's employment agreement, or the therapist may insist it be added to the company policy manual. |
| When providing contracted services to a local Board of Education (BOE) the occupational therapy practitioner completes documentation and billing on the BOE's system but makes an error. | Assuring that one provides accurate documentation and billing to an external agency/organization for services rendered on behalf of your organization. For example, any errors in the information submitted in the BOE's system must be corrected as soon as possible. |
| Instances when session notes or evaluation reports do not have a 1:1 correspondence to the coding of the occupational therapy services provided. The occupational therapy practitioner might be instructed by a supervisor that congruence between the type of service delivered, coded for billing purposes, and corresponding documentation to support the specific coded service is not important because reimbursement is by the hour or a flat rate per session, no matter the type of service provided. | Despite funding arrangements, the occupational therapy practitioner's documentation and billing must align with the specific services provided. |

intervention. Within school-based practice, two common scenarios for an occupational therapy screening include:

- Find and identify children with disabilities from birth through 21 years who might be eligible for special education and related services under the Child Find provisions of IDEA (P.L. 108–446, 2004; §300.111).
- Identify general education instructional strategies that might be helpful for children in the classroom. (Note: This is not for the provision of occupational therapy services under IDEA, which would require a full evaluation.)

When completing an occupational therapy screening to provide general education instructional strategies for a child, the therapist documents the referral source and reason for the request, followed by a brief occupational profile that focuses on participation in occupations (e.g., education, play, or self-care), as well as the contextual or environmental factors supporting or inhibiting participation (AOTA, 2021b). This information guides the assessment, recommendations, and plan. For example, the occupational therapist may recommend specific classroom-related strategies to improve a student's performance or engagement with educational lessons or materials. The occupational therapist collaboratively discusses the strategies with team members before officially documenting how and when strategies should be implemented. See Table 7.2 for a format to assist in documenting strategies and activities for general education implementation.

If the occupational therapist determines that the child needs monitoring or follow-up to support their general education, they review the documentation requirements (e.g., screening or evaluation) of the state regulatory and department of education policies. Parent notification and approval may be required.

## BOX 7.2 Service Contacts Requiring Documentation

- Direct service: daily treatment notes reflecting the provision of occupational therapy services to address goals identified on the IEP; See SOAP note section and modify as needed.
- Indirect service: comprehensive description of any professional contact, including:
  - Meetings with any member of the team
  - Collaboration, education, or training sessions related to suggested strategies, equipment usage, or specific safety plans, such as mealtime procedures for a child with significant oral motor concerns or an orthotic plan with the schedule, donning instructions, and skin integrity monitoring procedures
  - Other communications (e.g., phone calls, emails) made on behalf of the student
  - Advocacy efforts on behalf of the student or family

## TABLE 7.2 School-Based Collaboration Plan Template

Child's Name: ______________________ OTP and Contact Information: ______________________

Targeted Functional Outcome(s): ______________________

Teacher/Staff who have contributed to the discussion of how/when to implement OT suggestions: ______________________

| What school strategy will be implemented? | When and where will the strategy be implemented? | Who will implement the strategy? | Does the implementer need education on how to implement? If so, who will train the implementer? | Who needs to follow-up, and when, to see if the strategy is working well or needs to be modified? |
|---|---|---|---|---|
| | | | | |
| • What strategy will address the referral concern.<br>• Specifically describe the strategy/activity so that the person implementing the strategy/activity is clear on what is required.<br>• Remember that the OTP will not be present when the strategy/activity is implemented so the information needs to be very clear.<br>• NOTE: This is not a strategy/activity that OTP will provide. Rather, the OTP is asking a team member to implement. Remember language and words for the intended audience. | Be specific.<br><br>Think about where might be a natural context for this strategy to occur?<br><br>Think about the other activities that the implementer might be responsible for managing during that natural context and collaborate if this is the best time for implementation. | The OTP is not implementing the strategy or activity – rather, through collaboration, another team member is being asked to implement the strategy or activity.<br><br>Which team member would be most appropriate to implement the strategy or activity? | The OTP needs to be sure that the person implementing the strategy/activity is clear on what needs to occur. This section should outline how the OTP will train the teacher or staff member.<br><br>Remember to have the teacher or staff member demonstrate or verbally repeat back what they have heard so that everyone is clear on the expectations and specifics.<br><br>Be specific. | As the OTP, you will need follow-up with the person implementing your strategy. Based on the strategy outlined, when should there be an OTP follow-up? How often? One time or ongoing?<br><br>Be specific. |

 School-Based Collaboration Plan

**Evaluation.** An occupational therapy evaluation might be part of the initial evaluation to determine whether a child has a disability and is eligible for special education and related services or might be implemented after a child has been identified as eligible for special education and the educational team identifies occupational therapy as a possible related service (IDEA, 2004; §300.34) for the child to benefit from special education. Within this section, the term *evaluation* refers to an occupational therapy evaluation, which is different from the term evaluation or reevaluation within IDEA legislation to evaluate eligibility for special education and related services (IDEA, 2004; §1414).

Per IDEA (P.L. 108–446, 2004), an occupational therapy evaluation within school-based practice must be completed within the mandated timelines and requires parental consent (§300.300), including agreement with the identified assessment processes and tools to complete the evaluation. The occupational profile's comprehensive record review and interviews with team members are important as occupational therapy is a related service to assist the child in benefiting from the education provided by team members. The school-based model requires the occupational therapist to make assessment choices to identify the child's performance within the context of educational expectations, including highlighting affordances and barriers to successful engagement in the educational program (e.g., academics, recess, lunch, music, and extracurricular activities).

The assessment portion of the evaluation process might use a variety of standardized and nonstandardized methodologies to assess occupational performance and includes observing the student's performance within the classroom (§300.310). The occupational therapist (with input from the occupational therapy assistant) analyzes data related to occupations, performance skills, performance patterns, and/or context and makes clinical reasoning decisions based on whether and how the child's documented challenges adversely affect the student's ability to participate in or benefit from the educational program. The occupational therapy evaluative outcomes presented to the educational team for consideration focus on these questions:

- Does the student need skilled occupational therapy services to benefit from the educational program?
- How do the occupational therapy evaluation findings impact the student's involvement and progress in the general education curriculum?

If occupational therapy is recommended by the team, they identify the mode of occupational therapy service delivery to best meet the student's needs in the child's IEP. Occupational therapy intervention may include skilled, direct intervention, or indirect services to support the child, including context-specific suggestions, modification to the materials, teaching strategies, and processes of learning; and education/training for team members.

**Individualized Education Plan Goals and Objectives.** Occupational therapy as a related service within the school-based practice is documented along with other educational services on a student's IEP (IDEA, 2004; §1414). Within this legal document, objective, observable, and measurable goals are identified on an annual basis with consideration of the student's strengths, as well as the academic, functional, and developmental needs to benefit from or participate in their educational program and activities. Interprofessional goals are considered best practices where each team member supports the child's goals (AOTA et al., 2022).

Frolek Clark and Handley-More (2017, p. 68) outline a four-step process for school-based goal writing:

1. Gather information through the occupational profile (through collaboration with teachers and family) to establish the area of concern, baseline, and expected performance.
2. Define the desired performance, including when and where.
3. Identify the conditions.
4. Establish the criterion—how the team will know the performance has been met.

Another format, the SMART approach to writing goals and objectives, originated by Doran (1981) and slightly revised over the years, outlines the components of objectives: specific (e.g., who, what, where, when, and why), measurable, achievable/attainable, relevant/realistic, and time-related/time-bound. See Chapter 10 for goal setting and measuring outcomes.

The goals and objectives are documented on the IEP and may address occupations, such as self-help, independent living, social participation, and education. See Fig. 7.2 for a sample Goal Page of an IEP document. Postsecondary goals are required for children over 16 years (§1414) and are based on age-appropriate transition assessments focused on independent living skills, employment, education, and training. Occupational therapy practitioners must be aware of opportunities to collaborate in transition planning, particularly in preparing for future education, employment, independent living, and community/social inclusion (AOTA, 2017).

**Progress Reports, Annual Review, and Reevaluation.** Progress toward IEP goals is periodically measured and reported in concurrence with the schedule of the issuance of report cards, for example, written each quarter of the academic year (§1414); and the IEP is reviewed and revised by the team at least annually. Reevaluation of the student occurs at least every 3 years, termed a triennial evaluation, but can be more frequent as needed or requested. Occupational therapy practitioners communicate with team members when preparing progress, annual, or reevaluation reports, and collect data related to the student's progress toward IEP goals. See Chapter 10 for additional information related to measuring functional outcomes.

**Discharge Reports.** Occupational therapy practitioners prepare discharge reports when recommending a change in services. The occupational therapy discharge summary is similar to an annual progress report, or a reevaluation if occurring at the 3-year mark, but is more in-depth to document the services previously rendered, the impact on the child's educational achievement or functional participation, and the reason(s) for recommending termination of services. A child may be discharged from occupational therapy services for several reasons, including achievement of goals, no further need for occupational therapy services to meet their educational needs, or continued services are not likely to benefit the student. Children may be discharged from services if they are moving school districts or receiving therapy elsewhere.

The occupational therapist formally proposes discontinuation of occupational therapy services to the IEP team at the annual meeting, with prior written notification to the parent, for the team to discuss and make the final decision. Before the meeting, the occupational therapist collaborates and communicates with team members (including parents/caregivers) to ascertain other factors to consider when making a professional recommendation for discharge. This allows the occupational therapist to gain the perspectives of team members, ensure their observations are consistent across contexts, and confirm whether discharge is warranted. At the end of the discharge report, the therapist provides suggestions to support the student's ongoing success and, in some cases, indicators that might suggest the team reconsider the need for occupational therapy services.

## Early Intervention Services

Children under 3 years old receive occupational therapy services via different pathways. The first option is directly through medical facilities funded by the caregiver's medical insurance. Under medical insurance funding, the occupational therapist completes an evaluation and plan of care (POC), as described below under Medically-Based Services, and the child attends therapy at the outpatient clinic or outpatient unit of a hospital or health care system. The second option is through early intervention services under IDEA (Pub. L. 108–446), Part C within the natural context, such as the home or daycare.

Student: ______ Last Name, First Name DOB: ______ mm/dd/yyyy District: ______ Meeting Date: ______ mm/dd/yyyy

Pick 4 dates to show your quarterly updates between 1/2020 and 1/2021

| | | | | | ***Enter Dates for Evaluating and Reporting Progress in Boxes Below*** |
|---|---|---|---|---|---|
| ☐Academic/Cognitive | ☐Social/Behavioral | ☐Communication | ☑Gross/Fine Motor | ☐Postsecondary Education/Training | |
| ☐Self Help | ☐Employment | ☐Independent Living | ☐Health | ☐Other: (specify) | |

☐ **Check here if the student is 15 years of age.** (Note: Page 6, Transition Planning must be completed if this box is checked)

| 1 4/2020 | 2 6/2020 | 3 10/2020 | 4 1/2021 |
|---|---|---|---|
| 5 | 6 | 7 | 8 |

**Measurable Annual Goal* (Linked to Present Levels of Performance)#** ______

**Eval. Procedure:** 10
**Perf. Criteria:** H
**(%, Trials, etc.)** 3/3 objectives

Report Progress Below (Use Reporting Key)

| 1 | 2 | 3 | 4 |
|---|---|---|---|
| 5 | 6 | 7 | 8 |

Short Term Objectives/Benchmarks (Linked to achieving progress towards Annual Goal)

**Objective #1** ______

**Eval. Procedure:** 9
**Perf. Criteria:** G
**(%, Trials, etc.)** ex- 4/5

Report Progress Below (Use Reporting Key)

| 1 | 2 | 3 | 4 |
|---|---|---|---|
| 5 | 6 | 7 | 8 |

**Objective #2** ______

**Eval. Procedure:** 9
**Perf. Criteria:** G
**(%, Trials, etc.)** ex- 4/5

Report Progress Below (Use Reporting Key)

| 1 | 2 | 3 | 4 |
|---|---|---|---|
| 5 | 6 | 7 | 8 |

**Objective #3** ______

**Eval. Procedure:** 9
**Perf. Criteria:** G
**(%, Trials, etc.)** ex- 4/5

Report Progress Below (Use Reporting Key)

| 1 | 2 | 3 | 4 |
|---|---|---|---|
| 5 | 6 | 7 | 8 |

| **Evaluation Procedures** | | **Performance Criteria** | |
|---|---|---|---|
| 1. Criterion-Referenced/Curriculum Based Assessments | 7. Behavior/Performance Rating Scale | A. Percent of Change | F. Duration |
| 2. Pre and Post Standardized Assessment | 8. Smarter Balanced and CT Alternate Assessments | B. Months Growth | G. Successful Completion of Task/Activity |
| 3. Pre and Post Base Line Data | 9. Work Samples, Job Performance or Products | C. Standard Score Increase | H. Mastery |
| 4. Quizzes/Tests | 10. Achievement of Objectives *(Note: use with goal only)* | D. Passing Grades/Score | I. Other: (specify) |
| 5. Student Self-assessment/Rubric | 11. Other (specify) | E. Frequency/Trials | J. Other: (specify) |
| 6. Project/Experiment/Portfolio | 12. Other (specify) | | |

**Progress Reporting Key:** (indicating extent to which progress is sufficient to achieve goal by the end of the year) **M** = Mastered **S** = Satisfactory Progress – Likely to achieve goal **U**=Unsatisfactory Progress – Unlikely to achieve goal **N** = No Progress – Will not achieve goal **NI** = Not Introduced **O** = Other: (specify)

*Related to meeting the student's needs that result from the individual's disability, to enable the student to be involved in and make progress in the general curriculum, and to meet each of the student's other educational needs that result from the student's disability.

Page ___ of ___ Goal Pages

ED620, Revised February 2009a INDIVIDUALIZED EDUCATION PROGRAM 7

**Fig. 7.2** Sample goal page of the individual education plan (IEP).

IDEA Part C is a federal grant program implemented by each state to enhance the development of infants and toddlers with disabilities, to minimize their potential for developmental delay, and to recognize the significant brain development that occurs in the first 3 years of life (§1431). Early intervention (EI) services focus on infants and toddlers with disabilities under 3 years and their families. An infant or toddler with a disability is defined as a child who is experiencing a developmental delay or who because of a diagnosed condition has a high probability of experiencing a developmental delay.

The procedures for funding and providing support are outlined through federal law and implemented in each state through an identified lead agency (e.g., Department of Education, Department of Health). Each state coordinates and outlines how it will cover the costs of providing early intervention services. Some states cover all costs, some require partial payment by the family (typically on a sliding scale based on income), and other states access Medicaid or the family's private medical insurance.

**Evaluation for Eligibility.** The evaluation process to determine a child's initial and continuing eligibility needs to be timely, comprehensive, and multidisciplinary (§303.321). No single procedure may be utilized as the sole criterion for eligibility and procedures generally include the use of formal evaluation instruments, history and parent interviews, and gathering information from other sources to understand the full scope of the child's strengths and needs.

Occupational therapy practitioners are part of the multidisciplinary team tasked with evaluating children from birth until 3 years old to determine eligibility under IDEA Part C. Specific testing measures are outlined by each state's lead agency and can be supplemented by discipline-specific assessment tools. If the child has already been determined eligible for the federal program, discipline-specific assessment procedures are implemented when additional information is needed to assist the team in developing additional strategies. See Chapter 15 for descriptions of the IDEA Part C model of service delivery.

**Developing the Individualized Family Service Plan.** Documentation of IDEA Part C for children under 3 years and their families occurs via the **Individualized Family Service Plan** (IFSP). Components of the IFSP include:

- the child's current level of functioning (§303.344), such as physical, cognitive, communication, social-emotional, and adaptive; including strengths of the child and family
- family resources, priorities, and concerns
- expected outcomes which are written annually with a formal review every 6 months, keeping the following in mind:
  - Identify what the family should expect to see in 1 year.
  - Long-term goals are parent-driven, collaborative, and occupation-based.

    - Short-term behavioral objectives are functional and in the context of daily routines/occupations.
    - Goals and objectives should be written in family-friendly language.
    - Goals and objectives should be functional, measurable, and participation oriented.
- the steps and services to achieve the family's desired outcomes based on their strengths and needs and grounded in typical family routines

Completing an ecomap (McCormack et al., 2008), emphasizing that the early intervention team is concerned with the whole family and not just the child, and a routines-based interview (McMillan, 2010; McWilliam et al., 2009) are strategies to assist in the development of the IFSP. An ecomap outlines the family system to show team members the importance of people within the child's life. For example, see Fig. 7.3. Routines-based interviews are a method for collecting information on family routines so that team members can design effective intervention that works within each child's family system.

**Documenting Occupational Therapy Sessions.** The focus of occupational therapy services is to engage children in participation-based activities, within family routines, to promote occupational participation (e.g., rest and sleep, play, education, eating and mealtime, and social participation). Occupational therapy practitioners use collaborative, problem-solving, and coaching approaches to share information and ideas to support children's stated goals within the natural environment. They document and deliver occupational therapy services using family-centered care. Occupational therapy practitioners complete a visit note (also referred to as a progress note) describing what occurred during the occupational therapy session, how the child reacted, and suggestions for the family to implement to enhance skills until the next occupational therapy visit. Practitioners write notes that are professional, family-friendly, commensurate with the reader, and reflective of cultural humility (Agner, 2020) to engage and empower caregivers to meet their goals and priorities.

**Transition Planning.** When appropriate, the team identifies the steps planned for a transition from home-based to clinic-based and/or school-based services in the IFSP. The occupational therapy practitioner provides resources for community programs, as well as documentation outlining the therapeutic supports provided, outcomes achieved, current needs or expected needs within the new environment (e.g., adaptations and equipment to facilitate participation) and may include findings from recently administered assessments.

## Medically-Based Occupational Therapy Services

Medically-based pediatric occupational therapy services are financially supported by varying funding sources, each with their parameters for reimbursement of therapy services and thus each with their documentation rules and procedures to demonstrate the need for and the implementation of skilled occupational therapy services. For example, services may be paid for via commercial insurance, Medicaid state insurance, and state CHIP insurance for children from lower-income families. Although the format of documentation might vary, clinical documentation always includes reporting and interpreting assessment and intervention outcomes for the medical file, as well as demonstrating the practitioner's rationale for recommending skilled occupational therapy services (Sames, 2019).

**Diagnosis Coding.** Medically-based occupational therapy services are reimbursed based on the childs or youth's medical diagnosis. The World Health Organization's *International Classification of*

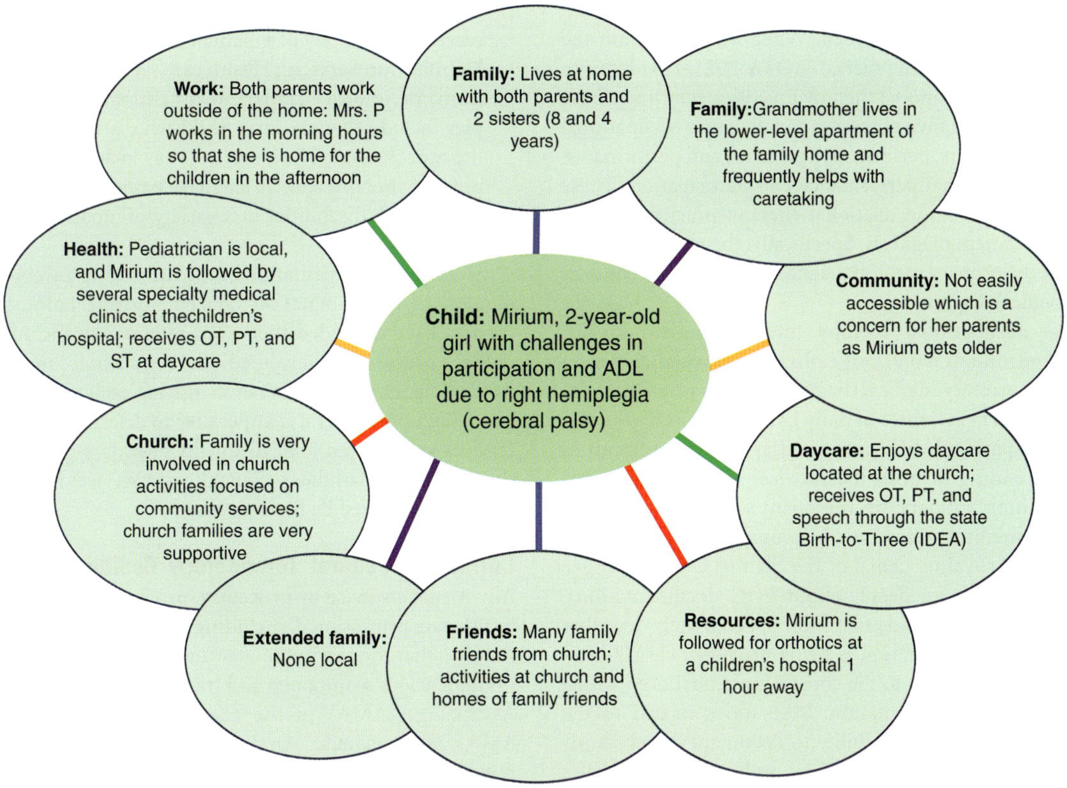


**Fig. 7.3** Sample EcoMap family system.

*Functioning, Disability and Health* (ICF) (WHO, 2001) provides standardized terminology related to health and health-related domains, function, and impact of disease, condition, or injury across health professionals. Terminology within the *Occupational Therapy Practice Framework* (AOTA, 2020a) is congruent with the ICF (WHO, 2001) concepts that the health, well-being, participation, and functioning of an individual occur in context. The *ICF-Children and Youth Version* (ICF-CY; WHO, 2007) provides insight into the impact of family, environment, participation, and the right for children with disabilities to have full enjoyment as a human right.

***International Statistical Classification of Diseases and Related Health Problems.*** The *International Statistical Classification of Diseases and Related Health Problems* (ICD), also published by WHO with periodic updates to reflect current health care changes, provides a system to report and code causes and consequences of human disease and death, or conditions impacting function. Based on WHO's 10th edition of ICD codes, the Center's for Disease Control and Prevention (CDC) created and annually updates the *International Classification of Diseases, 10th Revision-Clinical Modification* (ICD-10-CM; 2018) for reimbursement and resource allocation within the United States (U.S.). Thus, providing payer sources, other service providers, and team members with uniform information related to the diagnoses and conditions experienced by the clients served. HHS mandates that any U.S. entity covered by HIPPA for electronic health care communications/transactions, utilize the ICD coding system. The 11th edition (ICD-11) was released by the WHO in 2022. However, the National Center for Health Statistics, the Federal agency responsible for publishing ICD in the U.S., continues to maintain ICD-10-CM independently while the U.S. evaluates and considers the use of ICD-11 (National Committee on Vital and Health Statistics, 2023). The CDC provides an electronic source to search for applicable ICD-10-CM diagnosis codes (https://icd10cmtool.cdc.gov/?fy=FY2025).

The identified ICD-10-CM (2018) code, commonly referred to as the diagnosis code, is the first point of information reviewed by the medically-based payer source and needs to substantiate why skilled occupational therapy services are needed. While it is not within the occupational therapy standards of practice (AOTA, 2021a) to identify a medical diagnosis, the occupational therapy practitioner's clinical reasoning and analysis of evaluative outcomes can diagnose occupational challenges (e.g., client factors, performance patterns, and performance skills) impacting occupational performance and participation. These diagnoses, identified by the occupational therapy practitioner, are referred to as the treatment diagnosis. Specifically, the treatment diagnosis is not always the primary medical diagnosis, rather it is secondary to the primary medical diagnosis.

For example, occupational therapy intervention would not address Down syndrome (Q90.9) but rather a performance deficit associated with the primary medical diagnosis that is impacting the child's ability to perform activities of daily living, such as hypotonia (P94.2), or an occupational difficulty, such as feeding difficulties (R63.3). Accurate coding of both the medical and the treatment diagnosis or condition influencing the client's occupations, thus substantiating the medical necessity of occupational therapy services, can impact approval or denial of the Plan of Care (POC; see POC section below for more details about POC documentation). Practitioners use the diagnosis code that most appropriately describes the condition for which intervention is being provided, clearly linking the identified diagnosis code to the client's functional need which is reflected in the POC documentation. Regulations related to the occupational therapy practitioner's ability to document or substantiate treatment diagnoses are state-specific, as outlined in each state's Practice Act. Occupational therapy practitioners can avoid funding difficulty by communicating with the child's primary physician or pediatrician to document applicable ICD-11-CM codes and comorbidities impacting client performance.

Within pediatric practice, ICD-10-CM medical diagnosis codes indicating a developmental delay (e.g., R62.50 Other and unspecified lack of expected normal physiological development in childhood; R62.0 Delayed milestone in childhood), versus conditions caused by an incident or accident, require further investigation into the parameters of the payer source's coverage of developmental conditions. For example, some insurance plans specifically exclude developmental concerns as not medical in nature. After the occupational therapist analyzes evaluative findings, they can share and discuss the objective data with the primary physician or pediatrician to determine whether additional or refined diagnosis codes that might be covered by the payer source are warranted.

**Eligible Diagnoses.** Primary funding sources for medically-based coverage include commercial insurance carriers, such as insurance provided by employers to their employees or purchased by individuals through a state's marketplace under the Patient Protection and Affordable Care Act (ACA; 2010), and Medicaid. The introduction of the ACA was a turning point in coverage for medically-based occupational therapy for children with developmental concerns. The ACA identified Essential Health Benefits that all state plans must offer to receive federal monies to implement their programs. This was the introduction of habilitation versus rehabilitation as a covered benefit of insurance. To educate consumers about health services typically covered by health plans, the National Association of Insurance Commissioners (2010), an authoritative voice in the insurance industry, provided the following definitions:

- **Rehabilitation Services:** Health care services that help a person keep, get back, or improve skills and functioning for daily living that have been lost or impaired because a person was sick, hurt, or disabled. These services may include physical and occupational therapy, speech-language pathology, and psychiatric rehabilitation services in a variety of inpatient and/or outpatient settings.
- **Habilitation Services:** Health care services that help a person keep, learn, or improve skills and functioning for daily living. Examples include therapy for a child who is not walking or talking at the expected age. These services may include occupational therapy, physical therapy, speech-language pathology, and other services for people with disabilities in a variety of inpatient and/or outpatient settings.

Since the implementation of the Affordable Care Act and the introduction of the habilitation concept, private commercial insurance carriers have expanded their plan offerings to include these types of services previously considered "developmental" in nature and not a covered benefit. Therefore, investigating each potential client's insurance plan upon referral is imperative to determine whether habilitative services are covered and, if not, to provide a good faith estimate of therapy costs to families seeking therapy services for their children that will not be covered by their insurance.

**Current Procedural Terminology Coding for Patient Contact.** Any medical service or procedure provided by a physician and other health care professional, including occupational therapy practitioners, requires that the service be identified through the uniform, five-digit, numeric codes maintained and trademarked by the American Medical Association (AMA) in the *Current Procedural Terminology* (CPT; AMA, 2024) manual. An Editorial Panel authorized by the AMA, revises, updates, or modifies CPT codes, descriptors, and guidelines (AMA, n.d.). There are two seats on the editorial panel for health care professionals from the Health Care Professionals Advisory Committee, on which an AOTA representative sits. Therefore, facilities providing occupational therapy services monitor the Editorial Panel's activities for updates on approved therapy services and corresponding codes.

Physical Medicine and Rehabilitative (PM&R) codes are located in the 97000 section of the CPT manual (AMA, 2024). Each CPT code is designated as either a one-on-one, direct contact procedure in 15-minute increments; or an untimed procedure for direct therapy whereby the code is only billed once and has one reimbursement rate whether the procedure is provided for 20 minutes or 2 hours. See Table 7.3 for the common CPT codes for pediatric occupational therapy. Four codes (listed below) are identified as available in the CPT manual are not listed in Table 7.3 as they are either not generally funded by medical payers except for certain pediatric diagnoses (three codes) or are a recent addition (one code) with uncertain reimbursement success. Obtaining coverage for these CPT codes requires additional advocacy by the profession and/or a professionally persistent occupational therapy practitioner armed with current evidence to appeal denials for coverage.

- 97533 Sensory integrative techniques to enhance sensory processing and promote adaptive responses to environmental demands, direct (one-on-one) patient contact by the provider, each 15 minutes: A client with a diagnosis of autism spectrum disorder has a greater likelihood of getting approval for this intervention; otherwise, it is generally considered experimental.
- 97130 Therapeutic interventions that focus on cognitive function (e.g., attention, memory, reasoning, executive function, problem-solving, and/or pragmatic function): A client with a diagnosis related to head trauma with no prior cognitive difficulties has a greater likelihood of getting approval for this intervention.
- 96110 Developmental Screening: Screenings are not generally covered as an occupational therapy service under commercial insurance carriers or Medicaid; but might be covered under educationally-based services through Medicaid. Coverage is state-specific according to each state's Medicaid offerings and should be investigated for possible reimbursement.
- 97550-Caregiver training in strategies and techniques to facilitate the patient's functional performance in the home or community (e.g., activities of daily living [ADLs], instrumental ADLs [IADLs], transfers, mobility, communication, swallowing, feeding, problem-solving, safety practices) (without the patient present), face-to-face; initial 30 minutes: This is a newer code and successful reimbursement from the various payer sources, particularly for pediatric clients, remains unclear. Providing caregiver training while the child is present can be billed as the one-on-one intervention (e.g., 97535 Self-care/home management [e.g., ADLs] or 97530 Therapeutic activities) for each 15-minutes.

CPT codes for therapy services are also referred to as Level I codes. A second set of codes applicable to occupational therapy, referred to as Level II codes, include codes for supplies, products, and durable medical equipment such as E1130–E1161 for wheelchair specifications and L3806–L3904 for orthotics. Level II coding is referred to as the Healthcare Common Procedural Coding System CMS, 2022a.

The following categories highlight important points when deciding on which code(s) to bill, parameters regarding the number of codes you can bill per session length, and the rules for certain codes not to be billed on the same date of service.

***Current Procedural Terminology Evaluation Codes.*** In 2017, the AMA released new CPT codes for evaluation and reevaluation which were required for all HIPPA entities providing occupational and physical therapies for therapy services funded by commercial insurance, Medicaid, and CHIP. The evaluation code revision expanded coding to reflect low, moderate, or high-complexity evaluation procedures. The descriptive language in the occupational therapy evaluation codes recognized the importance of our profession, including implementation of an occupational profile (e.g., values, interests, patterns, needs, and priorities); assessment of performance deficits (i.e., occupations impacted by physical, cognitive, and psychosocial performance skills); and reasoning and decision-making to determine how these factors impact occupational performance.

**TABLE 7.3 Common Pediatric CPT Codes**

| CPT Code[a] | Description/Category |
|---|---|
| 97150 | Therapeutic Procedure(s), group (2 or more individuals); untimed |
| 97165 | OT evaluation—Low complexity; untimed |
| 97166 | OT evaluation—Moderate complexity; untimed |
| 97167 | OT evaluation—High complexity; untimed |
| 97168 | OT reevaluation; untimed |
| 97112 & 97113 | Developmental test administration (including assessment of fine and/or gross motor, language, cognitive level, social, memory, and/or executive functions) by standardized developmental instruments; 1st hour and each subsequent 30 minutes |
| 97110 | Therapeutic procedure; therapeutic exercise to develop strength and endurance, range of motion, and flexibility (one or more areas, each 15 minutes) |
| 97112 | Neuromuscular reeducation of movement, balance, coordination, kinesthetic sense, posture, and/or proprioception for sitting and/or standing activities (one or more areas, each 15 minutes) |
| 97113 | Aquatic therapy with therapeutic exercises (one or more areas, each 15 minutes) |
| 97140 | Manual therapy techniques, one or more regions, each 15 minutes |
| 97150 | Group therapeutic procedures |
| 97530 | Therapeutic activities, direct (one-on-one) patient contact (use of dynamic activities to improve functional performance), each 15 minutes |
| 97535 | Self–care/home management training (e.g., activities of daily living) and compensatory training, meal preparation, safety procedures, and instructions in the use of assistive technology devices/adaptive equipment) direct one-on-one contact, each 15 minutes |
| 97537 | Community/work reintegration training (e.g., shopping, transportation, money management, avocational activities and/or work environment/modification analysis, work task analysis) direct one-on-one contact, each 15 minutes |
| 97542 | Wheelchair management (e.g., assessment, fitting, training), each 15 minutes |
| 97760 | Orthotics management and training (initial encounter) |
| 97763 | Orthotic(s)/prosthetic(s) management and/or training, upper extremity(ies), lower extremity(ies), and/or trunk, subsequent orthotic(s)/prosthetic(s) encounter, each 15 minutes |
| 97755 | Assistive technology assessment |
| 92526 | Treatment of swallowing dysfunction and/or oral function for feeding; untimed |

[a]CPT Codes are registered and trademarked by the American Medical Association.

AOTA (2016) provided a detailed description of how to choose the appropriate evaluation code (i.e., low, moderate, or high complexity). This process involves determining the complexity of each component of the evaluation (i.e., occupational profile, assessment measures of performance, and clinical reasoning and decision-making). For billing purposes, the therapist selects the lowest complexity identified in any of the evaluation components. For example, if the therapist determined the occupational profile was low complexity; the assessment of performance was moderate complexity; and the clinical reasoning and decision-making was high complexity, the evaluation would only qualify for the low complexity evaluation CPT code. The high complexity evaluation CPT code can only be used if all three evaluative components are determined to be high complexity.

The complexity rating is not based on the expertise level of the therapist. Therefore, an evaluation that requires a seasoned therapist does not necessarily mean it is a highly complex evaluation. See Table 7.4 to assist when identifying the correct occupational therapy evaluation code. Case Example 7.2 Ayanna illustrates how to identify the appropriate evaluation code.

***Current Procedural Terminology Treatment Codes.*** Table 7.3 identifies treatment codes that are timed, such as 15 minutes of direct treatment for 97530 therapeutic activities or 97535 self-care; and untimed codes for direct treatment, such as 92526 oral motor for feeding, which are billed as one code per patient contact no matter the amount of time the occupational therapy practitioner provides the service.

Rules allow for timed and untimed codes to be billed during one treatment session. However, the rules for timed codes during one patient contact are a bit more complicated and depend on the funding source. Most payer sources follow CMS rules vs. AMA rules, but the rules for each client's payer source needs to be confirmed to assure compliance and correct coding. CMS and AMA rules are as follows:

- The CMS (2022a), governing all federal insurance programs (e.g., Medicaid for children and youth) and adopted by some commercial insurance carriers, follow the "8-minute Rule" which has two important features (1) Practitioners are not allowed to bill 15-minute units of service more than the total number of minutes provided. For example, if the child only received 45 minutes of service, you cannot bill more than three 15-minute units. (2) If 8 minutes are provided in the final 15-minute time block of the session, the last code can be billed. If 7 minutes are provided, another code cannot be billed. It is easiest to remember this rule as follows: the practitioner needs to complete each 15-minute block, before considering whether the final 15-minute block can be billed after satisfying 8 minutes of implementation.
- The AMA provided guidance on billing 15-minute timed codes in the CPT manual (AMA, 2024) which are different from the CMS rules. AMA outlined the concept of passing the midpoint of a 15-minute timed code—referred to as the "Greater than Midpoint" or "> 50%" rule. This calculation requires more specific tracking of the time that each intervention is provided. Specifically, the intervention provided must pass the 8-minute mark to be billed. For example, if you provided a 20-minute session, with 10 minutes of 97110 therapeutic exercise and 10 minutes of 97535 self-care, you could bill both codes, thus totaling two codes for that 20-minute session. Again, however, most funding sources do not follow this rule.

Case Example 7.3 Byron summarizes the differences between the CMS and AMA guidelines. See Table 7.5 on how to calculate the number of units to bill based on the total minutes the child received intervention following the CMS 8-minute Rule.

**TABLE 7.4 OT Evaluation CPT Code Checklist**

| Evaluation Code | Occupational Profile and Medical/Therapy History | Patient Assessment | Clinical Decision-making |
|---|---|---|---|
| Low complexity | ❑ occupational profile and **brief** history relating to presenting problem | ❑ **1–3 performance deficits** relating to **physical, cognitive, and psychosocial** skills resulting in activity limitations and/or participation restrictions;<br>**Performance deficits** relate to occupations that will be addressed in the plan of care (POC)—refer to OTPF-4 (2022, Table 2—Occupations, p. 30) | Low analytical complexity includes:<br>❑ **problem-focused** assessment(s)<br>❑ **no modification** of assessments or assessment tasks<br>❑ **no comorbidities** affecting occupational performance<br>❑ **limited** number of treatment options |
| Moderate complexity | ❑ occupational profile and **expanded** review of medical/ therapy records<br>❑ **additional** review of physical, cognitive, and psychosocial history related to current functional performance | ❑ **3–5 performance deficits** relating to **physical, cognitive, and psychosocial** skills that result in activity limitations and/or participation restrictions;<br>**Performance deficits** relate to occupations that will be addressed in the POC—refer to OTPF-4 (2022, Table 2—Occupations, p.30) | Moderate analytical complexity includes:<br>❑ **detailed** assessments<br>❑ **minimal to moderate modification** of assessments or assessment tasks<br>❑ **may have comorbidities** affecting occupational performance<br>❑ **several** treatment options |
| High complexity | ❑ occupational profile and **extensive** medical/therapy history review<br>❑ **Extensive** additional review of physical, cognitive, and psychosocial history related to current functional performance | ❑ **5 or more performance deficits** relating to **physical, cognitive, and psychosocial skills** that result in activity limitations and/or participation restrictions;<br>**Performance deficits** relate to occupations that will be addressed in the POC—refer to OTPF-4 (2022, Table 2—Occupations, p. 30) | High analytic complexity includes:<br>❑ **comprehensive** assessments<br>❑ **significant modifications** of assessments or assessment tasks<br>❑ **comorbidities** affecting occupational performance<br>❑ **multiple** treatment options |


Adapted from Brennan, C., & Glennon, T. J. (2017). *Occupational therapy checklist for CPT coding criteria.* American Occupational Therapy Association.

## CASE EXAMPLE 7.2 AYANNA

***Occupational Profile:*** Client is an 11-month-old female with no significant medical history; pregnancy and delivery were uneventful, and no medical conditions were reported. Pt. lives with both parents and a 2-year-old sister in the maternal grandparents' home. The mother self-referred after hearing an occupational therapist discuss infant feeding difficulties at the local library. Presenting concerns were a history of difficulty with bottle feeding and spillage with spoon feeding. Upon further interview, limited interest in play and having to fall asleep in the arms of certain caregivers were also highlighted as areas of concern.

***Assessment:*** The assessment included parent interview, clinical observations, *HELP 0–3 Checklist* (Furano et al., 2016), *Sensory Processing Measure—Toddler and Caregiver Self Report Forms* (Glennon et al., 2021), and observation of bottle/cup usage, spoon feeding, and play.

***Therapeutic Clinical Reasoning and Decision-making:*** Evaluative findings indicated co-regulation difficulties secondary to differing sensory processing patterns of caregiver and child, decreased play, decreased fine motor manipulation, and sensory over-responsivity impacting functional participation in age-expected occupations. See the following chart for the level of complexity for each of the evaluative components. The evaluation resulted in CPT Evaluation Code 97165 Low Complexity due to the low complexity rating of the occupation profile component of the evaluation process.

| Evaluation Code | Low Complexity | Moderate Complexity | High Complexity | Comments |
|---|---|---|---|---|
| Occupational profile and medical/therapy history | X | | | Brief history; no medical records to review relating to the presenting problem |
| Assessments | | | X | 5+ performance deficits to be addressed in the plan of care. Per OTPF-4 (2022, Table 2—Occupations, p. 30), these included: Sleep preparation, eating and swallowing; self-feeding (holding bottle, using a cup, finger feeding); play exploration; play participation; and family participation |
| Clinical reasoning & decision making | | X | | Minimal to moderate modification of tasks; no comorbidities; several intervention treatment options appropriate. |

## CASE EXAMPLE 7.3 BYRON—CMS VERSUS AMA CODING

Byron, an occupational therapist working in an outpatient hospital setting, was scheduled to provide services to a 3-year-old boy. After 20 minutes, the child vomited, and the session was discontinued. For the 20 minutes session, two interventions were provided: 12 minutes of 97530 therapeutic activities and 8 minutes of 97535 self-care.

According to AMA guidelines, Byron could bill the session as two 15-minute codes, one code for each intervention as both interventions were >50% of the 15 minutes required. However, this child's insurance plan followed CMS rules. Therefore, Byron could only bill one code for the 20-minute session because the 23-minute threshold for total time of intervention required to bill 2 units (requiring 15 minutes for the first code and at least 8 minutes for the second code) was not met. In this instance when billing one treatment code for CMS, Byron coded the intervention that occurred for most of the session (97530).

In a similar situation with another child, Bryon provided 8 minutes of 97110 therapeutic exercises, 8 minutes of 97530 therapeutic activities, and 8 minutes of 97535 self-care. Three codes could be billed for the 24 minutes of service according to AMA's > 50% rule, but again the child's insurance carrier followed CMS rules which only allowed two billable codes for the 24-minute session based on the total time the child received intervention.

**TABLE 7.5 CMS 8-Minute Rule Calculations**

| Minutes of Intervention Provided | @ 15 minutes per Unit | Total Units Billed |
|---|---|---|
| 1–7 | 0 | 0 |
| 8–22 | 15 | 1 |
| 23–37 | 30 | 2 |
| 38–52 | 45 | 3 |
| 53–67 | 60 | 4 |

***Current Procedural Terminology Coding Combinations.*** Another factor for correct billing of CPT codes is the code combinations the practitioner chooses to bill. To prevent payment for incorrect or improper billing, the National Correct Coding Initiative (NCCI) lists pairs of therapy codes that cannot be billed together on the same date of service. These limitations, called CPT pair edits, include (a) two Level I (CPT) codes for therapy intervention that cannot be billed together and (b) Level I and Level II (e.g., for durable medical equipment) code combinations that cannot be billed together. As each payer source has its own rules based on contractual arrangements with the provider organization, the occupational therapy practitioner discusses this concept with supervisors or administrators. This should also be discussed with the entire therapy team as there are instances when pair edits can be flagged and denied by the commercial insurance payer when the child receives therapies from multiple disciplines on the same day. If this occurs, appeals and additional paperwork are required.

There are times when the occupational therapy practitioner needs to alert the payer source that two codes not typically allowed together, but allowed in certain circumstances, were provided as two distinct services that did not overlap. In this situation, the addition of a Modifier 59 code is added to the billing statement. It is extremely important in this situation that session documentation is clear that two distinct, non-overlapping services were provided. See Box 7.3 for two examples of using Modifier 59 when coding/billing. An organization's EMR or health record system is typically programmed with pair edit limitations so when the occupational therapy practitioner clicks two codes that are not allowed together when billing, the system provides a pop-up alert to either choose a different code or add a Modifier 59 if allowed.

***Current Procedural Terminology Coding for Co-treatments.*** There are instances where two providers are present during a child's treatment session. While this might be considered optimal or a medically necessary intervention in certain situations, the time billed for services is limited to the amount of time the patient received therapy, rather than the amount of time practitioners provided intervention. For example, if both the occupational therapy practitioner and speech-language pathologist are

## BOX 7.3 Examples Using Modifier 59

- Ally, an occupational therapist with expertise in oral motor interventions, bills 92526 (oral motor for feeding) which is an untimed treatment code. She also billed 97110 (therapeutic exercises), a timed code (15 minutes of direct patient contact) but forgot to add Modifier 59. The insurance payer rejected the therapeutic exercise code as a pair edit – most likely because they interpreted exercises as part of oral motor interventions. Ally needed to resubmit her coding/billing, along with her session notes to demonstrate that she provided therapeutic exercises as a separate and distinct intervention from the oral motor purpose. Her notes documented that in addition to oral motor interventions on that day, she had also utilized therapeutic exercises to support Jose's fine motor skills (i.e., to a distinctly different body part).
- Roberto completed an OT evaluation which was coded as 97165 (Low Complexity), an untimed code. Roberto knew that the child did not require prior authorization for therapy intervention based on their diagnosis. After the evaluation was completed and the plan of care was conceptualized based on the caregiver's priorities, Roberto began treatment on the evaluation day. Roberto had the caregiver join the session to highlight and demonstrate the therapeutic strategies and activities so that they could immediately be implemented at home. Roberto billed 97530 (therapeutic activities; a timed code requiring 15 minutes of direct patient contact) as well as the evaluation code. Since an OT evaluation and therapeutic activities are listed as a pair edit, Roberto needed to use Modifier 59 to alert the insurance payer that the therapeutic activities were distinct from the evaluation process and the session notes clearly documented both the evaluative and treatment portions of the session.

present and providing therapy during a one-hour session, the patient is only billed for 1 hour, not 1 hour for occupational therapy and 1 hour for speech. This could be billed in any appropriate configuration (e.g., one hour for occupational therapy and no speech billed; half hour of occupational therapy and half hour for speech therapy).

## Requirements for Reimbursement in Medical Facilities

Reimbursement requirements for skilled, occupational therapy services within a medical model vary from payer to payer and, for pediatric occupational therapy services, are constantly evolving. For example, one commercial insurance plan might allow 97535 self-care, whereas Medicaid might deem it "not a covered service for children" under that specific state's Medicaid program. As a result, the details of each payer source's parameters for covered therapy services require monitoring to update documentation and coding procedures accordingly. This monitoring is critical to ensure that documentation provides the rationale for the purpose, value, and necessity of skilled occupational therapy services (AOTA, 2018), assure compliance if audited or during routine utilization management or review by the payer source, and assist the occupational therapy practitioner to navigate appeals if services are denied.

**Referral.** The occupational therapy process begins with the referral, and the referral information is the first document in the medical file related to occupational therapy services. In pediatric practice, a referral can come from various professionals who interact with children and youth. Professionals familiar with child development, such as daycare workers, often alert the caregiver to a child's difficulties with age-expected skills and occupational engagement and advocate that the caregiver seek professional intervention. Many local pediatric occupational therapy practices provide daycare centers with a referral form to streamline information sharing related to the child's difficulties (see Fig. 7.4 for a sample daycare referral form). If the occupational therapy practitioner is licensed in a state that allows "direct access" to occupational therapy, they may begin the occupational therapy evaluation process without a physician's referral. However, the occupational therapist should contact the primary physician or pediatrician to obtain the necessary documentation for medical insurance coverage.

**Evaluation.** The medically-based evaluation is intended to determine whether skilled occupational therapy services are warranted to address the client's needs, difficulties, and concerns related to performance in occupations. When documenting evaluative findings, the occupational therapist should be cognizant of and adhere to the payer's requirements for the presentation of evaluative findings. See Chapter 9 for a full discussion of the components of an occupational therapy evaluation. There are instances whereby a payer source requires completion of their paperwork/forms which may not allow for the level of detail that occupational therapists typically provide in pediatric practice. In these situations, it may be necessary and the therapist's professional obligation to provide supplemental information to describe the value of occupational therapy services for the child.

**Plan of Care and Authorization for Therapy Services.** Based on the evaluation results, when warranted, the occupational therapist collaboratively develops a POC (also called an intervention plan) with the caregiver and child. The POC document provides a clear rationale for the value and necessity of skilled occupational therapy services with clearly identified goals and short-term behavioral objectives. The POC is crafted based on the outcome of the comprehensive evaluation and typically includes:

- Occupational therapist's name, credentials, and state licensure number
- Rehabilitative/habilitative barriers (e.g., client factors, performance skills) to functional participation in needed occupations
- Goals and short-term behavioral objectives
- Frequency and duration of therapy to attain the short-term behavioral objectives

Be sure to understand the funding source's time expectation for the POC. For example, many insurance carriers will not approve therapy services for more than 90 days (3 months or 12 weeks) and, therefore, the plan outlines expectations for that specific period. Thereafter, subsequent plans for each 90-day period are submitted. However, some governmental or external funding agencies will allow 6-month or 1-year time frames for the goals and short-term behavioral objectives. In those cases, goals and short-term behavioral objectives correspond to the identified time frame.

Obtaining **prior authorization** from a commercial insurance carrier, governmental funding agency, or other funding source to financially support occupational therapy services is common. Prior authorization typically involves providing the evaluation results and POC for the child.

**Progress Note—Subsequent Plans of Care.** After the initial authorization period, the original POC based on evaluative results will need to be updated to obtain approval for services to continue. Each subsequent POC after the first POC is required to show progress, as well as document updated short-term behavioral objectives. The progress report clearly states the initial performance and the current level of functioning based on the identified goals and objectives. For example, if the therapist was authorized for a 3-month course of intervention by the insurance carrier, the progress note at the 3-month mark should include prior skill level and current performance. Clearly documenting the child's performance before and after within one document provides evidence of the change in functional performance.

During this process, avoid terms such as "age expected" or "age appropriate" as these are vague concepts and difficult to achieve within short timeframes. Be specific, with observable, measurable short-term behavioral objectives, and pay particular care in identifying objectives that can

Center for Pediatric Therapy
OT • Speech • PT

455 Post Road Suite 202
Darien, CT 06820
p 203.424.2584
f 203.202.7310

55 Walls Drive Suite 204
Fairfield, CT 06824
p 203.255.3669
f 203.255.1173

101 N. Plains Industrial
Wallingford, CT 06492
p 203.949.9337
f 203.284.3779

*Supporting children where they live, learn, and play.*

**Daycare Name:** ______________________ **Teacher:** ______________

**Daycare Address:** ______________________ **Phone:** ______________

**Child's Name:** ______________________ **DOB:** ______________

______________________________________________

**Parent Name** **Parent Signature** **Date**

## Please check this child's areas of concern.

### Gross Motor/ Postural Control

- ❑ Falls often, clumsy
- ❑ Delayed developmental milestones, such as rolling, sitting, crawling, or walking
- ❑ Frequently bumps into objects or other children
- ❑ Difficulty participating in movement games, such as Simon Says
- ❑ Difficulty with hopping, jumping, skipping
- ❑ Difficulty sitting still in chair or on the floor during circle time
- ❑ Frequently sits on edge of chair or falls off
- ❑ Frequently sits in W-sit position during circle time or floor play

### Fine Motor Coordination

- ❑ Awkward grasp patterns when picking up small objects
- ❑ Difficulty manipulating or drops small objects, such as beads or 1 inch blocks
- ❑ Awkward grasp pattern for crayon/marker
- ❑ Difficulty with coloring or drawing
- ❑ Difficulty copying or imitating age expected shapes/designs
- ❑ Awkward grasp pattern with classroom utensils or not using the utensil properly, such as spoon, scissors, or paint brush
- ❑ Doesn't have a preferred hand
- ❑ Difficulty with dressing, such as putting on coat, socks, or shoes
- ❑ Difficulty with zippers or snaps

### Sensory Function

- ❑ Difficulty adjusting to changes in routine
- ❑ In constant motion or "on the go"
- ❑ Avoids messy play, such as finger painting or gluing activities
- ❑ Difficulty calming self or settling down
- ❑ Chews on toys, collar, or sleeves often
- ❑ Pushes or shoves other children without malicious intent
- ❑ Distressed by everyday touch experiences, such as clothing or food textures
- ❑ Distressed by smells (e.g., food, paint, perfume) or sounds (e.g., toilet flushing) that others do not find annoying
- ❑ Seeks falling, crashing, or high intensity games more than other children
- ❑ Difficulty tolerating parties or a busy environment with lots of activity or noise
- ❑ Frequent meltdowns or outbursts
- ❑ Concerns with eating/feeding skills

### Speech and Language

- ❑ Vocalizes sounds or uses gestures instead of words
- ❑ Limited talking
- ❑ Others can't understand what he/she is saying
- ❑ Difficulty understanding directions
- ❑ Difficulty having a reciprocal conversation with peers
- ❑ Difficulty with social skills

**Fig. 7.4** Community infographics: (A) Back to school and (B) Creating a homework zone.

be mastered within the specific time frame authorized for reimbursement. For example, if the therapist completed an evaluation on a 2-year-old diagnosed with an autism spectrum disorder who was unable to follow any verbal directions during the evaluation session and is authorized for 3 months of intervention followed by a review, the short-term behavioral objectives need to be congruent with the 3-month time frame. Expecting the child to complete a three-step dressing task with minimal verbal prompting would not be realistic within 3 months given the baseline performance of not following any verbal instructions noted during the evaluation.

The therapist identifies the conditions and frequency for the target behavior. In subsequent plans of care, the conditions or criteria can be increased to show the progression of change and improvement in either the number of repetitions (criteria) or under what circumstances (conditions) progressively moving toward performing the target behavior within a more natural context. See Box 7.4 for an example plan documenting progressively difficult short-term behavioral objectives for a 3-month period.

**Appeal for Denial of Services.** An insurance company can issue a denial letter for a variety of reasons. For example, the initial authorization request as outlined in the POC can be denied as not necessary for the diagnosis stated; a subsequent POC can be denied to reflect that the number of visits requested does not match the insurance carrier's expected number of sessions for a specific diagnosis; a specific service provided, CPT coded, and submitted for payment can be denied per the patient's particular insurance plan coverage; the patient has reached their specific insurance plan's coverage limit for the number of allowable sessions; or the insurance carrier reviewer did not agree that skilled occupational therapy services were further warranted based on the diagnosis code, progress achieved to date, or some other reason. The following steps are suggested when appealing to insurance companies.

1. Be aware of the appeal timelines in the specific payer's contract or plan specifications as each payer source is different.
2. Carefully read the denial letter to ascertain the specific reason for denial as the denial reason guides the next steps. It is important to understand whether this is a policy issue (which might impact other children receiving occupational therapy services at the facility) or a child-specific issue.
    a. Policy issue: If, for example, the insurance company's policy does not cover occupational therapy services for children because they consider the child's needs to be developmental in nature, this requires the administrator at your company to reach out to an administrator or provider representative at the insurance company to discuss habilitative vs. rehabilitative therapy. While administrative channels are pursued, a letter of medical necessity (LOMN; see next section) should be submitted by the occupational therapist to the insurance reviewer outlining why this specific child's services should qualify as medical rather than developmental. This letter should not wait for the administrative channel to be pursued because the occupational therapist does not want to miss the appeal deadline.
    b. Child-specific issue: Have the support staff reconfirm insurance plan specifications for specific diagnoses covered, the number of sessions allowed per the policy, or any other child-specific reason stated in the denial. Obtain the policy information in writing to confirm the information that is being provided over the phone or check the insurance portal for specific policy statements. Keep track of dates and people with whom support staff have communicated with at the insurance company, and the specific information shared by the insurance company.
3. Determine whether it is a CPT coding issue. For example, was the wrong CPT code submitted (e.g., the occupational therapy practitioner coded 97533 sensory integration, and the insurance provider considers the treatment experimental) and the session needs to be recoded with another code that accurately reflects the intervention (e.g., 97530 therapeutic activities).

If the denial issue is child-specific and related to the reviewer not agreeing that skilled occupational therapy services are required, obtain assistance from the occupational therapy supervisor to craft an appeal letter which is considered an LOMN (see next section). Writing an appeal letter is often difficult when the occupational therapy practitioner's and family's emotions are running high due to the denial. Keep the reader's perspective in mind and consider how the reader (or reviewer) is likely to interpret the request (Sames, 2015). Keep a respectful and professional tone, without sounding condescending, and present a clear description of the child's status and need for services. Avoid professional jargon. Statements such as "[name] is unable to [skill] which is essential for [occupation/participation]" are important. For example, "Homer is unable to use his fingers to grasp objects which is essential for managing a spoon at mealtime and a toothbrush for proper dental care"; or "The caregiver, pediatrician, and team members (including the occupational therapy practitioner) are concerned from a safety perspective because Mercy's limited ability to swallow continues to result in choking incidents."

The appeal letter can also include a note from the primary physician, pediatrician, or other medical professional that monitors the child's medical status (e.g., neurologist). The occupational therapy practitioner needs to be persistent with follow-up communications, all in a timely manner as outlined in the denial paperwork from the insurance carrier.

If the appeal letter is not successful, the occupational therapist's professional judgment is that services are warranted, and the insurance carrier does not appear to be following accepted standards for reimbursement, the family can contact the state's insurance commissioner for further support. Filing a complaint with the insurance commissioner is a last resort, so it is essential that all appeals and procedures have been followed by the occupational therapist and the company providing the occupational therapy services.

**Letter of Medical Necessity.** A LOMN is often required to document the need for skilled occupational therapy services or equipment to a commercial insurance carrier or other funding source. The intent of the LOMN is to justify why a particular medical service or device is required to address barriers to skill acquisition. Assuring that the

### BOX 7.4 Plan of Care: Documenting Progressively Difficult Short-Term Behavioral Objectives

- Initial plan of care: Within a small, distraction-free environment with only the therapist and with *three* items within his reach (condition), Jose will follow the simple verbal direction "give me [blank]" (target behavior) at least *once* during the session for three out of four consecutive sessions (criteria).
- Subsequent plan of care—Criteria increased: Within a small, distraction-free environment with only the therapist and with three items within his reach (condition), Jose will follow the simple direction "give me [blank]" (target behavior) at least *three occurrences* during a session for three out of four consecutive sessions (criteria).
- Subsequent plan of care—Condition increased related to environmental factors: Within a small, distraction-free environment with only the therapist and with *six* items within his reach (condition), Jose will follow the simple verbal direction "give me [blank]" (target behavior) at least once during a session for three out of four consecutive sessions (criteria). In this example, only the condition increased; the target behavior (follow the verbal direction "give me") and the criteria (once during the session for three out of four consecutive sessions) did not increase. Yet, progress has been identified.

information provided is accurate and comprehensive will alleviate denials and/or delays in approval. Be aware of all timelines and follow-up if no responses have been received. If the LOMN is denied, follow the steps for appeal, being sure to adhere to all deadlines. See Box 7.5 for the information required in an LOMN.

**Intervention Session Notes.** Intervention documentation requirements, preferences, and "red flag" terminology, such as "age appropriate" language, are payer source-specific. Administrators at medically-based facilities providing services for children and youth can assist therapy staff to monitor the official requirements and unofficial preferences of each payer source. The pattern and flow of session notes that the reviewers at the payer source prefer is one area to keep track of when submitting paperwork. For example, "When postural stability was supported by sitting criss-cross on the floor and leaning against the wall, Ava utilized a tripod grasp to manipulate and engage 3 out of the 7 buttons on her sweater" is a full sentence that highlights the functionality of Ava's fine motor performance skills as well as the supports needed for occupational success. This information could also be written as "Pt. utilized tripod 3/7 buttons" which highlights performance skills, or components of the occupation. Occupational therapy practitioners often use more narrative, descriptive, client-centered language. Reviewers, however, specifically looking to determine whether progress is occurring to approve payment, can track 3/7 to 6/7 over subsequent treatment session notes more easily than scrolling through narrative sentences. In the end, the provider facility needs payment so that the child can get the services they need to functionally engage. Therefore, decisions on the format for treatment notes are decided by the provider organization where the occupational therapy practitioner provides therapy.

***S.O.A.P. Notes.*** The SOAP note format, Subjective–Objective–Assessment–Plan, provides organization when documenting a treatment session and highlights key concepts to remember. While this format is cumbersome and not always practical in a fast-paced facility, understanding the SOAP format allows any occupational therapy practitioner to modify based on payer source preferences and practical realities.

- Subjective: Subjective information cannot be measured. The focus is on the client's subjective experience, what the child says (Sames, 2019), perspective, feelings, and attitude toward their condition or the treatment (Gateley & Borcherding, 2017), for example: "I can't climb up." or "I did it!" If the child is nonverbal, the subjective portion can describe an observable action to reflect subjective communications, such as Mario smiled and looked at the practitioner after placing the puzzle piece correctly. For toddlers with limited language, observations of behaviors can be recorded, such as Hazel greeted this therapist with a huge smile and ran down the hall to the therapy room. It is also common to include caregiver perceptions. For example, when the occupational therapy practitioner picks up the child in the waiting area, a short conversation allows for the caregiver to share current status since the last visit. Comments such as "Kammy had a great week – she was able to get her shoes on twice!" or "Joey had a hard day but still wanted to come to occupational therapy." can be documented in the Subjective portion of the SOAP note.
- Objective: This is the data section that includes observable, measurable, and quantifiable information with functional participation overarching all observations. When documenting observable actions, be sure to include the level of assistance provided by the occupational therapy practitioner for the child to achieve occupational success. Include descriptors in the objective section of a SOAP note (e.g., the occupational therapy practitioner graded or adapted the task, modeled and provided moderate verbal prompts or minimal physical assistance) to support skilled intervention. This section can be lengthy. Practitioners may benefit from mentoring to refine observations and provide concise clinical documentation. Following are some recommendations for the Objective Section of the SOAP note:

### BOX 7.5 Letter of Medical Necessity (LOMN)

- General: Date of plan of care
- Patient: Name, date of birth, and diagnosis
- Insurance holder: name of person who is holding/purchasing the insurance plan, and corresponding member and group numbers.
- Referring physician: Name and contact information.
- Plan of Care (as an outcome of the comprehensive evaluation), including
  - Rehabilitative/habilitative barriers to functional participation in expected occupations
  - goals and short-term behavioral objectives
  - frequency and duration of therapy to attain the short-term, behavioral objectives.
- Therapeutic interventions required to attain the goals and objectives, and why those skilled services are medically necessary. This is generally the narrative portion of the LOMN. Considerations for the narrative portion of the LOMN include:
  - Each LOMN is specific to the requirements of the funding source. Therefore, knowing the funding source (check their website for covered services), the specific plan purchased by the caregiver of the child (call to confirm e.g., rehabilitative or habilitative coverage), and how the funding source views their role in financially supporting the therapy services.
  - Match your narrative to the language the funding source "understands." Therefore, you need to investigate the funding source's preferred functional outcome language (e.g., occupations such as tying shoes) or medical, client factor, or performance skills language (e.g., smaller components of the occupation such as motor control of the fingers to grasp an object).
  - It is also helpful to include addendums with research evidence for your proposed intervention(s) if you are proposing interventions that are considered experimental or not generally accepted.
- If the LOMN is to obtain funding for a specific medical device:
  - Outline the professionals on the medical team and how long each profession has been providing services.
  - List any other durable medical equipment devices that the patient currently utilizes (e.g., orthotics, visual or auditory supports, positional standers, or seating devices).
  - Include evaluative findings that support the need for the device/equipment.
  - Clearly describe the features of the device/equipment you are presenting for authorization and how the device will meet the needs of this specific patient (vs. generalities of how the device is helpful).
  - Be detailed in how the device will support the function or independence of the patient, how each requested accessory meets a functional need, and/or how the device assists the patient in meeting established goals of therapy. Illustrations of how an activity or functional task would be scaffolded by the device would be helpful.
- Summary section to highlight key points. Be clear, concise, and assertive yet professional. State that occupational therapy using evidence-based interventions that are considered best practice (but please be sure that you are accurate before you make this statement) is required to address the needs of the client to attain the skills to successfully complete or participate in expected functional occupations/tasks.
- Provide contact information for any questions or needed clarifications.
- Occupational therapy practitioner's name, credentials, and state licensure number
- If required, OT assistant's name and credentials and the state licensure number of the supervising occupational therapist.

- Begin note with a statement about the length, setting, and purpose of the treatment session, offering an introduction to where, what, for how long, and why concepts (Gateley & Borcherding, 2017).
- Focus on the where, what, and why concepts when CPT codes are utilized to document the length of the session.
- Illustrate both the skilled intervention and active patient participation (Sames, 2015) in an opening statement. For example, "Harry engaged in a variety of gross motor strengthening activities in the large therapy gym aimed at improving postural control to improve upright posture during mealtime." This sentence illustrates *what* is happening and *why* it was chosen as a therapeutic activity, aka strengthening to improve functional participation in an occupation. The sentence could also be reversed to emphasize occupation first. For example: "Harry worked on postural control to improve upright posture during mealtime through a variety of gross motor strengthening activities in the large therapy gym."
- Provide a statement briefly overviewing the child's strengths and challenges (e.g., "Client showed interest in moving throughout the session; she demonstrated decreased weight shifting and transitional movement patterns.").
- The detailed, observed performance/response to the intervention is presented in the objective section of the SOAP note. Presenting this information chronologically helps to illustrate how one therapeutic activity builds upon another to obtain functional participation in a specific activity.
- Presenting the information categorically in terms of areas of occupations, client factors, or performance skills is a more manageable approach, and full sentences are not required. For example, "Child reached for external support to maintain balance 4 times when traversing 1′ obstacle; unable to maneuver stand to crawl to enter the tunnel, attempted 5 times with success with moderate physical assistance; verbally stated the sequence but unable to complete w/o max gestural prompts and mod phys assist; decreased upper extremity strength limited ability to pull up onto elevated surfaces."

- Assessment: The assessment section includes a clinical appraisal of the client's performance, progress, and limitations based on the data in the Objective and Subjective sections. The assessment section is intended to provide an analysis of the client's potential and advocate for continued services. For the case above, the Assessment could include: "Harry was able to verbally outline the steps that his body needed to complete for transitional movement patterns and now only requires mod phys and max gestural prompting assistance to complete, and although he could not climb up, he was excited when he completed the task thus motivating him to continue attempts. Progress and positive reaction indicate potential for continued progress. Harry would benefit from continued occupational therapy to improve postural control and sitting stability as underpinnings to participation in mealtime and shoe tying."
- Plan: In many medically-based outpatient settings, "Continue POC as written" suffices because the plan outlines the frequency and duration of the recommended services. Gateley and Borcherding (2017), however, prefer repeating the specific information: "Jamal will continue occupational therapy for one hour per week to address postural control to support the occupations of sitting at mealtime, tying his shoes, performing table-top activities, and safely navigating the playground."

SOAP notes may provide a more specific POC if the child has an acute medical condition, a skill is emerging that requires particular attention, skills are changing weekly requiring frequent updates, or there is a need to contact other disciplines for an issue that emerged. There are also situations where the primary occupational therapist is out of the office and a covering occupational therapist reviews recent SOAP notes to understand the child's strengths, challenges, and goals. In this case, the therapist may provide a detailed "P" section. Some outpatient clinics have a treatment coverage form completed for each child so that the covering occupational therapist is fully informed about the status of intervention, what the child specifically enjoys so that the therapeutic relationship can begin on a positive note, what the current challenges might be at any point during the POC. (See Fig. 7.5 for a sample treatment coverage form.)

The SOAP note format may not be used by everyone in the organization. Occupational therapy practitioners determine whether a narrative of full sentences or medical shorthand may be used in the setting and the payer source requirements and preferences. However, the priorities for treatment session documentation are consistent. Each treatment note includes data presentation and analysis, a clear illustration that skilled intervention is required, and a notation of the client's reaction to successes in occupational engagement, including the caregiver's reaction. See Box 7.6 for pragmatic suggestions when completing CPT coding and narrative documentation.

**Discharge Plans.** **Discharge plans** are created upon completion of occupational therapy services. Occupational therapy services may be discontinued under the following conditions:

- Child has reached their goals and/or no further progress is expected.
- Rehabilitative potential is poor.
- The supports needed are currently implemented by another discipline.
- Home programs are in place and information sheets have been provided for maintaining skills.
- Child and family moving or will be receiving services elsewhere.

Discharge notes include the patient's status since the last progress note or POC, home programming, and referral information. There are certain situations where the discharge plan also includes suggestions for follow-up after a certain period. This might be the case when discharging, for example, a baby with a torticollis diagnosis who has completed the course of treatment but would benefit from a check-in at the 6-month mark post treatment to assure the spontaneous acquisition of skills without intervention. Infants discharged from the neonatal intensive care unit (NICU) require follow-up and home program suggestions. The discharge plan may include referral to an occupational therapist local to the family home, information describing hospital-based follow-up clinics for infants discharged from the NICU, information on signs to look for in the infant that might indicate the need for therapeutic support, home program suggestions, and other local resources to support the caregivers and family.

**Summary of Billing Compliance.** The provider organization's compliance administrator or therapy department supervisor should be familiar with each payer's coding rules; aware of AOTA official documents and resources applicable to legal, ethical, and professional implications of proper CPT coding/billing documentation for occupational therapy services; and establish an ongoing system to communicate specific information and updates with therapy staff. Information sheets (e.g., at each desk or computer station) with each payer source's requirements, expectations, preferences, and known patterns of utilization review help decrease errors or unfortunate word choices when documenting and coding services.

## Specific Requirements for Medicaid

The federal government's CMS oversees, legislates, and cofunds state government insurance plans, services, and programs provided to lower-income residents of that state. The program is considered an entitlement in that if one meets the state's eligibility criteria, they can enroll in the program. Each state implements and operates its Medicaid State Plan programs within the federal guidelines. State plans differ depending on their agreements, waivers, and amendments that define who is covered under the program beyond the federally identified mandatory populations, what services or programs

## TREATMENT COVERAGE

| | |
|---|---|
| Child's Name: | Tyson |
| Primary Therapist: | Tara |
| | |
| Day/Date/Time: | Saturday child; comes up from Brooklyn; 2 hour session |
| Able to Transition | Yes. But since he drives up for 1.5+ hours in the car, he sometimes falls asleep and so he might be a little shy when he first comes in the waiting room. Or sometimes he throws up in the car, in which case he will also be a little withdrawn. But once he's ready, he's ready. ☺ But if he's not ready (seems a bit shy), you can ask Tyson if he wants his father to come into the ballpit with him at the start of therapy. We invite mom or dad into the start of therapy on most Saturdays Tyson loves when someone comes into the therapy room as it gives him a chance to transition and he loves to show off his obstacle course skills which end with him jumping into the ballpit. But you will have to have a calm voice in order to keep the experience from getting escalated.... |
| | |
| Comments: | Tyson just turned 4 years old. His mother was just so excited that he actually understood that he was a new age and understood what a birthday party was all about.<br><br>Tyson has always come to the office when it is slow so he may escalate when others are around and playing. Although, he just got his first friend at school so he will be really into playing with others. This will be a good thing, just monitor his escalation.<br><br>Tyson's dad (Eric) loves his boy! A real hands-on dad. He's a bit of a mush when it comes to his son and takes great pride in Tyson's accomplishments**. So when you end the session, be sure to share what Tyson accomplished during the session.** He is also a high energy New Yorker, a marketing guy, a guy's guy, likes to rough-house with Tyson, and he is also a seeker! The difficulty is: Tyson is defensive. And while Tyson loves the physical engagement, I do think that it escalates him. And even if you can't see the escalation, I think that it does increase his internal arousal so be sure to have a calm voice to balance Eric and then you can do calming activities after his Eric leaves. |
| Precautions: | Tyson really only became aware of his body a few months ago so he is really into climbing. But he isn't all that safe so a close supervision for safety and remind him to protect his body. |
| | |
| Communication Skills: | Tyson's language is clear. However, you will see that decreased receptive language and motor planning his body particularly when you give complex body directions – you'll see it on his face that he is really trying to figure out what you said. So just be precise and clear with verbal directives, for example, during an obstacle course. It's also that Tyson is really just figuring out his body and how it can move in new, novel ways. You can almost see the wheels turning in his head. |
| | |
| Primary Areas of Concern: | 1) Trying to increase body awareness in space and motor planning – all while keeping him regulated and organized. Remember that *novelty, complexity, and intensity* all increase arousal so Tyson's central nervous system will already be a bit aroused because you are new to him.<br><br>Tyson loves deep touch pressure – he will often bury himself in the ballpit. There are times throughout the session when I will just have him relax under the pillows while I apply pressure. The regulates him well. |

**Fig. 7.5** Treatment coverage form.

| | |
|---|---|
| | You can also do Therapeutic Listening EASE #2. He will tell you if he doesn't like a song (I think some are too complex for him to process) so I will often repeat the first song a few times.<br><br>He likes the different obstacle courses that I ask him to complete. But it is challenging for him. But he loves it and takes great pride. So body transitions: up, down, through, jump off, climb over, etc. are good for him. |
| | 2) Then moving to visual motor activities for skill development. NOTE: He's a real splinter skill learner so I try not to skill train per se. For example, when I demonstrated his name with him one week, he completely got it and started drawing it on the coloring placemats when they went out to dinner. So, when you show it to him and "train" it, he typically gets it. This was great for his name but it was not a true reflection of his neuro-maturational level. So when I do visual motor tasks, I try to be different so that it doesn't end up as a splinter skill. I hope that makes sense. And, when he struggles (which he will if it is novel), speaking to him softly, encouraging, and helping voice will assist him….. just not too much talking as his brain will be trying to figure out the task and if you talk, you will disrupt his thinking pattern. Really, you'll see the confusion on his face. ☺<br><br>3) Recently, we have been trying to get him to eat healthier food. He just started eating a sandwich (cut up) that his parents send with him; and fruit. This is only about a month old and he did a lot of resisting in the beginning so if he resists you, no worries. When he is eating, I prompt him to move the food to right because he mostly chews on the left. He has a mushy mouth (low tone posture) so oral games are fine as well. |
| | |
| Helpful Hints: | Just have fun. He's a kid who loves the OT activities. Just try not to use too much language. |
| | |
| Tx/Activity Suggestions: | He is fine in any room but I would start in the small ballpit room. Make a small obstacle course that he can climb up/through in order to jump into the ballpit.<br><br>Throwing the puzzle or game pieces over the pillow pile is also really good for him. When you see him get tired, you can go hang out with him in the pillows and chat so that he gets a rest.<br><br>I recently did the lycra hammock with him and it's challenging. I would do it again but be careful to hold the sides up (firm/taught) as he is not really stable yet and might fall out. You can ask him to climb up from end to end – that's really challenging.<br><br>You can go into the big room as well but stay in one zone/area vs. using the whole room. Lots of jumping on the mattress pile (like a trampoline) – tell him to jump 10x and then crash into the ballpit. You can repeat this several times and at different times during the session. |
| | |
| Activities/ toys to avoid: | none; just watch for escalation and for that look on his face that says: I have no idea what I am supposed to do here; calm, caring voice; less talking as language is difficult for him to process. |

**Fig. 7.5 cont'd**

are provided beyond the mandatory services, and how providers are reimbursed for the delivery of outlined services (Center on Budget and Policy Priorities [CBPP], 2020; United States Department of Health and Human Services & CMS, n.d.-b). Although occupational therapy is federally identified as a covered service under Medicaid, it is not a required service and therefore provided at the discretion of each state (United States Department of Health and Human Services & CMS, n.d.-a). Occupational therapy practitioners must learn the features and requirements of eligibility, policy, services, and payment of their state's program.

### BOX 7.6 Pragmatic Suggestions for Coding and Narrative Documentation

- Daily session notes should follow the procedures set up by your funding agency, directly related to the ICD-10-CM diagnosis code for which you are providing intervention and support the CPT codes that you bill (if commercial insurance or Medicaid billing).
- Highlight the functional outcome in your session description. It is not enough to report that [blank] client factor increased or improved when [blank] intervention, level of support, or prompt was provided. Tell the story, paint the picture, and describe what function occurred (e.g., allowing [client] to complete [functional skill]), as well as the client's reaction to this achievement (Sames, 2015).
- Document your daily treatment notes in a timely manner. Avoiding or putting it off until "later" will only make remembering and organizing your thoughts more difficult. Get it done.
- Complete point-of-service documentation (POS; in real time, during the treatment session) only when it is reasonable and feasible. Discuss with the supervisor if there are sessions where POS documentation is not feasible and why (e.g., safety, decreased client independence to complete or engage in an activity while the occupational therapist is on the computer).
- Advocate for undisturbed, non-treatment time in your schedule for longer reports (e.g., evaluation, progress note, updated plans of care, discharge) as close to implementation of the services as possible. Consider time-efficient models of documentation, such as dictation for secretarial transcription, hand-held devices with templates, or a "master" document that can easily be modified for each client.
- Facility supervisors/administrators can provide additional support to specifically track diagnosis and CPT codes covered/allowable/authorized by various funding sources.
- Create a reference sheet for each payer source and post it at all computer stations; information should include the specific rules and procedures for coding/billing (including allowable number of units and CPT code combinations), note format, preferred terminology, and words/terms previously considered "red flags" (i.e., using sensory integration terminology when 97533 sensory integration is not covered).

### BOX 7.7 Readability of Health Information

Authors of content, particularly health-related content, want to ensure that their material will be understandable to the general population. In general, the number of words in a sentence and the number of syllables per word determine the ease of readability. The Flesch-Kincaid Grade Level analysis provides a score according to the US grade level. For example, a score of six means that a person with a sixth-grade reading level will be able to understand the written information. Microsoft Word has a readability feature tha allows authors to scan their Word document for the Flesch-Kincaid reading level. Several YouTube videos describe how to access the readability statistics features within Microsoft Word and provide the author with a Word Readability Report.

In addition to occupational therapy as a medically covered benefit, Medicaid can financially support occupational therapy services provided through, but not fully funded by, the Individuals with Disabilities Education Improvement Act (IDEA, 2004) federal legislation. Center for Medicaid and Medicare Services (United States Department of Health and Human Services, CMS, 2022b) highlights that schools are uniquely positioned to increase access to health care services and health quality through IDEA services outlined in a child's individualized educational program (IEP). Specifically, costs associated with providing medically necessary occupational therapy services as outlined in the IEP can be reimbursed by Medicaid for students enrolled in the Medicaid program (AOTA, 2017; United States Department of Health and Human Services, CMS, 2022b). When meeting the requirement that the intervention is related to the student's medical condition or disability, Medicaid funding for school-based occupational therapy allows local Boards of Education (BOE) to free up general education budgets for other educational initiatives (CBPP, 2017, 2018). When coding and billing Medicaid for school-based occupational therapy services, it is important to remember that most CPT codes require direct, one-on-one intervention. Therefore, common occupational therapy activities within school-based practice might not be billable to Medicaid. For example, attendance by the occupational therapy practitioner at an IEP meeting does not have a CPT code as it is not direct intervention to the student. Additionally, if the occupational therapy practitioner provides services to a group of children in school-based practice, the 97510 Group therapeutic procedure code must be recorded. The group CPT code is untimed and can only be billed once for the group session.

## Community-Based Practice

Occupational therapy practitioners create, promote, and implement programming to meet society's health and well-being needs through participation in meaningful activities (AOTA, 2020b). Essential skills to realize these professional initiatives include professional writing (e.g., proposals, grants, letters), comprehensive documentation of the occupational therapy process, and effective communication with a variety of community leaders (e.g., city or town officials, private and public organizations who have a mission to support children and their families/caregivers).

Occupational therapy practitioners may support access to service by securing community funding. They closely review the philosophy of the funding source, understand the types of programs the organization has already supported, and capitalize on how occupational therapy can support their future mission. Clearly highlighting and documenting how occupational therapy services support the philosophical mission and initiatives of the funding organization, entity, or department is critical. For example, the Healthy Cities initiative outlined by the World Health Organization (2022) might be a priority for a local government, philanthropic organization, or the local YMCA. This provides an ideal situation for occupational therapy practitioners to implement community-based programs to support the occupations of children and youth, including programs for health promotion, behavioral interventions, and health literacy.

Group and population services require different skills than individual services. The occupational therapy practitioners providing services within a community-based model to a group or population (considered the client) must engage with a population to determine their perceived needs, desires for support, and priorities. To address the needs of the group or population, practitioners begin by documenting findings from a needs assessment and capacity assessment. A **needs assessment** includes data on the group or population's current status, such as health trends, demographic and economic data, prevalence or concern for growth, and development risks. A **capacity assessment** identifies skills and resources that already exist that can be expanded upon.

Occupational therapy practitioners working in a community model pay attention to the health literacy of members. They use plain language (i.e., sixth-grade level) and pictures and limit the use of professional jargon to ensure that community members can access, understand, and utilize health-related information. Box 7.7 provides information on readability levels. They verify the community's languages and ensure that documentation is accessible to people who may not be able to read or have visual limitations. Documenting suggestions through clear and simple infographic material helps members access occupational therapy suggestions when the practitioner is not on site. See Fig. 7.6A and B for sample Community Infographics.

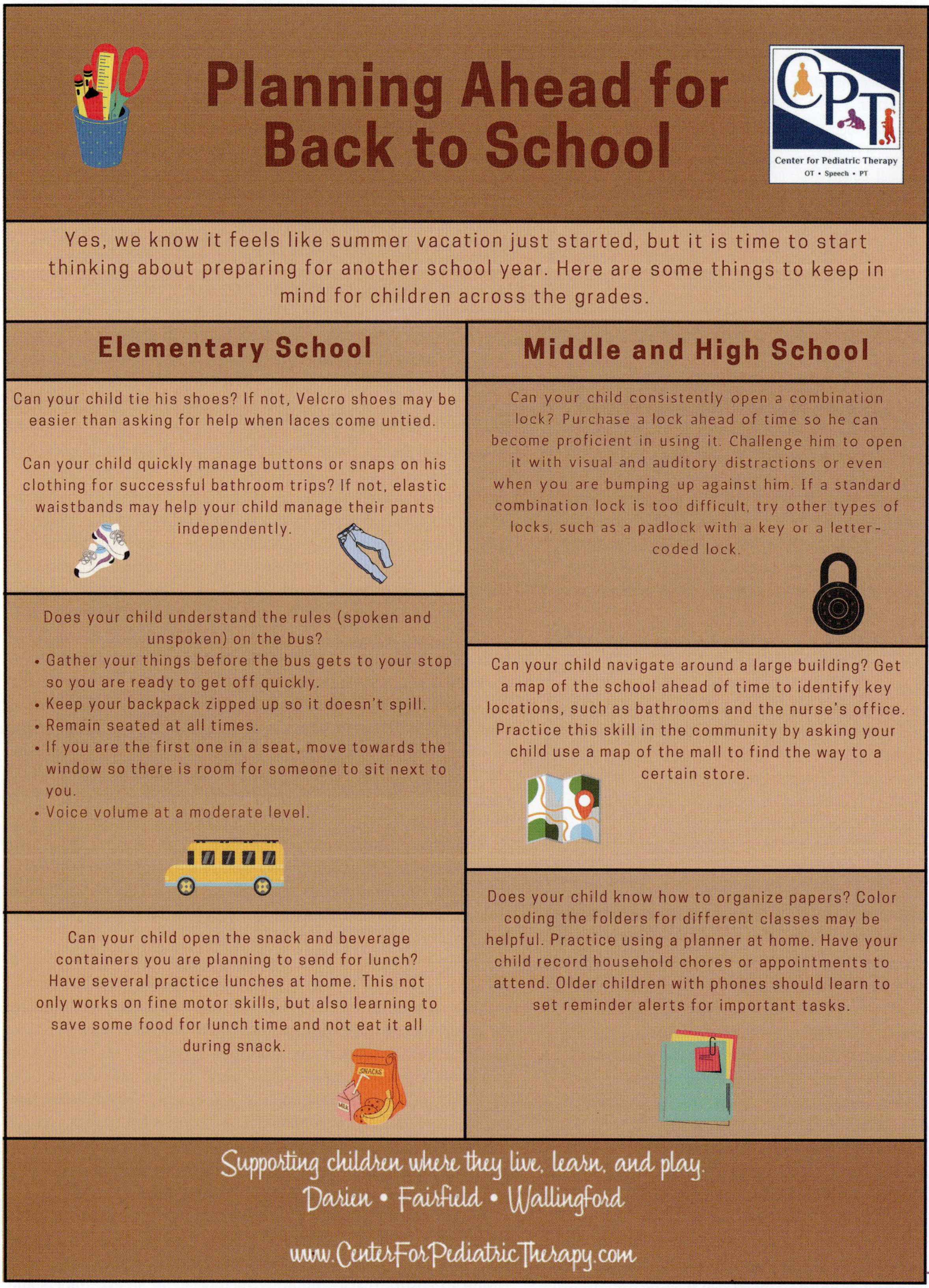


**Fig. 7.6** Community infographics: (A) Back to school and (B) Creating a homework zone.

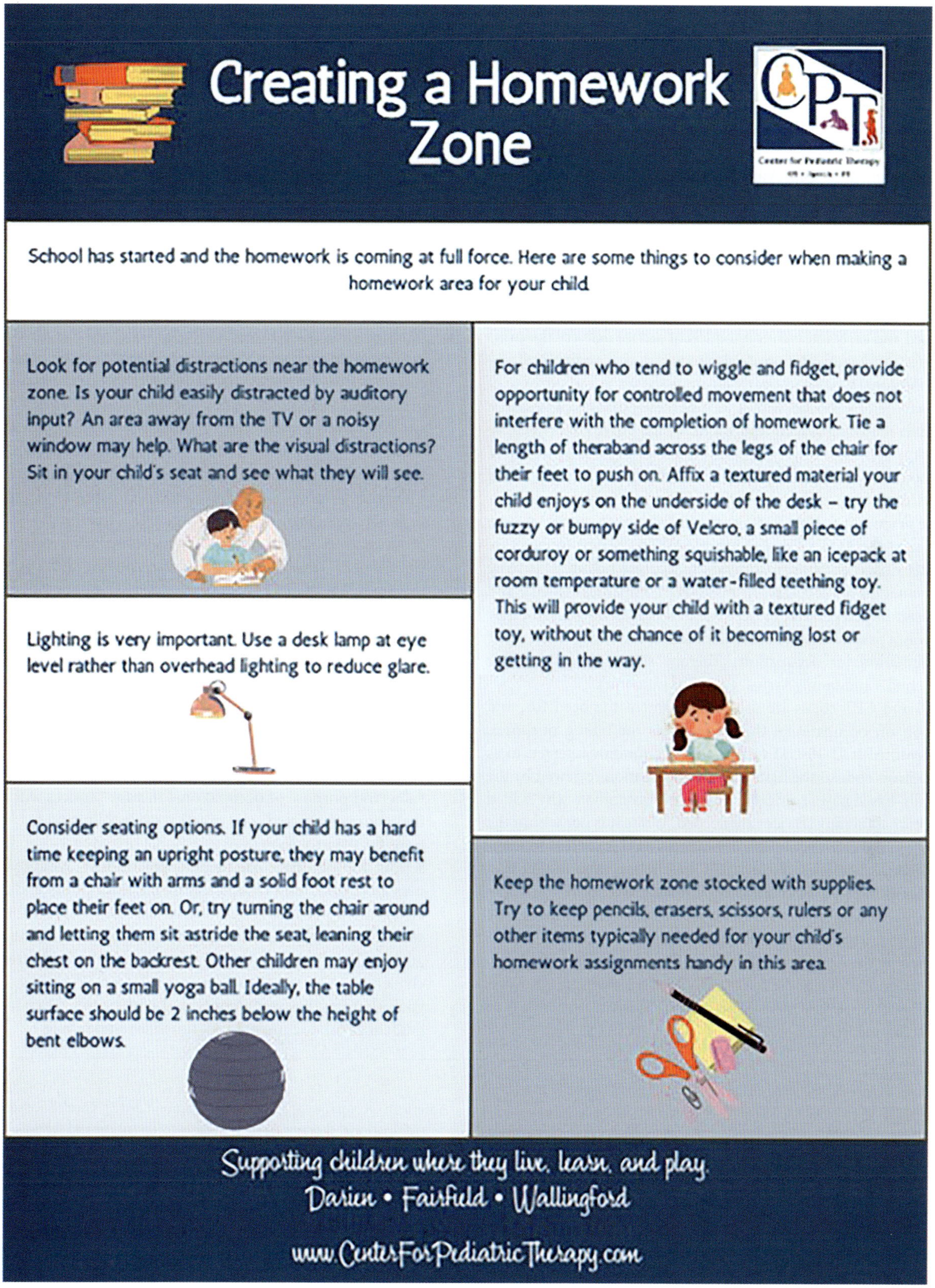

# Creating a Homework Zone

Center for Pediatric Therapy

School has started and the homework is coming at full force. Here are some things to consider when making a homework area for your child.

Look for potential distractions near the homework zone. Is your child easily distracted by auditory input? An area away from the TV or a noisy window may help. What are the visual distractions? Sit in your child's seat and see what they will see.

Lighting is very important. Use a desk lamp at eye level rather than overhead lighting to reduce glare.

Consider seating options. If your child has a hard time keeping an upright posture, they may benefit from a chair with arms and a solid foot rest to place their feet on. Or, try turning the chair around and letting them sit astride the seat, leaning their chest on the backrest. Other children may enjoy sitting on a small yoga ball. Ideally, the table surface should be 2 inches below the height of bent elbows.

For children who tend to wiggle and fidget, provide opportunity for controlled movement that does not interfere with the completion of homework. Tie a length of theraband across the legs of the chair for their feet to push on. Affix a textured material your child enjoys on the underside of the desk – try the fuzzy or bumpy side of Velcro, a small piece of corduroy or something squishable, like an icepack at room temperature or a water-filled teething toy. This will provide your child with a textured fidget toy, without the chance of it becoming lost or getting in the way.

Keep the homework zone stocked with supplies. Try to keep pencils, erasers, scissors, rulers or any other items typically needed for your child's homework assignments handy in this area.

Supporting children where they live, learn, and play.

Darien • Fairfield • Wallingford

www.CenterForPediatricTherapy.com

Fig. 7.6 cont'd

## SUMMARY

Proper documentation skills allow for effective professional communication, financial justification for skilled occupational therapy services, and clinical accountability for services rendered. Legal, ethical, and professional obligations are met when documentation provides a full and honest chronological accounting of services to support functional goals and objectives aimed at improving functional performance in desired or needed occupations. Narrative documentation and CPT coding/billing decisions within the medical model are scrutinized by payer sources to determine whether skilled occupational therapy intervention is warranted for the child's diagnosis, whether functional improvements are occurring within a reasonable time frame, and whether it meets the parameters outlined by the payer source for reimbursement. Within school-based and early intervention models of service delivery the principles of effective documentation are also required with particular attention to professional writing to clearly illustrate the value and purpose of occupational therapy services within each of these domains of pediatric practice while following federal regulations for the provision of occupational therapy services. AOTA provides a number of both general and specific resources to meet these documentation needs, including official documents, context-specific best practice publications, and webinars discussing the practicalities of providing services in context-specific arenas.

1. It is against the AOTA Code of Ethics (AOTA, 2020b) to fabricate or falsify documentation or provide inaccurate billing. Falsifying documentation for Medicare or insurance companies is illegal and may result in prosecution under state and federal laws a state may take away a practitioner's license to practice. Providing inadequate documentation for occupational therapy services may interfere with a child's and family's trust, care, and outcomes.
2. ICD-10 and CPT codes are used to document the need for, and provision of, occupational therapy services for billing purposes. The identified ICD-10-CM (2018) code, commonly referred to as the diagnosis code, is the first point of information reviewed by the medically-based payer source and needs to substantiate why skilled occupational therapy services are needed. While it is not within the occupational therapy standards of practice (AOTA, 2021a) to identify a medical diagnosis, the occupational therapy practitioner uses clinical reasoning to diagnose occupational challenges (e.g., client factors, performance patterns, and performance skills) impacting occupational performance and participation. These diagnoses, identified by the occupational therapy practitioner, are referred to as the treatment diagnosis. Specifically, the treatment diagnosis is not always the primary medical diagnosis, rather it is secondary to the primary medical diagnosis.
3. A variety of rules, regulations, and parameters guide the documentation and coding of occupational therapy services within medically-based occupational therapy practice. The federal government's CMS oversees, legislates, and cofunds state government insurance plans, services, and programs provided to lower-income residents of that state. Each state implements and operates its Medicaid State Plan programs within the federal guidelines. State plans differ in their coverage and services. Although occupational therapy is federally identified as a covered service under Medicaid, it is not a required service and therefore provided at the discretion of each state (United States Department of Health and Human Services & Centers for Medicare and Medicaid Services, n.d.-a). Primary funding sources for medically-based coverage include commercial insurance carriers, such as insurance provided by employers to their employees or purchased by individuals through a state's marketplace under the Patient Protection and Affordable Care Act (2010), and Medicaid. Practitioners document based on rules for coding using CPT codes, and the state and private insurance procedures. Some may have specific timelines, forms, and billing agreements.
4. The pragmatics of documenting the occupational therapy process (e.g., referral, diagnosis, evaluation, POC, treatment session notes, progress notes, denial appeals, letters of medical necessity, and discharge plans) involves providing clear, concise, and objective information in a way that others understand. The practitioner uses this information to make professional judgments regarding the child's services. The documentation provides a full and honest chronological accounting of services to support functional goals and objectives aimed at improving functional performance in desired or needed occupations.
5. Best practices for documenting educationally-based and early intervention occupational therapy services under Parts B and C of IDEA also require attention to professional writing to clearly illustrate the value and purpose of occupational therapy services within each of these domains of pediatric practice while following federal regulations for the provision of occupational therapy services. In a school setting the occupational therapy practitioner avoids jargon and uses more descriptors that illustrate the child's story and functional engagement in educationally-based activities. In early intervention settings, occupational therapy practitioners include the family's goals and insights and identify children and families' strengths and challenges. They avoid jargon and judgmental language and write goals that families can identify and understand. They follow state guidelines for documentation, timelines, and billing.

## REFERENCES

Agner, J. (2020). The issue is—Moving from cultural competence to cultural humility in occupational therapy: A paradigm shift. *American Journal of Occupational Therapy, 74* 7404347010.

American Medical Association. (n.d.). The CPT code process. https://www.ama-assn.org/about/cpt-editorial-panel/cpt-code-process

American Medical Association. (2022). *CPT® manual: Professional edition* (Author).

American Occupational Therapy Association. (2020b). AOTA 2020 occupational therapy code of ethics. *American Journal of Occupational Therapy, 74*(Suppl. 3) 7413410005.

American Occupational Therapy Association. (2018). Guidelines for documentation of occupational therapy. *American Journal of Occupational Therapy, 72*(Suppl. 2) 7212410010.

American Occupational Therapy Association. (2017). Guidelines for occupational therapy services in early intervention and schools. *American Journal of Occupational Therapy, 71*(Suppl. 2) 7112410010.

American Occupational Therapy Association. (2021a). Improve your documentation and quality of care with AOTA's updated occupational profile template. *American Journal of Occupational Therapy, 75*(Suppl. 2) 7502420010.

American Occupational Therapy Association. (2016). *New occupational therapy evaluation coding overview*. https://www.aota.org/~/media/Corporate/Files/Advocacy/Federal/Evaluation-Codes-Overview-2016.pdf.

American Occupational Therapy Association. (2020c). Occupational therapy in the promotion of health and well-being. *American Journal of Occupational Therapy, 74*(3) 7403420010p1–7403420010p14.

American Occupational Therapy Association. (2020a). Occupational therapy practice framework: Domain and process (4th ed.). *American Journal of Occupational Therapy, 74*(Suppl. 2) 7412410010p1–7412410010p87.

American Occupational Therapy Association. (2021b). Standards of practice for occupational therapy. *American Journal of Occupational Therapy, 75*(Suppl. 3) 7513410030.

American Occupational Therapy Association, American Physical Therapy Association, & American Speech and Hearing Association. (2022). *Joint statement on interprofessional collaborative goals in school-based practice.* https://www.asha.org/siteassets/ipp/joint-statement-on-interprofessional-collaborative-goals-in-school-based-practice-2022.pdf.

Center on Budget and Policy Priorities. (2017). *Medicaid helps schools help children.* https://www.cbpp.org/research/health/medicaid-helps-schools-help-children.

Center on Budget and Policy Priorities. (2018). *Medicaid works for children.* https://www.cbpp.org/research/health/medicaid-works-for-children.

Center on Budget and Policy Priorities. (2020). *Policy basics: Introduction to Medicaid.* https://www.cbpp.org/research/health/introduction-to-medicaid.

Department of Health and Human Services, & Centers for Medicare and Medicaid Services. (2022). *Healthcare common procedural coding system (HCPCS) level II coding procedures.* https://www.cms.gov/Medicare/Coding/MedHCPCSGenInfo/Downloads/2018-11-30-HCPCS-Level2-Coding-Procedure.pdf.

Doran, G. T. (1981). There's a S.M.A.R.T. way to write management's goals and objectives. *Journal of Management Review, 70*(11), 35–36. AMA Forum https://community.mis.temple.edu/mis0855002fall2015/files/2015/10/S.M.A.R.T-Way-Management-Review.pdf.

Family Education Rights and Privacy Act (1974), Pub. L. 93–380, 20 U.S.C. §1232g, 34CFR part 99 et seq.

Frolek Clark, G., & Handley-More, D. (2017). *Best practices for documenting occupational therapy services in schools.* AOTA Press.

Furano, S., O'Reilly, K., Hosaka, C. M., Inatsuka, T., & Zeisloft-Dalbey, L. (2016). *Hawaii Early Learning Profile: HELP Checklist 0-3.* Vort Corp.

Gateley, C. A., & Borcherding, S. (2017). *Documentation manual for occupational therapy: Writing SOAP notes* (4th ed.). Slack Inc..

Glennon, T. J., Ecker, C., Kuhaneck, H., Henry, D., & Parham, L. D. (2021). *Sensory Processing Measure – 2nd edition – infant, toddler, and caregiver forms.* Western Psychological Services.

Health Insurance Portability and Accountability Act (1996), Pub. L. 104–191, §264, 110 Stat. 1936.

Individuals with Disabilities Education Improvement Act (2004), Pub L. 108–446, 20 U.S.C. §1400-1482.

McCormack, K. M., Stricklin, S., Nowak, T. M., & Rous, B. (2008). Using eco-mapping to understand family strengths and resources. *Young Exceptional Children, 11*(2), 17–28.

McMillan, R. A. (2010). *Routines-based intervention: Supporting young children and their families.* https://brookespublishing.com/wp-content/uploads/2020/07/RBI-Excerpt.pdf.

McWilliam, R. A., Casey, A. M., & Sims, J. (2009). The routines-based interview: A method for gathering information and assessing needs. *Infants & Young Children, 22*, 224–233.

National Association of Insurance Commissioners. (2010). *Glossary of health insurance and medical terms.* https://content.naic.org/sites/default/files/inline-files/committees_b_consumer_information_ppaca_glossary.pdf.

National Committee on Vital and Health Statistics. (2023). *ICD-11 overview, key facts, history, and references.* https://ncvhs.hhs.gov/wp-content/uploads/2023/09/ICD-11-Overview-September-2023-508.pdf.

Patient Protection and Affordable Care Act. (2010). *Pub. L. 111–148, §3502, 124 Stat. 119, 124.*

Sames, K. M. (2019). Documentation in practice. In B. A. B. Schell, & G. Gillen (Eds.), *Willard and Spackman's Occupational Therapy* (pp. 572–582). Wolters Kluwer.

Sames, K. M. (2015). *Documenting occupational therapy practice* (3rd ed.). Pearson Education, Inc..

State of Connecticut v. (2019). *Therapy Unlimited, LLC and Catherine Risigo Wickline.* https://portal.ct.gov/-/media/AG/Press_Releases/2019/Therapy-Unlimited---Complaint-7-17-19.pdf?la=en.

United States Department of Education. (2021). *Family Educational Rights and Privacy Act.* https://www2.ed.gov/policy/gen/guid/fpco/ferpa/index.html.

United States Department of Health and Human Services. (2021). *HIPPA for professionals.* https://www.hhs.gov/hipaa/for-professionals/index.html.

United States Department of Health and Human Services, Centers for Medicare and Medicaid Services. (2022b). *CMCS Information Bulletin. Information on School-Based Services in Medicaid: Funding, Documentation and Expanding Services.* https://www.medicaid.gov/federal-policy-guidance/downloads/sbscib081820222.pdf.

United States Department of Health and Human Services, Centers for Medicare and Medicaid Services. (2022a). *Healthcare common procedural coding system (HCPCS) level II coding procedures.* https://www.cms.gov/Medicare/Coding/MedHCPCSGenInfo/Downloads/2018-11-30-HCPCS-Level2-Coding-Procedure.pdf.

United States Department of Health and Human Services Centers for Medicare and Medicaid Services. (n.d.-a). Mandatory & optional Medicaid benefits. https://www.medicaid.gov/medicaid/benefits/mandatory-optional-medicaid-benefits/index.html

United States Department of Health and Human Services - Centers for Medicare and Medicaid Services. (n.d.-b). Medicaid state plan amendments. https://www.medicaid.gov/medicaid/medicaid-state-plan-amendments/index.html

United States Department of Health and Human Services, Centers for Medicare and Medicaid Services, & Office of Management and Budget. (2012). *CMS 1500: Health insurance claim form.* https://www.cms.gov/Medicare/CMS-Forms/CMS-Forms/CMS-Forms-Items/CMS1188854.

United States Department of Health and Human Services, Health Sector Cybersecurity Coordination Center. (2022). *HHS Cybersecurity Programs: Electronic medical records in healthcare.* https://www.hhs.gov/sites/default/files/2022-02-17-1300-emr-in-healthcare-tlpwhite.pdf.

World Health Organization. (2022). *Creating healthy cities.* https://www.who.int/activities/creating-healthy-cities.

World Health Organization. (2001). *International classification of functioning, disability and health* (Author).

World Health Organization. (2007). *International classification of functioning, disability and health – children and youth version.* Author http://apps.who.int/iris/bitstream/handle/10665/43737/9789241547321_eng.pdf;jsessionid=E392964F329EC62C28AD1E711DE1E280?sequence=1.

8

# Developmental Trajectories

*Cheryl B. Lucas, Natasha Smet, and Aimee Piller*

## GUIDING QUESTIONS

1. What factors influence child development?
2. How do occupational therapy practitioners use knowledge of developmental milestones to inform practice?

## KEY TERMS

Abstract thinking
Adverse childhood experiences (ACEs)
Client factors
Construction play
Critical period
Environmental factors
Motor skills
Neuroplasticity
Object permanence
Personal factors
Primitive reflexes
Process skills
Social interaction skills
Universal design for learning

*Childhood means much more than just the space between birth and the attainment of adulthood. It refers to the state and condition of a child's life, to the quality of those years. It is a time for children to be in school and at play, to grow strong and confident with the love and encouragement of their family and an extended community of caring adults* (UNICEF, 2005).

## INTRODUCTION

Children have individual temperaments, abilities, and challenges. They require basic provisions such as adequate nutrition, physical shelter, and nurturing caretakers to promote their physical and mental health. Once these needs are met, most children with or without a diagnosed disability can participate in daily routines given adequate resources, contextual opportunities, and adult support. Most, but not all children follow an age-related, sequential course of development in all domains, and develop skills both horizontally across multiple domains and longitudinally within domains (See Box 8.1). Children follow an individual developmental growth trajectory that is predicated on a variety of factors both internal (e.g., genetics, health conditions, and social-emotional preferences) and external (e.g., culture, resources, and environment). Box 8.2 describes the concept of developmental trajectories.

## OCCUPATIONAL THERAPY PERSPECTIVE OF CHILD DEVELOPMENT

Occupational therapy practitioners working with children and youth view development on a continuum and consider a multitude of influences on development, such as family values, beliefs, customs, resources, situations, and environments. They practice cultural humility (see Chapter 4) by seeking to understand the beliefs, goals, expectations, and routines of the child within their family and environments that influence development. For example, not all families view independence as their child's primary goal in therapy (Petrenchik & King, 2013; Tomchek & Koenig, 2016). Occupational therapy practitioners view age ranges for achievements of milestones as guidelines rather than absolutes. They synthesize knowledge of human development (including theories), neuroscience, and occupational science (e.g., theories, principles of change, and philosophy) to address occupational engagement. Occupational therapy practitioners acknowledge that children and youth are influenced by a variety of factors (internal and external) and engage in a variety of occupations within changing environments. They partner with children, adolescents, and their family members, caregivers, peers, school personnel, and community organizations that interact with them to improve occupational performance in the settings in which children participate. The goal is not for children to achieve "typical" development but rather to actively participate in occupations and co-occupations they need to do, want to do, and are expected to do (Law et al., 1996; Rodger & Kennedy-Behr, 2017). See Case Example 8.1.

### Importance of Developmental Trajectories

The traditional approach to child development involved comparing typically developing children with children who were atypical in some way because of a diagnosis, an illness, or environmental deprivation. Development was measured as typical, delayed but following the typical sequence, or atypical. Contemporary approaches to child development consider the shape and rate of change of development over time, often using growth curve modeling. Researchers consider the complexity of human development and the myriad of influences on it to understand how development may be altered (Annaz et al., 2008; Knowland & Thomas, 2011; Murray et al., 2022).

Occupational therapy practitioners use contemporary research proposing developmental trajectories to understand the range of potential prognoses for children with a specific type of disability (Bjornson et al., 2020; Smits et al., 2019). They consider how intervention may alter the developmental trajectory of a child and how even a slight push or bump at an early age may have a progressively larger impact over time.

## BOX 8.1 Horizontal and Longitudinal Development

**Horizontal development** refers to development in multiple areas at the same time (Llorens, 1982). For example, infants develop head control, social trust, oral motor skills for feeding, and fine motor skills for holding objects. **Longitudinal development** refers to the development over time in one skill area. For example, in the motor area, children progress from supine to rolling, prone on hands, side lying, prop sitting, and independent sitting, and from creeping to crawling.

## BOX 8.2 Developmental Trajectories

A developmental trajectory describes a person's progression of behaviors over time. Examining the developmental progression of individuals within a population provides guidelines and information to support occupational therapy practice. Instead of comparing children's performance with the performance of typically developing children, researchers examine the performance over time of children from the population. For example, Jeffries et al. (2019) examined the developmental trajectories for range of motion, endurance, and muscle strength of children with cerebral palsy. Carretti et al. (2022) examined the developmental trajectories of working memory in children with Down syndrome. By understanding how the population performs over time, practitioners may create interventions to address the child's unique needs.

Research suggests a variety of factors influence child development and intervention alters developmental trajectories (Bentenuto et al., 2020; Darrou et al., 2010; Klintwall et al., 2015; Stuyvenberg et al., 2021).

### Factors that May Influence Developmental Trajectories

Child development is influenced by a variety of client, personal, and environmental factors (AOTA, 2020). **Client factors** include body structures and function, values, beliefs, and spirituality (AOTA, 2020). **Personal factors** include the child's background, and those areas that are unique features of the person (such as age, sexual orientation, gender identity, race and ethnicity, culture identification, social background, upbringing and life experiences, habits and patterns, psychological assets, education, lifestyle, other health conditions and fitness) (AOTA 2020). **Environmental factors** include the child's physical, social, and attitudinal surroundings (AOTA, 2020). Occupational therapy practitioners use professional reasoning to synthesize information regarding child development and information gained about the child's condition, goals, values, beliefs, and personal and environmental factors to create intervention using a developmental approach. Brofenbrenner (1997) viewed the relationships of environments to include relationships with caregivers, culture, community, and the geopolitical context as interacting to affect children's development (See Fig. 8.1). Occupational therapy practitioners view a child's occupational performance as dynamic and influenced by external and internal factors.

Personal, environmental, and child factors may support or hinder occupational performance. For example, caregivers who are responsive to their children promote child development (Fingerhut et al., 2013; Riley et al., 2017). The following section describes some factors—i.e., relationships, **adverse childhood experiences (ACEs)**, community, geopolitical structures and policies, and culture—that may influence child development and occupational engagement.

**Relationships.** Caregivers may include parents, grandparents, daycare providers, and foster parents who provide physical and emotional care for a child or youth. Early interactions with caregivers contribute to a child's emotional regulation, self-efficacy, and self-determination, which are important to occupational performance (Ikävalko et al., 2022). Appendix 8.1 provides a description of the development of emotional regulation. Adults foster behavioral self-regulation in children through coregulation, which occurs by providing children with warm, responsive adult relationships, structuring the environment for emotional safety to explore and learn at their own pace, and teaching and modeling self-regulation skills with opportunities for practice and feedback (Aubuchon-Endsley et al., 2020; Davel-Pickens & Pizur-Barnekow, 2009; Rosanbalm & Murray, 2017). Participation in co-occupations (engagement that has a distinct or overlapping meaning or purpose for two people) forms a foundation for emotional growth, increased autonomy, and intrinsic motivation leading to increased participation (Aubuchon-Endsley et al., 2020, 2021). Fig. 8.2A and B shows positive relationships between parents and their children, and Fig. 8.2C shows a grandfather interacting with his grandchild.

## CASE EXAMPLE 8.1 MARIA AND EMMA: HOW CONTEXTS AFFECT OCCUPATIONAL PARTICIPATION AND DEVELOPMENT

Maria is a 4-year-old child diagnosed with spastic cerebral palsy who uses a wheelchair for mobility. She lives with her parents, grandmother, and four older siblings in a third-floor, walk-up apartment in a metropolitan city. Maria is carried up the stairs by her father or mother. Maria attends her local Head Start program 4 days a week, where she gets occupational therapy (OT), physical therapy (PT), and speech therapy (ST) through IDEA from her public school.

Since it is difficult to carry her up and down the stairs, Maria has difficulty participating in community activities on the weekends with her family yet has much social interaction with siblings and other relatives. Emma, another 4-year-old child with cerebral palsy, also uses a wheelchair for mobility. She lives in a rural, one-story farmhouse with her grandparents in a rural community. She has access to leisure activities, a large backyard, and chores helping with the small animals and the garden. Emma does not socialize with neighbors, peers, or community members due to the lack of accessible transportation and the geographic distance between neighbors. She attends the local elementary preschool program where she receives OT, PT, and ST.

While Maria and Emma experience similar diagnoses and may have similar performance capacities, their development is affected by the contexts in which they live. The OT intervention sessions will reflect their individual needs and the contexts in which they live. Maria benefits from the socialization she gets from her siblings and relatives, and the resources of the city environment including the accessibility of adapted spaces such as transportation, playgrounds, and entertainment venues. However, her home setting not being wheelchair accessible, limits her engagement in participating in desired occupations and may limit her feelings of self-efficacy.

Emma on the other hand, has natural space readily available to her to explore but has limited opportunity to socialize with same-aged peers. She may require adaptations at home so that she can complete chores and engage in play outside. These may include adapted swings, ramps, and accessible pathways. Emma spends time with adults and may not have established important peer relationships needed for autonomy and feelings of self-efficacy.

**Critical Review:** These cases illustrate the contextual factors that transact with the child to determine OT intervention. The occupational therapist may also work with the families to determine the technological needs of each child. Both children are receiving services under the federal law of IDEA (2012) and may qualify for assistive technology for occupational performance and quality of life. They may also have medical insurance to provide additional services. OT will monitor the developmental trajectory of each child to ameliorate barriers to continued development.

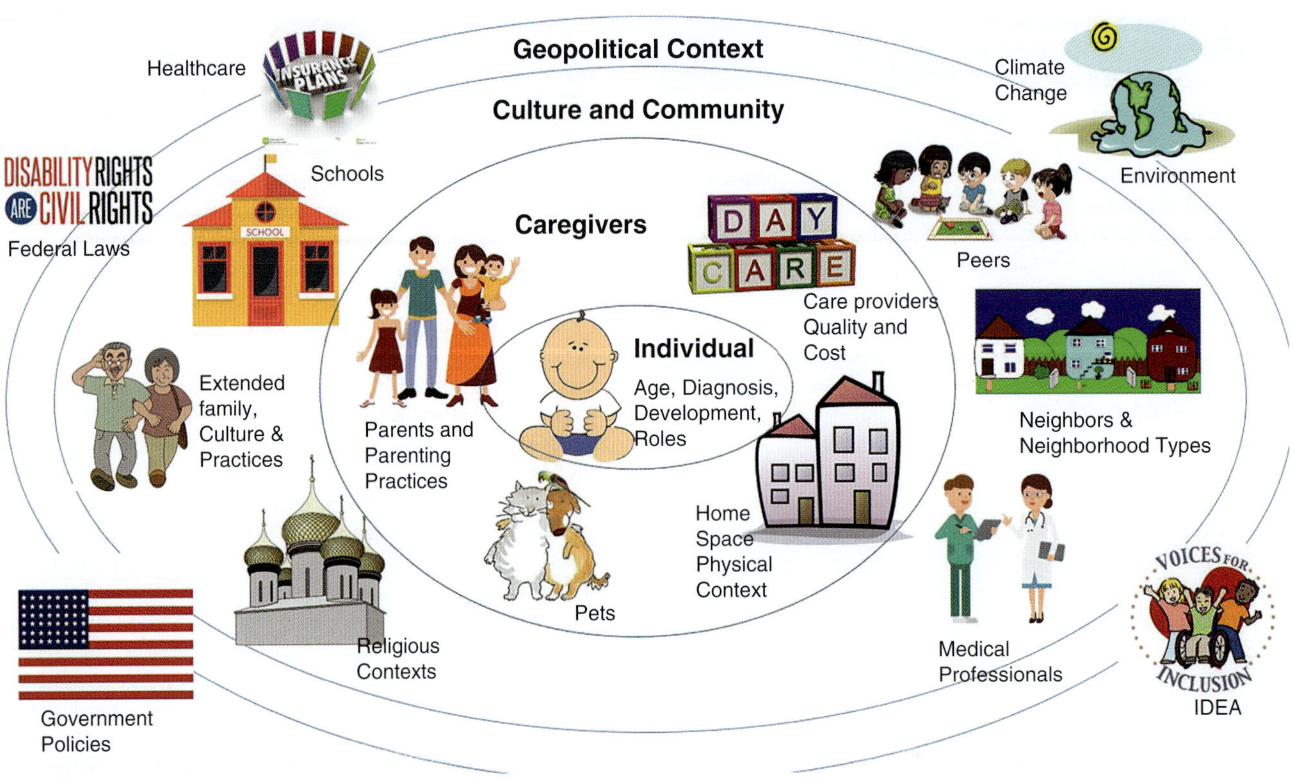


**Fig. 8.1** Contexts and transactional relationships affecting child development. A child's developmental trajectory is influenced by the many contextual factors that influence their performance and participation in chosen activities as illustrated in Bronfenbrenner's model (1997).

## APPENDIX 8.1 EMOTION REGULATION DEVELOPMENT

| Phases | Ages | Characteristics | Examples |
|---|---|---|---|
| Neurophysiologic modulation | Birth to 2–3 months | Modulation of arousal, activation of organized patterns of behavior. | Infants can self-soothe (e.g., with nonnutritive sucking) or respond quickly when soothed by parents. May be fussy or calm. Different routines of awake/sleep cycles. |
| Sensorimotor modulation | 3–9 months | Behavior depends on social or environmental stimuli or events. | Infants derive pleasure from sensorimotor play and seek sensory exploration. Some infants may have difficulty modulating sensory behaviors (e.g., may be sensory seeking). |
| Control | 12–18 months | Behavior demonstrates awareness of social demands. Toddler demonstrates compliance and self-initiated monitoring. | Toddler's behavior is goal-directed. They may show different levels of inhibition and compliance according to their understanding of consequences. |
| Self-control | 24–48 months | Child's behaviors are in accordance with social expectations. The child shows a developing sense of identity, and behaviors become more internally monitored. | Child demonstrates knowledge of social rules and conventions. Child has difficulty adapting to new demands but may visually check in with parent before acting. |
| Self-regulation | ≥36 months | Child develops behavioral flexibility according to the demands of the situation. They develop strategies for managing different situations. Child has self-awareness and can self-evaluate their actions. | Child may self-initiate cleanup. They become more flexible in their responses, such that child can adapt to unexpected events (e.g., parent leaving for a long time), primarily because communication and language have increased. |

Adapted from Kopp, C. B. (2009). Emotion-focused coping in young children. Self and self-regulatory processes. In E. A. Skinner, & M. J. Zimmer-Gembeck (Eds.). *Coping and the development of regulation.* 124. (pp. 33–46). New Directions for Child and Adolescent Development; Kopp, C. (1982). Antecedents of self-regulation: A developmental perspective. *Developmental Psychology,* 18, 199–214.

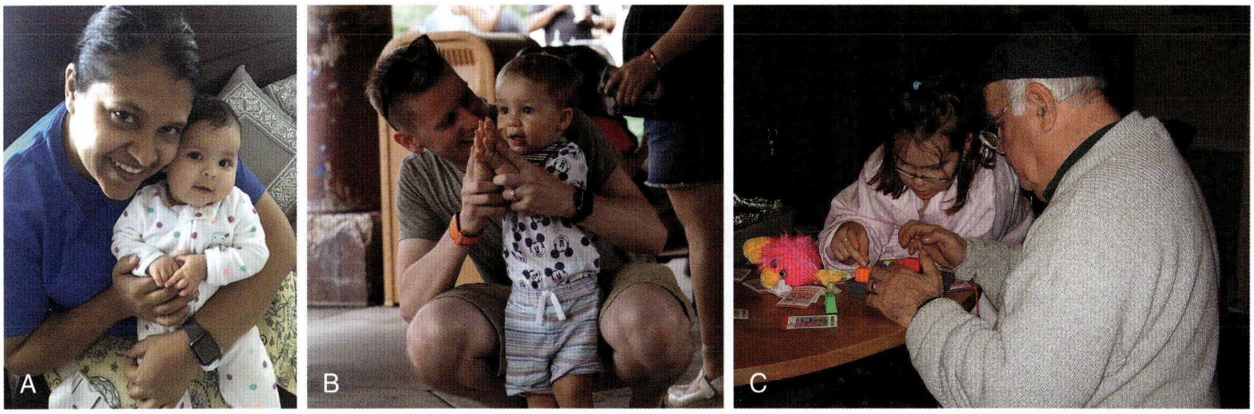


**Fig. 8.2** Relationships between caregivers and children. (A) Social-emotional development affects participation in all occupations. A child's ability to connect and communicate with others is necessary for health and wellbeing and begins with attachment to primary caregivers. (B) Children benefit from close relationships with family. This child enjoys social play with their father. (C) Children enjoy relationships with grandparents.

Appendix 8.2 describes the development of emotional regulation and related social behaviors.

**Adverse Childhood Experiences.** Children can be affected by adverse childhood experiences (ACEs), defined as traumatic events experienced by a child before the age of 18. Traumatic events include emotional/physical neglect or abuse, parental mental illness, parental separation or divorce, household domestic violence, substance abuse, and/or criminal activity. See Fig. 8.3 showing the ACE pyramid. The higher the ACE score, the worse the long-term health outcomes (Felitti et al., 1998; Monnat & Chandler, 2015). Trauma significantly impacts health, wellness, and the ability to safely engage in everyday roles, routines, and occupations (AOTA, 2018; Champagne, 2019).

Occupational therapy practitioners working with children and families play a role in identifying trauma that may influence a child's development and occupational performance (Petrenchik & Weiss, 2015). Practitioners support children and families who may have experienced trauma by empathizing, advocating, and collaborating with them. They often work with other professionals (e.g., social workers, counselors, and community support people) to support children and families.

**Community.** The community consists of institutions and people outside of the family structure, including peers, schools, neighborhoods, religious institutions, and transportation. Community environments may present opportunities or barriers to occupational participation. For example, communities may provide recreation facilities, such as playgrounds, pools, and open nature spaces that include hiking trails, lakes, and forests; and organizations, such as recreational sports teams, service groups, and community theater. Communities that value inclusion may have opportunities such as dance, soccer or baseball teams, horseback riding, boating, and swimming specifically designed for children with disabilities. Some communities offer spaces for safe play in neighborhoods, allowing children to develop friendships with diverse peers. Fig. 8.4 illustrates children playing soccer together in the community.

Schools are an important community space that can promote development and inclusion. Schools that actively engage parents in the educational process facilitate children's development through transactional relationships among parents, teachers, and community culture (Individuals with Disabilities Act [IDEA] 2012). Schools that value inclusion use Universal Design for Learning (i.e., principles to support learning for all in the classroom) and specialized services in the classroom to engage children. Box 8.3 provides an overview of Universal Design for Learning principles.

### APPENDIX 8.2 DEVELOPMENT OF EMOTION REGULATION AND RELATED SOCIAL BEHAVIORS

| Age | Emotion Regulation | Social Behaviors |
|---|---|---|
| 0–12 months | Self-soothes.<br>Learns to modulate reactivity.<br>Regulates attention.<br>Relies on caregiver for support during stressful situations. | Discriminates others' expressions.<br>Shows expressive responsiveness to stimuli.<br>Demonstrates different facial expressions. |
| 12–30 months | Shows increasing self-awareness.<br>Shows emerging consciousness of own emotional responses.<br>Can be irritable because of constraints and limits imposed when desiring to explore. | Expresses self-consciousness.<br>Shows shame, pride, and coyness.<br>Understands more language and emotions.<br>Expresses affective state. |

Adapted from Kopp, C. B. (2009). Emotion-focused coping in young children. Self and self-regulatory processes. In E. A. Skinner, & M. J. Zimmer-Gembeck (Eds.). *Coping and the development of regulation*, 124, (pp. 33–46). New Directions for Child and Adolescent Development. Saarni, C. (1999). *The development of emotional competence* (pp. 18–19). Guilford Press.

**Geopolitical Structures and Policies.** Geopolitical structures and policies affect the broader world in which children live. The geopolitical context may limit an individual's participation in living the life they choose based on broader contexts out of their immediate control (Silvestrini et al., 2019). For example, historical attitudes of racism, sexism, and ableism may covertly limit occupational participation. Fewer children of color achieve school completion, literacy, and math achievement, while more students of color are placed in special education settings (Children's Defense Fund, 2021).

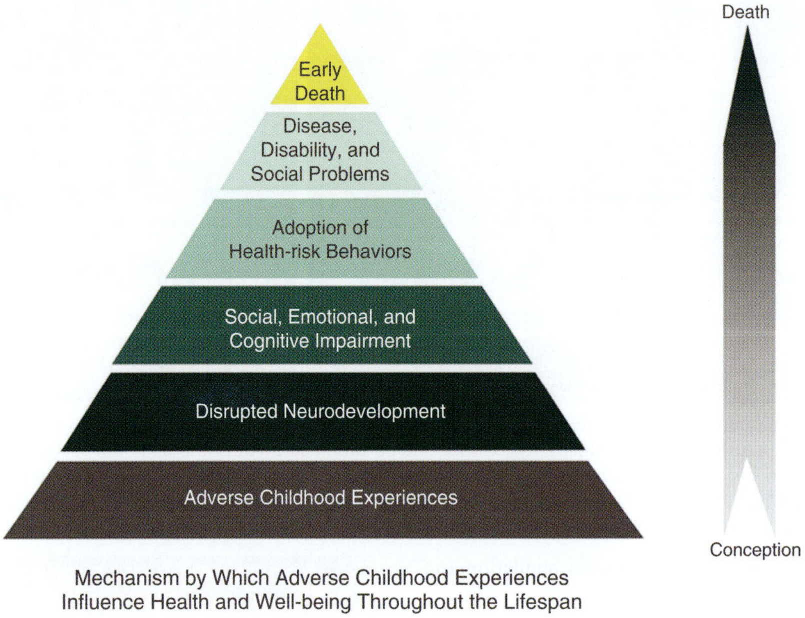


**Fig. 8.3** The adverse childhood experiences (ACEs) pyramid. https://www.cdc.gov/violenceprevention/aces/about.html (CDC, 2021).

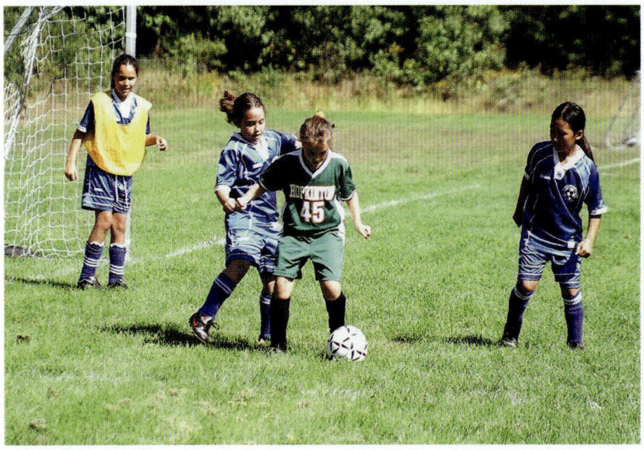

**Fig. 8.4** Popular play activities include ball play and outdoor sports (such as soccer).

Policies may support inclusion, such as the Individuals with Disabilities Education Act (IDEA, 2012), which requires that all students have access to free and appropriate education and the physical and social school environment and curriculum; and the Every Student Succeeds Act (ESSA, 2015), which mandates a basic level of education in the areas of literacy and math for future promotion to the workforce. Policies regarding access to health insurance for payment of necessary services and equipment, climate change, environmental pollutants, and access to healthy foods for nutrition are examples of broader geopolitical policies and attitudes affecting the human rights of children and occupational development (UNICEF, 2021; WHO, 2007).

Children's and families' health is affected by societal, environmental, and health policies. Physical health data show one out of five children in the United States lives in poverty, is food insecure, and collectively accounts for nearly 20% of the people living in homeless shelters (Children's Defense Fund, 2021). Fourteen percent of children and adolescents suffer from obesity, defined as a body mass index of 95th percentile or greater, leading to comorbid issues of asthma, type 2 diabetes, and sleep issues (Centers for Disease Control [CDC], 2018).

The National Center for Education Statistics (Irwin et al., 2022) reports that 22% of children during elementary and high school are bullied, while gun violence, including homicide and suicide, has become the leading cause of death of children and adolescents (Children's Defense Fund, 2021; U.S. Department of Health and Human Services, 2018). Long-term sequelae of these experiences include poor physical and mental health, limited school achievement, and a greater likelihood of chronic health conditions in adulthood (CDC, 2018).

**Culture.** Occupational therapy practitioners serve children and families who are culturally diverse, which is reflected in parenting and child-rearing practices (Tudge et al., 2018). Cultural practices include the routine activities common to the people of a culture and may reflect religion, traditions, economic survival, community organization, and regional ideology. A child's learning is highly influenced by participation in these cultural practices. Cultures vary in many aspects, such as the roles of women and children, family traditions, the importance of healthcare and education, and the view of interdependence versus autonomy. For example, the child in Fig. 8.5A thrives in a bilingual culture, and the child in Fig. 8.5B enjoys dressing in traditional ethnic clothing to celebrate cultural holidays.

Occupational therapy practitioners consider cultural practices and beliefs that may influence a child's developmental progression. For example, occupational therapists cautiously interpret findings from assessments regarding developmental milestones since many assessments have been standardized according to infants and children within the United States and Western Europe (CDC, 2010; Keller, 2017; Roopnarine & Davidson, 2015). This places some children at risk of being labeled as developmentally behind based on inaccurate or biased assessment items.

Children's developmental progression is influenced by cultural practices. For example, the rural Cameroonian Nso culture encourages independent walking at a young age. In this culture, the sooner children walk, the sooner they can join the farming community by helping with the chores required to maintain the home and sustain the family. Most middle-class European Americans value independence as a primary goal for their children. Parents in the United States

### BOX 8.3 Universal Design for Learning Guidelines

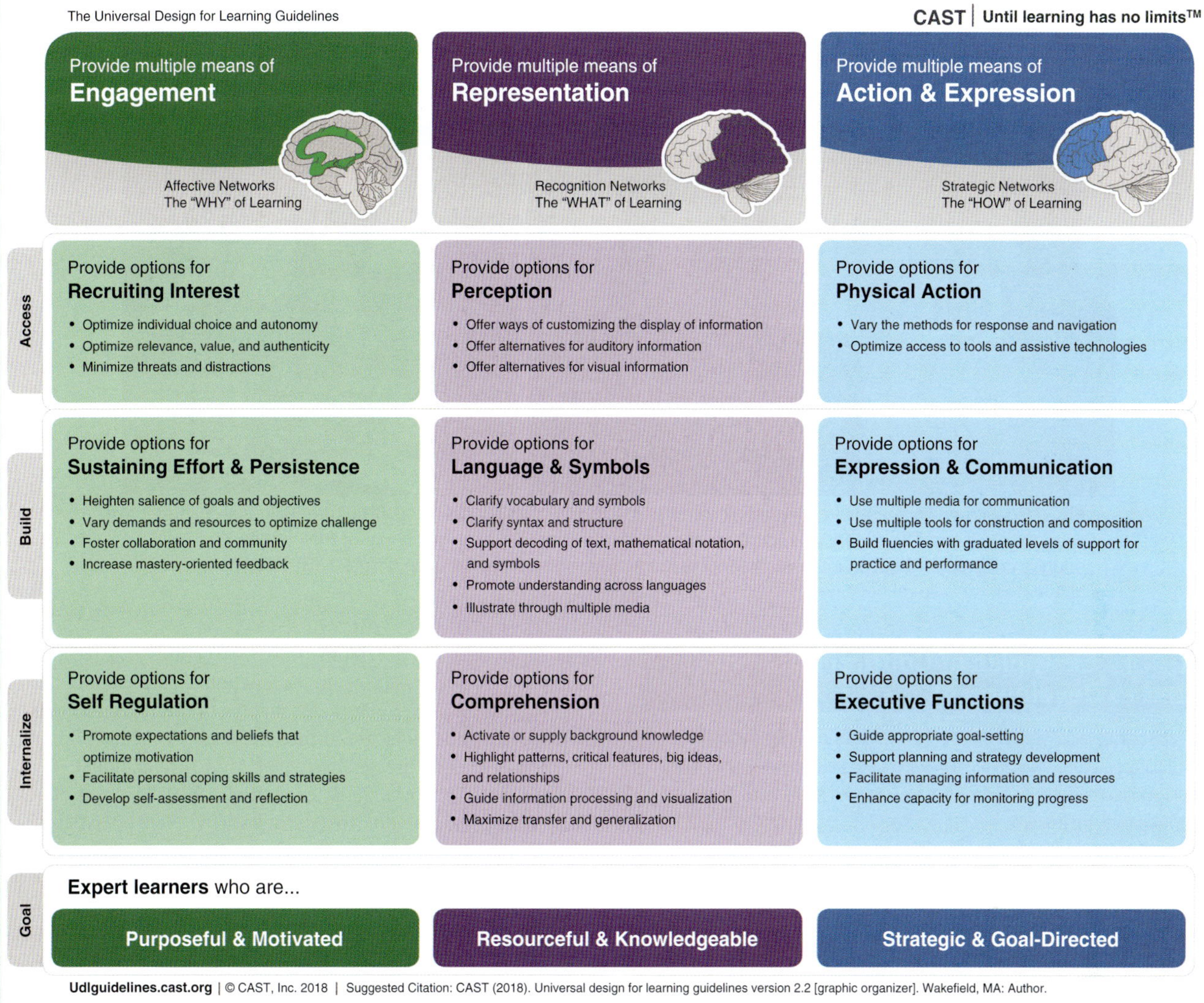


CAST (2018). *Universal design for learning guidelines version 2.2 [graphic organizer]*. Wakefield, MA: Author. http://udlguidelines.cast.org

encourage individuality, self-expression, and independence in their children's actions and thoughts (Pew Research Center, 2015). Families from Asian and Hispanic backgrounds often value interdependence and reliance on family members throughout the lifespan. Cultures that value interdependence over independence also value cooperation over competition. For example, many children of Asian and Hispanic backgrounds have been shown to be more cooperative in play than children from European American backgrounds (Farver et al., 1995; Trommsdorff, 2010). Box 8.4 illustrates important cultural influences and their impact on child development.

The social roles of young children are influenced by cultures, ethnicity, and community. In the United States, the importance of interaction with peers is stressed at young ages. Same-age peers become increasingly important through elementary school and dominate the social life of a teenager. In the United States and much of the world, children are grouped exclusively by age. These age groupings provide more play opportunities, but they also diminish opportunities for older children to teach and nurture younger children.

In Hispanic communities, for example, children spend almost all their time with siblings and other young relatives from a wide range of ages and primarily play with family members, including extended family. They socially participate in mixed-age groups, playing "on the edge" and watching intently until they can join in the play. Toddlers play with children of various ages, and they often play with older siblings. This enduring social network remains in place over time to care for, teach, and navigate children to adulthood (Trommsdorff, 2010). Interaction with children of varying ages provides older children the opportunity to practice teaching and nurturing young children and provides young children the opportunity to imitate older children.

Children may face barriers to engagement in meaningful and developmental occupations, however. Children born and living with disabilities such as cerebral palsy, autism spectrum disorder, Down syndrome, and other conditions may experience occupational alienation and deprivation due to the physical, social, and cultural contexts in which they live (Durocher et al., 2014). This has contributed to the focus on children's health and wellness worldwide (UNICEF, 2021). Occupational therapy practitioners consider the multitude of factors that influence development when designing interventions to enable children with disabilities to engage in meaningful activities within their communities.

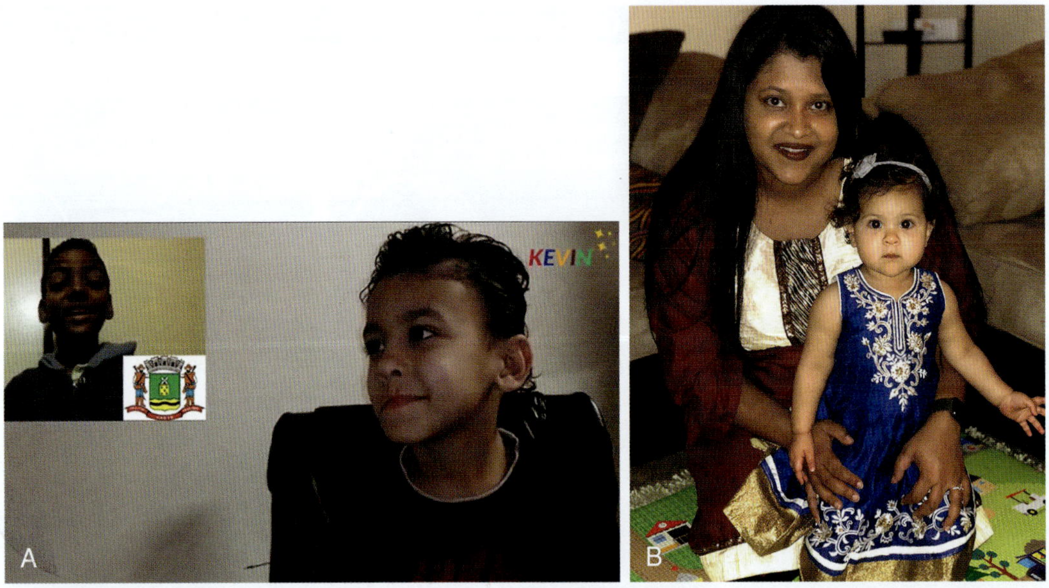


**Fig. 8.5** Children participate in their family culture. (A) Children thriving in a bilingual culture. Bilingual children span two cultures: The American culture of school and neighborhood and the culture of their family. This child bridges cultures through an internet channel teaching English to other Brazilian children. (B) This young child celebrates her cultural holidays dressed in traditional ethnic clothing.

**BOX 8.4 Examples of Cultural Differences Related to Development**

Infants' abilities develop because of the opportunities provided through one's culture. Their capabilities develop through transactions between the child's neurophysiological makeup and the culture that has provided affordances for occupational development. For example.

- In several rural or farming communities around the world, caregivers employ strategies and techniques within the first year of the child's life to promote early motor training (Keller et al., 2002).
- Rural African, Indian, and Caribbean cultures use regular infant massage to stimulate early motor movements as opportunities to advance motor skills. These infants tend to reach motor milestones earlier than their Western peers whose parents have not provided these opportunities (Adolph & Robinson, 2015).
- In the Nso culture, babies are wrapped and worn on the body, which provides rhythmic movement considered necessary for early motor development. When Nso babies are not worn on a caregiver's body, they are wrapped in sitting positions and placed in containers to advance their sitting abilities. The expectation is that these children will walk by 7 or 8 months. If walking is not achieved by that time, they are wrapped between bamboo poles and begin training under the supervision of family members, often siblings. Compared with middle-class German babies, Nso babies reach gross motor milestones several months earlier (Keller, 2017).
- In cultures where the infant's motor activity is restricted by practices such as being strapped to a Nez Perce cradleboard, a common practice in Native American culture, or a Tajikistani baby bound to a gahvora cradle, many infants still reach the milestones of motor development within the standard age expectations (Santrock, 2009).

## Occupational Performance and Development

Occupations are multisensory activities that require the use and integration of the central and peripheral nervous system as well as other body systems and structures. The child's experiences engaging in desired occupations produce new neurologic connections and structural changes allowing for continued development. Through both experience and development, new structures (e.g., cellular) and functions emerge, resulting in occupational performance changes. Occupations are powerful tools for shaping the brain over time as complex neural connections are formed among areas of the brain during multisensory goal-directed activities and occupational demands (Kleim, 2011; La Corte, 2008; Lane et al., 2019; Miller et al., 2021). These changes occur due to neuroplasticity. **Neuroplasticity** is the nervous system's ability to restructure and reorganize structures and connections in response to stimuli (Cramer et al., 2011). Three types of plasticity can be distinguished in the developing brain: experience-independent, experience-expectant, and experience-dependent (Kolb et al., 2013; Kolb et al., 2017). Box 8.5 defines each type.

Occupational therapy practitioners use knowledge of the progression of motor, processing, and social-interaction skills across the age span to design occupation-based interventions. They acknowledge that children develop at their own rates and that many factors influence the child's skills. **Motor skills** are involved when moving and interacting with objects and include mobility, coordination, strength, effort, and energy (AOTA, 2020). **Process skills** refer to those used in completing daily tasks and include energy, knowledge, temporal organization, organizing space and objects, and adaptation (AOTA, 2020). For example, process skills include choosing materials, understanding how to use tools, and adjusting one's approach to engage in the occupation. **Social interaction skills** refer to those needed to interact with other people and include physicality, information exchange, and relations with others (AOTA, 2020). Social interaction skills include language, gesturing, showing affect, and communicating one's needs (AOTA, 2020).

Occupational therapy practitioners use information about children's developmental progression to create effective intervention plans promoting occupational engagement. Understanding child development can inform activity choices, predict future milestones, and identify children's strengths and challenges. Practitioners may use knowledge of child development as a starting point to focus evaluation and questions for the occupational profile. Parents, caregivers, and family members seek information about child development to better understand their child's strengths and challenges, prepare for future

**BOX 8.5 Types of Neuroplasticity**

| Type | Definition | Example |
|---|---|---|
| Experience-independent | Neuronal changes that take place regardless of the environment and unfold over time. Neurons that are active together increase their connections, whereas those that are not active together weaken their connections (Kolb et al., 2017). | Children undergo brain growth (and neuronal growth) over time. |
| Experience-expectant | Changes in the organization of the brain from experiences that are universal to people within a certain window of development, such as light and sound | Infants and children will be exposed to a variety of sensory stimuli (such as light, movement, sound, and tastes) requiring that they process and respond promoting brain plasticity.<br>The auditory system may change based on the sounds the infant hears (Kolb et al., 2017). |
| Experience-dependent | Brain structure and function changes (i.e., neuronal changes) that occur because of the person's experience within their environment. Neuronal connections are modified by experience (Kolb et al., 2017). | Brain plasticity is stimulated when infants and children are exposed to opportunities to act (such as engaging in activities that require social, motor, and processing).<br>Children develop hand dominance with practice.<br>Changing the demands of the activity (such as with novel activities) stimulates brain activity.<br>Language, social interactions, and motor skills are dependent on environmental opportunities to practice. |

milestones, seek additional resources as needed, and instruct and support their child's development so that their child can engage in valued activities with family and friends.

Occupational therapy practitioners remind caregivers, parents, and teachers that children achieve milestones at different ages and at their own pace while also answering their questions and concerns. They use knowledge of the child's abilities and general child development to explain physical, social, and cognitive behaviors. The Centers for Disease Control (CDC, 2022) provides a milestone tracker and information to assist parents and practitioners. Box 8.6 describes the CDC Milestone Tracker. For example, a parent expresses concern that her 2-year-old child does not "play like the other children." The occupational therapist uses knowledge of the typical progression of play and considers the physical, motor, and cognitive aspects of play of 2-year-olds when evaluating the child. The practitioner inquires about the family's culture, expectations around play, opportunities for play, and environment. The therapist uses knowledge of child development (i.e., what does toddler play look like) along with information from multiple sources (e.g., environment, caregiver, observation, culture) to determine factors that may be influencing the child's play. Therefore, it is important that occupational therapy practitioners have a firm knowledge of typical developmental trajectories from prenatal to adolescence.

**BOX 8.6 CDC Developmental Milestone Tracker**

The Centers for Disease Control and Prevention (CDC) updated their developmental milestone checklists and parenting tips in 2022 to coordinate with the American Academy of Pediatrics Well Visits by Age. The milestones were updated based on current research and are based on the achievement of milestones by age of 75% of the children in that category. To access the child development page use the following link: https://www.cdc.gov/ncbddd/actearly/milestones/index.html. The CDC also offers a Milestone Tracker App to help parents promote development, which can be accessed at: https://www.cdc.gov/ncbddd/actearly/milestones-app.html.

## DEVELOPMENT: PRENATAL PERIOD TO ADOLESCENCE

### Prenatal Period

Healthy development in infancy, childhood, and adolescence begins in the intrauterine environment during pregnancy. A typical pregnancy lasts approximately 37–40 weeks and is often categorized into three stages or trimesters. The health of the mother, exposure and/or ingestion of beneficial or harmful substances by the mother and fetus, and access to prenatal care to monitor the mother and embryo's health play a role in the development of the central nervous system and other bodily systems of the fetus. Each trimester of pregnancy fosters specific growth in neurophysiological systems as summarized in Table 8.1. Infants who are born before 36 weeks or after 42 weeks are at risk for developmental concerns due to a disruption of gestational growth in the final weeks of pregnancy (Street & Bernasconi, 2020).

### Infancy

Infants demonstrate rapid brain growth, and by the age of 5 years, the brain reaches nearly adult size. The initial connections are laid down, and several experience-dependent changes give support to emerging individual differences in brain functioning (Cisneros-Franco et al., 2020; Gutman & Schindler, 2007). Although much development of the central nervous system is guided by gene expression, environmental influences and experiences take place in ideal brain development, which occurs during maturational stages known as critical periods. The **critical period** is the time during brain maturation when exposure to environmental stimuli and participation in occupations have a peak effect on development and learning, resulting in the child adapting to and responding to the environment in a functional way (La Corte, 2008; Nelson & Gabard-Durnam, 2020).

The newborn is well equipped with the capacity to form a strong bond with a caregiver and actively participate in the critical occupation of nursing. These innate capacities require rudimentary aspects of sensory integration that are built into the nervous system. However, even in this earliest period of development, environmental influences, such as maternal stress, can have a significant impact on the quality of sensory integrative development. Infants up to 2 years old are monitored for physical and motor growth to determine adequate nutritional intake, environmental stimulation, and psychosocial attachment to the caregiver.

**TABLE 8.1 Development of Sensory Systems**

| Period | Tactile/Proprioception | Vestibular | Gustatory | Olfactory | Auditory | Vision |
|---|---|---|---|---|---|---|
| **Prenatal** | Perioral area sensitive to stimulation by 7.5 weeks<br>Muscle spindle starts to differentiate<br>Clonus responses to stretch seen<br>Touching of face and mouth area becomes more frequent, starting at 10–12 weeks<br>Sensory nerve endings in place and functioning by 11 weeks<br>Touch is functional and fetal touches include rubbing eyelids and scratching the temple<br>Temperature discrimination at the end of the third trimester | Day 44: Primitive semicircular canal<br>Week 14: Sensory innervation completed<br>Week 16: Myelination completed<br>Vestibular systems are functional by weeks 17–21, but still developing<br>Semicircular canals reach adult dimension week 25<br>Organ of Corti<br>Complete week 30 | Week 4: Mouth begins to form tongue bud<br>Week 8: Mouth and tongue development completed<br>Week 20: Taste buds emerging<br>Weeks 26–28: Withdrawal response to bitter taste<br>Week 35: Differentiation between glucose and water is calming | Week 5: Nasal pits/plugs present<br>Nasal structure and components in place by week 8<br>Olfactory bulbs and sulci can be recognized after 30 weeks<br>Some olfactory perception by last trimester<br>fetuses learn odors from their pregnant mothers' diets | Week 4—First anatomical division<br>Week 24—System is structurally complete and functional<br>Cochlea, becomes functional by week 19, attains near adult size by week 23<br>By last trimester Will turn to auditory sounds<br>Can distinguish between the mother's voice and that of a female stranger | Day 22—eye formation begins, eyelids fused<br>Month 2—retinal differentiation<br>Weeks 6–8—optic nerve and cup being formed<br>Capable of perceiving light already by week 12 to 17<br>At 3 months—Precursors of rods and cones<br>At 22 weeks—all retinal layers present<br>At 23 weeks—immature rods and cones<br>At 24 weeks—myelination<br>At 25–26 weeks—All neurons of visual cortex present<br>Startle to light<br>At 28–40 weeks—General rapid ocular growth<br>Month 8—Iris sphincter develops<br>Month 9—retinal vessels reach the periphery<br>By 36 weeks—Awake visual alertness<br>Fetal eye movements are responsive to light in a way that is both systematic and independent of head movements |
| **Newborn** | Most mature system at birth | Functional at birth but continues to develop with motion against gravity, postural responses are learned and refined | Functional at birth<br>By day 3 to 6—differentiate between sweet, sour, and bitter and between breast milk and formula | Functional at birth newborns respond to new smells in the brain in similar ways as adults | Functional at birth<br>Newborns prefer to listen to a story that was read to them before birth rather than to other stories Prefer a melody that was played prenatally during the final weeks of pregnancy over other melodies | Development continues from 40 weeks gestation to 3–4 months postnatally to increase differentiation skills<br>Capable of perceiving light by weeks 12–17 |

Adapted from Alexandra Adam-Darque and others, fMRI-based Neuronal Response to New Odorants in the Newborn Brain, *Cerebral Cortex*, Volume 28, Issue 8, August 2018, Pages 2901–2907. Clark-Gambelunghe, M. B., & Clark, D. A. (2015). Sensory development. *Pediatric clinics of North America, 62*(2), 367–384. Fagard, J., Esseily, R., Jacquey, L., O'regan, K., & Somogyi, E. (2018). Fetal origin of sensorimotor behavior. *Frontiers in neurorobotics, 12*, 23. Johnson Chacko, L., Wertjanz, D., Sergi, C., Dudas, J., Fischer, N., Eberharter, T., & Handschuh, S. (2019). Growth and cellular patterning during fetal human inner ear development studied by a correlative imaging approach. *BMC Developmental Biology, 19*, 1–14. Purvis, B. (2005). The NICU Experience: Its impact and implications. Virginia Early Intervention Conference: Roanoke, VA – March 7-8. Retrieved http://www.infantva.org/documents/conf-PrenatalSensoryDevelopment.pdf. Reid, V. M., & Dunn, K. (2021). The fetal origins of human psychological development. *Current Directions in Psychological Science, 30*(2), 144–150. Stanley, N. G. (2004). Earlyneuro sensory visual development of the fetus and newborn. *Clinics in Perinatology*, 31(2), 199–216. Tristão, R. M., Lauand, L., Costa, K. S. F., Brant, L. A., Fernandes, G. M., Costa, K. N., & Lachmann, T. (2021). Olfactory sensory and perceptual evaluation in newborn infants: A systematic review. *Developmental Psychobiology, 63*(7), e22201.

**Reflexes.** In the immediate postnatal period, infants are assessed for the presence of primitive reflexes. Primitive reflexes are automatic survival responses necessary for the health and safety of the infant. Table 8.2 provides an overview of reflexes. Reflexes are predictable motor responses prompted by proprioceptive, tactile, and vestibular stimulation that are performed without conscious volition. These reflexes are present starting in the third trimester of pregnancy and persist after birth. Primitive reflexes often integrate within the first year of life. Persistence of reflexes after the first year of life may interfere with occupational performance. Fig. 8.6 shows an infant exhibiting the asymmetrical tonic neck reflex.

**Sensory.** The development of the sensory systems in the postnatal period includes touch, smell, and movement sensations important to the newborn infant, who uses these to maintain contact with a caregiver through nursing, nuzzling, and cuddling. Tactile sensations are critical in establishing a primary attachment relationship with a caregiver and fostering feelings of security in the infant (Bosmans et al., 2019). This is just the beginning of the important role that the tactile system plays in a person's emotional life because it is directly involved in making physical contact with others. Fig. 8.7 shows a caregiver and child enjoying movement and tactile sensations during play. Proprioception is also critical in the mother-infant relationship, enabling the infant to mold to the adult caregiver's body in a cuddly manner. Together, tactile and proprioceptive inputs set the stage for the eventual development of the body scheme, the brain's map of the body, and how its parts interrelate.

Although vestibular receptors are fully functional at birth, refinement of the vestibular system, particularly its integration with visual and proprioceptive systems, continues through childhood and early adolescence. Most caregivers who use rocking and carrying to soothe and calm the infant intuitively appreciate the influence of vestibular stimuli on the infant's arousal level (An, 2015). Experiences that activate the vestibular sense have other integrating effects on the infant. Being lifted into an upright position against the caregiver's shoulder increases alertness and visual pursuit (Weiner-Vacher, Hamilton, & Weiner, 2013). While being held in such a position, the infant's vestibular system detects the pull of gravity and begins to stimulate the neck muscles to raise the head off the caregiver's shoulder. This adaptive response reaches full maturation within 6 months. In the first month of life, head righting may be minimal and intermittent with much wobbling, but it will gradually stabilize and become firmly established as the baby assumes different positions (first when the baby lies in a prone position and later in the supine position).

The visual and auditory systems of the newborn are immature. The newborn orients to some visual and auditory inputs and is particularly interested in human faces and voices, although meaning is not yet attached to these sensations. Visually the infant is attracted to high-contrast stimuli, such as black-and-white designs, and the range of visual acuity for most stimuli is limited to approximately 10 inches. The infant's visual acuity and responsiveness to visual patterns expand dramatically over the first few months of life. During this time, the infant begins to sustain eye contact with the caregiver, further strengthening the bond between them.

Stimulation in each of the sensory systems potentially affects the infant's state of arousal. The infant's capacity to adapt to changing sensations is another important aspect of sensory integrative development: the development of self-regulation. It is relatively easy to overstimulate young infants, for example, with changes in water temperature, changes in body position, or an increase in auditory or visual stimuli (Schaaf & Anzalone, 2001). However, as sensory integration develops, older children are better able to self-regulate their responses to changing stimuli by initiating behaviors that facilitate calming and soothing (e.g., thumb sucking or cuddling with a favorite blanket) or exciting and energizing (e.g., jumping or singing). The process of self-regulation begins in the neonatal period and develops throughout early childhood.

By 4–6 months of age, a shift occurs in the infant's behavioral organization. The sensory systems have matured to the extent that the baby has much greater awareness and interest in the world. Additionally, connections among the vestibular, proprioceptive, tactile, and visual systems develop to provide a foundation for postural control. The infant begins to show a strong inner drive to raise the head and upper body against gravity as shown in Fig. 8.8. This drive is evident in much of the baby's spontaneous play. During the first 6 months after birth, a baby in a prone position shows gradually increasing extension from the neck down through the trunk as the arms gradually bear more weight to help push the chest off the floor. By 6 months of age, many infants spend much of waking playtime in the prone position with full active trunk extension, and most can sit independently, at least if propped with their own hands. These body positions usually are the infant's preferred positions for play. Head control is well established by 6 months of age and provides a stable base for control of eye muscles. The development of head control reflects the growing integration of vestibular, proprioceptive, and visual systems, which becomes increasingly important in providing a stable visual field as the baby becomes mobile.

The infant uses tactile and proprioceptive sensations to grasp objects, albeit with primitive grasps. Touch and visual information are integrated as the baby begins to reach for objects (Fig. 8.9). The infant has a strong inner drive to play with their hands by bringing them to midline while watching and touching them. Connections between the tactile and visual systems pave the way for hand-eye coordination skills. Midline hand play is a significant milestone in the development of bilateral coordination.

By now, neonatal reflexes no longer dominate behavior; the baby begins to exercise voluntary control over movements during play. The earliest evidence of motor planning is observed as the infant produces simple novel actions, that is, handling objects and initiating transitions from one body position to another. Although reflexes play a role in such actions (e.g., grasp and neck righting reflexes), the infant's actions have a goal-directed, volitional quality and are not stereotypically reflex-bound. The emergence of intentionality is a marker of the beginning of occupational engagement.

During the second 6 months after birth, tactile perception becomes further refined and plays a critical role in the child's developing hand skills. The infant relies on precise tactile feedback in developing a fine pincer grasp, which is used to pick up small objects. Proprioceptive information is also an important influence in developing manipulative skills, and now the baby experiments with objects using a variety of actions. These somatosensory-based adaptive responses contribute to the development of motor planning ability. Growing evidence indicates that these early sensory-motor experiences inform children about not only their own actions but also the actions of others (Libertus & Hauf, 2017). Further development of midline skills is also apparent as the baby easily transfers objects from one hand to the other and may occasionally cross the midline while holding an object.

Through the first year, auditory processing plays a significant role in the infant's awareness of the environment, especially the social environment. Auditory information is integrated with tactile and proprioceptive sensations in and around the mouth as the infant vocalizes. The fruits of this process begin to blossom in the latter half of this first year when the infant experiments with creating the sounds of the language used by caregivers. Vocalizations such as consonant-vowel repetitions ("baba" and "mamama") are common. Parents often attach meaning to these infant vocalizations and strongly encourage them, thus leading the infant also to attach meaning to these sounds. By their first

**TABLE 8.2 Reflex Development**

| Reflex or Reaction | Position (P) Stimulus (S) | Positive Response | Age of Onset to Integration | Lack of Integration or Onset |
|---|---|---|---|---|
| Rooting | P: Supine<br>S: Light touch on side of face near mouth | Opens mouth and turns head in direction of touch | Birth to 3 months | Interferes with exploration of objects and head control |
| Sucking/swallowing | P: Supine<br>S: Light touch on oral cavity | Closes mouth, sucks, and swallows | Birth to 2–5 months | Interferes with development of coordination of sucking, swallowing, and breathing |
| Moro | P: Supine, head at midline<br>S: Dropping head, more than 30 degrees extended | Arms extend and hands open; then arms flex and hands close; infant usually cries | Birth to 4–6 months | Interferes with head control, sitting equilibrium, and protective reactions |
| Palmar grasp | P: Supine<br>S: Pressure on ulnar surface of palm | Fingers flex | Birth to 4–6 months | Interferes with releasing objects |
| Plantar grasp | P: Supine<br>S: Firm pressure on ball of foot | Toes grasp (flexion) | Birth to 4–9 months | Interferes with putting on shoes because of toe clawing, gait, and standing and walking problems (e.g., walking on toes) |
| Neonatal positive support—primary standing | P: Upright<br>S: Being bounced several times on soles of feet (proprioceptive stimulus) | LE extensor tone increases, and plantar flexion is present<br>Some hip and knee flexion or genu recurvatum (hyperextension of the knee) may occur | Birth to 1–2 months | Interferes with walking patterns and leads to walking on toes |
| Asymmetrical tonic neck reflex | P: Supine, arms and legs extended, head in midposition<br>S: Head turned to one side | Arm and leg on face side extend; arm and leg on skull side flex (or experience increased flexor tone) | Birth to 4–6 months | Interferes with reaching and grasping, bilateral hand use, and rolling |
| Symmetrical tonic neck reflex | P: Quadruped position or over tester's knees<br>S:1. Flexed head<br>2. Extended head | 1. Arms flex and legs extend (tone increases)<br>2. Arms extend and legs flex (tone increases) | Birth to 4–6 months | Interferes with reciprocal crawling (children "bunny hop" or move arms and then legs in quadruped position) and walking |
| Tonic labyrinthine reflex | P:1. Supine, head in midposition, arms and legs extended<br>2. Prone<br>S: Position (laying on floor); being moved into flexion or extension | 1. Extensor tone of neck UE, and LE increases when moved into flexion<br>2. Flexor tone of neck UE, and LE increases when moved into extension | Birth to 4–6 months | Interferes with turning on side, rolling over, going from lying to sitting position, and crawling; in older children, interferes with ability to "hold in supine flexion" or assume a pivot prone position |
| Landau | P: Prone, held in space (suspension) supporting thorax<br>S: Suspension (usually), also active or passive dorsiflexion of head | Hips and legs extend; UE extends and abducts. Elbows can flex (typically used to determine overall development) | 3–4 to 12–24 months | Slows development of prone extension, sitting, and standing<br>Early onset (1 mo); may indicate excessive tone or spasticity |

**TABLE 8.2 Reflex Development—cont'd**

| Reflex or Reaction | Position (P) Stimulus (S) | Positive Response | Age of Onset to Integration | Lack of Integration or Onset |
|---|---|---|---|---|
| Protective extension UE—Parachute, downward forward, sideways, backward | P: Prone, head in midposition, arms extend above<br>S: Suspension by ankles and pelvis and sudden movement of head toward floor<br>P: Seated<br>S: Child pushed:<br>1. Forward<br>2. Left, right<br>3. Backward | Shoulders flex and elbow and wrist extend (arms extend forward) to protect head; infant catches self in directions pushed:<br>1. Shoulder flexes and abducts; elbow and wrist extend (arms extend forward)<br>2. Shoulder abducts, elbow and wrist extend (arms extend to side)<br>3. Shoulders, elbows, and wrists extend (arms extend backward) to protect head | 6–9 months and continues throughout life | Interferes with head protection when center of gravity displaced |
| Stagger LE—Forward, backward, sideways | P: Standing upright<br>S: Displacement of body by pushing on shoulders and upper trunk:<br>1. Forward<br>2. Backward<br>3. Sideways | Infant takes ≥1 steps in the direction of displacement. UEs often also have a protective reaction, with elbow, wrist, and fingers extending:<br>1. Shoulder flexes<br>2. Shoulder abducts and extends<br>3. Shoulder abducts | 15–18 months and continues throughout life | Interferes with ability to catch self when center of gravity displaced, causes trips and falls |
| Equilibrium—sitting | P: Seated, extremities relaxed<br>S: Hand pulled to one side or shoulder pushed | *Head righting: non–weight-bearing side*—trunk flexes; UE and LE abduct and internally rotate; and elbow, wrist, and fingers extend<br>*Head righting: weight-bearing side*—trunk elongates; UE and LE externally rotate; and elbow, wrist, and fingers abduct and extend. | 7–8 months and continues throughout life | Interferes with ability to sit or maintain balance when reaching for objects or displacing center of gravity |
| Standing | P: Standing upright, extremities relaxed<br>S: Body displaced by holding UE and pulling to side | *Head righting: non–weight-bearing side*—trunk flexes; UE and LE abduct and internally rotate; and elbow, wrist, and fingers extend.<br>*Head righting: weight-bearing side*—trunk elongates; UE and LE externally rotate; and elbow, wrist, and fingers extend and abduct | 12–21 months and continues throughout life | Interferes with ability to stand and walk and make transitional movements |
| Equilibrium or tilting—prone, supine | P: Prone or supine on a tilt board, extremities extended<br>S: Board tilted to left or right | *Head righting: non–weight-bearing side*—trunk flexes; UE and LE abduct; and elbow, wrist, hip, and knee externally rotate and extend<br>*Head righting: weight-bearing side*—UE and LE internally rotate and abduct and elbow, wrist, fingers, knee, and hip extend | 5–6 months and continues throughout life | Interferes with ability to make transitional movements, sit, and creep |

Adapted from Alexander, R., Boehme, R., & Cupps B. (1993). *Normal development of functional motor skills.* Therapy Skill Builders. Bly, L. (1994). *Motor skills acquisition in the first year: an illustrated guide to normal development.* Therapy Skill Builders. Fiorentino, M. R. (1981). *Reflex testing methods for evaluating CNS development* (2nd ed.), Charles C Thomas Publisher, Ltd.

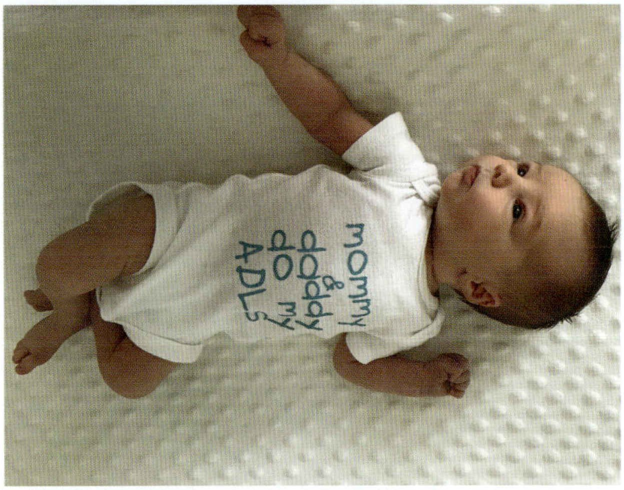


**Fig. 8.6** Baby demonstrates the asymmetrical tonic neck reflex (ATNR); the turn of the infant's head automatically elicits flexion of the upper extremity behind the head and extension of the lower extremity. The ATNR is meant as a reflexive, protective, response an infant makes when turning head toward an auditory or visual stimulus in the environment.

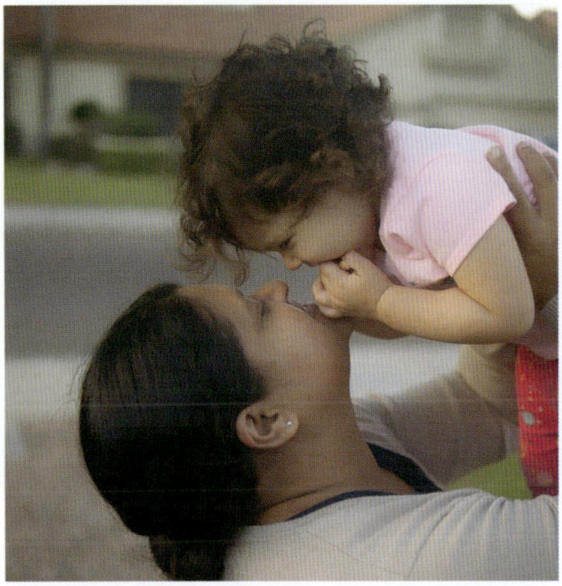

**Fig. 8.7** Tactile sensations play a critical role in incorporating feelings of security and comfort in the infant and are influential in emotional development and social relationships throughout the lifespan.

birthday, many infants have a small vocabulary of words or word-like sounds that they use meaningfully to communicate desires to caregivers. It is at the end of the first year that another wave of synaptic overproduction and pruning occurs so that by the age of 2 years, synaptic production in the occipital cortex is two times that of the adult brain.

As the child moves into the second year, the basic vestibular-proprioceptive-visual connections that were previously established continue to refine, resulting in growing finesse in balance and fluidity of dynamic postural control. Discrimination and localization of tactile sensations also become much more precise, allowing for further refinement of fine motor skills.

Increasingly complex somatosensory processing contributes to the continuing development of body schema (Rodrigues, 2020). Ayres (1972) in her seminal work hypothesized that as body schema becomes more sophisticated, so does motor planning ability. The child draws on

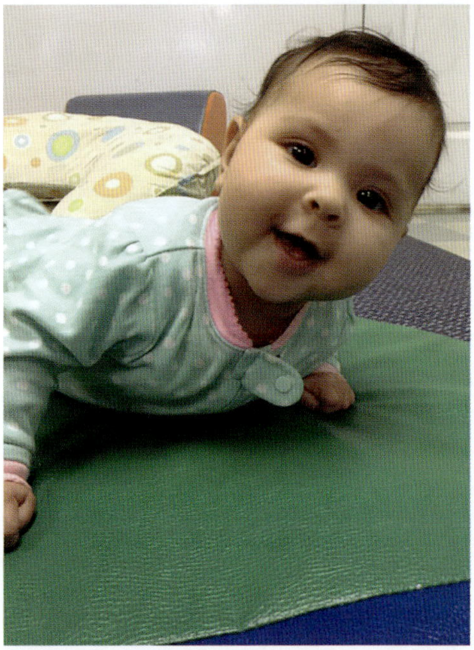

**Fig. 8.8** Infant playing prone against gravity picks up their head.

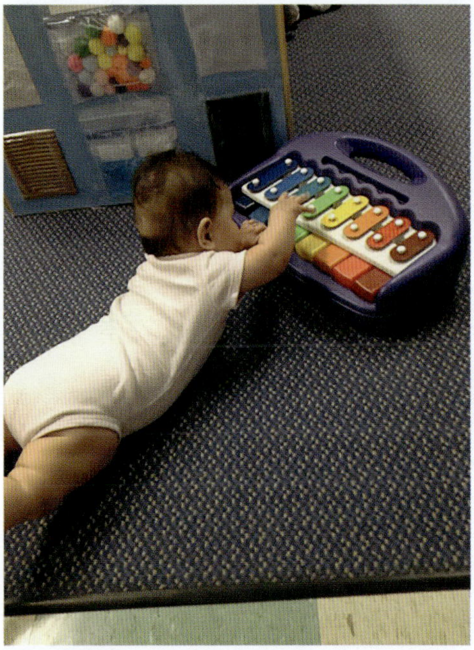

**Fig. 8.9** Infant in prone reaching for a toy during play.

knowledge of how the body works to program novel actions (Bardaglio et al., 2015) as shown in Fig. 8.10 as the toddler attempts to perform a somersault. Throughout the second year, the toddler experiments with many variations in body movements. Imitation of the actions of others contributes further to the child's movement repertoire. In experiencing new actions, the child generates new sensory experiences, thus building an elaborate base of information from which to plan future actions. For example, as infants gain postural control and bring their hands together, they hold a bottle (first with support from their caregiver, and eventually on their own). They become more skilled at holding, leading to drinking from a cup and bringing the cup to their mouth. Appendix 8.3 outlines the progression from bottle to cup drinking. Infants begin to feed themselves, first by raking small foods or putting

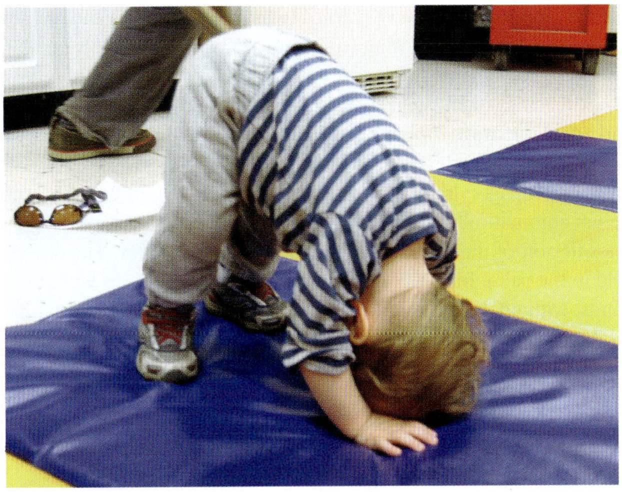

**Fig. 8.10** Toddler utilizing motor planning skills, vestibular processing, and body schema to experiment in motor play (e.g., try to perform a somersault).

## APPENDIX 8.3 SELF-FEEDING: BOTTLE TO CUP

| Age | Examples |
|---|---|
| 2–4 months | • Moves hand/hands up to the bottle/breast while feeding |
| 6–9 months | • Holds a bottle with both hands<br>• Uses a cup with help |
| 12–15 months | • Holds a cup with both hands<br>• Takes a few sips without help |
| 15–18 months | • Uses a straw |
| 2–3 years | • Drinks from a cup (no lid) without spilling |

Adapted from Case-Smith, J. (2005). *Occupational therapy for children* (5th ed.). Elsevier.

their hands (with food on it) in their mouths. As the infant's gross motor skills advance and they sit upright, their hand skills also advance so they can hold and bring to mouth, as well as their oral motor skills (to mouth, chew and eventually bite). Appendix 8.4 outlines the progression of self-feeding.

**Gross Motor.** The first movements of newborns appear to be reflexive; however, on closer examination, they reveal the ability to process and integrate sensory information. The neonate's movements contribute to perceptual development and organization and initiate their learning about the world. In the 2 months of life, the infant's sensory processing through response to gravity allows the infant to raise and move the head side to side when in a prone position and right the head when supported in sitting. Arms and legs move freely through space. By 4 months, with sustained prone positioning (tummy time), the child learns to move against gravity by pushing onto the elbow and forearms (CDC, 2022), lifting the head, and visually locating activities in the room. This ability to lift and sustain an erect-head position appears to relate to the infant's interest in watching the activities of others as well as improved trunk strength and stability. As the infant reaches 6 months, they gain more control against gravity to lift the head and trunk to move side to side on the forearms, and then on the hands (CDC, 2022). When supine, the infant actively kicks and brings the feet to the mouth. Over the next 6 months, this dynamic, postural stability prepares the infant to become mobile.

## APPENDIX 8.4 SELF-FEEDING

| Age | Examples |
|---|---|
| 6–9 months | • Wants to help with feeding<br>• Starts holding and mouthing large crackers/cookies<br>• Plays with spoon; grabs/bangs spoon; puts both ends in mouth |
| 9–13 months | • Finger feeds soft foods and foods that melt quickly<br>• Enjoys finger-feeding |
| 12–14 months | • Dips spoon into foods<br>• Moves spoon to mouth but is messy and spills |
| 15–18 months | • Scoops food with a spoon and feeds self |
| 18–24 months | • Wants to feed himself/herself |
| 2–3 years | • Stabs food with fork<br>• Uses spoon without spilling |
| 3–5 years | • Eats by himself/herself |

Adapted from Case-Smith, J. (2005). *Occupational therapy for children* (5th ed.). Elsevier.

A major transition occurs during the latter half of the first year. Infants become mobile in their environments, and by their first birthday, they can willfully move from one place to another, many walking while others creep or crawl. These locomotor skills are the product of the many adaptive responses in prior months, resulting in increasingly more sophisticated integration of tactile, proprioceptive, vestibular, and visual inputs. As the infant explores the environment, greater opportunities are generated for integrating a variety of complex sensations, particularly those responsible for developing body schemes and spatial perceptions. The child learns about environmental space and demands as well as the body's relationship to external space through sensorimotor experiences.

Rolling is the infant's first method of becoming mobile and exploring the environment. Initially, rolling is an automatic reaction of body righting; usually the infant first rolls from the stomach to the side and then from the stomach to the back. By 6 months, the infant rolls sequentially and can use this method of mobility to move across the room. Heavy or large infants may initiate rolling several months later and infants with hypersensitivity of the vestibular system (i.e., overreactivity to rotary movement) may avoid rolling entirely.

As an infant's vision and head control improve in the first 4 months, they become eager to view their environment from a supported sitting position. The newborn sits with a rounded back; the head is erect only momentarily. By 4 months, the infant can hold the head upright with control for long periods (CDC, 2022), moving it side to side with ease. Most 6-month-old infants sit alone by propping forward on their arms (CDC, 2022) using a wide base of support with the legs flexed. However, this position is precarious, and the infant easily topples when tilted. By 9 months an infant can sit independently (CDC, 2022) and play with toys using both hands rather than propping to support sitting.

As the infant masters sitting and has developed righting reactions, the infant may rise from a prone position by rotating (from a side-lying position) into a sitting position. The rotational pattern is important as it activates trunk muscles and requires the infant to cross the midline of the body. This important skill gives the infant the ability to progress by creeping to a toy, sitting, and playing. By 12 months, the infant can rise to sitting from a supine position, rotate and pivot when sitting, and easily move in between positions of sitting by pulling on furniture to stand.

The infant may first attempt belly crawling using both sides of the body together. However, reciprocal arm and leg movements are the most successful method of forward progression. Creeping (on the belly) leads to crawling (in quadruped). Infants first maintain a quadruped position, rock back and forth in this position, and then begin to crawl backward. By 7 months the infant moves from quadruped and back to sitting several times a day. They eventually crawl forward within the next few months. Crawling in a hands-and-knees posture requires more strength and coordination than belly crawling. The two sides of the body move reciprocally. In addition, shoulder and pelvic stability are needed for the infant to hold the body weight over the hands and knees. Mature, reciprocal hands-and-knees crawling also requires slight trunk rotation. Through the practice of crawling in the second 6 months of life, the child develops trunk flexibility and rotation. Most 10- to 12-month-old infants crawl rapidly across the room, over various surfaces, and up and down inclines.

Infants at 5 and 6 months of age delight in standing, and they gleefully bounce up and down while supported by their parents' arms. The strong vestibular input and practice of patterns of hip and knee flexion and extension are important to the development of full upright posture after 1 year. The infant prepares for a fully upright posture by standing against furniture or the parent's lap. A 12-month-old infant practices rising and lowering in upright postures while holding onto the furniture and can reach objects previously unavailable. This new level of exploration and increase in potential play objects motivates infants to practice standing. At this age, the infant also learns to shift the body weight onto one leg and to step to the side with the other. The infant soon takes small steps forward (CDC, 2022) while holding onto furniture or the parent's finger.

By 15 months the infant walks a few steps independently (CDC, 2022). Efforts toward unsupported forward movement through walking are short, erratic steps with a wide-based gait and arms held in high guard. All these postural and mobility skills contribute to the infant's ability to explore space and obtain desired play objects. By 18 months, the infant prefers walking to other forms of mobility, but balance remains immature, and the infant falls frequently. The infant continues to use a wide-based gait and has difficulty with stopping and turning. However, infants remain highly motivated to practice this new skill because walking brings new avenues of exploration and a sense of autonomy. Children begin climbing at 18 months and can climb onto chairs and furniture without assistance. When a child is 2 years of age they can run and navigate stairs, although they do not have full coordination and balance.

**Fine Motor.** Newborns move their arms in wide ranges, mostly to the side of the body, with exploratory movement patterns. By 2 months, the infant can open their hands briefly (CDC, 2022). In the first 3 months, the infant visually scans the environment and contacts objects with the eyes more than with the hands. By 4 months of age, an infant begins to coordinate hand and eye movements to swipe at toys and objects. This first pattern of reaching is inaccurate, but by 5 months, the accuracy of reaching toward objects increases greatly (Chin et al., 2019). The infant struggles to combine grasp with reach and may make several efforts to grasp an object held at a distance. However, the infant is skilled at bringing hands to mouth by 4 months of age (CDC, 2022), which serves for self-calming and prepares the infant to use the mouth to explore objects they will soon grasp. As postural stability increases, the infant learns to control arm and hand movements as a means of exploring objects and materials in the environment. By the time an infant is 6 months old, they can reach with one hand or both and smoothly and accurately extend the arm toward a desired object to grasp it (CDC, 2022). The infant also uses the mouth to explore objects and learn about the features of the objects. Infants progress from exploratory stage, as they learn to move their bodies and feel sensations to perceptual learning (transitional stages) that involve making voluntary movements and figuring out how they control their bodies to the skill achievement stage, where they can use movements in flexible and adaptable ways. Appendix 8.5 illustrates the progression through these stages for reach and grasp.

Grasp changes dramatically in the first 6 months. Initially, grasping occurs automatically when anything is placed in the hand and involves mass flexion of the fingers as a unit with the grasp reflex. The object is held in the palm. Infants 3–4 months of age squeeze objects within their hands, without involving the thumb. At 4–5 months of age, the infant exhibits a palmar grasp in which flexed fingers and an adducted thumb press the object against the palm. At 6 months, the infant uses a radial

### APPENDIX 8.5 REACH AND GRASP

| Stage | Age | Motor Actions |
|---|---|---|
| **Reach** | | |
| I. Exploratory | 1–3 months | Swipes at objects.<br>Reach is inaccurate.<br>Infant cannot combine reach and grasp. |
| II. Perceptual learning/ transitional stage | 3–6 months | Reaching becomes more accurate and direct.<br>Infant reaches to midline.<br>By 6 months, combines reach and grasp with two hands. |
| III. Skill achievement/ adaptability and flexibility | 6–9 months | Reaches with one or two hands.<br>Uses an accurate and direct reach.<br>Infants can change direction of reach midstream.<br>By 8–9 months, infants can reach in all directions in a smooth and efficient manner. They can combine reach and grasp and carry object through space. |
| **Grasp** | | |
| I. Exploratory | 3–5 months | First voluntary grasp begins between 2 and 3 months. Infant squeezes object with all fingers, thumb does not participate. Release is random, without voluntary control. Grasp is inefficient and infant cannot move objects in their hand. |
| II. Perceptual learning/ transitional stage | 6–12 months | Radial palmar and radial digital grasping patterns emerge. Infants actively use their thumb to grasp objects. An infant is unable to move an object within his hands but can transfer hand to hand and explore in their mouth. Voluntary release begins at 6-7 months. Infant awkwardly prehends small objects. |
| III. Skill achievement/ adaptability and flexibility | 12 months–2 years | By 12 months, infant demonstrates a pincer grasp; this grasp is precise by 18 months. By 18 months, demonstrates precision release. By 2 years, grasp is dynamic, allowing tool use. The child can use an object while holding it (toothbrush, spoon). Blended grasping patterns develop so the child can move an object while maintaining their grasp of the object. |

palmar grasp in which the first two fingers hold the object against the thumb. This grasp enables the infant to orient the object so that it can be easily seen or brought to the mouth. The infant secures small objects using a raking motion of the fingers, with the forearm stabilized on the surface.

Grasp changes rapidly from 7 to 12 months (Case-Smith, 2006). A radial digital grasp emerges in which the thumb opposes the index and middle finger pads. At approximately 9 months, wrist stability in extension increases, and the infant is better able to use the fingertips in grasping (e.g., the infant can use fingertips to grasp a small object, such as a cube or cracker). By holding objects distally in the fingers, the infant can move the object while it is in the hand; movement of objects within the hands allows the infant to explore them and use objects for functional purposes. A pincer grasp, with which the infant holds small objects between the thumb and finger pads, develops by 12 months. By this age, an infant is using a variety of grasp patterns for play and self-feeding (Wang et al., 2011).

In the second year of life, grasping patterns continue to be refined. Appendix 8.6 outlines the progression of fine motor manipulation skills. The child holds objects distally in the fingers, where holding is more dynamic. By the end of the second year, toddlers use a tripod grasp on utensils and other tools. They may also use other grasping patterns, depending on the size, shape, and weight of the object. For

## APPENDIX 8.6 FINE MOTOR MANIPULATION

| Age | Behaviors |
|---|---|
| Birth–6 months | Follows moving person with eyes<br>Develops accurate reach to object<br>Uses variety of palmar grasping patterns<br>Secures object with hand and brings to mouth<br>Transfers objects hand-to-hand<br>Examines objects carefully with eyes<br>Plays with hands at midline |
| 6–12 months | Mouths toys<br>Uses accurate and direct reach for toys<br>Plays with toys at midline; transfers hand to hand<br>Bangs objects together to make sounds<br>Waves toys in air<br>Releases toys into container<br>Rolls ball to adult<br>Grasps small objects in fingertips<br>Points to toys with index finger, user index finger to explore toys |
| 12–18 months | Holds crayon and makes marks; scribbles<br>Holds two toys in hand and toys in both hands<br>Releases toys inside containers, even small containers<br>Stacks blocks and fits toys into form space (places pieces in board)<br>Attempts puzzles<br>Opens and shuts toy boxes or containers<br>Points to pictures with index finger<br>Uses two hands in play, one to hold or stabilize and one to manipulate |
| 18–24 months | Completes four- to five-piece puzzle<br>Builds towers (e.g., four blocks)<br>Holds crayon in fingertips and draws simple figures (straight stroke or circular stroke)<br>Strings beads<br>Begins to use simple tools (e.g., play hammer)<br>Participates in multipart tasks<br>Turns pages of book |
| 24–36 months | Snips with scissors<br>Traces form, such as a cross<br>Colors in large forms<br>Draws circles accurately<br>Builds towers and lines up objects<br>Holds crayon with dexterity<br>Completes puzzles of four to five pieces<br>Plays with toys with moving parts |
| 3–4 years | Uses precision (tripod) grasp on pencil or crayon<br>Colors within lines<br>Copies simple shapes; begins to copy letters<br>Uses scissors to cut; cuts simple shapes<br>Constructs three-dimensional design (e.g., three-block bridge)<br>Manipulates objects within the hand |
| 4–5 years | Draws using a dynamic tripod grasp<br>Copies simple shapes<br>Completes puzzles of up to 10 pieces<br>Uses scissors to cut out squares and other simple shapes<br>Colors within the lines<br>Uses two hands together well, one stabilizing paper or object and the other manipulating object<br>Draws stick figure or may begin to draw trunk and arms<br>Copies own name<br>Strings small beads |
| 5–6 years | Cuts with scissors<br>Prints name from copy<br>Copies triangle; traces diamond<br>Completes puzzles of up to 20 pieces<br>Traces letters, begins to copy letters<br>Manipulates tiny objects in fingertips without dropping<br>Uses two hands together in complementary movements |
| 6–10 years | Good dexterity for crafts and construction with small objects<br>Bilateral coordination for building complex structure<br>Precision and motor planning evident in drawing<br>Motor planning evident in completion of complex puzzles |

## APPENDIX 8.7 PERCEPTUAL AND OBJECT MANIPULATION SKILLS

| Age | Perceptual Skill | Object Manipulation Skill |
|---|---|---|
| <6 months | Visually explores and mouths objects | Brings object to mouth |
| | Explores object textures by moving fingers back and forth | Begins to extend and move fingers together |
| 6–12 months | Explores objects with eyes and hands | Fingers and manipulates objects |
| | Discriminates hardness of object | Can tighten and loosen grip while holding an object |
| 12 months-3 years | Adjusts manipulation according to the object property | Moves an object from hand to hand |
| | Perceives object shape by moving between hands | Uses two hands to manipulate an object |
| >3 years | Identifies common objects using haptic perception (active touch) | Begins to demonstrate in-hand manipulation skills |
| | | Uses dynamic grasping patterns |

example, tools are held in the hand using first a palmar grasp and then a digital grasp. Blended grasping patterns develop toward the end of the second year, allowing the child to hold a tool securely in the ulnar digits while the radial digits guide its use.

Voluntary release of objects develops around 7–8 months of age. The first release is not precise and is characterized by full extension of all fingers. The infant becomes interested in dropping objects and practices release by flinging them from the high chair. By 10 months of age, objects are purposefully released into a container, one of the first ways the infant relates separate objects. As the infant combines objects in play, release becomes important for stacking and accurate placement. For example, 1-year-old children play by placing objects in containers, dumping them out, and beginning the activity again. Appendix 8.7 describes the development of perceptual and object manipulation skills.

By 15–18 months of age, the infant demonstrates the release of a food pellet into a small bottle and the ability to stack two cubes. Stacking blocks is part of relational play because the infant can control their arms in space, grasp with precision without support, and control release and has developed spatial relations and depth perception. The infant can also place large, simple puzzle pieces and pegs in the proper areas. At the same time, the child acquires the ability to discriminate between simple forms and shapes.

Children learn perceptual skills as they develop manipulative abilities (Schoder et al., 2020). They develop a perception of force so they can hold an object with the right amount of pressure (e.g., so cookies are not crushed before being eaten). Control of movements improves such that a child of 15 months can stack blocks. By 18 months the child can scribble and use a spoon. At 2 years, a child can manipulate buttons and knobs.

Bilateral hand skills (i.e., use of both hands together) can be observed when the 9-month-old infant bangs objects together and transfers items from one hand to another. Infants 12 months to 2 years develop skills to use both hands to play with objects. During this time, they use one hand to hold the object, while the other hand manipulates or moves the object. At 3 years, children can consistently use two hands in simultaneous, coordinated actions (e.g., using both hands to string beads or button a shirt) which results in improved performance in activities of daily living (ADLs) (Srinivasan & Bhat, 2019). See Appendix 8.8 for a description of ADL (i.e., dressing, feeding, bathing and grooming, and toileting) and instrumental activity of daily living (IADL) progression.

**Process Skills.** In the first 6 months, the infant learns about the body and the effects of its actions. At 2 months of age, infants watch their environment and follow people with their eyes as they move around the room. Infants can also look at a toy for several seconds and react to sounds within the environment. They focus their interest on actions with objects and the sensory input these actions provide. The infant learns through the primary senses: looking, tasting, touching, smelling, hearing, and moving. By 4 months of age, children begin to look at their own hands with interest and respond to the sound of voices by turning and making sounds in response (CDC, 2022). The infant enjoys repeating actions for their own sake and focuses on the action that can be performed with an object (e.g., mouthing, banging, shaking) rather than the object itself (Linder, 2008). By 8–9 months of age, the infant has an attention span of 2–3 minutes and combines objects when playing (e.g., placing a favorite toy in a container). At this age, children begin to understand **object permanence**; that is, they know that an object continues to exist even though they cannot see it (Bremner et al., 2015). They can also find a hidden sound and actively try to locate new sounds.

By 12 months of age, the infant increasingly understands the functional purpose of objects. They play with toys according to their function. The infant also demonstrates more goal-directed behaviors, performing with the intent of obtaining a specific result or goal. By 15 months, tools become important, and the infant uses play tools (e.g., hammers, spoons, shovels) to gain a further understanding of how objects work. Infants learn how objects work (e.g., how to activate a switch or open a door).

In the second year, the child can put together a sequence of several actions, such as placing small "people" in a toy bus and pushing it across the floor. Sequencing requires memory and attention span. The child's first sequential behaviors often imitate parent or sibling actions. As children learn to imitate, they engage in play sequences. By 15 months a child imitates other children during play and engages in simple pretend play (such as hugging a stuffed animal or doll). By 18 months, children imitate more complex actions of peers and adults, such as pretending to do chores (CDC, 2022). Appendix 8.9 provides an overview of cognitive and social skill development.

**Social Interaction and Play Skills.** Infants are born with the ability to see, hear, communicate (through crying and nonverbal expressions), and respond motorically through reflexes. An infant first demonstrates emotional regulation in the ease with which he or she feeds and sleeps. Problems in feeding, sleeping, toileting (urination, defecation), mobility, and play are concerns for overall health and interaction within the infant's environment. Babies learn to trust their caregivers and engage in carer–infant co-occupations. Infants learn to complete their occupations as caregivers set up environments that are meaningful and stimulating (Munier et al., 2008; Pierce et al., 2009).

The infant's emotional transition from the protective, warm womb to the moment of birth is a dramatic change. The primary purpose of the newborn's system is to maintain body functions (i.e., cardiovascular, respiratory, and gastrointestinal systems). As the infant

## APPENDIX 8.8 ACTIVITIES OF DAILY LIVING (ADLs) AND INSTRUMENTAL ACTIVITIES OF DAILY LIVING (IADLs)

| Age | Dressing | Feeding | Bathing/Grooming | Toileting | IADLs |
|---|---|---|---|---|---|
| 1–2 years | Doffs socks<br>Extends arms and legs to assist with dressing | Drinks from cup with lid<br>Finger-feeds self<br>Beginning to use spoon | Tolerates bathing and grooming tasks | Tolerates diaper changes. | Gives items when asked<br>Helps look for hidden items |
| 2–3 years | Doffs shoes, socks, pants<br>Buttons | Eats a variety of foods<br>Uses spoon, fork, and fingers to self-feed<br>Drinks from cup and straw | Tolerates hair care<br>Maintains posture during bathing | Maintain upright position on potty.<br>Indicates when wet/soiled. | Picks up toys |
| 3–4 years | Dons and doffs clothes (not including fasteners) | Uses utensils well<br>Drinks from cup without spillage | Washes hands<br>Gets into and out of bath safely<br>Spits out toothpaste | Bowl/bladder control during day<br>Indicates when needs to use bathroom and takes self to bathroom<br>Manages clothing and toilet sequence | Picks up belongings when asked<br>Understands safety<br>Gets items from pantry<br>Gets into and out of vehicle safely |
| 4–5 years | Dons and doffs clothing including simple fasteners (i.e., Velcro)<br>Unbuttons | Independent with self-feeding | Brushes hair with assistance<br>Obtains items for bath<br>Assists with set up for grooming (i.e., puts toothpaste on toothbrush) | Good bowl/bladder control<br>Independent in toileting sequence and hygiene | Gets snacks from kitchen |
| 5–6 years | Independent in dressing including most fasteners | Independent in self-feeding | Washes face<br>Brushes teeth<br>Completes bathing routine under supervision | Independent in toileting | Sets and clears the table with assistance<br>Understands what to do in an emergency (e.g., call 911)<br>Follows rules for safety shows stranger awareness |
| 6–7 years | Independent in dressing including all fasteners | Independent in self-feeding<br>Uses a knife to spread | Independent in bathing and grooming | Independent in toileting | Prepares simple snacks<br>Brings needed items to and from school<br>Unlocks and locks house<br>Follows basic road safety rules<br>Follows a safety plan |

Adapted from Roll, K. & Roll, W. (2013). *The REAL: The Roll evaluation of activities of life, user guide.* NSC Pearson.

matures, the focus shifts to increasing competence for interacting with the environment. An infant develops a sense of basic trust or mistrust that becomes a main theme in the infant's affective development and is highly dependent on the relationship with the primary caregivers. Appendix 8.10 outlines the development of attachment between an infant and a primary caregiver.

Toddlers are busy and active. They learn to feed themselves finger foods and use a spoon and fork. They begin to run, climb, walk up and down stairs, and kick a ball. Toddlers use functional communication to indicate their choices, wants, and needs to caregivers using words and gestures. They regulate their emotions and assert their temperament and personality as they approach situations and activities with caregivers or peers. Toddlers enjoy playing with toys for extended periods and engage in pretend play activities with dolls, household items, and cleanup activities.

Prosocial behaviors are an important part of development between the ages of 18 months and 2 years. Prosocial behaviors help a child develop empathy and perform tasks on behalf of others, rather than just to meet their own needs (Drummond et al., 2014). For example, they may assist in picking up toys, throwing trash away, or helping set and wipe the table. By the age of 3, a child can perform more complex chores such as sorting items as they put them away (Waugh et al., 2015).

Caregiver–infant bonding develops from experiences shared between caregiver and child over time. The infant responds differently to the parent's voice, usually quieting and demonstrating a calm affect. Although infants can cry to display discomfort from birth, they begin to express other emotions by 2 months, such as smiling and laughing. At this age, infants calm when they are picked up, look at faces, and seem happy when they see a caregiver. At 4 months of age, the infant smiles to get attention, chuckles, and attempts to get the attention of the caregiver by moving, looking, or making sounds. By 4–5 months, the infant vocalizes in tones that indicate pleasure and displeasure. By 5–6 months, the infant becomes interested in a mirror, indicating a beginning recognition of self. At 6 months, infants become more interactive with people in their environment. They know familiar people, laugh fully, and take turns making sounds with others. At 9 months of age, infants experience "stranger danger" and become fearful of strangers. They turn toward their name, show facial expressions, and

## APPENDIX 8.9 COGNITIVE AND SOCIAL SKILLS

| Age | Cognitive Behaviors | Social Behaviors |
|---|---|---|
| Birth–6 months | Repeats actions for pleasurable experiences<br>Uses hands and mouth to explore objects<br>Searches with eyes for sound<br>Bangs object on table<br>Integrates information from multiple sensory systems | Coos, then squeals<br>Smiles, laughs out loud<br>Expresses discomfort by crying<br>Communicates simple emotions through facial expressions |
| 6–12 months | Responds to own name<br>Recognizes words and family members' names<br>Responds with appropriate gestures<br>Listens selectively<br>Imitates simple gestures<br>Looks at picture book<br>Begins to generalize from past experiences<br>Acts with intention on toys<br>Takes objects out of container | Shows special dependence on mother<br>May show stranger anxiety<br>Lifts arms to be picked up Plays contentedly when parents are in room<br>Interacts briefly with other infants<br>Plays give and take<br>Responds playfully to mirror (laughs or makes faces) |
| 12–18 months | Acts on objects using a variety of schemas<br>Imitates model<br>Symbolic play with real props (e.g., pretends to drink with a cup)<br>Understands how objects work<br>Understands the functions of objects<br>Uses trial-and-error in problem-solving<br>Recognizes names of various body parts | Moves away from parent<br>Shares toys with parent<br>Responds to the facial expressions of others |
| 18–24 months | Links multiple steps together<br>Has inanimate object perform an action<br>Begins to use nonrealistic objects in pretend play<br>Continues to use objects according to functional purpose<br>Object permanence is completely developed | Expresses affection<br>Shows a wide variety of emotions: fear, anger, sympathy, and joy<br>Can feel frustrated<br>Enjoys solitary play, such as coloring, building<br>Engages in parallel play<br>Laughs when someone does something silly |
| 24–36 months | Combines actions into entire play scenario (e.g., feeding doll, then dressing in nightwear, then putting to bed)<br>Shows interest in wearing costumes; creates entire scripts of imaginative play<br>Matches pictures<br>Sorts shapes and colors<br>Plays house | Cooperative play: takes turns at times<br>Shows interest in peers, enjoys having companions<br>Begins cooperative play and play in small groups<br>Shy with strangers, especially adults<br>Engages in dialogue of few words<br>Can be possessive of loved ones |
| 3–4 years | Uses imaginary objects in play<br>Makes dolls and action figures carry out roles and interact with other toys<br>Categorizes and sorts objects<br>Shows a sense of humor | Attempts challenging activities<br>Prefers play with other children; group play replaces parallel play<br>Follows turn-taking in discourse and is aware of social aspects of conversation<br>Shows interest in being a friend<br>Prefers same-sex playmates |
| 4–5 years | Understands the rules to a game<br>Remembers rules with a few reminders<br>Makes up stories that involve role-playing with other children<br>Participates in goal-oriented, cooperative play with two or three other children<br>Participates in planning a play activity<br>Begins abstract problem-solving | Enjoys clowning<br>Sings whole songs<br>Role-plays based on parents' roles |
| 5–6 years | Reasons through simple problems<br>Bases play more on real life than on imaginary world<br>Participates in organized games<br>Uses complex scripts in play<br>Demonstrates deferred imitation<br>Sorts objects in different ways<br>Copies elaborate block structures | Participates in groups of two to four that play in organized, complex games<br>Has friends (same sex)<br>Enjoys singing and dancing; reflects meaning of words and music<br>Demonstrates understanding of others' feelings |
| 6–10 years | Abstract reasoning<br>Performs mental operations without need to try physically<br>Demonstrates flexible sddproblem-solving<br>Solves complex problems | Cooperative, less egocentric<br>Tries to please others<br>Has best friend<br>Is part of cliques<br>Is less impulsive, can regulate behavior<br>Has competitive relationships |

Data from Folio, M. R., & Fewell, R. R. (2000). *Peabody Developmental Motor Scales* (rev. ed.). Pro-Ed.; Knox, S. (2008). Development and current use of the Knox Preschool Play Scale. In L. D. Parham & L. Fazio (Eds.), *Play in occupational therapy for children* (2nd ed., pp. 55–70), Mosby; Linder, T. (2008). *Transdisciplinary play-based assessment* (rev. ed.). Brookes; Parks, S. (2007) *HELP Strands*. VORT Corporation.

## APPENDIX 8.10 DEVELOPMENT OF ATTACHMENT

| Phase Name | Age | Description |
|---|---|---|
| Orientation and Signals Without Discrimination of Figure | Soon after birth through 12 weeks, in some up to 6 months | Babies move and respond to stimuli in ways that elicit care and caregiver interest, but the infant does not discriminate between caregivers.<br>The infant behaviors lead to physical contact and warmth as well as nutrition.<br>The infant's sensory systems make it likely that the infant will respond to behaviors from the caregiver.<br>Early behaviors include crying, visual tracking, and looking at human faces, quieting to auditory stimuli, smiling, reaching, grasping, and clinging. |
| Orientation and Signals Directed toward one or more Discriminated Figures | Gradual shift occurs from 3 to 6 months, at different ages for different behaviors | More complex behaviors occur, and the infant establishes more control, for example, reaching for a caregiver and holding on to the caregivers clothing, hair, etc. The infant begins to discriminate the caregiver or caregivers who are most common and will display different behaviors to that person than others<br>Behaviors in this phase include stopping crying, smiling, or vocalizing upon appearance of a specific caregiver, crying when the caregiver leaves, actively seeking interaction with the caregiver.<br>Patterns of infant caregiver interaction during this phase lay the groundwork for later patterns of attachment. |
| Maintenance of Proximity to a Discriminated Figure by Locomotion | Beginning between 6 and 7 months and continuing through the 2nd–3rd year | During this phase, the infant is thought to be able to be truly attached to the primary caregiver or caregivers. When the infant is in a safe environment and with a caregiver who is sensitive to his or her cues, attachment develops. With the onset of some method of locomotion, the infant actively seeks proximity with the caregiver; in particular, there will be approach, especially after separation, or when distressed, using the caregiver as a base of exploration, and returning to the caregiver as a "safe place", clinging to the caregiver when scared or in discomfort, displaying wariness with a stranger and with novel and sudden events.<br>Between 6 and 24 months infants and toddlers become more wary of strangers. Readiness to form attachments to a primary attachment figure persists until at least 1 year, and although attachments can form later, it may be more difficult, and they are at risk of being less adaptive. By 18 months, most infants have an attachment to more than one "attachment figure" or caregiver but will focus on one primary person when that person is available.<br>Two-year-olds act similarly to 1-year-olds in terms of proximity to caregiver, and if the caregiver moves off, the toddler will stop exploring and reconnect with the caregiver; 2-year-olds will also be distressed by separation.<br>By age 3, most preschoolers will be willing to be left with other familiar people but may still be distressed if left alone.<br>Most 3- and 4-year-olds can wait for the return of their attachment figure, and they need less physical contact upon their return. They will seek brief proximity and then continue exploration.<br>Four-year-olds are not distressed by brief separation if they are aware of and had previously negotiated a plan for reunion. Older children tend to use less physical proximity and more behaviors such as eye contact, affect, conversation, and nonverbal behaviors to demonstrate their attachment. |
| Implications of the Partnership for the organization of attachment behavior | Preschool years | Ability to engage in a partnership of negotiating shared plans for proximity.<br>By age 4, the child is able to function in a partnership that is not as dependent on physical proximity, and physical contact and the availability of the attachment figure is most important over time. |

Please note that research in multiple countries and cultures has identified that attachment is a universal phenomenon. In most situations where an infant is in a safe environment, secure attachment develops, although the rates vary country to country. Although caregiver "sensitivity" is universally important, varied caregiver behaviors in different cultures may serve similar functions in varied contexts.

Based on Bowlby, J. (1982). *Attachment.* Basic Books. Marvin, R. S., & Britner, P. A. (1999). Normative development: The ontogeny of attachment. In J. Cassidy & P. R. Shaver (Eds.), *Handbook of attachment: theory research, & clinical applications* (pp. 44–67). The Guilford Press. Marvin, R. S., Britner, P. A., & Russell, B. S. (2016). Normative development: The ontogeny of attachment in childhood. In J. Cassidy & P. Shaver (Eds.), *Handbook of attachment: Theory, research, and clinical applications* (3rd ed., pp. 273–290). The Guilford Press. Mesman, J., van IJzendoorn, M. H., & Sagi-Schwarz, A. (2016). Cross-cultural patterns of attachment. In J. Cassidy & P. Shaver (Eds.), *Handbook of attachment: theory, research, and clinical applications* (3rd ed., pp. 852–877). The Guildford Press.

become upset when a caregiver leaves the room. They begin to express themselves with gestures such as raising their arms when they want to be picked up. At 1 year of age, infants play simple games like pat-a-cake and peek-a-boo, wave goodbyes, and say simple words like mama, dada, and no, and understand and respond to simple one-word commands (CDC, 2022).

In the second year of life, the child gains social interaction and communication skills. Caregivers remain the most important people in their lives. By 15 months a child imitates other children during play and shows preferences for toys. They are also affectionate toward trusted adults by giving kisses, hugs, and cuddling. They respond to more complex one-step commands, say one to two words or approximation of words, and point to get items they want or need. An 18-month-old's attention span increases and they can look at pages of a book with an adult. They may point to communicate with adults. The child begins to say a few more words other than mama and dada. By 2 years a child can point to requested items in a book, put two words together, and use more gestures for communication (CDC, 2022).

Toddlers play side-by-side with peers often, without verbally acknowledging each other. Although many infants play in a childcare center, the home provides the infant's first play environment. The crib is often a play environment, providing a place for comforting toys (e.g., music boxes and colorful mobiles). Other early play spaces include a play mat complete with multisensory pieces to allow for "tummy time on the floor," infant seats, car seats, swings, and baby carriages. Appendix 8.11 and Appendix 8.12 describe the play of infants, toddlers, and youth. Early exploratory play also occurs in the parent's or caregiver's arms as the infant is fascinated by the parent's face and clothing. At the same time, the infant feels safe and comforted by the parent's presence. At 18 months, the child moves further away from their caregiver but still looks back frequently to ensure the caregiver is present. Children at age 2 are interested in other children and a room of open spaces and they are likely to play next to each other (CDC, 2022).

In the second year of life, the child's environment may expand outside the home to the yard, sidewalk, neighbors' houses, extended families' homes, or previously unexplored spaces in the home. Some children have opportunities to play in their home's yard, the fenced-in areas of childcare centers, community spaces set up within apartment complexes, or wide-open spaces in rural areas. The child's increasing interest in visiting outdoor spaces provides important opportunities for sensory exploration.

## Preschool: 3–5 Years

Children in preschool learn to be independent in all self-care, mobility, and communication tasks in preparation for independence in elementary school. They can dress themselves independently, except for more complex fasteners, toilet with supervision for hygiene, and participate in a bedtime routine for sleep and rest (Chaput et al., 2015). Children begin to perform IADLs through simple household chores, such as putting dishes away in the sink, putting dirty clothes in the laundry, and assisting in chores like sweeping. They may help with simple chores, such as helping to stack rocks in the garden (Fig. 8.11) or picking apples with the family (Fig. 8.12). They become independent in community mobility tasks such as maneuvering around the playground, walking on the sidewalk, and getting in and out of the car seat. Appendix 8.13 describes the children's progression in completing chores.

In social participation, they expand their circle of engagement outside of their family. They learn to separate from their parents by taking a school bus or going to preschool and playing with peers in constructive ways. Play during this time becomes an interaction between doing and being as children and their caregivers learn about their interests, preferences, and skills. Beginning literacy skills are present as parents and teachers involve children in book reading, beginning coloring, and handwriting. The quality of the environments and interactions in this period of development may affect attentiveness, emotional regulation, and preparation for school entry (Gialamas et al., 2014).

**Construction play** is an important part of the preschool years that teaches children a variety of skills. At first, they demonstrate these skills by completing puzzles and toys with fit-together pieces (such as Legos and pop beads). Moreover, as children master simple

### APPENDIX 8.11 DESCRIPTION OF CATEGORIES OF EARLY PLAY

| Play Category | Age | Description | Examples |
|---|---|---|---|
| Sensorimotor | 2–4 months | Child explores objects, practices motor skills, enjoys sensory-motor exploration | Child bounces when held, bangs rattles, mouths toys |
| Relational | 6–10 months | Child relates one object to another | Child holds two objects, stacks blocks, places one object in or on another |
| Functional-conventional—discriminative: realistic object play | 10–12 months | Child relates object in a social, conventional manner; uses objects for functional (real) purposes | Child places toy phone on ear, stirs with spoon in cup |
| Symbolic: Pretend self; single play actions | 12–18 months | Child relates objects to self in pretend; one-step play actions | Child pretends to drink from a cup, brush own hair |
| Symbolic: Child as passive agent; substitute object play; multiple play actions | 18–24 months | Child extends familiar actions to dolls, figures; can use an object as a substitute for the actual object; carries out a sequence of two or more play actions | Child feeds doll, pretends to brush teddy bear's hair, puts doll in cart to ride; pretends that a block is an airplane or a car |
| Symbolic: Child as active agent; imaginary objects | 24–30 months | Child includes dolls or figure action in short scenario; pretends an action without the actual object. | Child pretends that teddy bear holds a cup, doll talks on the phone; drinks from an imaginary cup |
| Symbolic: Child uses imaginary objects in complex play actions | 30–36 months | Play is complex, with multiple steps in planned story | Child plans and carries out snack time with dolls; plays house in role as mother |

Adapted from Lifter, K. (2000). Linking assessment to intervention for children with developmental disabilities or at-risk for developmental delay: The developmental play assessment (DPA) instrument. In K. Gitlin-Weiner, A Sandgrund, & C. E. Schaefer (Eds.), *Play diagnosis and assessment* (2nd ed., pp. 228–251). Wiley; Takata, N. (1974). Play as a prescription. In M. Reilly (Ed.), *Play as exploratory learning* (pp. 209–246). Sage.

## APPENDIX 8.12 DEVELOPMENT OF PLAY

| Age Range | Type of Play | Play Behaviors |
|---|---|---|
| Birth–6 months | Exploratory | Sensorimotor play predominates<br>Social<br>Focused on attachment and bonding with parents |
| 6–12 months | Exploratory<br>Functional play (use toys according to their purpose) | Sensorimotor evolves into functional play<br>Social play with parents and others |
| 12–18 months | Relational and functional play | Engages in simple pretend play directed toward self (pretend eating, sleeping)<br>Links two or three schemas in simple combinations<br>Demonstrates imitative play from an immediate model |
| 18–24 months | Functional play | Multischema combinations<br>Performs multiple related actions together |
| 24–36 months | Symbolic play | Links multiple schema combinations into meaningful sequences of pretend play<br>Uses objects for multiple pretend ideas<br>Uses toys to represent animals or people<br>Plays out drama with stuffed animals or imaginary friends<br>Plays house, assigning roles to others, taking on specific roles |
| | Constructive play | Participates in drawing and puzzles<br>Imitates adults using toys |
| 3–4 years | Complex imaginary play | Creates scripts for play in which pretend objects have actions that reflect roles in real or imaginary life<br>May use complex scripts for pretend sequences; portrays multiple characters with feelings |
| | Constructive play | Creates art product without assistance<br>Works puzzles and blocks |
| | Rough and tumble play | Enjoys physical play, swinging, sliding board at playground, jumping, running |
| | Social play | Participates in circle time, games, drawing, and art time in preschool<br>Engages in singing and dancing in groups<br>Associative play: plays with other children, sharing and talking about play goal |
| 4–5 years | Games with rules | Begins group games with simple rules<br>Engages in organized play with prescribed roles<br>Participates in organized gross motor games such as kickball or "duck, duck, goose" |
| | Constructive play | Takes pride in products<br>Shows interest in the goal of the activity<br>Constructs complex structures |
| | Social play/dramatic play | Participates in role-play with other children<br>Participates in "dress up"<br>Tells stories<br>Continues with pretend play that involves scripts with imaginary characters |
| 5–6 years | Games with rules | Board games<br>Computer games<br>Competitive and cooperative games |
| | Dramatic play | Elaborate imaginative play<br>Role-plays stories and themes related to seasons or occupations<br>Emphasis is on reality<br>Reconstructs the real world in play |
| | Sports | Participates in ball play |
| | Social play | Participates in group activities<br>Organized play in groups<br>Goal of play (winning) may compete with social interaction at times |
| 6–10 years | Games with rules | Computer games, card games that require problem-solving and abstract thinking |
| | Crafts and hobbies | Has collections<br>May have hobbies |
| | Organized sports | Cooperative and competitive play in groups or teams of children<br>Winning and skills are emphasized |
| | Social play | Play includes talking and joking<br>Peer play predominates at school and home<br>Plays with consistent friends |

Adapted from Parks, S. (2007). *HELP Strands*. VORT Corporation; Linder, T. (2008). *Transdisciplinary play-based assessment* (rev. ed.). Brookes.

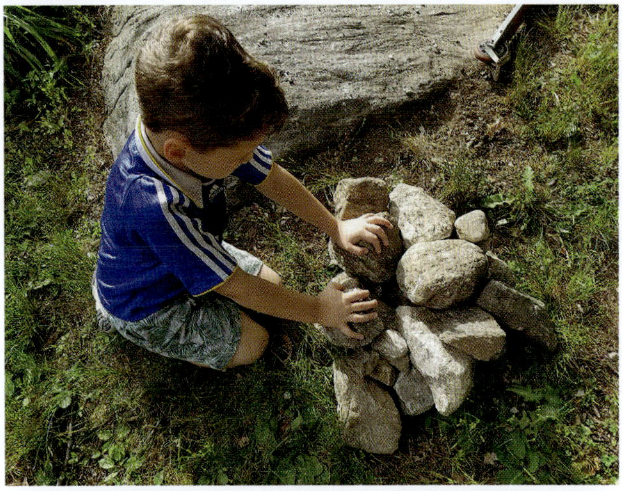

**Fig. 8.11** Preschool child stacking rocks as part of family chores.

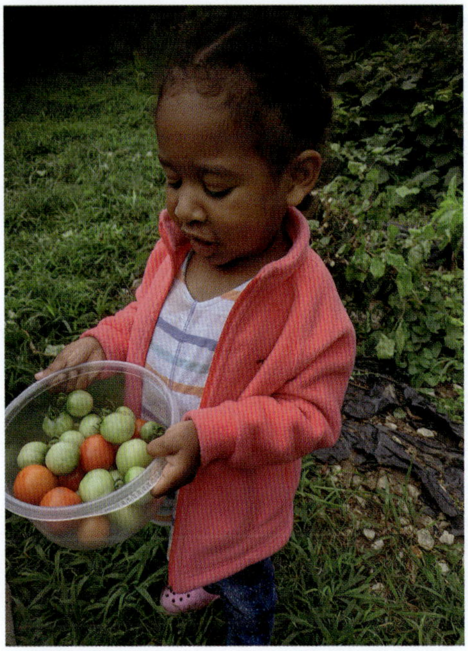

**Fig. 8.12** Preschool child picking apples with family.

construction, they become more creative. For example, a 4-year-old child can develop a plan to build a structure with blocks and then carry out the steps to complete the project. With instructions and a model, a 5-year-old child can make a simple art project or create a three-dimensional design (Barton, 2015). A 5-year-old child can also put together a 12-piece puzzle. Children value the final product, and they like to complete it and show it to others. Planning and designing involved in building and construction play helps the child develop spatial perception and object relationships which are foundational skills to academic performance.

Children 2–5 years of age are active and readily engage in rough-and-tumble play. They delight in movement experiences that provide strong sensory input. They enjoy activities such as running, hopping, skipping, and tumbling that are noncompetitive, without a goal, and rarely organized. Children enjoy movement as they play together.

During this period, children have strong inner drives to produce adaptive responses that meet complicated sensorimotor demands and interact with peers, as observed in the challenges posed by children's

### APPENDIX 8.13 CHORES FOR CHILDREN

| Age | Chore Examples | Chore Examples |
|---|---|---|
| 2–3 years | • Puts toys in toy box<br>• Stack books on shelf<br>• Place dirty clothes in laundry hamper<br>• Throw trash away | • Carry firewood<br>• Set the table<br>• Fetch diapers and wipes<br>• Dust baseboards |
| 4–5 years | • Feed pets<br>• Wipe up spills<br>• Put away toys<br>• Make the bed<br>• Straighten bedroom<br>• Water houseplants | • Sort clean silverware<br>• Prepare simple snacks<br>• Use hand-held vacuum<br>• Clear kitchen table<br>• Dry and put dishes away<br>• Disinfect doorknobs |
| 6–7 years | • Gather trash<br>• Fold towels<br>• Dust/mop floors<br>• Empty dishwasher<br>• Match clean socks | • Weed garden<br>• Rake leaves<br>• Peel potatoes or carrots<br>• Make salad<br>• Replace toilet paper roll |
| 8–9 years | • Load dishwasher<br>• Change lightbulbs<br>• Wash laundry<br>• Fold/hang clean clothes<br>• Dust furniture<br>• Spray off patio | • Put groceries away<br>• Scramble eggs<br>• Bake cookies<br>• Walk dog<br>• Sweep porches<br>• Wipe off table |
| 10–11 years | • Clean bathrooms<br>• Vacuum rugs<br>• Clean countertops<br>• Deep clean kitchen<br>• Prepare simple meal | • Mow lawn<br>• Bring in mail<br>• Do simple mending (i.e., hems, buttons)<br>• Sweep out garage |
| 12 and up years | • Mop floors<br>• Change overhead lights<br>• Wash/vacuum car<br>• Trim hedges<br>• Paint walls<br>• Shop for groceries w/list | • Cook complete dinner<br>• Bake bread or cake<br>• Do simple home repairs<br>• Wash windows<br>• Iron clothes<br>• Watch younger siblings |

Adapted from https://www.fatherly.com/news/a-montessori-chart-of-age-appropriate/

games and play activities. In the visual-motor realm, sophistication develops through involvement in crafts, drawing, painting, constructional play with blocks and other building toys, and video games. In fine motor tasks, children must efficiently coordinate visual with somatosensory information to guide eye and hand movements with accuracy and precision while maintaining a stable postural base (Pillar, 2022). During this time children become skilled with tools such as scissors, pencils, zippers, buttons, forks and knives, buckets, shovels, brooms, and rakes.

Many children begin to participate in occupations that present sensorimotor challenges such as soccer, softball, karate, gymnastics, playing a musical instrument, and ballet. They spend time learning to ride a bike and often use this first mode of transportation to be with friends (Fig. 8.13A or for exploring the playground (Fig. 8.13B). Children explore playground equipment by swinging, sliding, climbing, jumping, riding, pushing, pulling, and pumping. As children participate in these occupations, they frequently anticipate how to move in relation to changing environmental events by accurately timing and sequencing their actions (Cermak & Benson, 2020).

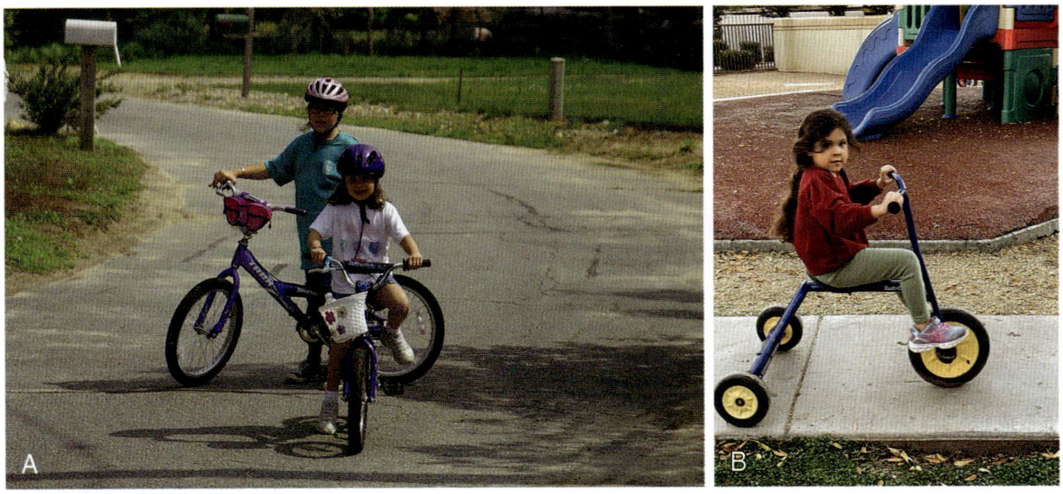

Fig. 8.13 Riding bikes is a favorite occupation of childhood that promotes physical, social, cognitive, and relationship development. (A) Children may enjoy biking with friends. (B) They may like to explore the playground on their own.

**Gross Motor.** Young children's motor function leaps forward during the preschool years. See the description of the progression of gross motor skills in Appendix 8.14. Between 2 and 3 years of age a child walks with an increased stride length and an efficient, well-coordinated, and well-balanced gait. Although children begin to run by 2 years, they exhibit true running (characterized by trunk rotation and arm swing) around 3–4 years of age. By 4 years of age, the child uses an adult-like walking pattern. By 5–6 years of age, children develop a mature running pattern, and they test their speed by challenging each other to races.

As mobility develops, children gain access to spaces previously unavailable to them. Running and stair climbing become possible, in part, because the child's balance and strength increase. They show emerging balance as the 2-year-old child briefly stands on one foot to kick a ball (CDC, 2022). By 5 years of age, the child can balance on one foot for several seconds and walk on a curb without falling. Jumping is first observed in 2-year-old children. This skill requires strength, coordination, and balance. By 3 years of age, the child can jump easily from a step. By 5 years of age, children have the strength and balance required to hop (CDC, 2022). Skipping is more difficult because it requires sequencing of a rhythmic pattern that includes a step and a hop. Children around 5 or 6 years of age have the coordination to skip. By 3 years of age, the child can pedal a tricycle but may run into objects. A 4-year-old child can steer and maneuver a tricycle around obstacles.

By 2.5 years of age, most children can catch a 10-inch ball. The first pattern of throwing involves a pushing motion, with the elbow providing the force for the throw. A 4-year-old child demonstrates more forward weight shift with throwing, increasing the force of the ball and the distance thrown. Kicking emerges by 2–3 years by 6 years of age children show accurate kicking to a target.

**Fine Motor.** Early childhood is a time of rapid improvement in fine motor and manipulation performance. Children develop advanced fine motor skills during the preschool years to engage in constructive and dramatic play and academics, including activities such as putting puzzles together, building towers, stringing small beads, using keys, and cutting out complex designs usually require dexterity, bilateral coordination, and motor planning.

Between 2 and 3 years of age a child uses both hands to screw and unscrew lids. They turn the pages of a book one at a time. At 3 years, children can string beads. By 4 years, children learn to move small objects efficiently within one hand (i.e., in-hand manipulation). A 4-year-old child can hold several small objects in the palm while moving individual pieces with the radial fingers (Pellegrini, 2009). In-hand manipulation requires isolated finger movement and easy movement of the thumb into opposition for pad-to-pad prehension. These skills require that the child accurately perceives the gentle force needed to manage small objects with the fingertips (Pellegrini, 2009).

With efficient in-hand manipulation, the preschool child learns the functional use of drawing and cutting tools. Most 4-year-old children hold a pencil with a static tripod grasp (i.e., with the pencil resting between the thumb and first two fingers) and use forearm and wrist movement to draw; however, by 5 years, a child demonstrates a mature, dynamic tripod (CDC, 2022). In this grasping pattern, children hold the pencil between the tips of the radial fingers and move it using finger movement. By controlling the pencil using individual finger movements, the child can make letters and small forms. Drawing with chalk provides additional proprioceptive input to improve hand strength and skills (Fig. 8.14).

Drawing skills progress from drawing circles to lines that intersect and cross in a diagonal (e.g., an X). The 4-year-old child begins to draw people with some recognizable details (CDC, 2022). Children 5 years of age often show a strong interest in drawing, which contributes to their imaginative play (Barton, 2015). They can draw detailed figures created in their imagination (i.e., monsters, fairies, and other fanciful creatures). Appendix 8.15 outlines the development of drawing skills.

The development of scissors skills follows the development of controlled pencil use. The first cutting skill, observed at 2–3 years, is snipping with alternating full-finger extension and flexion. Between 4 and 6 years, bilateral hand coordination, dexterity, and eye-hand coordination improve, enabling the child to cut out simple shapes. At 5–6 years, children can use scissors competently. They can cut accurately with isolated finger movements, simultaneous hand control, and well-developed eye-hand coordination (Bayley & Aylward, 2019; Folio & Fewell, 2000). See Appendix 8.16 for the progression of scissor skills.

## APPENDIX 8.14 GROSS MOTOR/ MOBILITY SKILLS

| Age | Behaviors |
|---|---|
| Birth–6 months | Lifts head (3–4 months), raises trunk when prone (4–6 months)<br>Kicks reciprocally when supine<br>Sits propping on hands<br>Plays (bounces) when standing with support from parents<br>Rolls from place to place |
| 6–12 months | Sits independently<br>Rolls from place to place<br>Independently gets into sitting position<br>Pivots in sitting position<br>Stands, holding on for support<br>Plays in standing when leaning on support<br>Crawls on belly initially, then crawls on all fours (10 months)<br>Walks with hand held (12 months) |
| 12–18 months | Sits in small chair<br>Plays in standing<br>Walks well, squats, picks up toys from the floor<br>Climbs into adult chair<br>Flings ball<br>Pulls toys when walking<br>Begins to run<br>Walks upstairs with one hand held<br>Pushes and pulls large toys or boxes on floor |
| 18–24 months | Runs, squats, climbs on furniture<br>Climbs on jungle gym and slides<br>Moves on ride-on toy without pedals (kiddy car)<br>Kicks ball forward<br>Throws ball at large target<br>Jumps with both feet (in place)<br>Walks up and down stairs |
| 24–36 months | Rides tricycle<br>Catches large ball against chest<br>Jumps from step or small height<br>Begins to hop on one foot |
| 3–4 years | Jumps, climbs, runs<br>Begins to skip and hop<br>Rides tricycle<br>Stands briefly on one foot<br>Alternates feet walking upstairs<br>Jumps from step with 2 feet |
| 4–5 years | Jumps down from high step; jumps forward<br>Throws ball<br>Hops for long sequences (4–6 steps)<br>Climbs on playground equipment, swinging from arms or legs<br>Throws ball and hits target<br>Skips for a long distance<br>Walks up and down stairs reciprocally |
| 5–6 years | Hops well for long distances<br>Skips with good balance<br>Catches ball with two hands<br>Kicks with accuracy<br>Stands on one foot for 8–10 seconds |
| 6–10 years | Runs with speed and endurance<br>Jumps, hops, skips<br>Throws ball well at long distances<br>Catches ball with accuracy |

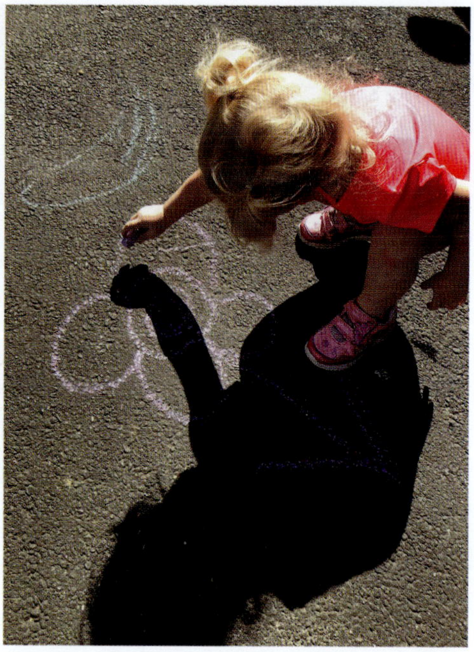

**Fig. 8.14** Opportunities for occupational creativity in a multisensory way (such as drawing on the sidewalk with chalk) that includes gross motor movements are important for skills integration.

**Process Skills.** Preschool children create symbolic representations of real-life objects and events during play. In addition, they begin to plan pretend scenarios in advance, organizing who and what are needed to complete the activity. Play becomes an elaborate sequence of events that is remembered, acted out, and later described for others. By 4 years of age, children recall and describe at least one event from the day (CDC, 2022). They also engage in role-play. For example, the child may act out the role of an adult, imitating actions remembered from an earlier experience. This form of role-play reflects the child's understanding of how roles relate to actions and how actions relate to each other (e.g., the child may role-play a grocery store clerk, displaying items for sale, taking money from the customer, and placing the money in a toy cash register). **Abstract thinking** begins in the preschool years between the ages of 2 and 3 as the child pretends that an object is something else (CDC, 2022). For example, the child may pretend a block is a doll bed; later the same block may become a telephone receiver or a train car.

In construction play (e.g., constructing train sets or building castles with Lego blocks), the child discriminates between object size and shape. Building in three dimensions requires spatial understanding and problem-solving skills. When building from a set of blocks, the child first categorizes and organizes the blocks. Next, the child solves the problem of how to fit them together to replicate a model or create the imagined structure.

Similarly, the emergence of drawing skills reflects cognitive abilities, motor planning, and perceptual skills. The 3-year-old child makes crude attempts to represent people and objects in drawings, especially when imitating drawings and simple shapes, such as circles. By 4 years, a child draws a recognizable person with at least three body parts (CDC, 2022), This develops further as the child demonstrates the ability to select salient features and represent them on a two-dimensional surface. At 5 years, the child's drawing is more refined, more realistic, and better proportioned. By this age, pictures begin to tell stories and reflect the child's emotions (Zakaria et al., 2020). By 5 years, a child can identify the letters of their name and write a few of them (CDC, 2022).

## APPENDIX 8.15 DEVELOPMENT OF DRAWING SKILLS

| Age | Developmental Skills |
|---|---|
| 2–3 years | Makes scribbling marks on paper that are without symbolic meaning (exploratory phase). Repetitious marks. |
| 3–4 years | Interprets drawing after it has been produced. Shapes emerge from scribbling. |
| 4–5 years | Draws an image, draws with intent a picture that represents an object, person, or event. Picture has shapes and distinct elements. It may be disordered, incorrect sizing, but has some semblance to intent. Draws a human figure with 4–7 features. |
| 5–6 years | Draws a human figure with 8–11 features. |

From Ziviani, J., & Wallen, M. (2006). The development of graphomotor skills. In A. Henderson & C. Pehoski (Eds.), *Hand function in the child* (2nd ed., pp. 217–238). St. Louis: Mosby.

## APPENDIX 8.16 DEVELOPMENT OF SCISSOR SKILLS

| Age | Developmental Skills |
|---|---|
| 1.5–2 years | Explores scissors, begins to hold scissors; may attempt to open and close the scissor blades with two hands |
| 2–2.5 years | May open and close the scissor blades in the air, and possibly make one simple snip at the paper. |
| 2.5–3 years | Opens and closes scissors with the entire hand and makes simple snips at the paper. |
| 3–3.5 years | Starts to make jagged snips across a piece of paper, (approximately 6 inches long). |
| 3.5–4 years | Cuts across straight lines and curved lines within ¼ inch of a thick guideline. Cuts out simple circles while using his/her helper hand. |
| 4.5–5 years | Starts to cut out shapes, like squares and triangles while using the helper hand. |
| 5–6 years | Can cut a variety of complex shapes, within a ¼ inch of a guideline. |

Adapted from Exner, C. E. (2007). Development of Hand Skills. In J. Case-Smith (Ed.) Occupational Therapy for Children (5th ed., pp. 287–306). Elsevier Inc. Teaford, P., Wheat, J., Baker, J. (Eds). (2010). HELP 3-6 Assessment Strands [Curriculum Based Assessment, 2nd Edition]. VORT Corporation. Warshaw, S. (2007). HELP strands 0-3 [Curriculum Based Assessment]. VORT Corporation.

**Social Interaction and Play Skills.** Children 4–5 years of age explore beyond the environment, discovering new activities. They seek new experiences to learn about the environment and explore. Through these activities, the child learns to question, reason, and find solutions to problems. Language and communication also increase. Between 2- and 3-year children have about 50 words and are starting to use a noun and a verb together. They can answer simple questions and say their name. By 4 years, children speak in complete sentences and can recall events of the day. They can identify colors. By 5 years, a child can count to 10, attend to a story or art craft for 5–10 minutes, understand basic units of time such as today and tomorrow, and retell a simple story (CDC, 2022).

The development of autonomy provides a foundation for the child's imagination. The young child explores the world through the senses. Although play can be reality-based, it includes fantasy, wishes, and role-play. As attention increases, children organize their play for longer periods. They can filter nonrelevant information and shift attention from one activity to another based on interests (Parham & Mailloux, 2020).

Preschool-age children's social skills and social participation develop as they gain independence from caregivers and begin to engage with more unfamiliar adults and peers. Between 2 and 3 years of age a child begins playing with other children rather than just playing next to them. By 3 years the child notices other children in the environment and initiates play with them. Between 2 and 3 years of age, children become interested in showing off their skills and may often say "Look at me!" They can follow simple routines. At 3 years, children can calm down after approximately 10 minutes when a parent leaves. They can engage in at least two back-and-forth communication exchanges and up to three exchanges by age 5. By age 4, children engage in more advanced pretend play and may pretend to be something else, like playing teacher or dog. They may ask to play with other children even if that child is not in their immediate environment. Children at 4 years old show empathy by comforting others when they are sad and have developed a sense of danger, avoiding dangerous situations and activities. By age 5, children follow rules during play and enjoy singing and dancing (CDC, 2022). Appendix 8.17 describes the development of friendship skills.

**Context.** Children can change their behavior based on different environments at 4 years of age (CDC, 2022). By the age of 5, their outdoor environment has expanded beyond the areas around the home and childcare center. A variety of outdoor environments offer space for rough-and-tumble play and provide the child with new opportunities for learning (and generalizing) the skills they have achieved. Although adult supervision remains essential, the entire neighborhood and natural environments, i.e., woods, rock formations, dirt may become the child's playground.

Preschool children experience new environments. Preschool classrooms usually have centers for different types of activities (e.g., creating art, listening to stories, playing games, pretend play). In addition, community groups sponsor a variety of indoor activities (e.g., preschool gymnastics and organized play programs) in which children can participate. Although structured play through organized games and activities is important for children to learn routines, follow directions, and cooperate with other children, unstructured free play is essential to the development of motor, sensory, social, and problem-solving skills (Lee et al., 2020).

Environments offer children the opportunity to adapt play skills learned at home to the constraints of new spaces. For example, the child who climbs and slides down the stairs at home learns to climb a 6-foot ladder and slide down the slide in the neighborhood park. Parks and playgrounds also provide the child with new surfaces that challenge balance and equipment that offers intense vestibular experiences.

Children often respond by instinctively exploring new spaces (e.g., hallways, cupboards, corners, furniture). Exploring the features of an environment can help orient children to the spaces that surround them, promote perceptual learning, and provide an understanding of the play possibilities in that environment. Based on sensory preferences, arousal levels, and activity levels, children may choose stimulating environments that are full of activity or prefer quiet spaces (Tomchek & Koenig, 2016). Spaces outside in nature or quiet spaces can be organizing and calming to some children, as illustrated in Fig. 8.15.

## APPENDIX 8.17 FRIENDSHIP SKILLS

| Age | Friendship Skills Examples |
|---|---|
| 1 year | • Looking, smiling, touching, imitating |
| 1–2 year | • Plays with others<br>• Can do fun things<br>• Identifies friend by name |
| 3–5 years | • Does things that please others<br>• Plays well in a twosome<br>• Approaches others to join |
| 5–7 years | • Helps and looks after others<br>• Takes others' feelings into account<br>• Sees others' viewpoints |
| 8–10 years | • Plays fair - follows the rules<br>• Talks and shares interests<br>• Talks and listens to others<br>• Forms groups with similar interests |
| 10–12 years | • Trusts others and is trustworthy<br>• Shares confidences<br>• Negotiates<br>• Respects one another |
| 12–18 years | • Understands others and who they understand<br>• Talks to others about feelings or problems<br>• Talks about personal and social issues<br>• Supports one another |

Adapted from Atwood, T. (2013). *Understanding and teaching friendship skills.* http://www.tonyattwood.com.au/index.php/publications/by-tony-attwood/archived-papers/75understanding-and-teaching-friendship-skills

## Middle Childhood: 6–10 Years

Although 6-year-old children continue to enjoy imaginative play, they begin to structure and organize their play. See Box 8.7 Piaget's game classification that corresponds to stages of cognitive development. By the time a child is 7 or 8 years old, structured games and organized play predominate. Games with rules are the primary mode for physical and social play. Groups of children organize themselves, assign roles, and explain (or create) rules to guide the game they plan to play. The goal of the game now competes with the reward of interacting with peers, and children become fascinated with the rules that govern the games they play.

Between 7 and 8 years, children do not understand that rules apply equally to everyone involved in the game, and they are often unable to place the rules of the game above the personal need to win (Florey & Greene, 2008). However, breaking the rules may incur criticism from peers, who also acknowledge the importance of rules at this time. By 9 and 10 years of age, children are more conscientious about obeying rules. They also learn to negotiate the rules of a game and construct their own rules.

In middle childhood, children are expected to actively engage in educational activities necessary for reading, writing, and comprehension of academic subjects. Leisure activities involve others such as video games, card games, and structured participation in organizations such as Boy/Girl Scouts of America. Middle school children are independent in advanced self-care routines and participate in IADLs such as making simple meals without appliances; community mobility, including walking to school; household chores such as taking care of pets, sweeping, emptying the dishwasher, making the bed; and outside chores such as raking, watering plants, and weeding (Rossman, 2002) (Fig. 8.16). They become comfortable in their roles as students, peers, family members, siblings, and community members.

In middle childhood, the child's play environment is now large and complex; more activities take place in the neighborhood and at school. The school's playground supports both social and physical play

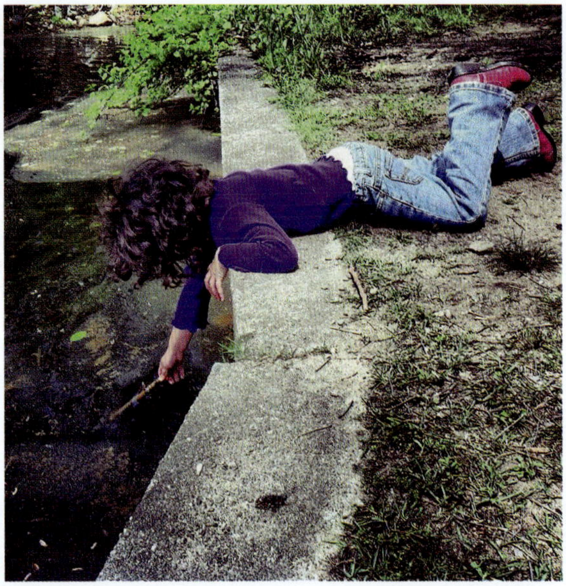

**Fig. 8.15** Child lying on the ground and playing in a stream during exploratory free play. Spaces in nature that allow children to explore quietly (such as playing with a stick in the water) can be calming to some children.

### BOX 8.7 Piaget's Stages of Cognitive Development as Expressed in Children's Games

**Practice (Sensorimotor Exploratory) Games**

Inia is a 5-year-old who enjoys running around the house and hiding from her 4-year-old sister. They like to roll around the floor bumping into each other and sometimes crawling over each other. They do not have rules or structure for this game which they play daily and sometimes outside as they tumble down a hill.

**Symbolic Games**

Inia and her sister love playing with toy animals and small cars. They spend time making roads, towns, and events in their sandbox and carry out stories. The toy animals may work together to "save someone" or reach a goal. Some days the animals are trying to prevent the other from getting the "prize." This game also lacks structure.

**Games With Rules**

The sisters often play games of "Go Fish" and "Let's Go Fishing." Inia knows most of the rules, plays cooperatively, takes turns, and knows how the game ends. She must make the game easier for her sister to play.

**Summary**

Although these classifications of play reflect different cognitive levels, children play at all three levels over an extended period. These play categories also have different goals and outcomes for the child's performance across developmental domains. All three play categories can be social play, object play, or both.

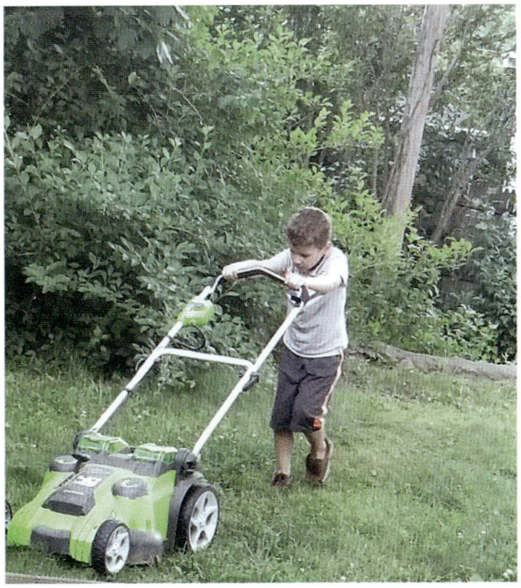

Fig. 8.16 Children can complete a variety of instrumental activities of daily living (IADLs) that encourage participation in family "work," self-competence, and responsibility (such as mowing the lawn).

for small groups of children. Play occurs on ball fields and in community centers, amusement parks, and sports arenas. Organized activities may be sponsored by school or community groups (e.g., YMCA, recreation centers, after-school programs, sports programs). By middle childhood, children maneuver through all environments (e.g., rough terrain, busy city streets). School-age children engage in activity in neighborhood streets and backyards, with bicycle races and spontaneous street hockey games. They may explore the woods and go on adventures in nearby parks to find areas unexplored by others (Lim et al., 2017). Although supervision by adults is still needed at times, intermittent supervision usually suffices (Barker et al., 2014; King et al., 2003). Children often become involved in organized, structured leisure activities at this age.

Creating craft and art projects continues into middle childhood as children show an increased ability to organize, solve problems, and create from abstract materials. However, adults may have to organize materials and identify steps for arts and crafts projects. Children in middle school value the final product. Playing with computers and video games is popular and may dominate play in middle childhood into adolescence (Halbrook et al., 2019; Nabawy et al., 2016).

Children at this age learn to cooperate but also to compete (Florey & Greene, 2008). They are now interested in achievement through play, and they recognize and accept an outside standard for success or failure and criteria for winning or losing. With competition in play comes risk-taking and strategic thinking.

During this period children enthusiastically grapple with motor-planning challenges posed by games such as jump rope, jacks, skateboarding, and hopscotch. Children gain skills with timing and sequencing, developing the ability to organize their behavior into complex sequences over longer time frames. This allows them to become more autonomous in daily routines, such as getting ready for school in the morning, completing homework and other school projects, and performing household chores (Larson, 2004).

**Gross Motor.** During elementary school years, children refine previously acquired skills by increasing speed, the precision of movement, and strength. They spend hours practicing their favorite physical activities, including sports, to attain mastery. Children ride bicycles, scale fences, swim, dance, skate, and jump rope. Although motor capabilities are highly varied for this age group, strength, endurance, balance, and coordination improve throughout middle childhood, providing children with the agility to participate in physical activities with proficiency.

**Fine Motor.** By middle childhood, children are efficient in tool use (e.g., scissors, tweezers) and precise drawing skills. They can competently handle and manipulate materials (e.g., fold, sort, adhere, cut) with competency. Children who are 8- and 9-year draw using appropriate proportions and accuracy. They write faster and with accuracy (Lin et al., 2017). They show improved speed, strength, and precision with construction skills, manipulation, and tool use.

**Process Skills.** In middle childhood, children can relate past events to the future and comprehend how situations change over time. Thinking is more flexible and abstract. The child reasons and solves problems by understanding variables and weighing pertinent factors before making decisions. Children now have a clear understanding of the difference between fantasy and reality, and they choose to move from one to the other.

Children between 8 and 9 years of age recognize that different solutions can be used to solve problems. They may arrive at answers through abstract reasoning rather than concrete trial-and-error. At this age, children can pay attention to more than one physical characteristic at a time and systematically put elements together. Children discriminate perceptual aspects of objects by size or shape. They also understand the relationship of the whole to the parts, and they imagine pieces as parts of a whole. With this understanding, they become more competent in organizing tasks and time. Children 9–10 years of age can give instructions to others and tell stories in detail.

By middle childhood, children learn to combine tasks and routines into complex games and competitive sports. Because numerous rules are needed to play sports or video games, the child understands the need to combine the rules into a complete game. To participate in the activity successfully, the child also understands when rules apply and when rules can be negotiated. Children also engage in computer games. Through virtual reality games, children in this age group may achieve a sense of power, feelings of accomplishment, and the ability to develop social strategies (Silcock et al., 2014).

## Adolescence: 10–24 Years

The period of adolescence has changed over generations and is dependent on geopolitical and social contexts. Adolescents seek peer friendships and support as they establish their own identity, prepare for adulthood, and change as they go through puberty. They enjoy spending time with other teens as shown in Fig. 8.17A and they may want to try out new activities such as surfing (Fig. 8.17B). The onset of puberty (hormonal stages of change) has emerged at younger ages while older adolescents continue to be dependent on parents for educational and economic needs for a longer period of time than past generations. Age at marriage and/or childbirth is later (Sawyer et al., 2018). Recently, child and adolescent health researchers have proposed an extension of the adolescent period beginning at 10 years of age and ending later, at 24 years of age. The extension of the adolescent age range is appropriate given access to US healthcare and other social services. College students in the United States, for example, can remain on their parents' health care plans until age 26 or graduation from college. This economic dependency is helpful for students, as paying privately for healthcare is now a requirement for attendance at

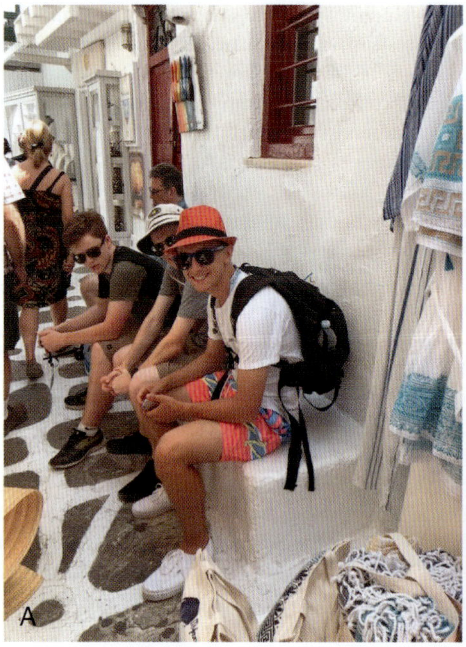
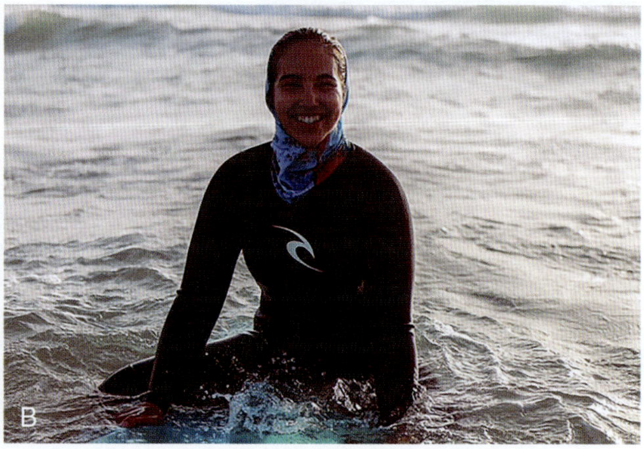

**Fig. 8.17** (A) Adolescents enjoy "hanging out" with each other. (B) They may also seek new adventures such as surfing as a way to better understand themselves and establish new interests.

higher education institutions. Special populations of adolescents may also be limited in healthcare, health access, and educational services. This includes adolescents with identified disabilities, those who have immigrated to the United States, may or may not have legal status, speak English as a second language, adolescents in foster care who are emancipated from the system at age 18 if not adopted, adolescents who identify as lesbian, gay, bisexual, transgender, or queer (LGBTQ+), and adolescents who are currently in the juvenile justice system (National Research Council/Institute of Medicine, 2008). Adolescents with developmental disabilities can transition out of high school services at 21 years of age due to the federal requirements of the IDEA (2012). They require specialized plans for transition from high school into community settings for work and/or higher education (IDEA, 2012; Lindsay et al., 2018).

Adolescence is a period of developmental transition characterized by neurophysiological, psychological, and cognitive changes. Adolescents undergo changes in sleep behaviors, and experience fluctuations of their hormonal and emotional states. While every child is slightly different, Appendix 8.18 reports the American Academy of Sleep Medicine's guidelines for the amount of sleep recommended by age. It is a time for more complex social behaviors, greater novelty seeking, and emotional instability. Adolescence is a critical period to develop patterns of physical and mental health for continued quality of life throughout the lifespan (U.S. Department of Health and Human Services, 2018).

There is continuous refinement and maturation of the brain's neural circuitry (Semple et al., 2013). Brain development allows for improved decision-making, complex social behaviors, and executive function (Guyer et al., 2018). Adolescents begin to develop enhanced abstract thinking, executive functioning, and abilities to problem-solve more quickly.

This is an interesting stage of development; however, as cognitive skills grow, so do levels of sensation seeking and decreased impulse control making this time precarious for safe and independent exploratory experiences (Murty et al., 2016)

## APPENDIX 8.18 SLEEP RECOMMENDATIONS FOR CHILDREN BY AGE

| Age | Recommended | May Be Appropriate | Not Recommended |
|---|---|---|---|
| Newborns<br>*0–3 months* | 14–17 hours | 11–13 hours<br>18–19 hours | Less than 11 hours<br>More than 19 hours |
| Infants<br>*4–11 months* | 12–15 hours | 10–11 hours<br>16–18 hours | Less than 10 hours<br>More than 18 hours |
| Toddlers<br>*1–2 years* | 11–14 hours | 9–10 hours<br>15–16 hours | Less than 9 hours<br>More than 16 hours |
| Preschoolers<br>*3–5 years* | 10–13 hours | 8–9 hours<br>14 hours | Less than 8 hours<br>More than 14 hours |
| School-aged Children<br>*6–13 years* | 9–11 hours | 7–8 hours<br>12 hours | Less than 7 hours<br>More than 12 hours |
| Teenagers<br>*14–17 years* | 8–10 hours | 7 hours<br>11 hours | Less than 7 hours<br>More than 11 hours |
| Young adults<br>*18–25 years* | 7–9 hours | 6 hours<br>10–11 hours | Less than 6 hours<br>More than 11 hours |

Retrieved from https://sleepfoundation.org/excessivesleepiness/content/how-much-sleep-do-babies-and-kids-need

Adolescence is a time of separation from primary caretakers leading to the development of adult and peer relationships outside of the family unit. Adolescents are independent in self-care tasks, household chores, laundry, and cooking simple meals. Adolescents are expected to be organized in the management of their daily school routine, complete homework assignments independently, and participate in all school environments such as the classroom, cafeteria, outside spaces, gym, art, and music. They have functional mobility (including the use of public transportation, car pick-up services, and driving) for getting to and from school, friends' homes, and community locations. The use of cell phones is the primary means of communication for adolescents and most feel this helps them stay connected to peers and caregivers (Ballarato et al., 2018; Frisson & Eggermont, 2015; Pew Research Center, 2018) (Fig. 8.18). Adolescents also spend time on social media which may have positive and negative effects on their self-image and self-esteem. Table 8.3 describes the positive and negative effects of social media.

Also during this period, youth enter puberty and experience a variety of changes associated with maturation and emerging sexuality. Occupational therapy practitioners working with children and adolescents use knowledge of developmental milestones (See Table 8.4) associated with sexuality and intimacy to support healthy development. Adolescents with developmental disabilities and chronic health conditions may experience early or late onset of puberty (Linkie & Hattjar, 2012; National Center on the Sexual Behavior of Youth, n.d.). Additionally, they are more likely to experience romantic or sexual debut later than their peers without disabilities (Penwell Barnett & Maticka-Tyndale, 2015). However, people with disabilities still report an interest and eventual engagement in similar sexual occupations as those without disabilities (Wiegerink et al., 2011).

Adolescents spend much of their time outside of school, forming peer and romantic relationships, and getting involved in afterschool activities such as sports teams, clubs, and community activities that reinforce their occupational identities (Mazurek & Kanne, 2010; Nippold et al., 2005). For some students this involves exploration of volunteer and paid work in settings such as dog shelters, daycare centers, landscaping, retail stores, and coffee shops. Others take care of family members such as younger siblings or provide translation services for grandparents and other family members. For some late adolescents, living back at home with their parents is an opportunity to gain economic footing before finding an independent living situation (Finn, 2016; Pew Research Center, 2015). For students who are still supported primarily by parents through college, late adolescence continues to be a time for work exploration, career development, and job acquisition as they begin their transition to adulthood.

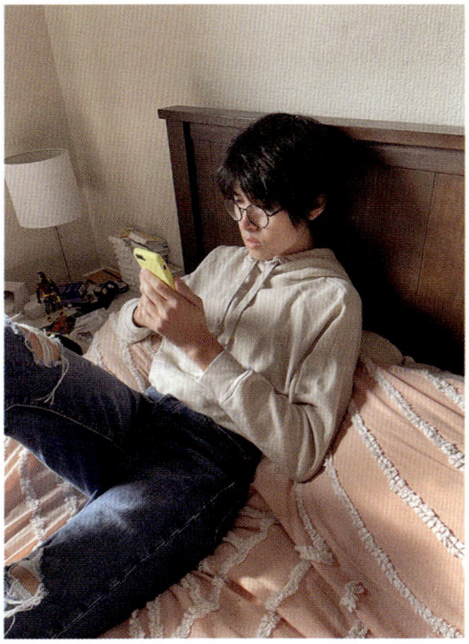

**Fig. 8.18** Cell phone use is a large part of teenage life. Teenagers should be encouraged to shut off all electronics 1 hour before bed to improve sleep.

**TABLE 8.3 Effects of Social Media on Teens Adolescents 13–19 Years of Age**

| Positive Effect 31% | Negative Effect 24% |
|---|---|
| Connecting with family and friends | Bullying/spreading rumors |
| Easier to get news and information | Harms relationships, lack of contact |
| Meeting others with same interests | Unrealistic view of others' relationships |
| Keeps you entertained and upbeat | Causes distraction/addiction |
| Self-expression | Peer pressure |
| Getting support from others | Causes mental health issues |

Adapted from Pew Research Center, Internet and Technology (2018). *Teens, social media and Technology, 2018.*

**TABLE 8.4 Sexuality and Intimacy: Milestones**

| Age Range | Occupations Associated With Sexuality and Intimacy | Role of Occupational Therapy Practitioners |
|---|---|---|
| Infancy and toddlerhood (0–2 years) | • Rely on parents for sexual health management<br>• Reflexive responses associated with self-exploration<br>• Development of language for anatomical vocabulary<br>• Curiosity about their own genitals<br>• Comfortable with own nudity<br>• Awareness of gender norms<br>• Parallel play | • Parent education to promote hygiene with diapering<br>• Parent education to use anatomically correct names for body parts<br>• Parent education to explain necessary touch (e.g., "I am going to clean your anus during this diaper change to help keep you clean")<br>• Parent education, individual and group intervention to promote parallel play as a stepping stone to more collaborative play with others |
| Preschool (3–5 years) | • Interested in own and others' bodies<br>• Behave in accordance with gender norms and social expectations<br>• Imitation play (e.g., playing house, playing doctor)<br>• Increased curiosity about others' body parts and reproduction<br>• Continued comfort with their own nudity | • Parent education to respond with simple, but honest answers to questions about bodies and reproduction<br>• Parent education, individual and group intervention to promote imitation play<br>• Parent education regarding boundaries<br>• Offering and respecting child's choice while creating safe boundaries for children in therapy sessions |

**TABLE 8.4 Sexuality and Intimacy: Milestones—cont'd**

| Age Range | Occupations Associated With Sexuality and Intimacy | Role of Occupational Therapy Practitioners |
|---|---|---|
| School age (6–11 years) | • Puberty management (i.e., menstrual hygiene management)<br>• Self-exploration (masturbation)<br>• Looking at others who are nude<br>• Enhanced understanding of gender and societal norms related to sexuality and intimacy<br>• Developing infatuations or "crushes"<br>• Initiating conversations about sexual activities<br>• Some may engage in sexual activities (e.g., kissing, touching others' genitals).<br>• Some may initiate intimate partner relationships. | • Parent education to prepare children with disabilities for puberty<br>• Strategies to promote independence in puberty management (e.g., Social Stories, practice with pad and paint for appropriate hygiene, etc.)<br>• Education for clients and parents about private vs. public (e.g., Social Stories)<br>• Continue educating on child's rights to their own bodies<br>• Continue offering and respecting child's choice while creating safe boundaries for children in therapy sessions |
| Adolescents (12–18 years) | • Increased interest in friends over family<br>• Intimate partner relationships<br>• Beginning to develop understanding of risks, consequences, etc. associated with sexual activities and intimate partner relationships<br>• Beginning to express one's sexuality<br>• May engage in sexual activities<br>• May engage in family planning (i.e., contraception)<br>• Increased independence in sexual health management (i.e., initiation of gynecological visits or prostate exams) | • Continue educating on child's rights to their own bodies<br>• Continue offering and respecting child's choice while creating safe boundaries for children in therapy sessions<br>• Facilitate child in recognizing healthy and unhealthy relationships<br>• Facilitate sexual self-advocacy |

Resources: Kellogg, N. (2010). Sexual behaviors in children: Evaluation and management. *American Family Physician, 82*, 1233–1238. Larsson, I., & Svedin, C. G. (2002). Sexual experiences in childhood: Young adults' recollections. *Archives of Sexual Behavior, 31*(3), 263–273. Mandel, A. & Datner, E. (2017). Sexual behaviors in children with developmental disabilities. *Journal of Alternative Medicine Research, 9*(3), 257–283. Mesman, G. R., Harper, S. L., Edge, N. A., Brandt, T. W., & Pemberton, J. L. (2019). Problematic sexual behavior in children. *Journal of Pediatric Health Care, 33*(3), 323–331. National Sexual Violence Resource Center. (2013). *It's time… to talk about it! Talk early, talk often. Prevent sexual violence: An overview of healthy childhood sexual development.* Retrieved from www.nsvrc.org/saam.

## SUMMARY

Infants, toddlers, and adolescents develop occupations, performance skills, and abilities over time (longitudinally) and within specific performance skills (horizontally). Development is not linear as once proposed, but rather it is influenced by the child's internal factors and the natural environment and social contexts in which they participate. Understanding developmental milestones provides occupational therapy practitioners with guidelines but is not the only measurement of the child's performance and progress. As advocates and change agents for children with a wide range of abilities and strengths, occupational therapy practitioners guide the infant, child, and adolescent along the developmental trajectory. They promote occupational participation, role competence, and access through environmental adaptations, skills acquisition, and engagement in meaningful activities. Occupational therapy practitioners provide intervention so children may progress along their developmental path, leading to long-term opportunities for self-determination, quality of life, and occupational engagement.

1. Practitioners consider many factors that may influence child development, such as the child's background and environmental factors as well as the unique features of the person (AOTA, 2020). They acknowledge the influence of relationships, experiences, community, policies, and culture on child development.
2. Occupational therapy practitioners use knowledge of developmental milestones as part of a broad view of development. They view the achievement of milestone ages cautiously, realizing that children progress at different rates; however, they use knowledge of the sequences of development to identify possible areas to target in intervention. Occupational therapy practitioners engage children in occupations, such as play, to promote neuroplasticity. Occupations are powerful tools for shaping the brain over time.

## REFERENCES

Adolph, K. E., & Robinson, S. R. (2015). Motor development. In L. S. Liben, U. Müller, & R. M. Lerner (Eds.), *Handbook of child psychology and developmental science: Cognitive processes* (pp. 113–157). John Wiley & Sons Inc.

American Occupational Therapy Association. (2020). Occupational therapy practice framework: Domain and process (4th ed.). *American Journal of Occupational Therapy, 74*(Suppl. 2) 7412410010.

American Occupational Therapy Association. (2018). AOTA's societal statement on stress, trauma, and posttraumatic stress disorder. *American Journal of Occupational Therapy, 72*(Suppl. 2) 7212410080p1–7212410080p3.

An, S. J. (2015). The effects of vestibular stimulation on a child with hypotonic cerebral palsy. *Journal of Physical Therapy Science, 27*(4), 1279–1282.

Annaz, D., Karmiloff-Smith, A., & Thomas, M. S. C. (2008). The importance of tracing developmental trajectories for clinical child neuropsychology. In J. Reed, & J. Warner-Rogers (Eds.), *Child neuropsychology: Concepts, theory and practice* (pp. 7–18). Wiley Blackwell.

Atwood, T. (2013). *Understanding and teaching friendship skills.* http://www.tonyattwood.com.au/index.php/publications/by-tony-attwood/archived-papers/75understanding-and-teaching-friendship-skills.

Aubuchon-Endsley, N. L., Gee, B. M., Devine, N., Ramsdell-Hudock, H. L., Swann-Thomsen, H., & Brumley, M. R. (2020). A cohort study of relations among caregiver–infant co-occupation and reciprocity. *Occupational Therapy Journal of Research: Occupation, Participation and Health, 40*(4), 261–269.

Aubuchon-Endsley, N. L., Gee, B. M., Ramsdell, H. L., Devine, N., Swann-Thomsen, H. E., Burgett, N., & Brumley, M. R. (2021). Observing and promoting normative developmental outcomes: Reciprocity is key. *The Open Journal of Occupational Therapy, 9*(3), 1–12.

Ayres, A. J. (1972). Sensory integration and learning disorders. *Western Psychological Association.*

Ballarato, G., Volpi, B., Marzilli, E., & Tambelli, R. (2018). Adolescent internet abuse: A study on the role of attachment to parents and peers in a large community sample. *Biomedical Research International, 2018*(14), 1–10.

Bardaglio, G., Marasso, D., Magno, F., Rabaglietti, E., & Ciairano, S. (2015). Team-teaching in physical education for promoting coordinative motor skills in children: The more you invest the more you get. *Physical Education and Sport Pedagogy, 20,* 268–282.

Barker, J., Semenov, A., Michealson, L., Provan, L., Snyder, H., & Munakata, Y. (2014). Less-structured time in children's daily lives predicts self-directed executive functioning. *Frontiers in Psychology, 5.*

Barton, G. (2015). Arts-based educational research in the early years. *International Research in Early Childhood Education, 6*(1), 62–79.

Bayley, N., & Aylward, G. (2019). *Bayley scales of infant development* (4th ed.). Pearson Assessments. https://www.pearsonassessments.com/.

Bentenuto, A., Bertamini, G., Perzolli, S., & Venuti, P. (2020). Changes in developmental trajectories of preschool children with autism spectrum disorder during parental based intensive intervention. *Brain Sciences, 10*(5), 289.

Bjornson, K., Fiss, A., Avery, L., Wentz, E., Kerfeld, C., Cicirello, N., & Hanna, S. E. (2020). Longitudinal trajectories of physical activity and walking performance by gross motor function classification system level for children with cerebral palsy. *Disability & Rehabilitation, 42*(12), 1705–1713.

Bly, L. (1994). *Motor skills acquisition in the first year: An illustrated guide to normal development.* Therapy Skill Builders.

Bosmans, G., Sanchez-Lopez, A., Finet, C., & De Raedt, R. (2019). Attachment-related attention bias plays a causal role in trust in maternal support. *Journal of Experimental Child Psychology, 185,* 176–190.

Bremner, J. G., Slater, A. M., & Johnson, S. P. (2015). Perception of object persistence: The origins of object permanence in infancy. *Child Development Perspectives, 9,* 7–13.

Carretti, B., Meneghetti, C., Doerr, E., Toffalini, E., & Lanfranchi, S. (2022). Developmetnal trajectories of spatial-sequential and spatial-simultaneous working memory in Down syndrome. *Journal of Intellectual Disability Research, 66*(pt. 1–2), 81–93.

Case-Smith, J. (2006). Hand skill development in the context of infants' play: Birth to 2 years. In A. Hendersen, & P. Pehoski (Eds.), *Hand function in the child: Foundations for remediation* (pp. 117–142). Mosby.

Case-Smith, J. (2005). *Occupational therapy for children* (5th ed.). Elsevier Inc.

CAST. (2018). *Universal design for learning guidelines version 2.2.* Wakefield, MA: Author. [graphic organizer] http://udlguidelines.cast.org.

Cermak, S. A., & Benson, T. A. (2020). Praxis and Dyspraxia. In A. C. Bundy, & S. L. Lane (Eds.), *Sensory integration theory and practice* (5th ed.) (pp. 115–150). F. A. Davis.

Centers for Disease Control and Prevention. (2010). Racial and ethnic differences in breastfeeding initiation and duration, by state. *United States: National Immunization Survey,* 2004–2008.

Centers for Disease Control and Prevention. (2018). *Technical notes for statistics tables: National health interview summary 2016.* https://www.cdc.gov/nchs/nhis/SHS/tables.htm.

Centers for Disease Control and Prevention. (2021). *ACE pyramid: Mechanism by which adverse childhood experiences influence health and well-being throughout the lifespan.* https://www.cdc.gov/violenceprevention/aces/about.html.

Center for Disease Control and Prevention. (2022). *CDC's developmental milestones.* https://www.cdc.gov/ncbddd/actearly/milestones/index.html.

Champagne, T. (2019). Trauma and stressor-related disorders. In C. Brown, G. Stoffel, & J. Munoz (Eds.), *Occupational therapy in mental health: A vision for participation* (2nd ed.). F.A. Davis Company.

Chaput, J., et al. (2015). Associations between sleep patterns and lifestyle behaviors in children: An international comparison. *International Journal of Obesity, 5*(Suppl. 2), S59–S65.

Children's Defense Fund. (2021). *The State of America's Children, 2021 Report.* https://www.childrensdefense.org/wp-content/uploads/2021/04/The-State-of-Americas-Children-2021.pdf.

Chin, L., Noonan, C., Hoffmann, M., & Lockman, J. (2019). Development of infant reaching strategies to tactile targets on the face. *Frontiers in Psychology, 10,* 9.

Cisneros-Franco, J. M., Voss, P., Thomas, M. E., & de Villers-Sidani, E. (2020). Critical periods of brain development. *Handbook of Clinical Neurology, 173,* 75–88.

Cramer, S. C., Sur, M., Dobkin, B. H., O'Brien, C., Sanger, T. D., Trojanowski, J. Q., Rumsey, J. M., & Vinogradov, S. (2011). Harnessing neuroplasticity for clinical applications. *Brain, 134*(6), 1591–1609.

Darrou, C., Pry, R., Pernon, E., Michelon, C., Aussilloux, C., & Baghdadli, A. (2010). Outcome of young children with autism: Does the amount of intervention influence developmental trajectories? *Autism, 14*(6), 663–677.

Davel-Pickens, N., & Pizur-Barnekow, K. (2009). Co-occupation: Extending the dialog. *Journal of Occupational Science, 16,* 151–156.

Drummond, J., Paul, E. F., Waugh, W. E., Hammond, S. I., & Brownell, C. A. (2014). Here, there and everywhere: Emotion and mental state talk in different social contexts predicts empathic helping in toddlers. *Frontiers in Psychology, 5.*

Durocher, E., Gibson, B., & Rappolt, S. (2014). Occupational justice: A conceptual review. *Journal of Occupational Science, 21*(4), 418–430.

Every Student Succeeds Act, 20 U. S. C. § 6301 (2015). https://www.congress.gov/bill/114th-congress/senate-bill/1177

Exner, C. E. (2007). Development of hand skills. In J. Case-Smith (Ed.), *Occupational therapy for children* (5th ed.) (pp. 287–306). Elsevier Inc.

Farver, J. M., Kim, Y. K., & Lee, Y. (1995). Cultural differences in Korean-and Anglo-American preschoolers' social interaction and play behavior. *Child Development, 66,* 1088–1099.

Felitti, V. J., Anda, R. F., Nordenberg, D., Williamson, D. F., Spitz, A. M., & Marks, J. S. (1998). Relationship of childhood abuse and household dysfunction to many of the leading causes of death in adults. The Adverse Childhood Experiences (ACES) Study. *American Journal of Preventative Medicine, 14*(4), 245–258.

Fingerhut, P., Piro, J., Sutton, A., Campbell, R., Lewis, C., Lawji, D., & Martinez, N. (2013). Family-centered principles implemented in home based, clinic-based, and school-based pediatric settings. *American Journal of Occupational Therapy, 67*(2), 228–235.

Finn, K. (2016). Young adults at home: Independence, intimacy, and intergenerational relationships in shared family space. In R. Vanderbeck, & T. Skeleton (Eds.), *Families, intergenerationality, and peer group relations* (pp. 1–17). Springer.

Fiorentino, M. R. (1981). *Reflex testing methods for evaluating CNS development* (2nd ed.). Ltd: Charles C Thomas Publisher.

Florey, L. L., & Greene, S. (2008). Play in middle childhood. In L. D. Parham, & L. Fazio (Eds.), *Play in occupational therapy for children* (2nd ed.) (pp. 279–300). Mosby.

Folio, M. R., & Fewell, R. R. (2000). *Peabody developmental motor scales-2* (2nd ed.). Pearson Assessments. https://www.pearsonassessments.com/.

Frisson, E., & Eggermont, S. (2015). The impact of daily stress on adolescent depressed mood: The role of social support seeking through Facebook. *Computers in Human Behavior* (44), 315–325.

Gialamas, A., Sawyer, A., Mittinty, M., Zubrick, S., Sawyer, M., & Lynch, J. (2014). Quality of childcare influences children's attentiveness and emotional regulation at school entry. *The Journal of Pediatrics, 165,* 813–819.

Gutman, S. A., & Schindler, V. P. (2007). The neurological basis of occupation. *Occupational Therapy International*, *14*(2), 71–85.

Guyer, A. E., Perez-Edgar, K., & Crone, E. A. (2018). Opportunities for neurodevelopmental plasticity from infancy through early adulthood. *Child Development*, *89*(3), 687–697.

Halbrook, Y. J., O'Donnell, A. T., & Msetfi, R. M. (2019). When and how video games can be good: A review of the positive effects of video games on well-being. *Perspectives on Psychological Science*, *14*(6), 1096–1104.

Ikävalko, M., Sointu, E., Lambert, M. C., & Viljaranta, J. (2022). Students' self-efficacy in self-regulation together with behavioural and emotional strengths: Investigating their self-perceptions. *European Journal of Special Needs Education*, *38*(4), 558–572.

Individuals with Disabilities Education Act. (2012). 20 U.S.C. 1400, et seq. P.L., 101–476.

Irwin, V., Wang, K., Cui, J., & Thompson, A. (2022). *Report on indicators of school crime and safety: 2021 (NCES 2022-092/NCJ 304625)*. Washington, DC: National Center for Education Statistics, U.S. Department of Education. https://nces.ed.gov/pubsearch/pubsinfo.asp?pubid=2022092.

Jeffries, L. M., Fiss, A. L., McCoy, S. W., Bartlett, D., Avery, L., & Hanna, S. (2019). Developmental trajectories and reference percentiles for range of motion, endurance, and muscle strength of children with cerebral palsy. *Physical Therapy*, *99*, 329–338.

Keller, H. (2017). Culture and development: A systematic relationship. *Perspectives on Psychological Science*, *12*(5), 833–840.

Keller, H., Yovsi, R. D., & Volker, S. (2002). The role of motor stimulation in parental ethnotheories: The case of Cameroonian Nso and German women. *Journal of Cross-Cultural Psychology*, *33*, 398–414.

King, G., Law, M., King, S., Rosenbaum, P., Kertoy, M., & Young, N. (2003). A conceptual model of the factors affecting the recreation and leisure participation of children with disabilities. *Physical & Occupational Therapy in Pediatrics*, *23*, 63–90.

Kleim, J. A. (2011). Neural plasticity and neurorehabilitation: Teaching the new brain old tricks. *Journal of Communication Disorders*, *44*, 521–528.

Klintwall, L., Eldevik, S., & Eikeseth, S. (2015). Narrowing the gap: Effects of intervention on developmental trajectories in autism. *Autism*, *19*(1), 53–63.

Knowland, V., & Thomas, M. (2011). Developmental trajectories in genetic disorders. D. Fidler (Ed.). *International Review of Research in Developmental Disabilities*, *40*, 43–73.

Knox, S. (2008). Development and current use of the Knox Preschool Play Scale. In L. D. Parham, & L. Fazio (Eds.), *Play in occupational therapy for children* (2nd ed.) (pp. 55–70). Mosby.

Kolb, B., Harker, A., & Gibb, R. (2017). Principles of plasticity in the developing brain. *Developmental Medicine and Child Neurology*, *59*, 1218–1223.

Kolb, B., Mychasiuk, R., Muhammad, A., & Gibb, R. (2013). Brain plasticity in the developing brain. *Progress in Brain Research*, *207*, 35–64.

Kopp, C. (1982). Antecedents of self-regulation: A developmental perspective. *Developmental Psychology*, *18*, 199–214.

Kopp, C. B. (2009). Emotion-focused coping in young children. Self and self-regulatory processes. In E. A. Skinner, & M. J. Zimmer-Gembeck (Eds.), *Coping and the development of regulation* (Vol. 124) (pp. 33–46). New Directions for Child and Adolescent Development.

La Corte, L. F. (2008). New and expanded concepts in neurophysiology, psychology, and sociology complementary to Llorens' developmental theory: Achieving growth and development through occupation for neonatal infants and their families. *Occupational Therapy in Mental Health*, *24*(3/4), 201–343.

Lane, S., Mailloux, Z., Schoen, S., Bundy, A., May-Benson, T., Parham, D., Smith-Roley, S., & Schaff, R. (2019). Perspective neural foundations of Ayres Sensory Integration®. *Brain Science*, *9*(7), 153.

Larson, E. A. (2004). Children's work: The less-considered childhood occupation. *American Journal of Occupational Therapy*, *58*, 369–379.

Law, M., Cooper, B., Strong, S., Stewart, D., Rigby, P., & Letts, L. (1996). The person-Environment-Occupation Model: A transactive approach to occupational performance. *Canadian Journal of Occupational Therapy*, *63*(1), 9–23.

Lee, R. L. T., Lane, S. J., Tang, A. C. Y., Leung, C., Louie, L. H. T., Browne, G., & Chan, S. W. C. (2020). Effects of an unstructured free play and mindfulness intervention on wellbeing in kindergarten students. *International Journal of Environmental Research and Public Health*, *17*(15), 5382.

Libertus, K., & Hauf, P. (2017). Motor skills and their foundational role for perceptual, social, and cognitive development. *Frontiers in Psychology*, *8*, 301.

Lim, C., Donovan, A., Harper, N., & Nayor, P. (2017). Nature elements and fundamental motor skill development opportunities at five elementary school districts in British Columbia. *International Journal of Environmental Research and Public Health*, *14*, 1279–1292.

Lin, Y. C., Chao, Y. L., Wu, S. K., Lin, H. H., Hsu, C. H., Hsu, H. M., & Kuo, L. C. (2017). Comprehension of handwriting development: Pen-grip kinetics in handwriting tasks and its relation to fine motor skills among school-age children. *Australian Occupational Therapy Journal*, *64*(5), 369–380.

Linder, T. W. (2008). *Transdisciplinary play-based assessment* (2nd ed.). Baltimore, MD: Paul H. Brookes.

Lindsay, S., Chan, E., Cancelliere, S., & Mistry, M. (2018). Exploring how volunteer work shapes occupational potential among youths with and without disabilities: A qualitative comparison. *Journal of Occupational Science*, 1–15.

Llorens, L. A. (1982). Application of a developmental theory for health and rehabilitation. *AOTA*.

Marasso, et al., (2017).

Mazurek, M., & Kanne, S. (2010). Friendship and internalizing symptoms among children and adolescents with ASD. *Journal of Autism and Developmental Disorders*, *40*, 1512–1520.

Miller, L. J., Marco, E. J., Chu, R. C., & Camarata, S. (2021). Sensory processing across the lifespan: A 25-year initiative to understand neurophysiology, behaviors, and treatment effectiveness for sensory processing. *Frontiers in Integrated Neuroscience*, *15* 652218.

Monnat, S. M., & Chandler, R. F. (2015). Long term physical health consequences of adverse childhood experiences. *The Sociological Quarterly*, *56*(4), 723–752.

Munier, V., Myers, C. T., & Pierce, D. (2008). The power of object play for infants and toddlers. In L. D. Parham, & L. Fazio (Eds.), *Play in occupational therapy for children* (2nd ed.) (pp. 219–250). Mosby.

Murray, A. L., Hall, H. A., Speyer, L. G., Carter, L., Mirman, D., Caye, A., & Rohde, L. (2022). *Developmental trajectories of ADHD symptoms in a large population-representat.*

Murty, V. P., Calabro, F., & Luna, B. (2016). The role of experience in adolescent cognitive development: Integration of executive, memory, and mesolimbic systems. *Neuroscience & Biobehavioral Reviews*, *70*, 46–58.

Nabawy, A., Moawad, G., & Ebrahem, G. (2016). The relationship between the use of technology and parent-adolescents social relationship. *Journal of Education and Practice*, *7*, 168–178.

National Research Council/Institute of Medicine. (2008). *Committee on adolescent health care services and models of care for treatment. Adolescent health services: Missing opportunities.* National Academies Press.

Nelson, C., & Gabard-Durnam, L. (2020). Early adversity and critical periods: Neurodevelopmental consequences of violating the expected environment. *Trends in Neuroscience*, *43*, 133–143.

Nippold, M., Duthie, J., & Larsen, J. (2005). Literacy as a leisure activity: Free time preferences of older children and young adolescents. *Language, Speech, and Hearing Services in Schools*, *36*, 93–102.

Parham, L. D., & Mailloux, Z. (2020). Sensory integration. In H. M. Kuhaneck, & J. O'Brien (Eds.), *Case-Smith's occupational therapy for children and adolescents* (8th ed.) (pp. 515–549). Elsevier.

Parks, S. (2007). *HELP strands*. Palo Alto, CA: VORT Corp. https://www.vort.com/product.php?productid=2.

Pellegrini, A. D. (2009). *The role of play in human development*. Oxford University Press.

Petrenchik, T., & King, G. (2013). Pathways to positive development: Childhood participation in everyday places and activities. In M. Bazyk, & M. Arbesman (Eds.), *Mental health promotion, prevention and intervention with children and youth* (pp. 71–94). AOTA Press.

Petrenchik, T., & Weiss, D. (2015). *Childhood trauma.* American Occupational Therapy Association School Mental Health Committee [Fact Sheet]. https://www.aota.org/~/media/Corporate/Files/Practice/Children/Childhood-Trauma-Info-Sheet-2015.pdf.

Pew Research Center, Internet and Technology. (2018). *Teens, Social Media and Technology. 2018.* http://www.pewinternet.org/2018/05/31/teens-social-media-technology-2018/pi_2018-05-31_teenstech_0-03/.

Pew Research Center, Social and Demographic Trends. (2015). *Parenting in America: Children's Extracurricular Activities.* http://www.pewsocialtrends.org/2015/12/17/5-childrens-extracurricular-activities/#on-a-typical-day-a-vast-majority-of-children-watch-tv-or-play-video-gamesHYPERLINK. *http://www.pewsocialtrends.org/2015/12/17/parenting-in-america/" \o.* http://www.pewsocialtrends.org/2015/12/17/parenting-in-america/.

Pierce, D., Munier, V., & Myers, C. (2009). Informing early intervention through an occupational science description of infant-toddler interactions with home space. *American Journal of Occupational Therapy, 63,* 273–287.

Pillar, A. (2022). Defining trauma informed care in OT [poster]. *American Journal of Occupational Therapy, Vol. 76*(Suppl. 1).

Purvis, B. (2005). *The NICU Experience: Its impact and implications.* Roanoke, VA: Virginia Early Intervention Conference. http://www.infantva.org/documents/conf-PrenatalSensoryDevelopment.pdf. March 7-8.

Riley, B., Hardesty, L., Butler, A., Kimmelman, A., Gardner, K., & Miceli, A. (2017). How do pediatric occupational therapists implement family-centered care? *American Journal of Occupational Therapy, 71*(4_Suppl. 1) 7111505155p1.

Rodger, S., & Kennedy-Behr, A. (Eds.). (2017). *Occupation-centered practice with children: A practical guide for occupational therapists* (2nd ed.) Wiley-Blackwell.

Rodrigues, M. R. (2020). A new definition of body schema with respect to body-centered vs. external frames of reference. *Acta Scientific Neurology,* 3(11), 92–100.

Roll, K., & Roll, W. (2013). *The REAL: The Roll evaluation of activities of life, user guide.* NSC Pearson.

Roopnarine, J. L., & Davidson, K. L. (2015). Parent-child play across cultures: Advancing play research. *American Journal of Play, 7*(2).

Rosanbalm, K., & Murray, D. (2017). *Caregiver co-regulation across development: A practice brief (OPRE Brief # 2017-80). Office of planning, research, and evaluation, Administration for children and families.* US Department of Health, and Human Services.

Rossman, M. (2002). *Involving children with household tasks: Is it worth the effort?* University of Minnesota. https://ghk.h-cdn.co/assets/cm/15/12/55071e0298a05_-_Involving-children-in-household-tasks-U-of-M.pdf.

Saarni, C. (1999). *The development of emotional competence.* Guilford Press, 18–19.

Santrock, J. W. (2009). Child development. In J. W. Santrock (Ed.), *motor, sensory, and perceptual development.* The McGraw-Hill Companies. 160–160.

Sawyer, S., Assopardi, P., Wickremarathne, D., & Patton, G. (2018). The age of adolescence. *The Lancet Child and Adolescent Health, 2,* 223–228.

Schaaf, J. R., & Anzalone, M. (2001). Sensory integration with high-risk infants and young children. In S. S. Roly, E. I. Blanche, & R. C. Schaaf (Eds.), *Understanding the nature of sensory integration with diverse populations* (pp. 385–408). Therapy Skill Builders.

Semple, B. D., Blomgren, K., Gimlen, K., Ferriero, D. M., & Noble-Hauesslein, L. J. (2013). Brain development in rodents and humans: Identifying benchmarks of maturation and vulnerability to injury across species. *Progress in Neurobiology, 106–107,* 1–16.

Silcock, M., Hocking, C., & Payne, D. (2014). Childhood constructions of contemporary technology: Using discourse analysis to understand the creation of occupational possibilities. *Journal of Occupational Science, 21,* 357–370.

Silvestrini, M. S., Silva, C. R., da Silva, A. C., & Prado, A. (2019). Occupational therapy and culture: Ethical-political dimensions and resistances. *Brazilian Journal of Occupational Therapy, 27*(4), 929–940.

Smits, D. W., Gorter, J. W., Riddell, C. A., Voorman, J. M., Rosenbaum, P. L., Palisano, R. J., & Ketelaar, M. (2019). Mobility and self-care trajectories for individuals with cerebral palsy (aged 1–21 years): A joint longitudinal analysis of cohort data from The Netherlands and Canada. *The Lancet Child & Adolescent Health, 3*(8), 548–557.

Srinivasan, S. M., & Bhat, A. N. (2019). Differences in means-end exploration between infants at risk for autism and typically developing infants in the first 15 months of life. *Developmental Psychobiology, 61,* 203–215.

Street, M. E., & Bernasconi, S. (2020). Endocrine-disrupting chemicals in human fetal growth. *International Journal of Molecular Sciences, 21*(4), 1430.

Stuyvenberg, C. L., Brown, S. E., Inamdar, K., Evans, M., Hsu, L. Y., Rolin, O., … Dusing, S. C. (2021). Targeted physical therapy combined with spasticity management changes motor development trajectory for a 2-year-old with cerebral palsy. *Journal of Personalized Medicine, 11*(3), 163.

Teaford, P., Wheat, J., & Baker, J. (Eds.). (2010). *HELP 3-6 assessment strands* (2nd ed.) VORT Corporation.

Tomchek, S. D., & Koenig, K. P. (2016). *Occupational therapy practice guidelines for individuals with autism spectrum disorder.* AOTA Press, The American Occupational Therapy Association, Incorporated.

Trommsdorff, G. (2010). Culture and development of self–regulation. *Social and Personality Psychology Compass, 4*(4), 282–294.

Tudge, J. R. H., Martins, G. D. F., Merçon-Vargas, E. A., Dellazzana-Zanon, L. L., Piccinini, C. A., & Freitas, L. B. L. (2018). Children, families, and communities in Brazil: A cultural-ecological approach to child-rearing values and practices. In M. Fleer, & B. van Oers (Eds.), *International Handbook of early childhood education.* Springer.

United Nations International Children's Emergency Fund [UNICEF]. (2005). Childhood under threat: The state of the world's children. *Childhood defined.* https://www.unicef.org/sowc05/english/childhooddefined.html.

United Nations International Children's Emergency Fund [UNICEF]. (2021). *The State of the World's Children 2021.* https://www.unicef.org/reports/state-worlds-children-2021.

U.S. Department of Health and Human Services, Office of Adolescent Health. (2018). *Adolescent development.* https://www.hhs.gov/ash/oah/adolescent-development/index.html.

Wang, T., Howe, T.-H., Hinojosa, J., & Weinberg, S. (2011). Relationship between postural control and fine motor skills in pre-term infants at 6-12 months adjusted age. *American Journal of Occupational Therapy, 65,* 695–701.

Warshaw, S. (2007). *HELP 0–3 assessment strands.* VORT Corporation.

Waugh, W., Brownell, C., & Pollock, B. (2015). Early socialization of prosocial behavior: Patterns in parents' encouragement of toddlers' helping in an everyday household task. *Infant Behavior and Development, 39,* 1–10.

World Health Organization (WHO). (2007). *International classification of functioning, disability and health, version for children and youth.* World Health Organization.

Zakaria, M. F., Yunus, F., & Mohamed, S. (2020). Examining self-awareness through drawing activity among preschoolers with high socioemotional development. *Southeast Asia Early Childhood Journal, 9*(2), 73–81.

Ziviani, J., & Wallen, M. (2006). The development of graphomotor skills. In A. Henderson, & C. Pehoski (Eds.), *Hand function in the child* (2nd ed.) (pp. 217–238). Mosby.

# 9

# Evaluation and Assessment in Pediatrics

*Heather Miller Kuhaneck, Jane Clifford O'Brien, Megan C. Chang, Pamela K. Richardson, Susan Spitzer, and Susan Cahill*

## GUIDING QUESTIONS

1. What is the process of evaluation for children and youth?
2. How do occupational therapists prioritize areas to evaluate and assess while creating an evaluation plan?
3. What are the primary purposes of evaluation and assessment?
4. How do specific assessments inform occupational therapy evaluation?
5. What are the types of assessments occupational therapists use to understand occupational performance of children and youth?
6. How do occupational therapists use information on test measurement including reliability and validity in practice?
7. What specific considerations must be made by the occupational therapist to evaluate each occupation, as well as specific skills and client factors?

## KEY TERMS

- Activity analysis
- Adaptability
- Adaptive response
- Agency
- Assessment
- Behavior support plan
- Evaluation
- Fiberoptic endoscopic evaluation of swallowing
- Flexibility
- Frames of reference
- Functional behavioral analysis
- Growth mindset
- Ideation
- Inner drive
- Interview-based assessment
- Ipsative assessment
- Just right challenge
- Neural plasticity
- Norm-referenced assessment
- Occupational profile
- Occupation-centered models of practice
- Praxis
- Professional reasoning
- Prospectivity
- Reliability
- Screening
- Self-regulation
- Sensory discrimination and perception
- Sensory modulation
- Sleep disorders
- Sleep disturbance
- Sleep problems
- Somatodyspraxia
- Standardized tests
- Upright modified barium swallow study
- Validity
- Variance
- Video fluoroscopic swallow study

## INTRODUCTION TO OCCUPATIONAL THERAPY EVALUATION FOR CHILDREN AND YOUTH

The occupational therapy **evaluation** is "the comprehensive process of obtaining and interpreting data necessary to understand the person, system or situation … Evaluation requires synthesis of all data obtained, analytic interpretation of that data, reflective clinical reasoning, and consideration of occupational performance and contextual factors" (AOTA, 2020b, p. 76; Hinojosa et al., 2014). The therapist completes the comprehensive evaluation to identify child and family strengths and also to understand the factors interfering with the child's ability to do those things they want or need to do. The process of an occupational therapy comprehensive evaluation typically consists of the occupational profile and the analysis of occupational performance. Within that process, therapists make decisions regarding what to evaluate and assess based on the purpose of the evaluation.

**Assessment** refers to a specific tool or procedure used to collect information about the child, their occupations, performance skills and patterns, client factors, and the contexts and environments where the child performs occupations (AOTA, 2020b; Hinojosa et al., 2014). While best practice in evaluation suggests the use of multiple methods of data gathering, the choice of an assessment tool depends upon the practice setting and the scope of the evaluation. Table 9.1 describes the evaluation, screening, assessment and reevaluation process.

**TABLE 9.1 Terms and Definitions Associated With Evaluation**

| Terms | Definitions |
|---|---|
| Evaluation | The process of collecting and interpreting data to make decisions about whether a child would be benefit from occupational therapy services. The process includes the examination of occupations, performance skills, performance patterns, client factors, and contexts/environments. |
| Screening | A process used to determine whether a child would benefit from a more comprehensive evaluation to determine if occupational therapy (or other services) would be beneficial. |
| Assessment | A tool or procedure used to collect information about the child, the occupations the child engages in, the child's performance skills and patterns, the child's client factors, and the contexts and environments where the child performs occupations. Assessment tools and procedures may be standardized or nonstandardized and can be used during screening, evaluation, or reevaluation. |
| Reevaluation | The ongoing process of collecting and interpreting data to refine and revise the occupational therapist's understanding of the child's strengths, needs, and priorities for therapy. |

Hinojosa, J., Kramer, P., & Crist, P. (2010). Evaluation: Where do we begin? In J. Hinojosa, P. Kramer, & P. Crist (Eds.), *Evaluation: Obtaining and interpreting data* (3rd ed, pp. 1–20). AOTA Press.

**TABLE 9.2 Occupational Therapy Aspects of Evaluation**

| Aspects of Evaluation | Definition | Examples |
|---|---|---|
| Occupations | Activities that children engage in during daily life (i.e., activities of daily living, instrumental activities of daily living, rest and sleep, education, work, play, leisure, and social participation) | • Feeding/eating<br>• Dressing<br>• Playing kickball during recess<br>• Completing a math assignment |
| Performance skills | Observable goal-directed actions that contribute to occupational engagement | • Motor skills<br>  • Gripping a writing utensil<br>  • Coordinating two sides of the body to use scissors<br>  • Transporting toys to the toy box<br>• Process skills<br>  • Sequencing the steps to tying shoes<br>  • Organizing school supplies<br>  • Responding to the signal to change classes<br>• Communication and interaction skills<br>  • Taking turns on the swing at park<br>  • Positioning self within an appropriate distance next to peers at library story time<br>  • Expressing anger appropriately at school |
| Performance patterns | Integrated habits, routines, rituals, and roles that shape performance and participation in occupations | • Automatically writing assignments down in a planner<br>• Following a sequence of steps to get ready for bed each night<br>• Attending a weekly prayer service<br>• Behavioral expectations associated with a member of a sports team |
| Client factors | Values/beliefs, body structures, and body functions that influence occupational performance and participation | • Shifting attention between chatting with a classmate and listening to a teacher<br>• Awareness of one's body position as it goes down a slide<br>• Recognizing letter shapes |
| Contexts/environments | The social, built and natural surroundings where occupations take place | • Home<br>• School/classroom<br>• Therapy clinic<br>• Playground<br>• Shopping mall<br>• Scout meeting |

Material modified from: American Occupational Therapy Association. (2020b). Occupational therapy practice framework: Domain and process (4th ed.). *American Journal of Occupational Therapy, 74*(Suppl. 2), Article 7412410010

Each evaluation is individualized based on the purpose for the evaluation, the client's concerns, the setting, and the current situation of child and family. A comprehensive evaluation of a child requires the use of a variety of methods such as caregiver or teacher interview, child self-report, observation of performance using the skill of activity analysis, and the use of standardized and nonstandardized assessment tools. See Table 9.2 for a description of the varied aspects of an occupational therapy evaluation.

Occupational therapists use **professional reasoning** (also referred to as therapeutic or clinical reasoning) to create an appropriate evaluation plan for each situation. While an initial evaluation is typically the first step in occupational therapy, therapists may reevaluate or explore areas in depth after the initial evaluation. The reasoning process for evaluation planning is dynamic and continual as practitioners get to know children and their families.

**BOX 9.1 The Role of the Occupational Therapy Assistant in Evaluation**

Occupational therapy assistants contribute to the evaluation process by performing services within their legal and professional scope of practice. After demonstrating competency, they can administer specific assessments, provide verbal and written reports of the assessments, and analyze a child's occupational performance (AOTA, 2020a). They provide the information to the occupational therapist who interprets the findings and uses the information in the evaluation (AOTA, 2020a).

The roles and responsibilities of the occupational therapist and the occupational therapy assistant are complimentary during the evaluation process. The occupational therapist directs all aspects of the evaluation process, including determining need for services, domains to be addressed, client's goals and priorities, assessment tools to administer, and tasks that can be delegated to the occupational therapy assistant (AOTA, 2020a). While the occupational therapist interprets the data to create the intervention plan, the occupational therapy assistant may contribute by completing assessments (once service competency is achieved), gathering information via observation, and interviewing children, family, and team members. For the purposes of this chapter, we use the term therapist throughout, while acknowledging that there are portions of the evaluation that can be completed by the occupational therapy assistant. See Box 9.1 for the role of the occupational therapy assistant in an evaluation.

Occupational therapists document the results of the evaluation using approved formats specific to the setting (see Chapter 7). While formats differ, evaluation reports include clear, objective descriptions of children's behaviors, plain language so parents can understand findings, and data that support the therapist's hypotheses leading to the intervention plan. Best practice is to complete strengths-based documentation that provides important and helpful information for the family and client rather than a laundry list of things the child cannot do.

## THE OCCUPATIONAL THERAPY EVALUATION PROCESS FOR CHILDREN AND YOUTH

Occupational therapists evaluate children by completing an occupational profile and analysis of occupational performance, the results of which are synthesized to inform the intervention plan (Hinojosa et al., 2014). The focus of the evaluation is to determine the child's occupational strengths, challenges, and goals and to identify supports and barriers to health, well-being, and participation (AOTA, 2020b, p. 21). Occupational therapists consider the practice setting (see Chapter 6) and the child's occupational needs when evaluating children. The evaluation process may include a **screening** or consultation to determine the need for a full occupational therapy evaluation (AOTA, 2020b; Hinojosa et al., 2014).

The evaluation process includes completing the occupational profile, selecting methods of assessment and specific assessment tools, administering assessments, making observations, interpreting data, synthesizing information, and if warranted, developing an intervention plan (AOTA, 2020b). During the evaluation process, occupational therapists create rapport, engage children and their families, and both gather and give information simultaneously (Woods & Lindeman, 2008).

### Gathering While Also Giving

It is likely while beginning an initial evaluation for occupational therapy that the caregiver(s) may have little understanding or prior knowledge of occupational therapy. They may not be familiar with the processes common to occupational therapy such as family-centered care, shared collaborative goal setting, or the importance of natural environments and occupation as opposed to contrived tasks. Their prior exposure to healthcare is likely primarily within the medical model, and they may be accustomed to the doctor as the individual who will diagnose and tell them what to do. Therefore, it is critical that as the occupational therapist begins the process of gathering information FROM the family that the therapist also provides information TO the family (Woods & Lindeman, 2008).

Caregivers need to understand the practitioner's expectations of them and their role in the therapy process. They need to understand why the occupational therapist is asking certain things, so they can learn to become a better informant as therapy progresses. Sharing why you are asking each question begins the process of helping the caregivers understand the role of occupational therapy and the types of things practitioners want to know about.

See Box 9.2 for an example of this form of communication.

**BOX 9.2 One Example of Gathering AND Giving Information**

We are going to ask you questions about your typical day, your family routines, and your child's favorite activities. We are asking these questions because as we work together to provide activities to promote your child's development, we want to embed those activities into the things you are already doing in your day, so as not to add extra work or stress for your family, and so you can use the natural opportunities you have in your day to encourage your child's learning.

Adapted from Woods and Lindeman (2008).

**TABLE 9.3 Example Interview Questions for Initial Stage of Evaluation**

| Information to Be Obtained | Example Question |
|---|---|
| Interests, values | What do you like to do at school? At home? At the park?<br>What games do you like to play?<br>Which toys do you like to play with?<br>Who do you like to play with?<br>What do you like to learn about? |
| Occupational strengths | What are you good at? |
| Occupational weaknesses; potential areas to address in therapy | What is difficult for you to do? What can I help you do better? |
| The impact of the environment on occupational performance and participation | What would you like to learn how to do?<br>Where do you like to study? Play? Eat?<br>Where is it hard to study? Play? Eat? |

### The Occupational Profile

The evaluation process begins with an **occupational profile** to understand the child's and family's perspective, occupational history and experiences, patterns of daily living, interests, values, needs, and relevant contexts (AOTA, 2017a, 2020b). As therapists learn about the child's interests, motivations, and occupational performance, they begin to target selected occupations for a more thorough evaluation. For example, a child who is referred for developmental delays to early intervention may exhibit feeding delays that require a more in-depth evaluation. Occupational therapists gather occupational profile information by reviewing charts and interviewing children and families to learn about the unique situation of the child and family. Table 9.3 provides questions that may be included in the occupational profile.

While using a structured format to obtain needed information, occupational therapists provide a comfortable and welcoming conversation that allows families to express themselves. For an example of an occupational profile, see Fig. 9.1.

## Analysis of Occupational Performance

The occupational therapist completes an *analysis of occupational performance* that "identifies the child's ability to effectively complete desired occupations" (AOTA, 2020b, p. 22). The occupational therapist uses all data collected to gain a perspective of the child's strengths, challenges, goals, and resources and to determine how these factors influence the child's ability to participate in occupations. They use information from the occupational profile to determine specific occupations and contexts to address. The therapist analyzes the demands of the occupation or activity to identify supports and barriers to the child's engagement (AOTA, 2020b). The occupational therapist may use this information to further examine factors that influence the child's occupational performance by observing the child engaging in the activity and/or selecting and administering specific assessments.

It is important to examine multiple factors that influence occupational performance as the evaluation will be used to create the hypotheses and the intervention plan. Incomplete or inaccurate evaluations may lead to poorly conceived intervention plans that are not effective. For example, if the therapist quickly evaluates a child and determines that their behavioral outbursts are within the typical range, without exploring other factors (such as pain, sensory discomfort, communication difficulties, feeding issues, or learned behaviors), the child's needs will not be adequately addressed. If this same therapist quickly jumps to the conclusion that the child's behavioral outbursts are learned behaviors, they may fail to investigate sources of pain. Therefore,

**Occupational Profile Template**

**Name:** Nicholas

**Age:** 4

**Why is the client seeking service, and what are the client's current concerns relative to engaging in occupations and in daily life activities? (This may include the client's general health status.)**

Nicholas was brought to occupational therapy by his mother for concerns related to: 1) social participation at home and at daycare and 2) age-appropriate self-care skills (e.g., donning/doffing coat and snow pants; brushing teeth).

**In what occupations does the client feel successful, and what barriers are affecting his or her success?**

Nicholas reports that he enjoys playing in the bathtub and at the water table at daycare. Nicholas frequently chooses to play with his family's dog when he has free time. Nicholas eats a variety of different foods and follows his bedtime routine without difficulty. When playing with peers at daycare, Nicholas struggles with taking turns with preferred toys and sometimes has difficulty regulating the use of repetitive behaviors. For example, when Nicholas and peers are playing with cars, Nicholas sometimes engages in repetitive behaviors that include spinning wheels, lining cars, up and making motor noises. When he engages in these behaviors, he will not share the cars with his peers. Sometimes his peers become disinterested and walk away. Other times, they become angry and try to take the toys from Nicholas. If a peer tries to take a car away from Nicholas, he will hit and push them. Nicholas takes off his socks and shoes but demonstrates decreased coordination and increased difficulty putting on/taking off his coat and snow pants at daycare.

**What are the client's values and interests?**
Nicholas reports that he enjoys spending time with his family and his family's dog. Nicholas reports that he loves playing in water and is always excited to go to swimming lessons. Nicholas reports that he enjoys listening to audiobooks and when stories are read aloud.

**What is the client's occupational history (i.e., life experiences)?**
Nicholas lives at home with his parents, his infant sister, and his family's dog. Nicholas was born full-term and without complications. Both of his parents work full-time and Nicholas attends daycare five days a week. Nicholas is brought to daycare at 7:00 AM and gets picked up around 6:00 PM.

**What are the client's patterns of engagement in occupations, and how have they changed over time?** Nicholas has been going to daycare since he was 9 months old. He began swimming lessons approximately 6 months ago. There have been no major disruptions in Nicholas's patterns of engagement.

**What are the client's daily life roles? (Patterns can support or hinder occupational performance.)** Nicholas is a son, a brother, a daycare student, peer, and pet owner. The performance patterns that Nicholas uses at meal times and when playing with his dog support his role performance. The performance patterns that Nicholas uses at bedtime and playing with peers hinder his role performance.

**Fig. 9.1, cont'd**

**What aspects of the client's environments or contexts does he or she see as:**

| | Supports to Occupational Engagement | Barriers to Occupational Engagement |
|---|---|---|
| **Physical** | Daycare<br>Home environment | |
| **Social** | Family; familiar peers; supportive daycare teachers | |
| **Cultural** | | |
| **Personal** | | Repetitive behaviors sometimes limit opportunities for social participation |
| **Temporal** | Able to follow family and classroom routines | |
| **Virtual** | | |

**Client's Priorities**

**Consider: occupational performance—improvement and enhancement, prevention, participation, role competence, health and wellness, quality of life, well-being, and/or occupational justice.**

- Increase social participation during free play at daycare
- Improve dressing

**Fig. 9.1** Sample occupational profile.

occupational therapists complete thorough evaluations of children and reflect upon their findings to synthesize the information based on the purpose of the evaluation, specific client needs, research, past experiences, and data obtained regarding the child and their situation.

## PURPOSES OF EVALUATION

Evaluation is one of the most necessary and complex functions the occupational therapist completes. The process of evaluation allows the therapist to collaborate with the child and family to establish whether there is a need for occupational therapy and, if so, to establish goals and determine intervention methods. Data from evaluation serve as a foundation for decision-making at each stage of the therapeutic process. The way the occupational therapist approaches evaluation and frames the child's strength and challenges often establishes the child's occupational therapy trajectory and may contribute to larger conversations related to diagnoses and eligibility for services and supports at home, school, and in the community or to determine the effectiveness of interventions for a specific population. Occupational therapists conduct evaluations for the purposes of (1) screening; (2) determining the scope and frequency of occupational therapy services; (3) setting goals and developing intervention plans; and (4) documenting progress toward therapy goals.

Occupational therapists evaluate children who have diverse conditions, occupational performance challenges, and home situations. They must gather the information quickly, efficiently, and comprehensively and in agreement with setting policies and standards. To effectively evaluate a child within the allowable time frame requires careful planning.

## CREATING AN EVALUATION PLAN

Occupational therapists observe, analyze, assess, and create hypotheses during the evaluation to address children's challenges within a variety of settings. Understanding the many factors that influence children's occupational performance is complex and therefore requires a structured, systematic approach toward the evaluation. Important decisions need to be made about the specific aspects of the comprehensive evaluation. For example, the therapist makes decisions regarding completing a chart review, interviewing people in the child's life, observing the child in different settings, and what assessments to administer. The therapist decides where the various portions of evaluation will occur and what role the occupational therapy assistant will play in the evaluation process. These decisions are made based on careful consideration of the practice setting, the referral information, the identified needs or concerns, the purpose of the evaluation, and selected models of practice and frames of reference. Table 9.4 provides examples of how occupational performance or participation concerns lead to hypotheses. The occupational therapist uses these hypotheses to make decisions on further assessment of skills, patterns, client factors, which informs selection of assessment tools or strategies.

### Prioritizing for the Evaluation Plan

While occupational therapists complete comprehensive evaluations, they prioritize their choices related to interviewing, observing, and completing assessment tools. There is not enough time to evaluate *everything*, nor is there typically a need. One of the first decisions is whether to use a top-down or bottom-up approach to the evaluation process.

**Top-Down and/or Bottom-Up Approach.** As a profession, occupational therapy has moved toward the adoption of a top-down approach to evaluation (Brown & Chien, 2010; Kennedy et al., 2012; Weinstock-Zlotnick & Hinojosa, 2004). A therapist using a top-down approach begins the evaluation process by gaining an understanding of the child's level of participation in daily occupations and routines with family, caregivers, and peers. They examine specific skills and client factors later. Case Example 9.1 shows the evaluation planning process using the top-down approach.

TABLE 9.4 **Evaluation Planning Example**

| Occupational Performance or Participation Concern | Hypothesis (Potential Reason Why Child Is Having Occupational Performance or Participation Deficit) | Performance Skill, Performance Pattern, Client Factor of Interest | Assessment Tool or Strategy |
|---|---|---|---|
| Social participation at daycare | It is possible that Nicholas's delayed communication skills are affecting his social participation at daycare. | Communication and interaction skills | Transdisciplinary Play-Based Assessment (Linder et al., 2008) |
| | It is possible that some of Nicholas's performance patterns affecting social participation are associated with differences related to sensory processing. | Sensory processing | Sensory Processing Measure (Parham et al., 2021) |
| Donning/doffing coat and snow pants | It is possible that Nicholas is demonstrating difficulty with donning/doffing shirts and pants due to decreased motor skills or limited understanding how to sequence task. | Motor and process skills | Observation of donning coat and snow pants at daycare while getting ready for outside playtime; focus on motor and process skills as outlined by the AOTA occupational therapy practice framework (2020b) or following a specific frame of reference |

### CASE EXAMPLE 9.1 A TOP-DOWN APPROACH TO EVALUATION

Hazim, an occupational therapist working in a community clinic, receives a referral for a 10-month-old boy, Chris, who has Down syndrome that reads, "evaluate and treat." Hazim knows that children with Down syndrome take longer to develop feeding, play, self-care, mobility, and social participation skills.

Hazim plans to interview the family to discover their concerns and priorities and to evaluate the child using a *top-down approach* by observing Chris playing, eating a snack, and taking off his shoes, socks, hat, and coat. Hazim decides to use the Person-Environment-Occupation-Performance (PEOP) model to structure the occupational profile and ensure that he understands the family's goals, concerns, routines, expectations, and environment. The PEOP model emphasizes the interactions between person, environment, and occupations as contributing to occupational performance. It is important to analyze how each element of the model supports or hinders a child's ability to engage in desired activities.

Hazim analyzes Chris' performance during play and interactions with his parents to identify strengths and challenges, understand Chris' motivations, and create a rapport with the child and family. Next, the parents provide Chris a snack (from home) using their cups and utensils, and special chair. This allows Hazim to analyze the environment, social interactions, and child's feeding skills. As Hazim considers the child's strengths and challenges, family values and routines, and the environment, he can create individualized meaningful intervention to promote occupational participation. This approach allows Hazim to build upon the child's strengths. Using a top-down approach allows the therapist to engage the child in meaningful activities, which can be easily practiced at home. This promotes carryover and allows the family to be an active part of the entire process.

Alternatively, a therapist using a *bottom-up* approach first evaluates specific skills or client factors in an attempt to understand what might be limiting a child's performance skills and occupational performance. Often the decisions about which skills and client factors to assess are related to the child's diagnosis and expected areas of difficulty. In this type of approach, the therapist might examine strength and range of motion (ROM) or manipulation skills first. The assumption is that deficits in these skills may hinder performance in functional tasks such as coloring or buttoning and therefore limit performance in broader occupations including activities of daily living (ADLs) and education. See Box 9.3 for a comparison of bottom-up and top-down approaches to evaluation.

Both types of evaluation approaches may be important in understanding the child's occupational performance (Hackett, 2010; Kennedy et al., 2013; Lalor et al., 2016; Weinstock-Zlotnick & Hinojosa, 2004). Generally, therapists move between these two approaches during the evaluation process. Beginning with a top-down approach may allow the therapist to prioritize which skills or factors require further evaluation. For example, when evaluating the child's occupational performance, the therapist may observe the child eating a snack with no difficulty. The parents also report no concerns with feeding and eating. In this case, there is no need to conduct a bottom-up evaluation of the components involved in feeding. Conversely, if the child coughs and spits up his snack or the parents express concerns with feeding, the occupational therapist may decide to further evaluate aspects of feeding and eating. It is possible that the results of a top-down approach could differ from those obtained from a bottom-up approach and vice versa, depending on the assessment methods selected and the informant (Kennedy et al., 2013; Lalor et al., 2016).

**Additional Considerations to Guide Evaluation Planning.** Occupational therapists use professional reasoning to guide their evaluation planning decisions. They begin by using knowledge of the practice setting, the type of information that needs to be gathered, the reason for referral, safety concerns, family concerns, child's condition, and the influence of the funding source for the evaluation. They structure and plan for the evaluation using occupation-centered models of practice and frames of reference. By integrating knowledge of models and frames of reference, they plan to evaluate a child's skills and abilities to understand the factors influencing the child's challenges.

***Practice Setting and Type of Information to Be Gathered.*** Occupational therapists work in a variety of settings (see Chapter 6) that influence evaluation planning and priorities. Therapists use knowledge of the setting and its vision and mission to inform the evaluation process. The mission of hospitals is to address and treat medical concerns of children. Therefore, occupational therapists working in hospitals prioritize medical concerns, recovery, and safety upon discharge when planning for the occupational therapy evaluation. They also plan for the likely need to rely on a parent or caregiver's report when evaluating a child in a hospital setting.

## BOX 9.3 Using a Bottom-Up or a Top-Down Approach for Evaluation

An occupational therapist working in an outpatient clinic often gets new referrals for children over the summer. Tomorrow the therapist will meet Adam for the first time. The information that was obtained during the clinic's intake interview with Adam's mom is as follows:

Adam is a 7-year-old boy. Adam's mother has concerns related to his motor development. She reports that Adam just completed first grade, has many friends, and is a proficient reader. Adam likes math and doing science experiments. He enjoys playing with action figures and video games. Adam's mother indicates that he has an immature pencil grip and trouble tying shoes. She also shares that Adam is a "butter fingers" and frequently spills when trying to pour milk in cereal in the morning.

The occupational therapist has 90 minutes scheduled with Adam tomorrow and needs to plan the evaluation session. The occupational therapist has developed a hypothesis that fine motor strength and dexterity may be limiting Adam's participation. The occupational therapist considers whether to use a bottom-up approach to evaluation or the more preferred top-down approach. To make this decision, the occupational therapist writes down the steps that could be taken with either approach. The following table outlines the steps that might be used in both approaches.

| Bottom-Up Approach to Evaluation | Top-Down Approach to Evaluation |
|---|---|
| ***Occupational Profile***<br>Interview with Adam and his mother | ***Occupational Profile***<br>Interview with Adam and his mother |
| ***Analysis of Occupational Performance***<br>1. Assessment of muscle strength (manual muscle testing, grip strength, pinch strength, maintaining specific gross motor postures)<br>2. Observational assessment of hand and dexterity skills (hand muscle integrity, web space, arches, thumb abduction and adduction, finger opposition, in-hand manipulation, translation).<br>3. Administration of the BOT-2 fine motor subtests (i.e., fine motor precision, fine motor integration, manual dexterity upper-limb coordination) and comparison to norms. | ***Analysis of Occupational Performance***<br>1. Observe Adam in ADLs and specific tasks he is reported to have difficulty with such as tying shoes, drawing a picture for his mother, pouring apple juice from jug into three cups, pass out napkins, open package of crackers, pass out one cracker to each person, eat snack, and clean up (collect snack item, throw away trash, put cups in sink, put crackers in cabinet).<br>2. Consider how modifications of tasks or environments might support Adam's performance (e.g., ask him to pour another cup of juice while standing on a step stool so that he can see over the counter).<br>3. Consider the influence of his interests and belief in his abilities. Ask him about his preferences for activities and about how he feels about his performance.<br>4. Administer Child Occupational Self-Assessment (COSA) (to better understand child's perspectives). |
| ***Additional Observations***<br>As Adam completes the testing, the therapist notes his difficulties, and discovers hat he has delays in fine motor skills compared to others his age. She hypothesizes that these delays result in functional performance deficits. | ***Additional Observations***<br>During the functional tasks, Adam reports that his hands get tired at school, and the therapist notices that he is unable to open one of the snack packages. The therapist hypothesizes that he has weakness in his hands and then decides to assess this as well. |
| ***Interpretation of Results***<br>Adam has specific fine motor deficits and fine motor delays for his age, and these fine motor deficits cause difficulties with occupational performance. | ***Interpretation of Results***<br>Adam has difficulty with functional tasks with fine motor components, and this is interfering with his school performance. His difficulties are also harming his motivation and weakening his self-efficacy.<br>However, he also does demonstrate some weakness in his hands and fingers that might be contributing to these deficits.<br>The top-down approach focuses on the functional performance first, only assessing client factors that are necessary to better understand the performance. This approach may also reveal how Adam feels about his performance and how it is affecting his sense of competency at school and during play. The occupational therapist may get a better understanding of Adam's strengths (interests, motivations, and activities) using a top-down approach to design effective intervention. |
| ***Resulting Type of Intervention***<br>This type of evaluation leads to intervention designed to address specific client factors or skills. | ***Resulting Type of Intervention***<br>Difficulties with performance might be addressed through changes to the environment, the task, or by increasing Adam's skills. The therapist addresses Adam's sense of competence and achievement by providing him with challenges that he can achieve.<br>There may be specific activities that Adam enjoys and wants to complete that will provide him with a sense of achievement that will also strengthen his hands and fingers. |

For example, a therapist working in a hospital setting with a child in the cardiac unit who receives a referral may prioritize planning for the evaluation to include observations of endurance over assessing specific developmental skills. In contrast therapists working in a home health setting, may plan to observe children in their own environment and emphasize participation in daily activities and therapists working in school settings prioritize planning to evaluate the child's ability to engage in their education. A therapist in the school setting who receives a referral for a child specifically for handwriting concerns will likely plan an evaluation that might include gathering work samples and completing standardized handwriting assessments.

Each setting may dictate policies regarding the timing of the evaluation, and occupational therapists must be aware of the time allotted for the evaluation process and consider this when selecting the assessment tools and methods for collecting information. Pragmatically, therapists also must consider the space and assessments that will be available to them during the evaluation as they are planning.

The specifics of the practice setting factor into the planning process in other ways as well. For example, in the school setting, the therapist is typically unable to observe certain activities and skills (such as bathing or perhaps toothbrushing), so they may therefore decide to ask about bathing in a caregiver interview if the therapist believes this information is important. A therapist completing the evaluation in the home is able to observe ADL skills more readily and therefore might plan to ask different interview questions.

In some practice settings, it is quite easy to interview caregivers and siblings, whereas in others, it can be much more difficult. In the school setting, it is easy to interview a teacher, but in an outpatient clinic setting, speaking with a teacher may be much more difficult. When planning the evaluation, the therapist considers the entirety of the information gathering that needs to occur and then specifically determines who will be interviewed and which activities will be directly observed by the therapist and which information can be gathered by interview or questionnaire.

***Reason for Referral.*** Referrals may come from physicians, teachers, parents, and other healthcare professionals depending upon the setting. Referrals to occupational therapy vary in specificity, requiring occupational therapists to communicate with referral sources for clarification if needed. The referral may indicate specific areas to address based upon the setting. For example, the therapist may receive a specific referral for an orthosis for a child in acute care. They may also receive a general referral to "evaluate and treat." In early intervention the referral may be about determination of developmental level. The therapist considers the referral source and specifications, along with all of the other areas discussed in this section, to finalize the evaluation plan prior to meeting the clients. Priority referrals would be those concerning safety or client needs that are time sensitive, such as a referral for someone post surgery who needs immediate attention.

***Safety.*** When planning for an evaluation, occupational therapists select assessments to address safety concerns identified in the referral (e.g., child is gagging when feeding; falling; unaware of safety; not following verbal directions). If a safety concern is identified during the referral process, it may impact scheduling of the evaluation (sooner rather than later) and will affect the selection of methods and tools to ensure that the safety concern is thoroughly understood by the occupational therapist. If evaluation time is limited, it may mean that other areas do not get thoroughly evaluated immediately.

***Family and Child Concerns and the Child's Condition.*** For the purposes of evaluation planning, the occupational therapist often prioritizes family concerns in selecting what to assess and with what methods. Caregiver concerns may not be clear from the initial referral, and at times a therapist may need to call the family prior to completing the evaluation to gather more information to plan the evaluation properly. If possible, at this stage, occupational therapists also seek to understand the child's concerns or perspectives; however, further investigation regarding child concerns often occurs once the evaluation is being completed rather than during the planning stage. Typically, the therapist will know the child's diagnosis or condition and may use that knowledge to hypothesize about potential areas of importance to plan to evaluate.

***Funding Source.*** Funding sources (e.g., private healthcare insurance policies, private pay, federal government, Medicare) have different guidelines and regulations for services that differ among settings. For example, occupational therapists working in school settings follow laws related to the child's participation in school. Therapists working in home health settings may adhere to early intervention policies and bill Medicare, state insurance, or private insurance companies. Children may receive services as part of their parents' military benefits, employee benefits, or state early intervention programs. Each setting adheres to policies and procedures regarding funding.

These funding sources often dictate how long the occupational therapist has to complete the evaluation and may also dictate specific types of assessments or tools that will be covered and paid for. The therapist factors this information into the planning process for the evaluation. If the therapist needs longer than the time allotted by the funding source, they must discuss it with the family. If the therapist must complete an evaluation in a shortened time frame, that creates an even greater need for careful prioritization for which information to focus on first. Also, any specific assessment method that may not be covered must be carefully discussed with the caregivers before completing the evaluation so as not to leave the family with larger bills than they intended.

**Using Theory to Guide Evaluation Planning.** In the planning process, occupational therapists use theory to determine which interview questions to ask and of who, what, and where to observe, and what specific assessments to complete. Occupational therapy theories are applied in practice through occupation-centered models of practice and frames of reference. Therefore, understanding models of practice and frames of reference are central to the evaluation process. There are several ways to view conceptual practice models (Ikiugu et al., 2019; Kielhofner, 2004; Wong & Fisher, 2015). We chose to describe them as occupation-centered models of practice and frames of reference (Wong & Fisher, 2015).

***Occupation-Centered Models of Practice.*** Occupation-centered models of practice provide the structure to evaluate children and youth while explaining the interactions between person, environment, and occupation. Practice models guide evaluations to allow occupational therapists to delve deeply into the occupations of childhood. Using an occupation-centered model of practice broadens the scope of occupational therapy practice with children and youth.

The following occupation-centered practice models—Model of Human Occupation (MOHO) (Kielhofner, 2008; Taylor et al., 2024), Person-Environment-Occupation-Performance (PEOP) (Bass et al., 2017; Baum et al., 2015; Christiansen et al., 2015), Canadian Model of Occupational Participation (CanMOP) (Egan & Restall, 2022), and Occupational Adaptation (OA) (Grajo, 2017; Schkade & Schultz, 2003)—are used in pediatric practice and allow therapists to consider multiple factors to develop occupation-centered intervention plans. A brief overview of the elements of the model and guiding principles is provided in Table 9.5. Readers are encouraged to explore each model in more depth to enhance occupational therapy practice with children and youth. Case Examples 9.2A and 9.2B demonstrate the use of two different models of practice to guide evaluation.

***Frames of Reference.*** Frames of reference (FORs) define occupational challenges in terms of function and dysfunction, provide principles for intervention, and suggest specific strategies and techniques to intervene with children and youth. The techniques and strategies are based on theoretical principles that explain phenomena that are important to pediatric occupational therapy interventions. Occupational therapists may use a specific frame of reference (e.g., developmental, biomechanical, sensory integration) when planning and while completing an evaluation. For example, they may select the biomechanical frame of reference

**TABLE 9.5 Occupation-Centered Model of Practice**

| Model (Current Reference) | Authors | Elements |
|---|---|---|
| **Kielhofner's Model of Human Occupation (MOHO)** | | |
| Taylor et al. (2024) | Dr. Gary Kielhofner | Volition<br>Habituation<br>Performance capacity<br>Environment |
| ***Guiding principles***<br>1. Occupational actions, thoughts, and emotions emerge out of the dynamic interaction of volition, habituation, performance capacity, and environmental context.<br>2. Change in any aspect of volition, habituation, performance capacity, and/or the environment can result in change in the thoughts, feelings, and actions that make up one's occupation.<br>3. Volition, habituation, and performance capacity are maintained and changed through what one does and what one thinks and feels about doing.<br>a. A particular pattern of volition, habituation, and performance capacity is maintained so long as the underlying thoughts, feelings, and actions are consistently repeated in a supporting environment.<br>b. Change requires that novel thoughts, feelings, and actions emerge and be sufficiently repeated in a consistent environment to coalesce into a new organized pattern (Kielhofner, 2008; O'Brien & Wolske, 2024). | | |
| **Person-Environment-Occupation-Performance (PEOP)** | | |
| Baum et al. (2015) | Dr. Caroline Baum<br>Dr. Charles Christiansen<br>Dr. Julie Bass | Person<br>Environment<br>Occupation<br>Performance |
| ***Guiding principles***<br>• The narrative (personal story) guides the development of an occupational profile and understanding of the client's perspective.<br>• Collaboration involving client input to guide decision-making, goal setting, and intervention planning is essential.<br>• PEOP emphasizes the active "doing" of occupational performance<br>• Occupational performance supports and enables participation in everyday life, which contributes to overall well-being (health, satisfaction, and quality of life) (Baum et al., 2015).<br>• It emphasizes the relationships among person factors, environmental factors, and occupations that support performance and participation.<br>• Client-centered practice (the client's choices, interests, and contexts) drive decision-making, goal setting, and intervention planning. | | |
| **New Canadian Model of Occupational Performance and Engagement (CanMOP)** | | |
| (Egan & Restall, 2022) | Canadian Association of Occupational Therapists | Person (spirituality is core)<br>Environment<br>Occupation |
| ***Guiding principles***<br>• Client-centered practice is a collaborative practice between the client and therapist that facilitates enabling occupations.<br>• Occupational engagement and experience are important for life satisfaction.<br>• A client's occupational performance also includes the level of importance and satisfaction with performance.<br>• Limitations within the person or an unsupportive environment decrease occupational performance.<br>• Limited occupational opportunities lead to decreased occupational engagement.<br>• Cognitive, affective, and physical factors interact within an environment for occupational performance. Change in one component results in change in another.<br>• Occupational therapy practitioners enable occupation by identifying gaps between desired and actual occupational participation and intervening. | | |
| **Occupational adaptation (OA)** | | |
| Grajo (2017) | Dr. Janette Schkade<br>Dr. Sally Schultz<br>Dr. Lenon Grajo | Press of mastery (occupational challenges, responses, role demands, roles)<br>Contexts (physical, social, cultural, temporal, personal, virtual)<br>Occupational adaptation<br>Occupational participation |
| ***Guiding principles***<br>• The person is an occupational being who has a desire to master his or her environment (by participating in occupations).<br>• The occupational environment demands mastery from the person. These demands enable or restrict participation in occupations.<br>• The person's level of mastery and the environment's level of demand for mastery create occupational roles and role demands or expectations, occupational challenges, and responses from the person (referred to as press for mastery).<br>• To navigate the press of mastery, the person goes through the process of occupational adaptation.<br>• During participation in occupations within an occupational environment, a person may experience an occupational performance breakdown. The person may respond adaptively or dysadaptively to a performance breakdown.<br>• The occupational therapist elicits an adaptive response from the client. The occupational therapist enables the client to participate in occupations, facilitates the environment, and uses occupations to empower the occupational adaptation process (Grajo, 2017). | | |

## CASE EXAMPLE 9.2 APPLYING OCCUPATION-CENTERED MODELS OF PRACTICE

### A. Kielhofner's Model of Human Occupation

Sienna is a 12-month-old girl with hydrocephalus and developmental delay. The occupational therapist uses MOHO to structure the occupational therapy evaluation. The therapist interviews the parents using questions generated from MOHO theory to learn about the child's volition (e.g., interests, motivations, goals), habituation (e.g., habits, routines, and roles), performance capacity (e.g., child's strengths and challenges, lived experience), and the environment. The therapist observes her playing and assesses her using the Pediatric Volitional Questionnaire (PVQ) (Basu et al., 2008) and clinical observations (e.g., manual muscle testing, range of motion, and endurance in sitting). The therapist summarized the evaluation findings as follows:

#### Volition

Sienna's parents would like her to "do things that children enjoy, such as play." They are concerned about her "difficulty sitting upright and feeding." She smiled when moving in her stroller. She scored low on the PVQ, demonstrating limited curiosity or interest in objects, people, or noises.

#### Habituation

Sienna is dependent on family for feeding, dressing, and daily routines. She spends the day with her mother.

#### Performance Capacity

Sienna does not indicate her needs or interests. Her parents reported that Sienna laughed occasionally and made eye contact. She did not turn to sound or reach for objects. Sienna was unable to lift her head or sit upright without trunk and head support. She showed inconsistent tracking. Sienna exhibits poor postural control, lack of voluntary movement patterns. She responded to movement in her stroller by smiling.

#### Environment

Sienna lives in an apartment in the city with her parents and grandparents. She is an only child. They live close to hospitals, grocery stores, and a shopping area. They take Sienna outside daily to the park and for walks (she is in a stroller).

#### Synthesis (Strengths and Challenges)

Sienna's parents report that she laughs occasionally and makes eye contact. Limited voluntary movement, hearing, and vision interferes with Sienna's ability to explore the environment, play, and engage in activities of interest. Sienna is unable to explore her environment to engage in developmental activities. She is currently dependent on family for feeding, dressing, and daily routines.

#### Goals for Therapy

The occupational therapist uses therapeutic reasoning to conceptualize how to best meet Sienna and her family's needs to develop her ability to choose, select, and engage in play activities despite limited motor and sensory abilities (vision and hearing). Since Sienna is not exhibiting curiosity or interest, the occupational therapist hypothesizes that she must first determine how to interest Sienna in play and socialization. The occupational therapist wants to understand what motivates, interests, and gives Sienna pleasure (volition). The occupational therapist feels Sienna will benefit from being able to act upon her environment. For this reason, she develops the following goals:

1. Sienna will activate a switch toy purposefully three times during a 30-minute play session.
2. Sienna will select between two switch-activated toys two times during a 10-minute play session.

#### Using MOHO to Support Professional Reasoning

Goal 1 targets volition (one's interests or curiosity) and performance capacity (ability to voluntarily move extremity). Goal 2 targets volition (choice and motivation) and allows her parents to engage in play with Sienna. Once she is able to choose between two objects, she can engage in a variety of activities of her choice (habituation). This will allow her to act freely and develop more interests and belief in her skills (personal causation) for play.

### B. Canadian Model of Occupational Performance (CanMOP)

Trey is a 6-year-old boy in the first grade who has right hemiplegia. Trey is having difficulty in school, getting ready for recess, eating with his friends at lunch, and "keeping up with schoolwork." The occupational therapist working in the school system observed Trey in the classroom and at recess. She used the CanMOP to structure the evaluation and Canadian Occupational Performance Measure to structure the interview with the parents and Trey.

#### Person

*Spiritual:* Trey loves being outside and spends the weekends playing in the woods with his brother for hours. He is close with his parents and cousins who live nearby. He likes people and has many friends.

*Cognitive:* Trey follows verbal directions and communicates clearly. He writes with his left hand but does not always use his right hand as an assist.

*Physical:* Trey has difficulty with bilateral tasks secondary to right hemiplegia. He walks independently, although falls frequently when hurrying. Trey takes longer to perform movements, and his movements are often inaccurate.

*Affective:* Trey stated he enjoys playing outside with his friends, and he wishes he could keep up with them when they run ahead. He states schoolwork is hard for him, and lately, he "can't get ahead of it."

#### Occupation

*Self-care:* Trey dresses himself but needs help with fasteners, zipping, and tying his shoes. He feeds himself and uses a fork and a spoon. Sometimes he eats quickly to go outside and spills.

*Productivity:* At home, he helps his mother get dinner ready and puts away his dishes. He plays outside with his brother and then does his homework, although he does not like to.

*Leisure:* Trey is not involved in sports or recreational activities, since he lives too far away and his parents cannot afford the costs. He was in a soccer league, but it is now very competitive, and he cannot keep up with peers.

#### Environment

*Physical:* Trey lives in a rural environment with outdoor space.

*Social:* Trey lives with his older brother (9 years old) and parents in a two-story home that is 3 miles from the school. He plays with his cousins and says he has friends at school. Parents report financial concerns and stress since his mother recently lost her job. They state they cannot help Trey with his homework, and they feel bad it has been so stressful lately. They would like for Trey to feel successful at school. They cannot afford to transport him to recreational activities.

*Institutional:* Trey's teacher noticed that Trey is behind at school and not keeping up. He has friends at school. The school is well equipped, and Trey feels comfortable there.

*Familial:* Trey's mother lost her job recently, and the family is experiencing financial difficulties. His father works at a local corner store and recently increased his hours to working nights (to help with finances).

#### Synthesis (Strengths and Challenges)

Trey likes being with people and enjoys being outside with his friends, brothers, and cousins. He follows directions and communicates clearly. Trey helps at home with some chores. Trey exhibits challenges keeping up with schoolwork and is frustrated that he cannot keep up with his friends (which may be due to motor difficulties related to right hemiplegia). Trey is not involved in recreational activities currently. He has difficulty with bilateral motor tasks, some coordination challenges, but generally can complete activities using his left hand. His family is experiencing financial difficulties.

#### Goals for Therapy

1. Trey will use a large keyboard to complete writing assignments in the classroom.
2. Trey will use organizational strategies, adaptive equipment, and coping strategies to complete his schoolwork with peers.
3. Trey will report improved satisfaction with his participation in leisure activities (such as the recreation after school program).
   - Trey will participate in after school "daily games" program X 4 days a week with peers provided by the recreational department free to residents. (The games include hula hooping, flying kites, dancing, red light–green light, where the goal is to have fun.)

#### Using CanMop to Support Professional Reasoning

Goals 1 and 2 address his school performance. The occupational therapist will teach Try keyboarding skills, organizational and coping strategies, and provide adaptive equipment as needed. As Trey experiences more success at school he may feel improved self-determination which may support his confidence level, allowing him to preserve when things get difficult. Goal 3 addresses his desire to engage with friends outside of school, while being successful and considering his family's current financial difficulties and transportation challenges. It also allows the therapist to consult with the recreation staff to support Trey's participation. The Canadian Model of Occupational Performance (CanMop) encourages therapists to examine multiple factors that influence occupational performance, outside of motor.

**TABLE 9.6 Frames of Reference Used With Children and Youth**

| Frame of Reference | Description | Principles | Strategies and Techniques |
|---|---|---|---|
| Developmental | Identifies the level of motor (gross, fine, and oral), social, emotional, and cognitive skills in which a child engages and targets intervention to help the child advance. | • Development occurs over time and across areas.<br>• The typical developmental sequence of skills is interrupted due to illness, trauma, or birth condition.<br>• Gaps in development can be affected by physical, social, emotional, or traumatic events.<br>• Occupational therapy can help fill in those gaps.<br>• Repetitive practice of developmental skills as the child is able to master them provides experiences that promote brain plasticity and learning.<br>• Promotes practice of skills in a developmental sequence and at the level just above where the child is functioning (Llorens, 1982). | • Engage child in activities at the leve they are successful and introduce the next step or level.<br>• Challenge child to engage in tasks that are slightly above their abilities.<br>• Use activities that match child's interests and developmental level.<br>• Grade activities so they are slightly more challenging.<br>• Allow for repetition of activities so child feels mastery. |
| Biomechanical | Based on concepts of kinesiology, this FOR evaluates and intervenes regarding range of motion (ROM), strength, and endurance. This approach focuses on the physical limitations that interfere with the child's ability to engage in occupation. | • Improving ROM through passive and active means can increase functional mobility required for activities and movement.<br>• Joint ROM influences movement. The ability to move in directions within certain degrees of motion is due to the bony structure and the integrity of the surrounding tissues.<br>• Preventing or reducing contractures or deformities will enhance movement and function.<br>• Increasing strength can promote stability and balance for successful engagement in activity.<br>• Muscle strength refers to the ability of a muscle to produce the tension necessary for posture and movement against resistance.<br>• To increase strength, the muscle must be overloaded to the point of fatigue, which recruits more motor units and causes hypertrophy and hyperplasia of glycolic type II fast-twitch muscle fibers (Rybski, 2024a).<br>• Energy is needed for a person to produce the required intensity or rate of effort over time for an activity or exercise.<br>• Endurance is sustained effort of muscles.<br>• To increase endurance, submaximal exertion will require adaptation to stress, resulting in hypertrophy and hyperplasia of oxidative type I slow-twitch muscle fibers and increased function in the cardiorespiratory systems (Rybski, 2024a).<br>• Decreasing pain enables clients to engage in occupations.<br>• Pain reduction is based on gate theory: Local stimulation of nonpain-mediated sensory afferents close the gate at the spinal cord level, thereby preventing further transmission of pain impulses (Rybski, 2024a).<br>• Every pain has a source, and the intervention must be directed toward and influence that source. | • Orthoses (to enforce rest until structures are healed).<br>• Positioning (to enforce rest until structures are healed).<br>• To increase ROM, a stretch force must be applied to the tissue that is beyond the current ROM to elongate the collagen fibers in soft tissues (heat, relaxation, pass ve stretch, and active stretch) (Rybski, 2024a).<br>• Edema and tissue integrity (including elevation, compression, temperature control, AROM, and edema mobilization).<br>• Duration, velocity, and type of muscle contraction required (Rybski, 2024a).<br>• Pain control modalities: Ice massage, cold packs, acupressure, and self-massage (Rybski, 2024a).<br>• Progressive or resistive exercise to recruit more motor units causes hypertrophy and hyperplasia of glycolytic type II muscle fibers. (i.e., weighted exercises, Theraplast, Theraputty, and overhead tasks like dressing) (Rybski, 2024a). |
| Motor control/ motor learning | Motor control examines how one directs and regulates movement, whereas motor learning theory describes how children learn movements. This approach is based on dynamic system theory that many factors influence movement and must be considered in intervention (O'Brien, 2015). | • The interaction among systems is essential to adaptive control of movement.<br>• Motor performance results from an interaction between adaptable and flexible systems.<br>• Dysfunction occurs when movement patterns lack sufficient adaptability to accommodate task demands and environmental constraints.<br>• Because task characteristics influence motor requirements, practitioners modify and adapt the requirements and affordances of tasks to help children succeed.<br>• Children develop improved neural pathways when they repeat meaningful, whole (occupation) tasks in the natural environment.<br>• Motor learning occurs as children repeat motor tasks that are intrinsically motivating, meaningful, and for which they can problem solve. | • Whole versus part: Engage child in occupation or whole activities. Part tasks may be used periodically but should not be emphasis of occupational therapy session.<br>• Variability: Engage child in activities that require variable adjustments to movements (such as distance to catch ball, moving body to reach in different planes).<br>• Meaningfulness: Engage child in meaningful activities of which they have choice and show an interest. Have a variety of activities available for child to choose. Children perform better when they are motivated to complete the task and it is something meaningful to them. Take the time to get to know the child.<br>• Implement motor learning strategies of feedback, practice, demonstration, and mental imagery. (See Chapter 29 for more details.) |

| Frame of Reference | Description | Principles | Strategies and Techniques |
|---|---|---|---|
| Rehabilitation | The rehabilitation approach allows a person to return to previous occupations with compensations and adaptations. It provides a more immediate return by changing how the person completes occupations, including the use of adaptive equipment. This top-down approach focuses on client's strengths and adapts tasks to compensate for limitations. | • Adapting task methods substitutes for loss of ROM, strength, use of one side of the body, limited vision, decreased endurance, inadequate stability, or to minimize the effects of spasticity and can simplify work and conserve energy (Rybski, 2024b).<br>• Adapting task objects or using adaptive/assistive devices or orthotics compensates for lack of reach, ROM, grasp, strength, vision, use of one side of the body, and loss of mobility to allow children to engage in proper positioning and overcome barriers (architectural, physical, or social/emotional) for occupational participation (Rybski, 2024b).<br>• Changing the context by modifying the environment will provide access to transportation, home, public and private facilities, work, and recreational activities so the child can participate in desired occupations (Rybski, 2024b). | • Teaching and learning (new ways of completing daily tasks).<br>• Changing the task (adapting methods or procedures; adapting the objects, using adaptive devices or orthotics).<br>• Change the context of occupations so client can succeed through:<br>• Environmental modifications<br>• Training caregiver or family<br>• Adapting (transportation, mobility, and positioning)<br>• Energy conservation<br>• Work simplification<br>• Adapted dressing methods<br>• Wheelchair mobility<br>• Preventing further disability (Rybski, 2024b) |
| Neurodevelopmental treatment (NDT) | Technique developed by Karel and Berta Bobath to help children with functional limitations due to neuropathology, primarily children with cerebral palsy. The goal of NDT is to help children perform skilled movements more efficiently so they can carry out life skills. | • The goal of NDT intervention is to improve overall function in daily tasks by increased active use of the trunk and involved extremities.<br>• Intervention is individualized and focused on functional outcomes.<br>• The OT practitioner may attempt to normalize muscle tone before and during functional movement.<br>• The OT practitioner analyzes musculoskeletal limitations interfering with movement and function.<br>• The OT practitioner facilitates normal movements that are meaningful to children.<br>• Intervention emphasizes quality of movement (e.g., accuracy, quickness, adaptability, and flexibility) and reproducibility of movement.<br>• Experience is the driving force for children. New activities build on previous sensorimotor experiences.<br>• Target postural control and movements by using key points of control. Proximal points of control (e.g., hips, trunk, pelvis) provide more support to children, whereas distal points of control (e.g., head, hands, feet) require children to perform more of the movement.<br>• The OT practitioner engages children in "typical" movement and repetition using new movement patterns to develop new neural pathways.<br>• Children's motivation and active problem-solving is considered when developing therapy goals and intervention activities. | • OTs begin with knowledge of typical movement.<br>• OTs use therapeutic handling techniques and key points of control to facilitate normal postures so that children "feel" typical movement patterns (Coker-Bolt, 2016).<br>• Inhibition and facilitation techniques to prepare muscle tone for activity (such as slow rolling, weight-bearing, fast movement, brushing).<br>• Handling techniques include using gentle guiding from OT to facilitate weight shift, protective extension, righting reactions, and equilibrium. |
| Ayres Sensory Integration (ASI) | Sensory integration is the organization of sensory input to produce an adaptive response; a theoretical process and intervention approach; addresses the processing of sensory information from the body and the environment; includes modulating discriminating, and integrating, sensory information to produce meaningful adaptive responses (see Chapter 27) | • Sensory input can be incorporated into activities systematically to elicit an adaptive response.<br>• Registration of meaningful sensory input is necessary before an adaptive response can be made.<br>• An adaptive response contributes to the development of sensory integration.<br>• Better organization of adaptive responses enhances the child's general behavioral organization.<br>• More mature and complex patterns of behavior emerge from consolidation of simpler behaviors.<br>• The more inner-directed a child's activities are, the greater is the potential for the activities to improve the neural organization. | • Create multisensory activities that require child to make an adaptive response and use active as opposed to passively applied vestibular, proprioceptive, and tactile input.<br>• Adjust the intensity of the activities to facilitate the "just right challenge."<br>• Collaborate with the child to create fun and challenging activities.<br>• Set up the environment to provide necessary sensory input and allow choice.<br>• Monitor the child's reactions carefully.<br>• Challenge praxis through novel activities to promote an adaptive response. See Chapter 27 for further explanation of ASI intervention, with fidelity and specific sensory techniques based on ASI FOR. |

*Continued*

**TABLE 9.6 Frames of Reference Used With Children and Youth—cont'd**

| Frame of Reference | Description | Principles | Strategies and Techniques |
|---|---|---|---|
| Behavioral (includes applied behavior analysis) | Behavior is reinforced with a reward. | • Positive reinforcement increases the likelihood that a behavior will be repeated.<br>• Children will stop behaviors that are ignored or receive negative reinforcement.<br>• Stimulus in the environment results in a response (behavior). | • Identify steps and behaviors that are interfering with child's daily activities. Determine what may be causing behaviors (such as sensory, positioning, and communication).<br>• Identify reinforcers and rewards.<br>• Develop behavioral support plan.<br>• Include child in plan and caregivers.<br>• Collect data regarding behaviors.<br>• Provide positive reinforcers that can be easily provided.<br>• Give reinforcers regularly at first and then intermittently.<br>• See Chapter 25. |
| Cognitive | Emphasizes assisting the child to identify, develop, and use cognitive strategies to perform daily occupations effectively.<br>Based on Bandura's (1996) work on importance of self-efficacy and establishing goals to motivate child to achieve. | Improved performance results from the dynamic interaction of the child's skills with the parameters of the task in the context in which it needs to be performed (Missiuna et al., 2001).<br>Child learns strategies to use in multiple situations and feels empowered that he/she has developed solutions, thereby is likely to repeat the strategy. | • Create activities to increase child's repertoire of cognitive strategies.<br>• Focus on activities to improve child's ability to select, monitor, and evaluate the use of strategies.<br>• Identify global problem-solving strategies.<br>• Task analysis.<br>• Anticipation of child's difficulties.<br>• Exploration and selection of task-specific strategies.<br>• Application of strategy.<br>• Evaluation of effectiveness (Missiuna, 1998).<br>• OT helps child develop strategies and self-evaluate.<br>See Chapter 26 for information on cognitive orientation to daily occupational performance (CO-OP) model. |
| Cognitive behavioral | Cognitive behavioral approach suggests that one's thoughts, and feelings (emotions, moods, and psychological responses) influence behaviors within the environment. | Behavior associated with mental illness is maintained by cognitive factors.<br>Changing one's cognitive thoughts and beliefs results in change in behaviors. | • Identify the thoughts and beliefs (such as negative self-talk) that affect performance or motivation.<br>• Help child reframe negative self-talk to promote performance and motivation to engage in occupations.<br>• OTs engage children in activities, such as role play, social stories, and novel activities to challenge children to explore and succeed.<br>• OTs encourage children to evaluate performance and problem solve.<br>• Techniques may include breathing exercises, graded activity, and systematic desensitization. |

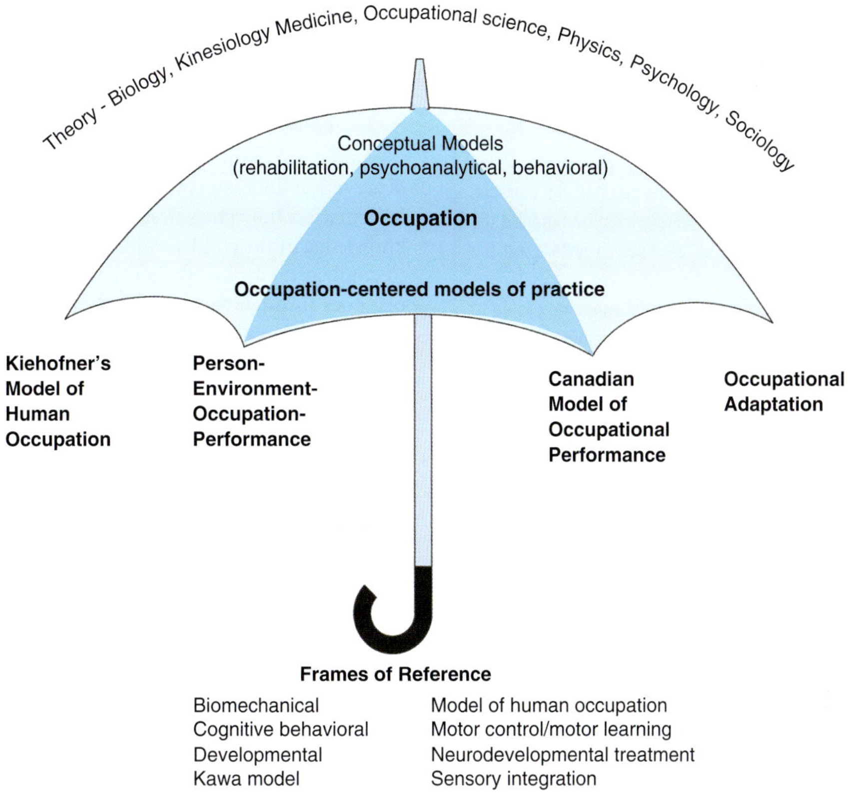


**Fig. 9.2** The umbrella of occupation: A conceptual diagram of the relationship between theories, occupation, models of practice, and frames of reference. (Adapted from MacRae, N., & Jane O'Brien (2001). OT 301 Foundations of occupational therapy. University of New England. In Jane Clifford O'Brien & B. Conners (2024). *Introduction to occupational therapy* (6th ed., p. 230). Elsevier.)

for a specific client and then decide to prioritize gathering information regarding physical factors such as ROM, endurance, and strength that interfere with the child's engagement in self-care. Each frame of reference identifies factors that may influence the child's performance. An overview of selected pediatric frames of reference is provided along with a description of the principles and strategies that inform intervention. Table 9.6 provides an overview of the frame of reference, guiding principles, and strategies.

***Combining Models and Frames.*** Fig. 9.2 illustrates the relationship between theory, occupation-centered models of practice, and frames of reference. Occupational therapists may combine models and frames of reference in practice. However, they use knowledge of the principles, strategies, and techniques to determine if the frames of reference work together. They understand the research supporting each model and frame of reference to evaluate the child's occupational performance, select assessments, create their hypotheses, and plan intervention. They consider the value of using the frame of reference or model of practice (Ikiugu et al., 2019). For example, if using CanMOP (CAOT), occupational therapists likely use the Canadian Occupational Performance Measure assessment tool (Law et al., 2005) and ask children or parents to describe their performance satisfaction. The occupation-centered model provides the structure and framework for the evaluation. It is typically not necessary to use two occupation-centered models of practice together, but practitioners may use multiple frames of reference.

A frame of reference is like a pair of glasses you can take on and off. The pair of "glasses" that is being used at any one time alters the occupational therapist's view. Occupational therapists have many different "glasses" or lenses with which to view a client's behavior. Just as reading, distance, and sunglasses each alter a person's view of the world slightly, so too does the choice of frame of reference. And just as someone could put on more than one pair of glasses at a time (although this would look silly), a therapist can use more than one frame of reference at a time, as will be illustrated later in the chapter. Occupational therapists may also use both a model and a frame of reference. See Case Example 9.3 that shows how a therapist uses a model and frame of reference together to organize the evaluation process.

### Finalizing the Evaluation Plan

During the planning process for the evaluation, the therapist considers the referral, the setting, the client's diagnosis and condition, and other information that is available at this early stage to hypothesize about possible challenges the client might have. The therapist considers multiple factors to eventually decide upon which documents to review, who to interview and what questions to ask, what to observe (and where and when) and what specific assessments to complete. Once the therapist has a plan in mind for this evaluation, they also consider the best time of day to complete specific portions of the evaluation and, if there are multiple options available, where to complete portions of the evaluation as well. Is a small room better, a larger space, or one that has specific features available? Ideally, children are observed and assessed in quiet child-friendly spaces, with age-appropriate toys or items. However, sometimes they are observed and assessed in busy spaces that may influence the evaluation findings.

## IMPLEMENTING THE EVALUATION PLAN

At the appointed time and place, the therapist must be prepared with the selected assessment tools and questionnaires, items or toys needed for observations, and a record sheet or format the therapist will use to document findings in preparation for later analysis and report writing (see Chapter 7). However, the therapist also needs to be prepared to

### CASE EXAMPLE 9.3 APPLYING OCCUPATION-CENTERED MODEL OF PRACTICE WITH FRAME OF REFERENCE

Karesa is a 6-year-old child with juvenile rheumatoid arthritis referred to occupational therapy for evaluation due to limited range of motion and pain interfering with her ability to play and engage in daily activities. The occupational therapist uses Person-Environment-Occupation-Performance (PEOP) model to organize the evaluation, along with a biomechanical frame of reference to understand the child's physical challenges.

The therapist uses PEOP to create questions for the occupational profile to understand the child's narrative (personal story), while examining the types of occupations (tasks and roles) that are meaningful to her within her family (environment). Sample questions are listed.

**Person**

- What do you do when you have trouble with your hands?
- What do you like to do?
- Who do you play with?
- What's it like at school?
- What is it like being you?
- What do you want to do?

**Occupation**

- What activities are the most fun for you to do?
- What activities are hard for you to do? Why?
- Are you able to play with your friends the way you want to?

**Environment**

- Where do you like to play?
- What is your classroom like?
- Who helps you out?

After learning from the child and parents through the interview, the therapist uses the *biomechanical frame of reference* to more closely evaluate person factors, such as range of motion, pain levels, strength, and endurance that support or interfere with Kareesa's ability to feed, dress, bathe, complete homework, and engage in sports. The therapist uses techniques from the biomechanical frame of reference regarding movement, stretching, and compensating to avoid pain and increase endurance while integrating information about the child's motivations, values, routines, and supports. The therapist considers the contexts in which Kareesa needs to perform (e.g., school, home, community) to determine how to advocate for services. This example illustrates the use of an occupation-centered model of practice to structure one's assessment of a child's situation along with a frame of reference (biomechanical) to address the child's needs.

change the plan, add additional methods, or skip planned activities or tools once the therapist actually meets the child and family. The therapist's initial hypotheses may be wrong, or the child may come to the evaluation in a state that is not conducive to their best performance, or the child may be afraid and refuse to complete planned activities. The therapist must plan but also be prepared to throw the plan away and try alternative methods.

Typically, the occupational therapist begins the evaluation with an interview. Occupational therapists delve more deeply into the reason for referral when they interview the caregiver(s) or teacher. They allow the interviewees to elaborate, define, and provide additional information regarding what led to the referral and how their specific concerns, as illustrated by the child's behaviors, resulted in a referral. For example, the therapist examines what the child does that warranted an evaluation regarding "poor handwriting." In this case, the referral elicits additional questions regarding the reason the child has poor handwriting, academic history, and child's performance level in school. The therapist inquires about the onset of the issue and inquires about any other conditions that may affect the child's educational performance.

As the occupational therapist collects information through direct observation and assessments, they filter their observations with the information they have already gathered from others, as well as their knowledge of the child's condition, and their own clinical experience to confirm their observations and assessment findings. As the therapist goes through the process, they may revisit aspects of the evaluation to further examine and confirm or disprove their hypotheses.

Gathering information from multiple sources allows the occupational therapist to make confident decisions supporting the child and family. For example, an occupational therapist working in an outpatient early intervention setting received a referral for a 12-month-old infant for "developmental delays." During the evaluation, they learned that the infant's corrected age was 10 months; the infant was born at 30 weeks. The parent expressed no concerns with feeding and eating. The therapist observed a small infant who took frequent naps during the session. They asked the parent to feed the child and noted the child had difficulty managing milk from a bottle, coughed, and that the parent cut the nipple of the bottle to make it larger. The parent reported they were not feeding the infant pureed foods but put some rice cereal in the bottle. The therapist observed feeding challenges although the family did not indicate this during the interview. This example illustrates the importance of evaluating the child using multiple sources.

At any point in the process, the evaluation plan may change. New concerns may arise that were not noted on the referral and therefore were not planned for. For example, during an interview a parent may report the child shows poor body awareness, is impulsive, and falls a lot. A teacher may note the child pushes children, and while they do not mean to hurt others, they cannot do this at school. The occupational therapist decides on the spot to gather more information about this concern. These type of last minute changes in plan may necessitate additional or altered assessment strategies.

## EVALUATION METHODS

Occupational therapists evaluate children through a variety of methods including interview, observation, occupation and activity analysis, and specific measurement tools (i.e., assessments).

### Interview

Interviewing is the one of the primary sources to understand a child's occupational performance and levels of participation while engaging in occupations. Interviews provide an opportunity for occupational therapists to understand a child and others' perception of the child's abilities and family routines and values, as well as to identify and discuss issues on a personal level. Some assessments are interview based, so occupational therapists need to be trained to ask questions and probe for information strategically. Information obtained from an interview is usually an in-depth exploration of a child and a family's culture and desires. Pediatric occupational therapists may interview the child, the caregiver(s), teacher, and/or other adults who are working with the child and therefore can use the process to establish therapeutic relationships and bonding with the child and family (Taylor, 2020).

**Using Interview-Based Assessment.** Occupational therapists can utilize **interview-based assessments** to obtain necessary information. The Canadian Occupational Performance Measure (COPM;

Law et al., 2005), Child Occupational Self-Assessment (COSA; Kramer et al., 2014), and the School Setting Interview (SSI; Hemmingsson et al., 2005) are examples of semistructured interviews that provide rating scales. Each of these measures strives to understand the child and family's views and can be used across all developmental stages for children as young as 4 or 6 years old (Kramer et al., 2014; Law et al., 2005). However, some children younger than 8 years may have trouble identifying difficulties in their daily activities. Therefore, when a child is not capable of expressing their thoughts and concerns, parents or caregivers are interviewed to elicit their concerns and gain their perspectives. Kramer et al. (2014) found that children as young as 4 years old could express their perceptions of their abilities. The COSA (Kramer et al., 2014) manual provides tips on interviewing young children to hear their perspectives. Children appear to provide a source of information that differs from that provided by parents, teachers, and direct observation (Kennedy et al., 2012; Lalor et al., 2016).

Semistructured interviews allow occupational therapists to understand occupations that are important to the child and the family. The interview process develops a partnership between the child and family and facilitates the process of identifying difficulties of the child's daily activities. Occupational therapists explain the process and reason for the interview and build rapport with the child and parent. The occupational therapist may decide to take notes during the interview. They ask for permission to take notes and let the child and caregiver know that they will use the notes to remind them of the important aspects of the session. Occupational therapists learn to multitask as they interview parents while watching a child play and potentially incorporate observation into probing questions. To multitask effectively, therapists become familiar with the questions and required forms to adhere to the instructions. Cue cards may help an inexperienced occupational therapist conduct the interview and observations more smoothly.

**Interview Strategies.** Interviewing is most effective when it takes place in a comfortable and supportive environment, and this may allow children and adolescents to present a different point of view from their parents or caregivers. In the interview environment, occupational therapists can demonstrate a confident, assertive, and emotionally self-protective character, which may reduce children and parents' anxiety (Taylor, 2020). Taylor (2020, p. 245) suggests 15 interpersonal guidelines when conducting an interview.

1. Creating a confidential and protective environment
2. Conveying a take-charge attitude
3. Assessing vulnerabilities and sensitivities
4. Orienting the client to the process and requesting consent
5. Rephrasing, reordering, or asking questions creatively (if the protocol permits)
6. Detecting and respecting the client's boundaries
7. Listening well
8. Responding (nonverbally or verbally) to a response
9. Responding therapeutically
10. Never apologizing for interview length or the questions
11. Checking in and acting as an emotional buoy
12. Knowing when to stop
13. Redirecting hyperverbal or tangential clients
14. Spotting and clarifying ambiguities and contradictions in content
15. Summarizing, seeking feedback, and establishing closure

When communicating with children, especially younger children, occupational therapists use language that matches the child's comprehension levels, which may require that they rephrase questions or answers. This promotes greater understanding and lets the child know that the therapist has heard them. In addition, the child's responses can lead the practitioner to ask further probing questions. Probing questions are used with caution, as this may expose children or caregivers to their vulnerability. Occupational therapists remain sensitive to reading cues, so they can detect and respect children and their families' boundaries. Box 9.4 provides more tips for interviewing children and adolescents.

Occupational therapists assess emotional reactions and behaviors during the interview and use impressions and intuition as guides to discontinue the interview. When encountering situations such as children or caregivers showing aggressive behaviors, being verbally hostile, or being emotional for an extensive time, practitioners may stop the interview and reschedule it at another time (Taylor, 2020).

**BOX 9.4 Strategies for Interviewing Older Children and Adolescents**

1. Begin the session by clarifying the purpose of the interview in terms that are meaningful to them.
2. Be sensitive to their physical and emotional needs throughout the interview.
3. Promote interaction by asking open-ended questions and guide them to participate fully in the conversation.
4. Through careful questioning, attempt to understand their values and beliefs.
5. Carefully plan when to take notes, preferably after the interview or when the child is involved in another task.
6. Remain positive in your approach and realistic in the information you provide the child and parent.
7. Be flexible throughout the interview, responding sensitively to the child's questions and need for information. If you cannot answer a question, let them know, and develop a plan to find the needed information.
8. Use effective verbal and nonverbal communication skills. Often nonverbal communication can override verbal information.
9. Avoid the use of therapy and medical jargon. If technical terms are used, be sure they are explained adequately at the child's level.
10. Be mindful of therapeutic use of self and show respect and empathy.

## Activity Analysis

**Activity analysis** is recognized as a process of examining the essential components of an activity to identify its demands and opportunities for therapeutic intervention (Crepeau et al., 2014; Hersch et al., 2005; Kuhaneck, Spitzer, et al., 2010; Mosey, 1986; O'Brien & Soloman, 2022; Polatajko et al., 2000; Thomas, 2015). Specifically, as depicted in Table 9.7, occupational therapists analyze the steps of the activity as well as the activity's requirements for body structures, body functions, and performance skills; context; and personal relevance in relation to the individual's interests and goals (AOTA, 2020b). Activity analysis is widely applied in pediatric populations for diverse occupations including ADLs, instrumental activities of daily living (IADLs), schoolwork, play, and leisure (e.g., Kuhaneck, Spitzer, et al., 2010; Mills & Chapparo, 2017; Orentlicher & Case, 2018; Weaver, 2015). Occupational therapists use activity analysis findings to match activities to client needs and strengths (Mosey, 1986; O'Brien & Soloman, 2022).

A *general activity analysis* refers to an analysis of the generic properties of an activity as it is typically performed including steps, materials, context, activity demands, and possible meanings (AOTA, 2020b; Creighton, 1992; Crepeau et al., 2014; Hersch et al., 2005; Kuhaneck, Spitzer, et al., 2010; O'Brien & Soloman, 2022; Polatajko et al., 2000). A general activity analysis identifies the core elements of an activity,

**TABLE 9.7 Elements of Activity Analysis in Pediatric Occupational Therapy**

| Activity | Context | Personal Relevance |
|---|---|---|
| • Steps<br>• Objects used<br>• Required body structures<br>• Required body functions<br>  • Cognitive, emotional, and other mental functions<br>  • Visual functions<br>  • Proprioceptive, touch, and other sensory functions<br>  • Joint function<br>  • Muscle strength and endurance<br>  • Muscle tone and movement functions<br>  • Other body functions<br>• Required performance skills<br>  • Postural stability<br>  • Coordination and other motor skills<br>  • Locating and functional use of materials<br>  • Adjusting, accommodation, and other process skills<br>  • Social interaction skills | • Time<br>• Location/space<br>• Sensory environment<br>• Social environment<br>• Social-cultural meanings and standards | • Values and motivation: Attempts and resistance<br>• Spirituality and meaning: Affect and emotional responses |

*Note:* Based on the Occupational Therapy Practice Framework (AOTA, 2020b), with modifications to reflect the most common aspects of pediatric practice.

which provide a base for comparative assessment of a client's performance. An example of a general activity analysis is provided in Box 9.5.

**Client-Focused Activity Analysis and Occupational Analysis.** A *client-focused activity analysis* refers to a highly individualized analysis of the personal way in which an activity or occupation is performed in real-life contexts by a specific individual. Each general activity may be performed with a range of common variations (Box 9.6) or specific individualized variations (Box 9.7). A client-focused activity analysis allows occupational therapists to analyze the unique features of how the activity is done and its personal meaning (Crepeau et al., 2014; Mosey, 1986). The term *client-focused activity analysis* is designed to encompass analysis of both current and potential occupations. If the activity is an occupation, then the *terms occupation analysis, occupational analysis*, or *occupation-based activity analysis* (Crepeau et al., 2014; O'Brien & Soloman, 2022; Thomas, 2015) are also applicable. See Box 9.8 for an example of how an experienced occupational therapist implicitly applies activity observation and analysis during an evaluation.

### Observation

As information obtained from an interview is typically based on other's perceptions of the child; it is important for occupational therapists to observe behaviors to see if their observations match those perceptions. Observation occurs from the moment the therapist and child meet and occurs throughout the evaluation. The occupational therapist uses observational skills to evaluate the child's occupational performance; analyze skills needed to engage in the occupation and examine contextual factors that support or hinder their performance; and further explore the impact on engaging in occupations. Occupational therapists can observe children in play or while engaging in their preferred occupations in natural or supported environments.

**Observation Strategies.** Pediatric occupational therapists develop observation skills to gather objective data on the quantity, quality, frequency, and duration of the child's performance. Dunn (2000) proposed that skilled observation is one of the essential tools for occupational therapy practice and described the following key competencies required to conduct skilled observations: (1) do not interfere with the natural course of events; (2) pay attention to the physical and social features of the environment that support or limit a child's performance; and (3) record the child's behavior in observable and neutral terms. When skilled observations are used in the evaluation process, occupational therapists select a systematic, objective recording procedure so that data collected are accurate and reliable. Those just entering the field may have difficulty remembering their observations and benefit from keeping notes in a format that will be understandable at a later time. Occupational therapists practice their observation skills so that they can recognize key behaviors or patterns and identify the meaning of those behaviors within the demands of the task and environment. Therapists entering the field of pediatric occupational therapy may seek out master clinicians and mentors who are willing to help them develop their observation skills.

### Screening Tools and Methods

Screening refers to the use of brief assessment tools and interviews for the purpose of determining if the child needs a full occupational therapy evaluation. For example, a therapist may screen all children entering a preschool to identify those who might need further evaluation. Infants who are at high risk for developmental delays may be referred for an occupational therapy screening as part of their follow-up. Screening often includes an interview with parent or caregiver to determine if there are any concerns, for observation to confirm information, and for short assessments (such as a neurological, developmental, sensory, or feeding/eating).

## ASSESSMENT USING TESTS AND MEASURES

A variety of assessment tools exist to measure concepts of interest to children and their families (see Appendix A). Some tools are used in screening; others assessments are observational; some assessments provide scores and information to assist with diagnosis and others measure progress. Occupational therapists select assessments to address the child's unique situation and challenges and to better understand the child's strengths and challenges. The tool(s) chosen should be appropriate for the evaluation purpose.

### Purpose of the Evaluation Related to Selection of Assessment Tool

An evaluation typically occurs for one of four purposes: (1) screening; (2) determining the need for and then the scope and frequency of occupational therapy services; (3) setting goals and developing intervention plans; and (4) documenting progress toward therapy goals. Within those broad categories, there are additional purposes requiring specific types of assessment methods. Assessments are the tools used to gather data.

## BOX 9.5 General Activity Analysis of Donning a Jacket

Note: This activity analysis is written for someone with right-hand dominance.

| Steps | Activity Demands | Context |
|---|---|---|
| 1. Hold top of jacket, inside facing, with left hand. | • Objects: Jacket<br>• Body structures: Left arm and hand<br>• Body functions:<br>  • Emotional function: Regulated to control body.<br>  • Visual function: Discriminate jacket and visual markers on the top, inside of jacket (e.g., hood, collar, label, etc.).<br>  • Cognitive functions: Recognize the need to locate the top of the jacket; understand that the visual markers indicate the top of jacket; insight for reason to put on a jacket.<br>  • Proprioceptive function: Adjust force to accommodate for weight of jacket.<br>  • Touch function: Tolerate tactile sensations from jacket's fabric.<br>  • Joint function: Moderate range and stability in left upper extremity (UE) joints.<br>  • Muscle functions: Good strength (left shoulder flexors and extensors, elbow extension and flexion, finger extensors and flexors, wrist extensors) and mild endurance to reach, grasp, and hold weight of jacket against gravity.<br>  • Movement functions: Voluntary control for reach, grasp, and sustained left UE position.<br>Performance skills:<br>  • Postural stability: Hold body upright in standing or sitting.<br>  • Coordination and other motor skills: Minimal coordination to target jacket.<br>  • Locating and functional use of materials: Locate jacket and use it on upper body as expected.<br>  • Adjusting, accommodation: Must be able to adjust grasp if not initially at top of jacket. | Time: During cold seasons; prior to going outside; approximately 10 seconds to complete.<br>Location/space: Various locations, enough space to extend arms.<br>Sensory environment: Cold temperatures or room temperature (in preparation for going outside).<br>Social environment: Adults may remind and direct children to put on their jackets.<br>Social-cultural developmental meanings and standards: By elementary school, most children are able and expected to put on their own jackets. Kindergarteners may need assistance with zippers.<br>Personal context: May include desire to protect oneself from the weather, keep oneself comfortable, be independent, and present oneself with a neat appearance. |
| 2. Place right hand into jacket's right arm hole. | • Body structures: Both upper extremities.<br>• Body functions:<br>  • Visual function: Discriminate right-side arm hole, which is correctly located on left.<br>  • Cognitive functions: Recognize the need to locate specific arm hole; understand that the visual markers indicate the correct arm hole.<br>  • Proprioceptive function: Body awareness to recognize which arm hole will fit correctly.<br>  • Touch function: Tolerate tactile sensations from jacket's fabric; discriminate sensation from arm hole.<br>  • Joint function: Moderate range and stability in left UE joints. Minimal range and stability in right UE joints.<br>  • Muscle functions: Good strength (left shoulder flexors, elbow extension and flexion, finger flexors, wrist extensors); fair strength (right shoulder flexors and horizontal adduction, elbow extension/flexion, wrist extension); and mild endurance to sustain hold of jacket's weight against gravity.<br>  • Movement functions: Voluntary control for right arm to cross body midline and bilateral control.<br>Performance skills:<br>  • Coordination and other motor skills: Minimal coordination is required to target hand to arm hole.<br>  • Adjusting, accommodation: Must be able to adjust UE movements if hand misses arm hole. | |
| 3. Push right arm through sleeve until hand is out. | Body structures: Both upper extremities.<br>Body functions:<br>• Cognitive functions: Recognize the need to sustain movement.<br>• Proprioceptive function: Adjust force to push through arm hole.<br>• Touch function: Discriminate when hand has gotten through arm hole.<br>• Joint function: Good range in left elbow flexion and right elbow extension; moderate stability in left wrist and hand joints.<br>• Muscle functions: Good strength (left elbow flexion, right elbow extension, right horizontal abduction; trunk); minimal endurance needed.<br>• Movement functions: Voluntary control for left arm to cross body midline and bilateral control to sustain left UE position.<br>Performance skills:<br>• Coordination and other motor skills: Bilateral coordination required to use both arms together. | |

*Continued*

## BOX 9.5 General Activity Analysis of Donning a Jacket—cont'd

| Steps | Activity Demands | Context |
|---|---|---|
| 4. Pull jacket up over right shoulder. | Body structures: Left upper extremity.<br>Body functions:<br>• Visual function: Discriminate jacket edge.<br>• Cognitive functions: Recognize the need to locate and pull up jacket.<br>• Proprioceptive function: Adjust force to pull over shoulder.<br>• Touch function: Tactile discrimination for awareness of jacket adequately onto shoulder.<br>• Joint function: Left shoulder horizontal adduction range; moderate stability in left UE joints.<br>• Muscle functions: Good strength (left elbow flexors, finger flexors, wrist radial deviators; trunk) and minimal endurance to sustain for few seconds.<br>• Movement functions: Voluntary control for reach, grasp, and crossing midline for left UE.<br>Performance skills:<br>• Coordination and other motor skills: Minimal coordination.<br>• Adjusting, accommodation: Must be able to adjust UE movements if jacket slips down or out of hand. | |
| 5. Reach left arm behind back to locate left arm hole. | Body structures: Left upper extremity.<br>Body functions:<br>• Cognitive functions: Recognize the need and remember to reach behind to locate other arm hole<br>• Proprioceptive function: To perceive where left arm is without looking.<br>• Touch function: Discriminate jacket material from other clothing; discriminate arm hole from other parts of jacket.<br>• Joint function: Good range in left shoulder internal rotation, elbow flexion, finger extension/flexion. Minimal joint stability.<br>• Muscle functions: Fair strength (left shoulder internal rotators, elbow flexors, finger extensors/flexors); good strength in wrist extension, trunk flexors/extensors. Minimal endurance to reach briefly.<br>• Movement functions: Voluntary control for moving left UE.<br>Performance skills:<br>• Postural stability: Need to hold body upright.<br>• Coordination and other motor skills: Minimal coordination is required to reach jacket.<br>• Adjusting, accommodation: Must be able to adjust reach until hand reaches arm hole. | |
| 6. Push left arm through the left arm hole. | Body structures: Left upper extremity.<br>Body functions:<br>• Cognitive functions: Recognize the need to sustain movement.<br>• Proprioceptive function: Awareness of left arm position and adjustment of force to push through arm hole in relation to the space available.<br>• Touch function: Discriminate when hand has gotten through arm hole.<br>• Joint function: Good range and stability in left elbow extension.<br>• Muscle functions: Good strength (left elbow extensors, left shoulder external rotation and flexion); minimal endurance needed.<br>• Movement functions: Voluntary control for left arm.<br>Performance skills:<br>• Coordination and other motor skills: Minimal coordination required. | |
| 7. Pull front of jacket to straighten as needed. | Body structures: Both upper extremities.<br>Body functions:<br>• Visual function: Discriminate front edges of jacket.<br>• Cognitive functions: Recognize the need to locate the front of the jacket, insight for straightening a jacket.<br>• Touch function: Discriminate front edges of jacket from other clothing.<br>• Joint function: Moderate elbow flexion range, good range in finger extensors and flexors. Good stability in finger, wrist, and shoulder joints.<br>• Muscle functions: Good strength (elbow extensors, finger flexors, trunk extensors). Minimal endurance for brief grasping.<br>• Movement functions: Voluntary control for reach and grasp.<br>Performance skills:<br>• Postural stability: To maintain upright position despite the movements.<br>• Coordination and other motor skills: Bilateral coordination to use two hands simultaneously. | |

## BOX 9.5 General Activity Analysis of Donning a Jacket—cont'd

| Steps | Activity Demands | Context |
|---|---|---|
| 8. Adjust collar and hood as needed. | • Body structures: One or both upper extremities.<br>• Body functions:<br>• Cognitive functions: Understand that adjusting the collar/hood may be more comfortable and/or socially expected; recognize the need to locate the collar/hood.<br>• Proprioceptive function: Awareness of arms relation to jacket when behind.<br>• Touch function: Tactile sensation of rolled collar or hood inside jacket; discriminate rolled collar/hood from other parts of jacket or other clothing.<br>• Joint function: Moderate range and stability in shoulder flexion, abduction, and internal rotation, elbow flexion, finger extension and flexion, wrist flexion and extension.<br>• Muscle functions: Good strength (shoulder flexors abductors, finger extensors and flexors, wrist flexors and extensors); fair strength in external rotation and elbow flexion; minimal endurance to hold arms up for 5–10 seconds.<br>• Movement functions: Voluntary control for reach, grasp, and sustained arm position.<br>Performance skills:<br>• Coordination and other motor skills: Fine motor coordination to unroll collar.<br>• Adjusting, accommodation: Continual feeling and adjusting until collar/hood are straightened. | |

## BOX 9.6 Considerations of Common Variations for Donning a Jacket

- Where is the jacket kept (e.g., hook, hanger, floor, cubby, backpack, back of chair)? Is the jacket kept in the same place?
- Is the jacket turned inside out or right-side out?
- What if the client uses a heavy coat, a long raincoat, a slick parka, or a cardigan sweater?
- What if the client uses his or her right hand to hold the jacket and to place left hand in the armhole first (as most left-handers do)?
- What if the client is wearing a long-sleeved shirt and does not want the sleeves to bunch up?
- What if the client wants or needs to zip or button up the jacket?

Occupational therapists consider the purpose of the evaluation, the information they want to gather, and the child's needs when deciding on the appropriate assessment. Different assessment tools are best for the varied evaluation purposes. The specific types of assessment tools are described below.

One purpose of evaluation may be to determine the child's qualification for services and assist in the determination of a diagnosis through use of *normative scores* that compare the child's performance with that of an age-matched sample of children. Standardized tests are frequently used to determine if a child has developmental delays or functional deficits significant enough to qualify the child for remedial services such as occupational therapy. Many funding agencies and insurance providers use the results of standardized testing as one criterion in deciding whether a child will receive occupational therapy intervention. In school-based practice, standard scores are used to determine eligibility for special education and may be helpful for further identifying specific student problems that may indicate that the involvement of an occupational therapist is appropriate. Funding approval for special services may depend on documentation of a predetermined degree of delay or deficit in one or more developmental or academic domains, and standardized test results are an important component of this documentation. The results of standardized testing performed by occupational therapists, when used in conjunction with testing done by other professionals, can help physicians or psychologists arrive at a medical or educational diagnosis.

A second purpose of evaluation is to document a child's status. This can include developmental levels, functional skills, and the child's level of participation in home, school, and community activities. Many funding and service agencies require periodic reassessment to provide a record of a child's progress and to determine if the child continues to qualify for services. Standardized testing is often a preferred way of documenting progress because the results of the most current assessment can be compared with those of earlier ones. Periodic formal reassessment can also provide valuable information to the occupational therapist working with the child. Careful examination of a child's test results can identify areas of greatest and least progress. This can assist the occupational therapist in prioritizing intervention goals. Many parents are also interested in seeing the results of their child's periodic assessments. Standardized tests used in periodic assessments must be chosen carefully so that areas of occupation or performance skills addressed in the intervention plan are also the focus of the standardized testing.

A discussion about the child's progress in areas that may not be measured by standardized testing should accompany the discussion of test performance. Structured or unstructured observations of the child's play, academic, social, and/or self-care performance; interviews with the caretaker or teacher about the child's home or school routine; the developmental, educational, and medical histories; and a review of pertinent medical or educational records are equally important components of the assessment process. Case Example 9.4 illustrates these concepts.

There are several issues that may occur with re-assessment. While it is certainly important to document a child's progress, it is essential for occupational therapists to be aware of the retesting period. Repeating the testing too soon may result in a practice effect, which should be avoided. If the occupational therapist is not sure about the period, they should review the user manual, which often provides such information.

Another issue is using *norm-referenced* tests. As the child gets older, the comparison group also gets older, so even if a child makes progress, the results may still show as delayed in comparison. When this is the case, the occupational therapist should discuss in the documentation the child's progress from admission as well as comparing to the age-related norm groups.

## BOX 9.7 Case Study: Client-Focused Activity Analysis of Ani's Jacket Donning

Ani is a third grader with mild cerebral palsy. She is a pleasant and cooperative child. She has just been transitioned to full inclusion in a regular education classroom with resource specialist services for math and curriculum modifications. The classroom aide assists Ani with self-care at school.

Because the team would like Ani to increase independence with self-care at school to increase inclusion, they have requested an occupational therapy evaluation. The occupational therapist interviews her father and teacher who specify that Ani needs help with donning her jacket, managing her clothing for toileting, opening food containers, eating neatly, and using her backpack. In preparation for school observations, the occupational therapist conducts several general activity analyses including the one in Box 9.5 for donning a jacket. For the classroom visit, the occupational therapist also prepares to observe and inquire about common factors that may be involved in Ani's performance (Box 9.6). Based on observations, supplemented with interviews, the occupational therapist adjusts the general activity analysis into a client-focused activity analysis of Ani's jacket donning, which is presented here. An additional column indicates where Ani's performance differs from the activity demands as well as personal relevance.

| Steps | Activity Demands | Context | Client Relevance and Performance |
|---|---|---|---|
| 1. Grasp top of jacket, inside facing with left hand. | • Objects: Jacket.<br>• Body Structures: Left arm and hand.<br>• Body functions:<br>  • Emotional function: regulated to control body; handle corrective feedback from classroom staff.<br>  • Visual function: Discriminate jacket and visual markers on the top, inside of jacket (e.g., hood, collar, label, etc.).<br>  • Cognitive functions: Recognize the need to locate the top of the jacket, understand that the visual markers indicate the top of jacket, insight for reason to put on a jacket.<br>  • Proprioceptive function: Adjust force to accommodate for weight of jacket.<br>  • Touch function: Tolerate tactile sensations from jacket's fabric.<br>  • Joint function: Moderate range and stability in left UE joints.<br>  • Muscle functions: Good strength (left shoulder flexors and extensors, elbow extension and flexion, finger extensors and flexors, wrist extensors) and mild endurance to reach, grasp, and hold weight of jacket against gravity.<br>  • Movement functions: Voluntary control for reach, grasp, and sustained left UE position.<br>• Performance skills:<br>  • Postural stability: Hold body upright in standing or sitting.<br>  • Coordination and other motor skills: Minimal coordination to target jacket.<br>  • Locating and functional use of materials: Locate jacket and use it on upper body as expected.<br>  • Adjusting, accommodation: Must be able to adjust grasp if not initially at top of jacket.<br>  • Social interaction skills: Respond to adult directions. | Time: During cold seasons; prior to going outside.<br>Location/space: In walkway next to desk.<br>Sensory environment: Room temperature (in preparation for going outside). High degree of auditory and visual stimuli from the other students' transitioning to leave the classroom.<br>Social Environment: Classroom staff remind the class to put on their jackets before going outside. Staff compliment her on following directions. As Ani starts step 2 with the jacket upside down, the aide quickly turns and holds the jacket so the top inside is facing Ani and tells her, "Do it this way."<br>Social-cultural meanings and standards: Most children are able and expected to put on their own jackets. | Values and motivation: Attempts immediately (self-directed).<br>Spirituality and meaning: Smiles with positive statements from staff, may want to please aide.<br>Time: Takes 1 minute to complete (with adult assistance), finishing after other students have begun walking out of class.<br>Adjusting, accommodation: Does not adjust grasp to accommodate for jacket being upside down.<br>Visual function: No signs of visually discriminating top of jacket. |

## BOX 9.7 Case Study: Client-Focused Activity Analysis of Ani's Jacket Donning—cont'd

| Steps | Activity Demands | Context | Client Relevance and Performance |
|---|---|---|---|
| 2. Place right hand into jacket's right arm hole. | • Body structures: Both upper extremities.<br>Body functions:<br>• Visual function: Discriminate right-side arm hole, which is correctly located on left.<br>• Cognitive functions: Recognize the need to locate specific arm hole, understand that the visual markers indicate the correct arm hole.<br>• Proprioceptive function: Body awareness to recognize which arm hole will fit correctly.<br>• Touch function: Tolerate tactile sensations from jacket's fabric, discriminate sensation from arm hole.<br>• Joint function: Moderate range and stability in left UE joints. Minimal range and stability in right UE joints.<br>• Muscle functions: Good strength (left shoulder flexors, elbow extension and flexion, finger flexors, wrist extensors); fair strength (right shoulder flexors and horizontal adduction, elbow extension/flexion, wrist extension); and mild endurance to sustain hold of jacket's weight against gravity.<br>• Movement functions: Voluntary control for right arm to cross body midline and bilateral control.<br>• Performance skills:<br>  • Coordination and other motor skills: Minimal coordination is required to target hand to arm hole.<br>  • Adjusting, accommodation: Must be able to adjust UE movements if hand misses arm hole. | Social environment: In response to Ani's error, the aide holds the jacket to show the correct arm hole as she instructs Ani by saying, "No, this one." | Visual function: Discriminates an (incorrect) arm hole.<br>Cognitive functions: Recognizes the need to locate an arm hole (but not the correct one); follows verbal directions.<br>Proprioceptive function: Does not use correct arm hole.<br>Touch function: Does not discriminate feeling of wrong arm hole.<br>Joint function: Left UE joint function not demonstrated.<br>Muscle functions: Left UE strength not demonstrated; right horizontal adductor strength not demonstrated.<br>Movement functions: No crossing of body midline; uses only right upper extremity.<br>Adjusting, accommodation: Does not self-adjust for incorrect arm hole. |
| 3. Push right arm through sleeve until hand is out. | • Body structures: Both upper extremities.<br>• Body functions:<br>  • Cognitive functions: Recognize the need to sustain movement.<br>  • Proprioceptive function: Adjust force to push through arm hole.<br>  • Touch function: Discriminate when hand has gotten through arm hole.<br>  • Joint function: Good range in left elbow flexion and right elbow extension; moderate stability in left wrist and hand joints.<br>  • Muscle functions: Good strength (left elbow flexion, right elbow extension, right horizontal abduction; trunk); minimal endurance needed.<br>  • Movement functions: Voluntary control for left arm to cross body midline and bilateral control to sustain left UE position.<br>• Performance skills:<br>  • Coordination and other motor skills: Bilateral coordination required to use both arms together. | Social environment: The aide continues to hold the jacket until hand is out. | Cognitive function: Identified alternative movement of shoulder flexion for gravity to assist in pulling jacket on arm.<br>Joint function: Left UE joint function not demonstrated; good range in right shoulder flexion.<br>Muscle functions: Demonstrates good strength (right elbow extension, shoulder flexion; trunk).<br>Movement functions: No crossing body midline, only uses right upper extremity.<br>Coordination and other motor skills: Bilateral coordination not demonstrated.<br>Adjusting, accommodation: Adjusted movement for gravity to compensate for not using left UE. |

Continued

**BOX 9.7 Case Study: Client-Focused Activity Analysis of Ani's Jacket Donning—cont'd**

| Steps | Activity Demands | Context | Client Relevance and Performance |
|---|---|---|---|
| 4. Reach left arm behind back to locate left arm hole. | • Body structures: Left upper extremity.<br>• Body functions:<br>  • Cognitive functions: Recognize the need and remember to reach behind to locate other arm hole.<br>  • Proprioceptive function: To perceive where left arm is without looking.<br>  • Touch function: Discriminate jacket material from other clothing, discriminate arm hole from other parts of jacket.<br>  • Joint function: Good range in left shoulder internal rotation, elbow flexion, finger extension/flexion. Minimal joint stability.<br>  • Muscle functions: Fair strength (left shoulder internal rotators, elbow flexors, finger extensors/flexors); good strength in wrist extension, trunk flexors/extensors. Minimal endurance to reach briefly.<br>  • Movement functions: Voluntary control for moving left UE.<br>• Performance skills:<br>  • Postural stability: Need to hold body upright.<br>  • Coordination and other motor skills: Minimal coordination is required to reach jacket.<br>  • Adjusting, accommodation: Must be able to adjust reach until hand reaches arm hole. | Social environment: After several attempts by Ani, the aide then holds the jacket with arm hole open until she puts her hand inside. | Cognitive function: May not know that pulling jacket over right shoulder makes it easier to do this step.<br>Proprioceptive function: Does not reach far enough (may not perceive where left arm is without looking).<br>Touch function: Discriminates that she has not touched jacket and needs to continue reaching.<br>Joint function: Left elbow flexion range not demonstrated. Demonstrated mild joint stability in left shoulder.<br>Muscle functions: Left elbow flexor strength not demonstrated.<br>Movement functions: Voluntary control for moving left UE while maintaining greater stability due to skipping step.<br>Postural stability: Turns body in circles with slight rotation to left.<br>Adjusting, accommodation: Does not change movements or accommodate steps despite lack of success.<br>Sequencing: Skipped step of pulling jacket over right shoulder, thereby making it more difficult to reach other arm hole. |
| 5. Push left arm through the left arm hole. | • Body functions:<br>  • Cognitive functions: Recognize the need to sustain movement.<br>  • Proprioceptive function: Awareness of left arm position and adjustment of force to push through arm hole in relation to the space available.<br>  • Touch function: Discriminate when hand has gotten through arm hole.<br>  • Joint function: Good range and stability in left elbow extension.<br>  • Muscle functions: Good strength (left elbow extensors, left shoulder external rotation and flexion); minimal endurance needed.<br>  • Movement functions: Voluntary control for left arm.<br>• Performance skills<br>  • Coordination and other motor skills: Coordination required to keep from bumping into surroundings. | Social context: Aide picks up items Ani knocks off desk. | Spirituality and meaning: Smiles and comments, "I did it" (suggesting achieving independence in this activity is meaningful for her).<br>Cognitive function: Understands this to be end of activity as she turns to leave afterward.<br>Proprioceptive function: Lack of awareness of available body space (knocking items off desk).<br>Touch function: No signs of recognition of bumping into items on desk.<br>Coordination: Bumped arm into surrounding items.<br>Adjusting, accommodation: Does not attempt to adjust jacket even though she rubs the jacket against her face with her shoulders and when asked, responds it "doesn't feel good." |

Note: End of activity.

Based on this activity observation and analysis, Ani's occupational therapist identifies:

- Strengths supporting her performance with donning a jacket: motivation to participate and be independent, handles corrective feedback from classroom staff, good motivation, values positive statements from staff, follows verbal directions, adequate cognitive understanding of task
- Possible barriers for difficulties with donning a jacket independently: sequencing, visual perception, crossing midline, bilateral coordination, postural control, adjusting and accommodating, proprioceptive function

These possible barriers indicate areas for further assessment whether through observation or standardized assessments. Ultimately, all of Ani's evaluation results will be integrated to create more comprehensive hypotheses about Ani's occupational needs.

## BOX 9.8 CASE STUDY: ACTIVITY OBSERVATION AND ANALYSIS OF CUTTING ON A LINE FOR JACK

Jack is a 5-year-old kindergartener diagnosed with ADHD and an anxiety disorder. Since moving to stable housing and starting school 2 months ago, Jack has been gaining more self-control and managing his anger better overall. However, the teacher still struggles with managing Jack's resistance and angry outbursts for any activity that requires the use of scissors, pencils, or crayons, such as worksheets and crafts. The IEP team agrees to refer him for an occupational therapy evaluation to determine the nature of these challenges and how to best address them. As part of this evaluation, the occupational therapist plans to observe Jack in class participating in these activities of concern. To prepare, the occupational therapist mentally references general activity analyses such as the following one for cutting on a line with scissors.

| Steps | Activity Demands | Context |
|---|---|---|
| 1. Pick up scissors with handles proximal to body using dominant hand. | 1. Object: Scissors.<br>2. Body structures: Hand and fingers.<br>3. Body functions:<br>• Emotional functions: Regulated to control body.<br>• Visual function: Determine orientation and handles of scissors.<br>• Cognitive functions: Recognize or remember that scissors are used for cutting and used by one hand.<br>• Proprioceptive function: Adjust adequate force for lifting scissors.<br>• Touch function: Discrimination grip on handles for slight adjustments of grip.<br>• Joint function: Moderate stability of wrist, thumb, and forearm; minimal range of UE.<br>• Muscle functions: Fair strength in shoulder flexors and extensors, elbow extensors and flexors, finger extensors (second and third); good strength in wrist extensors, finger flexors (second and third), thumb abductors, flexors, and adductors (opposition), forearm supinators; mild endurance.<br>• Movement functions: Voluntary control for reach, grasp, and sustained UE position.<br>4. Performance skills:<br>• Postural stability: Hold body upright while sitting.<br>• Coordination and other motor skills: Fair coordination to adjust UE and accurately target handles of scissors; three-jaw chuck grasp.<br>• Locating: Where scissors are stored.<br>• Accommodation: Slight to maintain successful grasp. | Time: Less than 10 seconds to complete.<br>Location/space: Classrooms and homes; usually seated at a table; need enough space to move arms ("elbow room").<br>Sensory environment: Adequate lighting needed.<br>Social environment: Adults may direct children to cut within academic or craft activities.<br>Social-cultural developmental meanings and standards: By 4 years of age, most children are able to cut within ½" of a straight line but may not yet demonstrate hand dominance, with refined skill developing especially over the next 2 years.<br>Potential personal context: May include desire to be independent, create aesthetically pleasing products, please teachers or parents. |
| 2. Pick up paper with nondominant hand. | 1. Objects: Paper with line.<br>2. Body structures: Second hand and fingers.<br>3. Body functions:<br>• Visual function: Discriminate edge of paper.<br>• Cognitive functions: Understand that the paper is used in this activity.<br>• Proprioceptive function: Use light force of nondominant hand to prevent wrinkling or ripping paper; good awareness to sustain grasp of scissors and position of dominant UE.<br>• Touch function: Discrimination of edge of paper provides information for slight adjustments in grasping.<br>• Joint function: Moderate stability of wrist, thumb, and forearm; minimal range of UE.<br>• Muscle functions: Fair strength in shoulder flexors and extensors, elbow extensors and flexors, finger extensors (second and third); good strength in wrist extensors, finger flexors (second and third digits), thumb abductors, flexors, and adductors (opposition), forearm supinators; mild endurance.<br>• Movement functions: Voluntary control for reach, grasp, and sustained bilateral UE positions.<br>4. Performance skills:<br>• Coordination and other motor skills: Fair coordination to adjust UE and accurately target edge of paper; bilateral coordination to sustain different position with dominant UE; three-jaw chuck grasp.<br>• Locating: Where paper is stored.<br>• Accommodation: Slight for correct positioning of paper. | |

*Continued*

## BOX 9.8 CASE STUDY: ACTIVITY OBSERVATION AND ANALYSIS OF CUTTING ON A LINE FOR JACK—cont'd

| Steps | Activity Demands | Context |
|---|---|---|
| 3. Open scissors. | 1. Body functions:<br>• Visual function: Minimal to provide feedback about movement.<br>• Cognitive functions: Recognize or remember how scissors work.<br>• Proprioceptive function: Significant to adjust force for opening scissors midway, good awareness to sustain grasp of paper and position of nondominant UE.<br>• Touch function: Discrimination of handles provides information for slight adjustments to minimize slippage.<br>• Joint function: Moderate stability of shoulder, wrist, fingers, thumb, and forearm; moderate range of thumb CMC joint.<br>• Muscle functions: Good strength in finger extensors (second and third digits) and thumb abductors, extensors, and adductors; fair strength throughout UE (for isometric contractions); mild endurance.<br>• Movement functions: Voluntary control for thumb movement and sustained UE position.<br>2. Performance skills:<br>• Coordination and other motor skills: Fair coordination to adjust UE and accurately target edge of paper; bilateral coordination to sustain grasp of paper with nondominant UE.<br>• Accommodation: Slight for any slippage of handles. | |
| 4. Place paper in between open scissor blades, aligned with printed line. | 1. Body functions:<br>• Visual function: Discrimination of edge of paper, depth perception of scissor opening, tracking and saccades of moving paper edge and scissors.<br>• Cognitive functions: Recognize or remember paper and specifically line must fit between the scissor blades; attend to objects and movements.<br>• Proprioceptive function: Maintain steady force to prevent wrinkling or ripping paper; grading of force and body awareness to meet at midline (not over- or undershoot movement).<br>• Touch function: Discrimination of edge of paper provides information for slight adjustments in grasping to prevent slippage.<br>• Joint function: Moderate stability of bilateral shoulder, wrist, thumb, fingers, and forearm; minimal range of bilateral UE.<br>• Muscle functions: Fair strength throughout bilateral UE (for isometric contractions) and shoulder internal rotators; mild endurance.<br>• Movement functions: Voluntary control for bilateral shoulder internal rotation and sustained UE position.<br>2. Performance skills:<br>• Coordination and other motor skills: Bilateral coordination to move both UEs together symmetrically.<br>• Accommodation: Slight to align paper with open scissor blades. | |
| 5. Squeeze scissors closed and move forward, keeping blades aligned with lines of shape. | 1. Body functions:<br>• Visual function: Spatial and depth perception to align scissor blades with line on paper, discrimination to see both line and scissor blades.<br>• Cognitive functions: Attend specifically to line on paper and body movements.<br>• Proprioceptive function: Awareness to maintain bilateral UE positioning and grade movement of arms to prevent wrinkling or ripping paper.<br>• Touch function: Discrimination of paper and scissor handles provides information for slight adjustments in grasping to prevent slippage.<br>• Joint function: Moderate stability of bilateral shoulder, wrist, thumb, fingers, and forearm; minimal range for dominant finger flexion (second and third digits), dominant elbow extension, dominant shoulder flexion, dominant thumb abduction-flexion-adduction (opposition), nondominant elbow flexion, nondominant shoulder extension.<br>• Muscle functions: Fair strength throughout bilateral UE (for isometric contractions); good strength in finger flexors (second and third digits), thumb abductors, flexors, and adductors (opposition); mild endurance.<br>• Movement functions: Voluntary control for grasp, bilateral control and sustained UE position.<br>2. Performance skills:<br>• Coordination and other motor skills: Significant bilateral coordination for differential use of both UEs together; pace grasping action of dominant UE to time with nondominant UE positioning of paper.<br>• Accommodation: Slight to align paper with open scissor blades. | |

## BOX 9.8 CASE STUDY: ACTIVITY OBSERVATION AND ANALYSIS OF CUTTING ON A LINE FOR JACK—cont'd

| Steps | Activity Demands | Context |
|---|---|---|
| 6. Repeat steps 5–7 until complete. | Additional process skills: Notice and adjust nondominant hand placement on paper to accommodate performance; continue action until end of line; terminates at end of line. | |

Jack's occupational therapist then observes him at school during a simple classroom cutting activity with straight lines on a worksheet and makes the following notes:

- Goes to table with other children
- Does not pull chair up to table
- Sits on side of chair
- Picks up paper with right hand with arm pronated
- Picks up scissors from bin with left hand in backward orientation (pointing toward body) without supinating forearm
- Opens scissors
- Attends visually to watch scissors
- Puts paper between blades cutting several inches from line
- Crumples paper as he snips it
- Says "bad"
- Drops scissors and paper
- Therapist modifies:
- Emotional element: encourages and reassures ("I like how hard you are working. Sometimes cutting can be a little tricky, can I help you try again?")
- Sequencing objects: moves paper out of reach until he first grasps scissors
- Proprioceptive-tactile function for tool positioning: holds blades of scissors with handles proximal to him
- Says "yes"
- Picks up scissors with right hand
- Pronates both arms
- Puts paper between blades aligning within 1/16" of printed line
- Crumples paper with left hand (transitions into palmar grasp)
- Rips paper as he closes blades on the line (full elbow extension and 90-degree shoulder flexion of right)
- States "it's stupid"
- Drops paper and scissors on table
- Teacher tells him, "Good work, Jack. Keep going."
- Pushes paper and scissors away
- Leaves to look at book
- Other children have finished cutting and gluing the items on their worksheets within 1/4" accuracy and placed them in the teacher's bin

Jack's occupational therapist mentally compares these observations with the general activity analysis and determines:

- Strengths supporting his performance with cutting: motivation to initiate and perform at expected standard; responsiveness to encouragement and reassurance; adequate visual perception of printed line, edge of paper, and scissor handles; coordination for three-jaw chuck grasp; adequate hand strength; locating scissors; adequate cognitive understanding of standard use of scissors and expected standard for cutting performance
- Suspected barriers for cutting a line: sequencing, noticing and accommodating ineffective actions, proprioceptive function, calibrating force and speed of movement, emotional regulation (frustration tolerance)
- Questionable areas that require further assessment: tactile discrimination and joint/motor function for sustaining three-jaw chuck grasp on paper; joint range and strength for supination; hand dominance

To complete the evaluation, Jack's occupational therapist continues to assess both suspected barriers and questionable areas whether through observation or standardized assessments. All the evaluation results are integrated to create a comprehensive hypothesis about Jack's occupational needs as well as strengths.

A third purpose of evaluation is program planning. Standardized tests provide information about a child's level of function, and they help occupational therapists determine the appropriate starting point for therapy intervention. Most commonly, **criterion-referenced** standardized tests are used as the basis for developing goals and objectives for children and measuring progress and change over time.

**Types of Assessments.** Assessments can be nonstandardized or standardized. Nonstandardized assessments include observations, interviews, and checklists that have not been tested on populations. The results of nonstandardized assessments may inform intervention planning, but the scoring (if available) is viewed cautiously. Standardized assessments have established procedures, scoring, and interpretation guidelines. Standardized assessments include ipsative assessment, norm-referenced assessment, and criterion-referenced assessments.

***Ipsative Assessment.*** Ipsative assessment evaluates one's performance or perception against the prior evaluation outcomes. An **ipsative assessment** has standardized procedures for occupational therapists to measure the outcomes but does not have a norm or criteria with which to compare the results. Occupational therapists follow the instructed standardized methods for data collection and compare a child's results across time. Two common forms of ipsative assessment are interview- and observation-based assessments.

***Norm-Referenced Assessment.*** A **norm-referenced assessment** is developed by giving the test in question to a large number of children, usually several hundred or more. This group is called the *normative sample*, and norms, or average scores, are derived from this sample. When a norm-referenced test is administered, the performance of the child being tested is compared with that of the normative sample. The purpose of norm-referenced testing, then, is to determine how a child performs in relation to the average performance of the normative sample.

## CASE EXAMPLE 9.4 NORM-REFERENCED TESTING

Katelyn is a 5.5-year-old kindergarten student referred for occupational therapy assessment by her teacher, Mrs. Clark, who notes that Katelyn is having difficulty learning to write; she holds her pencil awkwardly and exerts too much pressure on the paper. On the playground, she has difficulty keeping up with her peers, falls frequently, appears uncoordinated, and has difficulty learning new motor skills. Her energy level is low. She is easily overwhelmed by typical classroom activity and often has emotional outbursts, which affect her ability to complete her work and interact with classmates.

The occupational therapist, David, spoke to Katelyn's parents and discovered that Katelyn received physical therapy as an infant because of low muscle tone and slow achievement of developmental milestones. Her parents were worried about her ability to cope with the increase in writing assignments in first grade and her social acceptance by other children.

David considered Katelyn's age (5.5 years) and the areas of concern (gross and fine motor skills and social adjustment) in choosing which standardized tests to use. He decided to administer the Peabody Developmental Motor Scales (PDMS-2), along with clinical observations of Katelyn's posture, muscle tone, strength, balance, motor planning, hand use, hand preference, attention, problem-solving skills, and visual skills. He asked Katelyn's teacher to complete the School Function Assessment to provide information on Katelyn's performance of functional school-related behaviors. In addition, he had the teacher complete the Sensory Processing Measure (SPM-2) Classroom Form to determine whether sensory processing problems were contributing to Katelyn's motor delays.

### Test Results

Katelyn's testing session was scheduled at midmorning to avoid possible effects of fatigue or hunger. She attended well, although she needed encouragement for the more challenging items. By the end of the session, she complained of fatigue, but David believed he got a representative sample of Katelyn's motor skills and that the scores obtained were reliable.

On the PDMS-2, Katelyn received a gross motor quotient of 81, placing her at the 10th percentile for her age. Her fine motor quotient was 76, placing her at the 5th percentile. In the gross motor area, ball skills were an area of relative strength, but she had difficulty with balance activities and activities involving hopping, skipping, and jumping. In the fine motor area, Katelyn used a static tripod grasp on the pencil, frequently shifting into a fisted grasp if the writing task was challenging. Based on the small number of visual-motor items on this test, visual perceptual skills appeared to be an area of strength, whereas tasks involving speed and dexterity were difficult.

David found that Katelyn had low muscle tone overall, particularly in the shoulder girdle and hands, and strength was somewhat decreased overall. Katelyn's endurance was poor. Motor planning difficulties were evident in the way she handled test materials and moved about the environment. She had difficulty devising alternate ways to accomplish tasks that were challenging for her and required manual guidance to complete some tasks.

David obtained a functional profile on the School Function Assessment based on Mrs. Clark's responses to the items on the test. On the scales of recreational movement, using materials, clothing management, written work, and task behavior and/or completion, Katelyn received scores below the cutoff for her grade level. Other scales were within grade-level expectations, with strengths in the scales of memory and understanding, following social conventions, and personal care awareness.

On the SPM-2, scores indicated that Katelyn had definite differences in visual, auditory, and body awareness. The scale confirmed that she could easily become overloaded by environmental stimuli.

### Observations and Recommendations

According to her scores on the PDMS-2, Katelyn had mild delays in her gross motor skills and mild to moderate delays in her fine motor skills. Although David believed that the PDMS-2 gave a good indication of what Katelyn could do under optimal circumstances (i.e., a nondistracting environment, individual attention and encouragement, and structuring of tasks to maximize success and minimize frustration), he also thought it did not represent the level of performance that would be seen over the course of a typical day.

In the classroom, David observed that Katelyn avoided motor activities and completed writing and drawing activities rapidly, resulting in poor quality of the end product. Her materials were disorganized, she required multiple reminders to complete tasks, and she became upset when unable to finish on time. Her School Function Assessment results indicated that her performance of tasks involving fine and gross motor coordination and task organization was below grade-level expectations.

Standardized testing, specifically the PDMS-2, School Function Assessment, and SPM, provided a helpful framework for David's assessment of Katelyn and gave specific information about areas of strength and difficulty. David made use of his clinical observations and information gathering from a variety of sources to recommend interventions he felt would be beneficial, efficient, and relatively easy to implement. The standardized scores helped him identify Katelyn's problems in fine and gross motor skills, and the test items provided activities that revealed the challenges Katelyn faced when performing motor tasks.

However, if David had simply relied on the standardized test scores, he would not have acquired the breadth of knowledge that led to his decision-making process for developing intervention options. This example illustrates the important roles of both standardized testing and other methods of data collection in arriving at meaningful and realistic conclusions about children's intervention needs and modes of service delivery.

---

Test developers generally attempt to include children from a variety of geographic locations, ethnic and racial backgrounds, and socioeconomic levels so that the normative sample is representative of the population of the United States, based on the most recent US census data. Generally, the normative sample is composed of children who have no developmental delays or conditions, although many tests include data from subsamples of clinical populations as a means of determining whether the test discriminates between children whose development is proceeding normally and those who have known developmental delays.

Norm-referenced tests address one or more areas of behavior. If the test evaluates more than one area, each area typically has one or more subtests. Items are chosen to represent a broad range of skills within these composite areas, and developers often will select the items that had the best discriminative ability between typical and atypical populations. Additionally, items are chosen to incorporate materials and activities that are reasonably familiar and typical for children of the age group being tested. A child's performance on an individual test item is not as important as the overall subtest or area score. However, it is important for the occupational therapist to observe the quality and characteristics of a child's performance on each item, as these qualitative observations provide important information to complement the obtained standard scores.

Norm-referenced tests have standardized protocols for administration and scoring. The tester must adhere to these protocols so that each test administration is as similar as possible to that of the normative sample. This is necessary to compare any child's performance fairly with that of the normative sample.

Sometimes the examiner must deviate from the standard protocol because of the needs of the child being tested. For instance, a child with visual impairments may need manual guidance to cut with scissors, or a child with cerebral palsy (CP) may need assistance stabilizing the shoulder and upper arm to reach and grasp a crayon. If changes are made in the standardized procedures, the examiner indicates this in the summary of assessment, and standard scores cannot be used to describe that child's performance in comparison with the normative sample.

Norm-referenced tests have specific psychometric properties. They have been analyzed by statisticians to obtain score distributions, mean or average scores, and standard scores. This is done to achieve the primary objective of norm-referenced tests: comparability of scores with the normative sample. A test under development initially has a much larger number of items than the final version of the test. Through pilot testing, items are chosen or rejected based partly on how well they statistically discriminate between children of different ages and/or abilities. Items are not chosen primarily for their relevance to functional skills. Consequently, most norm-referenced tests are not intended to link test performance with specific objectives or goals for intervention.

***Criterion-Referenced Assessment.*** A **criterion-referenced assessment**, by contrast, is designed to provide information on how children perform on specific tasks. The term *criterion-referenced* refers to the fact that a child's performance is compared with a criterion, or level of performance of a skill. The goal of a criterion-referenced test is to determine which skills a child can and cannot accomplish, thereby providing a focus for intervention. In general, the content of a criterion-referenced test is detailed and, in some cases, may relate to specific behavioral or functional objectives. The intent of a criterion-referenced test is to measure a child's performance on specific tasks rather than to compare the child's performance with that of their peers.

Many developmental checklists have been field tested and then published as criterion-referenced tests. Administration and scoring procedures may or may not be standardized on a criterion-referenced test. Many other criterion-referenced tests take the form of checklists, in which the specific performance needed to receive credit on an item is not indicated. Many therapist-designed tests for use in a facility or setting are nonstandardized, criterion-referenced tests.

Criterion-referenced tests are not subjected to the statistical analyses performed on norm-referenced tests. No mean score or normal distribution is calculated; a child may pass all items or fail all items on a test without adversely affecting the validity of the test results. The purpose of the test is to learn exactly what a child can accomplish, not to compare the child's performance with that of the peer group. This goal is also reflected in the test development process for criterion-referenced tests. Items are generally chosen based on a process of task analysis or identification of important developmental milestones rather than for their statistical validity. Therefore, the specific items on a criterion-referenced test have a direct relationship with functional skills and can be used as a starting point for generating appropriate goals and objectives for therapy intervention.

The characteristics of norm- and criterion-referenced tests are compared in Table 9.8. As is shown in the table, some tests are both norm and criterion referenced. This means that although the items have been analyzed for their ability to perform statistically, they also reflect functional or developmental skills that are appropriate for intervention. These tests permit the occupational therapist to compare a child's performance with that of peers in the normative sample, and they also provide information about specific skills that may be appropriate for remediation.

Standardized tests can also be categorized as performance based or self-report. *Self-report* tests collect data on the child's performance, behavior, or participation in daily activities and natural environments from adults such as parents, caregivers, teachers, or therapists who interact regularly with the child or from the child himself or herself. The advantage of self-report tests is that the score represents typical or usual behavior, performance, or participation based on multiple observations of the child in different times and places. The disadvantage of self-report tests is that respondents may not carefully read or understand the test instructions or may answer according to what they believe the evaluator wants to hear. Clarity of questions and criteria for respondent ratings is crucial to the quality of a self-report test. Test development procedures include data collection from potential respondents so that they can provide input to ensure that the test content is meaningful, and the items and procedures are easily understandable (Kramer et al., 2012). Careful instruction of respondents at the time of the evaluation can also facilitate accuracy of responses.

**Characteristics and Testing Mechanics.** In general, each type of assessment (interview-based assessment; observation-based assessment; performance-based assessment; and self-report or parent report questionnaire) has its unique testing mechanics, so therapists are

**TABLE 9.8 Comparison of Norm-Referenced and Criterion-Referenced Tests**

| Characteristic | Norm-Referenced Test | Criterion-Referenced Test |
|---|---|---|
| Purpose | Comparison of child's performance with normative sample | Comparison of child's performance with a defined list of skills |
| Content | General; usually covers a wide variety of skills | Detailed; may cover specific objectives or developmental milestones |
| Administration and scoring | Always standardized | May be standardized or nonstandardized |
| Psychometric properties | Normal distribution of scores; means, standard deviations, and standard scores computed | No score distribution needed; a child may pass or fail all items |
| Item selection | Items chosen for statistical performance; may not relate to functional skills or therapy objectives | Items chosen for functional and developmental importance; provides necessary information for developing therapy objectives |
| Examples | BSID-III; PDMS-2; BO-2; PEDI-CAT | PDMS-2, PEDI-CAT, HELP, gross motor function measure, SFA |

*BO-2*, Bruininks-Oseretsky Test of Motor Proficiency (2nd ed.) (Bruininks & Bruininks, 2005); *BSID-III*, Bayley Scales of Infant and Toddler Development (3rd ed.) (Bayley, 2006); *HELP*, Hawaii Early Learning Profile (Parks, 2004); *PDMS*, Peabody Developmental Motor Scales (Folio & Fewell, 2000); *PEDI-CAT*, Pediatric Evaluation of Disability Inventory Computer Adaptive Test (Haley et al., 1992); *SFA*, School Function Assessment (Coster et al., 1998).

required to follow the test user manuals and guidelines. As stated, standardized tests have uniform procedures for administration and scoring. These standard procedures permit the results of a child's tests to be compared either with the child's performance on a previous administration of the test or with the test norms developed by administration of the test to many children.

Standardized tests characteristically include a test manual that describes the purpose of the test (i.e., what the test is intended to measure). The manual should also describe the intended population for the test. For pediatric assessments, this generally refers to the age range of children for whom the test was intended, but it may also refer to specific diagnoses or types of functional impairments. Test manuals also contain technical information about the test, such as a description of the test development and standardization process, characteristics of the normative sample, and studies done during the test development process to establish reliability and validity data. Finally, test manuals contain detailed information about the administration, scoring, and interpretation of the test scores.

Another characteristic of standardized tests is that they are composed of a fixed number of items. Items may not be added or subtracted without affecting the standard procedure for test administration. Most tests have specific rules about the number of items that should be administered to ensure a standardized test administration. These rules may differ significantly from test to test.

A third characteristic of standardized tests is fixed protocol for administration. The term *fixed protocol for administration* refers to the way each item is administered and the number of items administered. This is not the place for occupational therapists' creativity. The manual dictates what should be done. Generally, the protocol for administration specifies the verbal instruction or demonstration to be provided, the number of times the instructions can be repeated, and the number of attempts the child is allowed on the item. For some tests, instructions for each item are printed in the manual, and the tester is expected to read the instructions verbatim to the child without deviating from the text. However, other tests allow for more freedom of instruction, especially when the test involves a physical activity.

**Scoring Methods.** Standardized tests also have a fixed guideline for scoring. Scoring guidelines specify what the child's performance must look like to receive a score on the item. Depending on the nature of the item, passing performance may be described using text, a picture, or a diagram.

Standardized tests are scored in several different ways. Scoring methods include *Z*-scores, *T*-scores, deviation intelligence quotient (IQ) scores, developmental index scores, percentile scores, and age-equivalent scores. Many of these scores are based on the normal distribution and standard deviations.

**Test Psychometrics.** Standardized assessments have been examined to determine their validity and reliability. It is the responsibility of the test developers to provide such information. It is the responsibility of occupational therapists who use these tools to comprehend the technical aspects of standardized tests related to their reliability and validity.

In classical testing theory, a measurement error is assumed, so the testing score reflects the true score and measurement error. When researchers develop a test, they examine the reliability to make sure it is close to the true score and minimizes the measurement error. It is thus important to know whether reliability was established in certain populations or samples.

The reliability of a test describes the consistency or stability of scores obtained by one individual when tested on two different occasions with different sets of items or under other examining conditions (Urbina, 2004). For instance, if a child is given a test and receives a score of 50 and 2 days later the child is given the same test and receives a score of 75, the reliability of the test is questionable. The difference between the two scores is called the error variance of the test, which is a result of random fluctuations in performance between the two testing sessions. Some amount of random error variance is expected in any test situation because of variations in such things as mood, fatigue, or motivation. Error variance can also be caused by environmental characteristics such as light, temperature, or noise. However, it is important that error variance caused by variations in examiners or by the characteristics of the test itself be minimal. Confidence in the scores obtained requires that the test have adequate reliability over a number of administrations and have low error variance.

Most standardized tests developers evaluate two or three forms of reliability. The three forms of reliability most commonly used in pediatric standardized tests are (1) test-retest reliability, (2) interrater reliability, and (3) standard error of measurement (SEM). Reliability scores are often presented in a correlation coefficient (*r*) or Cohen's kappa coefficient (*k*). They are used to examine how closely the tests are either at different times (test-retest), by different raters (interrater), or between subtests of test (split-half).

*Test-retest reliability* is a measurement of the stability of a test over time. It is obtained by giving the test to the same individual on two different occasions. In the evaluation of test-retest reliability for a pediatric test, the time span between test administrations must be short to minimize the possibility of developmental changes occurring between the two test sessions. However, the time span between tests should not be so short that the child may recall items administered during the first test session, thereby improving their performance on the second test session, which is also called learning or practice effect.

During the process of test development, test-retest reliability is evaluated on a subgroup of the sample. The size and composition of the subgroup should be specified in the manual. The *correlation coefficient* between the scores of the two test sessions is the measure of the test-retest reliability. A test that has a high test-retest reliability coefficient is more likely to yield relatively stable scores over time. That is, it is affected less by random error variance than is a test with a low test-retest reliability coefficient. When administering a test with a low test-retest reliability coefficient, the examiner has less confidence that the score obtained is a true reflection of the child's abilities. If the child were tested at a different time of day or in a different setting entirely, different results might be obtained.

*Interrater reliability* refers to the ability of two independent raters to obtain the same scores when scoring the same child simultaneously. Interrater reliability is generally measured on a subset of the sample during the test development process. This is often accomplished by having one rater administer and score the test while another rater observes and scores at the same time. The correlation coefficient calculated from the two raters' scores is the interrater reliability coefficient of the test. It is particularly important to measure interrater reliability on tests for which the scoring may require some judgment on the part of the examiner. In the test manuals, interrater reliability is often presented by Cohen's kappa or intraclass correlation coefficient.

Although the scoring criteria for many test items are specific on most tests, scoring depends to a certain extent on individual judgment, and scoring differences can arise among different examiners. A test that has a low interrater reliability coefficient is especially susceptible to differences in scoring by different raters. This may mean that the administration and scoring criteria are not stated explicitly enough, requiring examiners to make judgment calls on several items. Alternatively, it can mean that the items on the test call for responses that are too broad or vague to permit precise scoring.

Examiners can exert some control over the interrater reliability of tests they use frequently. It is good practice for examiners to check interrater reliability with more experienced colleagues when learning a new standardized test before beginning to administer the test to children in the clinical setting. Also, periodic checking of interrater reliability with colleagues who are administering the same standardized tests is a good practice.

For self-report tests, interrater reliability is generally not a meaningful indicator of the psychometric integrity of the test, because everyone who contributes information to the test does so based on knowledge of the child in a specific environment with unique demands and perceptions. However, because different raters may be evaluating the child on similar constructs, some agreement between ratings should be expected. This is known as cross-rater concordance and is a measure of the validity of the instrument rather than reliability.

No universal agreement has been reached regarding the minimum acceptable coefficient for test-retest and interrater reliability. The context of the reliability measurement, the type of test, and the distribution of scores are some of the variables that can be considered when determining an acceptable reliability coefficient. One standard used by several examiners is 0.80 (Urbina, 2004).

Not all tests have test-retest or interrater reliability coefficients that reach the 0.80 level. Lower coefficients indicate greater variability in scores. When examiners use a test that has a reliability coefficient below 0.80, scores must be interpreted with great caution. For example, if one subtest of a test of motor development has test retest reliability of 0.60, the examiner who uses it to measure change over time must acknowledge that a portion of the apparent change between the first and second test administration is a result of the error variance of the test.

When individual subtests of a comprehensive test have a low reliability coefficient, it is generally not recommended that the standard scores from the subtests be reported. Often the reliability coefficient of the entire test is much higher than that of the individual subtests. One reason for this is that reliability increases with the number of items on a test. Because subtests have fewer items than the entire test, they are more sensitive to fluctuations in the performance or scoring of individual items. When this occurs, it is best to describe subtest performance qualitatively, without reporting standard scores.

Standard scores can be reported for the total, or comprehensive, test score. Examiners should consult the reliability information in the test manual before deciding how to report test scores for individual subtests and for the test. The test-retest and interrater reliability coefficients reported in the manual are estimates based on the context and conditions used during test development and may vary when children are tested in different contexts or when examiners have differing levels of training and experience.

The *standard error of measurement (SEM)* is a statistic used to calculate the expected range of error for the test score of an individual. It is based on the range of scores an individual might obtain if the same test were administered several times simultaneously, with no practice or fatigue effects. Obviously, this is impossible; the SEM therefore is a theoretical construct. However, it is an indicator of the possible error variance in individual scores.

The SEM creates a normal curve for the individual's test scores, with the obtained score in the middle of the distribution. The child has a higher probability of receiving scores in the middle of the distribution than at the extreme ends. The SEM is based on the standard deviation of the test and the test's reliability (usually the test-retest reliability). Once the SEM has been calculated for a test, that value is added to and subtracted from the child's obtained score. This gives the range of expected scores for that child, a range known as the confidence interval. The SEM corresponds to the standard deviation for the normal curve: 68% of the scores in a normal distribution fall within one standard deviation on either side of the mean, 95% of the scores fall within two standard deviations on either side of the mean, and 99.7% of the scores fall within three standard deviations on either side of the mean. Similarly, a child receives a score within one SEM on either side of his or her obtained score 68% of the time; a score within two SEM of the obtained score 95% of the time; and a score within three SEM of the obtained score 99.7% of the time.

Consideration of the SEM is especially important when the differences between two scores are evaluated (e.g., when the progress a child has made with therapy over time is evaluated) (Urbina, 2004). If the confidence intervals of the two test scores overlap, it may be incorrect to conclude that any change has occurred. For instance, a child is tested in September and receives a raw score of 60. The child is tested again in June with the same test and receives a raw score of 75. Comparison of the two raw scores would seem to indicate that the child has made substantial progress. However, the scores should be considered in light of an SEM of 5.0. Using a 95% confidence interval (the 95% confidence interval is two SEM on either side of the obtained score), the confidence interval for the first score is 50–70, and the confidence interval of the second score is 65–85.

Generally, test manuals report the 95% confidence interval. As can be seen by the preceding equation, when the standard deviation of the test is high, or the reliability is low, the SEM increases. A larger SEM means that the range of possible scores for an individual child is much greater (i.e., a larger confidence interval), and consequently the degree of possible error is greater. This means that the examiner is less confident that any score obtained for a child on that test represents the child's true score.

**Validity.** Validity is the extent to which a test measures what it claims it measures (Urbina, 2004). For example, it is important for testers to know that a test of fine motor development measures fine motor skills and not gross motor or perceptual skills. The validity of a test must be established with reference to the use for which the test is being considered (Urbina, 2004). For instance, a test of fine motor development is probably highly valid as a measure of fine motor skills. It is less valid as a measure of visual motor skills and has low validity as a measure of gross motor skills.

The information on validity reported in test manuals has been obtained during the test development process. In addition, after a test becomes available commercially, clinicians and researchers continue to evaluate validity and to publish the results of their validation studies. This information about test validity can help examiners make decisions about appropriate uses of standardized tests. The four categories of validity are construct-related validity, content-related validity, criterion-related validity, and Rasch analysis.

*Construct-related validity* is the extent to which a test measures a theoretical construct. Some constructs frequently measured by pediatric occupational therapists include fine motor skills, visual perceptual skills, self-care skills, gross motor skills, and functional performance at home or school. One method of establishing construct validity involves investigating how well a test discriminates among different groups of individuals. For instance, a developmental test is expected to differentiate between the performance of older and younger children. Older children should receive higher scores than younger children, providing clear evidence of developmental progression with advancing age.

Because these tests are also intended to discriminate between typically developing children and children with developmental delays, children in specific diagnostic categories should receive lower scores than children with no documented deficits.

Factor analysis can be used as another method of establishing construct-related validity. Factor analysis is a statistical procedure for determining relationships between test items. In a test of motor skills that includes gross motor items and fine motor items, factor analysis is expected to identify two factors on which items showed the strongest correlation, one composed mostly of gross motor items and one composed mostly of fine motor items.

Another method of establishing construct-related validity requires repeated administration of a test before and after a period of intervention. For example, a group of children are given a test of visual-perceptual skills and subsequently receive intervention focused on improving those skills. They are then retested with the same test and the difference in scores is analyzed. A rise in test scores supports the assertion that the test measures visual perceptual skills and provides evidence of construct-related validity.

*Content-related validity* is the extent to which the items on a test accurately sample a behavior domain. For instance, to test self-care skills, it is impractical to ask a child to perform every conceivable self-care activity. A sample of self-care activities must be chosen for inclusion on the test, and conclusions can be drawn about the child's abilities based on the selected items. Examiners must have confidence that self-care skills are adequately represented so that accurate conclusions regarding the child's self-care skills can be made. Test manuals should show evidence that the authors have systematically analyzed the domain being tested. Content validity is established by review of the test content by experts in the field, who reach some agreement that the content is, in fact, representative of the behavioral domain to be measured.

*Criterion-related validity* is the ability of a test to predict how an individual performs on other measurements or activities. To establish criterion-related validity, the test score is checked against a criterion, an independent measure of what the test is designed to predict. The two forms of criterion-related validity are concurrent validity and predictive validity.

Concurrent validity describes how well test scores reflect current performance. The degree of relationship between the test and the criterion is described with a correlation coefficient. Most validity correlation coefficients range from 0.40 to 0.80; a coefficient of 0.70 or above indicates that performance on one test can predict performance on a second test. Concurrent validity is examined in the test development process to determine the relationship between a new test and existing tests that measure a similar construct.

In contrast with concurrent validity, *predictive validity* identifies the relationship between a test given in the present and some measure of performance in the future. Establishing predictive validity is a much lengthier process than establishing other forms of validity because often several years must elapse between the first and second testing sessions. The predictive validity of a test often is not well documented until it has been in use for several years.

One final point about criterion-related validity: the meaningfulness of the comparison between a test and its criterion measure depends on both the quality of the test and the quality of the criterion. Because no single measure of criterion-related validity provides conclusive evidence of the test's validity, multiple investigations should be undertaken. Important standardized assessments undergo extensive evaluation of validity after publication. The resulting information helps the test user decide when and with whom the test results are most valid.

### BOX 9.9 Things to Consider When Selecting a Test

- Child's age and test's age range
- Area of performance to be assessed and the coverage of the test items
- Time requirement and space available to administer the test
- Availability of all required materials to administer the test
- Therapist's competence level
- Psychometrics of the test
- Cost of the test
- Online or in-person administration

Validity is an important but sometimes elusive concept that rests on judgments by authors of the tests, users of the tests, and experts in the field. It is important to remember that validity is not absolute and that a test that is valid in one setting or with one group of children may not be valid for other uses. Test users must not assume that because a test has been developed and published for commercial distribution that it is universally useful and appropriate. An examiner applies their clinical knowledge and experience, knowledge of normal and abnormal development, and understanding of an individual child's situation when deciding whether test findings are a valid measure of the child's abilities.

See Appendix A for a list of assessments commonly used in occupational therapy. It may also be appropriate to consult other sources for information about a test. The Twenty-First Mental Measurements Yearbook (Carlson et al., 2021) and Tests in Print X (Anderson et al., 2022) publish descriptions and critical reviews of commercially available standardized tests written by testing experts. Box 9.9 lists items to inform test selection.

**Becoming a Competent Test User.** Occupational therapists need to develop skills to ensure competency in administering assessments. Preparation is key for an optimal test situation. Interview and observation are essential skills in administering a standardized assessment, so prior to using an assessment, occupational therapists must first develop solid skills in interview and observation.

Potential examiners can take specific steps to ensure that they administer and score a test reliably. These steps also help examiners interpret test results accurately so that they provide a valid representation of each child's abilities. The steps to becoming a competent user of standardized tests are summarized in Box 9.10. First, the occupational therapist needs to understand the structure of the test by reading the manual. It is important to study the test manual to obtain knowledge of the assessment, develop an understanding of the details in administering procedures and psychometric properties, as well as logistics to determine if this assessment is suitable for the child and/or clinical settings. Next, the occupational therapist observes and practices administration to make sure they have the correct setup and environment and can use the materials and testing procedures indicated in the user manual competently. In addition to administering and scoring techniques, the occupational therapist reviews the technical attributes of the test, paying close attention to the size and composition of the normative sample, reliability coefficients, validation data, and the intended population for the test. The examiner determines if the standardized administration procedures can be altered for children with special needs without compromising the findings. The occupational therapist determines how the scores should be reported and interpreted if the standardized procedure is changed.

**BOX 9.10 Steps to Becoming a Competent Test User**

1. Study the test manual.
2. Observe experienced examiners, and discuss your observations.
3. Practice administering and scoring the test.
4. Check interrater agreement with an experienced examiner.
5. Prepare administration and scoring cue sheets.
6. Prepare the testing environment, and make sure the setup adheres to the test manual.
7. Consult with experienced examiners about test interpretation.
8. Periodically recheck interrater agreement.

**Selecting and Preparing the Optimal Testing Environment.** The testing environment should meet the specifications stated in the test manual. Generally, the manual specifies a well-lighted room free of visual or auditory distractions. If a separate room is not available, a screen or room divider can be used to partition off a corner of the room. Testing should be scheduled at a time when the child is able to perform optimally. For young children, caregivers should be consulted about the best time of day for testing so that the test session does not interfere with naps or feedings. Older children's school or other activities should be considered in the scheduling of assessments. For instance, a child who has just come from recess or a vigorous physical education session may have decreased endurance for gross motor testing activities.

The test environment should be ready before the child arrives. Child-sized furniture that allows children to sit at a table and rest their feet flat on the floor and can comfortably reach items on the table should be used. If a child uses a wheelchair or other adaptive seating, they should be allowed to sit in the equipment during testing. Infants or young children generally are best seated on the caregiver's lap unless items on the test specify otherwise. The examiner places the test kit where they can easily access items but not where the child can see or reach the kit. Often a low chair placed next to the examiner's chair is a good place to put a test kit.

Most importantly, the examiner must be so familiar with the test that their attention can be focused on the child's behavior and not on the mechanics of administering the test. This is a critical part of preparation because much valuable information can be lost if the examiner is unable to carefully observe the quality of the child's responses because they instead must devote energy to finding test materials or looking through the test manual. In addition, young children's attention spans can be short, and the examiner must be able to take full advantage of the limited time the child is able to attend to the activities.

Familiarity with the test also allows the examiner to change the pace of activities if necessary. The child can be given a brief break to play, have a snack, or use the bathroom while the examiner interviews the caregiver or jots down notes. Most standardized tests have some flexibility about the order or arrangement of item sets, and an examiner who knows the test can use this to their advantage. Sometimes, because of the child's fatigue or behavior or because of time constraints, a test cannot be administered completely in one session. Most tests provide guidelines for administering the test in two sessions, and examiners should be familiar with these guidelines before starting to test.

**Advantages and Disadvantages of Standardized Testing.** Standardized tests provide occupational therapists and other professionals a more scientific approach to assessment. Statistically valid numeric scores from standardized testing provide credible evidence to the assessment process. Standardized tests have several characteristics that make them a unique part of the assessment inventory of pediatric occupational therapists. For example, they are tests that in general are well known and commercially available. This means that a child's scores on a test can be interpreted and understood by therapists in other practice settings or geographic locations.

*Standard scores* generated by standardized tests allow testers from a variety of professional disciplines to "speak the same language" when it comes to discussing test scores. For example, a child may be tested by an occupational therapist for fine motor skills, by a physical therapist for gross motor skills, and by a speech pathologist for language skills. All three tests express scores as T-scores. An average T-score is 50. The child receives a fine motor T-score of 30, a gross motor T-score of 25, and a language T-score of 60. It is apparent that although this child is below average in both gross and fine motor skills, language skills are an area of strength; in fact, they are above average. These scores can be compared and discussed by the assessment team, and they can be used to identify areas requiring intervention and areas in which the child has strengths.

Standardized tests can be used to monitor developmental progress. Because they are norm-referenced according to age, the progress of a child with developmental delays can be measured against expected developmental progress compared with the normative sample. In this way, occupational therapists can determine if children receiving therapy are accelerating their rate of development because of intervention. Similarly, children who are monitored after discharge from therapy can be assessed periodically to determine whether they are maintaining the expected rate of developmental progress or are beginning to fall behind their peers without the assistance of intervention.

Standardized tests can be used for program evaluation to determine response to intervention across many clients. Standard test scores can be subjected to statistical analysis to evaluate efficacy of interventions. These data can contribute to evidence-based practice and provide information about areas of strength and weakness in the intervention program that can be addressed through quality improvement processes.

However, standardized tests are not without their drawbacks. A standardized test cannot stand alone as a measure of a child's abilities. Clinical judgment, informal or unstructured observation, caregiver interviews, and data gathering from other informants are all essential parts of the assessment process. These less structured evaluation procedures are needed to provide meaning and interpretation for the numeric scores obtained by standardized testing.

Occupational therapists consider several other factors when using performance-based standardized tests. For example, a test session provides only a brief "snapshot" of a child's behavior and abilities. The child's performance during a 1-hour assessment in a clinic setting may differ from their performance daily at home or at school. Illness, fatigue, anxiety, lack of familiarity with materials, the room, or the tester can adversely affect a child's performance. The tester must be sensitive to the possible impact of these factors on the child's performance.

A competent tester can do a great deal to alleviate a child's anxiety about testing and ensure that the experience is pleasant. However, test situations are artificial and may not provide an accurate indication of how the child performs daily. Therefore, it is important for occupational therapists to speak to the child's parent, caregiver, or teacher at the time of testing to determine whether the observed behavior is truly representative of the child's typical performance. The occupational therapist considers the parent, caregiver, or teacher feedback regarding the test setting behaviors when interpreting and reporting findings.

Another concern about standardized tests is the rigidity of the testing procedures themselves. Standardized tests specify ways of administering test items and, in many cases, exactly what instructions the tester must give. In view of these administration requirements, children who have difficulty understanding verbal instruction (e.g., children with autism, hearing impairment, or attention-deficit disorder) or lack control of movement (e.g., muscle weakness, lack of coordination) may be disadvantaged on performance-based tests. Although this issue is not addressed by all standardized tests, some provide guidelines for administering the test under nonstandard conditions, and some are specifically designed to evaluate functional performance and participation of children with disabilities using performance- and observation-based formats.

It is important to reiterate that although it is permissible to alter the administration procedures of most performance-based tests to accommodate children's individual needs, the child's performance cannot be expressed as a standard score. Rather, the purpose of the testing is to provide a structured format for describing the child's performance. The test manual should always be consulted for guidelines on alterations in test procedures.

**Interpreting Performance.** Occupational therapists use knowledge of test properties, client factors, and contextual factors along with professional reasoning skills to draw conclusions about a child's performance based on the standard scores obtained. In addition to the guidelines and interpretation standards specified in the test manual, the examiner considers several other factors when interpreting an individual child's performance. Specifically, the occupational therapist interprets test results after considering the following questions:

1. How representative or typical was the child's response to the testing situation?
2. If the child did not perform optimally during testing, what influenced the child's performance?
3. Are the scores congruent with observations or reports by caregivers, teachers, or other professionals?
4. How closely do the test scores obtained by the occupational therapist concur with standardized or nonstandardized test results of other professionals or from previous testing?
5. What may be reasons for possible discrepancies?
6. Which strategies used during the testing were effective or ineffective in organizing, motivating, or facilitating the child's best performance?
7. Did the tests administered provide a complete picture of the child's occupational performance and participation, or is additional testing, observation, or interview required?

When a parent observes testing, the occupational therapist asks the parent if the child's performance was typical. The parent's judgment of the child's performance during testing can be included in the report of findings. The occupational therapist also examines how the child performed on different tests with other professionals or in other environments. For example, a child may perform differently on tasks requiring movement than those involving speech. Understanding the situations in which the child performs better can signify areas of strength. The occupational therapist analyzes the performance demands or expectations in various environments, characteristics, and environmental supports provided to the child; levels of tolerance for the child's behavior; and the child's ability in different developmental or performance domains (which may be identified when several disciplines are evaluating a child).

Evaluating and discussing the efficacy of management strategies can provide important information to augment test results and recommendations. These observations and findings may influence interpretation of test scores and provide insight into the child's needs. For more information about interpretation of results, please see Chapter 10.

**Ethical Consideration in Testing.** Pediatric occupational therapists who use standardized tests in their practice must be aware of their responsibilities to the children they evaluate and to their families. Urbina (2004) describes several ethical issues relevant to standardized testing, including (1) examiner competency, (2) client privacy, (3) communication of test results, and (4) cultural bias. See Table 9.9 for a description of these issues.

## SPECIFIC CONSIDERATIONS FOR EVALUATION OF OCCUPATIONAL PERFORMANCE

For each of the areas that a therapist may evaluate, there are specific considerations that may be uniquely important for that area of occupation. Each of the chapter authors from this edition, as well as some authors from the last edition, contributed their expertise to developing the content that follows. Additionally, there are specific assessment tools that authors have recommended for each of the areas, and those are provided in Appendix A. For a listing of all of the contributors to this chapter, please see Table 9.10.

## EVALUATION OF FEEDING AND EATING

Occupational therapists evaluate feeding and eating challenges that may result from lack of experience, medical conditions, sensory, physical, and psychosocial factors. Feeding and eating is essential to growth and development and tied closely to family culture, values, and traditions.

### Importance of Feeding and Eating for Child and Family Functioning

Feeding and swallowing difficulties can have significant health implications, including adverse effects on growth, nutrition, overall development, and general well-being. When infants or children have feeding challenges, it puts strain and stress on the caregivers and alters the dynamics of mealtime for all. Mealtime is often a social experience, involving family and friends. Therefore, feeding difficulties have the potential to alter family social participation as well.

### Common Challenges Associated With Feeding and Eating

Children develop difficulties with feeding, eating, and/or swallowing because of medical, oral, sensorimotor, and behavioral factors, either alone or in combination. A variety of medical conditions can influence a child's ability and willingness to participate in oral feeding. Some of the most common medical issues associated with feeding dysfunction include prematurity, neuromuscular abnormalities, structural malformations (such as cleft lip and/or palate), gastrointestinal conditions, visual impairments, and tracheostomies. In addition, therapists who specialize in feeding often see children who are experiencing gastroesophageal reflux disease, food allergies, oral motor difficulties, and behaviors related to foods.

**Gastroesophageal Reflux.** One example of a common medical condition impacting feeding is *gastroesophageal reflux disease* (GERD), when a child exhibits frequent or chronic vomiting after feeding. It is important to note that gastroesophageal reflux (GER) is a normal physiologic process that is not unusual for babies, and many infants spit up occasionally as their gastrointestinal system matures. This occasional spitting up or vomiting is not harmful to the baby and generally

**TABLE 9.9 Ethical Issues Regarding Testing**

| Ethical Concern | Important Considerations for Test Use |
|---|---|
| Examiner competency | Therapists responsibilities include:<br>• Know how to administer and score a test before using it.<br>• Know for whom the test is intended and for what purpose.<br>• Know when it is not appropriate to use a standardized instrument.<br>• Evaluate the technical merits of the test.<br>• Know how test characteristics may affect its administration and interpretation.<br>• Be aware of the many things that can affect a child's performance on a test, such as hunger, fatigue, illness, or distractions.<br>• Be aware of sources of test or examiner error.<br>• Draw conclusions about a child's performance on a test only after considering all available information about the child. |
| Client privacy | The privacy rule of the Health Insurance Portability and Accountability Act (HIPAA) mandates that:<br>• All recipients of healthcare services are notified of their privacy rights.<br>• Recipients have access to their medical information, including provision of copies at their request.<br>• Recipients be notified of any disclosure of medical information for purposes other than treatment or billing.<br>• For minor children, the parent or legal guardian must provide consent before initiation of any evaluation or intervention procedures.<br>• Verbal exchanges about the child should be limited. It is not acceptable to have a casual conversation about a child anywhere where others could overhear. |
| Communication of results | • Write evaluation reports in neutral language that is understandable to a nonprofessional, with a minimum of jargon.<br>• Use an objective tone, and state conclusions and recommendations clearly.<br>• Consider the characteristics of the person receiving the information when results are discussed.<br>• Be aware of the caregiver's level of education and, in the case of bilingual families, the level of proficiency with English.<br>• Have an interpreter available if needed.<br>• Be aware of the technical nature of some of the information so that the interpreter is one who is familiar with the testing and can offer information in an understandable and culturally meaningful way.<br>• Present information to family members sensitively, considering the anticipated emotional response.<br>• Provide opportunities for the caregivers to ask questions.<br>• Use an objective yet positive tone. |
| Cultural considerations | • Be aware that tests developed primarily on a white, middle-class population may not be valid when used with children from diverse cultural backgrounds.<br>• Be aware of factors that could influence how children from diverse cultures perform on standardized tests; for example, children who have not had experience with testing may not understand the importance of doing a task within a time limit or of following the examiner's instructions. They may not be motivated to perform well on tasks because the task itself has no intrinsic meaning to them. The materials or activities may be seen as irrelevant, or the child, having had no experience with the kinds of materials used in the tests, may not know how to interact with them.<br>• Establishing rapport may be difficult either because of language barriers or because of a cultural mismatch.<br>• Allow a caregiver or an interpreter to be present to put the child at ease. A caregiver can be questioned about the child's familiarity with the various test materials to help determine whether the child's failure to perform individual items is the result of unfamiliarity with the materials or of inability to complete the task.<br>• If possible, allow a caregiver to administer items, particularly those involving physical contact or proximity to the child to make the situation less threatening for the child. (If these adjustments are made, standard procedure may have been violated, and it may be inappropriate to compute a standard score).<br>• Consider developing "local norms" on frequently used instruments that reflect the typical patterns of performance among children of that culture. |

does not produce adverse effects on feeding or growth. The infant likely outgrows these symptoms over time as they gain postural control and stability, with maturation of the gastrointestinal system, and with the transition from a liquid diet to a balance of liquids and solids. GER becomes problematic, however, when spitting up and vomiting leads to concerns with the infant's or child's health (such as esophagitis) or ability to eat successfully (characterized as refusal, distress with eating, or low volume of intake), which in turn leads to poor growth or inadequate weight gain.

**Food Allergies.** Food allergies can influence a child's success with feeding due to discomfort and negative experience associated with eating. Some of the most common food allergies include milk, eggs, soy, wheat, peanuts/tree nuts, and fish/shellfish. The presence of food allergies may cause esophagitis, vomiting, skin rash, itchiness, abdominal pain, breathing difficulties, and/or discomfort during eating. These experiences may contribute to the child's unwillingness to eat and subsequent maladaptive behavior at mealtimes or may impact the child's learning to accept new or alternative food choices. Eosinophilic esophagitis is a chronic allergen-immune mediated disease that commonly causes children to have symptoms including abdominal pain, vomiting, feeding avoidance, and dysphagia (Menard-Katcher et al., 2014).

**Difficulties With Oral Motor Function.** Skills of sucking, suckling, and chewing are acquired sequentially in typical development and rely on intact anatomy and physiology. Competency in oral motor function for feeding is a requirement for safe and effective eating. Children

**TABLE 9.10 Chapter Contributors**

| Chapter Topic | Contributors |
|---|---|
| Feeding and eating | Kimberly Korth and Nancy Creskoff Maune |
| Rest and sleep | Jayne Shepherd and Carol Ivey<br>Jean S. Koketsu and Megan C. Chang |
| ADLs | Jayne Shepherd and Carol Ivey |
| IADL | Theresa Carlson Carroll, Ashley Stoffel, Mary Khetani, Winnifred Schultz-Krohn, and Vivian Villegas |
| Play | Helen Lynch and Alice Moore |
| Education | Colleen Schneck, Shirley Peganoff O'Brien<br>Gloria Frolek Clark, Meira L. Orentlicher, and Yvonne Swinth |
| Telehealth | Jana Cason |
| Leisure | Susan Bazyk |
| Social participation and community integration | Karen Ratcliff and Claudia List Hilton |
| Sexuality | Elizabeth Koss Schmidt, Jenn Soros, Jayne Shepherd, and Carol Ivey |
| Driving and community mobility | Melissa "Missy" Bell |
| Assessment of transition, work, and volunteerism | Elizabeth Pfeiffer and Andrew Persch |
| Assessment of behavior | Renee Watling |
| Cognition | Jolien van den Houten, Angela Mandich, Jessie Wilson, and Kaitlyn Carmichael |
| Challenges in sensory integration and sensory processing | L. Diane Parham Tigg and Zoe Mailloux |
| Motor control | Katherine Dimitropoulou and Patty C. Coker-Bolt |
| Assessment of hand skills, fine motor, and visual perceptual motor skill | Colleen Schneck, Aimee Piller, Mitchell Scheiman, Jenny Marie Dorich, and Karen Harpster |
| Assistive tech | Judith Weenink Schoonover and Elisa Wern |
| Mobility | Sandy Hanebrink and Jane Loscheider |

with medical diagnoses or developmental disabilities may fail to meet basic nutritional needs because of delayed or deficient oral motor and self-feeding skills. Oral motor dysfunction causing poor nutrition is associated with poor growth and adverse health outcomes. Children with oral motor challenges may exhibit food refusal or selectivity behaviors, vomiting, swallowing difficulty, prolonged mealtimes, poor weight gain, and failure to thrive.

**Difficulties With Tongue Function.** There are a variety of structural issues that can occur with the tongue that will impact feeding function. *Macroglossia* is a term used when the tongue is disproportionately large in comparison with the size of the mouth or jaw and is most often associated with conditions such as Down syndrome and Beckwith-Wiedemann syndrome. In mild cases of macroglossia, infants and children may require therapy to reduce tongue-thrusting movements, minimize anterior food loss during feeding, and improve control of saliva to decrease drooling. In more severe cases, surgery may be recommended to reduce the size of the tongue.

*Ankyloglossia*, also referred to as tongue tie, is a congenital oral anomaly that may decrease the mobility of the tongue and is caused by an unusually short, thick, or anterior attachment connecting the tongue to the floor of the mouth. Anterior tongue tie is the more common finding, with classic heart shape of the tongue tip and obvious restriction of tongue movement forward past the gums and upward toward the palate. This tongue tie presentation is often easier to visualize and treat; a mild anterior tongue tie may not result in significant restriction in ROM or function, and findings may not be relevant or require further consideration. Posterior tongue ties are more difficult to see and assess given their location, deeper in the mouth and further underneath the tongue, and treatment requires a more invasive surgical procedure to treat. Babies with limited range of tongue movement related to tongue tie should be further evaluated by a pediatric dentist or otolaryngologist (ENT) to determine the need for surgical release or intervention. There are several tongue assessment tools that are specifically created to evaluate tongue tie. Occupational therapists assess the functional impact of structural differences and collaborate with providers to best determine the need for additional intervention.

**Drooling.** Extensive drooling is called *sialorrhea*, and it is common in children with neurological disorders, such as CP (Dias et al., 2016; Speyer et al., 2019). Evidence suggests that for children with CP, it is caused by oral motor dysfunction rather than hypersalivation (Dias et al., 2016). Children who drool may experience irritated facial skin, unpleasant odor, increased oral and perioral infections, hygiene problems and need for frequent bib or clothing changes, dehydration, choking, and aspiration of saliva (Bittmann et al., 2022). Drooling is considered atypical or pathologic after the age of 4 years (Melo et al., 2021), and typical toddlers gain salivary "continence" by 15–19 months of age. Drooling may be caused by multiple factors including poor oral motor abilities, poor intraoral sensations, and difficulty swallowing the saliva (i.e., dysphagia).

**Challenging Behaviors.** It is not unusual for children with feeding challenges to demonstrate negative behaviors when approaching feeding activities. Challenging behaviors may include crying, pushing the spoon or cup away, and spitting. Children may eat only foods of a certain taste, texture, brand name, or color (Chistol et al., 2018). Some children may need to have a specific cup, utensil, or plate when eating. Behavioral problems are important to consider for children with feeding difficulties. Food refusal and/or food selectivity can be related to multiple factors including anxiety, hypersensitivities, behavioral rigidity, or behavior dysregulation. Selective eating may also be related to underlying medical causes, such as GERD, food allergies, and eosinophilic esophagitis (Menard-Katcher et al., 2014; Mukkada et al., 2010).

TABLE 9.11 **Functions of Oral Structures in Feeding**

| Structure | Parts | Function During Feeding |
|---|---|---|
| Oral cavity | Lips, hard and soft palates, tongue, fat pads of cheeks, upper and lower jaws, and teeth | Contains the food during drinking and chewing and provides for initial mastication before swallowing |
| Pharynx | Base of tongue, buccinator, oropharynx, tendons, and hyoid bone | Funnels food into the esophagus and allows food and air to share space; the pharynx is a space common to both functions |
| Larynx | Epiglottis and false and true vocal folds | Valve to the trachea that closes during swallowing |
| Trachea | Tube below the larynx supported by cartilaginous rings | Allows air to flow into bronchi and lungs |
| Esophagus | Thin and muscular esophagus | Carries food from the pharynx, through the diaphragm, and into the stomach; collapses at rest and distends as food passes through it |

Adapted from Wolf, L. S., & Glass, R. P. (1992). *Feeding and swallowing disorders in infancy: Assessment and management.* Therapy Skill Builders.

Other behaviors include *selective eating* (i.e., eating a small selection of foods), rigidity surrounding mealtime routines, inability to come to or remain at the table, challenges with social expectations of mealtimes, and difficulty trying new foods. Children who have autism may refuse foods that are a specific color, texture, or temperature and be less responsive to the social aspects of mealtimes, such as trying new foods, table manners, or responding to praise and positive reinforcement (Bourne et al., 2022; Carruth et al., 2004; Gale et al., 2011; Laud et al., 2009).

Children may develop fears and phobia-based avoidance associated with sensory aversions or choking (Bourne et al., 2022). If not addressed, children with severe food selectivity or food refusal may become progressively more restrictive in their food preferences, which may lead to nutritional deficiencies (Laud et al., 2009; Sharp et al., 2022; Zhu & Dalby-Payne, 2019). In more extreme reactions, children may develop gagging and vomiting behaviors in response to feeding activities.

***Gagging.*** Gagging may be observed during an evaluation or reported by parents as a concern when children are learning to eat. While it may not be unusual to see occasional gagging, frequent or persistent gagging is a concern (Bassi et al., 2004), and practitioners evaluate the etiology of the response to determine the appropriate technique to address this barrier.

Gagging may be caused by difficulty with oral management of foods and may be protective, sensory based (e.g., triggered by smell, visual cues, or textures), or an emotional response or method used to communicate discomfort or food preference. Children may gag in response to either nonfood- or food-related experiences. Gagging may be observed during oral hygiene, routine dental visits, and restorative care (Benfer et al., 2015).

***Sensory-Related Responses.*** Children with sensory issues may experience mealtimes as uncomfortable or unpleasant. Some infants may not tolerate the sensory input of being held, talked to, or rocked in combination with eating. Other children may have difficulty with the sensory properties of the foods, such as taste, texture, odor, or even the sounds of the foods as they are moved and chewed in the mouth. While many infants and young children enjoy putting things in their mouths and experiencing new sensations such as taste, smell, and the feel of food, infants and children who have difficulty processing sensations may experience these types of touch in the mouth as uncomfortable or even painful. They may react negatively to touch near or within the mouth and avoid experiences related to feeding and eating by turning away, restricting food variety, gagging, or having difficulty with varied food textures and tastes. *Oral hypersensitivity*, an adverse reaction to oral stimuli, may occur when children have received extensive medical interventions, such as endotracheal intubation, orogastric or nasogastric tube feeding, tracheostomy, or frequent oral suctioning. Early feeding problems experienced in infancy, such as GER or swallowing difficulties, can create negative associations between food consumption and sensory discomfort (Vandenplas et al., 2009). The child's sensory system becomes overprotective, and hypersensitivities may continue long after the noxious stimuli have been eliminated. Children with hypersensitivity may be less willing to explore food with their hands to finger-feed independently, or they may become upset with food that spills during attempts at spoon-feeding.

Children may also demonstrate poor oral sensory awareness and seek oral sensory stimulation by mouthing their hands, toys, or clothing. They may have limited awareness of drooling, overstuff their mouths when eating, or demonstrate preferences for specific alerting food textures or flavors. Children who exhibit low sensory registration may eat at a slow pace and require frequent cueing to persist with eating at mealtimes.

## Specific Areas of Assessment Regarding Feeding and Eating

Specialized knowledge is needed to competently assess oral feeding and swallowing. The therapist must understand and be comfortable with the anatomy and functions of all of the oral and pharyngeal structures, the cranial nerves related to oral motor function and swallowing, and the typical development of oral motor and swallowing abilities.

**Anatomy and Development of Oral Structures.** Intact oral structures are prerequisites for eating and drinking. Various aspects of oral motor development emerge as the child begins to control movements of the tongue, cheeks, and lips. The anatomic structures of the mouth and throat change in significant ways throughout fetal development and the first 12 months of life (Clark & Clark, 2018; Lau, 2015). The growth and development of the oral structures allow for increasingly mature feeding patterns, and children refine these patterns over the first few years of life.

The oral cavity houses the structures that enable successful management of foods and liquids during oral feeding via sucking, suckling, biting, mashing, chewing, and food bolus formation in preparation for swallowing. These structures consist of the mandible, maxilla, upper and lower lips, gums, cheeks, tongue, teeth, floor of the mouth, hard palate, soft palate, uvula, and anterior and posterior faucial arches. Table 9.11 outlines the functions of oral structures in feeding.

The newborn has a small oral cavity filled with the tongue and fat pads inside the cheeks. The small and tight oral cavity allows the child to grasp and easily compress the nipple during breastfeeding and achieve suction. The positive pressure of compressing the nipple and negative pressure created by the sucking movements of the jaw extracts liquid from the nipple. Thus, a full-term, healthy newborn is supported to suck successfully from a breast or bottle nipple. Between 4 and 6

TABLE 9.12 **Cranial Nerves Associated With Eating and Swallowing**

| Cranial Nerve | Type | Function |
|---|---|---|
| I (olfactory) | Sensory | Sensory fibers for smell |
| V (trigeminal) | Mixed | Sensory fibers from cheek, nose, upper lip, and teeth<br>Sensory fibers from skin over mandible, lower lip, and teeth<br>Motor fibers to the muscles of mastication |
| VII (facial) | Mixed | Sensory fibers from taste receptors to the anterior two-thirds of the tongue<br>Motor fibers to the muscles of facial expression and salivary glands |
| IX (glossopharyngeal) | Mixed | Sensory fibers from taste receptors on the posterior third of the tongue<br>Motor fibers to the muscles used in swallowing and to the salivary glands |
| X (vagus) | Mixed | Sensory fibers from the pharynx, larynx, esophagus, and stomach<br>Motor fibers to the muscles of the pharynx and larynx<br>Autonomic fibers to the smooth muscles and glands to alter gastric motility, heart rate, respiration, and blood pressure |
| XII (hypoglossal) | Motor | Motor fibers to the muscles of the tongue |

Adapted from Morris, S. E., & Klein, M. D. (2000). *Prefeeding skills* (2nd ed., p. 49, Table 4.2). Therapy Skill Builders.

months of age, the infant's oral structures begin to change, influenced by growth and by maturation of postural control and overall motor systems. The oral cavity becomes larger and more open, the tongue becomes thinner and more muscular, and the cheeks lose much of their fatty padding. With the increase in oral cavity space, the tongue, lips, and cheeks must provide greater control of liquid and food within the mouth to enable the infant to manage liquid without the structural advantages of early infancy.

During this time, the tongue gains mobility to include up and down movements, sucking patterns become more voluntary, and oral motor control begins to support pureed foods and the introduction of spoon-feeding. This maturation continues as the child grows and acquires teeth to allow for effective mastication and improved management of food textures. See online materials regarding dental development, care, and oral hygiene.

**Cranial Nerves.** Multiple cranial nerves support sensory and motor functions during oral feeding. Cranial nerves V, VII, and XII innervate the sensory-motor pathways required to suck and extract liquid from a nipple. Table 9.12 lists the cranial nerves associated with eating and swallowing.

**Pharyngeal Structures and Function.** The pharynx consists of distinct structures important to management of airflow for respiration and control of food or liquid during swallowing. The pharynx, composed of the nasopharynx, oropharynx, and laryngopharynx, plays an integral role in the proper timing of breathing and swallowing during oral feeding.

The structures in the infant's throat are near one another, and this anatomic relationship allows an infant to feed in a reclined position. At rest, the epiglottis and soft palate are in direct approximation, which aids in the controlled passage of liquid from the base of the tongue to the esophagus. During swallowing, the larynx elevates, and the epiglottis falls over the opening to the upper airway, and the bolus is directed toward the esophagus.

As the infant grows, the hyoid, epiglottis, and larynx descend, creating space between these structures and base of the tongue. The hyoid and larynx become more mobile during swallowing, elevating with each swallow. The greater complexity of the suck-swallow-breathe sequence leads to the need for greater coordination among these structures. There is an increased risk of aspiration during feeding in a reclined position, as the pull of gravity accelerates the flow of liquid into the entrance of the esophagus without the benefit of the "gate" previously provided by the opposed epiglottis and soft palate. During this time, children should be fed in a more upright position for bottle feeding, cup drinking, and as more advanced food textures are introduced. Fig. 9.3 depicts the anatomic structures of the mouth and throat.

**A Model for a Comprehensive Evaluation of Feeding and Swallowing.** Feeding problems are seldom attributable to a single cause and usually are the result of delays, impairments, medical concerns, or behavioral challenges in multiple areas. For example, children with severe sensory problems may have subsequent oral motor skill delays, and children with neuromotor impairments may experience swallowing disorders. Often, because of past feeding challenges, families modify routines, mealtime structure, and behavioral expectations, thus creating maladaptive contextual challenges, which must also be addressed. Fig. 9.4 provides a model for feeding evaluation that highlights the critical areas to evaluate and address during a multidisciplinary feeding evaluation. With this framework, each "petal" on the "flower" identifies specific contributing factors, and the watering can illustrates strengths that the child or family brings to the feeding process. Needs are outlined in terms of how to best promote progress with the child's feeding challenges. It is worth noting that the approach to healthcare and children with complex medical needs has evolved into specialized, multidisciplinary care clinics that collaborate to take care of the most complicated patients, or those with the most "petals" on their feeding flowers.

For infants, an important aspect of the feeding evaluation is the coordination of suck-swallow-breathe. Infants must coordinate a suck, swallow, and breathe pattern to efficiently take liquid from the bottle or breast. They begin by nonnutritive sucking, which involves sucking at a fast rate and sucking bursts (pauses) on pacifiers, fingers, or teething objects (Marcus & Breton, 2022a). Nonnutritive sucking is soothing and calming but does not provide the infant with nutrients. Nutritive sucking occurs at a slower rate and allows the infant to receive liquids from the bottle or breast. Breastfeeding is associated with significant health benefits for infants and for mothers. During bottle-feeding or breastfeeding, infants coordinate the suck, swallow, and breathe pattern. Full-term infants demonstrate a sucking pattern of 10–30 sucks in a burst (Mizuno & Ueda, 2006 in Marcus & Breton, 2022a). Infants may exhibit difficulty coordinating suck, swallow, and breathe patterns to effectively intake nutrients. They may have difficulty latching on to the bottle or breast. A study of more than 500 mothers (in the United States) found that 92% reported breastfeeding difficulties by day three (Wagner et al., 2013).

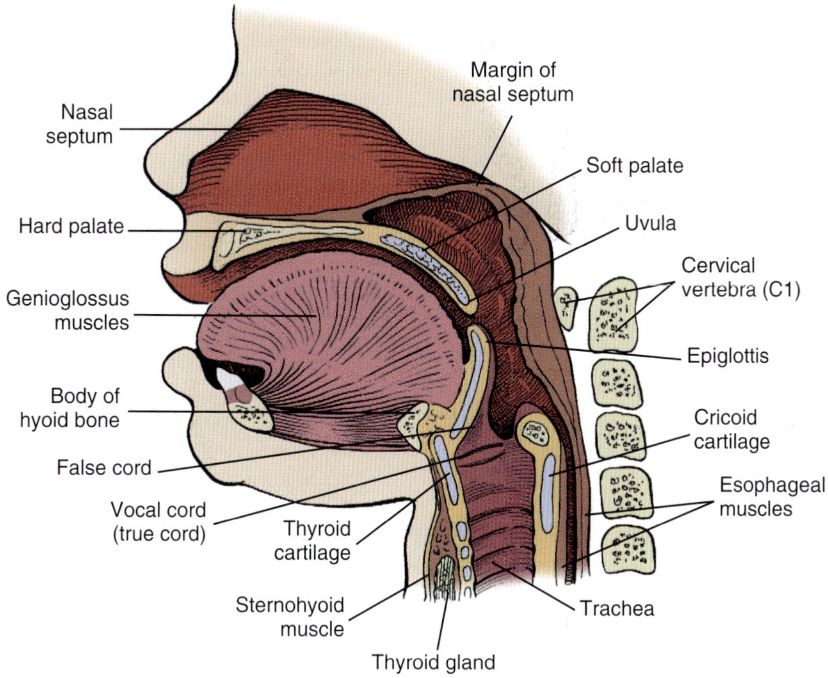


**Fig. 9.3** Anatomic structures of the mouth and throat.

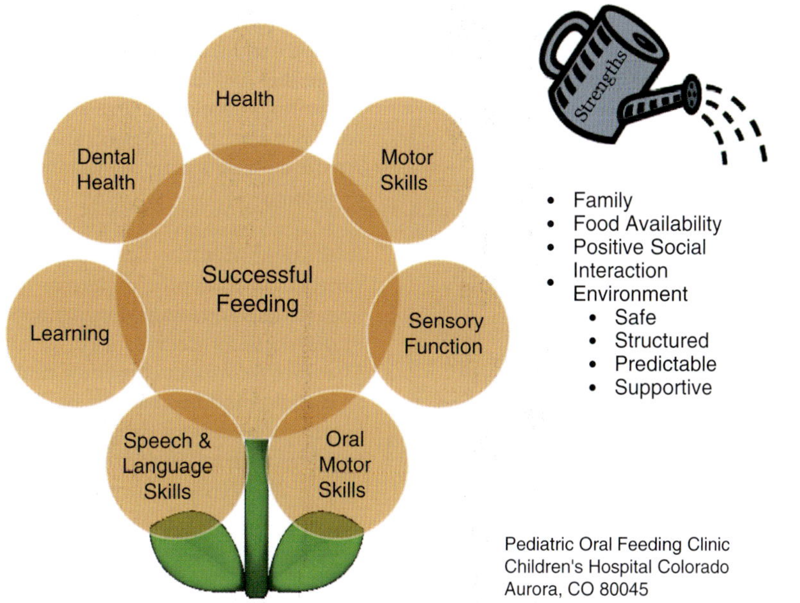


**Fig. 9.4** Feeding flower to guide feeding assessment.

**The Process of the Evaluation of Feeding and Eating.** Often the evaluation of feeding and eating begins with the caregiver completing intake paperwork that includes a developmental history and information about typical nutritional intake. The occupational therapist also gathers information through chart review to better understand the child's health and medical history. Caregiver interview includes detailed questions about the family's routines, goals, expectations, and typical feeding skills and abilities in the home, including their preferences and reactions. The occupational therapist observes the child feeding and eating and consults with the interprofessional team (e.g., physician, nurse practitioner, speech-language pathologist, nurse, dietician, medical specialists, lactation consultant, psychologist or psychiatrist, behavioral therapist, dentist) and family (AOTA, 2017b; Marcus & Breton, 2022a) to determine possible causes for eating and feeding dysfunction.

The occupational therapist obtains information about current feeding practices, cultural norms, social rules, and mealtime routines by asking the parents to describe the child's feeding over the course of a typical day. This open-ended inquiry allows the occupational therapist to identify potential areas of concerns that were not reported during the initial description of the child's feeding problems. Please see Box 9.11 for an outline to guide the evaluation process.

A discussion of the feeding problem from the parents' perspective is critical because it helps identify the primary concerns. For example, are the parents most concerned about weight gain, or is it the length of time required for feeding that poses a problem? Does the child seem to lose most of the food consumed during feeding (e.g., through poor oral control or through vomiting)? Is the child's behavior during feeding causing distress for the family during mealtimes? Although the parents' expressed

**BOX 9.11 Outline to Guild Feeding and Eating Evaluation**

**Interview Questions for Parents**

1. What questions would you like answered during this evaluation?
2. What specific concerns do you have about your child's feeding, growth, and/or development?
3. When did you first develop these feeding or swallowing concerns?

**Evaluation History**

1. Medical history
    1. Pregnancy, labor, and delivery
    2. Birth history
    3. Past surgeries and hospitalizations
    4. Therapies
    5. Past medical testing/results
    6. Medications
2. Feeding history
    1. Breast/bottle
    2. Spoon-feeding
    3. Solid food introductions

**Current Status**

1. Feeding schedule
2. Foods accepted/refused
3. Oral exam
    1. Structures
    2. Nonnutritive (oral play, tooth brushing, or drooling)
4. Development:
    1. Motor
    2. Communication
    3. Sensory
    4. Feeding observation
    5. Positioning (identify seating system)
    6. Food and beverages presented
    7. Nutritive oral feeding skills (by item)
    8. Mealtime behaviors (positive and problematic)
    9. Self-feeding (including utensils, cups, and any adaptive equipment used)
    10. Parent/child interactions
    11. Volume of intake
    12. Length of feeding

concerns become the focus of the subsequent intervention, the occupational therapist also considers concerns expressed by healthcare professionals (e.g., physicians or other health care providers) when developing a feeding plan.

The parents provide information about the child's development and feeding history, including feeding milestones. Obtaining this information helps the occupational therapist identify the root of the feeding problem such as long-standing sensory or behavioral issues that may have affected feeding. Inquiring about remediation strategies used with the child in the past may be helpful in identifying appropriate next intervention strategies. Parents whose child has been seen by other medical or therapy providers may have important information to share regarding interventions that worked and those that did not.

After the occupational therapist has completed a comprehensive interview, they form initial impressions about the child's feeding difficulties, the family's routines and structure around eating and mealtimes, or other areas that influence feeding and eating. The next step is to complete an evaluation of generalized muscle tone, neuromuscular status, sensory processing development, and general developmental level. Observations of movement initiation, play, and transition patterns allow the occupational therapist to observe muscle tone, sensory processing, and postural control. Low postural muscle tone can interfere with the ability to maintain upright posture and head and neck alignment. Hypotonicity or hypertonicity can lead to difficulty grading or sustaining oral motor patterns, uncoordinated breathing, drooling, decreased oral exploration, and limited self-feeding. Sensory processing difficulties may influence the child's ability to sit successfully for meals, progress with food textures, or accept other typical mealtime experiences.

Next the occupational therapist observes the child's oral structures, including symmetry, size, tone, and ROM of the outer oral structures, including the jaw, lips and cheeks, and then proceeding intraorally to the gums, teeth, hard and soft palates, and tongue. Nonnutritive skills are assessed, which may include how well the child manages their saliva, sucks on a pacifier, explores toys orally, or brushes their teeth.

The evaluator observes the child eating a snack or a meal with the parent or caregiver. The occupational therapist evaluates oral feeding abilities to learn more about mealtime routines, feeding practices, and social or behavioral interactions occurring during meals. Observing the parent–child interaction provides insight into the everyday context of feeding. For example, does the child send clear cues regarding readiness to eat, satiation, or food preferences? How does the parent respond to the child's verbal and/or nonverbal cues? Does the parent talk to the child? Does the child maintain eye contact with the caregiver while eating?

Observations of the parent-directed mealtime enable further assessment. The occupational therapist encourages the caregiver, when possible, to use the seating system, plates, utensils, and approach that are typically used at home. The parents are asked to bring foods for the evaluation that the child typically accepts at home, as well as foods that are more challenging for the child. Ideally, the occupational therapist observes the child's physical or mechanical abilities with the preferred feeding items and methods, while concurrently observing skills, behaviors, or responses that characterize the feeding difficulty with the challenging or nonpreferred foods or methods.

**Additional Medical Diagnostic Evaluations and Measures.** A variety of medical procedures may be recommended to further evaluate feeding and swallowing skills. See Table 9.13 for an overview of diagnostic procedures used for children with feeding disorders. The **video fluoroscopic swallow study** (VFSS), also commonly called an **upright modified barium swallow study** (UMBSS), is the radiographic procedure of choice for assessing the oral, pharyngeal, and upper esophageal anatomy and function during feeding and swallowing. The VFSS can identify aspiration or the risk of aspiration to inform treatment for infants and children with dysphagia. This evaluation can be helpful for detecting issues related to head and neck positioning, bolus characteristics, rate and sequence of feeding, and determining safe food or liquid consistencies. The results of the test help identify compensatory techniques that may be used to minimize the risk of aspiration and maximize eating efficiency.

The occupational therapist selects the types of food and liquid textures based on the child's current diet and level of feeding performance and mixes them with liquid, powder, or barium paste. The VFSS only captures a brief sample of swallowing; positioning, food or liquid amount, and order of presentation are up to the therapy team conducting the study. Typically, during this evaluation, radiation exposure is limited to 5 minutes or less, thus requiring occupational therapists to determine clinically the most important food and liquid textures to examine during this brief period.

The VFSS is used to analyze the swallow mechanism and is particularly important for children who aspirate or are at a high risk for aspiration because of motor, neurologic, developmental, or structural abnormalities. Clinical observations that may suggest swallowing problems include coughing, choking, loss of liquid or food from nose

**TABLE 9.13 Commonly Used Diagnostic Procedures for Children With Feeding Disorders**

| Test | Indications | Advantages | Limitations |
|---|---|---|---|
| Videofluoroscopic swallow study (VPSS); upright modified barium swallow study (UMBSS); videofluoroscopic swallow study | • Analyze the swallow mechanism<br>• Rule out aspiration<br>• Determine point of aspiration<br>• Identify safe food and liquid consistencies | • Fluoroscopy, not a single-picture X-ray<br>• Videotaped<br>• Upright position simulates feeding<br>• Primary feeder often presents food<br>• Familiar feeding utensils (bottle, cup, and spoon)<br>• Use of liquid, purée, and/or solid<br>• Lateral and anterior/posterior view<br>• Can determine when aspiration occurs<br>• Investigation of treatment options | • May be difficult to simulate normal feeding in radiology examination room<br>• Child must be able to swallow appropriate amount of barium<br>• Results reflect that particular date and time<br>• Study environment may increase child stress, resulting in aspiration<br>• Radiation exposure from fluoroscopy |
| Fiberoptic endoscopic evaluation of swallowing (FEES) | • Analyze the swallow mechanism<br>• Rule out aspiration<br>• Identify safe food and liquid consistencies<br>• Visualize anatomic structures during swallowing | • Allows variability in positioning the child during eating or drinking<br>• No X-ray radiation exposure<br>• Can be combined with traditional laryngoscopy | • Requires child to be awake and cooperative while having small tube inserted in the nose and pharynx while swallowing<br>• Often requires coordination between swallowing therapist and otorhinolaryngologist or ear, nose, and throat physician<br>• Visualization while swallow is occurring can be difficult because structures close and contract |
| Upper gastrointestinal (GI) series | • Diagnose structural abnormalities of the esophagus, stomach, or intestines, such as malrotation or stricture | • Clear contrast image of upper GI anatomy<br>• Documents gastroesophageal reflux (GER) events if they occur during study<br>• Observes esophageal motility and mechanism for stomach emptying | • X-ray radiation exposure<br>• Supine positioning<br>• Barium flow rate may not simulate bottle feeding<br>• Primary feeder often not present<br>• Limited accuracy in capturing or diagnosing GER |
| Esophageal pH probe | • Quantifies frequency, acidity, and duration of GER | • Prolonged evaluation of GER over 24 h<br>• Documents effect of movement, sleep, and meals on GER<br>• Documents frequency and severity of GER events<br>• Can be combined with other assessments, such as pulse oximetry, or documentation of choking episodes<br>• Established guidelines for normal and abnormal results | • Invasive procedure, often requiring overnight stay in a hospital<br>• May not correlate with clinical symptoms (e.g., coughing, vomiting, and wheezing) |
| Gastrointestinal (GI) endoscopy, esophagogastroduodenoscopy (EGD) | • Provides a direct view of GI tract to diagnose inflammation or structural abnormalities | • Direct observation of esophageal and stomach tissues for changes that may have occurred with chronic GER<br>• Tissue biopsies often studied for presence of eosinophils, which may indicate food allergies | • Invasive procedure, requiring anesthesia<br>• Presence of inflammation or abnormalities may not correlate with clinical symptoms (e.g., vomiting, other feeding problems)<br>• Cannot determine frequency of GER |

Adapted from Morris, S. E., & Klein, M. (2000). *Pre-feeding skills* (2nd ed.). Therapy Skill Builders.

while eating, increased congestion, wet vocal quality, and frequent occurrence of respiratory infections and/or pneumonias.

See Box 9.12 for a list of clinical criteria referral for a formal swallow evaluation. While a thorough history and feeding observation are critical, aspiration may be "silent," without cough or another observable cue. In addition, the ability to assess pharyngeal and/or esophageal function is not accurate or possible without instrumental evaluation of swallowing (such as a fluoroscopic, radiographic, or endoscopic procedure).

During the VFSS, the occupational therapist should distinguish aspiration from laryngeal penetration. Aspiration refers to food or liquid entering the airway before, during, or after a swallow. The presence of aspiration is an abnormal finding and may lead to chronic lung disease, pneumonia, and other medical problems. Laryngeal penetration describes the flow of food or liquid underneath the epiglottis into the laryngeal vestibule, but not into the airway. It does not pass through the vocal folds. The frequency and depth of laryngeal penetration may vary and may not always correlate to an increased risk of aspiration. Infants and children may have intermittent episodes of mild laryngeal penetration (also called epiglottic undercoating) during swallowing, which has not been found to increase the risk for aspiration. The presence of deep laryngeal penetration, characterized by food or liquid entering the laryngeal vestibule to the level of the vocal cords, is correlated to an increased risk factor for aspiration episodes.

**BOX 9.12 Clinical Indicators for Referral for Swallowing Evaluation**

- Increased congestion and/or wet vocal quality during or after eating
- Frequent occurrence of respiratory illnesses (pneumonia, bronchiolitis, prolonged colds, or asthma-like symptoms not well controlled)
- Difficulty weaning from oxygen or need for oxygen support on a frequent basis
- Significant neurological diagnosis and/or neuromotor involvement
- Coughing or choking on liquids and/or on other consistencies
- Oral motor dysfunction
- Prolonged mealtimes, such as longer than 30 minutes to feed because of oral motor issues
- Reliance on gastronomy tube (G-tube) feedings but is willing to eat something by mouth, and safety of oral feeding is questioned

Because the VFSS recording shows food traveling through the mouth and pharynx, the occupational therapist receives real-time, detailed information about the child's oral motor and pharyngeal function paired with clinical observations. The results of the VFSS identify the safety and appropriateness of oral feeding and guide the occupational therapist's recommendations (Stafler et al., 2022). These recommendations may include modified feeding positions and/or food and liquid textures for the parents to offer that result in optimal swallowing patterns without aspiration. Although the VFSS gives the occupational therapist important information and insight about the swallowing problem, it may not always be representative of the child's typical feeding in a more natural environment and is not usually the length or portion of a "meal." In addition, the VFSS does not determine etiology of refusal behaviors, and limited volume of intake during the study can make interpretation of the findings challenging.

A **fiberoptic endoscopic evaluation of swallowing** (FEES) also evaluates a child's swallow function. In contrast to the VFSS, the FEES uses a flexible endoscope with a light and camera that is inserted into a nostril and down the throat. With this evaluation, the camera records the pharyngeal swallow function from the inside as the child eats or drinks. This test allows for direct visualization of the larynx and pharynx to observe for penetration, aspiration, and residual material. The child must be awake and able to cooperate with drinking and eating while the endoscope is in place. Please see video examples of a VFSS and FEES provided in the supplemental Evolve material.

There are a variety of medical tests and procedures that may aid in diagnosing conditions that impact feeding. An upper gastrointestinal (GI) series is a common evaluation used to screen for anatomic differences, such as GI malrotation, stricture, vascular ring, and/or fistulas or pouches, which may cause vomiting and other feeding problems. An upper GI series can be helpful in evaluating the presence of GER. However, the upper GI series evaluates only one moment in time and, according to expert clinical guidelines, is not used to diagnose GER or to identify the severity (Vandenplas et al., 2009). The upper GI series does not provide optimal assessment of swallow function although it may document episodes of aspiration.

Medical providers may recommend an esophageal or pH probe to discover the presence and severity of GER. With this evaluation, a probe is inserted into the esophagus through the nose to monitor acid levels, typically over a 24-hour period. However, a pH probe test may be difficult to complete because it often requires an overnight stay in the hospital, and the probe may be poorly tolerated by young infants and children.

An endoscopy may be used to evaluate the esophagus, stomach, and duodenum, referred to as an esophagogastroduodenoscopy (EGD) or upper intestinal endoscopy. This test involves passing a flexible endoscope through the nose and visualizing the structures for the presence of esophagitis or other abnormalities. Tissue biopsies may be taken from the esophagus, stomach, or duodenum to evaluate for the presence of eosinophils. Eosinophils are present in abnormally large numbers when a child is experiencing food allergies. They contribute to esophagitis and discomfort during eating. The child must be sedated to complete an EGD. The nasal endoscopy is a procedure being explored for patients who meet criteria that do not require general anesthesia; current research is in progress using this procedure as an alternative and to minimize cumulative anesthesia exposure when serial evaluations are indicated (Friedlander et al., 2016).

## EVALUATION OF REST AND SLEEP

Sleep and rest involve three areas: preparation for sleep (sleep hygiene); participation in sleep; and rest (the activities that allow a child to relax while decreasing mental thinking and physical activity level) (AOTA, 2020b).

### Importance of Rest and Sleep to Client and Family Functioning

Sleep and rest are essential for a child's growth and well-being (Matricciani et al., 2019; Meltzer et al., 2021; Ramar et al., 2021; Spruyt, 2019; Williamson et al., 2020) because they allow children and their parents to restore energy for everyday occupations. During sleep, the muscles relax, and the brain processes the day's events. Sleep allows new neurological connections to form, is essential for memory consolidation, and impacts attention and focus. Sleep has even been associated with weight and obesity (Morrissey et al., 2020) and mental health (Short et al., 2019).

Inadequate sleep leads to a host of problematic outcomes (Li et al., 2021; Nelson et al., 2022; Williamson et al., 2020). When inadequate sleep occurs, cycles of REM (rapid eye movement) and NREM (non-rapid eye movement) sleep are shortened, and memory, muscle repair, and hormone release are stunted. Inadequate sleep may lead to fatigue, sleepiness, change in appetite, illness, difficulty learning, difficulty paying attention, inability to handle stress, and poorer cognitive and social skill development, which affect children's occupational performance. Inadequate sleep in adults may lead to greater risk for cardiovascular disease and coronary heart disease, falls, frailty, lung cancer, metabolic syndrome, and stroke. Chronic lack of sleep may also result in a propensity for mental health disorders (Alonzo et al., 2021; Li et al., 2021), and this may be a causal relationship (Scott et al., 2021).

When caregivers become sleep deprived because a child has difficulty sleeping, their ability to meet their own role expectations may be affected. Parents who are sleep deprived are more likely to report stress, irritability, reduced concentration, increased sleepiness during the daytime, and impaired sleep quality at night (Martin et al., 2019; Mindell et al., 2015). Caregiver mental and physical health may suffer as well when a child has extensive difficulties sleeping (Liu et al., 2021; Martin et al., 2021).

### Common Challenges Associated With Sleep

Difficulties with sleep may be labeled in a variety of ways (Kamara & Beauchaine, 2020). **Sleep problems** typically mean concerns with sleep such as sleeplessness, excessive daytime sleepiness, and parasomnias, and these are each typically considered to occur along a continuum of severity. A **sleep disturbance** is a combination of sleep problems and sleep disorders. The International Classification of Sleep Disorders has identified 7 major categories and more than 80 different types of sleep disorders (American Academy of Sleep Medicine, 2014). **Sleep disorders** in children are identified as bedtime resistance or difficulty falling asleep staying asleep (insomnia), irregularity of amount of time in sleep (sleep-wake cycle disruption), breathing disorders (sleep apnea),

**TABLE 9.14 Typical Amount of Sleep Required and Factors That May Impede Sleep by Age**

| Age | Amount of Sleep Needed | Naps | Factors to Consider When Child Has Sleep Problems |
|---|---|---|---|
| Newborn, 1–2 months | 12–18 hours<br>50–60 minutes REM-NREM cycle | Throughout day | No established sleep/wake cycle<br>Interrupted sleep related to feeding, comfort needs (diaper changes), medical procedures, sleep apnea alarms (if used), or too much sleep during the day<br>When asleep and put to bed, baby wakes up with change in position |
| 3–11 months | 12–18 hours | Three or four times daily, 30 minutes to 2 hours | Usually cannot sleep through the night without feedings until 6 months of age<br>70%–80% sleep through the night by 9 months<br>Separation anxiety interferes with sleep<br>Has not learned to self-soothe and is dependent on parents (needs to be drowsy or already asleep to be placed in crib)<br>May be insecure with attachment or always wants to engage with others |
| Toddler, 1–3 years | 12–14 hours | Once or twice daily (18 months once a day), 1–3 hours | Fewer naps needed<br>Needs independence<br>Anxiety about going to sleep (may relate to separation anxiety, inability to self-soothe, imagination, fear of being alone, nightmares)<br>Difficulty with transitions<br>Gets out of bed independently |
| Preschoolers 3.1–4.11 years | 11–13 hours | Once daily | Bed wetting<br>Nighttime fears or nightmares because of imagination developing (e.g., fear of being alone, the dark, tigers under the bed)<br>Peak age for sleepwalking and sleep terrors<br>Television watching too close to bedtime<br>Outgrown the need for naps and not sleepy when put to bed |
| School age, 5–10 years | 10–11 hours | 0 | Bed wetting (typical until age 7)<br>Medical issues: Tonsils enlarged, facial profile is convex, has cross bite, reflux, or medical procedure (e.g., positioning, suction)<br>Unaware of social cues for calming down to go to sleep<br>Increased demands for schoolwork or other extracurricular activities<br>More interest in computers and internet<br>Caffeine consumption or eating close to bedtime<br>Electronic use in the bedroom or too close to bedtime (e.g., computers, televisions, tablets, video games)<br>Erratic sleep schedule<br>Lack of understanding of the importance of healthy routines for sleep |
| Teens, 10.1–17 years | 8.5–9.25 hours | | Increased demands of school, work, social life, or other activities<br>Anxiety or emotional event during the day<br>Caffeine consumption or eating close to bedtime<br>Electronic use in the bedroom or too close to bedtime (e.g., computers, televisions, tablets, video games, smartphones)<br>Erratic sleep schedule especially weekend versus weekday nights<br>Internal clock of teens—like late nights and waking up later in the morning<br>Lack of understanding of importance for healthy routines for sleep |

*NREM*, Nonrapid eye movement; *REM*, rapid eye movement.
Collated from Mindell, J., & Owens, J. (2015). *Clinical guide to pediatric sleep: Diagnosis and intervention.* Wolters Kluwer. Sleep Foundation. (2024). Sleep hygiene. https://www.sleepfoundation.org/articles/sleep-hygiene; Sleep Foundation. (2020). The bedroom environment. https://www.thensf.org/how-many-hours-of-sleep-do-you-really-need/

sleepiness during the day (hypersomnia), nightmares or unusual experiences during sleep (parasomnias), or movement disorders or pains during sleep (e.g., restless leg).

Sleep disorders and disturbances are quite common in children (Kamara & Beauchaine, 2020; Matricciani et al., 2019; Trosman & Ivanenko, 2021; Williamson et al., 2019) and have been noted in typical children and children with a variety of disorders such as asthma, attention-deficit hyperactivity disorder (ADHD), autism spectrum disorder (ASD), allergies, diabetes, CP, epilepsy, sickle cell disease, obesity, cancer, or brain injury. Sleep problems occur in approximately 25%–30% of toddlers, 37% of school-age children, and 20% of adolescents (Ophoff et al., 2018).

## Specific Areas of Assessment Regarding Sleep

The National Sleep Foundation (2024) recommends regular sleep routines and patterns, with similar amounts of sleep each night. Table 9.14 describes the typical amount of sleep needed for children and youth at different ages and lists possible factors impeding sleep. The assessment of sleep often begins with a determination of the amount of sleep a client is getting each night.

To focus on the positive outcomes and importance of beneficial sleep, Buysse (2014) proposed the term "sleep health" defined as "a multidimensional pattern of sleep-wakefulness, adapted to individual, social, and environmental demands, that promotes physical and mental well-being. Good sleep health is characterized by subjective

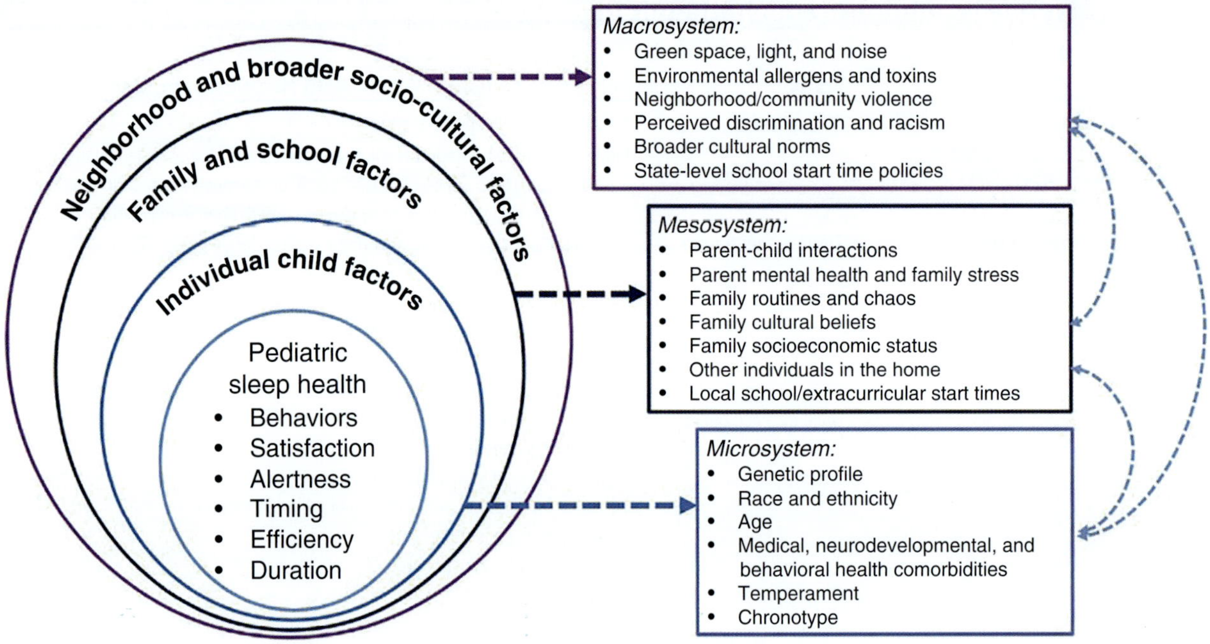


**Fig. 9.5** Socio-ecologic factors hypothesized to contribute to pediatric sleep health domains. (From Meltzer, L. J., Williamson, A. A., & Mindell, J. A. (2021). Pediatric sleep health: It matters, and so does how we define it. *Sleep Medicine Reviews*, *57*, 101425.)

satisfaction, appropriate timing, adequate duration, high efficiency, and sustained alertness during waking hours" (p. 12). Sleep health supports a child's occupational performance and their physical growth and ability to learn and behave. However, a variety of factors contribute to sleep health, many of which are out of a child's control (see Fig. 9.5).

Therapists may assess a child's sleep health. Sleep health for children is "characterized by subjective or caregiver-rated satisfaction, appropriate timing, adequate duration for age, high efficiency, sustained alertness during waking hours, and healthy sleep behaviors" (Meltzer et al., 2021, p. 12). The model initially developed by Buysee as adapted for pediatric use (Meltzer et al., 2021) considers six factors:

- Satisfaction with sleep
- Alertness during waking hours
- Timing of sleep
- Sleep efficiency
- Sleep duration
- Sleep-related behaviors

Each of these areas can be assessed through interviews with the caregivers or with children who are old enough to self-report.

When working with parents or caregivers, the occupational therapist assesses a child's activity level, sensory preferences, bedtime routines, sleep habits, and sleep environments to determine what may be hindering sleep. As always, it is important first to inquire about family routines and whether cultural considerations influence the sleep habits of the family or child. For example, some parents may sleep in the same room or bed with the infant or child; the infant may sleep in the family living area instead of a bedroom; or the infant may sleep with siblings in a room or in the same bed. Some parents place the sleeping baby in a hammock or in a tightly swaddled prone position. Box 9.13 provides some of the types of questions a therapist might ask during an assessment. Table 9.15 gives definitions of quality of sleep, assessment ideas, and questions to ask parents or caregivers to determine if a child has a sleep problem. Through careful and thorough evaluation of sleep, occupational therapists can provide important assistance to families (Gronski & Doherty, 2020).

### BOX 9.13 Questions for Assessment of Sleep

Asking caregivers questions about sleep is essential to begin to understand their values and understanding of sleep hygiene:

- Does your child or adolescent have regular sleep patterns (bedtime, nap times, and amount of uninterrupted sleep)?
- Where does the child or adolescent sleep?
- With whom or what (e.g., stuffed animal) does the child sleep?
- When is the child put to bed or to sleep?
- What are typical bedtime routines?
- How long does it take your child or adolescent to fall asleep?
- How do your child's sleep behaviors impact your sleep or the sleep of others in the household?

In addition to caregiver interviews, occupational therapists may consider the use of sleep questionnaires or sleep diaries, which are common methods of assessment (Kamara & Beauchaine, 2020). There are more than 300 different sleep questionnaires that are either caregiver or self-report (Meltzer et al., 2020). Therefore, the National Institutes of Health created a program to develop a new bank of sleep-related items and new measures called the Patient Reported Outcome Measurement Information System (PROMIS). The Pediatric Sleep Disturbance (SD) and Sleep-Related Impairment (SRI) measures have been made freely available for use (www.healthmeasures.net) (Meltzer et al., 2020).

## Additional Medical Evaluation of Sleep

Medical professionals may also request more intense measurement of sleep to diagnose sleep problems (Kamara & Beauchaine, 2020). Polysomnography measures brain wave, muscle, cardiovascular, and breathing activity during sleep by placing 16 electrodes on the body.

**TABLE 9.15 Sleep Quality Definitions and Assessments of Sleep for Children**

| Bears Algorithm (Measurement of Sleep Quality) | Definition | Assessment | Questions to Ask Parents, Caregivers, or Child | Possible Reasons for Sleep Issue |
|---|---|---|---|---|
| ***B***edtime or sleep latency | Time between trying to sleep and actually going to sleep | Sleep log<br>Routines used when going to bed<br>Consistent bedtime?<br>Nocturnal polysomnography or actigraphy<br>Sleep questionnaires | How long does it take your child to fall asleep?<br>Is your child resistant to go to bed or has difficulty going to bed?<br>Does he or she get out of bed frequently prior to sleeping?<br>Does he or she seem anxious when going to bed? | Lack of routines<br>Too early or too late to bed<br>Family discord<br>Social or emotional issues |
| ***E***xcessive tiredness during the day | Ability to stay awake during the day | Parent, child, or teacher questionnaire<br>Youth self-report<br>Actigraphy<br>Sleep questionnaires | Is your child hard to wake up in the morning?<br>Does your child fall asleep during the day outside of scheduled naps?<br>Does he or she complain of being tired, or is he or she drowsy, moody, irritable, and/or looks tired to you? | Not enough sleep<br>Irregular sleep<br>Sleep apnea<br>Illness<br>Stress or anxiety |
| ***A***wakenings at night | After going to sleep, number of times the child awakens at night | Sleep log by parents<br>Sleep log by youth, if able<br>Nocturnal polysomnography or actigraphy<br>Sleep questionnaires | Does your child wake up at night?<br>What interrupts his or her sleep?<br>How many times does he or she wake up?<br>Does he or she go back to sleep?<br>Does he or she sleep walk or talk? | Sleep terrors or nightmares<br>Environment is noisy or overstimulating<br>Lack of exercise during the day<br>Eating too close to bedtime<br>Restless leg syndrome<br>Illness |
| ***R***egularity and duration of sleep | Time child goes to sleep and amount of time sleeping (when sleep began and ended) | Sleep log by parents or youth, if able<br>Environmental assessment<br>Nocturnal polysomnography or actigraphy<br>Sleep questionnaires | How many hours does your child sleep?<br>Does he or she have a regular bedtime on weekdays and weekends?<br>What is the bedtime?<br>How many hours does your child sleep? | |
| ***S***noring | Amount and loudness of gasping, choking, or snoring while sleeping | Observation of parents while child sleeps<br>Reports of youth or sibling who sleeps in same room<br>Testing for sleep apnea<br>Sleep questionnaires | Does your child snore at night?<br>Does he or she gasp for air or choke while sleeping?<br>How often?<br>Is the snoring loud or has it changed? | Sleep apnea |
| ***M***ovement or sleep efficiency | Amount of movement during sleep (may have restless leg syndrome) | Observation of parents or siblings who sleep in same room<br>Report of youth, if able<br>Nocturnal polysomnography or actigraphy<br>Sleep questionnaires | When your child sleeps, are the legs restless or move a lot?<br>Are the covers in disarray?<br>Does your child change positions frequently when sleeping?<br>Does your child end up at the other end of the bed after being asleep? | Restless leg syndrome |

Adapted from National Sleep Foundation. (2013). *Children and sleep.* https://sleepfoundation.org/sleep-topics/children-and-sleep; Mindell, J., & Owens, J. (2015). *Clinical guide to pediatric sleep: Diagnosis and intervention.* Wolters Kluwer.

Fig. 9.6 demonstrates what this might look like for a child. For some children with sensory sensitivities, these procedures are invasive and difficult to tolerate. Actigraphy uses an actimeter that is worn on the wrist or sewn into clothing to measure circadian rhythms and muscle movements during sleep and wake periods.

## EVALUATION OF ACTIVITIES OF DAILY LIVING

According to AOTA (2020b), activities of daily living (ADLs) include bathing and showering, toileting, dressing, hygiene, and grooming, as well as additional areas that are described in separate sections in this chapter (feeding and eating, sexuality, for example).

### Importance of ADLs to Child and Family Functioning

Young children require adult assistance with ADLs but eventually acquire the ability to feed, dress, bath, groom, and carry through with daily routines. Children with disabilities may be delayed in developing ADLs, and some children may require lengthy periods of care from adults, perhaps for their lifetime, based on the severity of their disability and the level of dependency of the child

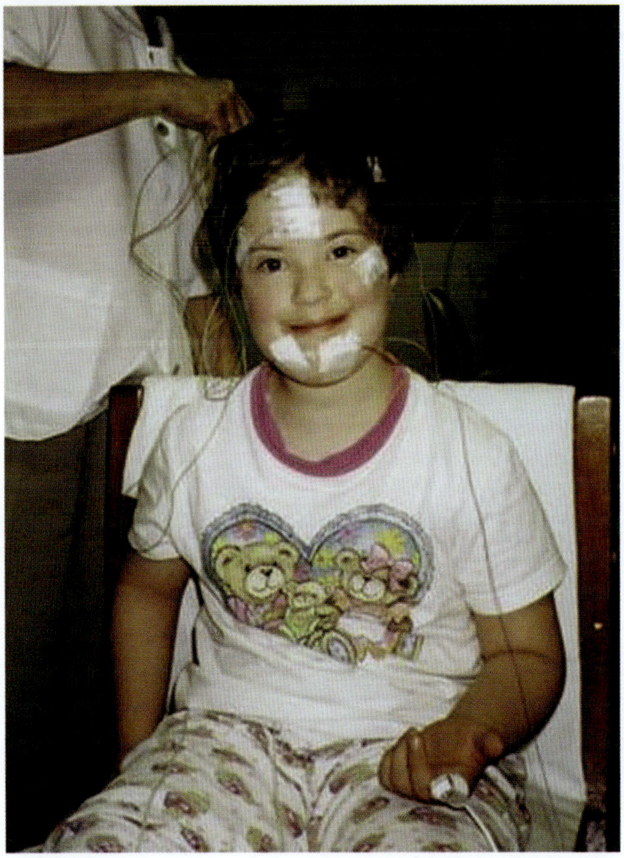

**Fig. 9.6** Child is having electrodes attached to have a nocturnal polysomnography test.

(Marsack-Topolewski, 2021; Marsack-Topolewski et al., 2021; Raina et al., 2005; Shattnawi et al., 2023). This lengthy course of caregiving has been called the "caregiver career" (Raina et al., 2004). Although there are many interrelated factors that predict caregiver wellness or distress, a child's level of independence with basic daily living skills is one of the factors (Bastawrous et al., 2015; Raina et al., 2005; Smith & Grzywacz, 2014).

### Common Problems Associated With ADLs

ADLs are complex activities that require a multitude of skills and abilities. Therefore, problems in any one area of function can hinder their performance, and as the severity of disability increases, independence with ADLs becomes more difficult. For example, cognitive deficits may make it difficult to properly sequence the steps of dressing oneself. Perceptual difficulties may hinder performance in terms of finding the proper clothing in a drawer or closet or in being able to tie one's shoes. Postural challenges may hinder independent dressing or bathing or may make it difficult to perform hygiene tasks after toileting. Bilateral and fine motor coordination difficulties also make dressing and hygiene more challenging. Sensory sensitivity may make dressing, toileting, bathing, and hygiene uncomfortable and distressing. However, performance in ADLs may also be highly affected by environmental or contextual factors, such as an inability to physically get to or into a rest room for example.

Cultural, class, and familial practices may differ in relation to the common occupational therapy goal for *independence* in the United States (Gross-Loh, 2013; Hamamura et al., 2013; Neff, 2003; Raeff, 2010). In some cultures and families, independence is not as highly regarded, nor is it required, while in others, children are much more independent than in the United States, and much earlier. The occupational therapist navigates these differences and focuses on family priorities, family concerns, and family expectations.

### Specific Areas of Assessment Regarding ADLs

As there are many possible areas to assess within the umbrella term of ADLs, whenever possible, the occupational therapist focuses on the specific activities of most importance to the family and child. Priorities will likely differ based on the practice setting; for example, there may not be a focus on showering at school. Similarly, priorities will vary based on the child's age.

### Comprehensive Evaluation of ADLs

A thorough evaluation of ADLs requires interviewing the caregivers and observing performance in natural settings if possible. Often ADL evaluation involves occupational analysis and observation. Certain activities, such as bathing or toileting, may not be able to be observed directly, and therefore, careful interviewing can be critical. Interview questions may be broad such as "tell me about your morning routine with your child," or they may be very specific and targeted such as "tell me more about what happens when you try to wash your child's hair." In many cases, assessment also includes the potential for adaptive equipment to improve performance and allow children to be more independent.

The goal of the evaluation of ADLs is to determine which ADLs the child is able to perform, either independently or with assistance or equipment, and which the child cannot complete. Then the therapist determines which of the challenging ADLs are most important for the family. The therapist then hypothesizes about and further identifies the causes of those challenges. This may at times require the use of specific assessments of skills or client factors (see Appendix A), for example if it appears that the difficulties with dressing skills are due to visual perceptual deficits.

When evaluating ADLs, occupational therapists consider the child's growth and potential development over time. For example, if a caregiver is currently able to bathe a very young child by carrying their child to the bathtub, the therapist considers the growth of the child over time and the potential future needs as the child becomes too large and heavy for the caregiver to do this safely. The therapist considers environmental issues, such as the need to go up a staircase to reach a bathroom, related to potential growth as well.

## EVALUATION OF INSTRUMENTAL ACTIVITIES OF DAILY LIVING

Instrumental activities of daily living (IADLs) include activities such as caring for others, driving and community mobility (discussed later in this chapter), financial management, health management and maintenance, home establishment and management, meal preparation and cleanup, care of pets, religious and spiritual activities, safety and emergency maintenance, and shopping. Many of these activities are primarily done by adults, although adolescents will begin engaging in some of these activities, and even younger children may begin to take on household chores.

### Importance of IADLs for Child and Family Functioning

Engagement in IADLs, as well as the ability to make autonomous decisions in adolescence that is supported by greater independence in IADLs, may lead to improved executive functions and greater self-determination (Richards et al., 2021; Taub & Werner, 2023; Tepper et al., 2022). Engagement in chores fosters a variety of skills that predispose youth to have better transitions to adulthood and better self-management of their health conditions (Mazzotti et al., 2021; Richards et al., 2021). Even in children as young as kindergarten age, performance of chores is associated with a variety of positive outcomes such as self-efficacy and prosocial behaviors (White et al., 2019). Therefore, IADLs are an important area of occupational therapy focus for both young children and adolescents.

Research on learning by observing and pitching in (LOPI) within indigenous communities suggests a variety of benefits for children, from this form of learning through doing (Coppens et al., 2014, 2016; Henne-Ochoa et al., 2020; Rogoff, 2014; Rosado-May et al., 2020). Learning by observing and pitching in occurs within a community structure where children contribute along with everyone else in the "work" of the family and community, with guidance from people in the community. The potential benefits to children when they are involved in a variety of household and community tasks with members of their community include learning language, specific skills, and to take initiative, collaborate, and innovate. Although not a common form of learning in the United States, children are typically very motivated to assist caregivers in this way, something that was noted decades ago in this country (Rheingold, 1982). In the United States, both youth engagement in IADLs and adult and youth expectations regarding required engagement vary between families, generations, and cultural backgrounds (Tamm et al., 2017; Vedder & Oortwijn, 2009).

### Common Challenges Associated With IADLs

IADLs are complex and can be affected by a variety of client factors, skills, and contextual issues. Although many of these issues can be addressed through interventions and adaptations, the basic idea or attitude that IADLs should even be an expectation for a child or youth can become a challenge. In the United States, there are typically significant differences in participation in IADLs by age. Occupational therapists consider age as they judge the relative importance between ADLs and IADLs in their practice (Shin et al., 2021). However, the research mentioned above suggests perhaps IADLs should be a focus much earlier than is typical.

Another potential attitudinal challenge related to IADLs is the negotiation between a youth's desire for more autonomy and independence and a caregiver's trust, fear, or willingness to support it (Han et al., 2022; Taub & Werner, 2023). In any given family, reduced autonomy may be because of caregiver rules and limitations or because of a youth's fear or even learned helplessness. For some families, parental attitudes and beliefs, and even overprotectiveness, may limit their promotion of their child's independence and self-determination (Arellano & Peralta, 2013).

When a child or youth has a disability, engagement in household chores and home management tasks also may vary by disability type and level of severity (do Amaral et al., 2014; Dunn & Gardner, 2013; Zhang, 2005). For some families, the challenges associated with particular engagement in IADLs for their child with severe disability may be too large a hurdle to manage given their resources. In other situations, contextual features of the environment present barriers.

### Specific Areas of Assessment Regarding IADLs

Interviews with caregivers and adolescents uncover family expectations, current level of participation and performance, and whether greater participation is a goal for the family or youth. Occupational therapists assess the child's engagement in IADLs by examining routines and the motor, process, and social interaction skills that support or hinder IADL engagement. They also examine the resources (e.g., equipment, community, supports) available to the child. For example, children who have motor difficulties may require adaptive equipment or modifications to assist with meal preparation. Children may need alternative forms of communication to express their needs when participating in IADLs such as shopping, meal preparation, or care of pets.

During the evaluation of IADLs, occupational therapists ask adolescents about their shopping behaviors. It is quite common for teens to have credit cards, shop independently, and even engage in problem shopping behavior (Grant et al., 2011). Teens also shop with peers and may be influenced in their shopping by these peer networks (Gentina & Bonsu, 2013). Youth with disabilities also want to engage in shopping with peers and find the mall a place to socialize; however, they face a variety of barriers to engagement (Dahan-Oliel et al., 2016). Adolescents are likely to also assist with food shopping and meal preparation at least some of the time (Vanderlee et al., 2018). Adults with autism report that grocery shopping is one of the aspects of home management in which they frequently engage, so this may be an important area of focus for occupational therapists (Shea et al., 2021).

Occupational therapists complete an occupational analysis to determine how the child engages in the IADL, which provides them with knowledge of the child's strengths and challenges to create an intervention plan. For example, a child may want to care for a pet (puppy). The therapist assesses the motor, processing, and social interaction skills required to care for a pet. The therapist works with the family to determine the family expectations and learn about the pet (e.g., is the pet trained?). The therapist conducts an occupational analysis of the skills and abilities needed to perform this IADL within the specific expectations and family setting. For example, the child's expectations change if they live in a family with other children also caring for the pet, versus if the pet will be the child's complete responsibility.

## EVALUATION OF EDUCATION

Occupational therapists working in school systems examine numerous factors related to learning, including environmental supports and barriers, and the requirements and expectations of others. This comprehensive approach to evaluation enables children of varying abilities to demonstrate their learning and succeed in school and also supports teachers in their work of educating children.

### Importance of Education for Child and Family Functioning

Education is often considered important for the economic benefit to society or as a way to produce good or ethical citizens or because it will allow someone to obtain employment or to bolster and improve society (Branson & Gross, 2014; Hanushek, 2020; Research.com, 2023; Roosevelt, 2008; Unicef, 2023). However, for an individual child, education is important for their development, to gain the ability to read, write, and think. It also provides the possibility for peer friendships and engagement in a variety of activities that can impact development of preferences and motivation.

The family has an important role in a child's education (Ceka & Murati, 2016). In particular, parental involvement and high parental expectations are related to academic achievement for typically developing children (Wilder, 2014). The relationships are more complex for students with disabilities, but parent expectations and involvement in their education remain important (Fishman & Nickerson, 2015; Flores de Apodaca et al., 2015; Newman, 2004). For families with children with disabilities, having a child in school can be stressful. For some families, parental involvement must become advocacy, as parents struggle to obtain the services they feel their child should receive (Burke et al., 2019; Burke & Hodapp, 2016; Goldman, 2020). The frequent advocacy needs may take a toll on caregivers and impact the family. In particular, the transition from early intervention services to school-age special education may be a difficult time for families (Douglas et al., 2022). Parents at times report limited communication regarding the special education services and a lack of collaboration with providers. Occupational therapists support family functioning with thoughtful interactions and advocacy for appropriate services at school.

## Common Challenges Associated With Education

Occupational therapists working in school settings often focus on traditional skill development, handwriting, and fine motor skills (Bolton & Plattner, 2020; Clough, 2019; Cramm & Egan, 2015; de Oliveira Borba et al., 2020). However, occupational therapy services in the schools can have a much broader focus (Ball, 2018; Bonnard & Anaby, 2016; Bonnard et al., 2022; Cramm et al., 2013; Frolek Clark & Polichino, 2021). Students in the schools have a variety of mental health needs and may struggle with executive functioning, making friends, and engaging in extracurricular activities. They may be bullied or isolated for being different.

School-based practice and educational services still often function from a deficit model, and full inclusion is not consistently the norm for students with disabilities (Sandoval & McKee, 2020). There is ample room for improvement in the provision of educational services that support inclusion, participation, and student strengths, starting with an occupational therapy evaluation that includes a wider range of performance than merely academics and handwriting.

## Specific Areas of Assessment Regarding Education

The occupation of education is broad and complex. Occupational therapists frame their evaluation based on student needs for formal educational participation. This information often comes from interviews with the teacher and the child's caregivers and from observations of the child in the classroom or other school environments.

Occupational therapists in the schools evaluate the child's performance both in academic and also in nonacademic activities, such as extracurricular, prevocational, or vocational activities. Occupational therapists evaluate executive function skills, self-regulation, and other global functions to examine the student's ability to perform in the educational setting. Depending on the specific areas of difficulty reported by those requesting the evaluation, the focus on the evaluation could be on reading and literacy tasks, math, social communication and interaction, play in the classroom or at recess, self-care for toileting or for physical education, and attention and behavior during school activities. Next there may be further specific assessment of the related underlying skills needed for school success, such as cognition, visual perception, and sensory processing. Any of these areas may be part of the occupational therapy school evaluation.

A child's social skills impact both academic and nonacademic aspects of education. For example, making friends, learning, and working in groups; adapting to school routines; and following rules can be impacted by one's ability to self-regulate. Children and adolescents who exhibit difficulty with social skills may demonstrate lack of respect toward peers, teachers, or school property. The development of social skills reinforces mental health and health promotion needs for school-based interventions. Social and emotional behaviors necessary for social development include self-awareness, self-management, social awareness, relationship skills, and responsible decision-making (Collaborative for Academic, Social, and Emotional Learning, 2015). Students need to see the value of why they must learn the skills, the impact of the skills, and how they fit into their learning. Social skills may be observed during lunch activities, recess, and hallway interactions of the student with peers, teachers, and other school personnel. Observations in the classroom, hallway, lunchroom, or at recess provide excellent sources of naturalistic data (Fig. 9.7). Table 9.16 provides an analysis of the motor and process skills needed for formal educational participation in academic, nonacademic, extracurricular, and vocational activities.

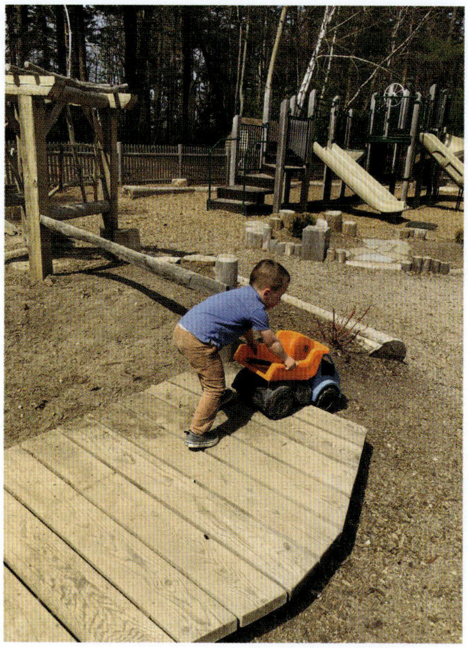

**Fig. 9.7** Observations of playground participation.

A student's skills are viewed along with student motivation, curiosity, and self-efficacy. Motivation is critical when performance difficulty exists. Self-efficacy is an important concept within ***mastery*** learning, to build a growth mindset and a belief in the learning process (Dweck, 2006; Komarraju & Nadler, 2013). A **growth mindset** is dynamic, developed through dedication and effort rather than a fixed view of one's abilities. A growth mindset allows the student to see challenges and failures as opportunities for learning and further developing their abilities, thus reinforcing self-efficacy.

**Self-regulation** is often viewed as the ability to manage and control emotions and behavior in response to a situation. Self-regulation requires emotional control and can be impacted by temperament and previous learned behaviors, along with motivation for the learning situation (Zimmerman, 2008; Zimmerman & Kitsantas, 2014). Martini et al. (2016) suggest *strategies* can be classified either as catalyst (i.e., changing the emotional or arousal state of an individual) or metacognitive, (i.e., higher-order thinking processes of self-monitoring). This is an important distinction when assessing a child's occupational performance.

Occupational therapists may use the term self-regulation differently than teachers. Therapists often view self-regulation from a sensory integrative theory approach rather than a cognitive behavioral approach to learning and performance. Occupational therapists plan strategies (based on children's sensory needs) to support students' self-regulation in the educational environment. It is important that they clarify how they are using the term to interprofessional team members (e.g., teachers, parents) (Martini et al., 2016).

Sensory processing abilities often impact a child's ability to participate within the classroom and throughout the school day (Chien et al., 2016; Dean et al., 2018). When difficulties in sensory processing exist, students may have poor coordination abilities in writing, moving about the classroom, and other physical activities, shy away from physical and social activities, and demonstrate a lack of resilience and adaptation in the school context. Underlying sensory processing problems may present as negative behaviors, with resultant embarrassment

**TABLE 9.16 Motor and Process Skills Needed During Formal Educational Participation**

| OTPF: Performance Skills | FORMAL EDUCATIONAL PARTICIPATION | | | | | | | | | |
|---|---|---|---|---|---|---|---|---|---|---|
| | ACADEMICS | | | | NONACADEMICS | | | EXTRACURRICULAR | VOCATIONAL | |
| | Scissors | Writing | Reading | Math | Recess | Lunchroom | Hallway | Sports or Dance | Prevocational | Vocational |
| **Motor skills** | | | | | | | | | | |
| Aligns | X | X | X | | | X | | | X | X |
| Stabilizes | | | | | X | X | X | X | X | X |
| Positions | X | X | X | X | | X | | X | X | X |
| Reaches | X | X | X | | X | X | | X | X | X |
| Bends | X | X | X | | X | X | | X | X | X |
| Grips | X | X | | | | X | | X | X | X |
| Manipulates | X | X | | | | X | | X | X | X |
| Coordinates | X | X | | | | X | | X | X | X |
| Moves | | X | | | | X | X | X | X | X |
| Lifts | X | X | X | | X | X | | | X | X |
| Walks | | | | | X | X | X | X | X | X |
| Transports | | | | | | X | X | | X | X |
| Calibrates | X | X | X | | X | X | X | X | X | X |
| Flows | X | X | | | | X | | X | X | X |
| Endures | X | X | X | X | X | X | X | X | X | X |
| Paces | X | X | X | X | X | X | X | X | X | X |
| **Process skills** | | | | | | | | | | |
| Paces | X | X | X | X | | X | X | X | X | X |
| Attends | X | X | X | X | | X | X | | X | X |
| Heeds | | X | X | X | | X | | | X | X |
| Chooses | X | X | | X | X | X | | X | X | X |
| Uses | X | X | | | X | X | | X | X | X |
| Handles | X | X | | | | X | | X | X | X |
| Inquires | | X | | X | | | | | X | X |
| Initiates | X | X | X | X | X | X | | | X | X |
| Continues | X | X | X | X | | | | X | X | X |
| Sequences | X | X | X | X | | X | | X | X | X |
| Terminates | X | X | X | X | X | X | X | X | X | X |
| Searches/locates | | | | | X | | | X | X | X |
| Gathers | | X | | | X | X | | X | X | X |
| Organizes | | X | X | | | X | | | X | X |
| Restores | | | | | | X | | | X | X |
| Navigates | | | | | | X | X | | X | X |
| Notices/responds | X | X | | | | X | | X | X | X |
| Adjusts | X | X | X | X | | X | | | X | X |
| Accommodates | X | X | X | X | X | X | | X | X | X |
| Benefits | X | X | X | X | X | X | | X | X | X |

and bullying by others. An important aspect of the assessment process is to consider tools for collaborating with teachers about the classroom sensory environment (Kuhaneck & Kelleher, 2015, 2018).

Knowledge of how underlying interoceptive body needs may impact behavior is also important for understanding a child's abilities with attention and learning (Mahler, 2019). Interoceptive awareness of internal body states, for example hunger, may contribute to behavioral outbursts, self-regulatory issues, and/or emotional withdrawal. By addressing sensory processing skill needs in the academic setting, students show better on-task behaviors, which allow them to focus for learning. Social interaction skills are also positively impacted in the classroom setting when underlying sensory processing needs are addressed (Swaminathan & Nandgaonkar, 2016). By facilitating student improvement in self-awareness of sensory needs, students can participate in problem-solving to support self-regulation needs in the school context. Self-regulation is typically assessed through observation of student behaviors and engagement in various activities throughout the day (e.g., recess, lunch time, classroom behavior.). Formal assessments for assessing self-regulation and sensory processing functions are listed in Appendix A.

Motor skill challenges can impact the student's participation in general classroom activities such as writing, using scissors, and other tool use, negotiating hallways during the changing of classes, recess, physical education, and participating in clubs or sporting events. The required fine motor and gross motor coordination skills for school tasks change over time, often impacting participation in differing activities during different grades (Bhat et al., 2011; Rosenberg et al., 2017) (Fig. 9.8). Occupational therapists examine the relationship of challenges within client factors and performance patterns that can impact a student's desire to attend school and fully participate in their student role. For example, students that have weak hand muscles may not want to take copious notes and miss information for learning. They may need adaptations for notetaking but forget to use them or not use the tools consistently. Prevocationally, students may need adaptations to successfully engage in potential job opportunities. Motor skill challenges may hinder skill development, needed for engagement in the transition from school to work (Juan & Swinth, 2010).

Students often show what they have learned through handwriting, although it need not be the only way to document learning. Occupational therapists frequently evaluate handwriting for students in the schools. They evaluate the following areas: domains of handwriting, legibility components, writing speed, and ergonomic factors. Assessment may also consider foundational skills: fine motor skills including in-hand manipulation, strength, and pencil grip; visual perception; visual motor integration; sensory skills including proprioception; and motor planning. To understand more fully the elements that interfere with a child's ability to produce text, the occupational therapist considers a student's performance skills, client factors, performance patterns, and contextual elements. Therapists also consider the teacher's perspective, the handwriting instruction methods, and the curricula requirements.

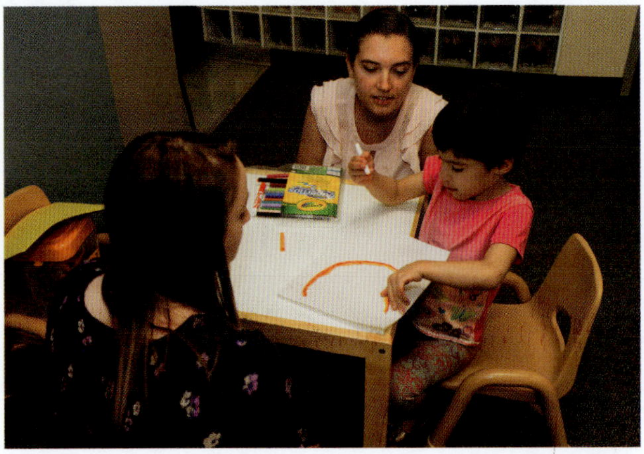

**Fig. 9.8** At young ages classroom activities often require fine and gross motor coordination skills for drawing, using two hands together in bilateral tasks, and sitting upright in a chair.

**Evaluation of Education Through Telehealth.** Normed questionnaire-based assessments and rating scales can be administered effectively through telehealth: synchronously using screen sharing or asynchronously through the publisher's online evaluation platform (Pearson, 2021a, 2022; WPS, 2022). For asynchronous administration, the occupational therapist inputs data about the child (e.g., gender, date of birth, age) into the online evaluation platform and provides a caregiver's email address. The caregiver receives an automated email from the assessment publisher with a secure link to complete the assessment through the publisher's online evaluation platform. Upon completion, the occupational therapist receives a notification and can access and electronically score the assessment. Additional features may be available to generate a report from the data or a list of therapeutic strategies aligned with specific assessment items (e.g., SPM Quick Tips). See Appendix A for information on specific tools that can be used in this manner.

Some performance-based assessments have digital assets that enable synchronous administration using screen sharing and skilled observation (Pearson, 2022; WPS, 2022). For other assessments, standardized administration can be completed synchronously using assessment materials (response forms or standardized materials) mailed to the caregiver prior to the evaluation. For example, for synchronous administration of the Beery-Buktenica Developmental Test of Visual-Motor Integration (6th ed.), Pearson recommends use of the original standardized response forms, a sharpened No. 2 pencil or ballpoint pen, an appropriately sized table and chair, and a peripheral camera (e.g., external camera or mobile device with camera) to clearly view the child's performance on tasks (Pearson, 2021c). A facilitator is recommended if the child is below a functional age of 5 years. Additional guidance is provided for the Beery VMI Full and Short Form, Visual Perception Supplemental Test Form, and Motor Coordination Supplemental Test Form (Pearson, 2021c). Similar telehealth guidance is available for other performance-based assessments.

Normative data for most normed performance-based assessments were collected through in-person administration using standardized materials. Any variance from the standardized assessment protocol, including telehealth administration, should be documented. Professional judgment is required to determine the impact of the telehealth administration on score interpretation and the capacity of the caregiver to assist in the standardized administration of the assessment (Pearson, 2021b). In cases wherein the telehealth administration of assessments, or subtests of assessments, may not allow for calculation of scores due to variance from the normed protocol, information gathered during the assessment can inform the evaluation and plan of care (Pearson, 2021b). Alternatively, a professional assessment facilitator may be trained to assist in standardized assessment administration under the guidance of the remote occupational therapist for some performance-based assessments requiring adherence to a normed protocol and use of standardized manipulatives (Pearson, 2021d).

***Copyright and Telehealth Occupational Therapy Assessment.*** Whether services are provided in-person or through telehealth, occupational therapists are obligated to adhere to copyright laws when providing standardized materials to clients. This may involve purchasing and mailing standardized response forms and stimulus books prior to administering telehealth occupational therapy assessments. If materials need to be returned to the practitioner, a stamped, self-addressed envelope should be provided when the materials are mailed to the caregiver. Unless explicitly permitted by the publisher, duplicating materials for use by scanning them onto a computer or making digital or photocopies is unethical and a violation of copyright law. Additionally, occupational therapists inform the caregiver during the informed consent process that taking video, photos, or screenshots of any assessment materials during the evaluation is a copyright violation (Pearson, 2021d).

***Set Up for Telehealth Assessment.*** It is important to determine if the client has access to the technology needed to complete the process through telehealth. In a telehealth service delivery model, consultation and screening may be completed through a combination of record review, caregiver interview using videoconferencing or phone, skilled observation through videoconferencing, and asynchronously with screening assessments completed through publishers' online evaluation platforms (Pearson, 2022; WPS, 2022).

Prior to the assessment, the occupational therapist communicates with the caregiver about the technology and materials needed to complete the assessment. For example, the child's screen size should be a minimum of 9.7 inches measured diagonally for assessments with onscreen visual stimuli (Pearson, 2021d). Occupational therapists inquire about the device being used by the client and follow the assessment publisher's guidelines for screen sharing digital components of the assessment. Devices used for telehealth occupational therapy assessment should be plugged directly into a power source to avoid loss of power due to battery depletion. The device should be turned on prior to the start of the assessment to allow time for any needed software updates to occur. Headsets worn by the practitioner and child may improve the ability to hear instructions and responses clearly. A headset may also improve attention to tasks by reducing environmental noises. However, benefits, availability, and the child's acceptance for wearing a headset should be considered (Pearson, 2021d).

The child's environment should have minimal distractions (e.g., the television or radio should be turned off, and the child's e-helper/caregiver should be the only person in the room with the child). The child should be positioned where there is adequate light for the practitioner to clearly see the child during the assessment. If lighting is inadequate or there are shadows impacting on screen visibility, the caregiver may open or close window shades, turn on overhead lights or lamps, or reposition the child in relation to the light source.

Request that seated activities (e.g., table-top activities, feeding, handwriting) occur at a table, with appropriate child-sized seating (high chair, booster seat, or chair) if available. A built-in camera on a desktop or laptop computer will provide a limited view. If available, a mobile device (electronic tablet or smartphone) can be used to provide alternate viewing angles during table-top and movement-based activities.

## EVALUATION OF PLAY

### Importance of Play to Child and Family Functioning

Play is important for child development and well-being (Ginsburg & Committee on Psychosocial Aspects of Child and Family Health, 2007; Milteer et al., 2012; Nijhof et al., 2018). Play brings joy and happiness to children and, as such, may also bring joy and happiness to the family unit. Family play and leisure have been associated with family well-being, family relationships, and positive affect (Coyl-Shepherd & Hanlon, 2013; Duff, 1996; Gil & Sobol, 2005; Levine, 1988).

**BOX 9.14 Toy Inventory**

Occupational therapists can share this toy inventory with parents to promote play and playfulness in the home. Parents often ask for ideas of gifts for their children before a child's birthday or holiday. This inventory may help educate others on the play needs of the child.

**Step 1**

Explain that "good toys" have the following qualities:

- Are appropriate for the child's age and developmental level
- Keep the child's interest
- Have longevity (in other words they are toys that will stand the test of time and can be used by the child in a variety of ways for years, such as Legos)
- Are safe and durable
- Stimulate learning

**Step 2**

Encourage parents to create a list of toys in their home by the following categories:

- Active toys (ride-on toys, outdoor or sports equipment)
- Manipulative toys (construction toys, puzzles, dressing toys, beads, blocks, bath toys, and sand or water toys)
- Make-believe (dolls, stuffed toys, puppets, role play, and transportation toys)
- Creative toys (musical toys, arts and crafts materials, digital music or tablet devices with creativity apps)
- Learning toys (games, specific-skill toys such as science models, computer or tablet devices with learning applications, books)

**Step 3**

Review toy inventory with the parent. Make suggestions for home play spaces and playthings that relate to the child's intervention goals.

### Common Challenges Associated With Play

There are a variety of possible difficulties that may be noted with play. Children may have difficulties creating ideas for play themes, motor planning actions for play activities, or physically manipulating toys and games with small pieces. Children may have behavioral challenges that make it hard to wait their turn or to share, or they may be unable to communicate clearly with peers to play certain games. There are a variety of potential difficulties with play; however, difficulties with imitation and difficulties with pretending are frequently noted. Additionally, there may be contextual factors that limit play such as lack of playthings, safe play spaces, and time allotted for play. Box 9.14 provides a toy inventory to examine playthings in the home.

### Specific Areas of Assessment Regarding Play

Play assessment includes identifying the types or forms of play children prefer, the play activities that are available to them, how playful they are, and also when, where, and with whom they play. Additionally, therapists seek to understand the child's experience with play and the meaning of play for that child. The evaluation of play involves informal as well as formal assessments that are carefully selected. Many tools designed to assess play may assess other skills such as fine motor skills, rather than play. The comprehensive play evaluation includes four components, outlined in Table 9.17.

The occupational therapist begins by using a top-down approach to explore the place of play in the family routine to gain an understanding of the child and family context and to gather an occupational profile for play. Having a general understanding of the characteristics associated with a child's diagnosis allows the therapist to look for potential areas

**TABLE 9.17 Components of a Comprehensive Play Evaluation**

| Evaluation Component | Occupational Therapist's Role | Play Tools and Considerations for Professional Reasoning |
|---|---|---|
| **Occupational profile** | Gather information on child and family play preferences, values, attitudes, and culture | Interviews and observations in ecologic settings |
| **Assessment of performance** | Assesses play occupation in context, including relevant play partners and play objects | Formal and informal tests; structured observations; use of video |
| **Assessment of environment** | Assesses physical environmental characteristics that hinder or support play occupation | Formal and informal tests; structured observations; use of video |
| **Analysis of performance** | Analyses play occupation strengths, challenges, and needs based on integration of insights gained | Use of professional reasoning including cultural sensitivity to understand play challenges and needs in ecologic contexts |

**TABLE 9.18 Potential Play Solutions based on Characteristics Associated with Childhood Conditions**

| Condition | Associated Characteristics | Potential Play Solutions |
|---|---|---|
| **Attention-deficit disorder** | • Short attention span<br>• Might be easily distracted<br>• Enjoys novelty<br>• Often impulsive | • Identify play preferences<br>• Explore strategies for making friendships<br>• Freedom to play outdoors<br>• Engaging in high impact play events such as trampolining and heavy work<br>• Encourage activities that can be achieved in a short timespan |
| **Autism** | • Likes repetitive behaviors<br>• Needs routines for successful engagement<br>• Enjoys objects and natural elements in environment<br>• Needs help to understand humor, jokes, or nonverbal communication | • Identify play preferences<br>• Explore strategies for making friendships<br>• Provide outdoor experiences for play that allow freedom to self-control play choices<br>• Use social stories when introducing new playgrounds or places for play |
| **Developmental coordination disorder/ dyspraxia** | • May prefer activities that do not involve a lot of manipulation<br>• Enjoys games or activities they can control themselves, not competitive | • Identify play preferences<br>• Explore strategies for making friendships<br>• Encourage more varied and intense outdoor play—large body movements |
| **Visual and hearing impairment** | • Needs time to orient and understand the physical layout and opportunities in the play environment | • Identify play preferences<br>• Explore strategies for making friendships<br>• Provide structured play opportunities with enhanced multisensory characteristics<br>• Support risk-taking at the just right level |

of play strengths and challenges to create play solutions (see Table 9.18 for examples).

The aim of the evaluation is to gather enough information to determine the child and family play preferences, values, and their sociocultural context. An ecologic assessment onsite in the child's home, school or community is an effective way to see what resources are available to the family in their physical and social environments. Cultural competence and sensitivity are crucial during this phase of evaluation to gain understanding of how cultural practices may influence play occupations and opportunities for the child (Hammell, 2013). See Table 9.19 for some questions to consider when examining play.

Based on the occupational profile, the therapist determines which play events or opportunities they want to observe more specifically to do an occupational analysis. Given that play is a freely chosen occupation that most often occurs when adults are not present, this makes conducting a play assessment challenging. Play is mostly assessed informally through observation, and most commonly, it involves unstructured observation (Bundy, 2011; Ray-Kaeser & Lynch, 2017). This is because observations in natural contexts allow the occupational therapist to consider the occupation in its entirety and as it happens, which contributes to the validity of the assessment (Bronfenbrenner & Morris, 2007).

Many play assessment tools examine aspects of play such as social or communication skills, but occupational therapists are interested in viewing play participation as an occupation (Romli & Wan Yunus, 2020). More than 24 play assessments exist (for examples, see Moore & Lynch, 2018 and Appendix A). A review of play assessments found eight occupational therapy tools with published results on psychometric properties (Romli & Wan Yunus, 2020). However, only three of the tools were commercially available (see Table 9.20). Efforts have been made to support test validity, and to reliably measure play in natural settings, despite the complexity of doing so (Bundy, 1993). For example, the Test of Playfulness (Skard & Bundy, 2008) uses video or observation of children playing in typical play contexts to determine a child's playfulness, and it has been used as an outcome measure in play-based intervention research (see for example, Kent et al., 2020). The Knox

**TABLE 9.19 Questions Relating to Cultural Values and Attitudes to Guide Evaluation of Play**

| | |
|---|---|
| For the parent/carer | • What does play mean to you, or your family?<br>• If you value play, how do you play at home with your child or as a family? Is there a type of play you do not agree with?<br>• What do you think of play with toys, online, outside in the community, in school, and in playgrounds?<br>• Is there a play challenge for your family, something you would love to be able to do with your child? |
| For the child | • If the child can talk with you, ask what they also think of play, what is their favorite thing to play, what do they dislike most, what would they love to play if they were allowed to do so, or if they had the ability?<br>• For nonverbal children, seek to observe them in a natural play event and gain insight and answers to these same questions.<br>• Asking an adult carer about the child's preferences will also provide more information. |
| For the therapist | • From the answers to the above questions, ask yourself, what do you know about the place of play in this family/community?<br>• Do you know the play preferences and needs of the child and family?<br>• How does this inform you about potential assessments, intervention approaches or goals you can establish to address play? |

**TABLE 9.20 Play Assessments**

1. Child-Initiated Pretend Play Assessment (ChIPPA) (Stagnitti, 2020)
2. Knox Preschool Play Scale (Knox PPS) (Knox, 2008)
3. McDonald's Play Inventory (MDPI) (McDonald & Vigen, 2012)
4. My Child's Play (Schneider & Rosenblum, 2014)
5. Play Assessment of Group Settings (PAGS) (Lautamo et al., 2005)
6. Play History Inventory (Behnke & Fetkovich, 1984)
7. Test of Playfulness (ToP) (Skard & Bundy, 2008)
8. Test of Environmental Supportiveness (TOES) (Bundy, 2009)

Preschool Play Scale (KPPS) scale is an observation tool that can be used in a natural preschool setting (Knox, 2008), and the child-initiated play assessment (CHIPPA) measures pretend play (Stagnitti, 2020). Other tools, such as My Child's Play questionnaire, are designed to gather information on the child's play to identify the child's play preferences through parent interview (Schneider & Rosenblum, 2014), while the McDonald Play Inventory includes the child's self-report as part of the assessment (McDonald & Vigen, 2012). Overall, few measures have been developed that evaluate play as an occupation or focus on evaluating the interrelated influences of environmental factors including the role of others and of the physical objects and spaces for play (Adolfsson et al., 2011). When selecting a tool to evaluate play, therapists consider how and what they want to measure and how they will identify any change in play participation as an outcome of the intervention.

Contemporary occupational therapy models emphasize the necessity of examining the contexts in which occupations occur (Kuhaneck, Spitzer, et al., 2010), and subsequently, occupational therapists have increasingly documented the importance of contextual features that influence children's play (Kuhaneck & Spitzer, 2023). Environmental features that support play and playfulness include physical safety, space for play, time for play, availability of developmentally appropriate and preferred play materials, and appropriate social interaction with either peers or adults (Kuhaneck, Burroughs, et al., 2010; Kuhaneck & Spitzer, 2023). The Test of Environmental Supportiveness, developed by Bundy (2009), examines the environmental supportiveness for playfulness and the fit between the player and the play environment. At a more universal level, Lynch et al. (2018) developed an audit tool of playgrounds to determine how the environment supported inclusive play. This has still to be advanced and progressed to determine its potential value.

Once the play assessments are completed, the therapist interprets the findings and synthesizes them into a play profile for the child, family, and community. They identify strengths and resources of the child, family, and community, as well as the needs arising and the play challenges. Once this is established, the practitioner and family create play goals, which requires consideration of sociocultural contexts and the child's right to play for the sake of play and not just for future skills or adulthood (Fahy et al., 2021; Lynch et al., 2020; O'Connor et al., 2021).

Supporting children's rights to play for the sake of play can be challenging. For example, in interviews with occupational and physiotherapists in Sweden, therapists talked of the pressure to work on skills for the future with the child, which meant ignoring current play needs for children and families (Nordström et al., 2023). However, if occupational therapists are to take an active role in implementing the right of the child to play, then this is an area of therapy that requires more commitment from an occupational justice perspective and can be included in the therapy goals alongside the more common focus on skill development.

## EVALUATION OF LEISURE

Children and youth participate in leisure activities, which include activities that are not required but for which they find meaning and enjoyment (AOTA, 2020b). They may engage in leisure alone, with family, or with groups of people. Families frequently engage in leisure activities together based on their family routines, culture, and interests. Occupational therapists view leisure as an important occupation for health and quality of life (Chen & Chippendale, 2018).

### Importance of Leisure to Child and Family Functioning

There is an important association between family leisure and positive family functioning that is observed across various countries and cultures (Buswell et al., 2012; Chen et al., 2019; Haanpää & Ursin, 2018; Hodge, et al., 2017, 2018; Zabriskie & Kay, 2013). Families that are satisfied with their leisure are satisfied with their family life (Agate et al., 2009). Children's well-being is influenced by the family's participation in leisure activities together, as are the relationships between parents or caregivers. Children and youth with disabilities want meaningful interactions with others and leisure experiences that improve their quality of life (Dahan-Oliel et al., 2012; Powrie et al., 2020; Willis et al., 2017).

### Common Challenges Associated With Leisure

Although participation in leisure is complex and affected by many factors, a primary issue with leisure participation for youth with disabilities is lack of access and opportunity, which is often related to the youth's level of independence (King et al., 2003; Sanches-Ferreira et al., 2019; Steinhardt et al., 2021). Specifically motor function, cognitive ability, and communication are important variables (Bult et al., 2011; Longo et al., 2020). Parents report a variety of difficulties accessing recreational opportunities for their child (Schleien et al., 2014) and even isolating experiences occurring while engaged in leisure (Hodge & Runswick-Cole, 2013).

### Specific Areas of Assessment Regarding Leisure

An occupational profile may be used initially to explore the young person's leisure interests and participation as well as to identify opportunities and barriers. This information can easily be obtained with informal interviews using open-ended questions such as "What do you do for fun after school and on weekends?" "Tell me about a typical weekend," "What are your favorite hobbies and interests?" and "What new leisure activity would you like to learn and do?" Informal interviews with the young person are critical for gaining their perspectives. Although several leisure inventories and assessments (see Appendix A) are available, taking the time to complete them may not be necessary when an adolescent indicates little or no leisure participation.

Evaluation also involves gathering information from other important "clients" including parents/caregivers and school and community providers. Conversations with parents/caregivers provide an opportunity to explore their priorities and concerns related to their child's leisure participation and perceptions of strengths and challenges. Although parents may have a sense of their child's interests, it is important to talk individually with the young person to gain their views. For example, when an occupational therapist used a picture interest inventory with a young girl with Down syndrome and intellectual impairment, she pointed to pictures of softball and camping. Her parents exclaimed, "We didn't think she was interested in these activities!" Based on this evaluation, the occupational therapist worked with the parents and young girl to find a local softball team and provided informal coaching to foster successful participation. The parents were excited to have their daughter be a part of a team and experience joy and success in participating. This example demonstrates how parents may make assumptions about their young person's interests or lack thereof. Communicating directly with the child fosters exploration and independent decision-making, which contributes to the development of autonomy.

Evaluation of the context is critical for gathering important information used during the intervention process. Whether the occupational therapist works in a school, clinic, or community, being aware of available leisure activities is essential in helping young people and families make informed choices. For example, occupational therapists can complete a leisure environmental scan in the young person's community. This involves searching for potential community-based options for participation in a wide array of areas including sports, outdoor nature activities, theater, arts and crafts, music, and cooking to name a few. Although this task may be time-consuming initially, a growing awareness of community resources will evolve over time as practitioners make leisure a part of their everyday work with youth.

Evaluation involves strategically tuning into youth at risk and exploring what they do for fun during free time. Evaluation also includes having an awareness of school and community leisure options and identifying those that might be a good fit for youth with developmental, physical, and/or mental health challenges. Visiting settings and meeting youth directors or coaches can serve a dual purpose of advocating for inclusion as well as assessing whether providers value inclusive participation and making accommodations to ensure success.

## EVALUATION OF SOCIAL PARTICIPATION

Social participation can be defined as "Activities that involve social interaction with others, including family, friends, peers, and community members, and that support social interdependence" (AOTA, 2020b, p. 34). This definition allows for overlap with other occupations if they occur with other people. This chapter focuses on the evaluation of friendships and community engagement. Table 9.21 provides a overview of social participation themes and their related aspects according to Mamas et al. (2021).

**TABLE 9.21 Social Participation Key Themes and Related Aspects**

| Key Themes | Related Aspects |
|---|---|
| 1. Level of friendships/ relationships | • Friendship network (size and composition)<br>• Mental friendships (trust and support) |
| 2. Type of contacts/ interactions | • Playing together<br>• Working together on tasks<br>• Participation in group activities<br>• (Un)acknowledged initiations<br>• Social isolation |
| 3. Social self-perception | • Self-perception of peer acceptance<br>• Satisfaction at school<br>• Social self-concept (understanding of one's self and others)<br>• Self-perception of social competence<br>• Loneliness |
| 4. Acceptance by classmates | • Attitudes of others within environment<br>• Social preference<br>• Social support (behaviors)<br>• Bullying<br>• Social rejection (social stigma) |

Adapted from Mamas et al. (2021) and Koster et al. (2009).

### Importance of Social Participation for Children and Families

Social connection is a basic and fundamental need for all humans and is related to their well-being (Xia & Hudac, 2023). Social participation is incredibly important for youth for their quality of life and physical health (DaWalt et al., 2019; Helseth & Misvaer, 2010; Holt-Lunstad, 2021; Holt-Lunstad et al., 2010). Alternatively, loneliness in children with neurodevelopmental disabilities is related to poorer mental health and behavior (Kwan et al., 2020). Whether one is discussing the *structural* aspects of social engagement, such as the size of one's social network, their number of social roles, and whether one lives alone or with others, or is more focused on the *functional* aspects of social life such as social support and resources, or examining the *quality* of social relationships such as satisfaction, each is linked to one's health or risk of poor health (Holt-Lunstad et al., 2017; Hostinar, 2015).

### Common Challenges Associated With Social Participation

For many individuals with disabilities, social stigma and the attitudes of others are barriers to social connection (Ditchman et al., 2016; Mueller, 2019). Similarly, the caregivers of youth with disabilities face stigma that impairs their mental health (Papadopoulos et al., 2019; Song et al., 2018), and these experiences of stigma in turn impact the social participation of the youth with disability (Lim et al., 2021). For autistic individuals, two of the most commonly reported barriers to social participation include their difficulty understanding social situations and specific challenging behaviors (Ghanouni et al., 2019). Finally, bullying is a frequently noted problem for children, but particularly for children with disabilities (Iyanda, 2022).

For families with young children with disabilities, the environment is often the most difficult barrier (Di Marino et al., 2018). For youth with physical disabilities, accessibility and transportation difficulties are common concerns (Bascom & Christensen, 2017; Bezyak et al., 2020; Moore et al., 2022). It is not uncommon for youth with physical disabilities such as CP to engage in minimal activities with friends or those other than family members (Kang et al., 2010). However, those with greater functional abilities in motor and communication skills appear to engage in activity outside the home with greater frequency and also to enjoy it more (Alghamdi et al., 2017).

### Specific Areas of Assessment Regarding Social Participation

Although in certain situations it may be necessary to evaluate specific client skills, it is critical that the occupational therapist take a broad view of social participation and focus most heavily on environmental barriers, attitudinal barriers, and policy issues related to social participation of those with disabilities, rather than focusing on trying to change the client's behaviors (Chen & Patten, 2021).

Initially, the therapist identifies what social participation activities are currently occurring and what the client would enjoy or prefer in relation to the amount, type, or level of participation. Evaluation might include gathering information about habits, routines, and the general level of social participation in which children engage through a variety of assessment measures (e.g., interview, self-report, rating scales, interest checklists, and observation). Additionally, using these types of tools and methods, the therapist gathers information about friendships or isolation and loneliness or social connection. See Appendix A for specific tools available to help in gathering this information.

There are a variety of important aspects or features of social participation that can be included in an occupational therapy evaluation. Based on the common barriers to participation discussed above, assessment may also include gathering information about accessibility of desired community spaces and activities and availability of preferred activities and transportation. Given the current focus on the importance of social connection for health, for all humans (Jordan, 2023), and the potential for social isolation of families with children with disabilities (Alsharaydeh et al., 2019; Currie & Szabo, 2020), it may be important to also discuss family perceptions of isolation and stigma as part of the evaluation. The high rates of bullying in youth with disabilities suggests that therapists should include questions related to bullying in the evaluation, and as it appears that engagement in extracurricular activities can reduce bullying, this is another important area to include (Haegele et al., 2020).

If necessary, occupational therapists assess the skills and client factors of the child, examining social interaction skills and behaviors. Several child development assessments have items reflecting social skill development. Occupational therapists may also choose to use assessment tools that are specific to social skills and social development. Social skills assessment includes information such as whether the child engages in activities with friends, prefers being alone or with others, establishes eye contact with others during interaction, understands nonverbal communication, displays and responds to humor, shares or takes turn, uses appropriate voice volume when talking with others, talks with others about their interests, or understands appropriate proximity when interacting with others. Occupational therapists may also choose from general assessments that include social information and specific assessments for social impairment. See Appendix A for a comprehensive list of these assessments.

## EVALUATION OF SEXUALITY

"Sexuality is a core characteristic and formative factor for human beings. It is a state of mind, representing our feelings about ourselves, what it's like to be male or female, how we relate to people of our own gender and those of the opposite gender, how we establish relationships, and how we express ourselves. It is basic to our sense of self" (MacRae, 2013). Sexuality is greater than merely sexual activity.

There are different pathways that adolescents take to sexual activity, and those pathways are related to family, religion, gender, and attitudes (Zimmer-Gembeck & Helfand, 2008). AOTA (2020b) describes sexual activity as including "the broad possibilities for sexual expression and experiences with self or others (e.g., hugging, kissing, foreplay, masturbation, oral sex, intercourse)" (p. 30). Occupational therapists evaluate children and youth's sexuality to identify barriers and supports to desired sexual activity.

### Importance of Sexuality for Youth and Families

While adult sexuality is commonly linked to well-being, the topic is more controversial when discussing teens and youth (Harden, 2014; Vasilenko et al., 2014; Vrangalova & Savin-Williams, 2011). Often adolescent sexuality is thought of as a risk factor for a variety of negative outcomes, particularly in those adolescents engaging in sexuality activity prior to age 16 (Prendergast et al., 2019; Zimmer-Gembeck & Helfand, 2008). However, research has also documented positive aspects of adolescent sexuality in terms of well-being (Harden, 2014; Vasilenko et al., 2014; Vrangalova & Savin-Williams, 2011).

Caregivers differ in their styles, their level of monitoring of their child's behavior, and their knowledge of, and reactions to, the sexual activity of an adolescent child, due to a variety of family factors such as caregiver education level, age, socioeconomic status, and the type of disability of their child (Coley et al., 2009; Deptula et al., 2010; Dewinter et al., 2016; Holmes et al., 2019; Huebner & Howell, 2003; Kaestle et al., 2021; Manor-Binyamini & Schreiber-Divon, 2019; Price & Hyde, 2009; Ream & Savin-Williams, 2005). This research as a whole suggests that strong family relationships and caregiver involvement are linked to better outcomes for adolescents in terms of safety and less risky sexual behavior. However, knowledge of and discussion of the adolescent's engagement in sexual activity can lead to family turmoil in some families and mental health challenges for the adolescent. This may be the case particularly in families of transgender youth (Pariseau et al., 2019). The time of transition for a family is extremely important.

### Common Challenges Associated With Sexuality

The development of children and youth's sexuality is a complex and lengthy process that begins when young children begin to learn about body parts and then explore their expression of gender (Holland-Hall & Quint, 2017). Children must learn about privacy and what is and is not acceptable for others to see or touch. Children who engage with media (likely most children in the United States) witness a large variety of sexual images and must learn to process those as well. When youth begin puberty, they must manage feelings of desire, hormonal changes and fluctuations, menstruation, and erections and all of the confusing peer interactions surrounding dating and relationships. The process can be stressful and can cause anxiety and depression, but ideally the adolescent or young adult eventually gains a way of bonding with others that is pleasurable and contributes to well-being and a positive sense of self.

It is common for people to have difficulty seeing individuals with a disability as sexual beings. This may be particularly true of caregivers

(Holland-Hall & Quint, 2017). However, adolescents and adults with disabilities are sexually active and have the same hormonal changes, desires, and need for connection as their nondisabled peers. They are, however, less likely to have appropriate sexual education and are more likely to be exploited or abused (Holland-Hall & Quint, 2017; Houtrow et al., 2021).

There are a variety of potential sexuality-related challenges for children and adolescents with disabilities (Holland-Hall & Quint, 2017; Houtrow et al., 2021). They may engage in masturbation in public places and need to be taught where and when it is acceptable. There may be a lack of awareness of knowledge about sexually transmitted diseases, and they may not recognize symptoms if they are infected. Adolescents may not fully understand the rules about consent and may get into trouble with authorities for behaviors considered stalking or assault. Adolescent girls may have difficulties managing menstruation because of their physical skills or because of a lack of understanding. Although sexual education is critical, caregivers may hold attitudes that make educating adolescents with disabilities more difficult (Ashcraft & Murray, 2017).

### Specific Areas of Assessment Regarding Sexuality

An occupational profile should include items that assist occupational therapists to evaluate relationships, knowledge, attitudes, skills, and satisfaction in sexual activities. See Box 9.15 The occupational therapist must consider the age and developmental stage of the child, the disability and underlying client factors that might influence engagement in sexual activity or management of changes with puberty, cognitive and language levels and ability to discuss sexuality, independence or dependence on others for self-care tasks, and the child's expressions of, preferences for, and desires around sexuality (Table 9.22). The evaluation also must include the caregivers and their perspectives regarding their child's romantic life and sexual activity and their hopes and fears for their child's future in this realm.

The majority of the evaluation of sexuality will occur through interview and observation. However, an important step in the process, particularly for minors, is to fully understand the caregivers' level of comfort with the discussion of certain matters with their child (Morawska et al., 2015; Robinson et al., 2017). It is important for the therapist to understand the laws and policies in their area before embarking on sexual evaluation or sexual education with a minor, as many families may not readily provide their consent (Brown, 2009). Managing confidentiality, autonomy, and rapport is a delicate balance with ethical, legal, and practical ramifications (Behnke & Warner, 2002). Once this aspect of the process has been attended to, the therapist may proceed with the occupational profile and consider including questions such as those in Boxes 9.15 and 9.16. In some cases, there may need to be observation of specific skills or simulation of specific activities to determine if the adolescent or youth has the physical or cognitive skill to engage in desired activities safely and to further determine needs for education and training.

### BOX 9.15 Interview Questions Regarding Sexuality

After obtaining permission to speak about these issues with a minor, and after asking the client if they are comfortable speaking about these areas, some potential questions to ask clients about sexuality include:

- Are you engaging in sexual activity? If so, are you satisfied with your experiences?
- Are you confident in your role as a sexual partner?
- What are you most concerned with regarding your sexuality and disability?
- Do you feel you have enough intimacy? Are you comfortable showing or expressing intimacy with or receiving from partners?
- Are you comfortable establishing or communicating sexual boundaries?
- Are you comfortable with obtaining the level of privacy you prefer?
- Are you comfortable communicating your needs or desires with partners?
- Are you experiencing pain or discomfort during sexual or intimate activities?
- Are you comfortable with knowing positions or how to engage in sexual or intimate activities safely?
- Do you feel your arousal or desire levels are matched or mismatched with your partners?
- Do you feel you understand sexuality and gender identity? Do you have any concerns or questions about your gender and sexual expression?
- Are you comfortable communicating about your gender pronouns?
- Do you feel a sense of attractiveness? Are you concerned about feeling attractive with ______ (ostomy bags of other externally worn medical devices or scars from medical procedures)?
- Are you concerned about relationships because your partners may not understand your illness, condition, or disability?
- Do you feel like your condition gets in the way of meeting partners' needs?
- Are you able to create an environment that is conducive to intimacy?
- Do you have concerns with creating, maintaining, or leaving intimate relationships?
- Are you able to access or navigate the environment or community to pursue intimacy and social connections?
- Are you able to maintain your sexual wellness through regular sexual health exams?
- Are you comfortable with choosing or using contraceptive options?
- Are you able to manage menstrual health and hygiene?
- Are you able to manage bowel/bladder during intimate activities?
- Are you able to find or use appropriate sexual wellness devices?
- Do you have any specific difficulties with any of the following?
  - Kissing
  - Holding
  - Cuddling
  - Intimate conversation
  - Intercourse
  - Positioning for intercourse
  - Application of "safe sex" devices, for example a condom

Adapted from Sherrick, M. (2004). Sexuality and the initial occupational therapy assessment for adults with physical disabilities. https://core.ac.uk/download/pdf/235073601.pdf; EnbyOT. (2023). The OT Sexual Assessment Framework. https://www.enbyot.com/using-the-ot-sexual-assessment-framework-as-a-guide-to-addressing-sexuality-and-intimacy-in-ot/.

## EVALUATION OF DRIVING AND COMMUNITY MOBILITY

Driving and community mobility are important occupations for developing independence, accessing resources, and engaging in work, hobbies, social events, and services. Adolescents value learning to drive, which provides them freedom. They may view earning a driver's license as an important accomplishment. The ability to get from one place to another (referred to as community mobility) includes walking, bicycling, or accessing and riding in buses, taxi cabs, ride shares, or other transportation systems (such as trains or subways) and is also valued. Although adolescents with disabilities face barriers, the range of mobility options available improve their chances for access and independence.

### Importance of Driving and Community Mobility

Driving and community mobility are valued occupations, often viewed as a "rite of passage" for adolescents that provides them with a sense

TABLE 9.22 **Typical Sexuality Concepts by Age**

| Age | Typical Behaviors or Concepts to Learn |
|---|---|
| Birth–2 years | Touches genitals for sensory pleasure<br>Experiences affection and touch<br>Questions about differences in bodies and bodily functions<br>Displays nudity (uninhibited) |
| 3–5 years | Shows interest in genitals of the opposite sex<br>Learns proper names of genitals (social demands)<br>Plays "show me" games with other children (e.g., playing doctor)<br>Understands that others should not touch his or her genitals<br>Learns that some behaviors are acceptable in public and others to be done in private (e.g., masturbation, undressing, or nudity)<br>Begins to learn privacy rights (e.g., close doors, knock and wait to enter, close blinds)<br>Begins to learn rules for touch and affection boundaries and authority figures<br>Questions where babies come from |
| 6–8 years | Understands "gender role" and expected behaviors (e.g., girls wear dresses)<br>Plays with friends in activities that explore sexuality and bodies<br>Knows differences between boys and girls<br>Names body parts correctly<br>Learns basic elements and language of reproduction and pregnancy<br>Learns about relationships (e.g., friends, mutual respect) and decision-making<br>Thinks about social responsibility<br>Understands appropriate and inappropriate social and sexual behaviors<br>Understands necessary (e.g., personal hygiene) and intimate touch<br>Begins to experience sexual identity and learns basics about sexual orientation<br>Avoids and reports sexual exploitation (understands necessary touch and intimate touch) |
| 9–12 years | Shows interest in social relationships; may want a girlfriend or boyfriend<br>Desires privacy and more independence<br>Discusses body image<br>Discusses sexuality within family<br>Understands personal boundaries and private masturbation and touch<br>Knows how to use refusal skills<br>Understands body changes that will occur during puberty (and any impact on his or her disease or disability)<br>Expresses curiosity about adult bodies (e.g., peeking at written materials and media, TV, movies, websites with sexual content)<br>Learns more about own sexual identity and orientation<br>Knows about reproduction and pregnancy<br>Learns about sexually transmitted diseases and the need to abstain from sexual intercourse<br>Avoids or reports sexual abuse (understands necessary touch and intimate touch) |
| 13–18 years | Is sensitive and private about body<br>Compares body with others and may be critical<br>Asks questions about changes occurring (physical and emotional)<br>Shows more interest in caring for body (e.g., hair, face, exercise)<br>Discusses sexuality and sexual identity with friends<br>Experiments with sexual orientation, activities, intimacy, and intercourse<br>Navigates social media about sexuality and learns ways to protect self<br>Uses preventive health care routinely (e.g., breast, gynecologic, testicular examinations)<br>Begins dating and learning about communication and love<br>Uses values to guide actions in intimacy<br>Expresses sexuality through dress, body movement, or intercourse<br>Understands reproduction, pregnancy, and birth control<br>Knows how to use contraceptives and prevent diseases (safe sex)<br>Asks for or is given genetic counseling or specific information about sexual activities related to their disability<br>Identifies and uses community sexual health services |

Adapted from Couwenhoven, T. (2001). Sexuality education: Building a foundation of healthy attitudes. *Disability Solutions, 4*(6), 1–8; National Sexual Violence Resource Center (NSVRS). (2013). An overview of healthy childhood sexual development. https://www.nsvrc.org/sites/default/files/2013-01/saam_2013_an-overview-of-healthy-childhood-sexual-development.pdf.

## BOX 9.16 Caregiver Questions Regarding Evaluation of Sexuality

During an evaluation of sexuality for an adolescent or youth, it is important to also include the caregivers. Questions that may be important to ask caregivers include:

- How comfortable are you in discussion with your child of topics related to puberty and sexuality?
- What are your family's beliefs regarding sexual activity in adolescence? What has your child been told in relation to engagement or abstinence?
- What level of sexual education have you already engaged in with your child? What do you feel was their level of understanding and comprehension?
- What are your hopes and dreams for your child's future relationships?
- What are your fears regarding your child's sexual activity?
- How experienced do you believe your child is at this time in terms of sexual activity?
- How has your family managed puberty?

of identity and freedom to make choices outside of the home. They allow teens to pursue interests and develop a sense of self apart from their family. These abilities also allow caregivers more freedom as well. Engaging parents in the process is an important element for promoting the driving process (Johnson et al., 2017).

Youth often use this newfound freedom to connect with others, work, engage in leisure, and access resources (such as food, health, and well-being). Youth with disabilities face barriers regarding driving and community mobility, resulting in challenges accessing community services that are necessary for health, development, and overall well-being. They may have to rely on others for assistance, limiting their options and affecting their life satisfaction. They may be unable to access driver education programs in their schools (Guerriere, 2019; McGill & Vogtle, 2001) or may find driver education stressful (Almberg et al., 2017).

### Common Challenges Associated With Driving and Community Mobility

Children and adolescents with disabilities experience challenges interfering with their ability to earn a driver's license to drive and move about their community. Family and caregivers may view the child or adolescent as unable to drive or be independent in the community. For example, teens with autism spectrum disorder get their license 1–2 years later than their same aged peers (Curry et al., 2018). Adolescents may experience cognitive, physical, or mental health challenges that make driving and community mobility challenging. For example, children with ADHD may experience difficulty attending to important environmental cues needed for safe driving. Teens with ADHD and autism may have difficulty with visual-motor integration, selective attention, mental flexibility, and decision-making in stressful driving situations (Classen et al., 2013; Ratzon et al., 2017). Children with intellectual disabilities may have difficulty with short-term memory, problem-solving, and executive functioning.

Physical challenges may interfere with a teen's ability to drive using both hands or feet. Teens may require alternate mobility devices that are not able to be transported on regular public transportation. The environment may present barriers for teens who require wheelchairs for mobility (e.g., no ramps, doors not wide enough, limited space to move, curbs preventing access). They may have vision or sensory challenges that interfere with daily activities and disrupt their ability to drive and move safely in the community. Mental health challenges, such as anxiety or depression, may interfere with a child's thought processes, making driving and community mobility challenging or even dangerous. Adolescents may exhibit poor judgment, difficulty reading environmental cues, or present as vulnerable and put themselves at risk in the community.

### Specific Areas of Assessment Regarding Driving and Community Mobility

Occupational therapists evaluate adolescents' driving and community mobility beginning with an occupational profile to understand the teen's values, personal history, routines, habits, and goals. Information should be gathered related to available private and public options for transportation, as well as the teen's preferences for type of mobility used.

Next, the therapist analyzes the youth's performance skills as they relate to accessing transportation to participate in the community and driving. They complete an occupational analysis specific to the adolescent to determine areas that support or interfere with the child's goals. Box 9.17 provides examples of client factors to assess to understand the client's driving and mobility needs.

Driving and community mobility require integration of cognitive and motor skills to make sound decisions, complete motor actions, and reflect upon those decisions. Adolescents use advanced cognitive skills when they use judgment, problem-solving, memory, and safety awareness to navigate a variety of environments. They must flexibly adapt to situations (such as a car suddenly stopping or a pedestrian veering into the street) and respond quickly and efficiently.

Driving also requires sensory integration. Drivers must judge the amount of force to use to turn the wheel to steer accurately and to use the gas and brake pedals smoothly. They must be able to reverse the motor action and the visual stimuli to back up while turned looking over one's shoulder or in the mirror, and they must be able to judge the speed of oncoming cars by the change in visual stimulus (car getting visually larger as it approaches). They must be able to manage noises, the motion of the car, and the intense visual stimuli (visual images rolling past in the peripheral vision and multiple moving objects in the central or focal visual area). They often use bilateral asymmetrical motions and accurate timing and sequencing of motion. Driving is a highly intense sensory-motor activity.

Youth also use physical strength, coordination, timing, and bilateral hand use to control the steering wheel, depress the accelerator, and apply the brake as needed. Adolescents use an internal body awareness to be able to drive without looking at their feet and to feel the motion of the car forward (and judge the speed). Driving and community mobility requires motor planning skills. Youth rely on tactile awareness to feel the buttons to operate the turn signal, look behind them when backing up, and pay attention to objects in front while driving. Additionally, they react quickly to situations to avoid collisions. When in the community, they react quickly to situations that require they change course or adjust their movements. Occupational therapists also conduct visual screenings and assess visual perceptual skills that are necessary for driving and navigating in the environment. Part of the driving and community mobility assessment includes safety awareness, ability to follow rules, and response to feedback. The practitioner assesses the adolescent's awareness of safety, risks, and their ability to understand the safety consequences.

The OT-FIRST clinical observation tool can be used to assess adolescents' driving readiness (Bell, 2022; Bell & Johns, 2022). OT-FIRST lists observations required for driving such as turning a wheel, applying pressure on pedals, remembering a sequence, understanding social gestures, and knowing what action to take quickly from road signage (Bell, 2022; Bell & Johns, 2022). The Sensory Processing Measure (2nd ed.; SPM-2) provides a driving form that assesses the impact of sensory processing challenges on driving, for those who

BOX 9.17 **Client Factors to Assess for Driving and Community Mobility**

| Client Factor | Definitions (AOTA, 2020b) | Examples of Driving and Community Mobility Observations |
|---|---|---|
| **Specific Mental Functions** | | |
| Higher-level cognitive | Judgment, concept formation, metacognition, executive functions, praxis, cognitive flexibility, insight | Problem-solving during daily tasks, safety precautions in the community, awareness of others, capable of changing plans and figuring out alternative solutions |
| Attention | Sustained shifting and divided attention, concentration, distractibility | Pays attention to surroundings, read signs, remains focused on tasks when multiple distractions, able to remain focused in unexpected situations (such as driving) |
| Memory | Short-term, long-term, and working memory | Remembers rules of road, directions, driving tasks, oriented to time and place |
| Perception | Discrimination of sensations (e.g., auditory, tactile, visual, olfactory, gustatory, vestibular, proprioceptive) | Identifies sounds and understands what they mean (e.g., siren signals pull over), sense of movement or speed in vehicle, awareness of body when driving so can visually attend to driving and press brake, feels hands on wheel, pressure of gas petal and feel of car moving, aware of size of vehicle for maneuvering, aware of self when in the community (able to walk past others at safe distance) |
| Thought | Control and content of thought, awareness of reality versus delusions, logical and coherent thought *(*Note: consider state laws in psychiatric cases)* | Aware of self and others, surroundings, and purpose of activity or event; able to engage in event with awareness and logical thought |
| Mental functions of sequencing complex movement | Mental functions that regulate the speed, response, quality, and time of *motor production, such as restlessness, toe-tapping, or hand wringing, in response to inner tension | Shows appropriate responses to environmental stimuli when driving or engaged in community mobility (such as on the bus), responds to situations, responds to driving events quickly and accurately (such as braking to avoid an accident, slowing down or waiting), able to wait for bus and board with others |
| Emotional | Regulation and range of emotions; appropriateness of emotions, including anger, love, tension, and anxiety; lability of emotions | Shows range of emotions appropriate to situation and circumstances, socially polite in community, expresses self differently to strangers and friends, emotions are consistent with situation |
| Experience of self and time | Awareness of one's identity (including gender identity), body, and position in the reality of one's environment and of time<br>*Note: Those who have not experienced normal movement may have spatial issues with driving* | Shows awareness of self, body, and time within the community; understands spatial awareness when engaged in community events and driving |
| **Global Mental Functions** | | |
| Consciousness | State of awareness and alertness, including the clarity and continuity of the wakeful state | Shows awareness of surroundings, community, others, and the environment; aware of driving conditions; dresses for the weather and situation |
| Orientation | Orientation to person, place, time, self, and others | Understands the event or outing, timing, and place; knows how to use transportation options |
| Psychosocial | General mental functions, as they develop over the life span, are required to understand and constructively integrate the mental functions that lead to the formation of the personal and interpersonal skills needed to establish reciprocal social interactions, in terms of both meaning and purpose | Engages in events that involve others and that they find interesting; engages with others per the event and within the community; enjoys the company of others and feels a sense of purpose; feels they have the skills to engage in the activity (self-efficacy) |
| Temperament and personality | Extroversion, introversion, agreeableness, conscientiousness, emotional stability, openness to experience, self-control, self-expression, confidence, motivation, impulse control, appetite | Shows a temperament to friends and others that allows them to engage in a variety of experiences; engages in activities with self and others that they find interesting and motivating; able to show self-control for driving and community mobility |
| Energy | Energy level, motivation, appetite, craving, impulse<br>*Note: Blood sugar pertains to driving and community mobility safety* | Level of energy matches the event or situation; level of energy allows a person to drive safely or access community transportation |
| Sleep | Physiologic process, quality of sleep | Children or youth get quality sleep and are rested so they can drive or engage in community mobility |

*Continued*

## BOX 9.17 Client Factors to Assess for Driving and Community Mobility—cont'd

| Client Factor | Definitions (AOTA, 2020b) | Examples of Driving and Community Mobility Observations |
|---|---|---|
| **Sensory Functions** | | |
| Visual functions | Quality of vision, visual acuity, visual stability, and visual field functions to promote visual awareness of environment at various distances for functioning | Children show adequate vision and visual processing skills to make sense of the environment for driving and community mobility |
| Hearing functions | Sound detection and discrimination; awareness of location and distance of sounds<br>*Note: New technology aides are valuable assets for drivers with hearing impairments* | Able to hear and understand what sounds mean and where they come from; for example, hearing a fire truck's siren coming from behind one's car and pulling over |
| Vestibular functions | Sensation related to position, balance, and secure movement against gravity | Sensing the movement of cars, public transportation, or walking |
| Proprioceptive functions | Awareness of body position and space<br>*Note: Accuracy is critical in driver operation of primary/secondary controls and accessories* | Understanding where one's body is without having to look to see; for example, being aware that one's feet are on the gas pedal or brake without looking |
| Touch functions | Feeling of being touched or touching; presence of sensation (numbness, paresthesia, hyperesthesia)<br>*Note: Pressure/force sensation is critical and discrimination of pedals for driving with feet* | Identifying how objects feel and being able to manipulate objects and know what they are by touch, such as feeling for a key inside one's purse |
| **Neuromusculoskeletal and Movement-Related Functions** | | |
| Joint mobility | Joint range of motion | Movement to access driving controls or to access public transportation; movement for sitting, standing, turning, holding objects |
| Joint stability | Maintenance of structural integrity of joints throughout the body; physiologic stability of joints related to structural integrity | Ability to stabilize joints so you can move others, such as sitting and using one's hands when driving; postural control to ambulate for community mobility |
| Muscle power | Strength | Strength is needed for many driving and community mobility tasks such as to sit upright and hold positions, walk, grasp, open doors, and walk upstairs |
| Muscle tone | Degree of muscle tension (e.g., flaccidity, spasticity, fluctuation) | Ability to voluntarily control one's muscle tension for functional movement needed for driving and community mobility |
| Muscle endurance | Sustainability of muscle contraction | Sitting endurance while driving; endurance for the activity and transportation to the activity |
| **Motor functions** | | |
| Motor reflexes | Involuntary contraction of muscles automatically induced by specific stimuli (e.g., stretch, asymmetrical tonic neck, symmetrical tonic neck)<br>*Note: *In some DRS cases, driving may not be indicated as safe or legal per state guidelines* | Responses to stimuli that produce reflex reactions, such as startle reflex, may interfere with quality of movements, interfering with driving and community mobility |
| Involuntary movement reactions | Postural reactions, body adjustment reactions, supporting reactions | Responses to changes in gravity support walking, movement, and mobility |
| Control of voluntary movement | Eye-hand and eye-foot coordination, bilateral integration, crossing of the midline, fine and gross motor control, *oculomotor function (e.g., saccades, pursuits, accommodation, binocularity) | Child or youth's ability to engage in coordinated movements required for driving and community mobility |
| Gait patterns | Gait and mobility in relation to engagement in daily life activities (e.g., walking patterns and impairments, asymmetric gait, stiff gait) | Ability to ambulate to engage in daily activities such as community mobility |

American Occupational Therapy Association. (2020b). Occupational therapy practice framework: Domain and process (4th ed.). *American Journal of Occupational Therapy, 74*(Suppl. 2), 7412410010; Bell, M. (2022). OT-FIRST method training for the OT practitioner. [Manuscript/Modules in Preparation].

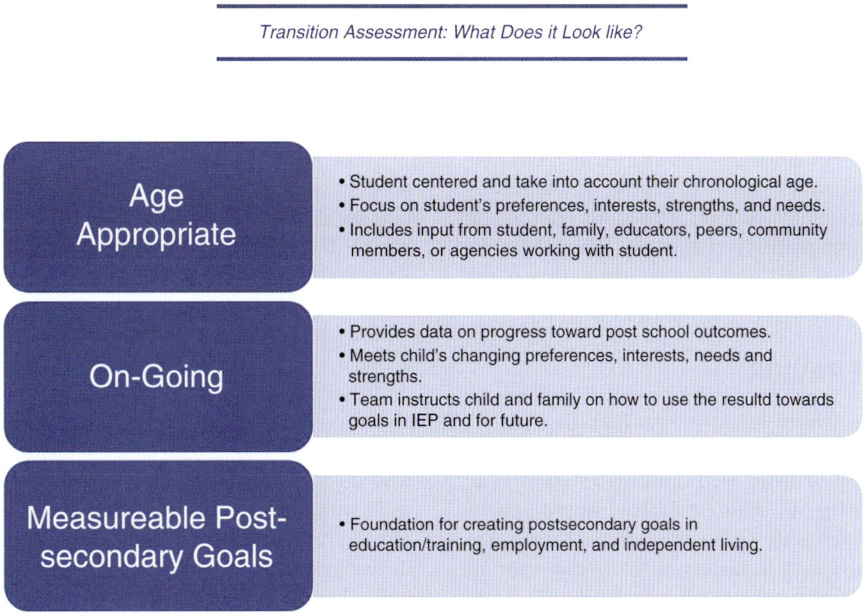


**Fig. 9.9** Transition assessment is an ongoing process that begins at or before 14 years and gathers information on children's strengths, challenges, motivations, and interests to support future life goals. (Adapted from Transition Improvement Grant (TIG). (2021). Age-appropriate transition assessments and resources. https://witig.org/wp-content/uploads/2017/10/Age-Appropriate-Assessment-Guide.pdf. Sitlington, P. L., Neubert, D. A., Begun, W. H., Lombard, R. C., & Leconte, P. J. (2007). *Assess for success: A practitioner's handbook on transition assessment* (2nd ed., pp. 2–3). Corwin Press.)

already have a license to drive. Occupational therapists who receive advanced training may assess adolescents on the road and make recommendations for modifications to vehicles. They must adhere to state licensure laws.

## EVALUATION OF TRANSITION TO WORK

Adolescents transitioning out of school to employment require planning to ensure the transition goes smoothly. "Transition assessment is an ongoing process of collecting information on the student's strengths, needs, preferences, and interests as they relate to the demands of current and future living, learning, and working environments. This process begins at age 14 or earlier and will continue until the student graduates or exits high school. Information from this process is used to drive the Individualized Education Plan (IEP) and transition planning process and contributes to the Summary of Performance (SoP) document detailing the student's academic and functional performance and postsecondary goals" (TIG, 2021; adapted from Sitlington et al., 2007, pp. 2–3). Effective transition planning is age appropriate, ongoing, and related to specific goals (Fig. 9.9). Occupational therapists have the knowledge and skills to contribute important information to the transition team (Trujillo et al., 2018).

### Common Challenges Associated With Transition to Work

In addition to the traditional performance skills and client factors addressed by occupational therapists working in the schools, adolescents with disabilities transitioning to work often require assistance with self-advocacy, self-determination, specific vocational skills, and a variety of soft skills related to work performance (Angell et al., 2019; Cooper et al., 2023). In addition, they must manage transportation to and from a job site, which may present barriers for some youth (Sabella & Bezyak, 2019). Students may also need assessment of habits and routines.

### Specific Areas of Assessment Regarding Transition to Work

Three primary questions: (1) "Where is the student presently?" (2) "Where is the student going?" and (3) "How will they get there?" form the basis of assessment to address an adolescent's transition to work. The practitioner assesses the youth's interests, preferences, and self-determination skills. They evaluate the child's strengths and abilities, the specific requirements of the work tasks, and the work environment and its accessibility and supports (Angell et al., 2019; Cooper et al., 2023; Khayatzadeh-Mahani et al., 2020; Trujillo et al., 2019). Common barriers to employment include social and communication skills, so these are also important areas to assess. In terms of the task, the occupational therapist will use activity and occupational analysis to investigate the work requirements and the adolescent's abilities in relation to those requirements. The therapist may assess the job site for accessibility and may investigate the attitudes of the workers to determine if they will be supportive or a hindrance.

Often the transition planning process includes formal assessment of areas such as adaptive behavior, independent living aptitude, interests, achievement, personality, preferences, career development, and self-determination (TIG, 2021). Informal measures are often used as well including interviews, questionnaires, observations, environmental assessment, curriculum-based assessment, and transition planning inventories. The National Technical Assistance Center on Transition: The Collaborative (https://transitionta.org/) provides a variety of resources to assist therapists and the team in providing effective transition planning, including assessment.

## ASSESSMENT OF PERFORMANCE SKILLS AND CLIENT FACTORS

Occupational therapists assess performance skills (i.e., goal-directed actions) and client factors (i.e., specific capacities, characteristics or beliefs that reside within the person) (AOTA, 2020b) to understand a child's challenges in occupational performance. They may use a top-down approach to assessment, by evaluating the child's occupational participation and moving to an analysis of the underlying client factor and skills that influence that participation. They may also use a bottom-up approach by examining client factors and skills first and then analyzing how these factors and skills influence occupational participation. The choice of where to start may depend on the setting, client's condition, child and family concerns, reason for referral, and therapist's experience. Of importance is that occupational therapists complete a holistic assessment that describes the many factors that influence occupational participation.

## ASSESSMENT OF BEHAVIOR

Challenging behaviors are defined as those behaviors that are not socially acceptable; can cause physical harm, disruption, or destruction; or can affect education or living environments (Matson et al., 2010; Petursdottir et al., 2010). All children display inappropriate or challenging behaviors at times as they grow through the various ages and stages of childhood, and such behaviors often are not cause for concern. However, attention must be given when such behaviors interfere with the child's ability to engage and participate in daily life activities, when they are disruptive to the engagement and participation of others, or when the behaviors place the child or others at risk for injury. Occupational therapists assess children whose behaviors interfere with their daily activities.

### Common Challenges Associated With Behavior

At least 10%–15% of children in early childhood programs have mild to moderate clinically significant behavior problems (Park & Scott, 2009), while the prevalence of problem and challenging behavior among individuals with diagnoses such as ASD ranges between 35.8% and 94.3% (Baghdadli et al., 2003; Jang et al., 2011; Matson et al., 2010). *Noncompliance* (doing other than what has been requested by an authority figure) is one of the top behavior concerns parents report to their pediatricians (Bryce & Jahromi, 2013; McMahon & Forehand, 2003). This is particularly interesting because noncompliance in itself is not a harmful behavior, even though it can be frustrating to an adult when their directive is not followed, and at times, it could place the child at risk, such as in issues of safety.

Challenging and problem behavior can take many forms. Passive behaviors such as noncompliance, withdrawal, avoidance, inattention, or lack of response are not overtly disruptive but still interfere with occupational performance and participation (Lipschultz & Wilder, 2017). Active behaviors such as direct refusal to engage, opposition, aggression toward people or property, or self-injurious behavior not only interfere with occupational performance and participation but can also be disruptive or harmful to self or others (Bryce & Jahromi, 2013; Matson et al., 2010). Both passive and active forms of challenging behavior can be difficult to manage and require attention and intervention by caregivers and service providers.

Decades of behavioral research have identified four primary purposes of challenging behavior: attention, alone/nonsocial, escape, and tangible (Foxx, 1996; Matson et al., 2010; Petursdottir et al., 2010). See Table 9.23 for examples of how the behaviors serve the child's purpose. The attention function is in effect when the behavior results in the individual receiving attention from or achieving reciprocal interaction with others, such as when a child receives teacher attention in response to acting out during class.

Behavior has an alone/nonsocial function when it results in the absence of any form of attention from others, including prompts for performance. An example of the alone/nonsocial function is a child who does not want to be called on by the teacher at school, so the child withdraws in class. The escape function results in an undesired object, event, or demand being removed from the child in response to the behavior, such as removing an assignment sheet from the student's desk when he displays self-injurious behavior. Finally, a behavior has a tangible function when the behavior results in the child obtaining a desired object or event, such as being allowed to continue using an iPad as a result of whining.

Some behaviorists recognize an additional function of behavior, often referred to as automatic reinforcement, that occurs via the sensory input received through self-stimulatory or stereotypic behaviors such as body rocking, finger flicking, bouncing on toes, or covering ears (Reese et al., 2005). Behaviors may have a single function or multiple functions. The most common co-occurring functions are attention along with either escape or tangible function (Matson et al., 2011).

### Specific Areas of Assessment Regarding Behavior

The term *behavior* refers to what a person does, including overt, observable actions, such as moving, talking, or playing a game, as well as covert, unobservable actions, such as thinking about something, experiencing emotion, or being confused. The domain of occupational therapy includes both overt and covert behaviors with concern for any behavior that interferes with occupational engagement.

Children's engagement in daily life experiences creates the building blocks for learning, growth, development, and productive occupation. When engagement in daily life is disrupted by challenging behavior, occupational therapists identify and intervene on those variables, influencing the individual's behavior and engagement patterns.

**TABLE 9.23 Functions of Behaviors and Examples**

| Function of Behavior | Examples of How Each Function Might Be Fulfilled |
|---|---|
| Attention | Verbal praise, smiles, eye contact, positive comments, joking, and joining in on what the child is doing |
| Alone/nonsocial | Absence of attention examples given above; allowed to seclude in study carrel, tent, or other hideaway; absence of questions, prompts to engage, or instructions to work |
| Escape | Removal of a task or performance demand, removal of a person, and removal of the student from the environment |
| Tangible | Acquire a snack, token, preferred activity, sticker, or prize |
| Sensory or automatic | Experience a visual, auditory, tactile, or vestibular input |

*Note*: Functions are best identified through analysis of the individual's behavior and systematic testing of the hypothesized function to determine its effect on the target behavior.

The appropriateness of a behavior is usually interpreted according to a social standard or expectation and is judged to be positive when it is in accordance with social expectations, or to be negative, problematic, or challenging when it does not conform to social norms or causes others in the vicinity to feel threatened or experience harm. For example, in a public school building, it would be deemed inappropriate and unacceptable for a student to leave the classroom and go to the playground when the teacher passes out a work assignment; however, the same behavior would be appropriate and desirable in response to the recess bell. Even behaviors such as playing with cars by lining them up along a seam in the carpet or carrying a Band-Aid everywhere and refusing to set it down, though not disruptive to the context or harmful to others, can be identified as challenging because they interfere with the child's occupational engagement and do not comply with social norms.

As the incidence of challenging and problem behaviors has increased, it has become increasingly expected that occupational therapists are knowledgeable about and skilled in addressing such behaviors among their clients. Much of what is known about challenging behavior and the strategies to facilitate behavior change has emerged from the fields of education and psychology. However, occupational therapists can use this information to provide therapeutic intervention to prevent and reduce challenging behaviors and diminish the negative impact of such behaviors on the child's occupational performance.

Uncovering the purpose is best accomplished by analyzing the antecedent and consequent variables surrounding the behavior and determining which are connected to the behavior in a manner that strengthens or sustains it (Dunlap & Fox, 2011). A process for making this determination is the **functional behavioral analysis** *(FBA)*. An FBA is a systematic process designed to identify the variables in the A-B-C relationship so that they can be analyzed to determine which ones are maintaining the behavior. Once the variables maintaining the behavior are identified, they can be targeted in intervention (Matson & Minshawi, 2006; Matson & Nebel-Schwalm, 2007). The FBA process involves five steps:

1. Team building and goal setting
2. Functional assessment of the behavior
3. Hypothesis formulation
4. Development of the comprehensive support plan
5. Implementation and outcome monitoring of the plan, including refining the plan as needed (Buschbacher & Fox, 2003)

During the first step of the FBA, a team of individuals gathers to address the challenging behavior. Ideally, the team includes the child's parents or caregivers as recognized experts on the child and as partners in the intervention process, along with other professionals who work with the child on a consistent basis. Occupational therapists should be part of the FBA process when they have personal knowledge of the child or adolescent and direct experience with the target behavior. The team collaborates to identify desired outcomes for the child (Buschbacher & Fox, 2003) as a foundation for addressing the behavior.

Step two involves the comprehensive functional assessment of the challenging behavior. Efforts focus on clearly and completely describing the behavior, the context(s) in which it occurs, the antecedents and consequences that maintain the behavior, and the functions of the behavior. The goal of this step is to understand the purpose of the behavior and conditions under which the behavior is most and least likely to occur. Data are systematically collected by interviewing people who have direct knowledge of the child and experience with the behavior, observing the child where and when the behavior is most likely to occur, reviewing records in which the behavior has been documented, and gathering information about contextual variables such as health or changes in other environments or activity schedules.

Third, a hypothesis about the behavior is formulated, including explicitly stating the antecedents, consequences, and function of the behavior. The hypothesis statement emerges from the information gathered in step two.

In the fourth step, a comprehensive **behavior support plan** *(BSP)* is developed that outlines the intervention(s) to be implemented. The BSP plan itself has four elements:

1. The functional assessment of behavior including hypothesized functions of the behavior
2. The specific individualized intervention strategies to be used
3. Strategies to be applied throughout the day
4. Evidence that the plan is consistent with the values and resources of the child receiving support and the persons providing support (Horner & Carr, 1997)

Fifth, the plan is implemented, outcomes data are collected, and the effect of the plan is evaluated. If the child is not progressing toward the outcomes identified in step one, the plan is modified, and outcome data are collected again.

## ASSESSMENT OF COGNITION

Cognition refers to the thought process and includes such skills as identification, awareness knowledge, association, problem-solving, and reflection. Cognition is a part of every occupation, and therefore, occupational therapists assess the child's cognitive skills as they relate to the child's ability to complete daily occupations. Occupational therapists measure aspects of cognition and specifically how that affects the child's ability to do those things they want to do. However, psychologists measure the child's cognitive levels typically with Intelligence Quotient (IQ). Educators work with children to advance their cognitive skills, whereas occupational therapists address engagement in daily activities. Therefore, occupational therapy goals focus on the child using cognition to complete daily living skills such as "the child will identify clothing appropriate for weather conditions."

### Common Challenges Associated With Cognition

Children with disabilities may experience difficulty at any level of cognition. Box 9.18 provides an overview of Piaget's stages of cognitive development. Children with intellectual disability, for example, may develop cognitive skills later than their peers. For example, toddlers may remain in the sensorimotor stage longer than their peers. School-age children with cognitive challenges may have difficulty remembering facts, sequencing steps, or following simple directions. Children with cognitive challenges may achieve milestones later than their peers and take longer to learn in class. Adolescents with cognitive challenges may be impulsive, less attentive to details, and unable to read people's cues. They may have difficulty problem-solving situations and show mental inflexibility. Children and youth with cognitive challenges may have difficulty generalizing to new situations. They may misunderstand jokes and experience difficulty communicating (in writing or orally). They may forget things, have difficulty organizing, and show difficulty with time management. They may require assistance for daily tasks. Many children and adolescents with cognitive challenges can live independently (with support) and find employment that is satisfying.

**BOX 9.18 Piaget's Stages of Cognitive Development**

| Stage (Age Range) | Description |
|---|---|
| Sensorimotor (Birth to 2 years) | Knows about the environment through movement and sensations |
| Preoperational (2–6 years) | Begins to think symbolically and uses words or pictures to represent objects; tends to be egocentric |
| Concrete operational (7–11 years) | Begins to think logically about concrete events and problems |
| Formal operations (11+ years) | Begins to think abstractly; reasons about hypothetical problems |

Adapted from Cherry, K. (2022). The 4 stages of cognitive development: Background and key concepts of Piaget's theory. https://www.verywellmind.com/piagets-stages-of-cognitive-development-2795457?.

## Specific Areas of Assessment Regarding Cognition

Occupational therapists assess how a child completes tasks, problem-solves challenges, and engages in daily activities. They observe cognition in everyday activities, such as watching a child play with a toy, put on their coat, and eat a snack. During the assessment, the occupational therapist observes the child completing age-appropriate activities that require sequencing, timing, motor planning, and problem-solving. Occupational therapists may complete a developmental assessment (see Appendix A), which provides an estimate of level of cognition. Box 9.19 lists cognitive skills and related questions that can be used to observe a child as part of a cognitive assessment.

Occupational therapists often combine cognitive interventions (such as Cognitive Orientation to daily Occupational Performance [CO-OP]) to address a child's motor skills and occupational performance. A variety of assessment tools can be used within the CO-OP approach to ensure meaningful goal selection, monitor skill acquisition, and demonstrate improvements in occupational performance. The tools discussed below have been well supported within the CO-OP literature, and their usefulness in demonstrating the outcomes of the intervention approach will be discussed. For further information on the standardized assessments, refer to Appendix A.

The daily activity log is a tool used to record the activities a child identifies as important over the course of a day. In CO-OP, the client is asked to complete the daily activity log, with the assistance of parents/significant others if necessary, thinking about a typical day. The completed daily activity log is used to provide the therapist with information on the client's typical day and is used to initiate the process of goal setting.

The Pediatric Activity Card Sort (PACS; Mandich et al., 2004) is a picture-based assessment used to determine the child's level of occupational engagement. The visual nature of the assessment is useful when setting client-centered goals with young clients, aligning with the key feature of the CO-OP approach. The PACS may be used to complement the daily activity log in the process of goal setting.

The Canadian Occupational Performance Measure (COPM; Law et al., 2005) is used within the CO-OP approach to identify the three client-chosen goals that are the focal point of the intervention. The therapist uses the information obtained from the daily activity log and the Activity Card Sort (ACS)/PACS to initiate the COPM interview and to help guide the questions asked to ensure that meaningful goals are identified. The COPM is administered prior to and after intervention to measure the child's perceived performance and satisfaction related to their chosen goals.

The Performance Quality Rating Scale (PQRS; Henry & Polatajko, 2003; Martini & Polatajko, 1998; Miller et al., 2001) is an observation-based rating scale used to measure performance and change in

**BOX 9.19 Assessing Cognition in Children Through Observation**

This is not an inclusive list but provides a start to evaluating cognition in children.

| Cognitive Skill | Questions to Guide Observations |
|---|---|
| Awareness | Does the infant notice things? People? Objects?<br>Do they seem curious? Interested?<br>Is the child aware that they are in a new environment?<br>Do they notice you? Toys? Sounds? Change in position? |
| Attention | How long does a child watch or engage in the activity?<br>Do they complete the action?<br>Are they purposeful in their focus? |
| Eye contact | Does the child look you in the eye? For how long?<br>Does the child acknowledge you? Others?<br>What does the child look at? |
| Reach for objects (initiative) | Does the child show initiative to reach for or get objects or people? How? |
| Socialization (smile, interact, notice) | Does the child smile, interact, or notice others?<br>Do they try to communicate with you? Others?<br>Do they read others' cues? Play with others? Show a sense of humor? |
| Memory (for familiar to unfamiliar) | Does the child remember daily routines? Do they remember facts from school? Requests from parents? Do they follow directions? |
| Naming object and recalling<br>Associating object | Can they identify objects? People? Places?<br>Can the child identify like objects? See similarities and differences? |
| Creating new things | Does the child use their imagination? Create new things? Tell stories? Play symbolically? |
| Synthesizing and problem-solving | Does the child figure things out? Summarize events? |
| Organizing multiple things | Can the child organize their homework? Sports activities? Interests? |
| Computing (math facts, word problems) | Can the child count, add, subtract, or do word problems? |
| Reading, writing | Can the child read? Identify letters and numbers? Write? |
| Measuring<br>Sequencing and timing | Can they measure? Follow recipes?<br>Does the child do things in order?<br>Can they time things to be ready on time? |

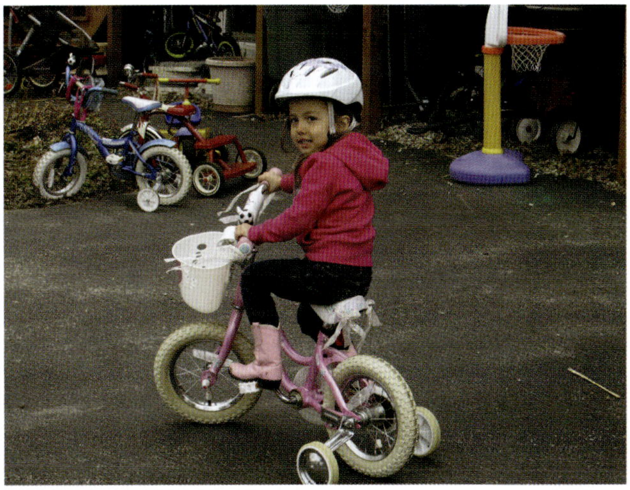

**Fig. 9.10** Adaptive responses help the child acquire skills such as riding a bicycle. Amelia's nervous system must integrate vestibular, proprioceptive, and visual information adequately for her to successfully steer the bicycle while it is moving.

performance. This assessment allows for the objective rating of the quality of the child's occupational performance before and after intervention.

Other assessments that are often used to determine changes after administering the CO-OP approach are the Movement Assessment Battery for Children (Movement ABC-2), the Bruininks-Oseretsky Test of Motor Proficiency (BOTMP), and standardized handwriting assessments. In addition, the Vineland Adaptive Behavior Scales (VABS) and Social Skills Rating Scales (SSRS) have been used to evaluate outcomes related to social, organizational, and ADL goals (Rodger et al., 2007, 2008; Thornton et al., 2016).

## ASSESSMENT OF SENSORY INTEGRATION AND SENSORY PROCESSING

Ayres used the term sensory integration to refer not only to the intricate synaptic connections within the brain but also to neural processes as they relate to functional behavior. Hence, her definition of *sensory integration* is the "organization of sensation for use" (Ayres, 1979, p. 5). The inclusion of the final clause "for use" ties sensory integration to occupation (Ayres, 1973, 1979, 2004). A child actively selects the sensations most useful at the time and organizes them in a way that facilitates accomplishing goals. This involves brain processes of sensory integration. When these processes are going well, the child also organizes a successful, goal-directed action on the environment, which is called an **adaptive response**. An adaptive response occurs when a challenge presented in the environment is successfully met. The adaptive response is possible because the brain has been able to efficiently organize incoming sensory information, which then provides a basis for action (Fig. 9.10). When a child makes an adaptive response that is more complex than any previously accomplished response, Ayres hypothesized that the brain attains a more organized state, and its capacity for further sensory integration is enhanced (Box 9.20). Adaptive responses come from within the child, who is an active doer, not a passive recipient. No one can force a child to respond adaptively, although a situation may be set up that is likely to elicit adaptive responses from the child. Children have a drive to develop sensory integration through adaptive responses. Ayres called this **inner drive** and speculated that it is generated primarily by the limbic system of the brain, a network of

### BOX 9.20 An Adaptive Response

Ayres provides the example of learning to ride a bicycle to illustrate an adaptive response (Ayres, 1979). The child must integrate sensations, particularly from the vestibular and proprioceptive systems, to learn how to balance on the bicycle. The vestibular, proprioceptive, and visual senses must accurately and quickly detect when the child begins to fall and then must be rapidly integrated with each other to produce motor reactions that counteract the direction of the fall. Eventually, often after many trials of falling, the child integrates sensory information efficiently enough to make the appropriate weight shifts over the bicycle to maintain balance. This adaptive response, and those that follow, enable the child to balance effectively to ride the bike. The child's nervous system has changed in how it integrates multisensory information to produce refined, dynamic balancing, so the child is now more adept at bicycle riding.

neural structures known to be critical in both motivation and memory (Ayres, 1979). Ayres designed therapeutic activities and environments to engage the child's inner drive and, in so doing, advance sensory integrative development and the child's occupational competence.

Ayres' tenet that change occurs in neural synapses and circuits as adaptive responses are made is based on understanding and appreciation of the brain's neural plasticity. *Plasticity* is the brain's ability to change, remodel, and reorganize with the outcome being a better ability to adapt to new situations (Demarin & Morović, 2014). **Neural plasticity** is the ability of experience to shape the development of neural circuits, both structurally and functionally, because of cellular and molecular neural activity (Berardi et al., 2015; Hübener & Bonhoeffer, 2014; Ostry & Gribble, 2016). Interesting and novel environments, such as those provided in studies of environmental enrichment, lead to significant increases in dendritic branching, synaptic connections, synaptic efficiency, and size of brain tissue (Sale et al., 2014; Scholz et al., 2015). These changes are most dramatic in the young and are likely a major mechanism of brain development, but changes occur throughout the lifespan (Berardi et al., 2015; Mandolesi et al., 2017; Sale et al., 2014; Scholz et al., 2015). Crucial elements of an enriched environment for animals and humans include active engagement with novel, meaningful, and challenging activities with both cognitive and motor components as well as social stimulation (Mandolesi et al., 2017; Sale et al., 2014). The brain's plasticity therefore makes it possible for an adaptive response to increase the efficiency of sensory integration at a neuronal level.

One of the basic propositions of Ayres' theory is that, because older parts of the brain integrate and filter information before it is relayed to the cortex, increased efficiency in structures such as the brainstem and thalamus enhance higher-order functioning (Ayres, 1973). Ayres emphasized the proximal, body-centered sensory systems (i.e., the vestibular, tactile, and proprioceptive systems) in her work with young children, because they lay a foundation for more complex developmental achievements. These systems mature early (Piontelli et al., 2015) and are seated in the lower central nervous system (CNS) centers (particularly the brainstem, cerebellum, and thalamus). Ayres reasoned that the refinement of primitive functions, such as postural control, balance, and tactile perception, provides a sensorimotor foundation for higher-order functions, such as intellectual and academic ability, behavioral self-regulation, and complex motor skills (e.g., those required in sports). Thus, the developmental process is one in which the primal body-centered functions serve as building blocks on which complex cognitive and social skills can be scaffolded.

Development, from a sensory integrative standpoint, occurs as the brain organizes sensory information and the child forms adaptive responses with increasing degrees of complexity to respond to and interact with early sensory experiences. Sensory integration enables adaptive responses to occur, which in turn promotes the development of sensory integration and the emergence of occupational engagement and social participation (Parham, 2002; Spitzer & Roley, 2001). As this process unfolds in infancy, the developing child begins to attach meaning to the stream of sensations experienced. The child becomes increasingly adept at shifting attention to what they perceive as intriguing and essential, tuning out that which is irrelevant to current needs and interests. As a result, the child can organize play behavior for increasing lengths of time and gains control in the regulation of emotions.

Inner drive leads children to search for opportunities in the environment that offer "just right" challenges to their emerging abilities and are aligned with their temperament and interests. These are challenges that are not so complex that they overwhelm or induce failure nor so simple that they are routine or uninteresting. The **just right challenge** (Ayres, 1972; Kuhaneck & Spitzer, 2024; Mack et al., 1982) is one that requires effort but is accomplishable and satisfying. Because there is an element of challenge, a successful adaptive response engenders feelings of mastery and a sense of oneself as a competent being.

The terms *sensory integrative problems*, *sensory integrative dysfunction*, and *sensory processing disorder* do not refer to one specific type of difficulty but to a heterogeneous group of patterns that emerge developmentally (i.e., not owing to traumatic brain injury) and are thought to reflect neural processing differences involving sensory and motor systems. Sensory integrative differences involve the CNS, rather than peripheral sensory functions, and therefore assume normal sensory receptor function (Bar-Shalita et al., 2014; Carriot et al., 2015; Parush et al., 1997). Thus, for example, when sensory integrative problems involving the vestibular system are discussed, these problems are generally thought to be based within the vestibular nuclei and its connections rather than the vestibular receptors (i.e., the semicircular canals, utricle, or saccule).

## Common Challenges Associated With Sensory Processing and Integration

Ayres and others found similar patterns of challenges across multiple studies involving diverse samples of children. Tables 9.24 and 9.25 summarize these studies and other studies of sensory integration patterns. Based on this body of research, four general categories of sensory integration differences are discussed: (1) sensory reactivity; (2) sensory discrimination and perception; (3) vestibular-bilateral function; and (4) praxis.

**Sensory Reactivity.** A *sensory reactivity* problem is synonymous with a *sensory modulation problem. Modulation* refers to CNS regulation of its own activity (Ayres, 1979). The term **sensory modulation** refers to the tendency to generate responses that are appropriately graded in relation to incoming sensory stimuli, rather than underresponding or over-responding to them. Children with sensory modulation problems experience difficulty reacting to sensory stimuli. They may over- or underreact. Please see Table 9.26 for definitions, descriptions, and examples of the types of problems associated with sensory reactivity.

**Sensory Discrimination and Perception.** **Sensory discrimination and perception** allow for refined organization and interpretation of sensory stimuli. *Discrimination* refers to the brain's ability to distinguish between different sensory stimuli, such as two points touched on the skin simultaneously. *Perception* is the brain's process of giving meaning to sensory information, as when the complex visual stimuli from a person's face are integrated and interpreted as a specific facial expression of emotion. Some types of sensory integrative disorders involve inefficient or inaccurate organization of sensory information (e.g., difficulty differentiating one stimulus from another or difficulty perceiving the spatial or temporal relationships among stimuli). For example, a child with a tactile perception problem may not be able to distinguish between a square block and a hexagonal block using touch only, without visual cues. Discrimination or perception problems can occur in any sensory system. Please see Table 9.27 for descriptions and observations of sensory perceptual issues.

**Praxis.** **Praxis** is the ability to conceptualize, plan, and execute a nonhabitual motor act (Ayres, 1979). Problems with praxis are often referred to as *dyspraxia* or *problems in motor planning.* When the term *dyspraxia* is used for children, it usually refers to a condition characterized by difficulty with motor planning that emerges in early childhood and cannot be explained by a medical diagnosis, developmental disability, or environmental constraint. Ayres hypothesized that tactile perception contributes to the development of an accurate and precise body scheme, which is necessary for planning new actions. Praxis problems may be manifested in different forms, not all of which are sensory integrative in nature (Ayres, 1989). **Somatodyspraxia** refers to a sensory integrative deficit that involves poor praxis and impaired tactile and proprioceptive processing. By definition, somatodyspraxia involves poor tactile perception in conjunction with signs of poor motor planning (Cermak, 1991).

The child with somatodyspraxia typically appears clumsy and awkward. They have difficulty performing novel motor activities, which often results in frustration. Transitioning from one body position to another or sequencing and timing the actions involved in a motor task may pose a great challenge. These children typically have difficulty relating their bodies to physical objects in environmental space. They often have difficulty accurately imitating the actions of others. Precision of movement may be poor, resulting in unintentional knocking down of toys or inefficient placement of materials and objects. Many of these children have difficulties with oral praxis, which may affect eating skills or speech articulation.

Some children with dyspraxia have problems with **ideation** (i.e., they have difficulty generating ideas of what to do in a novel situation or conceiving play possibilities when presented with unfamiliar toys or objects). When asked to simply play, without being given specific directions, they may not initiate any activity, or they may initiate activity that is habitual and limited or seems to lack a goal. They may respond by wandering aimlessly; performing simple repetitive actions such as patting or pushing objects around; randomly piling up objects with no apparent plan; or, for the more sophisticated child, waiting to observe others doing an activity and then imitating them rather than initiating a new activity independently. Language and the social environment play a role in the development of ideation (May-Benson, 2001).

For children with dyspraxia, skills that most children attain rather easily can be excessively challenging (e.g., donning a sweater, feeding oneself with utensils, writing the alphabet, jumping rope, completing a puzzle). These skills may be mastered only with high motivation on the part of the child, coupled with a great deal of practice, far more than most children require. Participation in sports is often embarrassing and frustrating, and organization of schoolwork may be a concern. Children who have somatodyspraxia and are aware of their deficits often avoid difficult motor challenges and may attempt to gain control over such situations by assuming a directing or controlling role

TABLE 9.24 Purpose, Methods, Results, and Contributions of Studies of Sensory Integrative Patterns

| Year | Author | Purpose | Instruments | Hypothesis | Analysis | Subjects | Results | Contributions to Theory |
|---|---|---|---|---|---|---|---|---|
| 1965 | Ayres, A. J. | To identify relationships among sensory perception, motor performance, and laterality in normal sample and children with perceptual problems. Establish construct and discriminant validity. | Early versions of the SCSIT, additional perceptual-motor and laterality tests. Also freedom from hyperactivity and tactile defensiveness. | That test results would identify factors for children with and without dysfunction. Normal and dysfunctional children will demonstrate different factors. | Thirty-three tests. Two behavioral parameters. Analysis of difference between group means. Q- and R-technique factor analysis. | $n=100$ dysfunctional. $n=50$ normal. Dysfunctional children had learning or behavioral disorders. | Tests discriminated between normal and dysfunctional groups. Five patterns were detected: Apraxia, dysfunction form and space perception, deficit bilateral integration, visual figure-ground perception, tactile defensiveness. | Established discriminant validity of early versions. Most children demonstrated more than one factor; therefore factors are related. Sensory integration clusters were not by sensory systems. Praxis and tactile functions are linked. Tactile defensiveness, hyperactivity, and distractibility are linked. Cognitive aspects are deemphasized. Eye-hand agreement is not discriminative. Empirical support for syndromes. |
| 1966a | Ayres, A. J. | To explore perceptual-motor relationships in a normal sample and compare with prior studies. Establish construct validity. | Frostig tests, early versions of the SCSIT. Also freedom from hyperactivity and tactile defensiveness. | That factors would emerge. | Seventeen tests. R-technique factor analysis (simplified matrix). | $n=92$. Formed normal distribution, 10% abnormal, three with mild cerebral palsy. | Praxis accounted for most variance. Motor planning, kinesthesia, tactile functions, motor accuracy, and bilateral coordination. Visual perception factor: Ayres space test and Frostig. | More support for praxis syndrome. Visual component without motor element. Perceptual-motor functions correlate as a whole in normative sample. Kinesthesia is closer to tactile than visual perception as in prior study. |
| 1966b | Ayres, A. J. | To provide an understanding of whether syndromes represent dysfunction or developmental lag. Establish construct validity. | Nearly the same as 1966a. | That variation in perceptual-motor abilities would be small in a group of typical children. | Sixteen tests. Two behavioral parameters. R-technique factor analysis. | $n=64$. Adopted, all normal on Gesell. | Visual motor ability accounted for most variation. Praxis and tactile perception were least variable. Hyperactivity, distractibility, and tactile defensiveness factor. Factors weak because of lack of variance in performance of normal children. | Suggested that low scores in praxis and tactile perception represent developmental deviation, not delay. Little systematic variation when tests given to normal children. Tactile defensiveness/hyperactivity may have a maturational component. |

Continued

TABLE 9.24 **Purpose, Methods, Results, and Contributions of Studies of Sensory Integrative Patterns—cont'd**

| Year | Author | Purpose | Instruments | Hypothesis | Analysis | Subjects | Results | Contributions to Theory |
|---|---|---|---|---|---|---|---|---|
| 1969 | Ayres, A. J. | To provide an in-depth analysis of dysfunctional patterns in children with learning handicaps. Establish construct validity. | Sixty-four tests and observations: SCSIT, psycholinguistic, intelligence, auditory, postural-ocular reactions, and academic achievement. | That brain functions involve several levels and will cluster accordingly. | Q-technique factor analysis. | *n* = 36. Educationally handicapped children. | Five factors identified: Auditory language sequencing; postural and bilateral integration; right hemisphere dysfunction; apraxia; tactile defensiveness. | Hints to left hemisphere dysfunction. |
| 1971 | Ayres, A. J. | To identify predictors of severity of sensory integrative syndromes. | Forty-eight tests and observations: SCSIT, psycholinguistic, intelligence, eye-hand usage, and postural responses. | That predictive equations would emerge. | Ten-step regression equations for each syndrome calculated. | *n* = 140. Educationally handicapped children. | Presence of more than one type of disorder was the norm. Prone extension best predictor of postural-bilateral integration. Imitation of postures best predictor of praxis. | Somatosensory and praxis are linked again. Elucidated best predictors of syndromes. As many children may have apraxia as have postural and bilateral coordination problems. |
| 1972 | Ayres, A. J. | To further analyze and refine factors. Establish construct validity. | Same as above. | That similar factors as presented previously would emerge. | R-technique factor analysis. | *n* = 148. Educationally handicapped children. | Six factors identified: Form and space perception; auditory language; postural-ocular; motor planning; reading, spelling, and IQ; hyperactivity and tactile perception. | Further confirmed left hemisphere dysfunction. Reconfirmed syndromes found in other samples of learning-disabled children. |
| 1977 | Ayres, A. J. | To further analyze interrelationships (add SCPNT) so that differential diagnosis can be further refined. | SCSIT, SCPNT, postural-ocular and lateralization measures, dichotic listening, ITPA, intelligence, academic achievement. Flowers-Costello (auditory). | That clusters would continue to be refined. | Series of R-technique factor analyses (not all measures entered each time). | *n* = 128. Learning-disabled children. | Five major domains identified: Somatosensory-motor planning, auditory-language, postural-ocular, eye-hand coordination, postrotary nystagmus. | Further elucidated nature of interhemispheric integration. Role of vestibular system was clarified. |

**TABLE 9.24 Purpose, Methods, Results, and Contributions of Studies of Sensory Integrative Patterns—cont'd**

| Year | Author | Purpose | Instruments | Hypothesis | Analysis | Subjects | Results | Contributions to Theory |
|---|---|---|---|---|---|---|---|---|
| 1987 | Ayres, A. J., Mailloux, Z., & Wendler, C. L. W. | To continue to attempt to differentiate types of sensory integration dysfunction.<br>New praxis tests as well as many of the tests that had been used in past studies. | SCSIT, SCPNT, selected ITPA test, sentence repetition.<br>Clinical observation of prone extension, supine flexion, ocular pursuits.<br>Preliminary versions of newly designed praxis tests: Sequencing praxis, praxis on verbal command oral praxis, and block-building test. | Is praxis a unitary function?<br>Would computer-generated clusters match those that had been identified clinically and through factor analysis? | Screen plot factor analyses, correlation coefficients.<br>Comparison of test profiles of children with diagnoses.<br>Use of computer-generated clusters. | $n$ = 182.<br>Learning or behavior disorders. | Praxis tests were related with one another.<br>Visual tests correlated with tactile tests.<br>Somatovisual-practic factor identified.<br>Tactile scores and praxis related; short duration postrotary nystagmus; statistical association with praxis. | Suggestion of a general somatopractic function.<br>Further verified close association of tactile score and praxis.<br>Computer-generated clusters were not meaningful. |
| 1989 | Ayres, A. J. | Factor analyses: To clarify the nature of the constructs measured by the sensory integration and praxis tests (SIPT). | SIPT (17 tests) | That factors related to those of the SCSIT would emerge. | Principal components analysis. | Three analyses: $n$ = 1750.<br>Normative sample.<br>$n$ = 125.<br>Learning or sensory integrative disorders.<br>$n$ = 293.<br>Combined sample of learning or sensory integrative disorders and matched children from normative sample. | Visuopraxis and somatopraxis factors emerged in all three analyses.<br>Bilateral integration and sequencing factor and praxis on verbal command factor seen only in dysfunctional sample.<br>Other factors related to vestibular and somatosensory processing were identified. | Expanded understanding of vestibular-bilateral disorders to include sequencing element.<br>Somatopraxis factor reinforced previous findings linking tactile perception and praxis.<br>Visuopraxis factor provided support for previous visual-motor linkages. |
| 1989 | Ayres A. J. | Cluster analyses: To assist in identifying children in need of different types of remediation or services. | SIPT (17 tests) | That meaningful diagnostic groupings would emerge. | Agglomerative cluster analysis, Ward's method. | $n$ = 293.<br>Same sample as above, combined dysfunctional and normative. | Six cluster groups identified: Low average bilateral integration and sequencing, generalized sensory integrative dysfunction, visuo- and somatodyspraxia, low average sensory integration and praxis, dyspraxia on verbal command, and high average sensory integration and praxis. | Children with and without dysfunction can be differentiated on the basis of SIPT profiles.<br>Identified specific SIPT profile that may be characteristic of left hemisphere dysfunction. |

*Continued*

TABLE 9.24 **Purpose, Methods, Results, and Contributions of Studies of Sensory Integrative Patterns—cont'd**

| Year | Author | Purpose | Instruments | Hypothesis | Analysis | Subjects | Results | Contributions to Theory |
|---|---|---|---|---|---|---|---|---|
| 2011 | Mailloux, Z., Mulligan, S., Roley, S. S., et al. | To explore relationships among modulation measures; examine low and high PRN as separate measures. | Eighteen test scores from the SIPT; subtests for directionality, laterality, and crossing midline; SPM items measuring sensory overresponsiveness; parent report of problems in attention. | That low PRN and measures of directionality, laterality, and crossing midline would be associated with measures of vestibular-bilateral integration; SPM items measuring sensory overresponsiveness would be more related to attention than other sensory or practic functions. | Exploratory factor analyses using Varimax and Promax rotations. | 273 children from a retrospective clinical sample. PRN scores fell primarily in the low to average range. | Four factors:<br>Visuo- and somatodyspraxia,<br>vestibular-bilateral integration and sequencing,<br>tactile defensiveness and attention, and tactile and visual discrimination. | Low PRN is related to vestibular and bilateral integration functions; tactile defensiveness is more strongly related to attention problems than to perception measures or praxis; measures of directionality, laterality, and crossing midline and modulation items other than for tactile defensiveness were not significant factors. |
| 2000 | Mulligan, S. | To explore subgroupings of children referred for SIPT testing and to provide information about the validity of the six cluster groups identified in the SIPT manual. | SIPT | That cluster groups similar to those identified by Ayres (1989) would emerge. | Agglomerative cluster analysis, Ward's method. | $n = 1961$ children assessed with the SIPT between 1989 and 1993. | Five cluster groups identified: Generalized sensory integration dysfunction and dyspraxia-severe, generalized sensory integration dysfunction and dyspraxia-moderate, low average bilateral integration and sequencing, and average sensory integration and praxis. | Demonstrated many similarities with Ayres's cluster analysis, with some differences.<br>Supports evidence of dyspraxia, bilateral integration and sequencing deficit, dyspraxia on verbal command, and more general dyspraxia.<br>More helpful in identifying degree of dysfunction rather than type, because this sample did not include a normative sample as did Ayres's analysis. |
| 1998 | Parham, L. D. | To examine whether sensory integrative measures are predictive of school achievement, when intelligence and other factors are taken into account, concurrently and over a 4-year period. | SIPT, converted into three factor scores: praxis, visual perception, and somatosensory.<br>Intelligence, reading, and math achievement.<br>Socioeconomic status. | That sensory integrative performance at ages 6–8 years is related to achievement concurrently and predictively 4 years later.<br>That sensory integrative performance at ages 10–12 is not related to achievement. | Multiple regression analyses. | $n = 91$, of whom 43 were identified as learning disabled.<br>Children were 6–8 years old initially and 10–12 years old at follow-up. | When controlling for IQ sensory integration: At ages 6–8, significantly correlated with math, but not reading; at ages 6–8, significantly predicted math and reading 4 years later; at ages 10–12, significantly predicted math and reading at same age.<br>Strong relationships between praxis and math achievement identified. | Supported the hypothesis that sensory integration, especially praxis, is related to achievement when taking IQ into account.<br>Sensory integration continues to contribute to achievement at middle school age. |

**TABLE 9.24 Purpose, Methods, Results, and Contributions of Studies of Sensory Integrative Patterns—cont'd**

| Year | Author | Purpose | Instruments | Hypothesis | Analysis | Subjects | Results | Contributions to Theory |
|---|---|---|---|---|---|---|---|---|
| 2011 | Mulligan, S. | To examine the validity of the PRN test as a measure of vestibular functioning and its relationship to variables measuring similar functions. | PRN, SWB, BMC, KIN, Mac, and PrVC from the SIPT. | That there would be a significant correlation between PRN and performance on SWB, BMC, KIN, and MAc.<br>That children with depressed PRN would score more poorly on SWB, KIN, BMC, and MAc.<br>That children with prolonged PRN would score lower on PrVC and that there would be a significant negative correlation between PRN and PrVC. | Pearson product moment correlations (SPSS version 17); analysis of variance. | 575 children with suspected SI problems extracted from 1000 data sets from WPS; S's were divided into three groups based on PRN scores (PRN-low, PRN-average, and PRN-high). | 1. There was a significant correlation between all pairs ($P < 0.05$).<br>2. Children with depressed PRN scored significantly lower on SWB, BMC, KIN, and MAc ($P < 0.001$).<br>3. Children with prolonged PRN did not score significantly lower on PrVC than children with average or depressed PRN. | Validates theory that low PRN can indicate a vestibular processing problem and that low PRN is associated with other vestibular-related functions such as difficulties in balance (SWB), coordination of both sides of the body (BMC), position awareness (KIN), and eye-head-hand coordination (MAc). Prolonged PRN was not particularly associated with low PrVC or other tests in this sample. |

*CFA*, Confirmatory factor analysis; *SIPT*, sensory integration and praxis tests; *SEM*, structural equation modeling.

TABLE 9.25 **Factors and Clusters Identified in Research**

| Author and Date of Study | Somatodyspraxia | Visual Perception and Visuomotor/ Visuopraxis | Vestibular, Postural, and Bilateral Integration | Auditory Language Functions | Somatosensory Perception | Tactile Defensiveness and Attention | Other Findings |
|---|---|---|---|---|---|---|---|
| Ayres, A. J. 1965 | Tactile tests<br>Motor planning<br>Eye pursuits | Frostig tests<br>Kinesthesia<br>Manual form<br>Perception<br>Ayres' space test | Right-left discrimination<br>Avoidance crossing midline<br>Rhythmic activities | Not tested | No specific factor | Hyperactive/ distractibleBehavior andtactile defensiveness | Figure-ground a separate factor<br>Eye-hand agreement not related to perceptual-motor dysfunction |
| Ayres, A. J. 1966a | Accounted for most variance<br>Motor planning<br>Tactile and kinesthesia<br>Motor accuracy<br>Figure-ground<br>Frostig tests | Figure-ground<br>Frostig spatial relations<br>Ayres' space test | | Not tested | No specific factor | Low association of tactile defensiveness with praxis factor | |
| Ayres, A. J. 1966b | | Frostig tests<br>Ayres' space test<br>Motor accuracy<br>Figure-ground | Integration of two sides of body and tactile perception | Not tested | No specific factor | Tactile defensiveness and hyperactivity; may be a maturational factor involved | |
| Ayres, A. J. 1969 | Tactile<br>Motor planning | Most SCSIT; visual tests not included in analysis<br>Possible right hemisphere dysfunction: Eye movement deficits, better right- than left-sided function | Bilateral integration<br>Postural reactions<br>Reading and language problems | Possible left hemisphere dysfunction: Auditory-language<br>Reading achievement<br>Auditory and visual-motor sequencing | No specific factor | Tactile defensiveness, hyperactivity, and attention related to each other, but not a distinct factor | |
| Ayres, A. J. 1972 | Motor planning<br>Hyperactivity<br>Tactile defensiveness (more emphasis on motor than tactile) | Poor praxis related to hyperactivity and tactile defensiveness | Poor ocular control<br>Excessive residual primitive postural responses<br>Relatively good left-hand coordination | Auditory language<br>Intelligence | Tactile perception and hyperactivity formed a factor separate from praxis | Tactile defensiveness and hyperactivity loaded with praxis | |
| Ayres, A. J. 1977 | Analysis 5: Imitation of postures<br>Composite tactile<br>Kinesthesia | Analysis 3: Four SCSIT visual tests<br>Manual form<br>Perception | Analysis 5: Prone extension<br>Composite postural<br>Flexion posture<br>Composite tactile<br>Kinesthesia<br>Bilateral integration symptom did not load | Analysis 5: Composite language (ITPA)<br>Dichotic listening<br>Flowers-Costello (auditory) | No specific factor | Not studied | |

| | | | | | | |
|---|---|---|---|---|---|---|
| Ayres, A. J. 1989 | Somatopraxis (oral praxis, postural praxis, graphesthesia)<br>Visuo- and somatodyspraxia cluster | Visuopraxis (constructional praxis, design copying, space visualization, and figure-ground) | Bilateral integration and sequencing (sequencing praxis, bilateral motor coordination, standing and walking balance)<br>Low average bilateral integration and sequencing cluster | Praxis on verbal command dyspraxia on verbal command cluster (high postratary nystagmus with low praxis on verbal command) | Somatosensory perception | Not studied |
| Mulligan, S. 1998 | Dyspraxia (oral praxis, postural praxis, and praxis on verbal command); also suggests generalized practice function underlying all other factors | Visual perceptual deficit (design copying, constructional praxis, space visualization, manual form perception, and figure-ground perception) | Bilateral integration and sequencing deficit (sequencing praxis and bilateral motor coordination) | Not tested | Tactile tests and kinesthesia | Not studied |
| Parham, L. D. 1998 | Somatopraxis is a powerful predictor of early and later math skills; predicts later reading skills | Visuopraxis is a predictor of early and later math skills; predicts later reading skills | Not studied | Not studied | Somatosensory perception related to early math but not reading | Not studied |
| Mailloux, Z., Mulligan, S., Roley, S. S., Blanche, E., Cermak, S., Coleman, G. G., Bodison, S., & Lane, C. J. 2011 | Some somatopraxis tests seen within the visuopraxis factor | Visuopraxis formed a distinct factor | PRN included as part of a bilateral integration and sequencing factor | Not tested | Tactile perception loaded with visual perception | Tactile defensiveness items loaded with signs of attention problems |
| Mulligan, S. 2011 | | | Association between depressed PRN and other signs of vestibular problems including balance, bilateral coordination, and eye-head-hand coordination, as well as poor proprioceptive awareness | | | |

*ITPA*, Illinois Test of Psycholinguistic Abilities; *SCSIT*, Southern California Sensory Integration Test; *SVCU*, space visualization contralateral use.

TABLE 9.26 **Problems With Sensory Reactivity**

| Type of Issue | Description | Observations | Impact on Participation |
|---|---|---|---|
| Limited sensory registration | • Often does not notice or "register" relevant environmental stimuli | • Often oblivious to touch, pain, movement, taste, smells, sights, or sounds<br>• Is not aware that the stimulus is present<br>• Usually more than one sensory system involved<br>• May not notice physical injury<br>• Potential for self-injurious behavior | • Participation may be severely limited by lack of awareness of people, objects, or sensations |
| Tactile defensiveness (Ayres, 1964, 1973, 1979) | • Hyperreactivity to ordinary touch sensations<br>• Light touch stimuli are aversive, especially in very sensitive body areas such as the face, abdomen, and palmar surfaces of the upper and lower extremities<br>• Generally, self-applied input is tolerated better than being touched by another person.<br>• Tactile stimuli may be especially threatening if the child cannot see the source | • Respond with irritation and discomfort to light touch stimuli, e.g., textures of clothing, textures of food, grass or sand against bare skin, glue or paint on skin, light brush of a person passing by, brushing hair or teeth<br>• Emotional responses to noxious stimuli often involve anxiety, distractibility, restlessness, anger, having a tantrum, aggression, fear, and distress<br>• Most feel comfortable with deep touch stimuli and may experience relief and feel calmed when deep pressure is applied | • Participation is often limited in self-care activities such as dressing, bathing, grooming, and eating<br>• Participation in classroom and play activities is often limited, e.g., finger painting, sand and water play, and crafts<br>• May avoid or become upset by activities that require proximity to others, such as playing near other children or standing in line<br>• Behavior is often misinterpreted as rejecting, demanding, or aggressive |
| [a]Gravitational insecurity (Ayres, 1979) | • Hyperreactivity to vestibular sensations involving linear movement, particularly sensations from the pull of gravity and from vertical movement through space | • Excessive fear during ordinary whole-body movement activities<br>• Moves very slowly and carefully through space<br>• Avoidance or refusal to use stairs, escalators, elevators, step stools, ladders, playground equipment that moves, and uneven or unpredictable surfaces<br>• Overwhelmed by changes in head position and movement, especially when moving backward or upward through space<br>• Fear of heights, even those involving only slight distances from the ground<br>• Many resist lifting feet off the ground<br>• Avoidance of tilting the head in different planes (especially backward) | • Participation in community activities may be severely limited when movement is involved<br>• Community mobility may be severely limited or stressful, e.g., refusal to use stairs or escalators, distress when lifted into a car, anxiety getting on and off bus or subway<br>• Participation with peers in games and sports may be very limited, walking or running on uneven ground, bicycle riding, ice skating, roller skating, skateboarding, skiing, and hiking<br>• Exploration of environment may be limited |
| Auditory/visual/olfactory and gustatory defensiveness | • Hyperreactivity to sounds, sights, smells, tastes | • Distress or discomfort with loud sounds, bright lights, strong smells or tastes, and excessive stimuli | • Limited or no participation in events such as birthday parties or community fairs and festivals<br>• Participation in classrooms and cafeterias very stressful due to sights, sounds, and smells<br>• Mealtime participation may be limited by smells and tastes of food, especially if food is not familiar |

[a]*Note:* A distinction is made between gravitational insecurity and a similar condition called *postural insecurity*. Postural insecurity refers to fearfulness of full body movement resulting from limited postural stability or motor control. The fears of children with postural insecurity result from a learned, realistic appraisal of their motor limitations, not a sensory reactivity problem per se.

**TABLE 9.27 Problems With Sensory Perception**

| Type of Issue | Description | Observations | Impact on Participation |
|---|---|---|---|
| Tactile perception | Difficulty interpreting the location, intensity, three-dimensional properties, or direction of movement of tactile stimuli precisely and efficiently | Difficulty localizing precisely where an object has brushed against them<br>Difficulty with stereognosis to manipulate an object that is out of sight—fine motor coordination is affected<br>May be seen along with problems with visual perception and motor planning | Hinders participation in play activities that require precise hand and finger movements, such as connecting pieces of constructional toys, or playing marbles<br>Difficulty participating in classroom and self-care activities that require precisely guided hand and finger movements, such as writing with a pencil, manipulating a spoon, or fastening buttons or snaps-<br>Participation may be stressful, requiring the child to compensate by visually guiding his or her actions during visual guidance for fine motor tasks |
| Proprioceptive perception | Difficulty interpreting body position and the position and movement of the muscles and joints | Appears clumsy and awkward<br>Relies on visual guidance of movement or on cognitive strategies<br>Uses too much or too little force in activities such as writing, clapping, marching, or keyboarding<br>May seek out excessive proprioceptive input, e.g., pushing, pulling, throwing, or jumping forcefully<br>Breaking toys, bumping into others, and misjudging personal space | Participation at school or in play with peers may be compromised by behaviors that get them into trouble because they are misperceived as intentionally disruptive<br>Participation in movement and sports activities may be hindered |
| [a]Visual perception | Difficulty interpreting features of visual stimuli such as shape, size, direction, and figure-ground relationships, despite adequate visual acuity | Difficulty with visual perception, visual spatial, visual construction, and/or visual-motor tasks<br>May affect motor functions such as grasp, balance, and locomotion | Participation in play activities may be limited, e.g., puzzles, building block activities, and crafts<br>Participation in academic activities at school may be affected, e.g., handwriting, art activities, projects requiring construction |
| [b]Auditory perception | Difficulty discriminating and interpreting sounds, but hearing is not impaired | Difficulty locating where sound is coming from<br>Difficulty with following directions<br>Difficulty understanding conversation<br>Difficulty focusing on sounds or words when background noise is present | Participation in social play may be affected due communication difficulties with peers<br>Participation in sports, games, and music or dance activities may be affected by inability to rapidly and accurately interpret temporal and spatial qualities of auditory cues<br>Participation in activities at home and in school may be compromised by difficulty understanding auditory cues and spoken instructions |

[a]*Note:* Problems with visual perception are commonly seen in children with sensory integrative difficulties, particularly when poor tactile perception or dyspraxia is present (Ayres, 1989; Ayres et al., 1987). A sensory integrative intervention approach is only appropriate for the child who demonstrates visual perception problems along with other indicators of sensory integrative difficulties. When other sensory integration issues are not present, the occupational therapist may choose to work with the child using another approach, such as visual perception training, use of compensatory strategies, or skill training in specific activities.

[b]Although auditory perception problems are not usually considered to be a type of sensory integrative condition when seen in isolation, difficulties with auditory perception and language development often coexist with signs of sensory integrative difficulties. If auditory perception problems are suspected, a clinical evaluation by a speech-language pathologist is indicated.

over others. Please see Table 9.28 for descriptions and observations of problems with praxis.

## Specific Areas of Assessment Regarding Sensory Processing and Integration

Assessment of sensory integration functioning is situated within a comprehensive evaluation of occupational performance when warranted. Assessment by the occupational therapist begins with a general exploration of the occupations of the child and family, focusing on their concerns and hopes in relation to the child's strengths and challenges. A variety of tools is needed to help the occupational therapist discern whether problems in sensory integration are relevant to the child's life situation, to understand the nature and scope of these difficulties, to consider how the difficulties may be offset by the child's talents and strengths, and to decide whether intervention should be recommended.

TABLE 9.28 **Problems With Bilateral Integration and Sequencing and Praxis**

| Type of Issue | Description | Observations | Impact on Participation |
|---|---|---|---|
| Problems in vestibular-bilateral integration | Inefficient processing of vestibular sensory information (related to head and body movement through space) needed for postural and ocular control, bilateral coordination, midline integration, optimal muscle tone for readiness to move, and balance | Jerky or disorganized eye tracking movements<br>Poor balance<br>Trouble assuming and maintaining an extensor position while prone<br>Frequent slouching or difficulty staying in an upright seated position for more than a few minutes at a time<br>Movement appears slightly floppy<br>Poor bilateral coordination<br>Difficulty with postural control during shifts in body midline<br>Frequent tripping or falling<br>Hesitance or avoidance of reaching across the body for an object<br>Hesitance or difficulty leaning forward or sideways to grasp an object out of reach | Difficulty participating in sports, dance, or play activities due to poor balance<br>Social participation is secondarily affected<br>Loss of place when looking up at the classroom board and then back down at a worksheet, affecting academic performance<br>Limited participation in activities that require remaining seated for an extended period of time<br>Trouble participating in activities that require coordination of both sides of the body such as pedaling a bicycle or tying shoes |
| Poor praxis | Difficulty coming up with an idea for how to move in a new way<br>Difficulty planning and performing a new sequence of movements to achieve a goal | Difficulty learning new motor skills<br>Lack of ideas about new ways to use an object or toy<br>Difficulty learning to dress self<br>Difficulty figuring out how to put on a new type of clothing<br>Imitates what others are doing, rather than initiating a new activity<br>Poor timing or sequencing of actions<br>Trouble manipulating objects, drawing, or building | Limited participation in sports<br>Limited participation in games that require moving in new ways<br>Limited participation in activities that require construction, such as building a pretend house with interlocking blocks<br>Difficulty developing independence in self-care skills such as dressing or bathing<br>Difficulty participating in arts activities that require new ways of moving or manipulating objects, such as dance, music, or drawing<br>Limited social participation due to difficulty joining others in an activity or coordinating actions to engage with others |

This type of evaluation requires a multifaceted approach because of the need to understand the child's presenting problems in relation to the family and environments in which that child participates. Assessment tools employed by occupational therapists using a sensory integration perspective include interviews and questionnaires, informal and formal observations, standardized tests, and consideration of services and resources available to and appropriate for the family. The American Occupational Therapy Association (AOTA), in partnership with the campaign called Choosing Wisely, has recommended that practitioners avoid using sensory interventions with children unless a specific assessment of sensory functioning has been conducted that indicates the existence of difficulties in sensory integration/processing (AOTA, 2018). Interventions must be directly linked to assessment results.

**Specific Assessment Tools and Measures.** Specific assessment of sensory functions may occur through a variety of means, but a comprehensive evaluation is crucial before beginning any intervention. See Appendix A for information about specific assessment tools.

## ASSESSMENT OF MOTOR CONTROL

Motor control refers to how a person activates muscles, coordinates movements, maintains positions, moves in and out of positions, manipulates objects, and uses their body for activities and is necessary to engage in all occupations. Motor control is dynamic and influenced by many systems (such as the child's body structures and functions, motivation, and determination), environment (including physical, attitudinal, cultural, and social aspects), and the task or activity itself (e.g., what is the child trying to do). Occupational therapists examine multiple factors to identify those that support or interfere with the child's ability to coordinate movements and do those things they want or need to do.

### Common Challenges Associated With Motor Control

Children with neurologic conditions, such as cerebral palsy (CP), traumatic brain injury, prematurity, or other conditions causing lesions in the brain, may present with motor control challenges as the result of abnormal muscle tone (hypertonicity, hypotonicity, or athetosis), which affects voluntary control, posture, timing, and quality of movements. Children with hypotonicity (such as children with Down syndrome) experience motor control challenges due to lack of postural control and difficulty recruiting muscles to complete actions. They experience slower reaction times resulting in less coordinated movements. Children with sensory integration dysfunction or developmental coordination disorder may also present with inefficient movement patterns, resulting in challenges with timing, sequencing, bilateral coordination, eye-hand control, or eye-foot control. They may exhibit challenges processing sensory stimuli causing delayed, absent, or inefficient movements that can present as poor balance, coordination, movement, and posture.

Motor control challenges interfere with infants' and children's play, coordination for feeding and eating, use of hands to manipulate objects, mobility, climbing, and walking. Children may have difficulty with handwriting, managing their classroom materials, and navigating the classroom environment. They may fall, bump into things, and tire easily. Their motor control challenges may interfere with their ability to reach and secure objects. They may achieve milestones while exhibiting poor quality of movement that interferes with tying their shoes, manipulating small objects, and producing efficient movements (such as required with riding a bike, jump roping, or engaging in sports).

## Specific Areas of Assessment Regarding Motor Control

Occupational therapists assess multiple systems to determine how person, task, and environmental factors influence motor control. Box 9.21 provides an outline with description of key aspects of motor control to support the therapist in making observations of the child's movement. Occupational therapists evaluate the child's **agency,** which is their ability to control aspects of the event or an activity through their own actions. This may be observed as the child's desire to move or interest in moving, reaching, grabbing, holding, and touching. Children may move in different ways to accomplish motor tasks that they want to do. Assessment of motor control includes an examination of how the child plans motor actions, known as **prospectivity** (Adolph, 2020; Adolph & Kretch, 2015). The therapist observes the child complete novel tasks (such as catching a ball, putting on a shirt, drawing letters, or completing an obstacle course) to determine how the child plans and executes movement. They observe the child's ability to move in a variety of ways (**flexibility**) and to problem solve for success, which illustrates **adaptability** flexibility and adaptability are key aspects of effective movement.

A thorough evaluation of the person factors that influence motor performance includes sensory, musculoskeletal, perception, cognition, and emotional factors. Assessment includes a physical evaluation of the child's musculoskeletal system to include physical appearance (such as symmetry and joints), ROM, strength, endurance, and sensory systems (e.g., visual, proprioceptive, vestibular, auditory). Occupational therapists can observe the child engaging in movements to assess their patterns and quality of movement as well as developmental milestones. They examine the child's postural control (in a variety of positions), balance, and use of extremities together (i.e., bilateral coordination). They observe the timing, sequencing, and accuracy of movements. They examine perceptual systems that allow the child to make sense of sensory stimuli to interpret distance, size, and their body position, which influence motor control (Adolph, 2020; Adolph & Young, 2021).

Cognition influences the child's desires to initiate movement, problem solve, engage in goal-directed tasks, and use a variety of movement strategies. Therapists examine the child's cognitive processing, which is observed as the child's ability regarding movement, tasks, and their environment. Occupational therapists also assess the child's emotional system or psychological state, which includes motivation, choice, self-efficacy, and self-determination, which play a role in the child's movement.

Examining how children engage in motor tasks provides insights into strategies that children may use to move. As therapists observe children, they analyze the motor and processing demands of the task, which can indicate the child's challenges (such as bimanual vs.

### BOX 9.21 Guidelines for Observing Motor Control

| Principles of Goal-Directed Movements | Indicators | Observation Notes |
|---|---|---|
| Agency | Children actively participate to select the task goal<br>Movements are voluntary, self-initiated, and generated to accomplish a goal<br>Children can detect and evaluate (are aware) of the outcomes of their motor actions<br>Children can detect the errors of their actions: explicitly state it or implicitly correct their strategies<br>Children actively participate to select the task goal<br>Movements are voluntary, self-initiated, and generated to accomplish a goal | |
| Prospectivity | Planning of movements and anticipating the task demands (e.g., shaping their grasp as they approach a cup in anticipation to grasp it)<br>Planning for anticipated consequences of their behavior (e.g., in a catch and throw game: timely repositioning of their arms/hands and body after a throw to receive the ball)<br>Accuracy of movement so that task is completed with ease<br>Timed coordination of movements allows for fluid movements<br>Ability to plan and carry out one, two-step, and multiple-step tasks | |
| Flexibility | Identify that motor strategies are not working<br>Stop motor strategies that do not work<br>Utilize effective motor strategies that can better accomplish the goal | |
| Adaptability | Children are able to carry out a task in a specific environment<br>Children's performance is significantly affected by changes in context (e.g., home, school, community, etc.) | |

unimanual). Occupational therapists assessing motor control evaluate the environmental contexts for the movement, which includes the physical, social, cultural, temporal, virtual and personal contexts in which movement occurs. Understanding the environmental contexts provides information on the child's expectations for movement and insight into adaptations and modifications that may support the child's movement, and it informs intervention planning.

A variety of assessments or evaluation tools provide objective measurements of the child's current level of motor skills and functioning for purposes of planning intervention and evaluating progress (see Appendix A). The evaluation process involves assessing body functions and structures (e.g., M-ABC, PDMS-2, VMI, BOT-2), skills for activity engagement (e.g., Abilihand-kids, Minnesota Handwriting Assessment), and participation levels (e.g., SFA, PEDI).

Occupational therapists may also observe children to better understand meaning. The Pediatric Volitional Questionnaire (Basu et al., 2008) and the Test of Playfulness (Skard & Bundy, 2008) provide observational assessments to measure interest, motivation, and approach toward activity (play). The Child Occupational Self-Assessment (COSA; Kramer et al., 2014) gathers information from the child to determine their level of interest in activities and measure their values (i.e., importance of activity) and perceived competency (i.e., how well they feel they perform the activity).

Occupational therapists analyze the task requirements in relation to person and environmental factors, so they can adapt the task to help the child successfully perform (Kolovelonis et al., 2012; Pless & Carlsson, 2000). The skilled occupational therapist considers all these contexts when analyzing a child's motor performance in the context of occupations. Careful analysis of the child's motor functioning in a variety of contexts (at least two) can reveal the child's strengths and weaknesses. The Test of Environmental Supportiveness (Bundy, 1999; Skard & Bundy, 2008) measures the influence of the environment on play and can provide occupational therapists with a structure when analyzing the play environment (see Appendix A). Most often occupational therapists informally assess the environment, with a focus on identifying the factors that seem to most influence the child's occupational performance.

## ASSESSMENT OF HAND AND FINE MOTOR SKILL

Children and youth of all ages use their hands and fingers daily. Infants use their hands and fingers to hold their bottle, grasp for items, touch people and objects, and point to things of interest to them. Young children pick up utensils, manipulate toys, button clothing, and manage classroom tools such as scissors. Adolescents use intricate fine motor skills for activities such as drawing, playing musical instruments, and playing video games. Fine motor movements may require precision (e.g., putting on makeup), strength (e.g., opening a jar), timing (e.g., playing piano), and accuracy (e.g., putting in earrings).

Fine motor skills are required to engage in most occupations, and therefore occupational therapists frequently assess this area. Occupational therapists typically perform one of two types of evaluation of hand function for children. One type is a developmental evaluation that examines abilities related to neurodevelopmental challenges. This type often takes place in a school or an outpatient facility. The second type is an evaluation due to an injury or traumatic event, or an orthopedic diagnosis, and this type might occur in an acute care hospital or a hand therapy clinic. The specific assessments used in each setting may vary. For example, pain and peripheral sensory function might commonly be assessed in a hospital or outpatient clinic but would occur less likely in a school setting during a comprehensive evaluation of educational performance.

### Common Challenges Associated With Hand and Fine Motor Skills

The more students use their hands and engage in fine motor skills, particularly in preschool and early elementary education, the more likely they are to participate with more variety, frequency, and independence in fine motor tasks (Gee Kee et al., 2014). Holding objects and manipulating objects, refinement of pinch, and hand strength impact dressing skills needed for gym class participation; the ability to open lockers as well as tool use of eating utensils, pencils, scissors, paintbrushes, and protractors (Ittyerah, 2013) should be evaluated. Tool use involves purposeful, goal-directed manipulation of a tool to interact with other objects or materials and is an essential method for interacting with the school environment. Proficient tool use is needed for participation in a variety of school, self-care, and play tasks.

### Specific Areas of Assessment Regarding Hand and Fine Motor Skills in Pediatric Hand Therapy

When administering a comprehensive evaluation, occupational therapists review the child's medical chart and interview the caregivers and child to guide the strategic elements and priorities of the evaluation process. The following sections describe the potential components to assess within an occupational therapy evaluation related to hand and find motor functioning.

**Pain.** Many children who are referred to hand therapy have pain. The occupational therapist screens for pain in the initial evaluation and continues to reassess pain throughout the course of care. The therapist uses the child's level of pain to guide the intervention plan. To assess the location of the child's pain, the occupational therapist asks the child to point to where they are experiencing pain. The occupational therapist interviews the child to further evaluate pain. Questions can help gauge if the pain is diffuse or localized and to determine the frequency and intensity of pain. To determine the quality of pain, the occupational therapist asks the child to describe their pain (i.e., sharp, dull, aching, burning, shooting, or hurting). This information can help the occupational therapist determine the appropriate intervention(s), as well as pertinent clinical findings that are reported to the referring clinician. Additionally, the child's responses can provide insight into the correct diagnosis. For example, tendonitis is often characterized by a sharp or shooting pain when using the upper extremity; generalized, aching joint pain is more typical in arthritis (Omoigui, 2007; Werner et al., 2005). The occupational therapist also asks the child how often and when the pain occurs. For example, the child may experience pain while performing specific activities or during certain periods of a day. Knowing the specific pattern of presentation guides the occupational therapist's recommendations for intervention. The intensity of pain can be quantified using a variety of self-report scales (Table 9.29). Quantifying the child's pain is valuable in determining the usefulness of therapeutic intervention to decrease pain. The occupational therapist uses a pain scale appropriate to the child's age and cognition.

Occupational therapists also ask questions to determine which strategies the patient and/or family have found helpful for managing the pain. Knowledge of all aspects of the child's pain guides the occupational therapist to determine the most appropriate intervention(s) to reduce and manage the child's pain so they can re-engage in those activities that are meaningful to them.

**Tenderness.** The occupational therapist screens for specific patterns of tenderness when a child reports pain. If the child reports pain as occurring in a specific location of the upper extremity (UE) in response to a clinician's manual examination, then the child is reported to have tenderness. A variety of special tests are used to

**TABLE 9.29 Pain Scales**

| Pain Scale | Age Range | Description |
|---|---|---|
| Faces pain scale—Revised (FPS-R) (Bieri et al., 1990; Hicks et al., 2001; Hunter et al., 2000; Spagrud et al., 2003) | 4–16 years | Therapist uses a card that has faces to describe pain. Child selects card that represents his or her pain. There are six faces, and each face represent a number from 0, 2, 4, 6, 8, and 10. |
| Oucher (Beyer, 1984; Beyer et al., 1992) | 3–12 years | This consists of two scales developed for children to rate pain level.<br>(1) The scale for younger children consists of six pictures of face to indicate pain intensity. The photographic scale should be used if the child is unable to count to 100 by ones or tens, if the child is unable to identify which of the two numbers is larger, or if the child can indicate a preference for using the photographic scale.<br>(2) The scale for older children consists of the numbers from 0 to 100. The numeric scale should be used if the child can count to 100 by ones or tens and can identify which of any two numbers is larger. There are five versions of the Oucher scale, based on ethnic background. |
| Visual Analog Scale (VAS) (De Jong et al., 2005) | 7 years to adult | The child or youth rates his or her pain using a visual representation of faces. |
| Numeric rating scale (Von Baeyer, 2009) | 6 years to adult | The child or youth rates his or her pain on a scale from 0 to 10, where 0 is no pain and 10 is the worst possible pain. |

assess specific patterns of tenderness in the UE to identify possible underlying structural concerns, such as ligamentous tear or inflamed tendon sheath. An example of a widely used assessment for tenderness is the Finkelstein's test for de Quervain tendonitis (Dawson & Mudgal, 2010; Flatt, 1994) The reliability of UE special tests is low (Marx et al., 1999; Prosser et al., 2011; Skirven et al., 2020); therefore, they should be used in conjunction with other clinical exam findings. The clinician considers the child's reported symptom pattern, strength, and ROM assessment to determine the most accurate clinical presentation.

**Skin.** The occupational therapist performs visual inspection of the skin at the evaluation, the start of treatment, and following therapeutic interventions. The skin's appearance provides information as to what therapeutic interventions may be necessary and how well a child is tolerating specific interventions.

If the child has undergone surgery or is recovering from a traumatic injury, they will likely have a healing wound or scar and require therapeutic intervention for wound or scar management. Children may also have skin color changes that can reflect circulatory compromise, indicating the need to change or discontinue intervention. In addition, occupational therapists monitor skin integrity regularly when providing interventions such as therapeutic taping or orthotic fabrication. Children may require a different intervention or a modification in orthotic design if compromised skin integrity is noted. Occupational therapists monitor children who report excessive pain or hypersensitivity for trophic changes because complex regional pain syndrome could be a concern warranting consultation with the referring physician.

Skin assessment is reported in subjective terms. When skin is noted to have compromised integrity, the following terms apply:

1. Color: red, white, blue, mottled (i.e., blotchy), or bruised
2. Quality: moist or dry
3. Temperature: cold or warm
4. Texture: calloused, macerated (i.e., moist, soft, and separated), or lacerated (i.e., cut)

The occupational therapist may also report if the skin has a rash or an abrasion.

When a child's skin has a wound or scar, the occupational therapist performs assessment at each treatment session to determine the effectiveness of the interventions being used for wound and scar management. Wound assessment includes notation of wound location, size, color, stage of healing, and exudate (i.e., drainage). Therapists closely monitor wounds for signs of infection (redness and edema in the wound bed and/or purulent [i.e., containing pus] drainage that is in excess of the inflammatory stage of wound healing) and notify the referring provider when they observe signs of a possible infection. When assessing a scar, the occupational therapist describes whether it is raised or flat, the size, height, location, pliability, and color. When a scar appears to be hypertrophic (raised or extending beyond the borders for the initial wound), and a formal assessment is needed, the occupational therapist may use the Modified Vancouver Scar Scale (MVSS) to measure changes in the four main scar characteristics (pigmentation, vascularity, pliability, and height) (Forbes-Duchart et al., 2007).

**Edema.** Edema is most common in cases of joint or tissue inflammation, such as arthritis or tendonitis, and in traumatic injury or postsurgical management of the UE. Occupational therapists may document edema using subjective terms, including:

- Amount: trace, minimal, moderate, or severe
- Quality: brawny (i.e., swollen and hard) or pitting (i.e., swelling in which an indentation persists after pressure is applied to skin and the pressure is released)
- Location: anatomic description of the area edema is covering.

More formal measurement of edema is recommended if (1) the amount of edema present is significant enough to limit the child's range of motion (ROM) or function, and (2) the child would benefit from interventions focused on controlling the edema. Location of edema dictates the measurement tool to be used. When the edema is localized to one or a few joints, circumferential measurements are most appropriate. Edema that covers the dorsum of the hand is best measured using the figure-of-eight method (Maihafer et al., 2003). In the figure-of-eight method, the occupational therapist wraps a tape measure through the palm of the hand and over the dorsum of the hand in a figure-of-eight pattern as depicted in Fig. 9.11. When the edema is more diffuse (i.e., throughout multiple joints in the hand and/or distal arm), the most accurate measurement is obtained using a volumeter (Fig. 9.12).

**Sensation.** Occupational therapists assess sensation to detect abnormal sensory patterns that require therapeutic intervention. Assessment

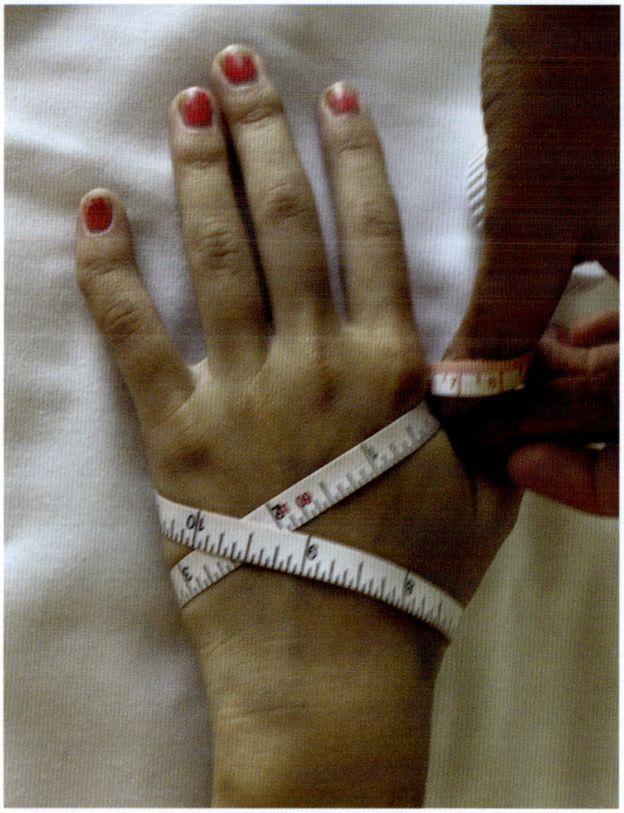

Fig. 9.11 Figure-of-eight method for measuring edema on the dorsum of the hand.

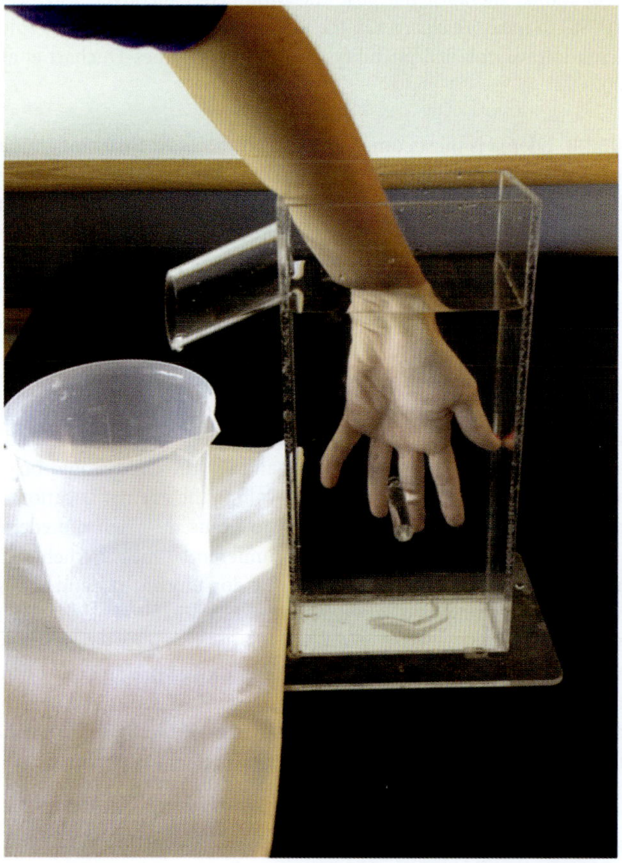

Fig. 9.12 Assessment of hand edema with a volumeter.

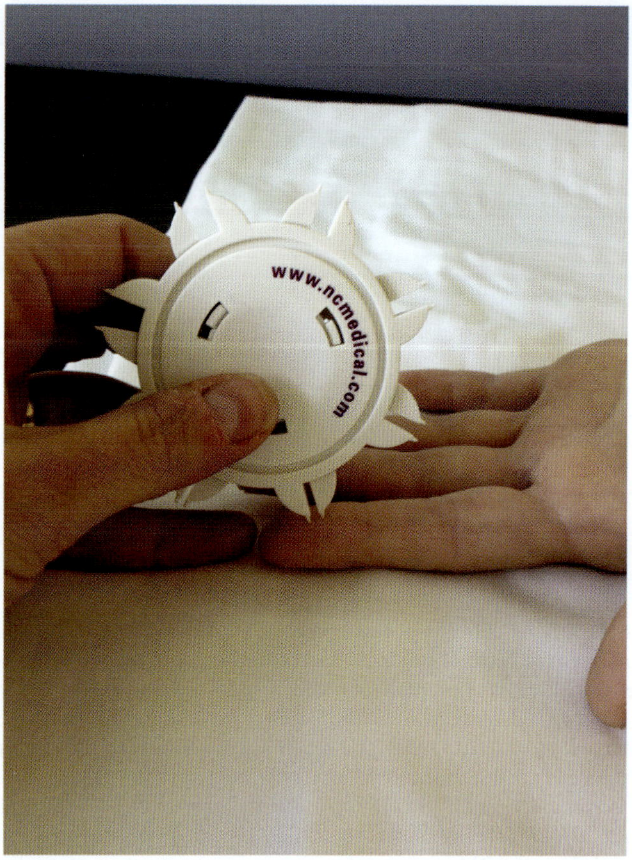


Fig. 9.13 Two-point discrimination assessment of hand sensation with the Disk-Criminator.

of sensation is important when peripheral nerve damage is reported or suspected or in cases in which extreme vascular changes have occurred. Information regarding a child's sensation is obtained through family interview, clinical observation, the wrinkle test, and other standardized assessments.

**Wrinkle Test.** The wrinkle test involves placing the child's hand in warm water for 30 minutes (van Barneveld et al., 2010). When a child has peripheral nerve impairment, fingertip wrinkling is absent or diminished compared with the unaffected hand. When sensory impairment improves, the typical wrinkling pattern returns. This is a particularly effective way to assess the presence of sensation in a child who is not able to report sensory symptoms.

**Hand Skills for Tool Use.** Observation and formal assessment of grip, strength, in-hand manipulation, and sensory-motor functions are necessary for evaluating tool use and handwriting. These underlying performance skills provide the foundation for engagement in many activities. An additional component of tool use is the role of the assisting hand. For example, in using scissors and eating, the assisting hand has an active role, while in writing and drawing the assisting hand primarily holds the paper.

**Two-Point Discrimination.** Two-point discrimination testing is used to assess the level of discriminative touch impairment. Therapists may use a standardized tool for assessing two-point discrimination, the two-point discriminator (Fig. 9.13) (Dellon, 1978). Occupational therapists also use Semmes-Weinstein monofilaments (SWMs) to evaluate touch discrimination. SWMs (Fig. 9.14) are used to quantify the level

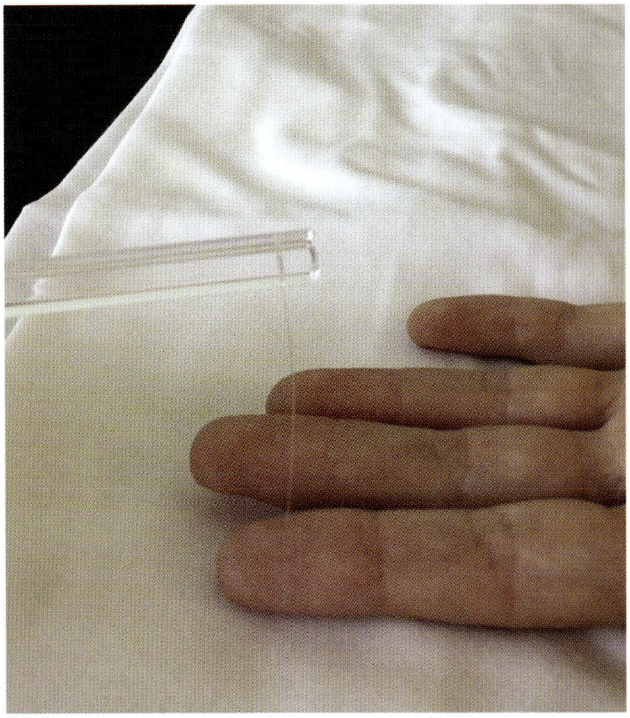

**Fig. 9.14** Assessment of hand sensation using Semmes-Weinstein monofilaments.

of abnormal sensory discrimination and pattern of impairment. To perform two-point discrimination or sensory assessment with SWMs, the child must be able to reliably report the sensory information he or she is feeling. When using the Disk-Criminator, the child reports whether one or two points are felt when touching the fingertip. With SWMs, the child must point to indicate whether or not and where they felt the monofilaments. For both assessments, the child must also feel at ease enough in the intervention setting to close their eyes while the test is being administered. When performing these assessments, the child places their hand palm facing up and the tester alternates touching the fingertips with the testing instruments. Two-point discrimination is highly related to the sensory function required to perform certain fine motor tasks (Dellon, 1978). Over time, reassessment with SWMs can document the progression of returning sensation (Tracey et al., 2012). For a child with sensory impairments, the interpretation scale for SWMs aids in identifying the specific level of impairment and in intervention planning. Children who have sustained a nerve injury are good candidates for using this assessment tool.

**Muscle Tone.** Children who have an underlying neurologic disorder typically have abnormal muscle tone in their affected UE. Muscle tone is assessed through the function and feel of the UE. The occupational therapist notes and describes the child's muscle tone. Generally, tone is described as normal muscle tone, diminished (or low) muscle tone (hypotonicity), or high muscle tone (hypertonicity). For example, a child who has spastic quadriplegic CP may have low muscle tone in core muscles and high muscle tone in his or her elbow flexors, pronators, wrists, and finger flexors. With children who have CP, the occupational therapist may use the Hypertonia Assessment Tool (HAT) to classify the type(s) of UE hypertonicity (Jethwa et al., 2010). The HAT allows the therapist to understand if the child's increased muscle tone is due to spasticity, dystonia, or rigidity, or if the child has mixed tone (Jethwa et al., 2010; Knights et al., 2014).

**Range of Motion.** Hand therapists complete a gross assessment of UE active range of motion (AROM), including shoulder, elbow, forearm, wrist, and digits. If limitations are noted in AROM, the therapist completes goniometric assessment of the limited ranges (Norkin, 2009; Reese & Bandy, 2009). When only one of the child's upper extremities is affected, goniometric assessment of the unaffected UE can be performed to use as a guide for the child's potential ROM and to establish plan-of-care goals. If there are no precautions that preclude assessing passive range of motion (PROM) (e.g., a recent fracture) and the child tolerates passive stretch, the occupational therapist also assesses the PROM in joints in which the child has AROM limitations. The occupational therapist notes the location and intensity of any pain the child reports during ROM assessment. This is particularly useful in cases of arthritis or other conditions in which pain is a primary symptom.

Limitations in ROM can be caused by joint tightness, tendon tightness, or scar adhesions. Occupational therapists may use the following techniques to determine if underlying factors are limiting ROM. If a child presents with similar measurements for AROM and PROM in the movement plane for the joint, they may have joint tightness. For example, a child with joint tightness in the proximal interphalangeal (PIP) joint would have 40° of active PIP flexion and only 40–45° of passive PIP flexion in the same digit. When a child has tendon tightness, the available AROM and PROM at a joint vary depending on the position of joints that are more proximal to the joints being tested. Tendon tightness may occur in the intrinsic or extrinsic muscles of the hand or both. One example of tendon tightness is extrinsic flexor tightness of the finger flexors that flex the PIP and distal interphalangeal (DIP) joints of the fingers, in which case the available AROM for PIP and DIP extension decreases as the angle of wrist extension increases.

ROM for the child who has sustained injury or undergone surgery can be limited when scarring adheres to soft tissue structures, such as the flexor tendons, and results in tightness. When scar adhesions limit joint ROM, the child will have a significant limitation in AROM at a joint while having near normal PROM at the same joint. Gaining a complete understanding of the biomechanics underlying the limitation in the ROM guides the occupational therapist in determining the appropriate intervention plan.

When a child presents with full PROM in a joint but limited AROM, they have muscle weakness. For example, the child may have full passive supination but active supination only to 30°. In this case the difference between PROM and AROM can reflect weakness of the muscle group (in this example, there is weakness in the supinator and/or biceps) or hypertonicity of the antagonist muscles (in this example, the pronators) that is the underlying cause of the limitation in AROM.

**Strength.** Impairments of the UE are often characterized by limitations in strength. Hand strength is most commonly assessed using a Jamar Dynamometer and pinch gauge (Molenaar et al., 2008). The strength of specific muscle groups in the hand and UE may also be assessed with manual muscle testing (Dekkers et al., 2014; Klingels et al., 2010).

For children who have sustained an injury to one UE, their strength on that side may be compared to that of their unaffected side to determine if weakness is contributing to functional limitations. Age-level normative data for grip and pinch strength are also available for children 3 and older (Tables 9.30–9.33) and can be useful to further determine the degree to which weakness is contributing to impairment (Häger-Ross & Rösblad, 2002; McQuiddy et al., 2015; Surrey et al., 2001). It is recommended that occupational therapists take three consecutive trials (Mathiowetz et al., 1984) of each measure for grip and

TABLE 9.30 **Grip Strength (Mean and SD) by Age, Hand, and Gender**

| | | MALES | | FEMALES | |
|---|---|---|---|---|---|
| **Age (y)** | **Hand** | **Kilograms** | **Pounds** | **Kilograms** | **Pounds** |
| 6 | R | 9.6±2.7 | 21.2±5.9 | 8.0±2.0 | 17.6±4.3 |
| | L | 8.8±2.2 | 19.4±4.9 | 7.3±2.1 | 16.2±4.7 |
| 7 | R | 11.7±3.0 | 25.8±6.6 | 10.8±2.9 | 23.7±6.5 |
| | L | 10.8±3.0 | 23.9±6.6 | 9.8±2.9 | 21.7±6.3 |
| 8 | R | 13.9±2.8 | 30.6±6.1 | 12.7±2.9 | 27.9±6.4 |
| | L | 12.9±2.4 | 28.4±5.2 | 11.4±2.5 | 25.1±5.6 |
| 9 | R | 15.2±3.7 | 33.6±8.1 | 17.0±3.3 | 37.6±7.3 |
| | L | 14.0±3.1 | 30.9±6.8 | 13.5±3.2 | 29.7±7.1 |
| 10 | R | 17.4±4.1 | 38.3±9.1 | 16.7±4.4 | 36.8±9.8 |
| | L | 15.8±3.3 | 34.9±7.3 | 15.2±4.6 | 33.5±10.2 |
| 11 | R | 20.9±4.4 | 46.1±9.6 | 20.5±4.4 | 45.3±9.8 |
| | L | 19.3±4.3 | 42.5±9.4 | 18.9±4.3 | 41.7±9.4 |
| 12 | R | 23.5±4.4 | 51.9±9.8 | 22.0±5.0 | 48.6±11.0 |
| | L | 21.2±4.0 | 46.7±8.8 | 19.6±4.3 | 43.2±9.5 |
| 13 | R | 27.1±7.0 | 59.7±15.5 | 23.5±49 | 51.9±10.8 |
| | L | 24.4±6.5 | 53.9±14.4 | 20.8±4.9 | 45.8±10.7 |
| 14 | R | 34.2±8.1 | 75.5±17.8 | 26.4±5.6 | 58.1±12.3 |
| | L | 31.7±8.1 | 69.9±17.8 | 24.2±5.5 | 53.4±12.1 |
| 15 | R | 33.5±9.3 | 73.9±20.5 | 27.2±5.7 | 60.0±12.5 |
| | L | 30.9±8.2 | 68.2±18.0 | 24.9±4.9 | 54.9±10.9 |
| 16 | R | 39.8±8.6 | 87.8±18.9 | 29.8±5.7 | 65.6±12.5 |
| | L | 37.5±8.1 | 82.6±17.9 | 27.2±5.2 | 60.0±11.5 |
| 17 | R | 42.9±8.3 | 94.6±18.4 | 27.8±5.7 | 61.3±12.5 |
| | L | 42.9±8.5 | 89.7±18.8 | 24.6±5.6 | 54.3±12.3 |
| 18 | R | 43.1±8.3 | 95.0±18.4 | 28.2±5.9 | 62.1±12.9 |
| | L | 39.9±7.3 | 87.9±16.2 | 26.4±6.0 | 58.1±13.2 |
| 19 | R | 45.5±8.8 | 100.2±19.4 | 29.3±6.2 | 64.6±13.6 |
| | L | 41.9±9.3 | 92.4±20.4 | 26.5±5.0 | 58.4±11.0 |

*L*, Left; *R*, right.
Data from McQuiddy, V. A., Scheerer, C. R., Lavalley, R., McGrath, T., & Lin, L. (2015). Normative values for grip and pinch strength for 6- to 19-year-olds. *Archives of Physical Medicine and Rehabilitation, 96*(9), 1627–1633.

the specific pinch strengths being assessed as this provides insight into the child's endurance. The three trials are averaged into one score.

It is important that children who are recovering from an injury or surgery have clearance for strength assessment prior to initiating, because during early stages of recovery strengthening may be contraindicated. Young children may be uncertain of the tools and methods for strength assessment, so showing them the tools and how they work first helps ensure they give their best effort. Therapists are advised to assess the unaffected side first to minimize guarding of the affected side during testing.

If the child is developmentally, cognitively, or physically unable to participate in formal strength assessment, then observation of their movement patterns during functional tasks can be useful to determine if impairments may be resulting from weakness. Children may use substitutional patterns, such as propping their proximal UE on a support to maximize strength. If AROM is noted to be greater in a gravity eliminated position compared to against gravity, weakness is likely present.

**Clinical Observation.** Observation of the child while engaged in age-appropriate and meaningful activities provides the occupational therapist with an understanding of how effectively the child uses the impaired UE. This may be particularly helpful to occupational therapists who are working with young children who are not able to report their functional skills and limitations or children who exhibit signs of neglect with the affected UE. The occupational therapist observes how the child spontaneously uses their affected UE during play and functional tasks to determine if skills are age appropriate. For infants and toddlers, it is helpful to assess the child's use of the UE during functional mobility while assessing gross motor skills (e.g., weight-bearing through the UE for positional changes).

Observing how the child positions and initiates use of the affected arm can provide the occupational therapist with insight into the child's true function in the affected arm. Occupational therapists observe the appearance of the child's affected arm, how the child holds the affected arm, and how the child spontaneously uses the affected arm for play or self-care activities. Observations such as the affected hand being less groomed than the unaffected (e.g., nails trimmed on the unaffected and long on the affected) or the child holding the affected arm in a protected position of shoulder adduction and internal rotation with the elbow flexed and hand held at the torso are indications that the child is protective of the affected arm and avoids using it.

For children with congenital differences of the UE and other conditions affecting UE function, such as CP or spinal cord injury, it is helpful to assess the type and efficiency of the grasping patterns used. The occupational therapist documents if the child can use a pinch grasp,

**TABLE 9.31 Tip Pinch Strength (Mean and SD) by Age, Hand, and Gender**

| | | MALES | | FEMALES | |
|---|---|---|---|---|---|
| **Age (y)** | **Hand** | **Kilograms** | **Pounds** | **Kilograms** | **Pounds** |
| 6 | R | 2.7±0.7 | 5.9±1.6 | 5.9±1.6 | 5.4±1.7 |
| | L | 2.6±0.8 | 5.7±1.7 | 5.7±1.7 | 5.3±1.8 |
| 7 | R | 3.0±0.8 | 6.7±1.8 | 6.7±1.8 | 6.3±1.6 |
| | L | 3.0±1.0 | 6.6±2.1 | 6.6±2.1 | 5.6±1.6 |
| 8 | R | 3.3±0.8 | 7.2±1.7 | 7.2±1.7 | 6.5±1.8 |
| | L | 3.1±0.7 | 6.9±1.6 | 6.9±1.6 | 5.7±1.6 |
| 9 | R | 3.6±1.0 | 7.9±2.1 | 7.9±2.1 | 7.7±1.8 |
| | L | 3.4±0.9 | 7.6±2.0 | 7.6±2.0 | 7.3±1.7 |
| 10 | R | 4.2±1.0 | 9.3±2.3 | 9.3±2.3 | 8.3±2.0 |
| | L | 3.9±1.0 | 8.6±2.2 | 8.6±2.2 | 7.8±2.0 |
| 11 | R | 4.0±1.0 | 8.9±2.3 | 8.9±2.3 | 8.4±2.4 |
| | L | 3.9±1.0 | 8.5±2.1 | 8.5±2.1 | 8.1±2.1 |
| 12 | R | 4.1±0.9 | 9.1±1.9 | 9.1±1.9 | 8.9±2.3 |
| | L | 3.8±0.9 | 8.4±2.0 | 8.4±2.0 | 8.2±2.3 |
| 13 | R | 5.0±1.3 | 11.1±2.8 | 11.1±2.8 | 9.6±2.3 |
| | L | 4.9±12 | 10.7±2.6 | 10.7±2.6 | 8.8±2.4 |
| 14 | R | 5.6±1.4 | 12.3±3.1 | 12.3±3.1 | 10.2±2.3 |
| | L | 5.3±1.3 | 11.7±2.9 | 11.7±2.9 | 9.6±2.4 |
| 15 | R | 5.4±1.5 | 11.8±3.3 | 11.8±3.3 | 9.8±2.4 |
| | L | 5.2±1.5 | 11.5±3.3 | 11.5±3.3 | 9.3±2.3 |
| 16 | R | 6.3±1.6 | 13.9±3.6 | 139±3.6 | 10.3±2.5 |
| | L | 5.8±1.4 | 12.7±3.1 | 12.7±3.1 | 9.6±2.2 |
| 17 | R | 6.5±1.8 | 14.4±3.9 | 14.4±3.9 | 10.8±3.1 |
| | L | 6.0±1.7 | 13.3±3.7 | 13.3±3.7 | 9.8±3.0 |
| 18 | R | 6.2±1.6 | 13.7±3.5 | 13.7±3.5 | 10.1±2.2 |
| | L | 5.9±17 | 13.1±3.7 | 13.1±3.7 | 9.4±1.9 |
| 19 | R | 6.5±1.7 | 14.3±3.8 | 14.3±3.8 | 10.6±2.2 |
| | L | 6.1±1.7 | 13.5±3.7 | 13.5±3.7 | 9.5±2.1 |

*L*, Left; *R*, right.
Data from McQuiddy, V. A., Scheerer, C. R., Lavalley, R., McGrath, T., & Lin, L. (2015). Normative values for grip and pinch strength for 6- to 19-year-olds. *Archives of Physical Medicine and Rehabilitation, 96*(9), 1627–1633.

spherical grasp, mass grasp, or any adaptive grasping patterns, such as a scissors grasp (i.e., grasping using finger adduction; Fig. 9.15). The occupational therapist assesses the child's lateral and/or palmar pinch to determine the child's capacity for tasks requiring a pinch grasp. When children have significantly limited thumb function, they may use an adaptive scissors grasp. The occupational therapist identifies which fingers the child uses for a scissors grasp and notes the efficiency of the grasp pattern. For instance, a child born with no thumb may use a scissors grasp of the index and middle finger. This preference to use the radial side of the hand for activities requiring fine motor dexterity suggests that the child is a good candidate for a pollicization (i.e., transplantation of the digit to the location of the thumb) of the index finger. On the contrary, children who use a scissors grasp of the ring finger and small finger stand to gain less function from an index finger pollicization given their preference for ulnar grasping patterns. The occupational therapist specifically evaluates whether the child can demonstrate a mass digital grasp and spherical grasp. A child with limited thumb function may have limited or no spherical grasping pattern present and have difficulty with activities that require active thumb palmar abduction, such as holding a ball in the hand. The occupational therapist determines the child's overall capacity for functional grasp with the affected hand and which factors may be limiting functional performance.

For children with a history of typical UE function who acquired an injury or condition affecting the arm or hand, the occupational therapist interviews the child and family to determine the child's prior level of UE function. As the child engages in play or self-care tasks, the occupational therapist can observe how the child uses the affected UE. Children can be highly adaptable in devising ways to work around their limitations. For example, the child may have switched to using the nondominant hand for writing, self-care, and play skills and may report minimal functional limitation yet have not returned to the baseline level of function. This provides the occupational therapist knowledge of the child's current level of function with the affected arm or hand compared with his or her baseline performance to guide long-term goals.

### Additional Assessment of Fine Motor Skills Related to Developmental Difficulties

For children who are being seen in occupational therapy outside of the realm of pediatric hand therapy, the occupational therapist may complete a different selection of fine motor assessments than those indicated above. For example, consideration of pain, edema, and ROM may not be necessary, whereas examination of in-hand manipulation skills, scissors skills, and ability to hold and use crayons and glue would be more likely. For slightly older children the focus of the

TABLE 9.32 **Lateral Pinch Strength (Mean and SD) by Age, Hand and Gender**

| | | MALES | | FEMALES | |
|---|---|---|---|---|---|
| Age (y) | Hand | Kilograms | Pounds | Kilograms | Pounds |
| 6 | R | 4.3±0.9 | 9.4±1.9 | 3.9±0.9 | 8.6±1.9 |
| | L | 4.3±0.8 | 9.5±1.7 | 3.9±0.9 | 8.5±2.0 |
| 7 | R | 4.9±1.0 | 10.9±2.2 | 4.5±0.9 | 10.0±2.0 |
| | L | 4.6±0.9 | 10.2±2.0 | 4.2±0.9 | 9.3±1.9 |
| 8 | R | 5.4±1.0 | 12.0±2.3 | 4.9±1.1 | 10.9±2.4 |
| | L | 5.2±0.9 | 11.5±2.0 | 4.6±1.0 | 10.2±2.1 |
| 9 | R | 5.4±1.3 | 12.0±2.8 | 5.3±0.9 | 11.7±2.0 |
| | L | 5.1±1.2 | 11.2±2.7 | 5.0±1.0 | 11.0±2.1 |
| 10 | R | 6.1±1.0 | 13.4±2.2 | 5.6±1.1 | 12.4±2.4 |
| | L | 5.6±1.0 | 12.4±2.2 | 5.3±1.0 | 11.6±2.3 |
| 11 | R | 6.6±1.0 | 14.6±2.1 | 6.4±1.0 | 14.2±2.3 |
| | L | 6.4±1.0 | 14.2±2.3 | 6.1±1.1 | 13.4±2.5 |
| 12 | R | 6.8±1.0 | 15.1±2.2 | 6.4±1.1 | 14.0±2.4 |
| | L | 6.7±1.0 | 14.7±2.1 | 5.9±1.0 | 13.0±2.2 |
| 13 | R | 7.9±1.5 | 17.4±3.3 | 6.8±1.2 | 14.9±2.6 |
| | L | 7.5±1.5 | 16.5±3.3 | 6.3±1.2 | 13.8±2.6 |
| 14 | R | 9.0±1.8 | 19.8±3.9 | 7.7±1.4 | 16.9±3.0 |
| | L | 8.6±1.8 | 18.9±3.0 | 7.1±1.1 | 15.6±2.5 |
| 15 | R | 8.8±2.0 | 19.4±4.3 | 8.0±1.2 | 17.7±2.7 |
| | L | 8.3±1.8 | 18.3±3.9 | 7.4±1.2 | 16.4±2.7 |
| 16 | R | 9.8±1.9 | 21.5±4.2 | 7.8±1.2 | 17.1±2.6 |
| | L | 9.3±1.7 | 20.5±3.8 | 7.3±1.0 | 16.2±2.2 |
| 17 | R | 10.3±1.8 | 22.8±3.9 | 7.7±1.6 | 16.9±3.5 |
| | L | 9.8±1.9 | 21.6±4.1 | 7.0±1.5 | 15.5±3.3 |
| 18 | R | 10.3±1.7 | 22.6±3.7 | 7.5±1.4 | 16.6±3.1 |
| | L | 9.8±1.6 | 21.5±3.5 | 6.9±1.2 | 15.2±2.7 |
| 19 | R | 10.3±1.8 | 22.6±4.0 | 7.7±1.1 | 17.0±2.5 |
| | L | 9.9±1.7 | 21.9±3.8 | 7.1±0/9 | 15.6±1.9 |

*L*, Left; *R*, right.
Data from McQuiddy, V. A., Scheerer, C. R., Lavalley, R., McGrath, T., & Lin, L. (2015). Normative values for grip and pinch strength for 6- to 19-year-olds. *Archives of Physical Medicine and Rehabilitation, 96*(9), 1627–1633.

assessment might be on handwriting and keyboarding abilities, ability to use a locker, and dressing and makeup skills. For more information on how to assess these areas, see the section on General Assessment of Developmental Status.

## ASSESSMENT OF VISION AND VISUAL PERCEPTUAL MOTOR SKILLS

Occupational therapists understand the importance of vision and visual perceptual skills to occupational performance. They work closely with vision specialists (e.g., opticians, optometrists, and ophthalmologists) to understand underlying causes of visual challenges.

### Importance of Vision and Visual Perceptual Motor Skills for Children and Youth

**Visual perception** is the total process responsible for the reception and cognition of visual stimuli. Vision is important for learning; it is more than just seeing. Children process visual information they take in from the environment and make sense of it by analyzing, interpreting, and associating the information with past experiences (Scheiman, 2011). These visual cognitive skills are used for extracting and organizing the visual information and integrating it with other sensory modalities and higher cognitive functions. Vision is also important for the development of hand skill, and particularly in developing new motor skills (Cermak, 2006). Vision enables children and youth to explore their environment. Children and youth use vision to explore their surroundings and learn.

### Common Challenges Associated With Vision and Visual Perceptual Motor Skills

Vision affects children and youth's ability to make sense of their environment. Children who have visual information processing challenges may experience difficulty with reading, observing cues, manipulating objects, and calculating distances, which may result in difficulty navigating within their environment. They may experience challenges in school leading to frustration or poor performance. They may have difficulty with dressing and understanding concepts (such as mental manipulation for puzzles, letters, and organization).

### Specific Areas of Assessment Regarding Vision and Visual Perceptual Motor Skills

Occupational therapists evaluate visual information processing skills, which include visual spatial, visual analysis, and visual motor integration. *Visual spatial skills* are the ability to make judgments about the location of objects in space in relation to one's own body. Areas that should be assessed include position in space, spatial relations, depth perception, and topographic orientation. *Visual analysis* skills determine the distinct features of visual forms, including size, shape, color, and orientation. *Visual analysis skill* components include visual discrimination, form constancy, visual figure-ground, visual closure,

**TABLE 9.33 Palmar Pinch Strength (Mean and SD) by Age, Hand, and Gender**

| | | MALES | | FEMALES | |
|---|---|---|---|---|---|
| **Age (y)** | **Hand** | **Kilograms** | **Pounds** | **Kilograms** | **Pounds** |
| 6 | R | 3.5±0.9 | 7.8±1.8 | 3.2±0.8 | 7.0±1.8 |
| | L | 3.4±0.7 | 7.6±1.6 | 2.9±0.8 | 6.5±1.7 |
| 7 | R | 3.7±0.8 | 8.2±1.7 | 3.5±0.8 | 7.7±1.8 |
| | L | 3.5±0.8 | 7.7±1.7 | 3.2±0.7 | 7.1±1.6 |
| 8 | R | 4.2±0.8 | 9.3±1.7 | 3.9±0.9 | 8.7±1.9 |
| | L | 4.1±0.6 | 9.1±1.4 | 3.6±0.9 | 8.0±1.9 |
| 9 | R | 4.5±1.1 | 10.0±2.5 | 4.7±1.0 | 10.3±2.1 |
| | L | 4.3±1.0 | 9.5±2.3 | 4.3±1.0 | 9.5±2.2 |
| 10 | R | 5.2±1.0 | 11.5±2.2 | 4.9±1.0 | 10.8±2.2 |
| | L | 4.8±0.9 | 10.5±1.9 | 4.5±1.0 | 9.9±2.2 |
| 11 | R | 5.4±1.0 | 12.0±2.2 | 5.5±1.1 | 12.2±2.4 |
| | L | 5.2±0.8 | 11.5±1.8 | 5.1±0.9 | 11.2±1.9 |
| 12 | R | 6.0±1.2 | 13.2±2.7 | 5.6±1.2 | 12.4±2.6 |
| | L | 5.8±1.1 | 12.7±2.5 | 5.2±1.0 | 11.5±2.3 |
| 13 | R | 6.8±1.4 | 14.9±3.0 | 5.9±1.2 | 13.1±2.6 |
| | L | 6.5±1.4 | 14.4±3.1 | 5.5±1.2 | 12.1±2.6 |
| 14 | R | 7.3±1.5 | 16.2±3.2 | 6.5±1.2 | 14.3±2.6 |
| | L | 6.9±1.7 | 15.3±3.8 | 5.9±1.1 | 13.0±2.4 |
| 15 | R | 7.7±2.0 | 16.9±4.3 | 6.6±1.0 | 14.5±2.2 |
| | L | 7.1±1.7 | 15.7±3.8 | 6.3±1.1 | 13.9±2.4 |
| 16 | R | 8.1±1.7 | 17.9±3.7 | 6.8±0.9 | 14.9±2.0 |
| | L | 7.7±1.5 | 16.9±3.2 | 6.1±0.8 | 13.5±1.8 |
| 17 | R | 8.8±1.9 | 19.3±4.1 | 6.6±1.2 | 14.6±2.7 |
| | L | 8.1±1.7 | 17.9±3.7 | 6.0±1.2 | 13.3±2.7 |
| 18 | R | 8.7±1.4 | 19.2±3.1 | 6.5±1.4 | 14.3±3.1 |
| | L | 8.1±1.5 | 17.9±3.3 | 6.0±1.2 | 13.3±2.7 |
| 19 | R | 9.1±1.8 | 20.1±3.9 | 6.6±1.1 | 14.5±2.4 |
| | L | 8.5±1.9 | 18.7±4.2 | 6.1±1.0 | 13.5±2.3 |

*L*, Left; *R*, right.

Data from McQuiddy, V. A., Scheerer, C. R., Lavalley, R., McGrath, T., & Lin, L. (2015). Normative values for grip and pinch strength for 6- to 19-year-olds. *Archives of Physical Medicine and Rehabilitation, 96*(9), 1627–1633.

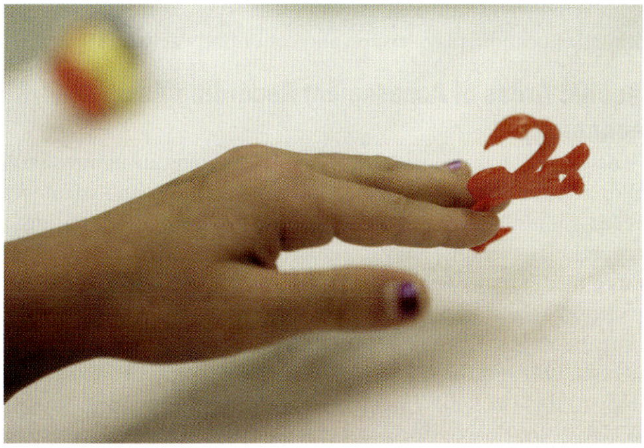

**Fig. 9.15** Example of a child using a scissors grasp of index finger and middle finger for fine motor prehension.

visual memory, and visualization. *Visual perception* is typically assessed in school through observations of reading, puzzle completion, and with assessment tools that require matching and discriminating shapes and objects. Throwing and catching a ball, cutting out a shape with scissors, and placing puzzle pieces and shapes in the correct spot are all examples of visual motor skills. Components of visual motor skills include vision, ocular motor abilities, sensory perception, movement, language, and motivation with attention and knowledge overarching perception. Handwriting is also a visual motor integration skill developed and used by school-age children.

**Vision Screening.** There are many instruments and vision screening methods that have been suggested for the pediatric population. In most school systems in the United States, visual screening is performed at least once during the child's elementary school years and sometimes on an annual basis. Also, many pediatricians periodically perform a vision screening. The problem with both the school and pediatrician-based vision screenings, however, is that the only aspect of visual function that is typically screened is visual acuity. However, visual acuity problems are not useful when screening for vision disorders that are related to occupation in children. Thus, occupational therapists screen for problems in visual efficiency and visual information processing, the two areas that the school nurses or pediatricians do not include in their screenings. Table 9.34 summarizes recommended vision screening tests for visual efficiency problems.

**Screening for Binocular Vision.** The most common binocular vision problem in the pediatric population is convergence insufficiency (Rouse et al., 1999). One of the key tests used to diagnose convergence insufficiency is the near point of convergence. In this test, the examiner moves an object toward the client's eyes and asks the client to try and maintain single vision for as long as possible. When the client reports double vision, examiners record the distance from the eyes and refer to this measurement as the near point of convergence break. The

**TABLE 9.34 Recommended Vision Screening Tests**

| Component to Be Screened | Element to Be Screened | Name of Test |
|---|---|---|
| Visual efficiency | Accommodation | • Convergence Insufficiency Symptom Survey (CISS)<br>• Accommodative amplitude (near point rod) |
| | Binocular vision | • Convergence Insufficiency Symptom Survey;<br>• Near point of convergence (near point rod) |
| | Eye movements | • Convergence Insufficiency Symptom Survey<br>• Northeastern State University College of Optometry (NSUCO) Eye Movement Test;<br>• Developmental eye movement test |
| Visual information processing | Visual spatial | • Garner reversal frequent test |
| | Visual analysis | • Test of Visual Perceptual Skills, 4th Edition (TVPS 4)<br>• Motor Free Visual Perception Test (MFVPT) |
| | Visual motor | • Developmental Test of Visual Motor Integration (DTVMI) |

practitioner then slowly moves the target away from the client until he/she reports single vision again. When the child reports single vision, the examiner records the distance from the child's eyes and records this as the *near point of convergence* recovery finding. The expected finding for any child is to be able to maintain single vision to a distance less than 6 cm from the eyes. So, the break should be less than 6 cm and the recovery less than 9 cm. Therapists should also assess pursuits and saccades. (See instructor resources in Evolve learning materials.)

**Visual Spatial Skills.** The Gardner Reversal Frequency Test: Recognition Subtest evaluates the existence, nature, and frequency of occurrence of receptive letter and number reversals (reversals that the child can recognize). In this test, the child is asked to mark off those letters and numbers that are written backward or reversed. This test gives information about the child's development of normal internal and external spatial concepts.

This test is appropriate for children 5–15 years old. When administering this test, it is important to seat the child so that they cannot observe books and other written material that may provide information about letter and number orientation. This is an untimed test, and children who have difficulty in this area may become frustrated by this task and take excessively long periods of time to complete the test. Because this test is used as a screening, occupational therapists may discontinue the test if it becomes clear after a short period of time that the child is struggling.

**Visual Analysis Skills.** The Test of Visual Perceptual Skills, 4th Edition (TVPS–4) can be used to evaluate visual analysis skills. The TVPS provides a separate score for each of the seven areas assessed. This allows a clinician to make decisions about treatment of each of these areas.

The TVPS–4 is designed to assess seven aspects of visual analysis skills including visual discrimination, visual spatial relationships, visual form constancy, visual figure-ground, visual closure, visual memory, and visual sequential memory. There are 18 items in each of seven perceptual areas. Norms are based on a nationally representative sample. In this edition of the test, more lower-level items were added to address the needs of younger or more impaired individuals, and norms now extend through 21 years of age, making the TVPS–4 useful for a wider range of pediatric clients. The TVPS–4 utilizes black-and-white line drawings, and children can respond verbally or by pointing to responses.

**Visual Motor Integration Skills.** Visual motor skills such as throwing and catching a ball or handwriting can be observed during classroom tasks, physical education, and recess. Assessments that require copying a picture, drawing a person, or writing in print or cursive are examples of tasks requiring visual motor skills (see Appendix A).

The Developmental Test of Visual Motor Integration (DTVMI) has well-developed normative data for ages 2 through 18 and can be used through adulthood as well. This test evaluates the child's ability to integrate visual information processing and fine motor skills by assessing his or her ability to accurately copy a visual stimulus. The child is presented with pictures of increasing complexity and is asked to reproduce the pictures as accurately as possible.

## ASSISTIVE TECHNOLOGY ASSESSMENT

Children and youth may benefit from assistive technology to enable them to participate in meaningful occupations. The assistive technology (AT) assessment is conducted (1) as part of an ongoing process linked to educational and/or therapeutic planning, (2) ideally by a team within the natural setting where the child engages in their occupations, (3) with trials using potential AT devices, and (4) with meaningful follow-through involving all team members (WATI Development Team, 2017). The goal of assessment is to understand the child and family's needs for AT that enables the child to participate in meaningful activities within their environment (such as feeding, dressing, bathing, education, play, leisure, and community activities).

### Specific Areas of Assessment Regarding Assistive Technology

AT assessments are considered fluid and ongoing in nature, and as children's needs change, a reassessment of the tools and adaptations needed should occur. Depending on the service delivery setting, an occupational therapist may conduct AT assessment independently or as a member of a team. A team approach to AT is considered best practice. The goal of AT is to enable children to participate in desired occupations. Occupational therapists assess a child's preferences, interests, and motivations along with social, spiritual, cultural, and family factors (including finances) that influence technology selection (AOTA, 2016; Kula, 2016; Watson et al., 2010). The child's participation in given activities, including how often and for how long the child engages in them, should be noted, along with any current AT in use and its effectiveness. Box 9.22 provides some guiding questions that may assist in evaluating a child's AT needs.

Occupational therapists consider many factors that contribute to selection of AT for children and youth. Box 9.23 provides a list of criteria to consider the user's perspective when evaluating AT. For example, the therapist considers whether the AT device significantly increases the child's level of participation, if the AT device will "grow" with the child, and whether a less complex device will meet the same

**BOX 9.22 Guiding Questions to Evaluate a Child for Assistive Technology (AT)**

**Motor**

- How does the child move? Sit? Rest?
- What movements are voluntary? Involuntary?
- Which body parts are capable of reliable, accurate, and controlled movement?
- Can the child be positioned adequately in and maintain an upright sitting posture?
- Is the child able to easily access the AT device?
- Does the child have sufficient ROM, finger dexterity, strength, and endurance?
- What is the child's overall endurance and strength?
- What is the child's level of independence in daily living skills?

**Sensory and Perceptual**

- Can the child hold objects in both hands? One hand?
- Can the child feel different shapes? Objects?
- Does the child pick out objects (toys) upon request? Can he identify objects by feel?
- Can the child attend to visual feedback on the monitor?
- Can the child respond to auditory directions? Feedback?
- What are the child's strengths and limitations in visual perception and visual motor skills?
- Does child follow objects with his eyes (visually scan)?
- Is the child easily distracted by visual stimuli?

**Cognitive and Communication**

- Does the child know "cause and effect"?
- Is the child able to scan for items?
- What is the child's cognitive level?
- What is the child's attention span?
- What are the child's receptive and expressive language skills and potential?
- What are the child's face-to-face and written communication needs?
- Can the child sequence multiple-step directions? One-step?

**Psychosocial**

- What does the child like to do? Which activities does the child enjoy?
- How does the child indicate wants and needs?
- Does the child want to use AT? Is he/she motivated and showing signs of pleasure when it is introduced?
- Does the AT device or system allow the child to do something he/she was not able to do?
- What is the child's and family's view of the AT device? Have they had adequate input into the process?
- Do persons interacting with the child and device feel positive about it? Are they able to understand how it is used?
- Is the child adequately challenged (motorically and cognitively) to succeed?
- Is the child successful? Do they show joy in their success?

**Context**

- Where will the child use the AT device?
- How can the AT device or interface be positioned for optimal use?
- Do classroom or home environments allow for safe and easy access to educational materials and use of the AT devices?
- Is the device portable? Can it be used in multiple environments?
- Has the child's and family's input been considered given multiple contexts?
- Where will the device be used (home, school, or community), and who will be assisting the child (if necessary)?
- What supports are available in the different contexts in which the child will be engaging with the AT? What barriers may limit success?
- Does the child have any previous experience with AT?
- Are the individuals who work with the child (family and professionals) willing and positive regarding the use of AT?
- What are the child's short- and long-term goals, and how does the AT device support these goals?

needs. It is also possible that a continuum of tools may be required depending on the circumstances or environment in which the device is being used. For example, a child who uses a dynamic screen voice output device may require an alternative means of communication (such as a laminated communication board) while in the bathtub. Decisions need to be made about whether the system is a reasonable and appropriate investment that will result in increasing independence, and the child, family, or institution should be provided objective and realistic information regarding investment in and use of AT. A trial period with different types of devices to determine the best AT solution is ideal. Trial periods help prevent the costly procurement of an incorrect device.

## ASSESSMENT OF MOBILITY

Occupational therapists address the mobility needs of children by assessing the child's strengths and challenges, occupational needs, and environment. Assessing mobility requires careful consideration of the child's current level of mobility with consideration for changes that may occur in the child's future. This requires the therapist to collaborate closely with the child and family, consider child and family preferences, and advocate for mobility that best meets the child's and family's needs.

### Common Challenges Associated With Mobility

The occupational therapist carefully considers all environments (e.g., home, school, community) where the child will be using a mobility device. Some home environments are fixed, meaning the family is unable to alter the condition (such as a rental). Families may not have the financial means to change the environment. The home may be on the third floor of a building with no elevator. As a result, consideration for multiple devices may be necessary. The ideal device for use at school and in the community may include a lighter, portable, or manual wheelchair with power assist or power add on options. The role of the occupational therapists(s) also includes advocating for and helping the client and the family to acquire all the recommended devices. The therapist provides necessary documentation and letters of medical necessity, helping identify alternate funding and equipment acquisition options when more than one device is needed beyond what insurance covers. Occupational therapists also advocate for environmental changes as disability rights laws afford. In other situations, the family may have plans to modify the environment, and the occupational therapist assists them in determining what is possible and needed to maximize use of the best equipment and to meet the child's needs at home, school, and in the community. See online resources for videos and learning resources.

The occupational therapist considers changes that the child may experience in the future, both expected and unexpected, when recommending equipment. For example, the therapist determines whether the system can be modified as the child gains new skills, grows, or changes physically. For example, a child with a progressive disability may be able to operate a joystick at the time the chair is ordered, but they may require other electronic options as their functional status changes and use of a joystick is no longer feasible. It may be economical to order options on equipment at initial purchase (rather than retrofit equipment later).

**BOX 9.23 Criteria for Evaluating Assistive Technology (AT) Devices Considering the User's Perspective**

1. *Effectiveness.* How much the device improves the user's living situation and enhances functional capability and independence
2. *Affordability.* The extent to which a person can purchase, maintain, and repair a device without financial hardship
3. *Reliability.* The degree to which a device is dependable, consistent, and predictable in its performance and levels of accuracy for a reasonable amount of time
4. *Portability.* The influence of the device's size and weight on the user's ability to move, carry, relocate, and operate it in varied locations
5. *Durability.* The extent to which a device delivers continued operation for an extended time
6. *Securability.* How well a consumer believes that a device affords physical control and is secure from theft or vandalism
7. *Safety.* How well a device protects the user, care provider, or family member from potential harm, bodily injury, or infection
8. *Learnability.* The ease of assembly, initial learning requirements, and time and effort to master use
9. *Comfort and acceptance.* The extent to which a user feels physically comfortable with the device and does not experience pain or discomfort with use; how aesthetically appealing the user finds the device and the user's psychological comfort when using it in private or public
10. *Maintenance and repairability.* The degree to which the device is easy to maintain and repair (by the consumer, a local repair shop, or a supplier)
11. *Operability.* The extent to which the device is easy to use, is adaptable and flexible, and affords easy access to controls and displays

From O'Rourke, P., Ekins, R., Timmins, B., Timmins, F., Long, S., & Coyle, E. (2013). Crucial design issues for special access technology: A Delphi study. *Disability and Rehabilitation: Assistive Technology.* http://informahealthcare.com/journal/idt

## Specific Areas Regarding Assessment of Mobility

The occupational therapist completes a thorough occupational profile using a top-down approach to understand the child's circumstances, needs, and preferences. They use knowledge of the child's occupational choices (i.e., those activities they want to do), physical, cognitive, and social strengths and challenges, and unique situations when examining mobility for occupational performance. The assessment considers much more than the child's physical strengths and challenges. After creating the occupational profile and completing the mat assessment and determining the child's strengths and challenges, the occupational therapist examines other needs that influence mobility, including additional environmental considerations (e.g., child's home, transportation availability, school, and community) and their occupational choices for where they are currently. For example, they consider the mobility needs of a toddler wanting to play at home versus a teen who wants to compete in adaptive sports and be independent in the community. Understanding a child's muscle tone, ROM, strength, and flexibility enables the clinician to determine the best secondary supports within the wheelchair to support growth and prevent secondary complications. Examples of secondary supports in a mobility device include lateral trunk supports, lateral hip supports, medial thigh supports, and anterior pelvic supports. (See Videos on Evaluation.)

Evaluating the child outside of their mobility device is critical to the evaluation and should be standard practice in all seating evaluations. The therapist considers the biomechanical forces of an individual's movements to determine what may be contributing to undesirable postures and limited function. Children using augmented means for mobility may develop scoliosis due to abnormal muscle use, pelvic positioning, poor trunk strength, and muscle tone. The findings from the mat assessment guide the clinician to determine optimal secondary supports to improve alignment for function, respiration, or digestion (Persson-Bunke et al., 2012). When documenting the secondary support, it is best practice to identify the location (medial, lateral, anterior, and posterior) and the anatomic structure supported. For example, posterior lateral trunk support would be a backrest that provides support along the client's back and sides for posture.

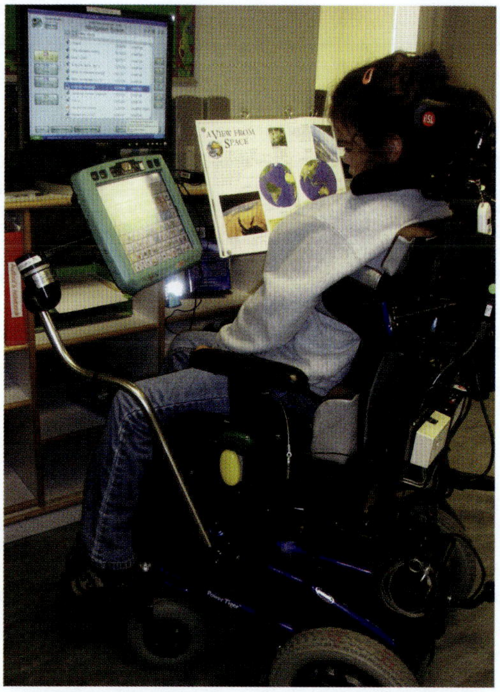

**Fig. 9.16** Girl in a power wheelchair with a head array, lateral supports, and a mounted alternative augmentative communication (AAC) device is seated in front of a computer.

Children with disabilities may also experience hip dislocation. The only successful positioning programs that have prevented dislocation are 24-hour positioning programs where the child's hips are always abducted (Pountney et al., 2009). The use of an abductor pommel will not, by itself, prevent hip dislocation. This is why the seating and mobility evaluation should be inclusive of all places the child spends time (bed, floor, commode/toilet, shower chair, etc.).

During the evaluation process, the occupational therapist works with a durable medical equipment provider to trial, or even lend, a power mobility device. Unfortunately, these devices may not be specifically designed for the child, requiring practitioners to make adjustments that must be considered in the recommendations. Equipment used during an evaluation should be in optimal working condition. The occupational therapist begins the intervention by test-driving the equipment to learn the forces and movements required to drive it, select the best speed for the client, and set any other adjustments, such as sensitivity of the controls, before the child comes in for the evaluation.

Depending on the child's medical needs, adaptations can be made for customized seating and for the addition of medical equipment like ventilators. Children that have mobility deficits may also have communication deficits. In this case, the team considers the alternative augmentative communication (AAC) device and how the child will use it (Fig. 9.16). Box 9.24 provides questions that may guide decisions regarding AAC and mobility devices.

## BOX 9.24 Questions to Guide Mobility Device Selection

**Questions for Mobility Device**

- Are the goals to provide functional and independent home, school, and community mobility, or are the goals to provide transitional mobility experiences so that the child can have new opportunities to learn how to move, explore, and interact within the environment?
- Which maneuverability features of the powered device are important in considering the various environments in which the device will be used (such as indoors in limited spaces in a classroom or home, outdoors over rough terrain, or on a playground)?
- What are the table heights the wheelchair must fit under at school, the home, and community?
- Is it necessary for the child to reach various heights in the wheelchair? Should a powered lift seat be considered?
- Will the child need the ability to tilt-in-space or recline?
- How will the child transfer into and out of the wheelchair?
- How will the mobility device be transported? Will it need to be disassembled to fit inside the trunk of a vehicle?
- If the wheelchair is to be transported in a van, is head clearance sufficient for the child when entering the vehicle, and can the wheelchair be secured to the van for transport?
- Will the environments need to be made accessible with ramps into doorways or powered lifts into vehicles?
- Will the child need an environmental control option included in the power wheelchair electronics for using the joystick or alternative access method to wirelessly access an alternative electronic device such as a speech-generating device or computer?

**Questions Regarding AAC and Mobility**

- Will the AAC be accessed through their drive control of the wheelchair?
- Will the user also be accessing a computer for school, work, or home, and if so, what type of accommodations do they need?
- How will they control the mouse functions or access the keyboard?
- Will they be integrating environmental and mobile device controls?
- When someone is accessing something besides driving through their wheelchair control, how will they get from driving to talking on their AAC device or using other devices or modes?
- Will the child be able to access the AAC and drive?
- Where and how will the AAC be positioned on the wheelchair?
- Will the additional equipment interfere with mobility?
- Does the AAC allow the child to communicate while driving the chair?

Successful use of mobility devices depends on the fit of the child to the device, which requires analysis of the features of the device, physical and social environments, client factors, and performance skills (Figs. 9.17 and 9.18). Readiness for powered mobility requires spatial relations and problem-solving (Furumasu et al., 2004; Tefft et al., 1999; Verburg, 1987), which must also be assessed.

The team determines the most accurate and efficient means for the child to access the device. The occupational therapist evaluates the position of the child and the access method. A careful analysis of the child's underlying factors (i.e., client factors) and performance skills is considered in determining how to structure the intervention. The therapist also considers contexts (environment, temporal, personal, and cultural), child and family goals, and the equipment.

The occupational therapist may also need to determine where and how a speech-generating device can be mounted to the child's wheelchair. Selection of a mounting bracket depends on the tube size of the wheelchair frame and where the mount can be attached.

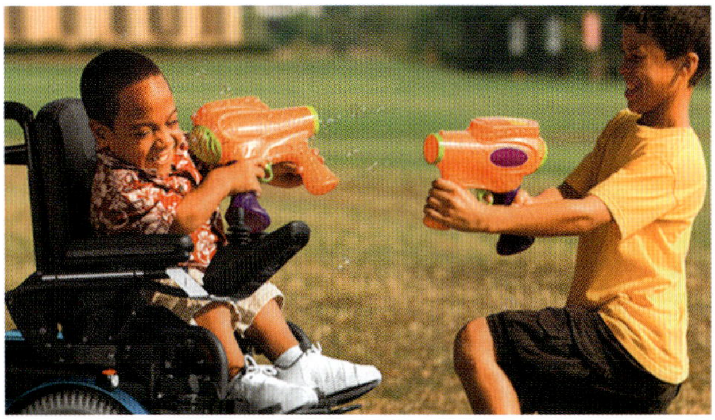

**Fig. 9.17** Young boy in a power wheelchair has a super-soaker water gun battle with a friend who on one knee kneels across from him. Power mobility enables motivated play in natural environments. (Courtesy of Permobil.)

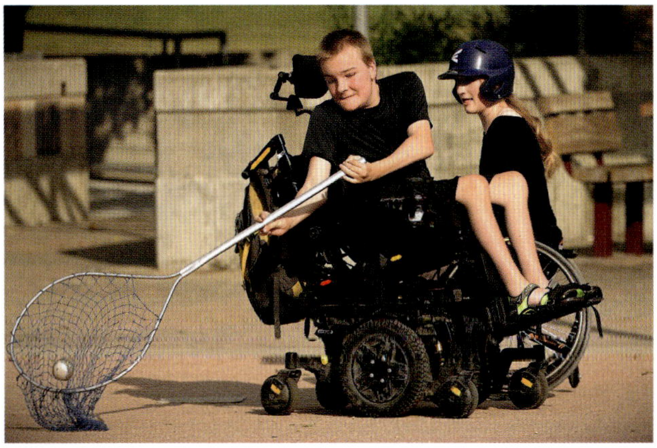

**Fig. 9.18** Teenage boy in mid-wheel drive power wheelchair playing softball, catches ball in fishing net with female player attempting to advance to base behind him in manual wheelchair wearing batter's helmet. (Photo credit with permission: Nick Nelson/Grand Forks Herald.)

Therapists carefully determine where to mount the speech-generating device to make certain the wheelchair is stable, and the child is able to move through doorways. Positioning the rear wheels too far forward may cause the wheelchair to tip when the communication device is mounted.

**Assessing to Select a Control Device.** Before selecting a switch to be used to control the mobility device, the occupational therapist first identifies the seating required to support access and then the most reliable movements the child can voluntarily use to access a switch, utilizing the least amount of active range and therefore energy expenditure. Children may have experience using a switch to operate a modified battery-operated toy or single-switch computer game, which requires one activation of the switch with a quick release. The child may be able to use the same movements for switch access to drive a power wheelchair, but most children will use an access method that requires them to maintain contact and activation on the switch during the time they are driving the power wheelchair and move off the switch in time for stopping (Fig. 9.19).

### Specific Assessment Tools and Measures

***Mat Assessment.*** The most effective way to assess the child's musculoskeletal status is through a mat assessment (Fig. 9.20). See Box 9.25.

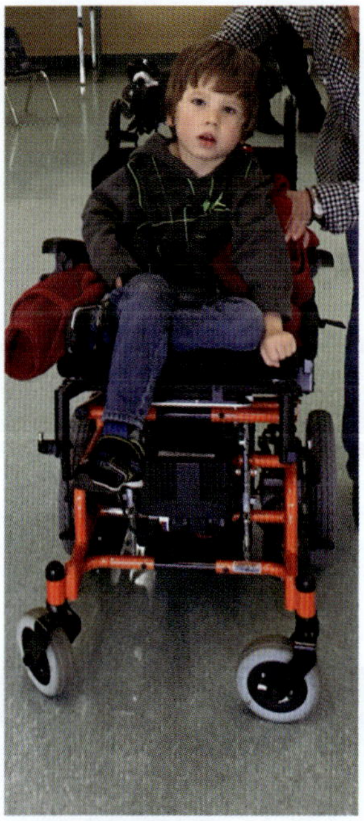

**Fig. 9.19** Starting with a single switch for access. (Courtesy of Adaptive Switch Laboratories [ASL].)

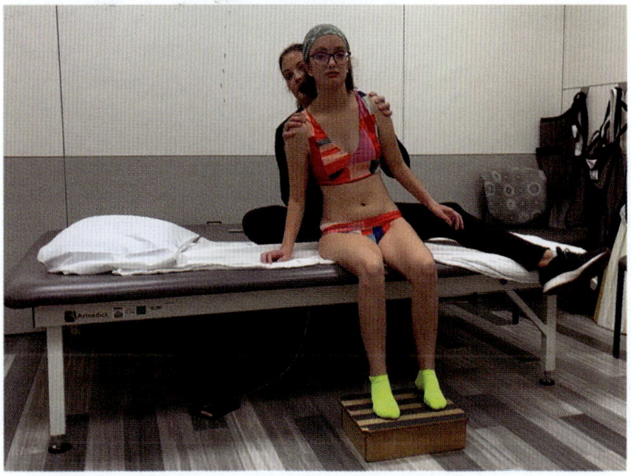

**Fig. 9.20** A mat assessment is critical to the seating assessment. Assess the person supine and sitting to identify any postural asymmetries and the influence of gravity.

***Home Visit.*** The assessment may include a visit to the home and a trial period where the child is able to use the equipment. Many insurance providers require documentation and evidence that the equipment fits in the home. Part of the assessment requires taking accurate anthropometric measurements of the client for fit of the mobility device, as shown in Video 32.2.

## GENERAL ASSESSMENT OF DEVELOPMENTAL STATUS

After completing an occupational profile, therapists often seek to identify those occupations, skills, and tasks that the child or youth can do. Understanding the developmental range for which the child accomplishes skills may guide the intervention process. Children achieve skills at different rates, but establishing the child's baseline for development within a range of skills (e.g., gross motor, fine motor, self-help, language, cognition, social participation, play) often informs occupational therapy intervention. Please see Chapter 8 for information on typical developmental skills at different ages.

**BOX 9.25 Mat Assessment**

1. Active and passive range of motion in hips, knees, ankles, and upper extremities and their effects on sitting posture (i.e., tight hamstrings)
2. Pelvic positioning including pelvic tilt, pelvic rotation, and pelvic obliquity in both supine and sitting and whether they are flexible into correction or require accommodation in the seating system
3. Spinal positioning including specifics of any scoliosis, kyphosis, or lordosis in both supine and sitting and whether they are flexible into correction or require accommodation
4. Sitting posture including trunk and head control
5. Spasticity and its effect on positioning
6. Skin integrity including any current or previous pressure injuries and any decreased sensation
7. Anthropometric measurements as taken by the equipment supplier (see attached form on Evolve site)

### Common Challenges Associated With Developmental Delays

When evaluating children with developmental delays, therapists should be aware of certain challenges that may be noted across multiple diagnoses. For example, children with developmental delays will often have atypical muscle tone, and some will have retained infant reflexes (see Chapter 8 for more information on infant reflexes). Some may demonstrate early indicators of sensory sensitivities or oral motor and feeding challenges.

Children with developmental delays may be delayed primarily in one or two areas of function or across all areas. Children may demonstrate peaks and valleys in performance or may have mastered specific "splinter skills" that are developmentally much higher than the rest of their skills. Therapists should note and be aware of the patterns of the child's strengths and difficulties.

### Specific Areas of Assessment Regarding Development

Therapists use a variety of developmental assessments (see Appendix A) as well as observations to investigate a child's current developmental level. Many of the developmental assessments include items related to multiple areas of development such as self-help, cognition, and fine and gross motor skill. Often these tools provide helpful scores to compare a child to other children, but therapists also observe the child's function to consider qualitative aspects of the child's performance that are not measured by test items. For example, an item that requires stacking 1-in wooden blocks may only score the number of blocks stacked, but it will not consider the way the child grasped the block, the accuracy of the child's release, or the ability to grade the force needed to do the task.

Therapists assess different skills depending on the age of the child. For this form of evaluation, it is critical that the therapist is familiar with the typical progression of developmental skills. Common areas of assessment for infants include feeding and oral motor skills, play skills and interaction with caregivers, ability to use the hands and fingers, and gross motor skills for lifting the body against gravity. Infants are also typically tested for their reflexes. Therapists adjust for prematurity typically up until age 2 when assessing a child who was born premature. There are a variety of adjusted age calculators available

## BOX 9.26 Calculating the Chronologic Age and Corrected Age

Many standardized tests require that the examiner calculate the child's exact age on the date of testing. The method for calculating both the chronologic and the corrected age is presented in the following.

### Calculating the Chronologic Age

First, the date of testing and the child's birth date are recorded in the following order:

| | Year | Month | Day |
|---|---|---|---|
| Date of testing | 99 | 6 | 15 |
| Birth date | 95 | 3 | 10 |
| Chronologic age | 4 | 3 | 5 |

Beginning on the right (the Day category), the day, month, and year of the child's birth date are subtracted from the date of testing. In the above example, the child's chronologic age is 4 years, 3 months, and 5 days at the time of testing.

The convention in calculating age is that if the number of days in the chronologic age is 15 or less, the month is rounded down. Therefore, in the above example, the child's age would be stated as 4 years, 3 months, or 4-3. If the number of days in the chronologic age is between 16 and 30, the month is rounded up. If the above child's chronologic age had been 4 years, 3 months, 16 days, the chronologic age would be expressed as 4 years, 4 months, or 4-4.

Sometimes, "borrowing" is necessary to subtract the birth date from the date of testing correctly:

| | Year | Month | Day |
|---|---|---|---|
| Date of testing | 99 | 6 | 15 |
| Birth date | 95 | 10 | 22 |
| Chronologic age | 3 | 7 | 23 |

Begin with the Day category. Twenty-two cannot be subtracted from 15 without borrowing from the Month category. One month must be borrowed and placed in the Day category. One month equals 30 days; 30 is added to the 15 days in the Date of testing, giving a total of 45. Twenty-two is subtracted from 45, leaving 23 days. Moving to the Month category, 1 month has been borrowed by the Day category, leaving 5 months. Because 10 cannot be subtracted from 5, 1 year must be borrowed from the Year category. One year equals 12 months; therefore 12 will be added to the 5 in the Month category for Date of testing, totaling 17. Ten is subtracted from 17, leaving 7 months. Moving to the Year category, 1 year has been borrowed by the Month category, leaving 98. Ninety-five can be subtracted from 98, leaving 3 years.

Therefore, this child's chronologic age is 3 years, 7 months, and 23 days. Using the rounding convention as discussed, the month is rounded up, giving a chronologic age of 3 years, 8 months.

### Calculating the Corrected Age

*Corrected age* is used for children who were born prematurely to "correct" for the number of weeks they were born before the due date. Generally, the age is corrected until the child turns 2 years of age, although this convention can vary. Given 40 weeks' gestation as full term, the amount of correction is the difference between the actual gestational age at birth and the 40 weeks' full-term gestational age. Therefore, a child born at 30 weeks' gestation is 10 weeks premature. Many practitioners consider 36 or 37 weeks or above to be full-term gestation; therefore, children with a gestational age of 36 weeks or above do not receive a corrected age. Because there is some variation in how and when corrected age is used, it is wise for the therapist to learn the procedures of his or her facility and to adhere to them when calculating corrected age.

If the expected due date and birth date are both known, subtracting the birth date from the due date yields an exact measurement of prematurity.

| | Year | Month | Day |
|---|---|---|---|
| Due date | 98 | 9 | 20 |
| Birth date | 98 | 6 | 12 |
| | — | 3 | 8 |

This child is 3 months, 8 days premature. To calculate corrected age, subtract the prematurity value from the chronologic age.

| | Year | Month | Day |
|---|---|---|---|
| Chronologic age | 1 | 1 | 25 |
| Prematurity | — | 3 | 8 |
| | — | 10 | 17 |

The child's corrected age is 10 months, 17 days, or, when rounded, 11 months.

online; however, see Box 9.26 for instructions on how to compute adjusted ages. Case Example 9.5 describes the initial evaluation of a 9-month-old infant with developmental delays.

Toddlers may be assessed for all of those areas above, with the addition of mobility skills of walking and attachment behaviors with the caregiver (willingness to explore and ability to be comforted by the caregiver when upset). The toddlers' play and interaction skills may now be observed with other children.

Preschool-age children will often be assessed for in-hand manipulation skills and related functional abilities such as being able to manage clothing fasteners. Assessment includes examination of rotation, translation, and shift, as well as the related skills of open web space, separation of the sides of the hand, and ability to isolate individual fingers. Preschoolers begin to snip and then cut with scissors, trace on a line, and start forming simple shapes for prewriting and then writing. Preschoolers draw simple human figures, imitate simple motions, match simple shapes, and start to have accuracy catching and throwing a ball.

School-age children will often be assessed for handwriting performance, attention and behavior, executive functions, and social participation with peers at recess, lunch, and outside of school. Some children will still require assessment of specific ADL skills, and shoe tying is a common area of difficulty. School-age children may be observed for a variety of sports-related skills and safe mobility in the hallways and outside. Frequently, school-age children will begin to be assessed for AT options to improve their independence. School-age children being seen outside of school may require assessment of praxis and sensory functions. See Case Example 9.6 for an evaluation for a school-age child with mental health and sensory-motor concerns.

## INTERPRETATION, SUMMARY, AND RECOMMENDATIONS

After all interviews, observations, and assessments have been completed, the occupational therapist, in collaboration with the child's team, interprets the assessment findings, prioritizes concerns, and develops initial recommendations to assist the child and family. If therapy intervention is warranted, the occupational therapist's intervention plan should be evidence based and include functional and measurable goals that are important to the child and family. Occupational therapists synthesize information from a variety of sources to interpret the evaluation findings to create meaningful client-centered intervention plans.

## CASE EXAMPLE 9.5 EVALUATION AND CLASSIFICATION: BEN

Ben is a 9-month-old infant referred for occupational therapy services because of developmental delay. His mother is concerned that he is "not moving like his older brother was at this age." He is just beginning to sit independently but has difficulty rolling because of "tightness" in the left arm and leg.

The occupational therapist completed a thorough evaluation including formal and informal assessment of body structures and function and development skills. The therapist administered the Grasping and Visual Motor Integration Subscales of the Peabody Developmental Motor Scales-2 (PDMS-2) and the Alberta Infant Motor Scales (AIMS).

On each of the assessments, Ben scored below average when compared to typical age peers. He did not reach and grasp with his left arm and did not bring both hands to midline to play. He did not use both hands to hold a sippy cup, and his mother reported difficulty putting on shirts and pants because of tightness in Ben's left arm and leg. The occupational therapist observed Ben's movement during play and noted that he had limited control of left arm and leg movement when transitioning out of sitting, rolling, or reaching for objects. He did not use his left arm for protective reactions forward or sideways. The therapist observed that his eyes were not aligned and his left eye drifted laterally.

The therapist reported the results to the referring pediatric neurologist. The neurologist ordered a magnetic resonance imaging (MRI) test to identify possible central nervous system lesion(s). The results of the MRI revealed that Ben had a lesion affecting the right primary motor cortex and internal capsule and the neurologist confirmed a diagnosis of spastic left hemiplegic cerebral palsy (CP).

## CASE EXAMPLE 9.6 ASSESSING MENTAL HEALTH AND SENSORY-MOTOR CHALLENGES

### Overview

Rhanny is a 9-year-old boy diagnosed with bipolar disorder and attention-deficit hyperactivity disorder (ADHD) and referred to occupational therapy and counseling for behavioral difficulties in the classroom. He currently is in a self-contained classroom due to his behavior difficulties. His teacher states he has aggressive behavior and refuses to do his work. His mother reports that Rhanny has difficulty following adult requests, socializing with friends, brushing his teeth, changing his clothes or wearing new clothes, or taking a shower. Rhanny also has difficulty with coordination and handwriting. Mother reported she has a history of depression.

### Observation

Rhanny followed directions during the initial evaluation with the occupational therapist, although he was aloof and did not engage in conversation. He completed the Bruininks-Oseretsky Test of Motor Proficiency (2nd ed.) (BOTMP-2), clinical observations, and the Developmental Test of Visual Performance (2nd ed.) (DTVP-2). The Sensory Processing Measure was completed by the parent. However, he refused to complete a handwriting sample toward the end of the evaluation. He wadded up the paper and threw the paper and pencil at the occupational therapist and said he was not going to do that. After negotiating with him, he copied the alphabet and a sentence. He had difficulty sequencing the alphabet and was not able to organize the letters to create a sentence and write it down on paper.

**Findings from Assessments** (scores that are bolded represent below age expectations).

#### *Bruininks-Oseretsky Test of Motor Proficiency*

Fine motor integration: 8
Manual dexterity: 12
Upper-limb coordination: 16
Bilateral coordination: **4**
Balance: **6**

#### *Developmental Test of Visual Performance*

General visual perceptual: 88
Motor visual perceptual: 98
Visual motor integration: **78**

#### *Sensory Processing Measure (areas that are bolded represent definate dysfunction)*

Vision: Some problems
**Tactile: Definite dysfunction**
**Proprioception: Definite dysfunction**
**Auditory: Definite dysfunction**
**Vestibular: Definite dysfunction**
**Praxis: Definite dysfunction**
**Social participation: Definite dysfunction**

### Assessment

Rhanny followed adult verbal directions for activities in which he could successfully complete and was cooperative in a one-on-one situation for 45 minutes. Rhanny demonstrated poor emotional regulation when frustrated with a task that was difficult for him. He showed poor coping behaviors (i.e., throwing things), which would lead to removal from the classroom. Rhanny had difficulty sequencing letters and organizing his thoughts for the handwriting assignment.

Rhanny shows difficulty processing sensory information (touch, movement, auditory, and taste/smell) that may interfere with his ability to attend and process information in the classroom. He exhibited difficulties with bilateral skills and balance and the complex tasks of visual motor integration. These findings suggest that his behavior difficulties may be in part due to sensory processing and executive functioning difficulties.

### Plan

Rhanny would benefit from occupational therapy to improve his ability to perform in the classroom. Specifically, therapy will focus on improving his self-efficacy for academic tasks (such as handwriting) and his ability to identify and control his emotional status so he can remain on task in the classroom. His difficulty processing sensory information may interfere with his activities of daily living (specifically grooming and hygiene). Goals for occupational therapy included improvement in toothbrushing, hygiene, grooming, and classroom behaviors.

### Occupational Therapy Intervention

After establishing a rapport with Rhanny, the occupational therapists created fun and interesting activities to promote self-efficacy. Since Rhanny exhibited many

## CASE EXAMPLE 9.6 ASSESSING MENTAL HEALTH AND SENSORY-MOTOR CHALLENGES—cont'd

difficulties in sensory processing, sessions began with proprioceptive activities to allow Rhanny to succeed and give him a sense of security. Activities such as animal walks, army crawling, and games requiring him to climb under tunnels reinforced his awareness of his muscles and joints. The occupational therapist targeted tactile activities to encourage toothbrushing. Using a cognitive behavioral approach, the occupational therapist worked to help Rhanny identify his goals and address how he could achieve them. Together, they emphasized positive self-talk and engaged in reappraisal.

After Rhanny made progress in engaging in varied sensory activities without showing signs of distress and began to label his emotions, the occupational therapist used behavior mapping to identify strategies and consequences for poor hygiene. Together, they developed scenarios. Rhanny received positive reinforcement from his mother, teacher, and peers on his newly groomed self, and he was able to note that made him feel better.

To address his behaviors in school, the occupational therapist took several routes. First, she worked with the teacher to make some classroom modifications (such as wearing headphones, providing a wiggle seat, and allowing Rhanny to get up and move periodically). The therapist addressed his skill in handwriting, challenging him so he could feel accomplishment but not overwhelming him. They also addressed his frustration tolerance and role-played how to handle difficult situations in the classroom. Meanwhile the occupational therapist collaborated with the parent and teacher to explain Rhanny's behaviors and develop strategies that would work for all. As they made changes that benefited Rhanny, the occupational therapist provided them with positive reinforcement (to promote their self-efficacy).

### Outcomes

As Rhanny experienced success in therapy and at home, his behavior changed at school. He began to complete his work and showed no aggressive outburst. He was placed back into the regular education classroom with only behavioral support. He showed positive self-efficacy by spontaneously praising himself. He showed a new confidence in himself as he wore new clothes, socialized with his peers, and verbalized how he was feeling.

## SUMMARY

A comprehensive pediatric occupational therapy evaluation should be based upon an occupation-centered model of practice, the use of appropriate frames of reference, and multiple methods of assessment. The specific selection of assessments relies upon the therapist's clinical reasoning, in relation to the child's age, diagnosis, the setting, the reason for referral, and the therapist's approach to evaluation (top-down vs. bottom-up). Therapists use knowledge of the benefits and the issues of concern regarding the use of standardized testing with children and youth with disabilities. They select tools with psychometric rigor that are appropriate for the specific child and situation.

1. The evaluation process for children and youth includes completing an occupational profile and then analyzing multiple factors that may influence occupational performance. Occupational therapy practitioners gather information through interview, observation, and administering assessment tools. The evaluation process includes synthesizing information about the child's condition, assessment findings, observations and interviews as well as an understanding of the child's environment, including cultural and family expectations and goals.
2. Occupational therapists prioritize the areas to assess based upon the reason for the referral for evaluation, the setting, and the child's and family's concerns and goals. They use professional reasoning throughout the process as they determine the assessments to use to understand the child's occupational performance strengths and challenges.
3. Occupational therapists conduct evaluations for the purposes of (1) screening; (2) determining the scope and frequency of occupational therapy services; (3) setting goals and developing intervention plans; and (4) documenting progress toward therapy goals.
4. Assessment tools are created to measure a variety of occupations, skills, client factors, body functions, and environments. Findings from specific assessments provide information related to a child's strengths and challenges that contribute to occupational performance. Assessments provide measures that inform intervention planning and can be used to create goals and measure a child's progress overtime. Findings from assessments contribute to decisions regarding the scope and frequency of occupational therapy services. Assessment scores are often needed for documentation and funding of services.
5. Assessments can be nonstandardized or standardized. Nonstandardized assessments include observations, interviews, and checklists that have not been tested on populations. Standardized assessments have established procedures, scoring, and interpretation guidelines. Standardized assessments include ipsative assessment, norm-referenced assessment, and criterion-referenced assessments.
6. Occupational therapists use information regarding reliability and validity to assist their selection of appropriate tools for various evaluation purposes.
7. The occupational therapist evaluates each occupation using the same process but focuses differently on the content of the evaluation based on the model of practice and frame(s) of reference chosen and the specific needs of the situation (child's diagnosis, age, and setting). After completing an occupational provide, the occupational therapist may decide to focus on the specific skills and client factors. Occupational therapy practitioners use professional reasoning which involves synthesizing scientific evidence, clinical experience, knowledge of the setting and environment, reason for the evaluation, and the child's and family's goals to make decisions regarding the evaluation.

## REFERENCES


Adolfsson, M., Malmqvist, J., Pless, M., & Granuld, M. (2011). Identifying child functioning from an ICF-CY perspective: Everyday life situations explored in measures of participation. *Disability and Rehabilitation, 33*(13–14), 1230–1244.

Adolph, K. E. (2020). An ecological approach to learning in (not and) development. *Human Development, 63*(3–4), 180–201.

Adolph, K. E., & Kretch, K. S. (2015). Gibson's theory of perceptual learning. *International Encyclopedia of the Social and Behavioral Sciences, 10*, 127–134.

Adolph, K. E., & Young, J. W. (2021). Learning to move in the real world. *Science, 373*(6555), 620–621.

Agate, J. R., Zabriskie, R. B., Agate, S. T., & Poff, R. (2009). Family leisure satisfaction and satisfaction with family life. *Journal of Leisure Research, 41*(2), 205–223.

Alghamdi, M. S., Chiarello, L. A., Palisano, R. J., & McCoy, S. W. (2017). Understanding participation of children with cerebral palsy in family and recreational activities. *Research in Developmental Disabilities, 69*, 96–104.

Almberg, M., Selander, H., Falkmer, M., Vaz, S., Ciccarelli, M., & Falkmer, T. (2017). Experiences of facilitators or barriers in driving education from learner and novice drivers with ADHD or ASD and their driving instructors. *Developmental Neurorehabilitation, 20*(2), 59–67.

Alonzo, R., Hussain, J., Stranges, S., & Anderson, K. K. (2021). Interplay between social media use, sleep quality, and mental health in youth: A systematic review. *Sleep Medicine Reviews, 56*:101414.

Alsharaydeh, E. A., Alqudah, M., Lee, R. L. T., & Chan, S. W. C. (2019). Challenges, coping, and resilience among immigrant parents caring for a child with a disability: An integrative review. *Journal of Nursing Scholarship, 51*(6), 670–679.

American Academy of Sleep Medicine. (2014). *International classification of sleep disorders: Diagnostic and coding manual* (3rd ed.). American Academy of Sleep Medicine.

American Occupational Therapy Association. (2016). Assistive technology and occupational performance. *American Journal of Occupational Therapy, 70*:7012410030.

American Occupational Therapy Association. (2017a). AOTA occupational profile template. *American Journal of Occupational Therapy, 71*(Suppl. 2):7112420030.

American Occupational Therapy Association. (2017b). The practice of occupational therapy in feeding, eating, and swallowing. *American Journal of Occupational Therapy, 71*(Suppl. 2):7112410015.

American Occupational Therapy Association. (2018). Five things patients and providers should question. http://www.choosingwisely.org/societies/american-occupational-therapy-association-inc/.

American Occupational Therapy Association. (2020a). Guidelines for supervision, roles, and responsibilities during the delivery of occupational therapy services. *American Journal of Occupational Therapy, 74*(Suppl. 3):7413410020.

American Occupational Therapy Association. (2020b). Occupational therapy practice framework: Domain and process (4th ed.). *American Journal of Occupational Therapy, 74*(Suppl. 2):7412410010.

Anderson, N., Schlueter, J. E., Carlson, J. F., & Geisinger, K. F. (Eds.). (2022). *Tests in print X*. Buros Center for Testing.

Angell, A. M., Carroll, T. C., Bagatell, N., Chen, C., Kramer, J. M., Schwartz, A., Tallon, M. B., & Hammel, J. (2019). Understanding self-determination as a crucial component in promoting the distinct value of occupational therapy in post-secondary transition planning. *Journal of Occupational Therapy, Schools, & Early Intervention, 12*(1), 129–143.

Arellano, A., & Peralta, F. (2013). Self–determination of young children with intellectual disability: Understanding parents' perspectives. *British Journal of Special Education, 40*(4), 175–181.

Ashcraft, A. M., & Murray, P. J. (2017). Talking to parents about adolescent sexuality. *Pediatric Clinics, 64*(2), 305–320.

Ayres, A. J. (1964). Tactile functions: Their relation to hyperactive and perceptual motor behavior. *American Journal of Occupational Therapy, 18*, 6–11.

Ayres, A. J. (1965). Patterns of perceptual-motor dysfunction in children: A factor analytic study. *Perceptual and Motor Skills, 20*, 335–368.

Ayres, A. J. (1966a). Interrelationships among perceptual-motor functions in children. *American Journal of Occupational Therapy, 20*(2), 68–71.

Ayres, A. J. (1966b). Interrelations among perceptual-motor abilities in a group of normal children. *American Journal of Occupational Therapy, 20*(6), 288–292.

Ayres, A. J. (1969). Deficits in sensory integration in educationally handicapped children. *Journal of Learning Disabilities, 2*(3), 44–52.

Ayres, A. J. (1971). Characteristics of types of sensory integrative dysfunction. *American Journal of Occupational Therapy, 25*(7), 329–334.

Ayres, A. J. (1972). Improving academic scores through sensory integration. *Journal of Learning Disabilities, 5*, 338–343.

Ayres, A. J. (1973). *Sensory integration and learning disorders*. Western Psychological Services.

Ayres, A. J. (1977). Cluster analyses of measures of sensory integration. *American of Journal of Occupational Therapy, 31*(6), 362–366.

Ayres, A. J. (1979). *Sensory integration and the child*. Western Psychological Services.

Ayres, A. J. (1989). *Sensory Integration and Praxis tests manual*. Western Psychological Services.

Ayres, A. J. (2004). *Sensory integration and the child* (2nd ed.). Western Psychological Services.

Ayres, A. J., Mailloux, Z., & Wendler, C. L. W. (1987). Development apraxia: Is it a unitary function? *Occupational Therapy Journal of Research, 7*(2), 93–110.

Baeyer, C. L. (2009). Children's self-report of pain intensity: what we know, where we are headed. *Pain Research and Management, 14*(1), 39–45.

Baghdadli, A., Pascal, C., Grisi, S., & Aussiloux, C. (2003). Risk factors for self-injurious behaviours among 222 young children with autistic disorders. *Journal of Intellectual Disability Research, 47*, 622–627.

Ball, M. A. (2018). Revitalizing the OT role in school-based practice: Promoting success for all students. *Journal of Occupational Therapy, Schools, & Early Intervention, 11*(3), 263–272.

Bandura, A., Barbaranelli, C., Caprara, G. V., & Pastorelli, C. (1996). Multifaceted impact of self-efficacy beliefs on academic functioning. *Child Development, 67*(3), 1206–1222. https://doi.org/10.2307/1131888

Bar-Shalita, T., Vatine, J. J., Yarnitsky, D., Parush, S., & Weissman-Fogel, I. (2014). Atypical central pain processing in sensory modulation disorder: Absence of temporal summation and higher after-sensation. *Experimental Brain Research, 232*(2), 587–595.

Bascom, G. W., & Christensen, K. M. (2017). The impacts of limited transportation access on persons with disabilities' social participation. *Journal of Transport & Health, 7*, 227–234.

Bass, J. D., Baum, C., & Christiansen, C. (2017). Person-environment-occupation-performance models. In J. Hinojosa, P. Krmer, & C. B. Royeen (Eds.), *Perspectives in human occupation: Theories underlying practice* (2nd ed.). FA Davis.

Bassi, G. S., Humphris, G. M., & Longman, L. P. (2004). The etiology and management of gagging: A review of the literature. *The Journal of Prosthetic Dentistry, 91*(5), 459–467.

Bastawrous, M., Gignac, M. A., Kapral, M. K., & Cameron, J. I. (2015). Factors that contribute to adult children caregivers' well-being: A scoping review. *Health and Social Care in the Community, 23*(5), 449–466.

Basu, S., Kafkes, A., Geist, R., & Kielhofner, G. (2008). *Pediatric Volitional Questionnaire (PVQ; Version 2.1)*. Model of Human Occupation Clearinghouse, Department of Occupational Therapy, College of Applied Health Sciences, University of Illinois at Chicago. https://moho-irm.uic.edu.

Baum, C. M., Christiansen, C. H., & Bass, J. D. (2015). Person-environment-occupation-performance (PEOP) model. In C. H. Christiansen, C. M. Baum, & J. D. Bass (Eds.), *Occupational therapy: Performance, participation, well-being* (4th ed.) (pp. 49–55). Slack.

Bayley, N. (2006). *Bayley scales of infant and toddler development (3rd ed.): Technical manual*. Harcourt.

Behnke, C. J., & Fetkovich, M. M. (1984). Examining the reliability and validity of the play history. *American Journal of Occupational Therapy, 38*(2), 94–100. https://doi.org/10.5014/ajot.38.2.94

Behnke, S. H., & Warner, E. (2002). Confidentiality in the treatment of adolescents. *APA Monitor on Psychology, 33*(4), 44.

Bell, M. (2022). *OT-FIRST method training for the OT practitioner*. [Manuscript/Modules in Preparation].

Bell, M., & Johns, C. (2022). *Feasibility study: Implementing the OT-FIRST methods and Clinical Observations Measurement Tool with young, novice drivers*. Poster Presentation www.safedrivingrehab.com/ot-first/.

Benfer, K. A., Weir, K. A., Bell, K. L., Ware, R. S., Davies, P. S. W., & Boyd, R. N. (2015). Clinical signs suggestive of pharyngeal dysphagia in preschool children with cerebral palsy. *Research in Developmental Disabilities, 38*, 192–201.

Berardi, N., Sale, A., & Maffei, L. (2015). Brain structural and functional development: Genetics and experience. *Developmental Medicine and Child Neurology, 57*, 4–9.

Beyer, J. E. (1984). *The Oucher: A user's manual and technical report*. The Hospital Play Equipment Co.

Beyer, J. E., Denyes, M. J., & Villarruel, A. M. (1992). The creation, validation, and continuing development of the Oucher: A measure of pain intensity in children. *Journal of Pediatric Nursing, 7*(5), 335–346 PMID: 1479552.

Bezyak, J. L., Sabella, S., Hammel, J., McDonald, K., Jones, R. A., & Barton, D. (2020). Community participation and public transportation barriers experienced by people with disabilities. *Disability & Rehabilitation, 42*(23), 3275–3283.

Bhat, A. N., Landa, R. J., & Galloway, J. C. (2011). Current perspectives on motor functioning in infants, children, and adults with autism spectrum disorders. *Physical Therapy, 91*(7), 1116–1129.

Bieri, D., Reeve, R. A., Champion, G. D., Addicoat, L., & Ziegler, J. (1990). The Faces Pain Scale for the self-assessment of the severity of pain experienced by children: Development, initial validation and preliminary investigation for ratio scale properties. *Pain, 41*, 139–150.

Bittmann, S., Luchter, E., Bittmann, L., Moschuring-Alieva, E., & Villalon, G. (2022). Current aspects of treatment options of chronic sialorrhea in children. *Journal of Clinical Medicine Research, 14*(6), 246–249.

Bolton, T., & Plattner, L. (2020). Occupational therapy role in school-based practice: Perspectives from teachers and OTs. *Journal of Occupational Therapy, Schools, & Early Intervention, 13*(2), 136–146.

Bonnard, M., & Anaby, D. (2016). Enabling participation of students through school-based occupational therapy services: Towards a broader scope of practice. *British Journal of Occupational Therapy, 79*(3), 188–192.

Bonnard, M., Hui, C., Manganaro, M., & Anaby, D. (2022). Toward participation-focused school-based occupational therapy: Current profile and possible directions. *Journal of Occupational Therapy, Schools, & Early Intervention*, 1–18.

Bourne, L., Mandy, W., & Bryant-Waugh, R. (2022). Avoidant/restrictive food intake disorder and severe food selectivity in children and young people with autism: A scoping review. *Developmental Medicine and Child Neurology, 64*(6), 691–700.

Branson, C. M., & Gross, S. J. (Eds.). (2014). *Handbook of ethical educational leadership* (1st ed.). Routledge. https://doi.org/10.4324/9780203747582.

Bronfenbrenner, U., & Morris, P. A. (2007). The bioecological model of human development. In W. Damon, R. M. Lerner, & R. M. Lerner (Eds.), *Handbook of child psychology*. https://doi.org/10.1002/9780470147658.chpsy0114.

Brown, E. J. (2009). When insiders become outsiders: Parental objections to public school sex education programs. *Duke Law Journal*, 109–144.

Brown, T., & Chien, C.-W. (2010). Top-down or bottom-up occupational therapy assessment: Which way so we go? *British Journal of Occupational Therapy, 73*. https://doi.org/10.4276/030802210X12682330090334.

Bruininks, R. H., & Bruininks, B. D. (2005). *Bruininks-Oseretsky Test of Motor Proficiency (2nd ed.; BOT-2)*. PsycTESTS.

Bryce, C. I., & Jahromi, L. B. (2013). Brief report: Compliance and noncompliance to parental control strategies in children with high-functioning autism and their typical peers. *Journal of Autism and Developmental Disorders, 43*, 236–243.

Bult, M. K., Verschuren, O., Jongmans, M. J., Lindeman, E., & Ketelaar, M. (2011). What influences participation in leisure activities of children and youth with physical disabilities? A systematic review. *Research in Developmental Disabilities, 32*(5), 1521–1529.

Bundy, A. (1993). Assessment of play and leisure: Delineation of the problem. *American Journal of Occupational Therapy, 47*, 217–222.

Bundy, A. (2011). Children: Analyzing the occupation of play. In L. Mackenzie, & G. O'Toole (Eds.), *Occupational analysis in practice* (pp. 133–146). Wiley-Blackwell.

Bundy, A. C. (1999). *Test of Environmental Supportiveness (TOES)*. Colorado State University.

Burke, M. M., & Hodapp, R. M. (2016). The nature, correlates, and conditions of parental advocacy in special education. *Exceptionality, 24*(3), 137–150.

Burke, M. M., Rios, K., & Lee, C. E. (2019). Exploring the special education advocacy process according to families and advocates. *The Journal of Special Education, 53*(3), 131–141.

Buschbacher, P. W., & Fox, L. (2003). Understanding and intervening with the challenging behavior of young children with autism spectrum disorder. *Language, Speech, and Hearing Services in Schools, 34*, 217–227.

Buswell, L., Zabriskie, R. B., Lundberg, N., & Hawkins, A. J. (2012). The relationship between father involvement in family leisure and family functioning: The importance of daily family leisure. *Leisure Sciences, 34*(2), 172–190.

Buysse, D. J. (2014). Sleep health: Can we define it? Does it matter? *Sleep, 37*(1), 9–17.

Carlson, J. F., Geisinger, K. F., & Jonson, J. L. (Eds.). (2021). *The twenty-first mental measurements yearbook*. Buros Center for Testing.

Carriot, J., Jamali, M., Brooks, J. X., & Cullen, K. E. (2015). Integration of canal and otolith inputs by central vestibular neurons is subadditive for both active and passive self-motion: Implication for perception. *Journal of Neuroscience, 35*(8), 3555–3565.

Carruth, B. R., Ziegler, P. J., Gordon, A., & Barr, S. I. (2004). Prevalence of picky eaters among infants and toddlers and their caregivers' decisions about offering a new food. *Journal of the American Dietetic Association, 104*(Suppl. 1), s57–s64.

Ceka, A., & Murati, R. (2016). The role of parents in the education of children. *Journal of Education and Practice, 7*(5), 61–64.

Cermak, S. A. (2006). Perceptual functions of the hand. In A. Henderson, & C. Pehoski (Eds.), *Hand function in the child: Foundations for remediation* (2nd ed.) (pp. 63–88). Elsevier.

Cermak, S. A. (1991). Somatodyspraxia. In A. C. Bundy, S. J. Lane, & E. A. Murray (Eds.), *Sensory integration: Theory and practice* (2nd ed.) (pp. 137–170). F. A. Davis.

Christiansen, C. H., Baum, C. M., & Bass, J. D. (Eds.). (2015). *Occupational therapy: Performance, participation, and well-being* (4th ed.) Slack.

Chen, C. Y., Lin, Y. H., Lee, C. Y., Lin, Y. K., Chen, W. I., & Shih, J. R. (2019). Family leisure and subjective well-being: Do patterns and timing matter? *Social Behavior and Personality: International Journal, 47*(9), 1–7.

Chen, S. W., & Chippendale, T. (2018). Leisure as an end, not just a means, in occupational therapy intervention. *American Journal of Occupational Therapy, 72*(4):7204347010p1–7204347010p5.

Chen, Y. L., & Patten, K. (2021). Shifting focus from impairment to inclusion: Expanding occupational therapy for neurodivergent students to address school environments. *American Journal of Occupational Therapy, 75*(3).

Chien, C. W., Rodger, S., Copley, J., Branjerdporn, G., & Taggart, C. (2016). Sensory processing and its relationship with children's daily life participation. *Physical & Occupational Therapy in Pediatrics, 36*(1), 73–87.

Chistol, L. T., Bandini, L. G., Must, A., Phillips, S., Cermak, S. A., & Curtin, C. (2018). Sensory sensitivity and food selectivity in children with autism spectrum disorder. *Journal of Autism and Developmental Disorders, 48*(2), 583–591.

Clark, M. B., & Clark, D. A. (2018). Oral development and pathology. *The Ochsner Journal, 18*(4), 339–344.

Classen, S., Monahan, M., & Wang, Y. (2013). Driving characteristics of teens with attention deficit hyperactivity and autism spectrum disorder. *American Journal of Occupational Therapy, 67*(6), 664–673.

Clough, C. (2019). School-based occupational therapists' service delivery decision-making: Perspectives on identity and roles. *Journal of Occupational Therapy, Schools, & Early Intervention, 12*(1), 51–67.

Coker-Bolt, P. (2016). Positioning and handling: A neurodevelopmental approach. In J. Solomon, & J. O'Brien (Eds.), *Pediatric skills for occupational therapy assistants* (4th ed.) (pp. 335–392). Elsevier.

Coley, R. L., Votruba–Drzal, E., & Schindler, H. S. (2009). Fathers' and mothers' parenting predicting and responding to adolescent sexual risk behaviors. *Child Development, 80*(3), 808–827.

Collaborative for Academic, Social, and Emotional Learning. (2015). https://casel.org/.

Cooper, O., Springer, C., & Elleman, B. (2023). Occupational therapy services for transition-age youth with moderate to severe disabilities: A scoping review. *Research Directs in Therapeutic Sciences, 2*(1).

Coppens, A. D., Alcalá, L., Rogoff, B., & Mejía-Arauz, R. (2016). Children's contributions in family work: Two cultural paradigms. *Families, Intergenerationality, and Peer Group Relations*, 1–27.

Coppens, A. D., Silva, K. G., Ruvalcaba, O., Alcalá, L., López, A., & Rogoff, P. (2014). Learning by observing and pitching in: Benefits and processes of expanding repertoires. *Human Development, 57*(2–3), 150–161.

Coster, W., Deeney, T., Haltiwanger, J., & Haley, S. (1998). *School Function Assessment*. Psychological Corporation/Therapy Skill Builders.

Coyl-Shepherd, D. D., & Hanlon, C. (2013). Family play and leisure activities: Correlates of parents' and children's socio-emotional well-being. *International Journal of Play, 2*(3), 254–272.

Cramm, H., & Egan, M. (2015). Practice patterns of school-based occupational therapists targeting handwriting: A knowledge-to-practice gap. *Journal of Occupational Therapy, Schools, & Early Intervention, 8*(2), 170–179.

Cramm, H., Krupa, T., Missiuna, C., Lysaght, R. M., & Parker, K. C. (2013). Broadening the occupational therapy toolkit: An executive functioning lens for occupational therapy with children and youth. *American Journal of Occupational Therapy, 67*(6), e139–e147.

Creighton, C. (1992). The origin and evolution of activity analysis. *American Journal of Occupational Therapy, 46*(1), 45–48.

Crepeau, E. B., Boyt Schell, B. A., Gillen, G., & Scaffa, M. E. (2014). Analyzing occupations and activity. In B. A. Boyt Schell, G. Gillen, & M. E. Scaffa (Eds.), *Willard & Spackman's occupational therapy* (12th ed.) (pp. 234–248). Lippincott Williams & Wilkins.

Currie, G., & Szabo, J. (2020). Social isolation and exclusion: The parents' experience of caring for children with rare neurodevelopmental disorders. *International Journal of Qualitative Studies on Health and Well-Being, 15*(1):1725362.

Curry, A. E., Yerys, B. E., Huang, P., & Metzger, K. B. (2018). Longitudinal study of driver licensing rates among adolescents and young adults with autism spectrum disorder. *Autism: The International Journal of Research and Practice, 22*(4), 479–488.

Dahan-Oliel, N., Shikako-Thomas, K., & Majnemer, A. (2012). Quality of life and leisure participation in children with neurodevelopmental disabilities: A thematic analysis of the literature. *Quality of Life Research, 21*, 427–439.

Dahan-Oliel, N., Shikako-Thomas, K., Mazer, B., & Majnemer, A. (2016). Adolescents with disabilities participate in the shopping mall: Facilitators and barriers framed according to the ICF. *Disability & Rehabilitation, 38*(21), 2102–2113.

DaWalt, L. S., Usher, L. V., Greenberg, J. S., & Mailick, M. R. (2019). Friendships and social participation as markers of quality of life of adolescents and adults with fragile X syndrome and autism. *Autism, 23*(2), 383–393.

Dawson, C., & Mudgal, C. S. (2010). Staged description of the Finkelstein test. *The Journal of Hand Surgery, 35*(9), 1513–1515.

Dean, E. E., Little, L., Tomchek, S., & Dunn, W. (2018). Sensory processing in the general population: Adaptability, resiliency, and challenging behavior. *American Journal of Occupational Therapy, 72*:7201195060.

De Jong, A. E., Bremer, M., Schouten, M., Tuinebreijer, W. E., & Faber, A. W. (2005). Reliability and validity of the pain observation scale for young children and the visual analogue scale in children with burns. *Burns, 31*(2), 198–204.

Dekkers, K. J. F. M., Rameckers, E. A. A., Smeets, R. J. E. M., & Janssen-Potten, Y. J. M. (2014). Upper extremity strength measurement for children with cerebral palsy: A systematic review of available instruments. *Physical Therapy, 94*(5), 609–622.

Dellon, A. L. (1978). The moving two-point discrimination test: Clinical evaluation of the quickly adapting fiber/receptor system. *The Journal of Hand Surgery, 3*(5), 474–481.

Demarin, V., & Morović, S. (2014). Neuroplasticity. *Periodicum Biologorum, 116*(2), 209–211.

de Oliveira Borba, P. L., Pereira, B. P., de Souza, J. R. B., & Lopes, R. E. (2020). Occupational therapy research in schools: A mapping review. *Occupational Therapy International, 2020*:5891978.

Deptula, D. P., Henry, D. B., & Schoeny, M. E. (2010). How can parents make a difference? Longitudinal associations with adolescent sexual behavior. *Journal of Family Psychology, 24*(6), 731.

Dewinter, J., Vermeiren, R. R. J. M., Vanwesenbeeck, I., & Van Nieuwenhuizen, C. (2016). Parental awareness of sexual experience in adolescent boys with autism spectrum disorder. *Journal of Autism and Developmental Disorders, 46*, 713–719.

Dias, B. L. S., Fernandes, A. B., & Filho, H. S. M. (2016). Sialorrhea in children with cerebral palsy. *Journal de Pediatria, 92*, 549–558.

Di Marino, E., Tremblay, S., Khetani, M., & Anaby, D. (2018). The effect of child, family and environmental factors on the participation of young children with disabilities. *Disability and Health Journal, 11*(1), 36–42.

Ditchman, N., Kosyluk, K., Lee, E. J., & Jones, N. (2016). How stigma affects the lives of people with intellectual disabilities: An overview. In K. Scior, & S. Werner (Eds.), *Intellectual disability and stigma: Stepping out from the margins* (pp. 31–47). Palgrave Macmillan. https://doi.org/10.1057/978-1-137-52499-7_3.

do Amaral, M. F., de França Drummond, A., Coster, W. J., & Mancini, M. C. (2014). Household task participation of children and adolescents with cerebral palsy, Down syndrome and typical development. *Research in Developmental Disabilities, 35*(2), 414–422.

Douglas, S. N., Meadan, H., & Schultheiss, H. (2022). A meta-synthesis of caregivers' experiences transitioning from early intervention to early childhood special education. *Early Childhood Education Journal*, 1–13.

Duff, S. E. (1996). A study of the effects of group family play on family relations. *International Journal of Play Therapy, 5*(2), 81–93.

Dunlap, G., & Fox, L. (2011). Function-based interventions for children with challenging behavior. *Journal of Early Intervention, 33*, 333–343.

Dunn, L., & Gardner, J. (2013). Household task participation of children with and without physical disability. *American Journal of Occupational Therapy, 67*(5), e100–e105.

Dunn, W. (2000). Best practice in occupational therapy in community service with children and families. Slack. In J. Case-Smith, & J. O'Brien (Eds.), *Occupational therapy for children* (6th ed.) (p. 208). Elsevier.

Dweck, C. S. (2006). *Mindset: The new psychology of success*. Random House.

Egan, M., & Restall, G. (Eds.). (2022). *Promoting occupational participation: Collaborative relationship-focused occupational therapy*. Canadian Association of Occupational Therapist Publications ACE.

EnbyOT. (2023). *The OT Sexual Assessment Framework*. https://www.enbyot.com/using-the-ot-sexual-assessment-framework-as-a-guide-to-addressing-sexuality-and-intimacy-in-ot/.

Fahy, S., Delicate, N., & Lynch, H. (2021). Now, being, occupational: Outdoor play and children with autism. *Journal of Occupational Science, 28*(1), 114–132.

Fishman, C. E., & Nickerson, A. B. (2015). Motivations for involvement: A preliminary investigation of parents of students with disabilities. *Journal of Child and Family Studies, 24*, 523–535.

Flatt, A. E. (1994). *The care of congenital hand anomalies* (2nd ed.). Quality Medical Pub., Incorporated.

Flores de Apodaca, R., Gentling, D. G., Steinhaus, J. K., & Rosenberg, E. A. (2015). Parental involvement as a mediator of academic performance among special education middle school students. *School Community Journal, 25*(2), 35–54.

Folio, M. R., & Fewell, R. R. (2000). *Peabody developmental motor scale (2nd ed.; PDMS-2)*. Pro-Ed.

Forbes-Duchart, L., Marshall, S., Strock, A., & Cooper, J. E. (2007). Determination of inter-rater reliability in pediatric burn scar assessment using a modified version of the Vancouver Scar Scale. *Journal of Burn Care and Research, 28*(3), 460–467.

Foxx, R. M. (1996). Twenty years of applied behavior analysis in treating the most severe problem behavior: Lessons learned. *The Behavior Analyst, 19*, 225–235.

Friedlander, J. A., DeBoer, E. M., Soden, J. S., Furuta, G. T., Menard-Katcher, C. D., Atkins, D., Fleischer, D. M., Kramer, R. E., Deterding, R. R., Capocelli, K. E., & Prager, J. D. (2016). Unsedated transnasal esophagoscopy for monitoring therapy in pediatric eosinophilic esophagitis. *Gastrointestinal Endoscopy, 83*(2), 299–306.e1.

Frolek Clark, G., & Polichino, J. (2021). School occupational therapy: Staying focused on participation and educational performance. *Journal of Occupational Therapy, Schools, & Early Intervention, 14*, 19–26.

Furumasu, J., Guerette, P., & Tefft, D. (2004). Relevance of the pediatric powered wheelchair screening test for children with cerebral palsy. *Developmental Medicine and Child Neurology, 46*(7), 468–474.

Gale, C., Eikeseth, S., & Rudrud, E. (2011). Functional assessment and behavioral intervention for eating difficulties in children with autism: A study conducted in the natural environment using parents and ABA tutors as therapists. *Journal of Autism and Developmental Disorders, 41*, 1383–1396.

Gee Kee, E., Chien, C., Rodger, S. A., & Copley, J. A. (2014). Examining the association between children's hand skill performance and participation in everyday life. *Journal of Occupational Therapy, Schools, & Early Intervention, 7*, 246–259.

Gentina, E., & Bonsu, S. K. (2013). Peer network position and shopping behavior among adolescents. *Journal of Retailing and Consumer Services, 20*(1), 87–93.

Ghanouni, P., Jarus, T., Zwicker, J. G., Lucyshyn, J., Chauhan, S., & Moir, C. (2019). Perceived barriers and existing challenges in participation of children with autism spectrum disorders: "He did not understand and no one else seemed to understand him". *Journal of Autism and Developmental Disorders, 49*, 3136–3145.

Gil, E., & Sobol, B. (2005). Engaging families in therapeutic play. In C. E. Bailey (Ed.), *Children in therapy: Using the family as a resource* (pp. 341–382). W. W. Norton & Company.

Ginsburg, K. R., & Committee on Psychosocial Aspects of Child and Family Health. (2007). The importance of play in promoting healthy child development and maintaining strong parent-child bonds. *Pediatrics, 119*(1), 182–191.

Goldman, S. E. (2020). Special education advocacy for families of students with intellectual and developmental disabilities: Current trends and future directions. *International Review of Research in Developmental Disabilities, 58*, 1–50.

Grajo, L. C. (2017). Occupational adaptation. In J. Hinojosa, P. Kramer, & C. B. Royeen (Eds.), *Perspectives in human occupation: Theories underlying practice* (2nd ed.). FA Davis.

Grant, J. E., Potenza, M. N., Krishnan-Sarin, S., Cavallo, D. A., & Desai, R. A. (2011). Shopping problems among high school students. *Comprehensive Psychiatry, 52*(3), 247–252.

Gronski, M., & Doherty, M. (2020). Interventions within the scope of occupational therapy practice to improve activities of daily living, rest, and sleep for children ages 0–5 years and their families: A systematic review. *American Journal of Occupational Therapy, 74*(2):7402180010p1-7402180010p33.

Gross-Loh, C. (2013). *Parenting without borders: Surprising lessons parents around the world can teach us.* Avery Press.

Guerriere, T. (2019). *Implications for providing access to driver's education for disabled students: Results of related health assessments.* Teachers College, Columbia University. https://academiccommons.columbia.edu/doi/10.7916/d8-t2gb-3g31.

Haanpää, L., & Ursin, P. A. (2018). Leisure participation and child well-being: The role of family togetherness. *Handbook of Leisure, Physical Activity, Sports, Recreation and Quality of Life*, 107–117.

Hackett, J. (2010). Top-down and bottom-up assessments. *British Journal of Occupational Therapy, 73*(4), 189.

Haegele, J. A., Aigner, C., & Healy, S. (2020). Extracurricular activities and bullying among children and adolescents with disabilities. *Maternal and Child Health Journal, 24*, 310–318.

Häger-Ross, C., & Rösblad, B. (2002). Norms for grip strength in children aged 4-16 years. *Acta Paediatrica, 91*(6), 617–625.

Haley, S., Coster, W., Dumas, H. M., Fragala-Pinkham, M. A., & Moed, R. (1992). *Pediatric Evaluation of Disability Inventory - Computer Adaptive Test (PEDI-CAT).* Pearson.

Hamamura, T., Xu, Q., & Du, Y. (2013). Culture, social class, and independence–interdependence: The case of Chinese adolescents. *International Journal of Psychology, 48*(3), 344–351.

Hammell, K. R. (2013). Occupation, well-being, and culture: Theory and cultural humility. *Canadian Journal of Occupational Therapy. Revue Canadienne D'ergotherapie, 80*(4), 224–234.

Han, C. S., Brussoni, M. J., & Mâsse, L. C. (2022). Parental autonomy support in the context of parent–child negotiation for children's independent mobility:'I always feel safer with my parents' to 'Boom! Bust down those walls!'. *The Journal of Early Adolescence, 42*(6), 737–764.

Hanushek, E. A. (2020). Education production functions. In *The economics of education* (pp. 161–170). Academic Press.

Harden, K. P. (2014). A sex-positive framework for research on adolescent sexuality. *Perspectives on Psychological Science, 9*(5), 455–469.

Helseth, S., & Misvaer, N. (2010). Adolescents' perceptions of quality of life: What it is and what matters. *Journal of Clinical Nursing, 19*, 1454–1461.

Hemmingsson, H., Egilson, S., Hoffman, O., & Kielhofner, G. (2005). *School Setting Interview (SSI), version 3.0.* Swedish Association of Occupational Therapists. https://moho-irm.uic.edu.

Henne-Ochoa, R., Elliott-Groves, E., Meek, B. A., & Rogoff, B. (2020). Pathways forward for Indigenous language reclamation: Engaging Indigenous epistemology and learning by observing and pitching in to family and community endeavors. *The Modern Language Journal, 104*, 481–493.

Henry, L., & Polatajko, H. J. (2003). Exploring the inter-rater reliability of the performance quality rating scale. *In Canadian Association of Occupational Therapy Conference*, Winnipeg MB.

Hersch, G. I., Lamport, N. K., & Coffey, M. S. (2005). *Activity analysis: Application to occupation* (5th ed.). SLACK Incorporated.

Hicks, C. L., von Baeyer, C. L., Spafford, P. A., van Korlaar, I., & Goodenough, B. (2001). *Faces Pain Scale-revised (FPS-R).* APA PsycTests. https://doi.org/10.1037/t05331-000.

Hinojosa, J., Kramer, P., & Crist, P. (2014). Evaluation: Where do we begin? In J. Hinojosa, & P. Kramer (Eds.), *Evaluation in occupational therapy: Obtaining and interpreting data* (4th ed.) (pp. 1–18). AOTA Press.

Hirshkowitz, M., Whiton, K., Albert, S. M., Alessi, C., Bruni, O., DonCarlos, L., Hazen, N., Herman, J., Adams Hillard, P. J., Katz, E. S., Kheirandish-Gozal, L., Neubauer, D. N., O'Donnell, A. E., Ohayon, M., Peever, J., Rawding, R., Sachdeva, R. C., Setters, B., Vitiello, M. V., & Catesby Ware, J. (2015). National Sleep Foundation's updated sleep duration recommendations: Final report. *Sleep Health: Journal of the National Sleep Foundation, 1*(4), 233–243. https://www.sleephealthjournal.org/article/S2352-7218(15)00160-6/abstract?_gl=1*kf1m64*_gcl_au*MjEwNDQ1NzEwNS4xNzM0NjMyODk2*_ga*MTA4NTM1NzA2OC4xNzM0NjMyODk2*_ga_4NJJ62HMGF*MTczNDYzMjg5NS4xLjEuMTczNDYzMjkwMS41NC4wLjA.

Hodge, C. J., Duerden, M. D., Layland, E. K., Lacanienta, A., Goates, M. C., & Niu, X. M. (2017). The association between family leisure and family quality of life: A meta–analysis of data from parents and adolescents. *Journal of Family Theory & Review, 9*(3), 328–346.

Hodge, C. J., Zabriskie, R. B., Townsend, J. A., Eggett, D. L., & Poff, R. (2018). Family leisure functioning: A cross-national study. *Leisure Sciences, 40*(3), 194–215.

Hodge, N., & Runswick-Cole, K. (2013). 'They never pass me the ball': Exposing ableism through the leisure experiences of disabled children, young people and their families. *Children's Geographies, 11*(3), 311–325.

Holland-Hall, C., & Quint, E. H. (2017). Sexuality and disability in adolescents. *Pediatric Clinics, 64*(2), 435–449.

Holmes, L. G., Strassberg, D. S., & Himle, M. B. (2019). Family sexuality communication for adolescent girls on the autism spectrum. *Journal of Autism and Developmental Disorders, 49*, 2403–2416.

Holt-Lunstad, J. (2021). The major health implications of social connection. *Current Directions in Psychological Science, 30*(3), 251–259.

Holt-Lunstad, J., Robles, T. F., & Sbarra, D. A. (2017). Advancing social connection as a public health priority in the United States. *American Psychologist, 72*(6), 517–530.

Holt-Lunstad, J., Smith, T. B., & Layton, J. B. (2010). Social relationships and mortality risk: A meta-analytic review. *PLoS Medicine, 7*:e1000316.

Horner, R. H., & Carr, E. G. (1997). Behavioral support for students with severe disabilities: Functional assessment and comprehensive intervention. *The Journal of Special Education, 31*, 84–104.

Hostinar, C. E. (2015). Recent developments in the study of social relationships, stress responses, and physical health. *Current Opinion in Psychology, 5*, 90–95.

Houtrow, A., Elias, E. R., Davis, B. E., Kuo, D. Z., Agrawal, R., Davidson, L. F., Ellerbeck, K. A., Foster, J. E. A., Fremion, E., O'Connor Leppert, M., Saunders, B. S., Stille, C., Vargus-Adams, J., Yin, L., Norwood, K., Coleman, C., Mann, M. Y., Simpser, E., Poon, J., Yeargin-Allsopp, M., & Kuznetsov,

A. (2021). Promoting healthy sexuality for children and adolescents with disabilities. *Pediatrics, 148*(1).

Hübener, M., & Bonhoeffer, T. (2014). Neuronal plasticity: Beyond the critical period. *Cell, 159*(4), 727–737.

Huebner, A. J., & Howell, L. W. (2003). Examining the relationship between adolescent sexual risk-taking and perceptions of monitoring, communication, and parenting styles. *Journal of Adolescent Health, 33*(2), 71–78.

Hunter, M., McDowell, L., Hennessy, R., & Cassey, J. (2000). An evaluation of the Faces Pain Scale with young children. *Journal of Pain and Symptom Management, 20*(2), 122–129. https://doi.org/10.1016/S0885-3924(00)00171-8

Ikiugu, M. N., Plastow, N. A., & van Niekerk, L. (2019). Eclectic application of theoretical models in occupational therapy: Impact on therapeutic reasoning. *Occupational Therapy in Health Care, 33*(3), 286–305.

Ittyerah, M. (2013). *Hand preference and hand ability*. John Benjamins Publishing Co.

Iyanda, A. E. (2022). Bullying victimization of children with mental, emotional, and developmental or behavioral (MEDB) disorders in the United States. *Journal of Child & Adolescent Trauma, 15*(2), 221–233.

Jang, J., Dixon, D. R., Tarbox, J., & Granpeesheh, D. (2011). Symptom severity and challenging behavior in children with ASD. *Research in Autism Spectrum Disorders, 5*, 1028–1032.

Jethwa, A., Mink, J., Macarthur, C., Knights, S., Fehlings, T., & Fehlings, D. (2010). Development of the Hypertonia Assessment Tool (HAT): A discriminative tool for hypertonia in children. *Developmental Medicine and Child Neurology, 52*(5), e83–e87.

Johnson, J. A., Jakubovski, E., Reed, M. O., & Bloch, M. H. (2017). Predictors of long-term risky driving behavior in the multimodal treatment study of children with attention-deficit/hyperactivity disorder. *Journal of Child and Adolescent Psychopharmacology, 27*(8), 747–754.

Jordan, M. (2023). The power of connection: Self-care strategies of social wellbeing. *Journal of Interprofessional Education & Practice, 31*:100586.

Juan, H. G., & Swinth, Y. (2010). As students become adults: The role of occupational therapy in the transition process. *Journal of Occupational Therapy, Schools, & Early Intervention, 3*(3), 255–267.

Kaestle, C. E., Allen, K. R., Wesche, R., & Grafsky, E. L. (2021). Adolescent sexual development: A family perspective. *The Journal of Sex Research, 58*(7), 874–890.

Kamara, D., & Beauchaine, T. P. (2020). A review of sleep disturbances among infants and children with neurodevelopmental disorders. *Review Journal of Autism and Developmental Disorders, 7*, 278–294.

Kang, L. J., Palisano, R. J., Orlin, M. N., Chiarello, L. A., King, G. A., & Polansky, M. (2010). Determinants of social participation—with friends and others who are not family members—for youths with cerebral palsy. *Physical Therapy, 90*(12), 1743–1757.

Kennedy, J., Brown, T., & Chien, C. W. (2012). Motor skill assessment of children: Is there an association between performance-based, child-report, and parent-report measures of children's motor skills? *Physical & Occupational Therapy in Pediatrics, 32*(2), 196–209.

Kennedy, J., Brown, T., & Stagnitti, K. (2013). Top-down and bottom-up approaches to motor skill assessment of children: Are child-report and parent-report perceptions predictive of children's performance-based assessment results? *Scandinavian Journal of Occupational Therapy, 20*(1), 45–53.

Kent, C., Cordier, R., Joosten, A., Wilkes-Gillan, S., Bundy, A., & Speyer, R. (2020). A systematic review and meta-analysis of interventions to improve play skills in children with autism spectrum disorder. *Review Journal of Autism and Developmental Disorders, 7*, 91–118.

Khayatzadeh-Mahani, A., Wittevrongel, K., Nicholas, D. B., & Zwicker, J. D. (2020). Prioritizing barriers and solutions to improve employment for persons with developmental disabilities. *Disability & Rehabilitation, 42*(19), 2696–2706.

Kielhofner, G. (2008). *Model of human occupation: Theory and application* (4th ed.). Lippincott, Williams & Wilkins.

Kielhofner, G. (2004). The organization and use of knowledge. In *Conceptual foundations of occupational therapy*(3rd ed.) (pp. 10–26). FA Davis.

King, G., Law, M., King, S., Rosenbaum, P., Kertoy, M. K., & Young, N. L. (2003). A conceptual model of the factors affecting the recreation and leisure participation of children with disabilities. *Physical & Occupational Therapy in Pediatrics, 23*(1), 63–90.

King, G. A., Law, M., King, S., Hurley, P., Hanna, S., Kertoy, M., & Rosenbaum, P. (2007). Measuring children's participation in recreation and leisure activities: Construct validation of the CAPE and PAC. *Child: Care, Health and Development, 33*(1), 28–39.

Klingels, K., De Cock, P., Molenaers, G., Desloovere, K., Huenaerts, C., Jaspers, E., & Feys, H. (2010). Upper limb motor and sensory impairments in children with hemiplegic cerebral palsy. Can they be measured reliably? *Disability & Rehabilitation, 32*(5), 409–416.

Knights, S., Datoo, N., Kawamura, A., Switzer, L., & Fehlings, D. (2014). Further evaluation of the scoring, reliability, and validity of the Hypertonia Assessment Tool (HAT). *Journal of Child Neurology, 29*(4), 500–504.

Knox, S. (2008). Development and current use of the Revised Knox Preschool Play Scale. In L. D. Parham, & L. Fazio (Eds.), *Play in occupational therapy for children* (pp. 50–70). Elsevier.

Kolovelonis, A., Goudas, M., & Dermitzaki, I. (2012). The effects of self-talk and goal setting on self-regulation of learning a new motor skill in physical education. *International Journal of Sport and Exercise Psychology, 10*(3), 221–225.

Komarraju, M., & Nadler, D. (2013). Self-efficacy and academic achievement: Why do implicit beliefs, goals, and effort regulation matter? *Learning and Individual Differences, 25*, 67–72.

Kramer, J., ten Velden, M., Kafkes, A., Basu, S., Federico, J., & Kielhofner, G. (2014). *Child Occupational Self-Assessment (COSA) version 2.2*. Model of Human Occupation Clearinghouse. Department of Occupational Therapy. University of Illinois at Chicago. https://moho.irm.uic.edu.

Kramer, J. M., Coster, W. J., Kao, Y. C., Snow, A., & Orsmond, G. I. (2012). A new approach to the measurement of adaptive behavior: Development of the PEDI-CAT for children with youth with autism spectrum disorder. *Physical & Occupational Therapy in Pediatrics, 32*, 34–47.

Kuhaneck, H. M., Burroughs, T., Wright, J., Lemanczyk, T., & Darragh, A. R. (2010). A qualitative study of coping in mothers of children with an autism spectrum disorder. *Physical & Occupational Therapy in Pediatrics, 30*(4), 340–350.

Kuhaneck, H. M., & Kelleher, J. (2015). Development of the classroom sensory environment assessment (CSEA). *American Journal of Occupational Therapy, 69*(6):6906180040p1–6906180040p9.

Kuhaneck, H. M., & Kelleher, J. (2018). The classroom sensory environment assessment as an educational tool for teachers. *Journal of Occupational Therapy, Schools, & Early Intervention, 11*(2), 161–171.

Kuhaneck, H., & Spitzer, S. (2023). *Making play just right: Unleashing the power of play in occupational therapy* (2nd ed.). Jones and Bartlett Learning.

Kuhaneck, H., & Spitzer, S. L. (2024). The importance of conceptual origins: The case of the just-right challenge. *American Journal of Occupational Therapy, 78*(4), 7804185110. https://doi.org/10.5014/ajot.2024.050619. PMID: 38889183.

Kuhaneck, H. M., Spitzer, S. L., & Miller, E. (2010). *Activity analysis, creativity and playfulness in pediatric occupational therapy: Making play just right*. Jones & Bartlett Learning.

Kula, L. (2016). Assistive technology solutions for school aged children. *Illinois Occupational Therapy Association Newsletter, 3*, 9–11.

Kwan, C., Gitimoghaddam, M., & Collet, J. P. (2020). Effects of social isolation and loneliness in children with neurodevelopmental disabilities: A scoping review. *Brain Sciences, 10*(11), 786.

Lalor, A., Brown, T., & Murdolo, Y. (2016). Relationship between children's performance-based motor skills and child, parent, and teacher perceptions of children's motor abilities using self/informant-report questionnaires. *Australian Occupational Therapy Journal, 63*(2), 105–116.

Lau, C. (2015). Development of suck and swallow mechanisms in infants. *Annals of Nutrition and Metabolism, 66*(Suppl. 5), 7–14.

Laud, R. B., Girolami, P. A., Boscoe, J. H., & Gulotta, C. S. (2009). Treatment outcomes for severe feeding problems in children with autism spectrum disorder. *Behavior Modification, 33*(5), 520–536.

Lautamo, T., Kottorp, A., & Salminen, A. L. (2005). Play assessment for group settings: A pilot study to construct an assessment tool.

*Scandinavian Journal of Occupational Therapy, 12*(3), 136–144. https://doi.org/10.1080/11038120510031798. PMID: 16389739.

Law, M., Baptiste, S., Carsell, A., McColl, M. A., Polatajko, H., & Pollock, N. (2005). *Canadian occupational performance measure* (4th ed.). CAOT Publications ACE.

Levine, J. B. (1988). Play in the context of the family. *Journal of Family Psychology, 2*(2), 164–187.

Li, J., Cao, D., Huang, Y., Chen, Z., Wang, R., Dong, Q., Wei, Q., & Liu, L. (2021). Sleep duration and health outcomes: An umbrella review. *Sleep and Breathing*, 1–23.

Lim, V. H. T., Chen, Y. W. R., Tseng, M. H., Bundy, A., & Cordier, R. (2021). The impact of caregiver stigma on real-life social experience of Taiwanese adolescents with autism spectrum disorder. *Autism, 25*(7), 1859–1871.

Linder, T. W., Anthony, T. L., Bundy, A. C., Charlifue-Smith, R., Hafer, J. C., & Rooke, C. C. (2008). *Transdisciplinary play-based assessment (2nd ed.; TPBA 2)*. Paul H. Brooks.

Lipschultz, J. L., & Wilder, D. A. (2017). Behavioral assessment and treatment of noncompliance: A review of the literature. *Education & Treatment of Children, 40*, 263–298.

Liu, R., Dong, H., Wang, Y., Lu, X., Li, Y., Xun, G., … Zhao, J. (2021). Sleep problems of children with autism may independently affect parental quality of life. *Child Psychiatry and Human Development, 52*, 488–499.

Llorens, L. A. (1982). *Application of developmental theory for health and rehabilitation*. American Occupational Therapy Association.

Longo, E., Regalado, I. C. R., Galvão, E. R. V. P., Ferreira, H. N. C., Badia, M., & Baz, B. O. (2020). I want to play: Children with cerebral palsy talk about their experiences on barriers and facilitators to participation in leisure activities. *Pediatric Physical Therapy, 32*(3), 190–200.

Lynch, H., Moore, A., Edwards, C., & Horgan, L. (2020). Advancing play participation for all: The challenge of addressing play diversity and inclusion in community parks and playgrounds. *British Journal of Occupational Therapy, 83*(2), 107–117.

Lynch, H., Moore, A., & Prellwitz, M. (2018). From policy to play provision: Universal design and the challenges of inclusive play. *Children, Youth, and Environments, 28*(2), 12–34.

Mack, W., Lindquist, J. E., & Parham, L. D. (1982). A synthesis of occupational behavior and sensory integration concepts in theory and practice, Part 1. Theoretical foundations. *American Journal of Occupational Therapy, 36*(6), 365–374.

MacRae, N. (2013). *Sexuality and the role of occupational therapy*. American Occupational Therapy Association. https://www.aota.org/About-Occupational Therapy/Professionals/RDP/Sexuality.aspx.

Mahler, K. J. (2019). *The interoception curriculum: A step-by-step framework for developing mindful self-regulation*. Mahler Autism Services.

Maihafer, G. C., Llewellyn, M. A., Pillar, W. J., Jr., Scott, K. L., Marino, D. M., & Bond, R. M. (2003). A comparison of the figure-of-eight method and water volumetry in measurement of hand and wrist size. *Journal of Hand Therapy, 16*(4), 305–310.

Mailloux, Z., Mulligan, S., Roley, S. S., Blanche, E., Cermak, S., Coleman, G. G., Bodison, S., & Lane, C. J. (2011). Verification and clarification of patterns of sensory integrative dysfunction. *American Journal of Occupational Therapy, 65*(2), 143–151. https://doi.org/10.5014/ajot.2011.00075

Mamas, C., Daly, A. J., Cohen, S. R., & Jones, G. (2021). Social participation of students with autism spectrum disorder in general education settings. *Learning, Culture and Social Interaction, 28*:100467.

Mandich, A., Polatajko, H., Miller, L., & Baum, C. M. (2004). *The Pediatric Activity Card Sort (PACS)*. Canadian Occupational Therapy Association.

Mandolesi, L., Gelfo, F., Serra, L., Monuori, S., Polverino, A., Curcio, G., & Sorrentino, G. (2017). Environmental factors promoting neural plasticity: Insights from animal and human studies. *Neural Plasticity, 2017*. https://doi.org/10.1155/2017/7219461.

Manor-Binyamini, I., & Schreiber-Divon, M. (2019). Parental perceptions of the sexuality of adolescents with intellectual disabilities. *Sexuality and Disability, 37*(4), 599–612.

Marcus, S., & Breton, S. (2022a). Development of oral-motor skills. In S. Marcus, & S. Breton (Eds.), *Infant and child feeding and swallowing: Occupational therapy assessment and intervention* (2nd ed.) (pp. 7–17). AOTA Press.

Marsack-Topolewski, C. N. (2021). Relationship between caregiver burden and basic and instrumental activities of daily living among compound and non compound caregivers. *Journal of Family Social Work, 24*(4), 299–319.

Marsack-Topolewski, C. N., Samuel, P. S., & Tarraf, W. (2021). Empirical evaluation of the association between daily living skills of adults with autism and parental caregiver burden. *PLoS One, 16*(1):e0244844.

Martin, C. A., Papadopoulos, N., Chellew, T., Rinehart, N. J., & Sciberras, E. (2019). Associations between parenting stress, parent mental health and child sleep problems for children with ADHD and ASD: Systematic review. *Research in Developmental Disabilities, 93*:103463.

Martin, C. A., Sciberras, E., Papadopoulos, N., Engel, L., Hiscock, H., Williams, K., Howlin, P., McGillivray, J., & Rinehart, N. J. (2021). Associations between child sleep problem severity and maternal well-being in children with autism spectrum disorder. *Journal of Autism and Developmental Disorders, 51*, 2500–2510.

Martini, R., Cramm, H., Egan, M., & Sikora, L. (2016). Scoping review of self-regulation: What are occupational therapists talking about? *American Journal of Occupational Therapy, 70*:7006290010.

Martini, R., & Polatajko, H. J. (1998). Verbal self-guidance as a treatment approach for children with developmental coordination disorder: A systematic replication study. *Occupational Therapy Journal of Research, 18*(4), 157–181.

Marx, R. G., Bombardier, C., & Wright, J. G. (1999). What do we know about the reliability and validity of physical examination tests used to examine the upper extremity? *The Journal of Hand Surgery, 24*(1), 185–193.

Mathiowetz, V., Weber, K., Volland, G., & Kashman, N. (1984). Reliability and validity of grip and pinch strength evaluations. *The Journal of Hand Surgery, 9*(2), 222–226.

Matricciani, L., Paquet, C., Galland, B., Short, M., & Olds, T. (2019). Children's sleep and health: A meta-review. *Sleep Medicine Reviews, 46*, 136–150.

Matson, J. L., Mahan, S., Hess, J. A., Fodstad, J. C., & Neal, D. (2010). Progression of challenging behaviors in children and adolescents with Autism Spectrum Disorders as measured by the Autism Spectrum Disorders-Problem Behaviors for Children (ASD-PBC). *Research in Autism Spectrum Disorders, 4*(3), 400–404.

Matson, J. L., & Minshawi, N. F. (2006). *Early intervention for autism spectrum disorders: A critical analysis*. Elsevier.

Matson, J. L., & Nebel-Schwalm, M. (2007). Assessing challenging behaviors in children with autism spectrum disorders: A review. *Research in Developmental Disabilities, 28*, 567–579.

Matson, J. L., Rivet, T. T., Fodstad, J. C., Dempsey, T., & Boisjoli, J. A. (2009). Examination of adaptive behavior differences in adults with autism spectrum disorders and intellectual disability. *Research in Developmental Disabilities, 30*(6), 1317–1325.

Matson, J. L., Sipes, M., Horovitz, M., Worley, J. A., Shoemaker, M. E., & Kozlowski, A. M. (2011). Behaviors and corresponding functions addressed via functional assessment. *Research in Developmental Disabilities, 32*(2), 625–629.

May-Benson, T. (2001). A theoretical model of ideation in praxis. In E. Blanche, S. Roley, & R. Schaaf (Eds.), *Sensory integration and developmental disabilities* (pp. 163–181). Therapy Skill Builders.

Mazzotti, V. L., Rowe, D. A., Kwiatek, S., Voggt, A., Chang, W. H., Fowler, C. H., Poppen, M., Sinclair, J., & Test, D. W. (2021). Secondary transition predictors of postschool success: An update to the research base. *Career Development and Transition for Exceptional Individuals, 44*(1), 47–64.

McDonald, A. E., & Vigen, C. (2012). Reliability and validity of the McDonald Play Inventory. *American Journal of Occupational Therapy, 66*(4), e52–e60. https://doi.org/10.5014/ajot.2012.002493. PMID: 22742701.

McGill, T., & Vogtle, L. K. (2001). Driver's education for students with physical disabilities. *Exceptional Children, 67*(4), 455–466.

McMahon, R. J., & Forehand, R. L. (2003). *Helping the noncompliant child: Family-based treatment for oppositional behavior* (2nd ed.). Guilford Press.

McQuiddy, V. A., Scheerer, C. R., Lavalley, R., McGrath, T., & Lin, L. (2015). Normative values for grip and pinch strength for 6- to 19-year-olds. *Archives of Physical Medicine and Rehabilitation, 96*(9), 1627–1633.

Melo, B., Araújo, R., Azevedo, M. J., Amorim, R., & Palhau, L. (2021). Management of sialorrhea in children. *Pediatric Oncall Journal, 18*. https://doi.org/10.7199/ped.oncall.2021.28.

Meltzer, L. J., Forrest, C. B., de la Motte, A., & Bevans, K. B. (2020). Clinical validity of the PROMIS pediatric sleep measures across populations of children with chronic illnesses and neurodevelopment disorders. *Journal of Pediatric Psychology, 45*(3), 319–327.

Meltzer, L. J., Williamson, A. A., & Mindell, J. A. (2021). Pediatric sleep health: It matters, and so does how we define it. *Sleep Medicine Reviews, 57*:101425.

Menard-Katcher, C., Henry, M., Furuta, G. T., Atkins, D., Maune, N. C., & Haas, A. M. (2014). Significance of feeding dysfunction in eosinophilic esophagitis. *World Journal of Gastroenterology, 20*(31), 11019–11022.

Miller, L. T., Polatajko, H. J., Missiuna, C., Mandich, A. D., & Macnab, J. J. (2001). A pilot trial of a cognitive treatment for children with developmental coordination disorder. *Human Movement Science, 20*, 183–210.

Mills, C., & Chapparo, C. (2017). Use of perceive, recall, plan, perform stage two cognitive task analysis for students with autism and intellectual disability: The impact of a sensory activity schedule. *Journal of Occupational Therapy, Schools, & Early Intervention, 10*(3), 232–253.

Milteer, R. M., Ginsburg, K. R., Council on Communications and Media, Committee on Psychosocial Aspects of Child and Family Health, Mulligan, D. A., Ameenuddin, N., Brown, A., Christakis, D. A., Cross, C., Falik, H. L., Hill, D. L., Hogan, M. J., Levine, A. E., O'Keeffe, G. S., Swanson, W. S., Siegel, B. S., Dobbins, M. I., Earls, M. F., Garner, A. S., McGuinn, L., Pascoe, J., & Wood, D. L. (2012). The importance of play in promoting healthy child development and maintaining strong parent-child bond: Focus on children in poverty. *Pediatrics, 129*(1), e204–e213.

Mindell, J. A., Li, A. M., Sadeh, A., Kwon, R., & Goh, D. Y. (2015). Bedtime routines for young children: A dose-dependent association with sleep outcomes. *Sleep, 38*(5), 717–722.

Missiuna, C. (1998). Development of "All About Me," a scale that measures children's perceived motor competence. *The Occupational Therapy Journal of Research, 18*(2), 85–108.

Missiuna, C., Mandich, A. D., Polatajko, H. J., & Malloy-Miller, T. (2001). Cognitive orientation to daily occupational performance (CO-OP): Part I—theoretical foundations. *Physical & Occupational Therapy in Pediatrics, 20*(2-3), 69–81.

Molenaar, H. M., Zuidam, J. M., Selles, R. W., Stam, H. J., & Hovius, S. E. (2008). Age-specific reliability of two grip-strength dynamometers when used by children. *Journal of Bone and Joint Surgery American Volume, 90*(5), 1053–1059.

Moore, A., & Lynch, H. (2018). Play and play occupation: A survey of paediatric occupational therapy practice in Ireland. *Irish Journal of Occupational Therapy, 46*(1), 59–72.

Moore, A., Lynch, H., & Boyle, B. (2022). Can universal design support outdoor play, social participation, and inclusion in public playgrounds? A scoping review. *Disability & Rehabilitation, 44*(13), 3304–3325.

Morawska, A., Walsh, A., Grabski, M., & Fletcher, R. (2015). Parental confidence and preferences for communicating with their child about sexuality. *Sex Education, 15*(3), 235–248.

Morris, S. E., & Klein, M. D. (2000). *Prefeeding skills* (2nd ed., p. 49). Tucson, Az: Therapy Skill Builders.

Morrissey, B., Taveras, E., Allender, S., & Strugnell, C. (2020). Sleep and obesity among children: A systematic review of multiple sleep dimensions. *Pediatric Obesity, 15*(4):e12619.

Mosey, A. C. (1986). *Psychosocial components of occupational therapy*. Rover.

Mueller, C. (2019). Adolescent understandings of disability labels and social stigma in school. *International Journal of Qualitative Studies in Education, 32*(3), 263–281.

Mukkada, V. A., Haas, A., Maune, N. C., Capocelli, K. E., Henry, M., Gilman, N., Petersburg, S., Moore, W., Lovell, M. A., Fleischer, D. M., Furuta, G. T., & Atkins, D. (2010). Feeding dysfunction in children with eosinophilic gastrointestinal diseases. *Pediatrics, 126*(3), e672–e677.

Mulligan, S. (1998). Patterns of sensory integration dysfunction: A confirmatory factor analysis. *American Journal of Occupational Therapy, 52*, 819–828.

Mulligan, S. (2000). Cluster analysis of scores of children on the Sensory Integration and Praxis tests. *Occupational Therapy Journal of Research, 20*, 256–270.

Mulligan, S. (2011). Validity of the postrotary nystagmus test for measuring vestibular function. *Occupation, Participation, and Health, 31*(2), 97–104.

National Sexual Violence Resource Center (NSVRS). (2013). *An overview of health childhood sexual development*. https://www.nsvrc.org/sites/default/files/2013-01/saam_2013_an-overview-of-healthy-childhood-sexual-development.pdf.

National Sleep Foundation. (2024). https://www.sleepfoundation.org/sleep-hygiene

Neff, K. (2003). Understanding how universal goals of independence and interdependence are manifested within particular cultural contexts. *Human Development, 46*(5), 312–318.

Nelson, K. L., Davis, J. E., & Corbett, C. F. (2022). Sleep quality: An evolutionary concept analysis. *Nursing Forum, 57*(1), 144–151.

Newman, L. A. (2004). A national study of parent involvement in education of youth with disabilities. In *Promising practices connecting schools to families of children with special needs* (pp. 25–39). https://files.eric.ed.gov/fulltext/ED489979.pdf.

Nijhof, S. L., Vinkers, C. H., van Geelen, S. M., Duijff, S. N., Achterberg, E. J. M., van der Net, J., Veltkamp, R. C., Grootenhuis, M. A., van de Putte, E. M., Hillegers, M. H. J., van der Brug, A. W., Wierenga, C. J., Benders, M. J. N. L., Engels, R. C. M. E., van der Ent, C. K., Vanderschuren, L. J. M. J., & Lesscher, H. M. B. (2018). Healthy play, better coping: The importance of play for the development of children in health and disease. *Neuroscience & Biobehavioral Reviews, 95*, 421–429.

Nordström, B., Lynch, H., & Prellwitz, M. (2023). Physio- and occupational therapists view of the place of play in re/habilitation: A Swedish perspective. *International Journal of Disability, Development and Education, 70*(2), 228–239.

Norkin, W. (2009). *Measurement of joint motion: A guide to goniometry* (4th ed.). FA Davis.

O'Brien, J. (2015). Application of motor control/motor learning to practice. In J. Case-Smith, & J. O'Brien (Eds.), *Occupational therapy for children and adolescents* (7th ed.) (pp. 193–219). Elsevier.

O'Brien, J., & Wolske, J. (2024). Examining the dynamics of human occupation. In R. Taylor, P. Bowyer, & G. Fisher (Eds.), *Kielhofner's Model of Human Occupation: Theory and application* (6th ed.). Wolters Kluwer.

O'Brien, J. C., & Soloman, J. W. (2022). *Occupational analysis and group process* (2nd ed.). Elsevier.

O'Connor, D., Lynch, H., & Boyle, B. (2021). A qualitative study of child participation in decision-making: Exploring rights-based approaches in pediatric occupational therapy. *PLoS One, 16*(12):e0260975.

Omoigui, S. (2007). The biochemical origin of pain--proposing a new law of pain: The origin of all pain is inflammation and the inflammatory response. Part 1 of 3--A unifying law of pain. *Medical Hypotheses, 69*(1), 70–82.

Ophoff, D., Slaats, M. A., Boudewyns, A., Glazemakers, I., Van Hoorenbeeck, K., & Verhulst, S. L. (2018). Sleep disorders during childhood: A practical review. *European Journal of Pediatrics, 177*, 641–648.

Orentlicher, M. L., & Case, D. (2018). Intervention for participation in IADLs and independent living for individuals with ASD. In R. Watling, & S. L. Spitzer (Eds.), *Autism across the lifespan: A comprehensive occupational therapy approach* (4th ed.) (pp. 287–303). AOTA Press.

Ostry, D. J., & Gribble, P. L. (2016). Sensory plasticity in human motor learning. *Trends in Neurosciences, 39*(2), 114–123.

Papadopoulos, C., Lodder, A., Constantinou, G., & Randhawa, G. (2019). Systematic review of the relationship between autism stigma and informal caregiver mental health. *Journal of Autism and Developmental Disorders, 49*, 1665–1685.

Parham, L. D. (1998). The relationship of sensory integrative development to achievement in elementary students: Four-year longitudinal patterns. *Occupational Therapy Journal of Research, 18*(3), 105–127.

Parham, L. D. (2002). Sensory integration and occupation. In A. C. Bundy, S. J. Lane, & E. A. Murray (Eds.), *Sensory integration: Theory and practice* (2nd ed.) (pp. 413–434). F. A. Davis.

Parham, L. D., Ecker, C. L., Kuhaneck, H., Henry, D. A., & Glennon, T. J. (2021). *Sensory processing measure (2nd ed.; SPMTM-2) [Manual]*. Western Psychological Services.

Pariseau, E. M., Chevalier, L., Long, K. A., Clapham, R., Edwards-Leeper, L., & Tishelman, A. C. (2019). The relationship between family acceptance-rejection and transgender youth psychosocial functioning. *Clinical Practice in Pediatric Psychology*, *7*(3), 267.

Park, K. L., & Scott, T. M. (2009). Antecedent-based interventions for young children at risk for emotional and behavioral disorders. *Behavioral Disorders*, *34*, 196–211.

Parks, S. (2004). *Inside HELP: Hawaii Early Learning Profile: Administration and reference manual.* VORT Corporation.

Pearson. (2022). *Staying connected through telepractice.* https://www.pearsonassessments.com/professional-assessments/digital-solutions/telepractice/about.html.

Parush, S., Sohmer, H., Steinberg, A., & Kaitz, M. (1997). Somatosensory functioning in children with attention deficit hyperactivity disorder. *Developmental Medicine and Child Neurology*, *39*(7), 464–468. https://doi.org/10.1111/j.1469-8749.1997.tb07466.x. PMID: 9285437.

Pearson. (2021a). *Telepractice and questionnaires or rating scales.* https://www.pearsonassessments.com/content/dam/school/global/clinical/us/assets/telepractice/guidance-documents/telepractice-and-questionnaires-or-rating-scales.pdf.

Pearson. (2021b). *Telepractice and the Bayley-4.* https://www.pearsonassessments.com/content/dam/school/global/clinical/us/assets/telepractice/guidance-documents/telepractice-and-the-bayley-4.pdf.

Pearson. (2021c). *Telepractice and the Beery VMI.* https://www.pearsonassessments.com/content/dam/school/global/clinical/us/assets/telepractice/guidance-documents/telepractice-and-the-beery-vmi.pdf.

Pearson. (2021d). *Telepractice and the BOT-2.* https://www.pearsonassessments.com/content/dam/school/global/clinical/us/assets/telepractice/guidance-documents/telepractice-and-the-bot-2.pdf.

Persson-Bunke, M., Hägglund, G., Lauge-Pedersen, H., Wagner, P., & Westbom, L. (2012). Scoliosis in a total population of children with cerebral palsy. *Spine*, *37*(12), e708–e713.

Pétursdottir, A. I., Esch, J. W., Sautter, R. A., & Stewart, K. K. (2010). Characteristics and hypothesized functions of challenging behavior in a community-based sample. *Education and Training in Autism and Developmental Disabilities*, *45*(1), 81–93.

Piontelli, A., Ceriani, F., Fabietti, I., Fogliani, R., Restelli, E., & Kustermann, A. (2015). Fetal sensory abilities. In *Development of normal fetal movements* (pp. 111–126). Springer.

Pless, M., & Carlsson, M. (2000). Effects of motor skill intervention on developmental coordination disorder: A meta-analysis. *Adapted Physical Activity Quarterly*, *17*(4), 381–401.

Polatajko, H. J., Mandich, A., & Martini, R. (2000). Dynamic performance analysis: A framework for understanding occupational performance. *American Journal of Occupational Therapy*, *54*, 65–72.

Pountney, T. E., Mandy, A., Green, E., & Gard, P. R. (2009). Hip subluxation and dislocation in cerebral palsy—A prospective study on the effectiveness of postural management programmes. *Physiotherapy Research International*, *14*(2), 116–127.

Powrie, B., Copley, J., Turpin, M., Ziviani, J., & Kolehmainen, N. (2020). The meaning of leisure to children and young people with significant physical disabilities: Implications for optimising participation. *British Journal of Occupational Therapy*, *83*(2), 67–77.

Prendergast, L. E., Toumbourou, J. W., McMorris, B. J., & Catalano, R. F. (2019). Outcomes of early adolescent sexual behavior in Australia: Longitudinal findings in young adulthood. *Journal of Adolescent Health*, *64*(4), 516–522.

Price, M. N., & Hyde, J. S. (2009). When two isn't better than one: Predictors of early sexual activity in adolescence using a cumulative risk model. *Journal of Youth and Adolescence*, *38*, 1059–1071.

Prosser, R., Harvey, L., LaStayo, P., Hargreaves, I., Scougall, P., & Herbert, R. D. (2011). Provocative wrist tests and MRI are of limited diagnostic value for suspected wrist ligament injuries: A cross-sectional study. *Journal of Physiotherapy*, *57*(4), 247–253.

Raeff, C. (2010). Independence and interdependence in children's developmental experiences. *Child Development Perspectives*, *4*(1), 31–36.

Raina, P., O'Donnell, M., Rosenbaum, P., Brehaut, J., Walter, S. D., Russell, D., Swinton, M., Zhu, B., & Wood, E. (2005). The health and well-being of caregivers of children with cerebral palsy. *Pediatrics*, *115*(6), e626–e636.

Raina, P., O'Donnell, M., Schwellnus, H., Rosenbaum, P., King, G., Brehaut, J., Russell, D., Swinton, M., King, S., Wong, M., Walter, S. D., & Wood, E. (2004). Caregiving process and caregiver burden: Conceptual models to guide research and practice. *BMC Pediatrics*, *4*, 1–13.

Ramar, K., Malhotra, R. K., Carden, K. A., Martin, J. L., Abbasi-Feinberg, F., Aurora, R. N., Kapur, V. K., Olson, E. J., Rosen, C. J., Rowley, J. A., Shelgikar, A. V., & Trotti, L. M. (2021). Sleep is essential to health: An American Academy of sleep medicine position statement. *Journal of Clinical Sleep Medicine*, *17*(10), 2115–2119.

Ratzon, N. Z., Lunievsky, E. K., Ashkenasi, A., Laks, J., & Cohen, H. A. (2017). Simulated driving skills evaluation of teenagers with attention deficit hyperactivity disorder before driving lessons. *American Journal of Occupational Therapy*, *71*:7103220010.

Ray-Kaeser, S., & Lynch, H. (2017). Occupational therapy perspective on play for the sake of play. In S. Besio, D. Bulgarelli, & V. Stancheva-Popkostadinova (Eds.), *Play development in children with disabilities* (pp. 155–165). De Gruyter.

Ream, G. L., & Savin-Williams, R. C. (2005). Reciprocal associations between adolescent sexual activity and quality of youth-parent interactions. *Journal of Family Psychology*, *19*(2), 171.

Reese, N. B., & Bandy, W. D. (2009). *Joint range of motion and muscle length testing* (2nd ed.). Saunders.

Reese, R. M., Richman, D. M., Belmont, J. M., & Morse, P. (2005). Functional characteristics of disruptive behavior in developmentally disabled children with and without autism. *Journal of Autism and Developmental Disorders*, *35*, 419–428.

Research.com. (2023). Why is education important to individuals and societies? https://research.com/education/why-is-education-important.

Rheingold, H. L. (1982). Little children's participation in the work of adults, a nascent prosocial behavior. *Child Development*, 114–125.

Richards, J., Nazareth, M., van Tilburg, M. A. L., Jain, N., Hart, L., Faldowski, R. A., Coltrane, C., Hooper, S. R., Ferris, M., & Rak, E. (2021). Engagement in household chores in youth with chronic conditions. Health care transition implications. *OTJR: Occupation, Participation and Health*, *41*(1), 6–14.

Robinson, K. H., Smith, E., & Davies, C. (2017). Responsibilities, tensions and ways forward: Parents' perspectives on children's sexuality education. *Sex Education*, *17*(3), 333–347.

Rodger, S., Ireland, S., & Vun, M. (2008). Can Cognitive Orientation to daily Occupational Performance (CO-OP) help children with Asperger's syndrome to master social and organisational goals? *British Journal of Occupational Therapy*, *71*(1), 23–32.

Rodger, S., Springfield, E., & Polatajko, H. (2007). Cognitive orientation for daily occupational performance approach for children with Asperger's syndrome: A case report. *Physical & Occupational Therapy in Pediatrics*, *27*(4), 7–22.

Rogoff, B. (2014). Learning by observing and pitching in to family and community endeavors: An orientation. *Human Development*, *57*(2–3), 69–81.

Romli, M., & Wan Yunus, F. (2020). A systematic review on clinimetric properties of play instruments for occupational therapy practice. *Occupational Therapy International*, *2020*, 1–19.

Roosevelt, E. (2008). Good citizenship: The purpose of education. *Teachers College Record*, *110*(14), 312–320.

Rosado-May, F. J., Urrieta, L., Dayton, A., & Rogoff, B. (2020). Innovation as a key feature of indigenous ways of learning: Individuals and communities generating knowledge. In *Handbook of the cultural foundations of learning* (pp. 79–96). Routledge.

Rosenberg, L., Moran, A., & Bart, O. (2017). The associations among motor ability, social-communication skills, and participation in daily life activities in children with low-functioning autism spectrum disorder. *Journal of Occupational Therapy, Schools, & Early Intervention*, *10*(2), 137–146.

Rouse, M. W., Borsting, E., Hyman, L., Hussein, M., Cotter, S. A., Flynn, M., Scheiman, M., Gallaway, M., & De Land, P. N. (1999). Frequency of convergence insufficiency among fifth and sixth graders. *Optometry and Vision Science*, *76*(9), 643–649.

Rybski, M. (2024a). Biomechanical approach. In *Kinesiology for occupational therapy*(3rd ed.) (pp. 323–366). Routledge.

Rybski, M. (2024b). Rehabilitation approach. In *Kinesiology for occupational therapy*(3rd ed.) (pp. 367–438). Routledge.

Sabella, S. A., & Bezyak, J. L. (2019). Barriers to public transportation and employment: A national survey of individuals with disabilities. *Journal of Applied Rehabilitation Counseling, 50*(3), 174–185.

Sale, A., Berardi, N., & Maffei, L. (2014). Environment and brain plasticity: Towards an endogenous pharmacotherapy. *Physiological Reviews, 94*(1), 189–234.

Sanches-Ferreira, M., Alves, S., Gomes, M., Santos, B., & Lopes-dos-Santos, P. (2019). Participation in leisure activities as an indicator of inclusion: A comparison between children with and without disabilities in Portugal. *European Journal of Educational Research, 8*(1), 221–232.

Sandoval, G. A., & McKee, A. (2020). When special education and disability studies intertwine: Addressing educational inequities through processes and programming. *Frontiers in Education, 5*:587045.

Scheiman, M. (2011). *Understanding and managing vision deficits: A guide for occupational therapists* (3rd ed.). Slack.

Schkade, J. K., & Schultz, S. (2003). Occupational adaptation. In P. Kramer, J. Hinojosa, & C. B. Royeen (Eds.), *Perspectives in human occupation: Participation in life* (pp. 182–221). Lippincott Williams, & Wilkins.

Schleien, S. J., Miller, K. D., Walton, G., & Pruett, S. (2014). Parent perspectives of barriers to child participation in recreational activities. *Therapeutic Recreation Journal, 48*(1), 61–73.

Schneider, E., & Rosenblum, S. (2014). Development, reliability, and validity of the My Child's Play (MCP) questionnaire. *American Journal of Occupational Therapy, 68*(3), 277–285. https://doi.org/10.5014/ajot.2014.009159. PMID: 24797191.

Scholz, J., Allemang-Grand, R., Dazai, J., & Lerch, J. P. (2015). Environmental enrichment is associated with rapid volumetric brain changes in adult mice. *NeuroImage, 109*, 190–198.

Scott, A. J., Webb, T. L., Martyn-St James, M., Rowse, G., & Weich, S. (2021). Improving sleep quality leads to better mental health: A meta-analysis of randomised controlled trials. *Sleep Medicine Reviews, 60*:101556.

Sharp, W. G., Silverman, A., Arvedson, J. C., Bandstra, N. F., Clawson, E., Berry, R. C., McElhanon, B. O., Kozlowski, A. M., Katz, M., Volkert, V. M., Goday, P. S., & Lukens, C. T. (2022). Toward better understanding of pediatric feeding disorder: A proposed framework for patient characterization. *Journal of Pediatric Gastroenterology and Nutrition, 75*(3), 351.

Shattnawi, K. K., Al Ali, N., Almanasreh, A. A. A., & Al–Motlaq, M. A. (2023). Caregiver burden among parents of children with chronic diseases: A cross–sectional study. *Journal of Clinical Nursing.*

Shea, L. L., Verstreate, K., Nonnemacher, S., Song, W., & Salzer, M. S. (2021). Self-reported community participation experiences and preferences of autistic adults. *Autism, 25*(5), 1295–1306.

Sherrick, M. (2004). Sexuality and the initial occupational therapy assessment for adults with physical disabilities. https://core.ac.uk/download/pdf/235073601.pdf.

Shin, J., Decker, B., & Blanchard, S. (2021). Instrumental activities of daily living in pediatric occupational therapy practice: A survey of current practice patterns and perceived importance. *Physical & Occupational Therapy in Pediatrics, 42*(1), 46–61.

Short, M. A., Bartel, K., & Carskadon, M. A. (2019). Sleep and mental health in children and adolescents. In *Sleep and health* (pp. 435–445). Academic Press.

Sitlington, P. L., Neubert, D. A., Begun, W. H., Lombard, R. C., & Leconte, P. J. (2007). *Assess for success: A practitioner's handbook on transition assessment* (2nd ed.). Corwin Press.

Skard, G., & Bundy, A. C. (2008). Test of playfulness. In L. D. Parham, & L. S. Fazio (Eds.), *Play in occupational therapy for children* (2nd ed.) (pp. 71–93). Elsevier.

Skirven, T. M., Osterman, A. L., Fedorczyk, J., Amadio, P. C., Felder, S., & Shin, E. K. (2020). *Rehabilitation of the hand and upper extremity*. Elsevier Health Sciences.

Smith, A. M., & Grzywacz, J. G. (2014). Health and well-being in midlife parents of children with special health needs. *Families, Systems & Health, 32*(3), 303.

Song, J., Mailick, M. R., & Greenberg, J. S. (2018). Health of parents of individuals with developmental disorders or mental health problems: Impacts of stigma. *Social Science & Medicine, 217*, 152–158.

Spagrud, L. J., Piira, T., & von Baeyer, C. L. (2003). Children's self-report of pain intensity: The Faces Pain Scale - Revised. *American Journal of Nursing, 103*(12), 62–64.

Speyer, R., Cordier, R., Kim, J. H., Cocks, N., Michou, E., & Wilkes-Gillan, S. (2019). Prevalence of drooling, swallowing, and feeding problems in cerebral palsy across the lifespan: A systematic review and meta-analyses. *Developmental Medicine and Child Neurology, 61*(11), 1249–1258.

Spitzer, S., & Roley, S. S. (2001). Sensory integration revisited: A philosophy of practice. In S. S. Roley, E. I. Blanche, & R. C. Schaaf (Eds.), *Understanding the nature of sensory integration with diverse populations* (pp. 3–27). Therapy Skill Builders.

Spruyt, K. (2019). A review of developmental consequences of poor sleep in childhood. *Sleep Medicine, 60*, 3–12.

Stafler, P., Akel, K., Eshel, Y., Shimoni, A., Grozovski, S., Mei-Zahav, M., Levine, H., Gendler, Y., Blau, H., & Prais, D. (2022). Videofluoroscopy compared with clinical feeding evaluation in children with suspected aspiration. *Acta Paediatrica, 111*(7), 1441–1449.

Stagnitti, K. (2020). *The Child-Initiated Pretend Play Assessment (2nd ed.; ChIPPA 2)*. Learn to Play. https://www.learntoplayevents.com/product/child-initiated-pretend-play-assessment-2-chippa-2-kit/.

Steinhardt, F., Ullenhag, A., Jahnsen, R., & Dolva, A. S. (2021). Perceived facilitators and barriers for participation in leisure activities in children with disabilities: Perspectives of children, parents and professionals. *Scandinavian Journal of Occupational Therapy, 28*(2), 121–135.

Surrey, L. R., Hodson, J., Robinson, E., Schmidt, S., Schulhof, J., Stoll, L., & Wilson-Diekhoff, N. (2001). Pinch strength norms for 5- to 12-year-olds. *Physical & Occupational Therapy in Pediatrics, 21*(1), 37–49.

Swaminathan, A., & Nandgaonkar, H. P. (2016). Effect of fostering self-regulation in children with attention deficit hyperactivity disorder. *Indian Journal of Occupational Therapy, 48*(3), 79–83.

Tamm, A., Kasearu, K., Tulviste, T., Trommsdorff, G., & Saralieva, Z. K. M. (2017). Helping parents with chores or going out with friends: Cultural differences in adolescents' responses to potentially conflicting expectations of parents and peers. *Journal of Adolescent Research, 32*(4), 456–478.

Taub, T., & Werner, S. (2023). Perspectives of adolescents with disabilities and their parents regarding autonomous decision-making and self-determination. *Research in Developmental Disabilities, 136*:104442.

Taylor, R., Bowyer, P., & Fisher, G. (2024). *Kielhofner's model of human occupation: Theory and application* (6th ed.). Wolters Kluwer.

Taylor, R. R. (2020). *The intentional relationship: Occupational therapy and use of self* (2nd ed.). FA Davis.

Tefft, D., Guerette, P., & Furumasu, J. (1999). Cognitive predictors of young children's readiness for powered mobility. *Developmental Medicine and Child Neurology, 41*(10), 665–670.

Tepper, D. L., Howell, T. J., & Bennett, P. C. (2022). Executive functions and household chores: Does engagement in chores predict children's cognition? *Australian Occupational Therapy Journal, 69*(5), 585–598.

Thomas, H. (2015). *Occupation-based activity analysis* (2nd ed.). SLACK Incorporated.

Thornton, A., Licari, M., Reid, S., Armstrong, J., Fallows, R., & Elliot, C. (2016). Cognitive orientation to (daily) occupational performance intervention leads to improvements in impairments, activity and participation in children with developmental coordination disorder. *Disability & Rehabilitation, 38*(10), 979–986.

TIG. (2021). Age-appropriate transition assessments and resources. https://witig.org/wp-content/uploads/2017/10/Age-Appropriate-Assessment-Guide.pdf.

Tracey, E. H., Greene, A. J., & Doty, R. L. (2012). Optimizing reliability and sensitivity of Semmes-Weinstein monofilaments for establishing point tactile thresholds. *Physiology & Behavior, 105*(4), 982–986.

Transition Improvement Grant (TIG). (2021). *Age-appropriate transition assessments and resources. https://witig.org/wp-content/uploads/2017/10/Age-Appropriate-Assessment-Guide.pdf.*

Trosman, I., & Ivanenko, A. (2021). Classification and epidemiology of sleep disorders in children and adolescents. *Child and Adolescent Psychiatric Clinics, 30*(1), 47–64.

Trujillo, C., Carr, M., & Poach, M. (2018). High school transition team members' perception of occupational therapy—conducted transition assessments. *American Journal of Occupational Therapy, 72*(4_Supplement_1):7211500052p1. https://doi.org/10.5014/ajot.2018.72S1-PO6042

Trujillo, C., Poach, M., & Carr, M. (2019). Exploring the applicability of occupational therapy transition assessments for students with disabilities. *World Federation of Occupational Therapists Bulletin, 75*(1), 71–77.

Unicef. (2023). https://www.unicef.org/education.

Urbina, S. (2004). *Essentials of psychological testing.* Wiley.

van Barneveld, S., van der Palen, J., & van Putten, M. J. (2010). Evaluation of the finger wrinkling test: A pilot study. *Clinical Autonomic Research, 20*(4), 249–253.

Vandenplas, Y., Rudolph, C. D., Di Lorenzo, C., Hassall, E., Liptak, G., Mazur, L., Sondheimer, J., Staiano, A., Thomson, M., Veereman-Wauters, G., Wenzl, T. G., & North American Society for Pediatric Gastroenterology Hepatology and Nutrition, & European Society for Pediatric Gastroenterology Hepatology and Nutrition. (2009). Pediatric gastroesophageal reflux clinical practice guidelines: Joint recommendations. *Journal of Pediatric Gastroenterology and Nutrition, 49*(4), 498–547.

Vanderlee, L., Hobin, E. P., White, C. M., & Hammond, D. (2018). Grocery shopping, dinner preparation, and dietary habits among adolescents and young adults in Canada. *Canadian Journal of Dietetic Practice and Research, 79*(4), 157–163.

Vasilenko, S. A., Lefkowitz, E. S., & Welsh, D. P. (2014). Is sexual behavior healthy for adolescents? A conceptual framework for research on adolescent sexual behavior and physical, mental, and social health. *New Directions for Child and Adolescent Development, 144*, 3–19.

Vedder, P., & Oortwijn, M. (2009). Adolescents' obligations toward their families: Intergenerational discrepancies and well-being in three ethnic groups in The Netherlands. *Journal of Comparative Family Studies, 40*(5), 699–717.

Verburg, G. (1987). Predictors of successful powered mobility control. In K. M. Jaffe (Ed.), *Childhood powered mobility: Developmental, technical and clinical perspectives Proceedings of the RESNA 1st NW Regional Conference:* (pp. 70–104). RESNA Press.

Von Baeyer, C. L. (2009). Children's self-report of pain intensity: What we know, where we are headed. *Pain Research and Management, 14*(1), 39–45.

Vrangalova, Z., & Savin-Williams, R. C. (2011). Adolescent sexuality and positive well-being: A group-norms approach. *Journal of Youth and Adolescence, 40*, 931–944.

Wagner, E. A., Chantry, C. J., Dewey, K. G., & Nommsen-Rivers, L. A. (2013). Breastfeeding concerns at 3 and 7 days postpartum and feeding status at 2 months. *Pediatrics, 132*(4), e865–e875.

WATI Development Team. (2017). Assistive technology assessment and consideration forms. http://www.wati.org/free-publications/assistive-technology-consideration-to-assessmen.

Watson, A. H., Ito, M., Smith, R. O., & Andersen, L. T. (2010). Effect of assistive technology in a public-school setting. *American Journal of Occupational Therapy, 64*, 18–29.

Weaver, L. L. (2015). Effectiveness of work, activities of daily living, education, and sleep interventions for people with Autism Spectrum Disorder: A systematic review. *American Journal of Occupational Therapy, 69*(5):6905180020p1–6905180020p11.

Weinstock-Zlotnick, G., & Hinojosa, J. (2004). Bottom-up or top-down evaluation: Is one better than the other? *American Journal of Occupational Therapy, 58*(5), 594–599.

Werner, R. A., Franzblau, A., Gell, N., Hartigan, A., Ebersole, M., & Armstrong, T. J. (2005). Predictors of persistent elbow tendonitis among auto assembly workers. *Journal of Occupational Rehabilitation, 15*(3), 393–400.

Western Psychological Services [WPS]. (2022). FAQ: Assessment telepractice. https://pages.wpspublish.com/telepractice-101.

White, E. M., DeBoer, M. D., & Scharf, R. J. (2019). Associations between household chores and childhood self-competency. *Journal of Developmental and Behavioral Pediatrics, 40*(3), 176–182.

Wilder, S. (2014). Effects of parental involvement on academic achievement: A meta-synthesis. *Educational Review, 66*(3), 377–397.

Williamson, A. A., Mindell, J. A., Hiscock, H., & Quach, J. (2019). Child sleep behaviors and sleep problems from infancy to school-age. *Sleep Medicine, 63*, 5–8.

Williamson, A. A., Mindell, J. A., Hiscock, H., & Quach, J. (2020). Longitudinal sleep problem trajectories are associated with multiple impairments in child well–being. *Journal of Child Psychology and Psychiatry, 61*(10), 1092–1103.

Willis, C., Girdler, S., Thompson, M., Rosenberg, M., Reid, S., & Elliott, C. (2017). Elements contributing to meaningful participation for children and youth with disabilities: A scoping review. *Disability & Rehabilitation, 39*(17), 1771–1784.

Wong, S., & Fisher, G. (2015). Comparing and using occupation-focused models. *Occupational Therapy in Health Care, 29*(3), 297–315.

Woods, J. J., & Lindeman, D. P. (2008). Gathering and giving information with families. *Infants & Young Children, 21*(4), 272–284.

Xia, M., & Hudac, C. (2023). Social connection constellations and individual well-being typologies: Using the loglinear modeling approach with latent variables. *Journal of Happiness Studies, 24*, 1–22.

Zabriskie, R. B., & Kay, T. (2013). Positive leisure science: Leisure in family contexts. In T. Freire (Ed.), *Positive leisure science: From subjective experience to social contexts* (pp. 81–99). Springer.

Zhang, D. (2005). Parent practices in facilitating self-determination skills: The influences of culture, socioeconomic status, and children's special education status. *Research and Practice for Persons with Severe Disabilities, 30*(3), 154–162.

Zhu, V., & Dalby-Payne, J. (2019). Feeding difficulties in children with autism spectrum disorder: Aetiology, health impacts and psychotherapeutic interventions. *Journal of Paediatric Child Health, 55*(11), 1304–1308.

Zimmer-Gembeck, M. J., & Helfand, M. (2008). Ten years of longitudinal research on US adolescent sexual behavior: Developmental correlates of sexual intercourse, and the importance of age, gender and ethnic background. *Developmental Review, 28*(2), 153–224.

Zimmerman, B., & Kitsantas, A. (2014). Comparing students' self-discipline and self-regulation measures and their prediction of academic achievement. *Contemporary Educational Psychology, 39*(2), 145–155.

Zimmerman, B. J. (2008). Investigating self-regulation and motivation: Historical background, methodological developments, and future prospects. *American Educational Research Journal, 45*(1), 166–183.

Visit Elsevier eBooks+ (eBooks.Health.Elsevier.com) to access additional resources.

# 10

# Data Interpretation, Goal Setting, and Outcome Measurement in Pediatrics

*Gloria Frolek Clark and Teresa May-Benson*

## GUIDING QUESTIONS

1. What do the scores from standardized assessments mean?
2. How do qualitative and quantitative data influence goal setting?
3. What is the process of setting goals in occupational therapy practice?
4. What are the similarities and differences between the Canadian Occupational Performance Measure (COPM), goal attainment scaling (GAS), and performance monitoring to measure pediatric outcomes?

## KEY TERMS

Age-equivalent scores
Fidelity
Goal attainment scaling (GAS)
Measures of central tendency
Measures of variability
Percentile scores
Qualitative data
Quantitative data
Rasch scores
Standard deviation
Standardized scores

## CONSOLIDATION AND INTERPRETATION OF DATA

When interpreting collected data, the occupational therapist examines the child's performance on standardized and nonstandardized assessments, observes their occupational performance, and considers information provided by other sources. The occupational therapist then uses therapeutic reasoning as part of the decision-making process to identify patterns of function/dysfunction as they relate to referral concerns, identifies which frame(s) of reference or occupational therapy models best fit the child's concerns and performance, and determines whether occupational therapy services would benefit the child.

Different types of data may be used in various ways to achieve these goals. Data are used to identify strengths and limitations, measure the child's progress, and provide insight into which underlying client factors may impact functional occupational performance. Further, data interpretation may influence the selection of intervention strategies and techniques as well as recommendations for home programs, school placement, and services.

### Interpretation of Standardized Assessment Data

Standardized measures report findings in various ways. First, the occupational therapist must be aware of whether the results of an assessment reflect typical or atypical performance. On some measures, the higher the score, the better the performance the child has in comparison to neurotypical peers. On other measures, a higher score reflects more dysfunction or the presence of undesirable traits.

Standardized scores will be reflected in one of a variety of formats. These include:

- mean scores and standard deviations
- standard z-scores
- standard t-scores
- scaled scores
- Rasch scores
- percentile scores and age equivalents

These **standardized scores** can all be converted from one to the other; the format depends on the test developer. In addition, some facilities or agencies require or prefer the use of one format over another. For instance, school systems tend to prefer the use of percentile scores. In addition, some assessments will include age equivalents. **Age-equivalent scores** provide a comparison of the child's performance to that of other children who score similarly. Age equivalents refer to the age at which other children perform similarly to the child under investigation. For example, if a 12-year-old child being evaluated scores 20 and the average score of an 8-year-old is 20, the child would have an age-equivalent score of 8 years. **Rasch scores** are also increasingly popular in standardized tests. These scores measure item difficulty relative to the child's ability.

### Measures of Central Tendency and Variability

Patterns of human performance on most standardized, norm-referenced tests follow a distribution referred to as the normal curve (or bell-shaped curve) (see Fig. 10.1). Scores derived from these types of tests provide information about how the designated child's performance compares with similar children when plotted on the normal bell curve. The scores derived from a bell-shaped curve distribution on a test are based on two important statistics, measures of central tendency and measures of variability.

**Measures of central tendency** indicate the middle point of the distribution of children's scores on an assessment. The mean and the median are the most used. A mean is essentially the average score—the sum of all scores divided by the number of scores. The median is the middle score when all scores are listed in rank order—half the scores are below the median and half are above it. The median is most often used when outlying or extreme scores are present in the distribution that could skew the mean score (Chan & Richardson, 2019).

**Measures of variability** include the variance and the standard deviation. Both rely on a normal distribution of scores and report how

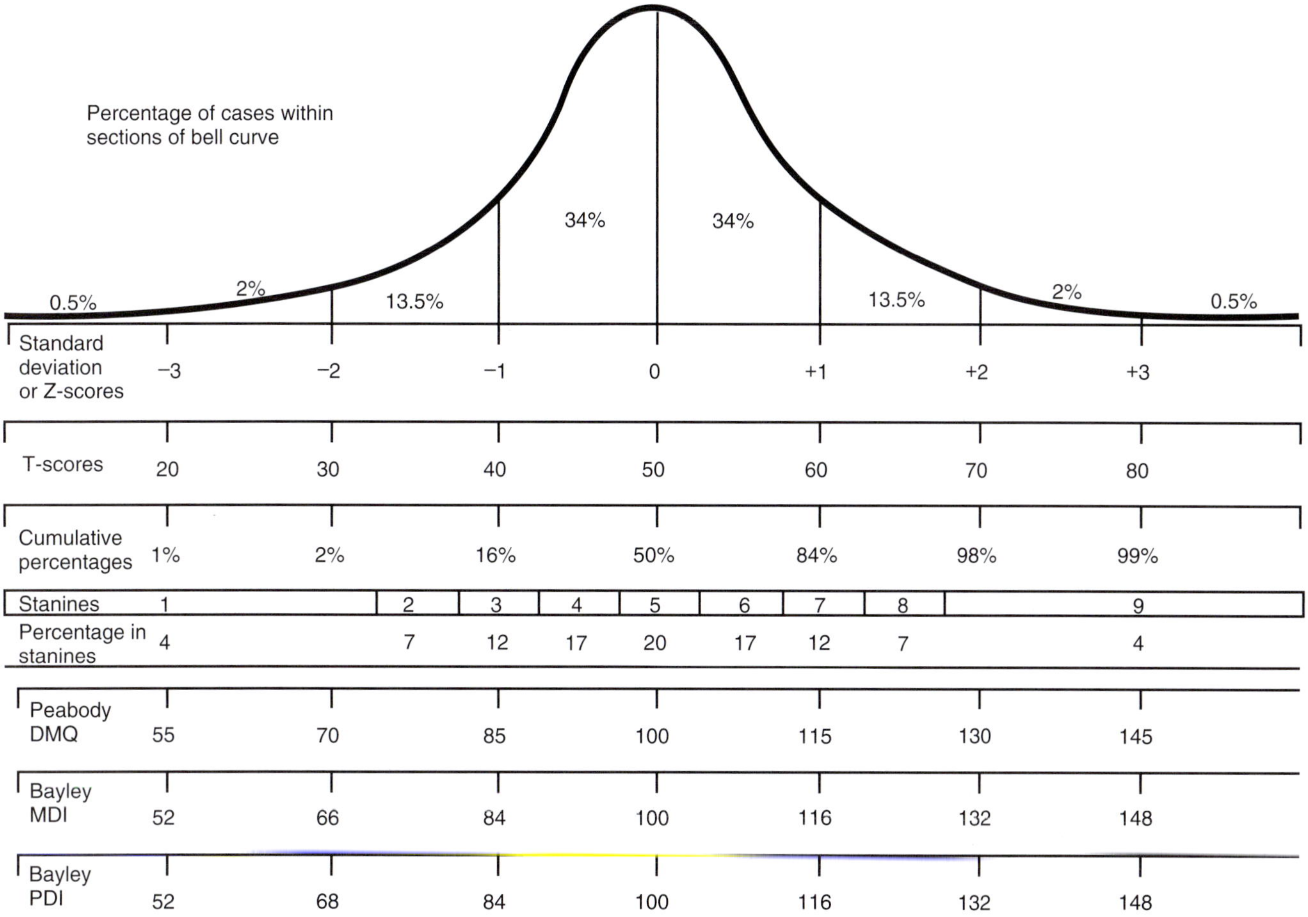


**Fig. 10.1** The normal curve and associated standard scores. The greatest number of people receive a score in the middle part of the distribution, with progressively smaller numbers receiving scores at either the high or the low end.

far group or individual scores deviate from the mean. *Variance* is the average of the squared deviations of scores from the mean and measures how far the score of an average child in a sample deviates from the group mean. The **standard deviation (SD)** reflects the variability in performance within a group of children and provides information on how far scores can be expected to vary from the mean. The SD is used to calculate many of the standard scores listed above. It is based on the placement of a given score on a bell curve, as illustrated in Fig. 10.1. In a normal bell curve distribution of scores, 68% of the scores fall within 1 SD of the mean (±1 SD); 95% of the scores are within 2 SDs of the mean (±2 SD); and 99.7% of the scores are within 3 SDs of the mean (±3 SD). Typical performance in occupational therapy practice is usually considered between ±1 SD of the mean. Scores below -1 SD typically reflect some level of difficulty that may or may not indicate functional performance problems. Scores below -2 SD, however, reflect definite difficulties that almost always reflect functional performance problems. However, these interpretations may vary by the test.

## Standard Scores

As noted above, the z-score and t-score, both based on the test mean and SD, are the most used **standard scores** in standardized testing. The z-score is computed by subtracting the mean for the test from the individual's score and dividing it by the SD. A negative value indicates that the z-score is below the mean for the test, and a positive value indicates that the z-score is above the mean (Chan & Richardson, 2019).

The t-score is derived from the z-score. In a t-score distribution, the mean is 50 and the SD is 10. All t-scores have positive values, but because the mean of a t-score distribution is 50, any number less than 50 indicates a score below the mean. A score of 40 or less typically indicates areas of difficulty. T-scores may be used when a test developer does not wish to have negative scores as outcomes of the assessment. They are also sometimes used when a test measures dysfunctional characteristics and only one end of the bell curve is significant to report. This is seen frequently in psychology tests that examine functions such as attention or behavior problems.

Scaled scores are frequently seen in standardized tests that examine developmental areas of performance. One familiar scaled score is the IQ test, which has a mean of 100 and an SD of either 15 or 16. These scores are obtained from tests such as the Stanford-Binet (Thorndike et al., 1986) or the Wechsler Intelligence Scale for Children (Weschler, 1991). On these tests, individuals with scores 2 SDs below the mean (IQs of 70 and 68) are considered to have an intellectual disability. Individuals with scores 2 SDs above the mean (IQs of 130 and 132) are considered gifted. Other developmental tests, such as the Peabody Developmental Motor Scales (PDMS-2; Folio & Fewell, 2000) and the Bayley Scales of Infant and Toddler Development (Bayley, 2006) also use scaled scores with a mean of 100 and an SD of 15 or 16. Children who receive scores 1 to 2 SDs below the mean (e.g., scores of 85 or 70) in one or more skill areas often need occupational therapy services (Chan & Richardson, 2019). Similarly, some tests or subsections of tests use scaled scores with a mean of 10 and a standard deviation of 3, with scores below 7 indicating challenges.

## Rasch Scores

**Rasch scores** are derived from assessments developed based on Rasch methodology. This includes tests such as the School Function Assessment (SFA; Coster et al., 1998), the Pediatric Evaluation of Disability Inventory-Computer Adaptive Test (PEDI-CAT; Haley et al., 2017) and the School Assessment of Motor and Process Skills (School AMPS; Atchison et al., 1998; Fisher et al., 2005). To use Rasch methodology (Coster, 1998), the construct being measured (e.g., activities of daily living) must be representable as a continuous function with measurement covering a full range of possible performance. The assessment (or an individual scale of the assessment) must measure only one characteristic (or construct) of performance. Each item on the assessment or scale therefore represents a sample of the characteristic being measured.

Rasch analysis methodology provides estimates of item difficulty independent of the sample of persons tested, and an individual's ability estimate is independent of the specific items tested. The Rasch model generated during test development provides a hierarchic ranking of items on the test from easiest to most difficult. With the items on the measure or the individual scale ranked along this continuum, a child's performance is assessed in relation to an item's difficulty rather than against a normative sample. The ranking of items therefore creates an expected pattern of mastery of items with more difficult items on the continuum expected to be mastered only after easier items have been learned. Therefore, occupational therapy practitioners who administer an assessment tool developed using Rasch methodology generally can assume that the most appropriate goals for intervention will be the items and/or skills immediately above the items successfully passed by the client. Occupational therapists can then develop interventions and generate recommendations directly from the child's observed and/or reported performance and participation (Chan & Richardson, 2019).

## Percentile Scores and Age Equivalents

Percentile scores and age-equivalent scores are used with some tests as an indicator of a child's performance relative to a normative group. These scores are not calculated from means and standard deviations but from raw scores. However, percentile scores can usually be translated into standard scores.

A **percentile score** is the percentage of people in a standardization sample whose score is at or below a raw score. A percentile score of 60, for instance, indicates that 60% of the people in the standardization sample received a score that was at or below the raw score corresponding to the 60th percentile. Although percentile rank scores can be easily calculated and understood, they have a significant disadvantage: The percentile ranks are not equal in size across the score distribution. Distances between percentile ranks are much smaller in the middle of the distribution than at the ends; consequently, improving a score from the 50th to the 55th percentile requires much less effort than improving a score from the fifth to the 10th percentile. As a result, an improvement in performance by a child functioning at the lower end of the score range may not be reflected in the percentile score the child achieves. Other standard scores are more sensitive at measuring changes in the performance of children who fall at the extreme ends of the score distribution (Chan & Richardson, 2019).

The ***age-equivalent* score** is the age at which a raw score is at the 50th percentile. The age-equivalent score generally is expressed in years and months, e.g., 4 years 3 months. It is a score that is easily understood by parents and caregivers who may not be familiar with testing concepts or terminology. However, age-equivalent scores have significant disadvantages. Although they may provide a general idea of a child's overall developmental level, it may be misleading to say, for example, that a 4-year-old is functioning at the 2.5-year level. The age-equivalent score may be an average of several developmental domains, some of which may be at the 4.5-year level and some at the 1.5-year level. Therefore, the child's performance may be highly variable and may not reflect that of a typical 2.5-year-old. In addition, the age-equivalent score represents only the score that a child at the same age who is performing at the 50th percentile would receive. A child who is performing within normal limits for their age but whose score is below the 50th percentile would receive an age-equivalent score below their chronologic age. This can cause parents or caregivers to conclude incorrectly that the child has delays. Age equivalents, then, are a type of standard score that can contribute to an understanding of a child's performance, but they are the least psychometrically sound, can be misleading, and should be used only with caution (Chan & Richardson, 2019).

## Interpretation of Nonstandardized Data

In addition to standardized assessments and standardized scores, the occupational therapist considers information gathered from personal reports of subjective experiences (such as quality of life, perceptions of performance, sense of self) as well as observations of physical changes, performance of skills and abilities, and changes in performance across contexts. Both qualitative and quantitative data collected in these conditions provide important information about a child's performance.

**Qualitative Data.** **Qualitative data** provide subjective information on how environmental factors or contexts influence everyday participation in both positive and negative ways (Hammel et al., 2015). Perspectives from the child, family, teacher, or others may provide insight into the child's performance. The Model of Human Occupation (Tham et al., 2017, p. 74) emphasizes *subjective experience* as providing insight into the person's lived experience and how it shapes how they perform (Kielhofner, 1995; Fisher et al., 2024). For example, a child who feels they are a good student will typically enjoy school and perform better than a child who feels they are "bad and not smart." Qualitative data may be collected by recording a child's observation, and include information from scales (e.g., pain scales), assessments [e.g., Child-Occupational Self-Assessment (Kramer et al., 2014); Short Child-Occupational Profile (Bowyer et al., 2008)], and interviews with the child and family. Fig. 10.2 shows a therapist gathering qualitative data. While some data may produce a number (such as pain scales), the child's perception of the pain, challenges, or supports

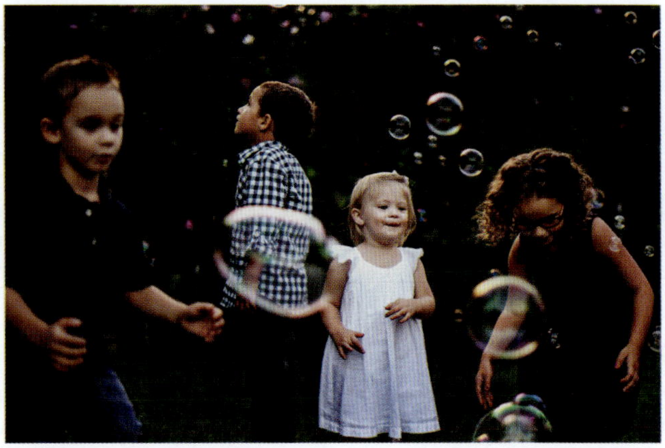

**Fig. 10.2** A child's reaction provides qualitative data regarding participation in a familiar activity. The occupational therapy practitioner observes their response and notes if the child appears to be cautious, or distressed, or expressing enjoyment. (katherine-hanlon-xaG8oaZD7ss-unsplash.)

is the focus. The occupational therapist considers differences and similarities in child and caregiver or teacher reports.

**Quantitative Data.** Quantitative data focus on quantity, amount, intensity, and/or frequency of behaviors during the child's performance. Data may be collected by recording time (e.g., how long it takes an infant to drink 4 ounces), distance (e.g., how far the child can push the broom during a prevocational task), frequency (e.g., the number of times the child hits a target), or results of a tool (e.g., pain scale, occupation-based performance measure). The occupational therapy practitioner collects baseline data and compares it to the expectations or desired outcomes of the parent, school, and child to develop meaningful goals. This type of data may provide insight into how specific behaviors, activities, or skills impact functional performance. Fig. 10.3 shows a child's mealtime which is a great context to gather quantitative data which can then be used to identify baseline and changes in the child's performance. Quantitative data provide easy, accurate, and objective measurement of behaviors and consequently, these measures are often used in goal setting.

## SETTING GOALS

Regardless of the work setting, occupational therapy practitioners are responsible and accountable for the documentation required by agencies, payment sources, and education laws, and to develop measurable goals and document the impact of occupational therapy on a child's health, well-being, engagement, and participation in their occupations and activities. To avoid confusion with the term "outcomes" used in early intervention services under the Individuals with Disabilities Education Improvement Act (IDEA, 2014) to describe child- or family-focused expectations and the term "outcomes" used by OTPF-4 (AOTA, 2020) to refer to the end of occupational therapy services (e.g., discharge or transition), this chapter uses the term "goal" to encompass measurable expectations collaboratively established by occupational therapists and others. Goals should address the child's current performance (baseline) and identify the expected performance (goal criteria). The process begins with identifying the concern, which often includes collaboration with a team of people (e.g., Individualized Family Service Plan, Individualized Education Program, teams within a healthcare agency) including the parent, child, and occupational therapist.

### Identify the Concern and Impact on the Child

During the occupational therapy evaluation process, concerns are identified that impact the child's health, well-being, and engagement in their occupations (AOTA, 2020). Collaborating with the child, family, and others to identify and prioritize the concerns is important for developing the goals and planning the intervention. Operationalizing the performance concerns is necessary for everyone to have the same idea about the outcome. For example, "child will dress self independently" may be interpreted differently (e.g., Does this mean tie shoes? Button coat?), whereas "child will put on a short sleeve pullover shirt, underwear, and elastic waist shorts independently" is less confusing.

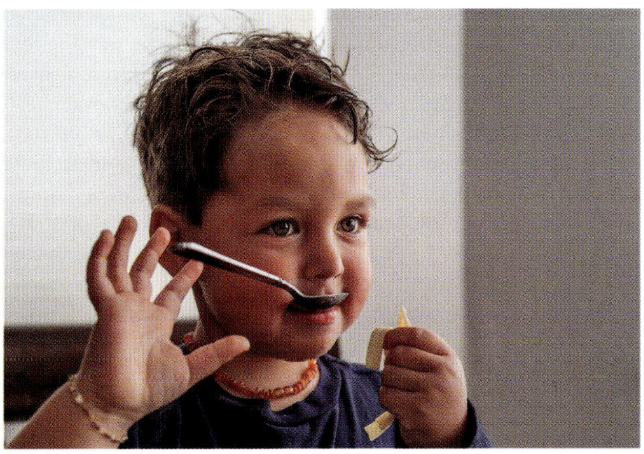

**Fig. 10.3** Mealtime provides quantitative data such as the number of times a child brings a spoonful of food to her mouth independently during a meal. (karo-kujanpaa-FpcoRCeKh1g-unsplash.)

### Establish Baseline and Expected Goals or Outcomes

Methods of collecting baseline data may vary by setting. Baseline performance may be established through observation, assessment tools, parent, caregiver, or teacher reports, and educational materials (e.g., journal or office behavior reports). Data collection within the natural or modified environments is consistent with occupational therapy values and purpose; however, services may be provided outside of the natural setting to address underlying factors and skills (AOTA, 2022).

### Define the Conditions, Actions, and Criteria for the Goal

Goals should be written clearly so parents and others understand the expectations. Typically, a goal includes the *conditions* (e.g., timeframe, having an adult nearby, using a modified device), *actions* (e.g., will sit, will demonstrate homeostasis, will write, will initiate conversation), and the criteria that indicate the goal has been met (e.g., 90% of attempts, three consecutive days, 4/5 attempts). Some settings require short-term and long-term goals; others require annual or short-term goals and benchmarks to measure the child's progress. When developing early intervention outcomes, the parent voice is typically included in the text. For example: parents are exhausted since their child is awake and crawls into their bed every night. They say "We want Roja to fall asleep and remain in his own bed through the night. Completion of the goal may be determined by the parents or based on the outcome criteria, in which case the therapist may ask, "How will we know this is met?" The parent's response is "When Roja can stay in his bed throughout the night for 5 nights." So it becomes, "Roja will fall asleep and remain in his own bed throughout the night for 5 consecutive nights." The use of the child, parent, teacher, or other's voice when collaboratively writing goals aligns with performance within the child's natural context. Measurable goals may be developed using qualitative or quantitative data. Table 10.1 provides examples of goals.

## MEASURING OUTCOMES IN PEDIATRICS

Unlike goals which are the long- or short-term statements of desired client performance, client outcomes are the result of the occupational

**TABLE 10.1 Examples of Measurable Goals**

| Based on Qualitative Data | Based on Quantitative Data |
|---|---|
| • Within 6 weeks, when asked, "Tell me one thing about mealtime that went well at home (or school)," child will describe one positive experience for 3 consecutive sessions.<br>• Within 2 months, when asked, "Tell me about something this week that upset you and how you handled it," child will describe using an appropriate cognitive or self-regulatory activity, 3 consecutive sessions. | • In 3 days during diaper changes, infant will maintain respiratory homeostasis, 90% of the time.<br>• In 3 months, child will independently feed self 75% of the meal twice daily for 3 consecutive days<br>• In 9 months, while washing hands, child will complete the preschool 6-step program, independently for 4/5 preschool days. |

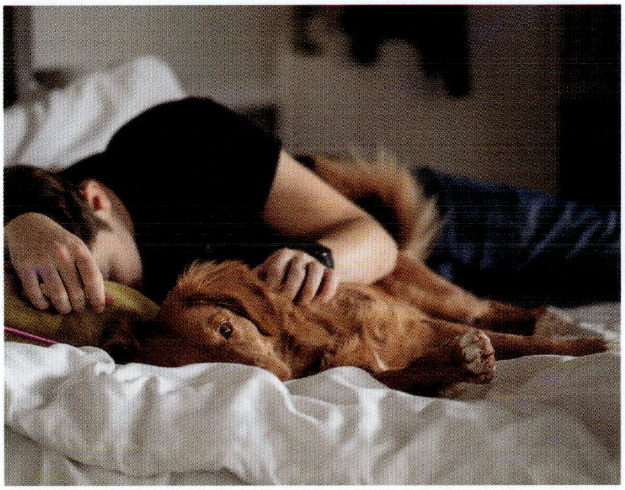

**Fig. 10.4** An occupational therapist may gather qualitative data from an adolescent (*how well* he slept) as well as quantitative data (*how long* he slept) to identify if sleep interventions are effective. (jamie-street-WvZ4dTE7dLI-unsplash.)

therapy process desired for transition or discharge from services and are "woven throughout the process of occupational therapy" (AOTA, 2020, p. 26). Outcomes may also refer to the larger end products of a given program, department, or therapeutic activity. These programmatic outcomes reflect the ability of the program to achieve its desired goals (e.g., reaching a given level of productivity and achieving a desired level of community outreach). These are distinct from client outcomes, although client outcome data may be collected as part of a programmatic review.

For client outcomes, the selection of individual outcomes and measures for those outcomes are identified early to determine the desired results of occupational therapy, plan future actions with the individual, family, or team, and evaluate intervention effectiveness. Outcomes should reflect aspects of improvement or enhancement of occupational performance and participation or prevention of challenges in those areas. Outcomes may also address other areas including health and well-being, quality of life, role competence, or occupational justice. Fig. 10.4 shows an adolescent who has difficulty sleeping at night which affects his schoolwork and after-school job. Outcomes may include improving a child's health (e.g., eating a variety of healthy foods for a child with food refusal) or improving the quality of a youth's life (e.g., enabling a teenager with mental health challenges to maintain an after-school job that enhances their self-determination). Modifications to these outcomes may occur during the intervention or reevaluation process as needs or contexts change (AOTA, 2020). Various measures may be used to evaluate the achievement of these individualized outcomes. This may include formal goal-setting measures such as Goal Attainment Scaling (GAS) or the Canadian Occupational Performance Measure (COPM). It may also include other types of data, such as observational behavioral counts, treatment notes, or parent reports. These data may be gathered at various points in time including throughout the intervention or at reevaluation.

## Data Gathering During Implementation of Intervention

Regular and frequent data collection about the child's performance informs professional judgment, determines if occupational therapy interventions are effective, and measures progress toward outcomes (Frolek Clark, 2016). Occupational therapy practitioners use the same methods that they used to collect baseline data to examine the child's progress during intervention. Fig. 10.5 shows a pre-school age child

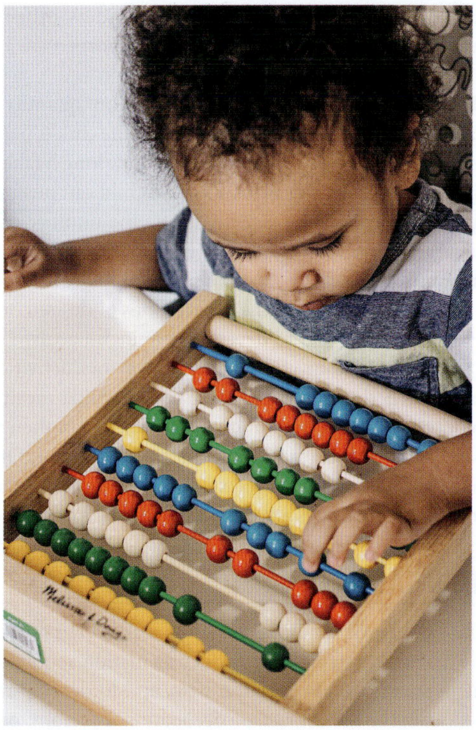

**Fig. 10.5** The parents wanted their preschool son to play with toys for at least 10 minutes. His baseline was 20 seconds before he would throw the toy and run off. Data were collected weekly by the parents and occupational therapist. He is now playing with toys for 7 minutes before running off. (luis-arias-ayH7wwVOtc0-unsplash.)

playing while the occupational therapy practitioner collects data to document progress. They collect data based on the intensity of the concern. For example, more intensive behaviors such as hitting others may need daily data collection, while self-care or literacy performance may be collected weekly. Data are recorded in the occupational therapy practitioner's professional contact reports (e.g., daily treatment notes) and may include visual displays (e.g., graphs, charts, data collection tables). The occupational therapy practitioner selects the type of data and format for recording and displaying the data to clearly show the child's progress toward desired outcomes. Specific methods of gathering and displaying information will be covered later in this chapter.

**Gathering Data About Intervention Fidelity.** Before gathering client data, the occupational therapy practitioner ensures that the intervention they are providing is consistent with the way the intervention was intended to be delivered, in other words, it is delivered with **fidelity** (Gresham et al., 2000). Fidelity measures evaluate the actual intervention provided to ensure that intervention protocols, home programs, and school programs are consistently and accurately followed as intended. Unless there is some mechanism for determining and measuring if the trained person is doing the activity or strategy correctly and with the expected frequency, there is no way for the therapist to judge the intervention's true effectiveness.

Changing or discontinuing an intervention based on performance data that suggests an intervention is ineffective, may be detrimental to the child if the intervention was not implemented properly. Therefore, occupational therapists create systems to measure the fidelity of intervention implementation. Occupational therapists may ask parents or teachers to record every time the activity was carried out by placing a checkmark on a calendar or recording on the program form. The occupational therapist uses their professional reasoning to determine when and how to provide information on intervention fidelity to individuals involved in implementing the intervention.

## Identify Methods of Gathering Client Outcome Data

Methods used to determine the child's status at evaluation should also be used to compare their status at discharge or transition. Objective outcome measures should be selected during the evaluation process that are valid, reliable, sensitive to change, consistent with targeted outcomes, consistent with the child or family's goals, and designed to predict outcomes (AOTA, 2020).

**Specific Tools.** Depending upon the setting, occupational therapists may select specific assessment tools that measure the child's performance as they complete occupations or activities (ideally within the child's natural routine and environment); that measure the child's client factors, performance skills, and performance patterns as they support or challenge participation and engagement in daily life skills; or that measure the supports and barriers within the child's contexts (AOTA, 2020). The COPM (COPM; Law et al., 2019) was designed specifically as an outcomes measure to compare the client's performance and satisfaction before and after intervention. Examples of other measures commonly used as assessment and outcome measures include the Pediatric Evaluation of Disability (PEDI; Haley et al., 1992; 2012) and Functional Independence Measure for Children (Wee-FIM; Uniform Data System for Medical Rehabilitation, 2016) and Short Child Occupational Profile (Bowyer et al., 2008).

***Canadian Occupational Performance Measure.*** The *COPM* (COPM, Law et al., 2019) is used to measure progress and outcomes in practice as well as research. The COPM can be used to identify problems within occupational performance, rate priorities, evaluate performance and satisfaction, assist with goal setting, and measure changes in occupational performance (Law et al., 2019).

The COPM is a five-step process. First the problem is defined by the client (e.g., child with parent or teacher assisting, if necessary). During this interview, they identify the person's strengths and challenges within three broad occupational performance areas (self-care, productivity, and leisure). Up to five problem areas are chosen by the client(s). The second, third, and fourth steps include rating using a 10-point scale (1 is not important at all to a 10, which is extremely important). The person rates these three questions: "How important is it to you to be able to do this activity" (Step #2 Importance); "How would you rate the way you do this activity now?" (Step #3 Performance); and "How satisfied are you with the way you do this activity now?" (Step #4 Satisfaction). Step 5 is the reassessment and repeats Steps two to four at the chosen time variable. Case Example 10.1 illustrates the use of the COPM to measure progress and outcomes in practice.

***Goal Attainment Scales.*** Goal attainment scales (GAS) was originally developed for use in mental health settings to measure individual and group responses to intervention and is now routinely used to measure intervention progress (Becker et al., 2000; Kiresuk & Sherman, 1968; Schlosser, 2004; Steenbeck et al., 2005). Goals are established at the start of the intervention and reflect a range of possible outcomes that are predicted to occur after a specified period. The child's performance is then rated at the designated time to determine progress. The advantage of GAS goals is that they reflect individualized functional changes that the client and/or family wish to see following intervention. GAS can capture small increments of change in areas that are not readily evaluated on standardized assessments. For example, GAS may be developed for a child whose family wants to improve the child's ability to eat a variety of foods or dress himself.

GAS provides a framework that allows objective measurement of individualized goals and provides quantifiable and individualized measures. Because GAS goals are written based on a distribution of predicted outcomes that is expected to follow a standard bell curve, they may be converted to standard t-scores which allows these individualized goals to be aggregated within and across clients. This makes GAS a particularly useful data source for programmatic reviews or evaluation of intervention effectiveness in addition to individual outcomes. While developing the GAS, occupational therapy practitioners

## CASE EXAMPLE 10.1 USING THE CANADIAN OCCUPATIONAL PERFORMANCE MEASURE (COPM) TO MEASURE PROGRESS AND OUTCOMES

Tisha is a 14-year-old with autism who struggles with socializing with classmates because of her poor personal hygiene and limited food range. She told her mother she hates not having any friends and kids saying she "stinks" or laughing because she gags at foods in the cafeteria. During the COPM interview, Tisha picked "eating more foods, hygiene, and friends" as her primary areas to address. Her current ratings (time 1 or $T_1$) are listed on the chart below.

Strategies to enhance Tisha's occupational performance were discussed with her for each of these areas, and an intervention program was implemented. While Tisha was making some progress in these areas, the occupational therapy practitioner documented in their notes how Tisha informally rated her performance and satisfaction. After 4 months, Tisha reported she had been invited to a sleepover at a classmate's house and was able to eat a slice of cheese pizza and popcorn without gagging. Two girls at the party asked if she wanted to hang out at the mall with them.

The occupational therapist asked Tisha to rate her performance and satisfaction in the three chosen areas. Her ratings are listed in the chart below under the $T_2$ scores. Changes are computed by subtracting $T_2$ from $T_1$ scores. Research from various studies and populations indicates a "change of two points or more on the COPM represents an important change" (Law et al., 2019, p. 17). Tisha's change in performance for Friends was 7, Hygiene 5, and Foods 6. Changes in satisfaction for Friends were 7, Hygiene 6, and Foods 6. These scores indicated important changes and were consistent with observed behaviors and were consistent with Tisha's reports. The therapist discussed Tisha's steady and ongoing progress with her and her family and discontinuing services. Discontinuation was discussed with Tisha and her family since her progress had been steady and ongoing. They agreed to discontinue occupational therapy services and continue to implement strategies at home, school, and community.

**TISHA'S SELF-SCORING ON THE COPM**

| Area | Importance | Performance $T_1$ | Satisfaction $T_1$ | Performance $T_2$ | Satisfaction $T_2$ |
|---|---|---|---|---|---|
| **Friends** | 10 | 1 | 1 | 8 | 8 |
| **Hygiene** | 8 | 2 | 2 | 7 | 8 |
| **Foods** | 8 | 1 | 2 | 7 | 8 |

monitor progress at specific periods after initiating occupational therapy intervention (e.g., monthly or at the end of the intervention). Occupational therapists who wish to measure the effectiveness of services across many individuals may use the Kiresuk-Sherman formula (Kiresuck et al., 1994) which converts raw GAS scores to T-scores (i.e., M = 50; SD = 10), which allow comparison of the scores across individuals.

The GAS measurement system as developed by Kiresuk et al. (1994) is based on a 5-point response scale. The expected outcome is listed as "0" with numbers ranging from "-2" (e.g., much less than expected outcome) to "+2" (e.g., much more than expected outcome). Occupational therapists using the GAS methodology must be trained in how to determine, write, and measure goals. This training is important to minimize bias and ensure the validity and reliability of the goal-setting and rating processes. Occupational therapy practitioners creating GAS measures should do the following:

(a). Create goals from objective data (e.g., observations) as well as subjective data (e.g., interviews, records)
(b). Operationally define the outcome criteria so that data can be recorded accurately and reliably throughout the process.
(c). Use an independent examiner to determine the attainment of the goal rather than persons involved in the treatment or goals-setting process.
(d). Determine whether an intervention was implemented as stated (Becker et al., 2000; Ottenbacher & Cusick, 1993).

Nine interrelated steps used to establish GAS (Ottenbacher & Cusick, 1993) are outlined below:

1. *Identify a general objective.*
   What is the overall program/client goal?
2. *Identify specific problem areas that should be addressed.*
   Identify observable, reportable components that can be used to measure performance.
3. *Specifically identify three to five behaviors or events that will indicate progress in Step 2.*
   Operationalize the terms so that measurable indicators of improvement are clearly defined.
4. *Determine the methodology that will be used to collect the necessary information. Identify how data will be collected (e.g., who, where, when).*
5. *Select the expected level of performance (professional judgment and client appraisal) to be attained after a specified time.*
   Determine realistic levels of performance that can be expected.
6. *Identify performance outcomes which reflect the four additional levels of the GAS scale of less improvement than expected (-1), much less improvement than expected (-2), more improvement than expected (+1) and much more improvement than expected (+2).*
   Focus on realistic outcomes—identify increments of progress that are achievable for each level on the scale.
7. *Assure that change in only one dimension is being measured.*
   Individual levels must reflect change in the same single dimension. For example, all levels measure change in frequency of performance of a behavior NOT one level measures frequency and the other duration of performance.
8. *Once the 5-point system has been set, determine if the intervals overlap or have gaps. Determine if behaviors and instructions for data collection are clear.*
   Review the scale to be sure there is no overlap and no gaps between criteria, definitions are clear, and instructions for data collection are easy to follow, e.g., frequencies are typically reported as a range of 1–3 seconds, 4–5 seconds, 6–8 seconds, etc.
9. *Determine the client's current status and when future evaluations are needed to document progress.*

This final step in the development of the GAS scale requires the selection of a time for evaluating the client's or program's outcomes. The frequency should consider the intervention provided, expected performance level, the child's rate of progress, and criteria from outside sources (e.g., third-party payers, education system).

See Box 10.1 for modifications to GAS that are not recommended for use, and Case Example 10.2, which shows how GAS can be used to create and measure meaningful client-centered goals for children in practice.

***Progress or Performance Monitoring.*** Progress or performance monitoring is often used within the educational system. This is a standardized method for collecting and reviewing data in a chart format to enhance student performance. This process may be used to identify children who are not responding to intervention, to quantify children's rate of responsiveness to the intervention, and to determine the effectiveness of the interventions (Fuchs & Oxaal, n.d.; National Center on Response to Intervention, January 2013).

Strengths of this system are the ability to visualize the child's performance over time, the ability to identify if the child is progressing at the rate needed to meet their goal on time, record changes to the intervention and observe ongoing results, and to identify need for extended year services due to regression (e.g., loss of skills over a break) and recoupment (e.g., time needed to relearn skills). Challenges include time to complete the process. The steps to monitor performance and a brief explanation are included in Table 10.2. Case Example 10.3 provides an example of monitoring a child's performance over time based on an expected rate of progress.

## EXAMINATION OF PROGRAMMATIC OUTCOMES

In addition to measuring and monitoring individual child intervention outcomes, occupational therapists may find it helpful to use performance monitoring data to evaluate the effectiveness and outcomes of a therapeutic program. The Early Childhood Outcomes data is one type of program outcome that is routinely evaluated.

### IDEA's Early Childhood Outcomes

In addition to intervention data collected by occupational therapy practitioners, the Office of Special Education (OSEP) requires teams to collect program outcome data and report to each state on specific child outcomes and family indicators for early intervention and preschool special education programs to OSEP. The outcomes include data on the percentage of children receiving services under the Individuals with Disabilities Education Improvement Act (IDEA, 2004) who

#### BOX 10.1 Modifications to GAS that are not recommended

Other authors have since modified the GAS scaling systems; however, these systems are not recommended for use as they invalidate the foundational theoretical concepts of normal distribution of scores that allow GAS scales to be combined within and across clients. Some individuals who have modified GAS include Steenbeck et al. (2005) who used a six-point scale where the expected level of outcome is listed as "0" but a level was added to allow for regression (-3). Ruble and colleagues (Ruble et al., 2012) modified the original 5-point scale whereby the "-2" level represented the baseline or present level of performance, "0" represented the expected level of outcome (e.g., the actual description of the written IEP objective is used) and "+2" was much more than expected. In this case, a child who improves their baseline (-2) toward the expected level of outcome (0), has progressed (-1). Both methodologies skew the distribution of scores to the lower end of the bell curve.

## CASE EXAMPLE 10.2 CREATING GOALS AND MEASURING PROGRESS USING GAS IN PRACTICE

Tessa is a 4-year-old female who loves to run and explore. She lives with her foster parents after being removed from her parents for exposure to drugs. Her foster parents sought outpatient occupational therapy services since Tessa was diagnosed with attention deficit disorder and does not play independently or sit at a table for fine motor activities.

The occupational therapist observed Tessa while playing with toys and fine motor materials that her foster parents stated she enjoyed most (e.g., stacking pegs and puzzles). The therapist documented the length of time Tessa sat and engaged with these materials. She played with one toy for 60 seconds before jumping up and running around the room. After a short break, she returned to the table where she played with another toy for 55 seconds. A third observation with a preferred toy indicated 60 seconds of engagement before throwing it to the floor and screaming (baseline: 60 seconds).

Tessa's preschool teacher expects children to play with toys or work independently at the table for 10–15 minutes. The parents and occupational therapist felt this was a realistic outcome for Tessa and they determined the goal of occupational therapy would be: *In 3 months, Tessa will sit and play/work with toys or fine motor materials for 7–10 minutes.* The occupational therapist used GAS to measure this outcome. A 5-point scale which incorporated her current performance at -2 and expected outcome at 0 was used (see chart below).

Tessa participated in weekly therapy. Data were collected each session relating to sitting and playing with fine motor materials. The foster parents carried out a home program offering practice opportunities with 90% fidelity each week. After 3 months, reevaluation data indicated that Tessa sat and played with toys for 17 minutes (+1 GAS) during the occupational therapy session. Parents stated Tessa played independently for almost 20 minutes (+2 GAS) at home if the television was not on to distract her. The preschool teacher also timed Tessa's sitting during classroom tabletop activities and found she sat for 18 minutes (+2 GAS). GAS provided a clear and objective way that was individualized for Tessa to measure the outcome of occupational therapy intervention.

**TESSA'S GOAL ATTAINMENT SCALE (BASED ON KIRESUK-SHERMAN, 1994)**
**BASELINE: -2**
**EXPECTED OUTCOME: 0**

| | | |
|---|---|---|
| +2 | Much more than expected outcome | Sit and play/work for ≥18 minutes |
| +1 | More than expected outcome | Sit and play/work for 14–17 minutes |
| 0 | EXPECTED outcome | Sit and play/work for 7–13 minutes |
| −1 | Less than expected outcome (baseline) | Sit and play/work for 2–6 minutes |
| −2 | Much less than expected outcome | Sit and play/work for ≤1 min |

**TABLE 10.2 Performance Monitoring Steps**

| Step | Action | Description |
|---|---|---|
| 1 | Defining and operationalizing the concern. | Clarify the concern regarding the child's performance (this is what will be measured) |
| 2 | Identifying the measurement strategy | Choose a strategy that is simple, time efficient, systematic, and can be collected at regular intervals to measure the child's performance concern (typically through timing or counting performance) |
| 3 | Gathering current baseline performance | Typically, 3–4 data points are collected within a short period. The median data point is considered the baseline measure. |
| 4 | Establishing a goal | Typically, the goal is related to the expected education-related performance at the end of the goal period (e.g., 6 months, school year) and is clear and concise so everyone understands what is hoped to be accomplished. |
| 5 | Creating a visual chart with a goal line | The visual representation of the data assists in decision-making. A goal line connects the baseline to the expected goal point and represents the rate of progress that is required for the child to reach the goal. |
| 6 | Creating a decision-making plan | Decision plans should be based on at least 6–10 data points (Christ & Silbergli, 2007; Shinn, good, & Stein, 1989). The four-point decision rule (White, 1985) is commonly for data collected weekly. |
| 7 | Collecting data during intervention and using for decision-making | Data should be collected at the same time and location. Based on the data, decisions are generally made to continue the intervention, change the intervention, or stop since the child has met their goal. |

demonstrate improvements in positive social-emotional skills; acquisition and use of knowledge and skills; and use of appropriate behaviors. Data collected may be used to support programming or service needs for children and families. States that are not progressing in their outcomes may be at risk of losing program funding. As members of the team, occupational therapists assist in the documentation of these outcomes. Data must be reliably collected to be a valid measure of the results of the intervention.

### Data for Programmatic Outcomes

Other programs may have outcomes that involve a discrete program such as a structured group (e.g., percentage of children that meet their goals), or it may reflect departmental outcomes (cost-effectiveness of a group intervention program). These types of larger program outcomes may be useful when justifying occupational therapy services as a programmatic service in schools, clinical settings, or third-party payors like insurance companies.

Programmatic outcomes differ from individual client outcomes in that they tend to focus on aspects of evidence-based practice related to client perspectives and experiences of the intervention and to practical administrative-oriented factors. They may address client or provider feelings about services, or reactions and satisfaction related to engaging in various aspects of the evaluation or intervention processes. These outcomes may also examine process factors such as how much time is involved in various steps of the occupational process, what services are utilized by clients, and when or how long are services utilized. This may include processes from referral to follow-up.

Data for programmatic outcome evaluation may be collected specifically to examine some aspect of program review, such as client satisfaction with services, or existing data from clinical records may be accessed (for example, billing records may be accessed to evaluate attendance, rate of absences, frequency, or duration of services). Further, client assessment data via reports or intervention treatment notes may be accessed to identify which functional goals are most often achieved among participants in a group, or how often goals of certain types (e.g., occupation-based goals like dressing vs. client

## CASE EXAMPLE 10.3 USING PERFORMANCE MONITORING TO VISUALIZE A CHILD'S PERFORMANCE OVER TIME

This case study takes the reader through the 7-step process of performance monitoring. Ty, a first grader, loves to run and jump in the classroom but screams when asked to sit at his desk or participate in classroom activities. After talking with the teacher, the parents agreed to an education evaluation to determine if Ty was eligible for special education and related services. As part of this team, an occupational therapist gathered data for the occupational profile by conducting interviews with the teacher and parent to identify Ty's current concerns regarding engaging in daily life activities, occupations that were successful or challenging, contextual factors that supported or inhibited engagement, and targeted outcomes for Ty. Their main concern within the domain of occupational therapy was Ty's inability to sit and perform fine motor tasks (e.g., cutting, writing, coloring). The occupational therapist observed Ty in the classroom during seated tasks and collected baseline data by recording the length of time Ty remained in his seat and worked on tasks after he was initially seated with the task. The time ended when he left the chair. Data were 20, 10, and 15 seconds (median score of 15 seconds). The score of three peers identified as "average" peers by the teacher was 18 minutes (median score). Based on the data, Ty's performance is considerably below that of his peers and interferes with learning and participation in his educational program.

The members of the IEP team shared their results and found Ty eligible for special education and several goals for Ty were developed including: "By 11/28/2022, after given a fine motor task in the classroom, Ty will sit on his chair and perform the fine motor activity for at least 15 minutes for 4/5 days". The team agreed occupational therapy services were necessary for Ty to benefit from his educational program. To monitor Ty's progress, the occupational therapist used Microsoft Excel to develop a chart (See Fig. 10.6). Data were charted in minutes. Therefore, Ty's 15 s baseline was converted to minutes (e.g., 15/60 = 0.25 min). A goal line was added (green line) to identify the rate of progress required for Ty to meet his goal. A goal line connects the baseline data point to the expected goal data point.

Occupational therapy intervention was implemented with data collected by the teacher and occupational therapist. After 3 weeks involving a structured routine including Ty's favorite and nonfavorite activities, data indicated Ty's performance was both above and below the goal line. Following the four-point decision rule (i.e., goal is met if four consecutive data points are above the goal line), a decision was made to continue the intervention. The vertical lines in Fig. 10.6 indicate when decisions were made. Data collected and reviewed 4 weeks later indicated ongoing progress with only one data point below the goal line. Intervention was continued. During the next 4 weeks, data indicated he did not stay in his seat. His teacher mentioned Ty was out of school with a fever and took a few days to get back into the routine. At the annual IEP meeting data indicated that Ty met and exceeded his IEP goal.

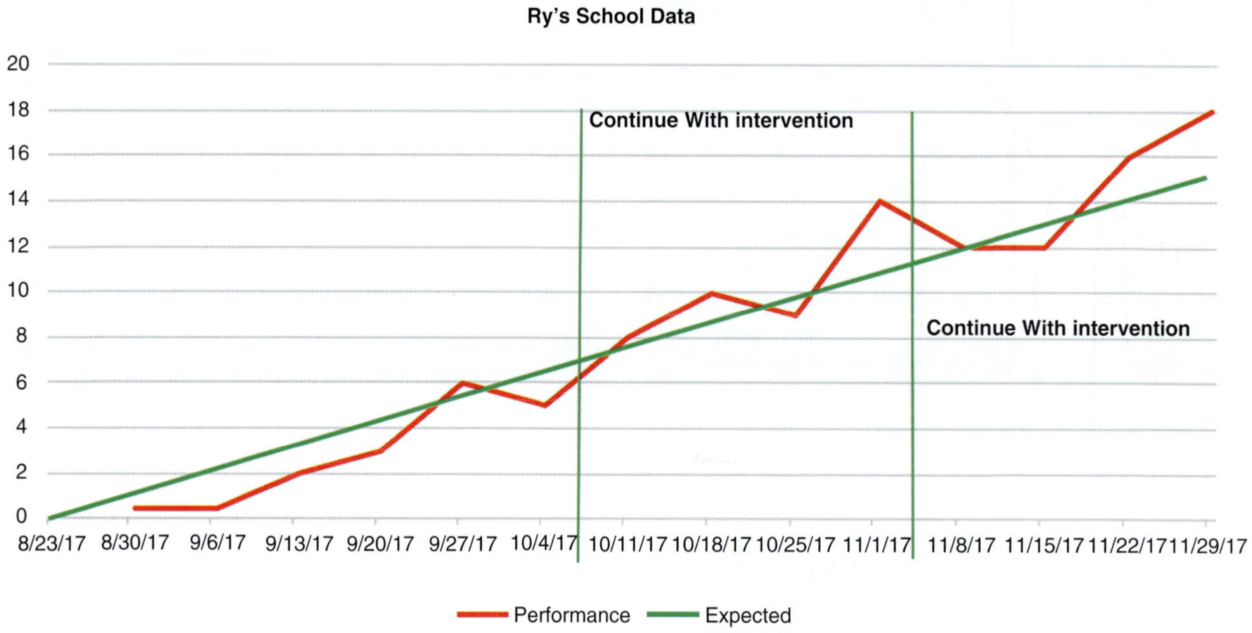


**Fig. 10.6** Ty's progress monitoring graph baseline.

factor goals like attention) are written for clients. Client goals such as GAS goals may provide particularly useful data for program review outcomes. Programmatic data is unique to the specific program under review and generally follows different guidelines for research review than human subjects' research. Regardless, all protections for deidentification of data and of the Health Insurance Portability and Accountability Act (HIPAA, 1996) rights of individuals must be followed if client data is accessed for program review purposes. These types of programmatic outcomes can help occupational therapy managers budget for their departments, justify services, guide staff in clinical reasoning, and focus service delivery. Occupational therapists can promote the collection of data for programmatic outcome reviews by incorporating some important strategies into their clinical practice.

First, occupational therapy practitioners or the department should establish protocols for data collection. They identify important programmatic outcomes that need to be examined and decide what data will be collected to measure those outcomes.

Second, they develop a process to collect consistent data. This includes using data from up-to-date treatment notes and clinical records. This may include establishing regular intervals for reassessment and consistent assessment measures to be used across clients and therapists. Goals for clients should be reevaluated at consistent and regular intervals. Goal writing systems should be consistent among the occupational therapy staff. It is important to report client outcomes in accessible formats, such as via an electronic medical records system or visual data reporting charts.

Third, a team of individuals needs to be designated to collect, analyze, report, and disseminate the results of the program review. Collecting and interpreting programmatic outcomes is just as important for supporting the evidence-based practice of occupational therapy as the examination of individual client intervention effectiveness.

## SUMMARY

Occupational therapy practitioners are responsible and accountable for providing efficient and effective evidence-based pediatric services across a variety of settings. Occupational therapists collect data from diverse sources and interpret assessment scores and observational data using clinical reasoning skills to determine intervention programs for their clients. Goals are developed collaboratively with the child, family, and various teams to enhance the child's health, well-being, engagement, and participation in daily life activities. Occupational therapy practitioners understand the importance of monitoring treatment integrity measures as well as gathering reliable and valid data to use in ongoing decision-making and program evaluation. During the child's evaluation, outcome measures are identified and later compared to data at the child's discharge or transition to determine the effectiveness of occupational therapy services. Occupational therapists also contribute to the achievement and data collection for program outcomes.

1. Scores from standardized assessments can be reflected as standard scores, percentile scores, age-equivalent scores, Rasch scores, mean scores, and standard deviations. The author of the assessment determines the scoring procedures and provides guidelines for how the scores are interpreted. For example, higher scores may reflect better performance or the presence of more dysfunction. Occupational therapy practitioners use therapeutic reasoning and knowledge of the assessment scoring and interpretation to understand the meaning of the scores from standardized assessments as they relate to the child's goals and occupational therapy intervention.
2. Qualitative data provides subjective information on how environmental factors or contexts influence the child's participation in everyday activities. Qualitative data provides information on the child's subjective experiences (i.e., lived experience) and provides insight from others (e.g., parents, peers, teachers) on the child's performance in a variety of settings. Quantitative focus on quantity, amount, intensity, and/or frequency of behaviors during the child's performance. This data provides insight into how specific behaviors, activities, or skills impact functional performance. Occupational therapy practitioners use both types of data to synthesize information to develop meaningful client-centered goals used to create intervention plans and measure client and program outcomes.
3. Occupational therapy practitioners engage in the goal-setting process by collaborating with the child, family, and others to identify and prioritize the child's concerns. They operationalize performance concerns by specifically identifying the behaviors that need to be addressed in therapy. They identify the child's baseline performance (e.g., where the child starts) and determine the expected goal or outcome. They define the conditions, actions, and criteria for the goal. Goals are written clearly, concisely, and in collaboration with the child and family.
4. The Canadian Occupational Performance Measure (COPM) is used to measure progress and outcomes in practice was well as research. The COPM can be used to identify problems with occupational performance, rate priorities, evaluate performance and satisfaction, assist with goal setting, and measure changes in occupational performance (Law et al., 2019). Goal Attainment Scaling (GAS) is a method to establish objective individualized goals that are quantifiable. GAS goals are written based on the standard bell curve. They can be confirmed to standard t-scores which allows the scores to be aggregated within and across clients so they can be used for programmatic reviews and measuring intervention effectiveness in addition to individual outcomes. Progress or performance monitoring is often used within educational systems. This is a standardized method for collecting and reviewing data in a chart format to enhance student performance. This process may be used identify children who are not responding to intervention, to quantify children's rate of responsiveness to intervention and to determine the effectiveness of intervention (Fuchs & Oxaal, n.d.; National Center on Response to Intervention, January 2013).

## REFERENCES


American Occupational Therapy Association. (2020). Occupational therapy practice framework: Domain and process-fourth edition. *American Journal of Occupational Therapy, 74*(Suppl. 2), S16.

American Occupational Therapy Association. (2022). Position Statement—inclusive environments: Home, work, public spaces, technology, and specialty environments. *American Journal of Occupational Therapy, 76*. https://www.aota.org/-/media/corporate/files/secure/practice/officialdocs/position/inclusive-environments_ajot_76s2001_prepublication-version.pdf.

Atchison, B. T., Fisher, A. N., & Bryze, K. (1998). Rater reliability and internal scale and person response validity of the school assessment of motor and process skills. *American Journal of Occupational Therapy, 52*, 843–850.

Bayley, N. (2006). *Bayley scales of infant and toddler development, motor scale* (3rd ed.). Psychological Corporation.

Becker, H., Stuifbergen, A., Rogers, S., & Timmerman, G. (2000). Goal Attainment Scaling to measure individual change in intervention studies. *Nursing Research, 49*, 176–178.

Bowyer, P. L., Kramer, J., Ploszaj, A., Ross, M., Schwartz, O., Kielhofner, G., & Kramer, K. (2008). *The short child occupational profile (SCOPE), Version 2.2.* Chicago, IL: The University of Illinois at Chicago.

Chan, M., & Richardson, P. (2019). Use of standardized tests in pediatric practice. In C. O'Brien, & H. Kuhaneck (Eds.), *Case-Smith's occupational therapy for children and adolescents* ($8^{th}$ ed.). St Louis: Elzevier.

Coster, W. J., Deeney, T., Haltiwanger, J., & Haley, S. (1998). *School function assessment.* San Antonio, TX: Psychological Corporation.

Coster, W. (1998). Occupation-centered assessment of children. *American Journal of Occupational Therapy, 52*, 337–344.

Fisher, A., Bryze, K., Hume, V., & Griswold, L. (2005). *School AMPS: School version of the assessment of motor and process skills* (2nd ed.). Three Star Press.

Fisher, G., Tham, K., Erikson, A., Fallahpour, M., & Wolske, J. (2024). Performance capacity and the lived body. In R. Taylor, P. Bowyer, & G. Fisher (Eds.), *Kielhofner's model of human occupation: Theory and application* (6th ed., pp. 72–92). Wolters Kluwer.

Folio, M. R., & Fewell, R. R. (2000). *Peabody developmental motor scales: Examiner's manual.* Pro-Ed.

Frolek Clark, G. (2016). Collaborating within the paces: Structures and routines. In B. Hanft, & J. Shepherd (Eds.), *Collaborating or student success: A guide for school-based occupational therapy* (2nd ed.) (p. 177207). AOTA Press.

Fuchs, L. S., & Oxaal, I. (n.d.). Progress monitoring: What, why, how, when, where. Presentation released by the National Center on Student Progress Monitoring. Retrieved from http://www.rti4success.org/pdf/progressmonitoringwhatwhyhowwhenwhere.pdf.

Gresham, F. M., MacMillian, D. L., Beebe-Frankenberger, M. D., & Bocian, K. M. (2000). Treatment integrity in learning disabilities intervention research: Do we really know how treatments are implemented? *Learning Disabilities Research & Practice, 15*, 198–205.

Haley, S. M., Coster, W. J., Dumas, H. M., Fragala-Pinkam, M. A., & Moed, R. (2012). Pediatric evaluation of disability inventory computer adaptive test. Available at: http://www.pedicat.com.

Hammel, J., et al. (2015). Environmental barriers and supports to everyday participation: A qualitative insider perspective from people with disabilities. *Archives of Physical Medicine and Rehabilitation, 96*(4), 578–588.

Health Insurance Portability and Accountability Act of. (1996). *Pub. Law 104-191, 42 U.S.C. § 300gg, 29 U.S.C. §1181–1183, and 42 U.S.C. §1320d–1320d9.*

Individuals with Disabilities Education Improvement Act of. (2004). *Pub. Law 108-447, 20 U.S.C. Code §1400-1482.*

Kielhofner, G. (1995). A meditation on the use of hands. *Scandinavian Journal of Occupational Therapy, 2*, 153–166.

Kiresuk, T., & Sherman, R. (1968). Goal attainment scaling: A general method for evaluating comprehensive mental health programmes. *Community Mental Health Journal, 4*, 443–453.

Kiresuk, T., Smith, A., & Cardillo, J. (1994). *Goal attainment scaling: Applications, theory, and measurement*. London: Erlbaum.

Kramer, J., ten Velden, M., Kafkes, A., Basu, S., Federico, J., & Kielhofner, G. (2014). *Child-occupational self-assessment (COSA) [version 2.2]. Model of human occupation clearinghouse, department of occupational therapy. College of applied health sciences*. University of Illinois at Chicago.

Law, M., Baptiste, S., Carswell, A., McColl, M., Polatajko, H., & Pollock, N. (2019). *Canadian occupational performance measure* (5th ed.). CAOT Publications.

National Center on Response to Intervention. (January 2013). *Progress monitoring brief #2 common progress monitoring graph omissions: Missing goal and goal line*. Washington, DC: U.S. Department of Education, Office of Special Education Programs, National Center on Response to Intervention.

Ottenbacher, K. J., & Cusick, A. (1993). Discriminative versus evaluative assessment: Some observations on goal attainment scaling. *American Journal of Occupational Therapy, 47*, 349–354.

Ruble, L., McGrew, J., & Toland, M. (2012). Goal attainment scaling as an outcome measure in randomized controlled trials of psychosocial interventions in autism. *J Autism Dev Disorders, 42*(9), 1974–1983.

Schlosser, R. (2004). Goal attainment scaling as a clinical measurement technique in communication disorders: A critical review. *Journal of Communication Disorders, 37*, 217–239.

Steenbeck, D., Meester-Delver, A., Becher, J. G., & Lankhorst, G. J. (2005). The effect of botulinum toxin type A treatment of the lower extremity on the level of functional abilities in children with cerebral palsy: Evaluation with goal attainment scaling. *Clinical Rehabilitation, 19*, 274–282.

Tham, K., Erickson, A., Fallophour, M., Taylor, R., & Kielhofner, G. (2017). Performance capacity and the lived body. In R. Taylor (Ed.), *Kielhofner's model of human occupation: Theory and application* (5th ed.) (pp. pp74–90). Wolters Kluwer.

Thorndike, R. L., Hagen, E. P., & Sattler, J. M. (1986). *Technical manual, Stanford-Binet intelligence scale* (4th ed.). Riverside.

Uniform Data System for Medical Rehabilitation. (2016). *The WeeFIM II® clinical guide* (UDS MR).

Wechsler, D. (1991). *Wechsler intelligence scale for children*. Harcourt.

# 11

# Interventions for Feeding and Eating

*Kimberly Korth and Nancy Creskoff Maune*

## GUIDING QUESTIONS

1. How do occupational therapy practitioners approach interventions for feeding and eating?
2. What specific interventions address feeding and eating challenges in children and youth?

## KEY TERMS

Aspiration
Dysphagia
Enteral or nonoral feeding
Environmental adaptations
Esophageal dysphagia
Fiberoptic Endoscopic Evaluation of Swallowing
Gastroesophageal reflux
Jaw control
Oral hypersensitivity
Oral phase
Oral preparatory
Oral propulsive
Pediatric feeding disorder
Selective eating or food refusal
Suck-swallow-breathe
Videofluoroscopic swallow study (VFSS)

## FEEDING AND EATING

Occupational therapy practitioners provide interventions for children with feeding, eating, and swallowing disorders to improve their participation in mealtimes and support their nutritional intake and growth. Feeding refers to setting up and bringing food to one's mouth, whereas eating requires manipulating the food (or fluid) in the mouth and swallowing (AOTA, 2020). To intervene in these occupations, practitioners must understand the typical development of feeding and eating (see Chapter 8) as well as the process of comprehensively evaluating feeding and eating (see Chapter 9).

A range of severity exists for pediatric feeding and eating challenges. Some infants or children may present with simple feeding challenges that can be addressed by occupational therapy, such as difficulty with bottle feeding or delayed oral motor skills. Other children may present with more significant feeding and eating difficulties, resulting in a diagnosis of Pediatric Feeding Disorder (PFD), which is defined as "*impaired oral intake that is not age-appropriate, and is associated with medical, nutritional, feeding skill, and/or psychosocial dysfunction*" and can be classified into acute (<3 months' duration) and chronic (≥3 months' duration; Goday et al., 2019). Children with PFD requiring feeding intervention may present with comorbidities and complex medical and nutritional needs. PFD is quite common, as suggested by a survey during 2009 to 2014 (Kovacic et al., 2021). The annual prevalence ranged from 1 in 23 to 1 in 37 in children under 5 years in two publicly insured cohorts and one privately insured cohort. See Chapter 9 for more on the evaluation of feeding disorders and the types of feeding disorders treated by occupational therapy practitioners. This chapter focuses on the approach to intervention for feeding and eating, as well as specific intervention strategies for each stage of the process, and intervention strategies to improve difficult behaviors related to feeding and eating.

### Feeding and Eating Interventions: Guiding Principles and Approach to Intervention

Interventions for feeding and eating, no matter the severity, involve a multidisciplinary approach that ensures the safety of the child. Occupational therapy practitioners work closely with families, physicians, nurses, dieticians, and nutritionists to create and implement feeding and eating interventions specific to each child's needs. They address multiple factors that may influence feeding and eating.

**Multidisciplinary.** To work effectively with children with feeding disorders, occupational therapy practitioners must collaborate with other healthcare professionals to create optimal intervention plans that also take into consideration these medical and nutritional concerns. Core interventionists on the team include psychology, nutrition, medicine, speech-language pathology, and occupational therapy. Evidence suggests that multidisciplinary approaches with these team members can lead to successful weaning from tube feedings, increased oral intake, improved mealtime behaviors, and reduced parenting stress (Sharp et al., 2010, 2017). The occupational therapy practitioner must keep in mind that planned intervention may need to be adjusted with goals for intake or nutrition, for example, such as promoting respiratory health or establishing growth.

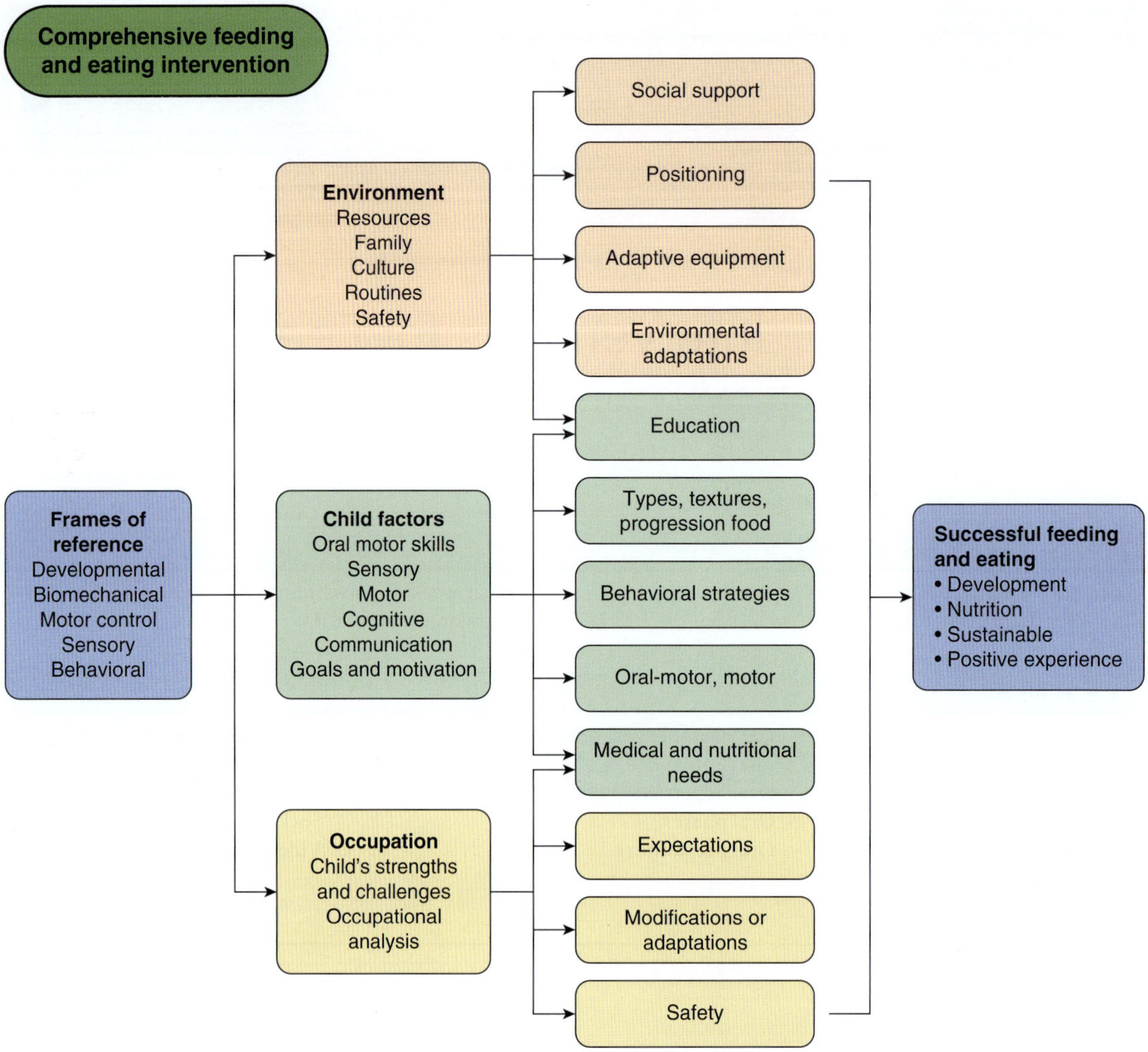


**Fig. 11.1** Diagram of comprehensive feeding intervention plan.

**Holistic.** Occupational therapy practitioners use a holistic approach when developing comprehensive intervention plans to address feeding and eating challenges as illustrated in Fig. 11.1. The practitioner considers the medical and nutritional needs of the child while intervening to address needs related to feeding and eating skills and psychosocial factors. The intervention plan is also tailored to the child's physical and developmental level. The plan is created in concert with the family's cultural beliefs, routines, and expectations. For families of children with feeding disorders, mealtimes may be quite stressful and the child's feeding difficulties may create negative experiences for caregivers, especially when there are ongoing problems with nutrition and growth. To address all of those potential areas, a comprehensive and individualized intervention plan includes a combination of approaches and recommendations regarding mealtime structure and set up, positioning, presentation of food, environmental adaptations, adaptive equipment, remediation, types, or textures of food, sensory or behavioral strategies, changes to family routines and expectations, and caregiver education and training, with safety always a primary concern (Andrew et al., 2012; AOTA, 2017; Boop & Smith, 2017; Desai et al., 2022).

**Focus on Safety.** Throughout the intervention process, occupational therapy practitioners follow a variety of safety guidelines. For example, they must follow universal precautions including washing hands frequently and wearing gloves to prevent the spread of infection during therapy activities involving food, mucus, or structures within the child's mouth (United States Department of Labor, 2018). They also must abide by any dietary restrictions for food allergies, metabolic disorders, diabetes, or other medical conditions. Since infants and children with feeding and eating challenges may have trouble managing liquid or food intake, they are at risk for aspiration, gagging, or choking. Occupational therapy practitioners recognize signs of distress or concerns for safety impacting overall health and readily communicate with the child's caregivers and healthcare team.

## APPROACHES TO ADDRESS FEEDING AND EATING DIFFICULTIES

A variety of treatment care models are used to treat children with feeding problems, including specialized inpatient programs, intensive outpatient programs, direct weekly therapy, feeding group therapy, telepractice, and periodic consultative services. Treatment strategies within these care models may be categorized in different ways, for example, by frame of reference or by intervention strategies used during treatment. Please see Table 11.1 for further discussion on care models and considerations associated with each approach. In the following section, the interventions will be presented by their intended outcome or function, in the order of (1) feeding and (2) phases of eating and swallowing.

TABLE 11.1 **Models of Care for Feeding Disorders**

| Model | Explanation | Benefits and Considerations |
|---|---|---|
| Specialized inpatient programs | Children are admitted to inpatient feeding programs with a multidisciplinary team. | Highest frequency of intervention with direct access to multidisciplinary specialists and providers. Programs may be disruptive to regular family routines (school/home), may be expensive, and often last for weeks/months depending on the facility. |
| Outpatient Therapy | Children receive feeding intervention in an outpatient facility, typically on a weekly basis. | Outpatient care is less disruptive for the family routines than inpatient care. Frequency can vary depending on child/family needs. This model can pose challenges for generalization of strategies and skill building, dependent on family's follow through with home program recommendations. |
| Intensive Feeding Therapy | Rather than traditional once or twice per week sessions, intensive therapy offers frequent (daily or more than once a day) intervention sessions for a specific duration of time. Typically offered in an outpatient facility. | The rationale for intensives supports the philosophy regarding increased frequency, to encourage greater improvement. It is important to consider cost, location, time commitment, family dynamics and specific referral criteria. |
| Group feeding therapy | Children of similar ages, developmental level, and/or social abilities are organized together. These groups provide unique opportunities for children to learn from each other through peer influence. | There are assumed benefits of group-based therapy due to most children's inherent desire to engage and interact with other children their same age. However, children who do not readily engage in imitation and are not socially motivated, may not benefit from the group therapy model. |
| Telehealth and consultative Feeding therapy | Telehealth involves the delivery of health-related services using virtual technology (See Chapter 23 for more on telehealth). | Specific benefits may include savings in travel time and cost for families, opportunities for "real life" observations and problem solving, timely parent coaching, and in some cases decreased stress for children related to remaining in their home environment for the therapy sessions. Telehealth may not be appropriate for children who have difficulty learning through a virtual platform, or for families with limited access to the necessary technology. |

## Interventions for Feeding

Feeding, the act of bringing food or drink to the mouth, requires a variety of sensorimotor skills that may be difficult for a child for a variety of reasons. Following the evaluation, the practitioner selects an appropriate method and model of intervention to address challenges based on the age and developmental level of the child. Feeding interventions may include activities to promote upright posture, grasp, release, motion of the entire upper extremity, and provision of adaptive equipment to bring food or beverages to the mouth.

**Adaptive Equipment for Feeding.** Adaptive equipment supports feeding and allows children to compensate for a sensorimotor impairment. There are a variety of pieces of adaptive equipment that may foster greater performance and independence. Children with upper extremity weakness or poor grasping skills may benefit from simple adaptations, such as a utensil with a lightweight, built-up handle (Fig. 11.2A) or a universal cuff (Fig. 11.2B). The universal cuff is a low-technology piece of equipment that helps a child grasp a spoon and fork with a palm strap that secures the utensil to the hand in a stable position. Utensils with shorter handles, curved handles, or larger grip diameters may help a child self-feed more independently. A nonskid place mat may help prevent the movement of the dish or bowl to compensate for uncoordinated arm movements. Some dishes also have a suction cup on the bottom to help secure them to the table. Children may have improved independence when self-feeding by using a scoop dish or a sectioned plate that has raised edges to allow them a surface to scoop against. A cup with a handle may help a child with poor fine motor skills to drink more independently. Cups with a wide base or cups with lids may help reduce spillage when the child is placing the cup on a table. Some children may benefit from a long straw placed into a cup that is secured in a cup holder, reducing the need to lift or move the cup with the hands.

Adaptive seating with a stable tray or table for increased arm stability can provide greater trunk and shoulder stability while decreasing the distance the child needs to move the utensil from the bowl to the mouth. Stabilizing the elbow on the table or tray can also help reduce the physical demands of self-feeding, extending the child's endurance. More complex options for severe impairments include a deltoid aid, mobile arm support, and an electronic feeding system activated by a simple push-button switch. Advanced feeding systems (such as robotic feeding devices) may be recommended for those with complex needs.

When encouraging self-feeding in children with visual impairments, occupational therapy practitioners recommend consistent orientation of food and drink on the place mat. For example, placing the cup in the two o'clock position next to the plate or placing foods in consistent locations in the dish may improve the child's awareness of the mealtime environment for improved independence. Contrasting colors with plates, cups, and place mats help children with visual discrimination (Ferrell, 2011). Adaptive equipment, such as the EATSY Adaptive Table Wear for the Visually Impaired, provides increased sensory cues, enabling improved independence for individuals with visual impairments. See online resources for more adaptive equipment resources.

**Activities to Promote Grasp, Release, and Active Range of Motion in the Upper Extremities for Feeding.** Using a biomechanical and developmental approach the practitioner seeks to improve a child's ability to pinch finger foods, grasp utensils, bottles, or cups, lift utensils, bottles, or cups off the surface, spear or pierce foods, scoop foods, successfully bring them to the mouth, and eventually progress to using utensils to cut food into pieces. Intervention activities are designed to address range of motion, strength, endurance, and coordination, while also addressing the occupation.

Motor control approaches focus on addressing movement through meaningful, whole, and repetitive practice. Occupational therapy practitioners using a motor control approach strive to use actual objects

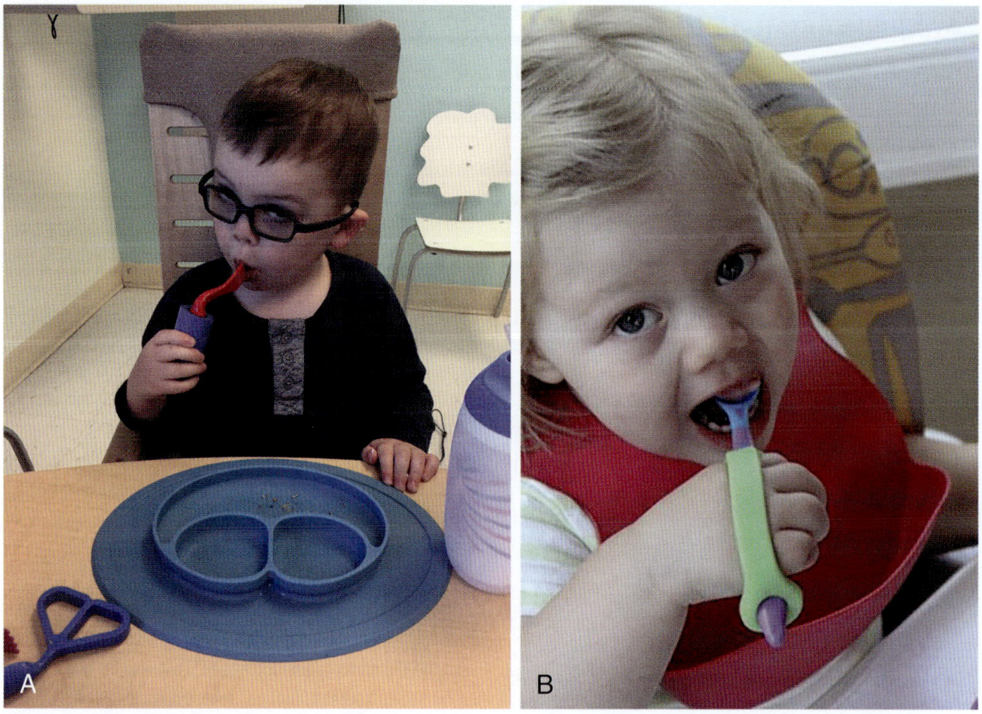

Fig. 11.2 (A) Child uses adaptive equipment for self-feeding (Pediatric Oral Feeding Clinic Children's Hospital Colorado) and (B) Child uses an EazyHold universal cuff to handle utensils for self-feeding.

(such as the child's high chair, utensils, plates, and cups) to provide additional cues to support the child's movements. It is best to use actual food and engage the child in feeding and eating activities at regular meal/snack times. The practitioner promotes meaningful repetition of movements through part and whole practice. Current research evidence supports the use of occupation-based interventions including repeated exposure and parent training to address feeding and eating issues (Kingsley & Clark, 2020). Practitioners adjust the activities to engage the child in motor challenges that are not too difficult for the child but present the just-right challenge. They use motor learning strategies, such as feedback, demonstration, coaching, practice, and problem-solving so children develop a sense of competence in their self-feeding abilities. Chapter 29 describes this approach in more detail.

## Phases of Eating and Swallowing

Occupational therapy practitioners provide intervention to address challenges with feeding and within the four phases of eating and swallowing (AOTA, 2017; Marcus & Breton, 2022a; Miller & Willging, 2003; Morgan et al., 2012). These include:

- The oral preparatory phase includes removing food or drink from the utensil or container, chewing, and forming a bolus.
- The oral propulsive phase where food and liquid are moved posteriorly through the oral cavity with the tongue.
- The pharyngeal phase when swallowing the food and liquid occurs, and the bolus moves through the pharynx.
- The esophageal phase where food or liquid moves toward the stomach through the esophagus.

## Interventions for the Oral Preparatory Phase

The oral preparatory phase requires postural and oral motor control. Interventions to improve a child's ability to remove food or drink from the utensil or container, chew, and form a bolus, include a variety of approaches such as proper positioning, improving the movement of the jaw, tongue, and lips, and using equipment to support improved performance. Occupational therapy practitioners must be aware that while interventions using oral motor therapy are common, there is limited evidence that they improve nutritional outcomes, caloric intake, pharyngeal motility, or airway protection (Gosa et al., 2017; Quitadamo et al., 2016; Rogers, 2004). Therefore, occupational therapy practitioners monitor children's progress regarding intervention plans closely and collaborate with team members to adjust plans as needed.

**Positioning for the Oral Preparatory Phase.** Oral motor activities require skilled movement and coordination of many small muscle groups, which are supported by postural stability. Midline positioning, with full support of head and body and gently flexed posture is ideal for young infants who are breast and bottle feeding. Optimal positioning for older children includes vertical head and trunk position, hip flexion greater than 90 degrees, knee flexion at 90 degrees, and feet supported on a flat surface. Children should have slight flexion at the trunk and neck to facilitate swallowing.

Infants may be supported in a few different positions. Side-lying on an incline in the caregiver's arms may be recommended for children who have difficulty coordinating sucking, swallowing, and breathing because the impact of gravity does not immediately draw the liquid into the pharyngeal space (Fig. 11.3). Once a baby reaches the age of 4 to 6 months (when anatomy changes are expected such as elongation through the neck) it is important to feed them in a more upright position. When bottle or breast feeding, infants may be supported in a semireclined or sitting position in the caregiver's arms to provide alignment and midline orientation. Positioning that includes lying down or propping the bottle on the young infant's chest is not recommended as it can pose an increased risk of choking. An infant seat (e.g., car seat, Tumble Form Feeder Chair, or Special Tomato Chair; Fig. 11 4A and B) may be adapted with small rolls to provide head and trunk support or slight shoulder protraction to help an infant hold his or her bottle. These positioning options allow the caregiver to have

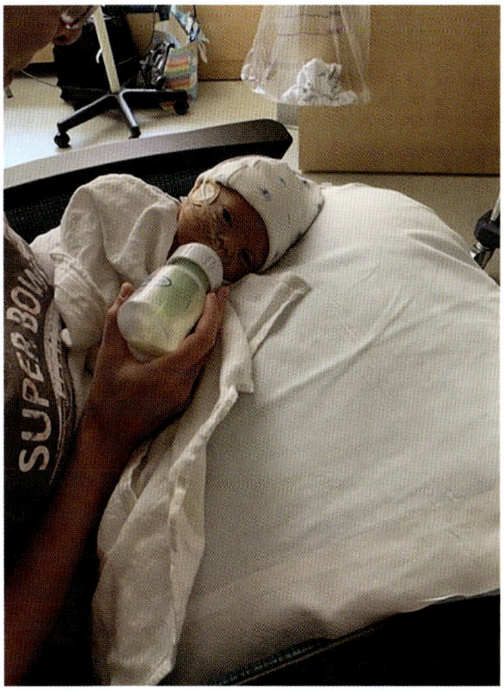

**Fig. 11.3** Feeding an infant in a semireclined side-lying position supports drinking from a bottle.

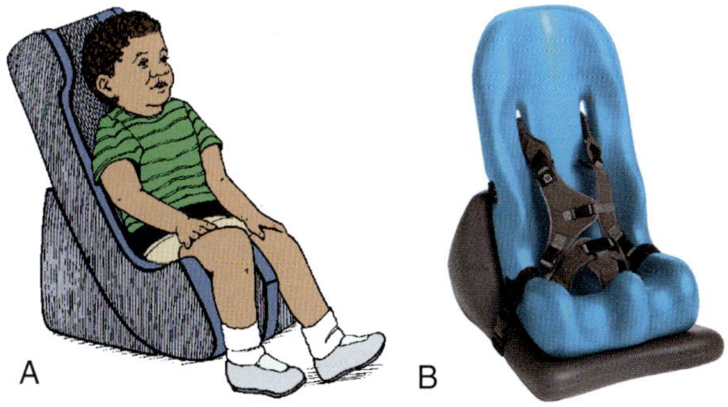

**Fig. 11.4** (A) Tumble form feeder chair and (B) Special tomato chair offer support and an adjustable feeding angle.

two hands free, creating opportunities to provide oral motor support. Please see Box 11.1 for additional information to consider related to infant breast- and bottle-feeding support.

Positioning changes may have an immediate impact on difficult oral motor problems, such as tonic bite and tongue thrust movement patterns. Positioning adaptations provide proximal support (support at the trunk) which influences distal movement and control (including oral motor control). Occupational therapy practitioners position the child's feet, legs, and pelvis to influence trunk stability. Postural control in the trunk muscles affects the child's head and neck position which in turn influences jaw movements. Finally, jaw stability and freedom of movement influence the child's tongue and lip control (Marcus & Breton, 2022b). Providing external support, stability, and alignment using positioning adaptations improves comfort, oral motor skills, and oral intake during mealtimes. Older infants and toddlers benefit from seated positioning options. A regular high chair provides trunk support and can be easily adapted with small towel rolls for additional foot support or lateral support (Fig. 11.5). The height of a standard high chair also allows caregivers to sit comfortably at the table next to the high chair, promoting social interaction between the child and family.

## BOX 11.1 Additional Considerations for Infant Feeding

### Bottle Feeding

When infants are referred for bottle feeding intervention, the occupational therapist must assess the baby's feeding efficiency and ensure that the feeding modality is the best match for the infant's oral motor skills. When supporting bottle feeding needs, the well-known Dr. Brown's brand offers a wide variety of nipple flow rates (from ultrapreemie to Y-cut) to support feeding efficiency needs. Depending on oral feeding skills, some infants may need a faster flow rate, while others may require a decreased flow. Positioning for feeding is another important consideration, as well as pacing and following the baby's cues regarding the need for breaks. Sucking skills, feeding efficiency, and state control are other aspects of bottle feeding that the OT may address. Infants benefit from regularly scheduled feedings at consistent times and locations from day to day. While a newborn infant may need to eat more frequently, eating on a predictable schedule helps establish the infant's daily rhythms and routines for beginning self-regulation.

### Breast Feeding

Breastfeeding is associated with significant health benefits for infants and mothers; however, it can be challenging to establish even healthy, full-term babies. Lactation consultants have specialized training and expertise to become breastfeeding specialists. In general, it is best to seek an evaluation with a lactation consultant to formally assess the mother-baby dyad and to address many common concerns such as painful nursing, cracked or bleeding nipples, positioning at the breast, latch, and over- or underproduction of breastmilk. There are opportunities for occupational therapy practitioners to collaborate with lactation consultants to support breastfeeding outcomes, and there is increasing interest and specialization among occupational therapy professionals to include breastfeeding and lactation in their scope of practice. In some cases, the baby may be typical and in other cases, the baby may present with anatomical differences (such as tongue tie or retracted jaw) or developmental differences (for example, poor state control, altered muscle tone, or weakness) that need to be addressed for breastfeeding to be successful.

The occupational therapy practitioner may be a valuable partner for the lactation consultant in specific situations. They may support mothers by partnering with lactation specialists to:

- Promote optimal positioning at the breast, including exploring different "holds" (such as cradle, cross cradle, or football hold) to allow the baby full support of head and body.
- Identify concerns for oral anatomy or sucking coordination.
- Outline a feeding schedule and routine that is age-appropriate and supports coregulation.
- Provide information on infant state control, calming strategies, and environmental considerations.
- Explore bottle feeding to supplement breastfeeding, if indicated.
- Provide mother strategies to care for herself (e.g., nutrition, rest, support) to support daily routines and care of infant.

There are continuing education courses offered that are focused on the role of occupational therapy in supporting breastfeeding. Additional learning is recommended for practitioners to gain knowledge and skills in this specialty area of practice. Please see additional online resources.

Children may require adaptive seating such as a wheelchair or an adaptive stroller (e.g., Kid Kart, Rifton chair), to provide optimal support during feeding (Fig. 11.6). Lateral trunk or arm supports, pelvic strap or seat belt, pommel, headrests, specialized chest straps, or a tray may provide more stability for the pelvis, trunk, and head. For example, children with cerebral palsy experience muscle tone challenges that may lead to poor trunk control, postural stability, and poor head control resulting in feeding and eating challenges that include lack of food retention, poor food mastication, delayed swallowing, breathing incoordination, and respiratory

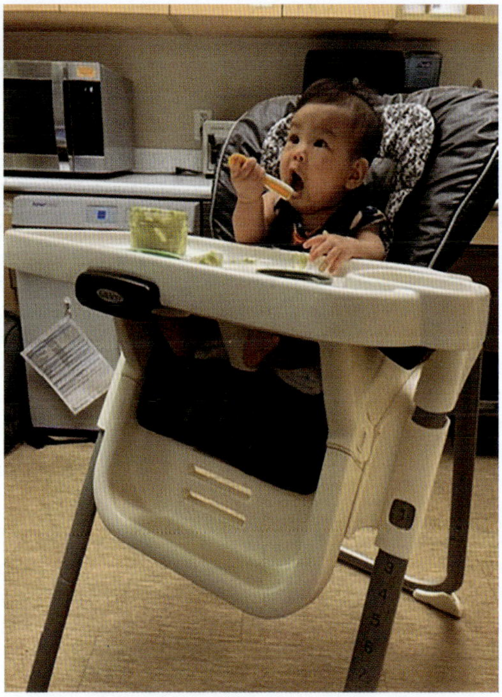

**Fig. 11.5** Toddler sits on a folded towel for optimal positioning for feeding in the highchair.

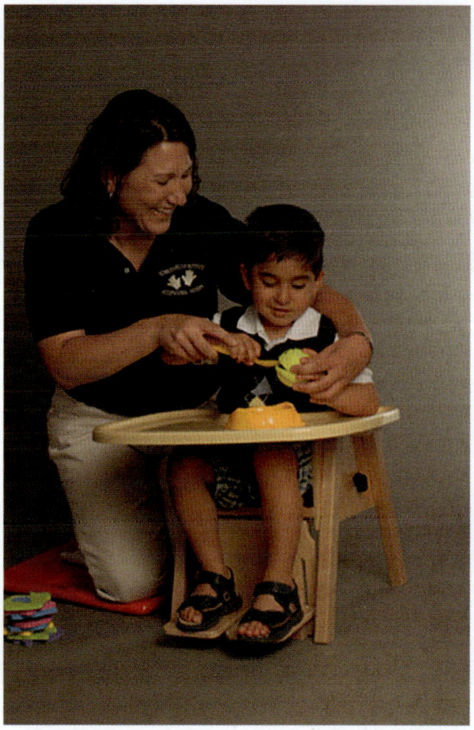

**Fig. 11.6** Adaptive positioning provides a firm base of support to the trunk and feet during self-feeding.

challenges (Acar et al., 2022). A well-supported and slightly flexed head position may reduce abnormal movement patterns such as a tonic bite in response to a stimulus, with difficulty opening or relaxing the jaw, or strong tongue thrust, in which the tongue forcefully protrudes beyond the border of the lips during oral feeding activities (Beckman, 2000).

**Interventions to Improve the Oral Motor Skills Required of the Oral Preparatory Phase.** Oral motor challenges may affect lip closure, tongue movements, biting, and chewing, and poor coordination of oral movements may result in spillage, drooling, coughing, choking, and aspiration. The practitioner addresses oral motor strength including tongue, lips, cheek, and jaw. Anatomical differences of the face and mouth are also important to consider when supporting oral motor skill development, such as cleft lip and palate (illustrated in Fig. 11.7). Please see Box 11.2 for further details regarding treatment for children with cleft lip and palate. Additional information is also available online. The occupational therapy practitioner in Fig. 11.8 engages children in varied intervention activities for the oral preparatory phase.

***Interventions for the Lips and Cheeks.*** Problems affecting the lips and cheeks may include structural differences (such as a cleft), abnormal tightness, or weakness. A child may demonstrate lip or cheek retraction, making it difficult for the child to assume or sustain lip closure. Adequate lip closure and lip seal are needed for sucking and to assist the child with oral control to prevent anterior spillage during feeding. It is difficult to swallow with retracted lips and cheeks because the lips are unable to seal the oral cavity to create pressure to propel the food bolus into the pharyngeal cavity. Although evidence is not strong (Howe & Wang, 2013), slow perioral and intraoral cheek elongation may promote lip closure before initiating functional activities with whistles or with spoon-feeding.

***Interventions for the Tongue.*** Tongue size, position, range of motion, strength, and coordination are critical considerations to support successful oral feeding. Children may demonstrate immature forward-backward tongue movements during feeding, poor dissociation of the tongue from the jaw, poor tongue lateralization to control textured food over the molar surfaces, or difficulty using the tongue to gather food after chewing and to form a bolus to swallow. Occupational therapy practitioners may engage the child in activities to facilitate tongue movements, such as encouraging the child to make silly faces in a mirror or lick lollipops, frosting, or whipped cream from the corners of the mouth or within the cheeks. Stimulating the sides of the tongue and inside the cheeks with a Nuk brush or oral motor tool may also encourage tongue lateralization, as needed for chewing and food gathering. Children with tongue thrust may benefit from oral motor activities to facilitate tongue lateralization, which can be encouraged by placing the spoon or food bolus to the sides of the mouth, rather than at the midline (Beckman, 2000).

***Interventions to Support the Jaw.*** Children may exhibit jaw weakness that results in an open-mouthed posture at rest, drooling, food loss during feeding, difficulty chewing a variety of foods, and poor stabilization when drinking from a cup. Jaw weakness and instability also affect lip closure for spoon-feeding and control during swallowing. Practitioners facilitate jaw strength through a variety of nonnutritive or nutritive activities. Nonnutritive strengthening activities may include sustained biting or repetitive chewing on a resistive device. Fig. 11.9 illustrates a child engaging in a jaw-strengthening activity. Nutritive jaw-strengthening activities include biting or chewing on fruits or vegetables encased in a mesh pouch or progressive resistive activities with a variety of solid or chewy foods placed over the molar surfaces (Gosa et al., 2017). Children may practice chewing foods encased in a mesh or silicone feeding bag to experience repetitive chewing with less risk of gagging or choking. For safety reasons, practitioners do not offer food (even for oral motor practice) that the child is unable to chew and swallow safely. If needed, external jaw support can be provided by the occupational therapy practitioner whose index finger is placed below the mandible and the thumb is placed on the anterior chin. Providing jaw support while sitting beside the child with the arm around the back of the child's neck may allow the occupational therapy practitioner to provide additional stability for the child to maintain adequate head alignment (Fig. 11.10).

Efficient cup drinking requires more mature jaw control than bottle feeding. One reason for difficulty transitioning from the bottle to the cup can be related to poor jaw stability. To help children prepare

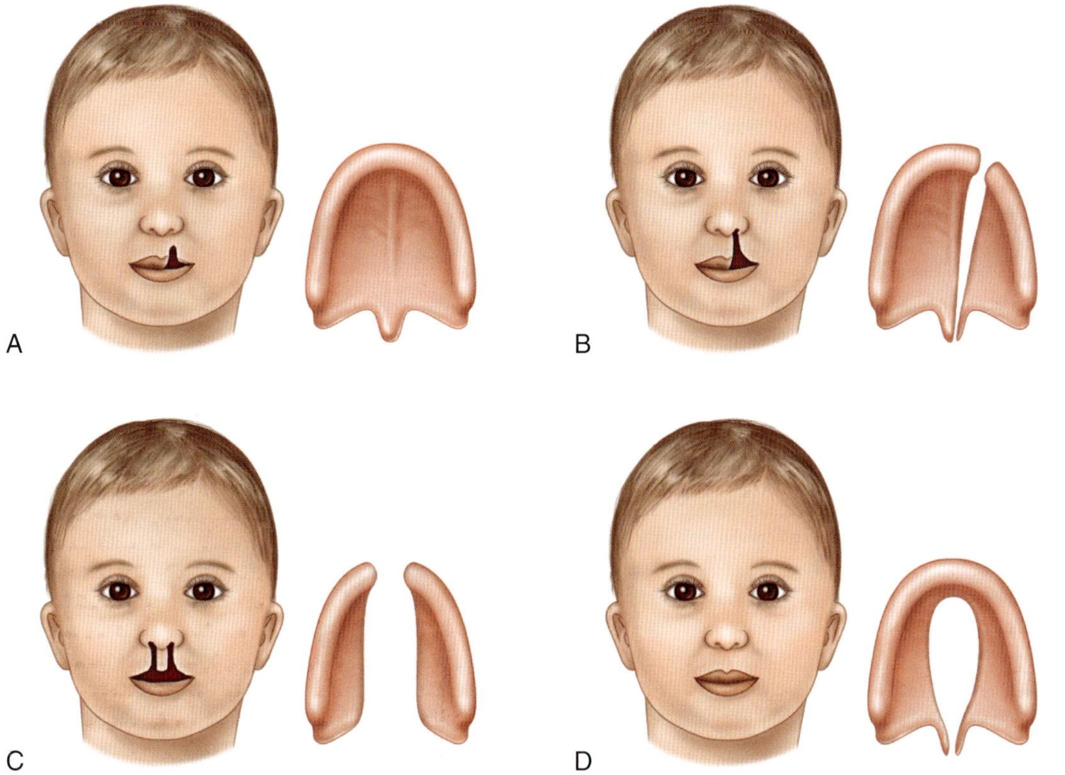


**Fig. 11.7** Cleft lip and palate. (A). Unilateral cleft lip. (B). Unilateral cleft lip and palate. (C). Bilateral cleft lip and palate (D). Cleft palate. (From Silvestri, L. S. (2018). *Saunders comprehensive review for the NCLEX-RN examination* (7th ed.). Elsevier.)

for cup-drinking activities, occupational therapy practitioners may initially work on jaw stability and mouth closure through positioning, handling, and oral motor activities (Rosenfeld-Johnson, 2005).

***Interventions for Chewing.*** Chewing abilities are formed as part of a developmental continuum through early feeding experiences. Infants develop initial chewing abilities through gumming and mashing with their tongue, which is most successful with foods that are dissolvable or soft. Once teeth begin to emerge the child has an increasing ability to bite and chew foods of varying textures (Wilson et al., 2021). Please see Box 11.3 for further details regarding dentition.

Children with difficulty chewing may need adaptations to their diet so that the texture of offered food matches their oral motor skill development. Modifications to food consistencies may also be appropriate to allow the child to practice chewing while minimizing the potential for choking or adverse feeding experiences. While the category of meltable solids tends to include many snack foods, this texture category provides a safer alternative to practice chewing as the foods easily dissolve with saliva.

**Interventions to Support Reduce the Oral Control Required for Drinking.** Providing alternatives to traditional methods of drinking and eating may reduce the oral motor demands on a child and allow for better performance. For example, infants that have a weak suck, limited endurance, and/or an anatomic difference, such as an oral cleft, may benefit from an adaptive bottle system (e.g., Medela Special Needs Feeder, Dr. Brown's Zero-Resistance Specialty Feeding System, Pigeon Baby Nursing Bottle for Cleft Lip/Palate). A child first learning to drink from a straw may do better with a short or small straw. Small straws require less oral suction and may deliver a smaller liquid bolus that is easier to control in the mouth. An adaptive straw drinking system such as the Honey Bear Squeeze Bottle can be used to help teach a child to drink from a straw, given that the liquid reservoir is designed to be squeezable to assist with liquid delivery into the child's mouth. When liquid is pulled into the straw with a one-way valve, it does not fall back into the cup if the child loses suction, allowing the child to put forth less effort and achieve flow.

Sippy cups are easier for some children to use for drinking and are commercially available in a variety of styles. They may have hard plastic spouts or soft spouts and permanent or removable nonspill valves. They may be fast-flowing, with little suction required, or slower-flowing, requiring more oral suction. Occupational therapy practitioners carefully consider how the sippy cup properties affect the child's oral motor control and swallowing. A spouted cup may initially make it easier for a child to suck the liquid or form a bolus in the mouth. Cups with nonspill valves in the lid require stronger lip closure and oral suction abilities and may be more difficult to use for children with neuromuscular impairments or anatomical differences such as cleft palate. U-shaped cut-out cups (such as Flexi Nosey Cups, Fig. 11.11) help to maintain a neutral head position when drinking liquid. When drinking from a cup with a spout, the child may need to tilt the head back, which may create additional difficulties if the child has extensor posturing, poor head control, or pharyngeal swallowing problems. The use of a cut-out cup may help reduce head and neck extension and allow the occupational therapy practitioner to easily observe the flow of liquid and the child's mouth movements during drinking activities. Clear cut-out cups allow the occupational therapy practitioner or caregiver to see liquid entering the child's mouth easily when they are providing physical assistance for drinking activities.

Children may benefit from the slower flow of thickened liquids when first learning to drink from a cup to compensate for limited oral control or swallowing abilities. Children often bite on the rim or spout of the cup to gain jaw stability. They also may push the cup into the corners of their lips or rest their tongue on the rim of the cup for additional stability and sensory input. These patterns should decrease over time as the child becomes more skilled in managing liquids from a cup.

## BOX 11.2 Cleft Lip and Palate

Occupational therapy practitioners recommend compensatory positioning, adaptive feeding techniques, and specialized bottles for young infants with cleft lip or palate. Feeding the child in a more upright position (>60 degrees) may help improve milk transfer to the posterior oral cavity. Cheek and/or lip support may be recommended to help with gentle closure of a cleft lip to improve latching or suction during feeding. A variety of specialized bottles and nipples are available that use up-and-down compression movements (rather than suction) or allow the caregiver to squeeze the bottle to help extract and transfer milk. The Special Needs Feeder (previously called the Haberman Feeder) has a long, soft nipple and one-way valve that can deliver milk with little to no oral suction required (Miller, 2011, Fig. 11.6). The longer length of the nipple helps deposit the liquid toward the back of the mouth, beyond the cleft. This specialty feeding system has a feature to allow the feeder to assist with milk transfer in synchrony with the infant's sucking efforts. Dr. Brown's Infant Paced Feeding Valve can be inserted into any standard Dr. Brown's bottle/nipple system to improve an infant's ability to use compression to extract milk from the bottle. Positioning adaptations and specialized bottle systems are often recommended as a first approach. Infants with severe cleft lip and palate may require additional medical interventions, such as a nasal trumpet, palatal obturator, or nasoalveolar molding (Bessell et al., 2011; Grayson & Maull, 2005).

While breast/bottle feeding and nutritional challenges are usually the first obstacles for babies born with clefts, it is important to provide anticipatory guidance regarding introduction to spoon feeding, cup drinking, and approach to care before and after surgical repair. Many surgical protocols include avoiding the use of nipples, spoons, straws, and spouted cups immediately following palate surgery to protect the area of repair. The infant should have practice with alternative means for eating before planned procedures, such as practice with open cups or nonvalved rimmed sipper cups, or the Medela SoftFeeder. The TenderCare Feeder is also an alternative feeding option for infants when more traditional cup options are not successful.

After surgical repair of a cleft, occupational therapy practitioners may perform scar massage, initiate therapy activities to reduce oral hypersensitivity, and reassess the oral feeding method. Some children may have ongoing problems with food or liquid entering the nasal cavity during oral feeding. Interventions for this problem include evaluating which food or liquid textures are more challenging for the child, alternating bites of food with sips of liquid, suggesting more upright positioning during feeding, and recommending smaller-sized bites of food or sips of liquid. Please see online resources for further foundational content on the diagnosis of Cleft Lip and Palate.

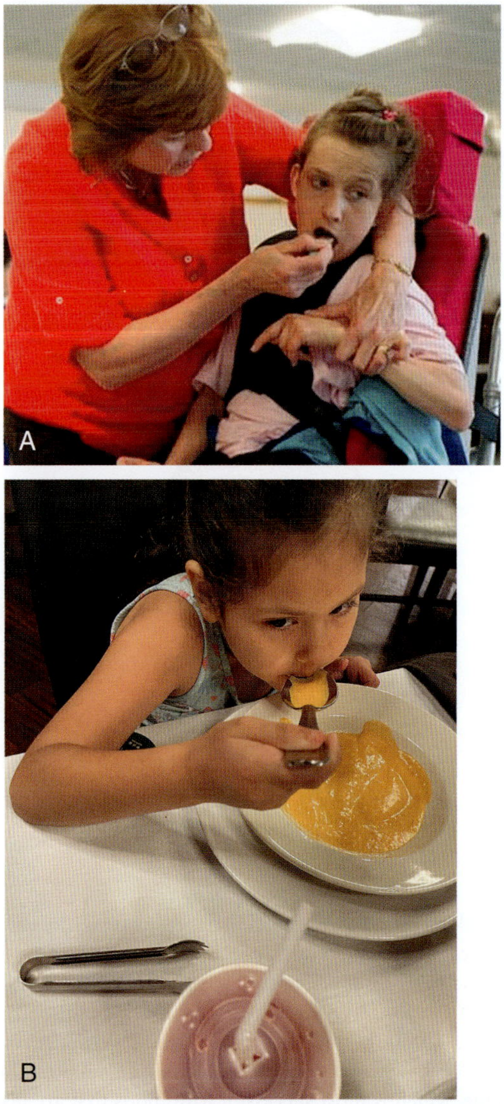

Fig. 11.8 (A) Practitioner is working on placement of foods on the side of the mouth. (B) Child is working on lips closure and oral control with a thick soup.

**Interventions to Improve Oral Control and Reduce Drooling.** Different therapeutic methods for addressing chronic drooling have been described in the scientific literature, including the use of scopolamine transdermal patch, botulinum toxin A injections, and surgical treatments of duct ligation, relocation, or excision in the salivary glands, however, there is no consensus on the ideal strategy of treatment, and there may be negative consequences of these procedures that target decreased saliva production (Hung et al., 2021; Melo et al., 2021; Silva et al., 2022; You et al., 2022).

Other interventions to control drooling include oral-motor activities to promote lip closure and tongue movements, such as encouraging lateral and rotary movements of the tongue by chewing or licking food items placed on the sides of the mouth. Intervention may also include training on sensory awareness. Oral motor and sensorimotor exercises have been found to be effective in reducing drooling (Awaad et al., 2023; Myles, 2020).

### Interventions for the Oral Propulsive Phase

During the oral propulsive stage, the tip of the tongue touches the hard palate just behind the upper teeth, while the posterior tongue drops so that the back of the oral cavity opens. The tongue then expands contact with the palate from anterior to posterior, moving upwards and squeezing the bolus back into the pharynx. Tongue weakness or incoordination can impair bolus formation and transport, leading to retention of food in the oral cavity and may impact swallow initiation. Therefore, intervention for this phase primarily focuses on the tongue, in terms of mobility and coordinated function. Please see the sections above for strategies to support interventions for the tongue.

### Interventions for the Pharyngeal Phase

Children with pharyngeal dysphagia may have difficulty swallowing, which presents with coughing, gurgly voice, wet breathing, and multiple swallows (Benfer et al., 2015). Difficulty swallowing may result in aspiration. **Aspiration** is defined as the entry of a foreign substance below the vocal cords into the trachea. Box 11.4 lists signs of aspiration. Clinical signs of aspiration may require assessment with an instrumental evaluation of swallowing, such as a **videofluoroscopic swallow study** (VFSS) or **fiberoptic endoscopic evaluation of swallowing (FEES)**. Please see Chapter 9 for information on swallow evaluation.

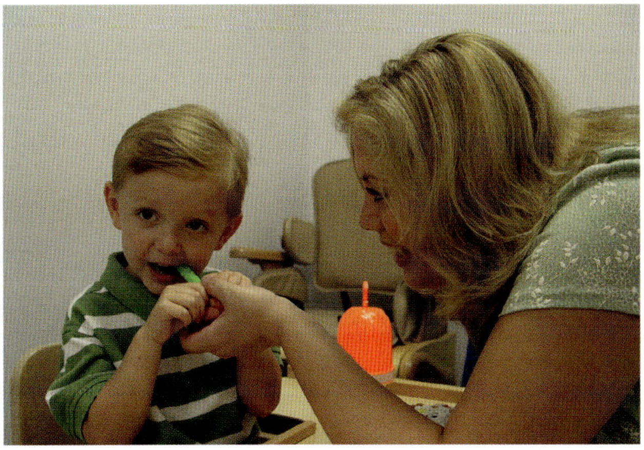

**Fig. 11.9** Using a resistive device for nonnutritive jaw strengthening.

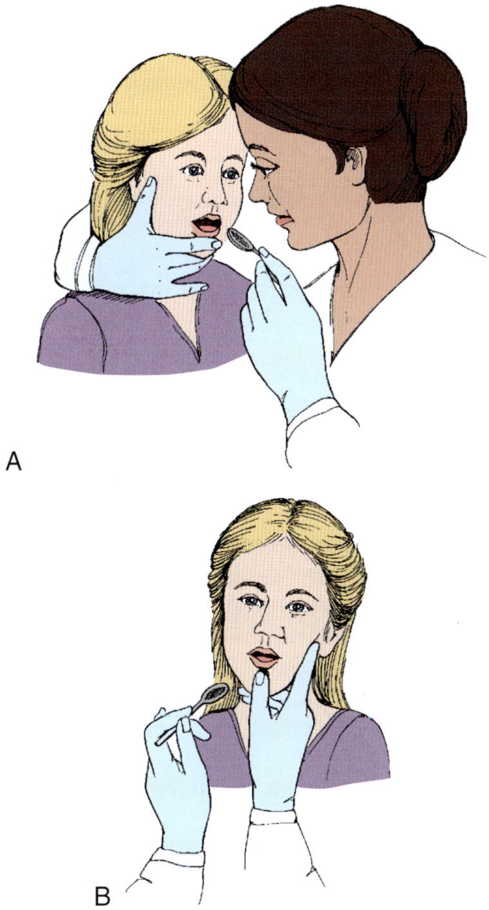

**Fig. 11.10** Jaw control and oral support. (A) From the side. (B) From the front.

Occupational therapy practitioners may address aspiration or pharyngeal dysphagia by using the data from an instrumental evaluation of swallowing to suggest changes to positioning, the method of presenting foods and liquids, and adjusting the food or liquid consistency to mitigate aspiration. In some cases, aspiration is silent and cannot be detected during clinical observations. Because of the potential medical complications resulting from chronic aspiration and the limited number of effective treatment options, alternative, nonoral feeding methods such as tube feeding may be required for some children.

### BOX 11.3 The Role of Dentition in Oral Feeding

Dentition or tooth development is essential to support the successful management of solid food textures. Dental anomalies and oral health can greatly impact a child's willingness and ability to eat. Whether these anomalies are acquired or congenital, they can play a significant role in the occupational therapy intervention plan. For example, atypical dental development (missing teeth or malocclusion) may require modification of food textures to enable effective breakdown of food. Dental decay may limit a child's interest in meals due to pain associated with chewing. This decay may also lead to the need for dental extractions, with additional implications for learning and success with the mechanics of eating. Oral hygiene, including tooth brushing and flossing, is a daily living activity that is essential to support oral and overall health.

Occupational therapy practitioners can support the child and family in developing positive tooth brushing and flossing routines that will facilitate success with this self-care task. There is a wide range of readily available tools to help support caregivers, such as a 3-sided toothbrush, Infadent, ARK probe, NUK brush, vibrating/electric toothbrush, visual timer, songs, and connections to pediatric dentists.

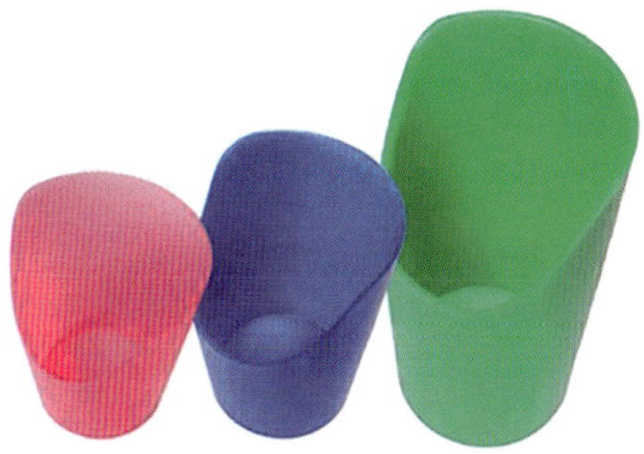

**Fig. 11.11** Flexi Nosey cups. (*Source*: ARK Therapeutic.)

### BOX 11.4 Clinical Indicators for Referral for Swallowing Evaluation

- Congestion and/or wet vocal quality during or after eating
- Frequent occurrence of respiratory illnesses (e.g., pneumonia, bronchiolitis, prolonged colds, asthma-like symptoms not well controlled)
- Difficulty weaning from oxygen or need for oxygen support frequently
- Significant neurological diagnosis and/or neuromotor involvement
- Coughing or choking on liquids and/or on other consistencies
- Oral motor dysfunction
- Prolonged mealtimes, such as longer than 30 minutes to feed because of oral motor issues
- Reliance on gastronomy tube (G-tube) feedings but is willing to eat something by mouth and safety of oral feeding is questioned.

**Changes to Positioning to Support Optimal Swallowing and Reduce Likelihood of Aspiration.** Supportive positioning can have a major impact on the child's swallowing abilities. A chin tuck position may be recommended when the child has delayed swallow initiation. One way to achieve a more natural chin tuck position is to encourage the use of a straw, straw sipper cup, or straw-style sports bottle. There are many options that can be age-appropriate choices across the lifespan. During a VFSS, a delay in swallow initiation is characterized as pooling of food or liquid in the pharyngeal space located close to the opening of the larynx. When the child is positioned with a slight chin tuck, the laryngeal opening may become smaller, reducing the risk of penetration or aspiration when there is a delay (Arvedson & Brodsky, 2002). Occasionally, a chin tuck position may be contraindicated for young infants who have laryngomalacia or tracheomalacia (softening of the cartilage in the larynx or trachea) because their soft tissues may be more prone to collapse (Ruark, 2007). A side-lying position for infants may be an appropriate adaptation, specifically for young infants with vocal cord dysfunction. In general, when children are nearing 6 months of age, it is important to consider a more upright drinking position due to typical growth and changing anatomy which impacts swallow function (Morris & Klein, 2000). Occupational therapists need to make individualized positioning recommendations based on a comprehensive assessment and, when available, information obtained from a VFSS..

**Changes to the Presentation of Foods and Liquids.** Some children require multiple swallows to clear one bite of food. If a child is unable to complete a subsequent or "dry" swallow in response to a verbal prompt, an empty spoon offered in the same way as a bite of food may stimulate oral movements to prompt a second swallow. Occupational therapy practitioners may also provide recommendations for the pace of oral feeding to allow the child sufficient time to swallow all the food between each bite. More difficult foods, liquids, or self-feeding activities may need to be limited or presented within the first few minutes of a meal session when the child is less fatigued. Children may also benefit from smaller bites of food or sips of liquid. This modification can be achieved using a controlled-flow cup or straw, a smaller diameter straw, single discrete sips, a slow-flow bottle system, or a smaller spoon.

**Modifications to Food and Liquid Consistency.** The International Dysphagia Diet Standardization Initiative (IDDSI, 2019) established by the American Dietetic Association provides standardized terminology and guidelines for food texture modifications in dysphagia management. Many institutions use the dysphagia diet framework and testing methods in practice (IDDSI, 2019, Fig. 11.12; Box 11.5). Other programs use descriptive language and characterize foods based on the oral motor mechanics required, such as "meltable solids" which melt or dissolve with saliva. Some practitioners use common descriptors for food textures, such as "stage 3," "junior," or "ground." Box 11.6 provides a list of foods and their properties.

Practitioners working with infants and children recommend food textures and types of foods to support a child's safe swallowing and may recommend modifications to the thickness of liquid to compensate for a variety of swallowing, oral motor, and oral sensory deficits. Different consistencies of liquid present different demands. Thin liquids offered from an open cup are the most difficult to control during swallowing because they move so quickly. Children with dysphagia may not be able to coordinate swallowing thin liquids, and aspiration events are more common with thin liquids when evaluated with VFSS (Bulow et al., 2003; Friedman & Frazier, 2000; Miller & Willging, 2003). Room temperature water is the most challenging liquid, as it moves the fastest, is odorless, colorless, and relatively tasteless, providing minimal feedback to the mouth and pharynx when swallowing. Thickened liquid is easier to control as it moves more slowly in the mouth and allows the child more time to organize a bolus for effective swallowing, without early spillage into the pharyngeal cavity. Box 11.7 provides descriptions of liquid consistencies.

A variety of foods and products can be used to thicken liquids, including SimplyThick, Gelmix, and Purathick. The IDDSI Flow Test (IDDSI, 2019) is an objective measurement for the liquid thickness that requires the use of Luer-Lok syringes and a device for measuring time such as a phone or stopwatch. Fig. 11.13 describes this testing method. Additionally, see online resources. Some commercial thickeners may present challenges in maintaining the desired liquid thickness over time or may result in a gritty consistency, which may impact palatability for drinking. The US Food and Drug Administration (FDA) has issued warnings and precautions for the use of xanthan gum thickeners with young infants, premature infants, and older children who have a history of necrotizing enterocolitis (Beal et al., 2012; United States Food and Drug Administration, 2012). Necrotizing enterocolitis (NEC) is a serious medical condition related to necrosis of tissue in the intestines or bowel. The team of medical and/or dietary providers must closely monitor the child's response to thickening,

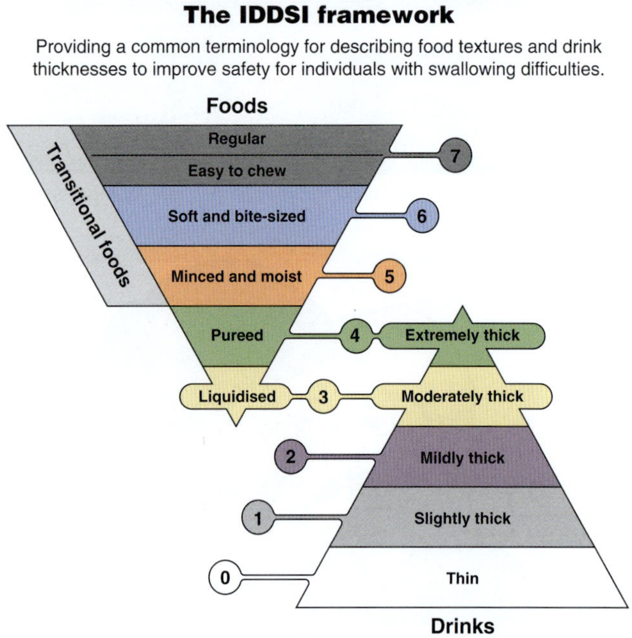


**Fig. 11.12** International dysphagia diet standardization initiative framework. (From IDDSI. (2019). *International dysphagia diet standardization initiative: A global initiative to improve the lives of over 590 million people worldwide living with dysphagia.* Retrieved from: http://www.iddsi.org)

## BOX 11.5 International Dysphagia Diet Standardization Initiative (IDDSI) Levels of Food

Texture for Dysphagia Management.

**Level 3 Liquidized:** Thin pureed foods such as stage 2 baby foods or the consistency of honey which drip slowly or in dollop through the tines of a fork.

**Level 4 Pureed:** Pureed foods that are homogeneous, cohesive, or pudding-like substance. Pureed foods do not dollop or drip continuously through fork tines.

**Level 5 Minced and moist:** Cohesive, moist, semisolid foods that may require some chewing. Level 5 foods also include ground or minced meats and fork-mashed soft fruits and vegetables.

**Level 6 Soft and meltable:** Soft and bite-sized small pieces of meltable and soft-solid foods that require more chewing ability (than level 5), such as crackers, breads, cooked vegetables, soft fruits, and meats.

**Level 7 Easy to chew:** Everyday foods, of soft/tender textures that may range in bite sizes. Teeth and chewing skills are required to break down these foods.

**Level 7 Regular:** No food restriction and includes fruit with skins, hard or crunchy vegetables, nuts, tough meats such as beef or pork steak, and foods that are sticky or dry.

*Source*: IDDSI. (2019). *International dysphagia diet standardization initiative: A global initiative to improve the lives of over 590 million people worldwide living with dysphagia.* Retrieved from: http://www.iddsi.org

the volume of liquid intake, and hydration to ensure that the child is meeting daily fluid and nutrition requirements.

Regular fruits and vegetables, baby foods, yogurt, and pudding may be blenderized to make thickened smoothies or shakes for older children. Dried infant cereals or mashed potato flakes may be added to thicken pediatric formula or nonhuman milk. Of note, infant cereals are not effective in thickening expressed human breast milk because the starches contained in the cereal are broken down by the amylase in breast milk, quickly returning the milk to a thin liquid. It is difficult to create recipes for standard viscosities due to the variable thickness of these foods, but it is possible to evaluate the viscosity of each finished product, using IDDSI testing. Each thickener has different sensory, nutritional, and thickening properties, all of which should be considered in an occupational therapist's recommendations in collaboration with the child's medical team.

### Interventions for the Esophageal Phase

Children who have a history of esophageal phase swallow problems may have difficulty advancing to higher food textures because of decreased esophageal motility or function. Some examples of conditions that can impact the esophageal phase include upper esophageal sphincter dysfunction, gastroesophageal reflux, esophageal strictures, and eosinophilic esophagitis (Morgan et al., 2012). Children with structural anomalies of the esophagus are at increased risk for aspiration during swallowing, food refusal behaviors, delayed transition to textured foods, and poor esophageal motility (Baird et al., 2015). Esophageal motility describes how quickly foods and liquids move through the esophagus and empty into the stomach. Liquids and smooth, runny foods empty into the stomach more quickly than thick, fibrous, or more solid foods.

Occupational therapists may recommend adapting food textures to maximize oral intake, alternating bites of food with sips of liquid to help clear the esophagus, slowing the pace of feeding, or encouraging a subsequent dry swallow after each bite of food to help compensate for delayed esophageal motility (Friedlander et al., 2016). Children with eosinophilic esophagitis (EoE; a chronic allergic/immune condition of the esophagus, where the esophagus becomes inflamed and does not contract properly) may benefit from modifications to the order of food presentation to promote effective or comfortable swallowing (Menard-Katcher et al., 2014; Mukkada et al., 2010). Case Example 11.1 provides a case study that illustrates common concerns and management of eosinophilic esophagitis.

**BOX 11.6 Properties of Foods for Children With Oral Motor Difficulties**

**Recommended Foods**

- Even consistency
- Increased density and volume
- Thick (liquids)
- Foods with uniform texture
- Food that stays together (will not break up in the mouth)
- Easy to remove and suck
- Foods that dissolve quickly (such as crackers)

**Contraindicated Foods**

- Multiple textures and consistencies (e.g., tacos, vegetable soup, stews, salads)
- Sticky (e.g., peanut butter)
- Greasy (e.g., fried foods)
- Tough (e.g., red meat, processed meats, diced fruit)
- Fibrous and stringy (e.g., celery, citrus fruits, raw vegetables)
- Food with skins (raw fruits, peanuts)
- Spicy (pepper and horseradish)
- Seeds and nuts (plain or in breads and cakes)
- Thin liquids (e.g., water, broth, coffee, tea, apple juice)
- Foods that liquefy quickly (e.g., Jell-O, ice cream, and watermelon)
- Foods that break up in the mouth (e.g., some cookies and flaky pastries)
- Hard, crunchy (e.g., carrots)

## INTERVENTIONS TO REDUCE FEEDING AND EATING REFUSAL

Infants, children, and youth may present with behaviors that challenge feeding and eating, such as refusing foods or being very selective about

**BOX 11.7 Liquid Consistencies (From Thinnest to Thickest) for Dysphagia Management**

**Level 0 Thin:** Liquid that is the consistency of water or juice. Many formulas and milk products have a slightly higher viscosity than that of liquids; however, they are still considered thin liquids. Soup broth and foods that melt such as popsicles are also considered thin liquids.

**Level 1 Slightly thick:** Level 1 liquids were previously referred to as half nectar thick. They are thicker than water, but still thin enough to flow through a straw.

**Level 2 Mildly thick:** Level 2 (previously referred to as nectar thick) liquids are the consistency of tomato juice and include many natural fruit nectars (e.g., apricot nectar, pear nectar) and some pre-made yogurt smoothies.

**Level 3 Moderately thick:** Liquid that is the consistency of honey, which drips slowly or in dollops through the tines of a fork.

**Level 4 Extremely thick or pureed:** Liquids that are the consistency of pudding or yogurt, which do not drip, dollop, or flow though the tines of a fork.

*Source*: IDDSI. (2019). *International dysphagia diet standardization initiative: A global initiative to improve the lives of over 590 million people worldwide living with dysphagia.* Retrieved from: http://www.iddsi.org

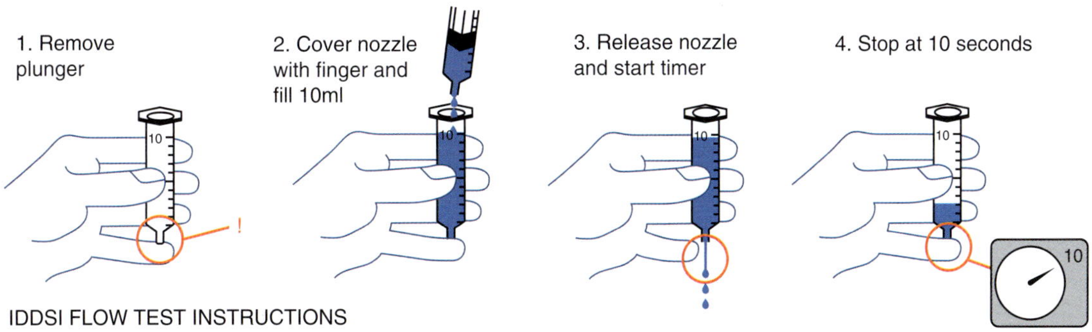


**Fig. 11.13** The IDDSI flow test to classify liquid thickness. (From IDDSI. (2019). *International dysphagia diet standardization initiative: A global initiative to improve the lives of over 590 million people worldwide living with dysphagia.* Retrieved from: http://www.iddsi.org)

## CASE EXAMPLE 11.1 FEEDING CONSIDERATIONS WITH EOSINOPHILIC ESOPHAGITIS

Sally is a 5-year-old girl with long-standing challenges with eating, including coughing, gagging, and vomiting while eating. She has not experienced these symptoms when drinking or eating pureed food (such as applesauce), and she prefers eating a soft diet. When younger, the physician diagnosed Sally with over 30 food allergies. She has outgrown many of these allergies (based on recent testing) but she is reluctant to add food to her diet. During the occupational therapy evaluation, Sally and her mother reported the following feeding challenges:

- Sally often complains of food sticking in her throat, and that the food "won't go down."
- She avoids solid foods, especially food that requires chewing (e.g., chicken, steak, raw carrots) or anything with a peel or skin (e.g., apples, grapes, and blueberries).
- She needs to have a glass of water to sip on while she is eating. She drinks water after most bites of food.
- She is a slow eater, chews "forever," and is often the last person at the table. It takes Sally 45 to 60 minutes to eat each meal.
- She does not like to try new foods and she currently eats a limited variety of foods.
- Her mother reported that mealtimes are stressful. They are frustrated with her resistance to trying new or nonpreferred foods. Her mother prepares Sally a different meal from the family. The family becomes frustrated with how long it takes Sally to eat, and Sally does not like being pushed to eat faster.
- Sally's gag response is easily triggered, such as when she tries to swallow a bigger bite of food, or when it feels like the food is not moving when she swallows. If she gags, she might vomit, and she is fearful of eating with peers or outside of her home because she is worried about gagging and vomiting in public.
- Sally loves ketchup and ranch dressing, and she adds sauces and dips to her food.

The occupational therapist completed a developmental screening, which did not reveal any developmental differences in terms of muscle tone, strength, balance, fine motor, gross motor, or self-help skills. She observed Sally and her mother eating lunch. Sally's demonstrated coordinated oral motor skills. She was able to lick, bite, chew, and suck from a straw. She did not show any clinical signs of pharyngeal swallow dysfunction, such as cough or wet vocal quality, and Sally's respiratory health history was unremarkable. Sally's mother did not report any challenges regarding sensory development and the therapist did not observe sensory seeking or sensory avoidance behaviors. Sally's mother described her as an active girl who enjoys riding her bike, jumping on the trampoline, and doing arts and crafts projects. She was socially interactive, cooperative, and answered questions clearly. Sally made eye contact and expressed her likes and dislikes. She was curious and asked about other people who entered space.

The occupational therapist referred Sally to a Pediatric Gastroenterologist to assess suspicion for esophageal swallow dysfunction. An upper endoscopy and biopsy confirmed the diagnosis of eosinophilic esophagitis. Along with medication and a tailored diet to treat this disease, Sally received specific feeding recommendations from the occupational therapist to support her eating and mealtime participation. These recommendations included suggestions to promote comfortable swallowing, such as taking small bites and chewing well, using dips and sauces as lubricants for food, and using a drink during mealtimes to help wash food down. Other strategies were related to food modification, preparing, and offering softer food textures, and avoiding the foods that consistently got "stuck." The practitioner provided Sally and her parents ideas for helping Sally learn to try new foods, and practice eating in different environments, such as at a restaurant and at a friend's house. The therapist answered questions about the diagnosis and provided information and strategies to support the family's routines.

the foods they will eat (Blisset & Harris, 2002). Problem-feeding behaviors (see Chapter 9) can arise over time and require behavioral interventions.

### Interventions to Improve Behaviors Related to Feeding and Eating

Occupational therapy interventions may include creating opportunities for positive interactions and associations by grading and adapting tasks and expectations. using positive reinforcement to increase desired behaviors, and ignoring or redirecting undesired behaviors (Caldwell et al., 2018, 2020). Research suggests that positive reinforcement combined with ignoring or redirection of inappropriate behaviors improves oral intake and self-feeding skills (Gronski & Doherty, 2020; Sharp et al., 2022). It is not recommended to use food as a reinforcer, as this may create further negative associations with foods. Toys or activities that are used to praise a child for positive eating behaviors should not be readily available outside feeding sessions so that the child is motivated to earn the item during mealtimes.

Problematic feeding and eating behaviors may be addressed with techniques such as systematic desensitization or cognitive behavioral therapy (CBT; Zhu & Dalby-Payne, 2019). **Systematic desensitization** targets feeding behaviors by slowly exposing children to new or nonpreferred foods at their comfort level, with the encouragement of playful food interactions that can ultimately increase a child's variety of accepted foods (Zhu & Dalby-Payne, 2019). CBT addresses the child's feelings, thoughts, and behaviors (Bloomfield et al., 2019) and targets their mood or anxiety. Children who have a psychosocial eating disorder such as avoidant/restrictive food intake disorder (AFRID) may benefit from this approach (Bryant-Waugh, 2019; Bryant-Waugh et al., 2018). Box 11.8 provides a brief description of AFRID.

Box 11.9 provides examples of specific behavioral strategies to manage problem behaviors during feeding and eating. These strategies are supported by extensive research (Bell et al., 2021; Caldwell et al., 2018, 2020; Chistol et al., 2018; Clark & Kingsley, 2020; Cravener et al., 2015; Desai et al., 2022; Gronski & Doherty, 2020; Howe & Wang, 2013; Huston et al., 2019; Johnson et al., 2015, 2019; Nicklaus, 2016; Sharp et al., 2017; Van den Engel-Hoek et al., 2017). See Chapter 25 for further discussion on approaches to managing challenging behaviors.

Parents may report challenging and disruptive mealtimes with frustration and anxiety as the child's refusal or selectivity contributes to caregiver stress (Beaudry-Bellefeuille et al., 2021; Bourne et al., 2022; Milano et al., 2019). Therefore, parents may benefit from education on strategies to promote hunger cues, increase food variety, limit access to less nutritious foods, and create structure within the meal to establish positive eating patterns. Box 11.10 provides information on hunger and appetite.

### Intervention to Address the Sensory Aspects of Feeding and Eating

Occupational therapy practitioners may address oral hypersensitivity using a sensory approach. A sensory approach includes the use of deep touch pressure and proprioception to reduce sensitivities, along with opportunities for gradual oral sensory exploration through play and positive experiences to reduce oral hypersensitivity (Boggs & Ferguson, 2016; Marcus & Breton, 2022b). Children with oral hypersensitivity may also benefit from generalized calming strategies such as slow linear rocking before oral stimulation. Infants may be encouraged to soothe themselves with hand-to-mouth activities or a pacifier. Practitioners may

### BOX 11.8 Avoidant Restrictive Food Intake Disorder

Avoidant Restrictive Food Intake Disorder (ARFID), has been identified within the DSM-5 (The Diagnostic and Statistical Manual of Mental Disorders, fifth edition) to help further understand and support treatment approaches when working with children who have concerns for food selectivity. ARFID has specific diagnostic criteria, in which the feeding difficulty is not better explained with another physical or mental health disorder, or the severity of the feeding difficulty exceeds what is routinely associated with their condition or disorder (Milano et al., 2019).

Children diagnosed with ARFID clinically present with a range of concerns. Treatment approaches vary and depend on the child's individual presentation. Three primary feeding behaviors associated with ARFID include selectivity, poor appetite, and fear of feeding (Milano et al., 2019). Children with long-standing, untreated picky eating concerns are more likely to develop ARIFD. According to the National Eating Disorders Association, many children with ARFID also have a co-occurring anxiety disorder.

The treatment for children with ARFID includes multidisciplinary care to address psychosocial challenges, nutrition, and potential need for medical monitoring. Occupational therapy practitioners work with team members to support treatment goals. Bryant-Waugh (2019) suggests, the aim of intervention may be to "minimize physical or nutritional risk through behavioral change and/or to help the individual learn to manage their own anxiety about trying new foods or extending their dietary intake" (p. 562). There is evolving research and program development for the treatment of children with ARFID that offer opportunities for the occupational therapy practitioners to explore.

### BOX 11.9 Behavioral Interventions for Feeding and Eating Refusal or Selectivity

- Positive reinforcement
- Gradual progression and shaping of behaviors
- Repeated exposure to foods during positive experiences (e.g., play)
- Incorporating nonfood rewards into daily routine and intervention
- Parent and caregiver training
- Modeling by parents and caregivers
- Offering choices and turn-taking to help a child feel a sense of control and increase their willingness to participate in mealtimes.
- Collaboration between child, family, and occupational therapy practitioner
- Emphasizing child's strengths
- Promoting self-determination and self-efficacy throughout the intervention

### BOX 11.10 Hunger and Appetite

People often use the terms hunger and appetite interchangeably, but they are different. Hunger is a biological need to eat, a complex system of physical and hormonal signals that informs the body's physiological need for food (Davis, 2018). Hunger is the body's way of telling a person that they need to eat to maintain homeostasis and fuel their body to maintain bodily functions. Appetite is a desire to eat because of external cues, such as seeing, smelling, or thinking about food. Appetite is created by the environment. For example, expecting food at certain times out of routine can lead to developing an appetite in anticipation of eating. External factors such as stress can decrease a person's appetite even if physiological hunger is present (Austin et al., 2009). Children with feeding issues may have interruptions in both the experiences of hunger and appetite.

One myth regarding hunger and "picky" eating or low volume of intake is that if a child is hungry enough, they will eat. This approach does not hold true, especially for children with developmental delays, physical disabilities, or other health concerns (Milano et al., 2019). Although tube feeding is effective in providing the necessary energy and nutrients when children do not eat enough by mouth, it can hinder the child's motivation to eat related to the interpretation of hunger and satiety cues as well as developing appetite (Wright et al., 2011). There are inpatient and outpatient programs for weaning patients from tube feeding to eating by mouth. Many gaps have been identified in terms of data on the best methods for weaning children off enteral feedings (Edwards et al., 2016), however, most programs recognize the role of hunger and appetite in supporting success. Several studies have shown that clinical hunger provocation can be an effective short-term intervention for weaning young children from tube feeding (Hartdorff et al., 2015; Edwards et al., 2016; Krom et al., 2020). With medical and dietary guidance, hunger provocation can be achieved by withholding tube feeding and/or with the use of appetite-enhancing medications. More research is needed to better understand how to promote the natural processes of hunger, satiation, and appetite when children are faced with eating difficulties.

playfully engage children in sensory play using textured objects, teethers, or vibrating toys that children hold or mouth. Using a sensory approach, the child would not be forced to experience an unpleasant sensation to "get used to it." Rather children are given opportunities to accept varied experiences as their tolerances improve. Children may benefit by engaging in routines and strategies (such as sensory diet strategies) before mealtimes to provide their bodies with the sensory input they need to improve their overall attention to a task. For example, a child may benefit from engaging in activities that provide proprioceptive input to the muscles and joints (such as hopping) that help them focus and engage in mealtime. See Chapters 27 and 28 for more on sensory approaches.

The practitioner also considers the sensory properties of food, including taste, texture, temperature, and the internal sounds associated with chewing. Children with lower sensory awareness may respond positively to cold foods or foods with strong flavors, including tangy, salty, or sour foods. Bland, room temperature, or slightly warm foods may be more acceptable for children with oral hypersensitivity. Practitioners make one change in sensory property at a time and provide the child with opportunities to experience comfort with the change.

The sensory properties of the environment matter as well. Environmental distractions may affect a child's skills. **Environmental adaptations** such as limiting the sensory stimuli in the environment may allow infants and children to focus on the task of feeding and eating. A calm sensory environment can be created with dim lights, reduced noise, soft or rhythmic music, and limited interruptions.

## INTERVENTIONS TO ADD NEW FOODS AND TEXTURES TO THE CHILD'S DIET

Occupational therapy practitioners often create feeding programs that consider the child's current feeding status in combination with behavioral and sensory strategies to increase the number and variety of foods and food textures the child eats. They create plans to reduce food selectivity by providing sequential (and graded) progressions and specific intervention activities that incorporate aspects of desensitization along with an understanding of sensory processing.

Several approaches include sensory exploration of foods and the concept of food chaining, which was developed by Fraker et al. (2007). In food chaining, the child begins with a preferred food, and gradually accepts new foods that are like the preferred food in all aspects but one. Considering color, shape, texture, and smell, the practitioner changes one aspect at a time. See Box 11.11 for an example of food chaining. The Positive Eating Program (PEP) is a framework that can be used

## BOX 11.11 Food Chaining

Food chaining is the process of beginning with a familiar accepted food (such as french fries) and changing it slightly, so the child increases their food choices. The following example shows the food chaining progression from French fries to carrots, with descriptions of the properties considered in the progression. The practitioner began with the child's favorite food, French fries. Making sure to keep the warm salty taste of the child's favorite food, the practitioner made sweet potato fries, using the same shapes. As the child became accustomed to this taste, they added butternut squash fries, which are the same color as sweet potato, but taste different. As the child experimented with these tastes, the clinician played a game with the child with all three types of fries ("name that fry"). His parents made the fries at home to reinforce the child's progress. Next the practitioner changed the shape and they tried roasted butternut squash. To make this appealing, they placed it in a small decorative bowl of the child's favorite color. They used this strategy to progress to roasted carrots and then steamed carrots.

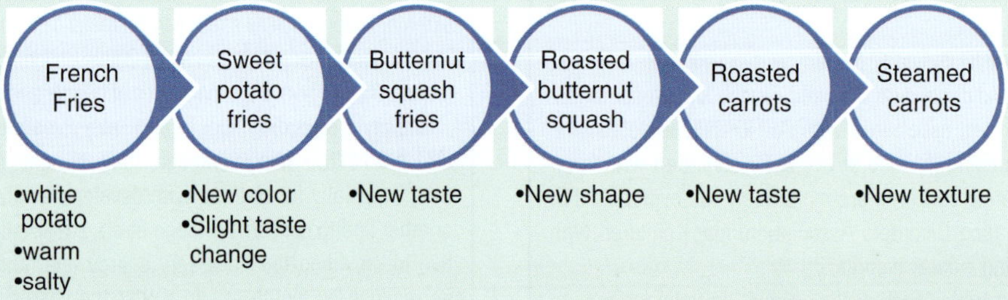


to provide feeding intervention for children with behavioral and/or sensory-based feeding difficulties (Boggs & Ferguson, 2016). This program incorporates theories of sensory processing and behavioral learning. Food chaining is also noted as an important component of the PEP.

The practitioner may also consider a playful approach to food while engaging children in sensory exploration of the various properties of the foods to build comfort and familiarity with the foods that are being targeted. This strategy can help prepare children to participate in family mealtimes, feed themselves, and add new foods to their accepted diet.

In addition to systematic desensitization and sensory food exploration, opportunities for seeing other people eating and engaging with a variety of food can facilitate learning about new or nonpreferred foods. Caregivers, siblings, peers, and therapists can all be models; an important part of a home program includes opportunities for the child to eat with others to capture these learning experiences.

## INTERVENTIONS FOR TRANSITIONING FROM NONORAL FEEDING TO ORAL FEEDING

Children with medical, oral, sensorimotor, and/or behavioral challenges may require supplemental **enteral or nonoral feeding** support to meet their nutritional needs for adequate growth and development. Enteral feeding support may be delivered temporarily via nasogastric, or less commonly, via orogastric feeding tubes. For children needing sustained enteral nutrition support (longer than a few weeks or months), healthcare providers often recommend a gastrostomy tube (G-tube). A jejunal tube (NJ, GJ, or J-tube) may be needed when a child does not accept traditional feeding (Fig. 11.14). Children who receive nonoral feeding are at risk for motor and sensory impairments related to limited feeding experiences (Scarborough et al., 2006). Transitioning from nonoral to oral feeding is a gradual process and may require engagement in oral sensory activities, oral feeding skill development, consistent practice at mealtimes, and behavioral intervention. Occupational therapy practitioners consult with family, medical, and dietary providers throughout the process.

Occupational therapy practitioners design interventions to create positive social and oral exploration experiences daily and ultimately link these pleasurable experiences with the sensation of hunger satiation. Children with a history of aspiration or when oral feeding is not medically safe may suck on a pacifier or engage in mouth play with teethers, spoons, and toys during nonoral feedings. They may benefit from play to touch and explore their face and mouth, make sounds, give kisses, or blow whistles or bubbles. Families are encouraged to treat tube feedings as mealtimes and to include their child in mealtime routines (such as sitting with the family at the table). Please see Box 11.12 for a discussion on tracheostomies and considerations for oral feeding. Flavors or tastes of foods may be gradually introduced by dipping a finger, pacifier, spoon, or toy into juice, formula, or puréed foods. As the child begins to advance oral intake skills, occupational therapy practitioners collaborate with physicians and dietitians to determine appropriate schedule changes and reductions in nonoral nutrition when possible. Case Example 11.2 describes the occupational therapy activities and goals for Cooper who is transitioning from a G-tube to oral feedings.

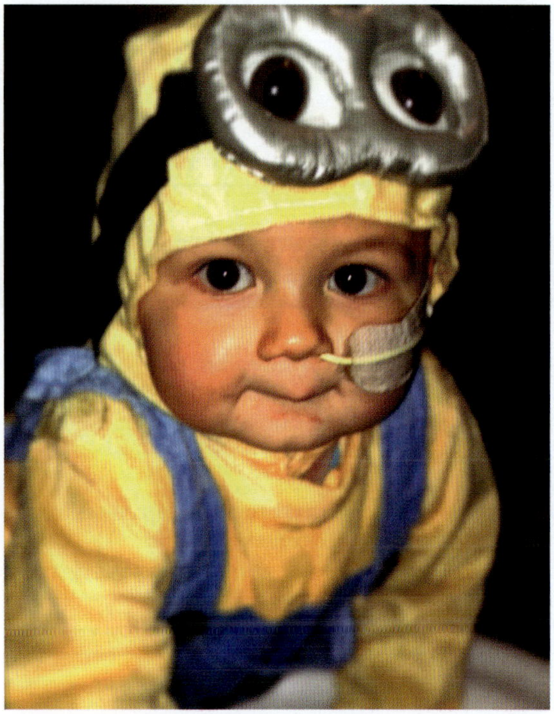

**Fig. 11.14** Child with a nasogastric tube.

Some tube-fed children may never experience typical feelings of hunger and satiety. Specialized tube feeding schedules such as overnight feedings or continuous feedings may impact these sensations.

Of note, children who have a J-tube are unable to receive bolus feedings due to the delivery of nutrients into the intestines, rather than the stomach, impacting hunger. Please refer again to Box 11.9 for information on hunger and appetite. Some feeding programs use the strategy of hunger provocation as a tool to promote hunger to help children wean themselves with oral feedings with close medical monitoring (Edwards et al., 2016; Hartdorff et al., 2015; Krom et al., 2020; Wright et al., 2011).

## BOX 11.12 Tracheostomies and Considerations for Oral Feeding

Children who have a tracheostomy often require nonoral feeding methods. The risk and complications of aspiration are significantly increased in a child with a tracheostomy because of the fragility of the respiratory system (Abraham & Wolf, 2000). Increased risk of aspiration may occur in children with a tracheostomy, related to the changes in pressure created by the new opening in the laryngeal cavity or poor laryngeal mobility. Children with a tracheostomy may be ready for nutritive stimulation when they can manage their own saliva without frequent suctioning and can tolerate a speaking valve or cap, which may help create more normalized pharyngeal swallowing coordination (Gross et al., 2003). Occupational therapy practitioners collaborate with physicians and complete comprehensive assessments of swallowing prior to initiating nutritive oral feeding activities in children with a tracheostomy. Before receiving medical clearance for oral feeding, children with a tracheostomy will benefit from nonnutritive oral exploration and mouth play activities when oral feeding is not possible (Fig. 11.15).

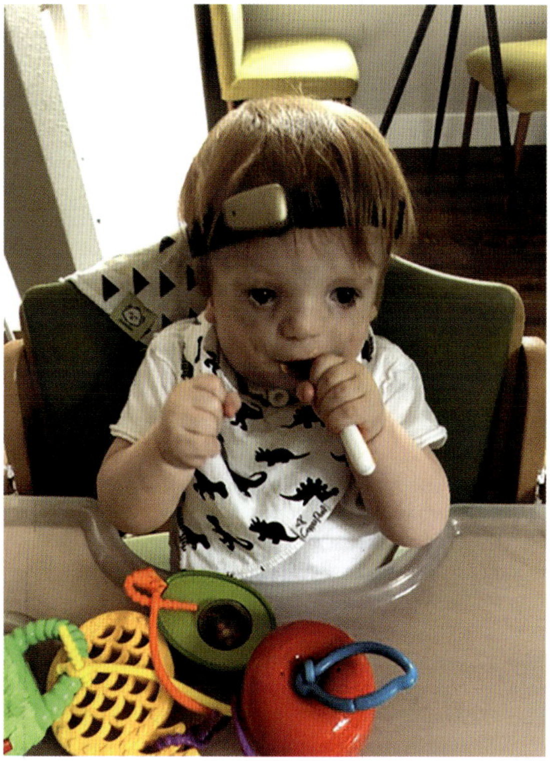

**Fig. 11.15** Child with tracheostomy engaging in oral exploration.

## CASE EXAMPLE 11.2 COOPER, A CHILD WHO IS FED BY G-TUBE

Cooper is a 2-year-old boy referred for a feeding evaluation due to his parents' concerns regarding gagging, choking, and food refusal. He has long-standing difficulties with growing and has a gastrostomy tube (G-tube) for supplemental nutrition. Currently, Cooper relies on his G-tube for most of his calories, however he is willing to eat small portions of preferred foods (goldfish crackers, veggie sticks) while watching his favorite videos on television. He continues to be interested in oral exploration with toys and his parents state that he puts "everything" in his mouth.

Cooper has little interest in trying to use a spoon, but he can feed himself with his fingers independently. He drinks sips of water from a straw cup, with occasional coughing reported, however he refuses to drink formula or milk. Cooper receives physical therapy through early intervention services for delayed motor milestones and low muscle tone. He was referred for a speech-language evaluation since he does not yet use single words or respond to simple requests and directions.

Review of Cooper's medical history revealed that Cooper was born full term, weighing 8 pounds, 4 ounces. Challenges during the newborn period included: low muscle tone, weak suck, gastroesophageal reflux (GER), and slow growth. Despite close follow-up by a gastroenterologist and medical treatment for GER, Cooper experienced frequent gagging and vomiting and over time self-limited his intake by bottle to 2 ounces at a time. Due to limited intake and growth concerns, Cooper's medical team elected to introduce pureed foods at 4 months of age to supplement growth, improve reflux symptoms, and support Cooper's feeding development. Due to Cooper's low muscle tone and delayed motor skills, his parents held him in their arms in a semireclined position for spoon-feeding. He responded to purees with an increase in gagging and refusal and began to cry at every attempted meal. At 6 months of age, a G-tube was placed to support Cooper's intake and growth, while still encouraging him to eat by mouth.

Once the G-tube was placed, Cooper was fed continuous feedings overnight. His parents offered him food and his formula during the day, but he showed little interest in eating orally during waking hours. Cooper was included in family mealtimes, and he reached for his parents' food. To preserve Cooper's limited interest, they gave him any food that he wanted, without hesitation. During this period, Cooper showed an increase in gagging, choking, and spitting out food, despite motivation to try his parents' foods. He would gag or vomit if his parents pushed him to take a bite of pureed food. As a result, Cooper no longer wanted to participate in family meals and began to resist when requested to sit in the highchair at the table. His feeding difficulties created a stressful environment around mealtimes for both Cooper and his parents. Since Cooper was not eating or drinking much volume, his parents did not insist that he continue to participate in family meals, that he follow a schedule, or sit at the table to eat.

The occupational therapist completed a feeding evaluation that revealed that Cooper's feeding development was impacted by his medical history, developmental delays, negative experiences with eating and altered daily living schedule (feeding and eating patterns). The therapist summarized Cooper's challenges as follows:

- There are persistent concerns for gastrointestinal health with GER and constipation managed by a GI specialist.
- Cooper was not referred for an instrumental evaluation of swallowing due to low suspicion for pharyngeal dysphagia. He has a good pulmonary health history and lack of significant clinical indicators (such as persistent coughing or choking when drinking) to suggest that swallow dysfunction is a contributing factor.
- His feeding schedule is not consistent with typical toddler's feeding regime as he is fed all night long and grazes on small amounts of snack foods and water during the day.
- Persistent gagging, vomiting, and learned oral hypersensitivity with feeding experiences and tooth brushing are noted.
- Lack of oral feeding experience, typical mealtime experiences, and self-feeding opportunities have resulted in delayed oral motor skills and limited self-feeding abilities.
- Cooper has developed maladaptive mealtime behaviors, including not staying at the table, refusal of most foods offered, pushing foods away, need for video distraction, gagging, crying, and occasional vomiting.
- Global developmental delays and low muscle tone are limiting typical progression of feeding skills.
- Stressful family mealtimes have resulted from Cooper's behaviors and long-standing feeding challenges.

Continued

## CASE EXAMPLE 11.2 COOPER, A CHILD WHO IS FED BY G-TUBE—CONT'D

### Intervention Considerations

**Creating a Team:** It was important to partner with Cooper's GI physician and a pediatric dietitian to begin the process of transitioning G-tube feedings to a more typical toddler feeding schedule. These specialists provided input on issues related to tolerance, bolus feeding, and optimal nutrition. The long-term goal was to establish a schedule for meals and snacks (by tube and by mouth) during the day that aligned with his family's daily routines and was appropriate for his age. Cooper's primary care physician continued to monitor his overall health, growth and development during the process and the occupational therapist updated them on Cooper's progress. The team recommended the family establish regular appointments with a pediatric dentist to support Cooper's ability to tolerate oral care and hygiene through tooth brushing and routine dental visits. The occupational therapist collaborated with Cooper's physical therapist to promote foundational skills that supported sitting at the table, participation in eating, and self-feeding.

**Mealtime Environment Considerations:** In an effort to promote a healthy balance of self-care, work, and play the therapist and family collaborated to create a predictable and consistent schedule for Cooper and his family. His schedule provided opportunities for structured mealtimes, time for supportive developmental activities and learning, and protected optimal time for sleep. While hunger was one consideration to promote Cooper's intake, the team presumed that providing meals and snacks (including G-tube feedings) on a planned basis would create natural periods of hunger and satiety consistent with typical development. In general, the occupational therapist recommended that G-tube feedings be paired with eating by mouth, with the entire meal completed in a 20–30-minute period. Cooper needed a consistent, designated place to sit (such as the highchair or booster seat) and to eat with the family so that he could learn from the social context of mealtimes. All distractions, such as toys, books, videos, and television, were removed from the table and Cooper's attention was directed to foods, people at the table, and the mealtime routine.

**Motor Considerations:** Cooper has low muscle tone throughout, and while he sat independently, his posture and alignment were best when he was provided with additional support from the highchair, with five-point harness, tray, and footrests in place. This gave him support so that Cooper was able to engage in exploration of foods, utensils, and self-feeding development. Remaining seated while eating and drinking is the safest practice for children and the family modeled this "rule" to help Cooper stay at the table for supervised meals and snacks. Based on his success with self-feeding when given proximal support, the therapist trialed adaptive feeding equipment including utensils with broad handles, suction cup bowl, and sippy cup with handles. Outside of mealtimes, the therapist paid attention to Cooper's gross and fine motor skill acquisition. The therapist engaged Cooper in play activities to promote stability and mobility, graded motor control, and precise motor movements. The therapist created gross motor play through crawling, climbing, and jumping. The therapist played activities to promote fine motor skills by activities such as: dump and fill play using play kitchen, puzzles with knobs, stringing large beads and pointing or poking with an isolated index finger.

**Oral Feeding Considerations:** Cooper needed to develop oral motor skills for improved feeding efficiency to allow him to progress his diet successfully. The occupational therapist designed activities to promote lip pursing, mouth closure and tongue retraction. He benefitted from gaining skilled tongue mobility to allow his tongue to adeptly move food from midline to the side, maintain food on the lateral gums, gather and retrieve food in preparation for swallowing. The therapist provided food textures that matched his oral motor skills and created opportunities for developing skilled chewing. The therapist avoided food textures which may have increased the likelihood of gagging and/or choking. Based on his delayed chewing development, the ideal solid food textures offered included meltable solids and soft solids. These foods were safer to offer as first foods, as they dissolve with saliva or change shape/size easily and pose reduced risk for choking. Cooper's success with eating these textures decreased episodes of spitting out food, gagging and choking, and reduced negative experiences paired with eating. Attention to specific oral motor patterns and skills were supported with use of nonnutritive oral motor toys and tools such as: chewy tubes, NUK brushes, whistles and/or blow toys. As Cooper's oral intake increased, his reliance on tube feeding was reduced, as guided by his medical team.

Oral sensory factors were considered in conjunction with oral motor considerations. Cooper presented with low muscle tone and decreased responsivity. He engaged in general mouthing of nonfood items but did not discriminate oral exploration. Cooper did not appear to notice anterior loss of saliva or food/drink from his mouth, as when drinking from his cup. The therapist used toys and activities to engage Cooper in oral motor play. In addition, the occupational therapist chose to increase sensory input by targeting touch, smell, taste, temperature, and texture. Cooper responded well to using an electric toothbrush, for example, which provided vibration, and he gravitated toward high flavor foods in therapy, like lemon pudding.

**Global Sensory Considerations:** Cooper's sensory development is influenced by his low muscle tone and overall developmental delays, since he has not engaged in the variety of play and exploration as age-matched peers. The occupational therapy plan included activities to promote optimal arousal level and postural stability for Cooper to best attend and learn during mealtimes. While playing with food at meals is not usually recommended, it is important to allow children to explore foods by touching, engaging, and interacting with foods with their hands to support typical sensory learning that is inherent in learning to feed oneself. As Cooper developed his self-feeding skills there were natural opportunities for the occupational therapist to further assess and promote his sensory processing development.\

**Behavior Considerations:** Eating is a learned activity, and Cooper's feeding profile reflects medical and feeding experiences which are in turn influenced by his developmental challenges. Since infancy, he learned that eating can be uncomfortable, unsatisfying, and even painful at times. Cooper's parents made accommodations in their approach to feeding him, such as using the television and allowing grazing, which have inadvertently reinforced maladaptive behavior patterns. For Cooper to learn positive mealtime behaviors, a consistent structured approach to eating was recommended, which included a schedule, establishing "rules" for mealtimes (such as remaining seated in the highchair), and eating with Cooper. Behavioral and cognitive strategies are effective in shaping behavior and improving eating. Cooper's therapy plan included the use of behavioral strategies of praise and clapping as positive reinforcement for tasting a new food, and intentional ignoring of spitting out foods as negative punishment.

**Parent Education:** Parent education was integrated throughout Cooper's treatment to help his parents understand the many facets of his feeding difficulties. To be successful, Cooper's home program was realistic, helpful, and effective. Partnering with his parents included opportunities for problem solving, prioritization of goals, and information sharing, to make progress with Cooper's feeding development and intake.

### Discharge Status

At discharge, Cooper followed a full daytime feeding schedule, with most of his nutritional intake by mouth. His G-tube was now used at the end of breakfast, lunch, and dinner to provide small volumes of supplemental feedings to support his growth. The dietitian had a plan for discontinuing tube feeding and monitoring his growth. Cooper accepted a narrow range of pureed foods, meltable solids and some soft solid foods. He developed oral motor skills to bite, move food to the side and chew with his mouth closed. Gagging was infrequent and only triggered with large bites. Importantly, the gagging no longer resulted in vomiting. Cooper participated in mealtimes by sitting in his highchair, using his hands to pick up finger foods, and practicing with a spoon. Of importance, he learned to drink his pediatric formula from a cup, which was a critical factor supporting his potential for transitioning off tube feeding. Cooper's parents planned to continue to follow the approach and techniques outlined in his home program to promote his ongoing learning and feeding skill development.

## SUMMARY

Occupational therapy practitioners address children's feeding and eating challenges by collaborating with families and team members to create child and family-centered intervention plans. They use a variety of strategies and support practice decisions with evidence:

1. Occupational therapy practitioners address feeding and eating in children by creating comprehensive intervention plans that address the child's nutritional needs and the family's needs and that promote greater occupational performance with feeding and eating. They determine the child's developmental level and conditions that affect feeding and eating and use knowledge of motor, sensory, and processing skills in combination with the family's routines and expectations to address feeding and eating challenges, including poor intake, nutritional concerns, food aversions, poor oral motor skills, and disruptive mealtime behaviors. They work closely with other professionals (e.g., physicians, nutritionists, dieticians, nurses) and caregivers to create and monitor the child's progress and safety.
2. Occupational therapy practitioners create occupation-based interventions that focus on engaging children and families in eating and feeding at the child's current level and in consideration of their medical status and environmental resources. Specific strategies may address the ability to bring foods and liquids to the oral cavity, manage food and liquids during the oral phase, or swallow successfully. In addition, interventions address behavioral aspects of food selectivity, sensory reactions to feeding and eating, and the process of transitioning from nonoral feeding to feeding.

## REFERENCES

Abraham, S. S., & Wolf, E. L. (2000). Swallowing physiology of toddlers with long-term tracheostomies: A preliminary study. *Dysphagia*, *15*, 206–212.

Acar, G., Ejraei, N., Turkdoğan, D., Enver, N., Öztürk, G., & Aktaş, G. (2022). The effects of neurodevelopmental therapy on feeding and swallowing activities in children with cerebral palsy. *Dysphagia*, *37*(4), 800–811.

American Occupational Therapy Association. (2020). Occupational therapy practice framework: Domain and process (4th ed.). *American Journal of Occupational Therapy*, *74*(Suppl. 2), 7412410010.

American Occupational Therapy Association. (2017). The practice of occupational therapy in feeding, eating, and swallowing. *American Journal of Occupational Therapy*, *71*(Suppl. 2), 7112410015.

Andrew, M. J., Parr, J. R., & Sullivan, P. B. (2012). Feeding difficulties in children with cerebral palsy. *Archives of Disease in Childhood. Education, Practice Edition*, *97*, 222–229.

Arvedson, J. C., & Brodsky, L. (2002). *Instrumental evaluation of swallowing. Pediatric swallowing and feeding: Assessment and management* (2nd ed.). In Albany, NY: Singular/Thomson Learning.

Austin, J., et al. (2009). Hormonal regulators of appetite. *International Journal of Pediatric Endocrinology*, *141*(53).

Awaad, H. M., Aly, M. G., & Kamal, H. M. (2023). Kinesio taping versus oromotor training on drooling in children with spastic cerebral palsy: Comparative study. *The Egyptian Journal of Hospital Medicine*, *91*(1), 4462–4467.

Baird, R., Levesque, R., Bimbaum, R., & Ramsay, M. (2015). A pilot investigation of feeding problems in children with esophageal atresia. *Diseases of the Esophagus*, *28*, 224–228.

Beal, J., Silverman, B., Bellant, J., Young, T. E., & Klontz, K. (2012). Late onset necrotizing enterocolitis in infants following use of a xanthan gum-containing thickening agent. *The Journal of Pediatrics*, *161*(2), 354–356.

Beaudry-Bellefeuille, I., Pomoni, M., Welch, A., Moriyon-Iglesis, T., Suarez-Gonzalez, M. S., & Ramos-Polo, E. (2021). Multidisciplinary approach to assessment and intervention of feeding problems in children with autism spectrum disorders: A clinical perspective. *Irish Journal of Occupational Therapy*, *49*(2), 77–83.

Beckman, D. (2000). *Oral motor assessment and intervention.* Charlotte, NC: Presented at the oral motor assessment and intervention I conference.

Bell, L. K., Gardner, C., Tian, E. J., Cochet-Broch, M. O., Poelman, A. A. M., Cox, D. N., Nicklaus, S., Matvienko-Sikar, K., Daniels, L. A., Kumar, S., & Golley, R. K. (2021). Supporting strategies for enhancing vegetable liking in the early years of life: An umbrella review of systematic reviews. *American Journal Clinical Nutrition*, *113*, 1282–1300.

Benfer, K. A., Weir, K. A., Bell, K. L., Ware, R. S., Davies, P. S. W., & Boyd, R. N. (2015). Clinical signs suggestive of pharyngeal dysphagia in preschool children with cerebral palsy. *Research in Developmental Disabilities*, *38*, 192–201.

Bessell, A., Hooper, L., Shaw, W. C., Reilly, S., Reid, J., & Glenny, A. M. (2011). Feeding interventions for growth and development in infants with cleft lip, cleft palate, or cleft lip and palate. *Cochrane Database of Systematic Reviews*, *2*, 1–23.

Blisset, J., & Harris, G. (2002). Behavioral intervention in a child with feeding problems. *Journal of Human Nutrition and Dietetics*, *15*, 255–260.

Bloomfield, B. S., Fischer, A. J., Clark, R. R., & Dove, M. B. (2019). Treatment of food selectivity in a child with avoidant/restrictive food intake disorder through parent teleconsultation. *Behavior Analysis in Practice*, *12*(1), 33–43.

Boggs, T., & Ferguson, N. (2016). A little PEP goes a long way in the treatment of pediatric feeding disorders. *Perspectives of the ASHA Special Interest Groups*, *13*(1), 26–37.

Boop, C., & Smith, J. (2017). The practice of occupational therapy in feeding, eating, and swallowing. *American Journal of Occupational Therapy*, *71*(S2), 7112410015p1+.

Bourne, L., Mandy, W., & Bryant-Waugh, R. (2022). Avoidant/restrictive food intake disorder and severe food selectivity in children and young people with autism: A scoping review. *Developmental Medicine and Child Neurology*, *64*, 691–699.

Bryant-Waugh, R. (2019). Avoidant/restrictive food intake disorder. *Child and Adolescent Psychiatric Clinics of North America*, *28*(4), 557–565.

Bryant-Waugh, R., Micali, N., Cooke, L., Lawson, E. A., Eddy, K., & Thomas, J. J. (2018). Development of the Pica, ARFID, and Rumination Disorder Interview, a multi-informant, semi-structured interview of feeding disorders across the lifespan: A pilot study for ages 10 – 122. *International Journal of Eating Disorders*, *52*, 378–387.

Bulow, M., Olsson, R., & Ekberg, O. (2003). Video radiographic analysis of how carbonated thin liquids and thickened liquids affect the physiology of swallowing in subjects with aspiration on thin liquids. *Acta Radiologica*, *44*, 366–372.

Caldwell, A. R., Skidmore, E. R., Bendixen, R. M., & Terhorst, L. (2020). Examining child mealtime behavior as parents are coached to implement the Mealtime PREP intervention in the home: Findings from a pilot study. *British Journal of Occupational Therapy*, *83*(10), 631–637.

Caldwell, A. R., Skidmore, E. R., Raina, K. D., Rogers, J. C., Terhorst, L., Danford, C. A., & Bendixen, R. M. (2018). Behavioral activation approach to parent training: Feasibility of promoting routines of exploration and play during mealtime (mealtime PREP). *American Journal of Occupational Therapy*, *72*, 7206205030.

Chistol, L. T., Bandini, L. G., Must, A., Phillips, S., Cermak, S. A., & Curtin, C. (2018). Sensory sensitivity and food selectivity in children with autism spectrum disorder. *Journal of Autism and Developmental Disorders*, *48*(2), 583–591.

Clark, G. F., & Kingsley, K. L. (2020). Occupational therapy practice guidelines for early childhood: Birth-5 Years. *American Journal of Occupational Therapy*, *74*(3), 7403397010p1–7403397010p42.

Cravener, T. L., Schlechter, H., Loeb, K. L., Radnitz, C., Schwartz, M., Zucker, N., Finkelstein, S., Wang, Y. C., Rolls, B. J., & Keller, K. L. (2015). Feeding strategies derived from behavioral economics and psychology can increase vegetable intake in children as part of a hone-based intervention: Results of a pilot study. *Journal of the Academy of Nutrition and Dietetics, 115*(11), 1798–1807.

Davis, J. (2018). Hunger, ghrelin and the gut. *Brain Research, 1693*, 154–158.

Desai, H., Lauridson, S., Nguyen, M., Ornelas, E., & Schomberg, J. (2022). Feeding skill and behavior changes in children with complex feeding disorders following therapy in an intensive multidisciplinary feeding program. *Perspectives of the ASHA Special Interest Groups, 7*, 1156–1165.

Edwards, S., Davis, A. M., Bruce, A., Mousa, H., Lyman, B., Cocjin, J., Dean, K., Ernst, L., Almadhoun, O., & Hyman, P. (2016). Caring for tube-fed children: A review of management, tube weaning, and emotional considerations. *Journal of Parenteral and Enteral Nutrition, 40*(5), 616–622.

Ferrell, K. (2011). *Reach out and teach: Helping your child who is visually impaired learn and grow.* American Foundation for the Blind Press.

Fraker, C., Fishbein, M., Walbert, L., & Cox, S. (2007). *Food chaining: The proven 6-step plan to stop picky eating, solve feeding problems, and expand your child's diet.* Da Capo Press.

Friedlander, J. A., DeBoer, E. M., Soden, J. S., Furuta, G. T., Menard-Katcher, C. D., Atkins, D., Fleischer, D. M., Kramer, R. E., Deterding, R. R., Capocelli, K. E., & Prager, J. D. (2016). Unsedated transnasal esophagoscopy for monitoring therapy in pediatric eosinophilic esophagitis. *Gastrointestinal Endoscopy, 83*(2), 299–306.e1.

Friedman, B., & Frazier, J. B. (2000). Deep laryngeal penetration as a predictor of aspiration. *Dysphagia, 15*, 153–158.

Goday, P. S., Huh, S. Y., Silverman, A., Lukens, C. T., Dodrill, P., Cohen, S. S., & Phalen, J. A. (2019). Pediatric feeding disorder: Consensus definition and conceptual framework. *Journal of Pediatric Gastroenterology and Nutrition, 68*(1), 124.

Gosa, M. M., Carden, H. T., Jacks, C. C., Threadgill, A. Y., & Sidlovsky, T. C. (2017). Evidence to support treatment options for children with swallowing and feeding disorders: A systematic review. *Journal of Pediatric Rehabilitation Medicine, 10*(2), 107–136.

Grayson, B. H., & Maull, D. (2005). Nasoalveolar molding for infants born with clefts of the lip, alveolus, and palate. *Seminars in Plastic Surgery, 19*(4), 294–301.

Gronski, M., & Doherty, M. (2020). Interventions within the scope of occupational therapy practice to improve activities of daily living, rest, and sleep for children ages 0–5 years and their families: A systematic review. *American Journal of Occupational Therapy, 74*(2), 7402180010p1–7402180010p33.

Gross, R. D., Mahlmann, J., & Grayhack, J. P. (2003). Physiologic effects of open and closed tracheostomy tubes on the pharyngeal swallow. *Annals of Otology, Rhinology, and Laryngology, 112*, 143–152.

Hartdorff, C. M., Kneepkens, C. M., Stok-Akerboom, A. M., van Dijk-Lokkart, E. M., Engels, M. A., & Kindermann, A. (2015). Clinical tube weaning supported by hunger provocation in fully-tube-fed children. *Journal of Pediatric Gastroenterology and Nutrition, 60*(4), 538–543.

Howe, T. H., & Wang, T. N. (2013). Systematic review of interventions used in or relevant to occupational therapy for children with feeding difficulties ages birth–5 years. *American Journal of Occupational Therapy, 67*(4), 405–412.

Hung, S. A., Liao, C. L., Lin, W. P., Hsu, J. C., Guo, Y. H., & Lin, Y. C. (2021). Botulinum toxin injections for treatment of drooling in children with cerebral palsy: A systematic review and meta-analysis. *Children, 8*(12), 1089.

Huston, P. L., Dempster, R., & Garbacz, L. (2019). Cognitive and behavioral strategies for the treatment of feeding disorders in adolescents. *Perspectives of the ASHA Special Interest Groups, 4*, 1498–1506.

IDDSI. (2019). *International dysphagia diet standardization initiative: A global initiative to improve the lives of over 590 million people worldwide living with dysphagia.* Retrieved from: http://www.iddsi.org.

Johnson, C. R., Brown, K., Hyman, S. L., Brooks, M. M., Aponte, C., Levato, L., Schmidt, B., Evans, V., Huo, Z., Bendixen, R., Eng, H., Sax, T., & Smith, T. (2019). Parent training for feeding problems in children with Autism Spectrum Disorder: Initial randomized trial. *Journal of Pediatric Psychology, 44*(2), 164–175.

Johnson, C. R., Foldes, E., DeMand, A., & Brooks, M. (2015). Behavioral parent training to address feeding problems in children with autism spectrum disorder: A pilot trial. *Journal of Developmental and Physical Disabilities, 27*, 591–607.

Kingsley, K. L., & Clark, G. F. (2020). Occupational therapy interventions for children ages birth-5 years. *American Journal of Occupational Therapy, 74*(5), 7405390010p1–7405390010p4.

Kovacic, K., Rein, L. E., Szabo, A., Kommareddy, S., Bhagavatula, P., & Goday, P. S. (2021). Pediatric feeding disorder: A nationwide prevalence study. *The Journal of Pediatrics, 228*, 126–131.

Krom, H., de Meij, T. G. J., Benninga, M. A., van Dijk-Lokkart, E. M., Engels, M., Kneepkens, C. M. F., Kuiper-Cramer, L., Otten, M. G. M., van der Sluijs Veer, L., Stok-Akerboom, A. M., Zilverberg, R., van Zundert, S. M. C., & Kindermann, A. (2020). Long-term efficacy of clinical hunger provocation to wean feeding tube dependent children. *Clinical Nutrition, 39*(9), 2863–2871.

Marcus, S., & Breton, S. (2022a). Development of oral-motor skills. In S. Marcus, & S. Breton (Eds.), *Infant and child feeding and swallowing: Occupational therapy assessment and intervention* (2nd ed.) (pp. 7–17). AOTA Press.

Marcus, S., & Breton, S. (2022b). Difficulty transitioning to purees, solid foods, and cup drinking. In S. Marcus, & S. Breton (Eds.), *Infant and child feeding and swallowing: Occupational therapy assessment and intervention* (2nd ed.) (pp. 77–106). AOTA Press.

Melo, B., Araújo, R., Azevedo, M. J., Amorim, R., & Palhau, L. (2021). Management of sialorrhea in children. *Pediatric Oncall Journal, 18*(3), 71–76.

Menard-Katcher, C., Henry, M., Furuta, G. T., Atkins, D., Maune, N. C., & Haas, A. M. (2014). Significance of feeding dysfunction in eosinophilic esophagitis. *World Journal of Gastroenterology, 20*(31), 11019–11022.

Milano, K., Chatoor, I., & Kerzner, B. (2019). A functional approach to feeding difficulties in children. *Current Gastroenterology Reports, 21*(10), 51.

Miller, C. K. (2011). Feeding issues and interventions in infants and children with clefts and craniofacial syndromes. *Seminars in Speech and Language, 32*(2), 115–126.

Miller, C. K., & Willging, J. P. (2003). Advances in the evaluation and management of pediatric dysphagia. *Current Opinion in Otolaryngology and Head and Neck Surgery, 11*, 442–446.

Morgan, A. T., Dodrill, P., & Ward, E. C. (2012). Interventions for oropharyngeal dysphagia in children with neurological impairment. *Cochrane Database of Systematic Reviews, 10*, CD009456.

Morris, S. E., & Klein, M. D. (2000). *Pre-feeding skills* (2nd ed.). Tucson, AZ: Therapy Skill Builders.

Mukkada, V. A., Haas, A., Maune, N. C., Capocelli, K. E., Henry, M., Gilman, N., Petersburg, S., Moore, W., Lovell, M. A., Fleischer, D. M., Furuta, G. T., & Atkins, D. (2010). Feeding dysfunction in children with eosinophilic gastrointestinal diseases. *Pediatrics, 126*(3), e672–e677.

Myles, D. (2020). *Critical review: The effectiveness of oral sensorimotor therapy in the treatment of drooling in children with cerebral palsy.* https://www.uwo.ca/fhs/lwm/teaching/EBP/2019_20/Myles.pdf.

Nicklaus, S. (2016). Complementary feeding strategies to facilitate acceptance of fruits and vegetables: A narrative review of the literature. *International Journal of Environmental Research and Public Health, 13*(11), 1160.

Quitadamo, P., Thapar, N., Staiano, A., & Borrelli, O. (2016). Gastrointestinal and nutritional problems in neurologically impaired children. *European Journal of Paediatric Neurology, 20*(6), 810–815.

Rogers, B. (2004). Feeding method and health outcomes of children with cerebral palsy. *The Journal of Pediatrics, 145*(2), S28–S32.

Rosenfeld-Johnson, S. (2005). Assessment and treatment of the jaw. *Talk tools innovative therapists international*, 1–185.

Ruark, M. M. J. (2007). Best practices for behavioral management of pediatric dysphagia. *Pediatric Feeding and Dysphagia Newsletter, 7*, 1–5.

Scarborough, D. R., Boyce, S., McCain, G., Oppenheimer, S., August, A., & Strinjas, J. N. (2006). Abnormal physiological responses to touch among children with persistent feeding difficulties. *Developmental Medicine and Child Neurology, 48*(6), 460–464.

Sharp, W. G., Jaquess, D. L., Morton, J. F., & Herzinger, C. V. (2010). Pediatric feeding disorders: A quantitative synthesis of treatment outcomes. *Clinical Child and Family Psychology Review, 13*(4), 348–365.

Sharp, W. G., Silverman, A., Arvedson, J. C., Bandstra, N. F., Clawson, E., Berry, R. C., … Lukens, C. T. (2022). Toward better understanding of pediatric feeding disorder: A proposed framework for patient characterization. *Journal of Pediatric Gastroenterology and Nutrition*, *75*(3), 351.

Sharp, W. G., Volkert, V. M., Scahill, L., McCracken, C. E., & McElhanon, B. (2017). A systematic review and meta-analysis of intensive multidisciplinary intervention for pediatric feeding disorders: How standard is the standard of care? *The Journal of Pediatrics*, *181*, 116–124.

Silva, J. P. S., Faria, L. V., Almeida, R. C., Medeiros, Y. L., & Guimarães, L. D. A. (2022). Effectiveness and safety of botulinum toxin in comparison with surgery for drooling in paediatric patients with neurological disorders: A systematic review. *British Journal of Oral and Maxillofacial Surgery*, *60*(5), e691–e701.

United States Department of Labor. (2018). *Occupational Safety and Health Administration*. https://www.osha.gov.

United States Food and Drug Administration. (2012). *FDA expands caution about SimplyThick*. Retrieved from: https://wayback.archive-it.org/7993/20170722060115/. https://www.fda.gov/ForConsumers/ConsumerUpdates/ucm256250.htm.

Van den Engel-Hoek, L., Harding, C., van Gerven, M., & Cockerill, H. (2017). Pediatric feeding and swallowing rehabilitation: An overview. *Journal of Pediatric Rehabilitation Medicine*, *10*(2), 95–105.

Wilson, E., Simione, M., & Polley, L. (2021). Paediatric oral sensorimotor interventions for chewing dysfunction: A scoping review. *International Journal of Language & Communication Disorders*, *56*(6), 1316–1333.

Wright, C. M., Smith, K. H., & Morrison, J. (2011). Withdrawing feeds from children on long term enteral feeding: Factors associated with success and failure. *Archives of Disease in Childhood*, *96*(5), 433–439.

You, P., Strychowsky, J., Gandhi, K., & Chen, B. A. (2022). Anticholinergic treatment for sialorrhea in children: A systematic review. *Paediatrics and Child Health*, *27*(2), 82–87.

Zhu, V., & Dalby-Payne, J. (2019). Feeding difficulties in children with autism spectrum disorder: Aetiology, health impacts and psychotherapeutic interventions. *Journal of Paediatrics and Child Health*, *55*(11), 1304–1308.


## FURTHER READING


Cohen, M. S., Zhuang, L., Simons, J. P., Chi, D. H., Maguire, R. C., & Mehta, D. K. (2011). Injection laryngoplasty for type 1 laryngeal cleft in children. *Otolaryngology—Head and Neck Surgery*, *144*(5), 789–793.

Cooper–Brown, L., Copeland, S., Dailey, S., Downey, D., Petersen, M. C., Stimson, C., & Van Dyke, D. C. (2008). Feeding and swallowing dysfunction in genetic syndromes. *Developmental Disabilities*, *14*, 147–157.

Gisel, E. (2008). Interventions and outcomes for children with dysphagia. *Developmental Disabilities Research Review*, *14*, 165–173.

Jackson, A., Maybee, J., Moran, M. K., Wolter-Warmerdam, K., & Hickey, F. (2016). Clinical characteristics of dysphagia in children with Down syndrome. *Dysphagia*, *31*(5), 663–671.

Jadi, J., Hyder, S., Rodriguez Ormaza, N. P., Twer, E., Phillips, M., Akinkuotu, A., & Reid, T. D. (2021). Evaluation of complications and weight outcomes in pediatric cerebral palsy patients with gastrostomy tubes. *American Journal of Surgery*, *28*, 31–34.

Lively, E. J., McAllister, S., & Doeltgen, S. H. (2021). Characterizing international approaches to weaning children from tube feeding: A scoping review. *Journal of Parenteral and Enteral Nutrition*, *45*(2), 239–250.

Park, J., Thoyre, S. M., Pados, B. F., & Gregas, M. (2019). Symptoms of feeding problems in preterm-born children at 6 months to 7 years old. *Journal of Pediatric Gastroenterology and Nutrition*, *68*(3), 416–421.

Raatz, M., Ward, E. C., Marshall, J., & Burns, C. L. (2019). Developing the system architecture for conducting synchronous paediatric feeding assessments via telepractice. *Journal of Telemedicine and Telecare*, *25*, 552–558.

Raatz, M., Ward, E. C., Marshall, J., & Burns, C. L. (2021). Evaluating the use of telepractice for bottle-feeding assessments. *Children*, *8*, 989.

Schwarzenberg, S. J., Hempstead, S. E., McDonald, C. M., Powers, S. W., Wooldridge, J., Blair, S., Freedom, S., Harrington, E., Murphy, P. J., Palmer, L., Schrader, A. E., Shiel, K., Sullivan, J., Wallentine, M., Marshall, B. C., & Leonard, A. R. (2016). Enteral tube feeding for individuals with cystic fibrosis: Cystic fibrosis foundation evidence-informed guidelines. *Journal of Cystic Fibrosis*, *15*(6), 724–735.

Snider, L., Majnemer, A., & Darsaklis, V. (2011). Feeding interventions for children with cerebral palsy: A review of the evidence. *Physical & Occupational Therapy in Pediatrics*, *31*(1), 58–77.

Speyer, R., Cordier, R., Kim, J. H., Cocks, N., Michou, E., & Wilkes-Gillan, S. (2019). Prevalence of drooling, swallowing, and feeding problems in cerebral palsy across the lifespan: A systematic review and meta-analyses. *Developmental Medicine & Child Neurology*, *61*(11), 1249–1258.

Wolf, L. S., & Glass, R. P. (1992). *Feeding and swallowing disorders in infancy: Assessment and management*. Tucson, AZ: Therapy Skill Builders.

12

# Intervention to Improve Sleep and Rest

*Jean S. Koketsu and Megan C. Chang*

## GUIDING QUESTIONS

1. Why do occupational therapy practitioners address sleep and rest in children and adolescents?
2. What factors affect participation in sleep and rest for children and adolescents?
3. What are the sleep recommendations for children and teenagers in terms of amount and timing?
4. What intervention strategies and approaches are used to promote healthy sleep and rest?

## KEY TERMS

**Bedtime routines**
**Circadian rhythm**
**Environmental factors**
**Personal factors**
**Rest**
**Sleep**
**Sleep hygiene**
**Social and relational factors**

## INTRODUCTION TO SLEEP AND REST

Unlike occupations that may be optional, all humans must sleep and rest (Tester & Foss, 2018). Sleep and rest are described as activities to "support healthy, active engagement in other occupations" (AOTA, 2020, p. 32). Although both sleep and rest are categorized under restorative occupations in the most recent version of the Occupational Therapy Practice Framework (OTPF; AOTA, 2020), they are not the same.

**Sleep** is a reversible state where one is perceptually disengaged from and unresponsive to the environment (Carskadon & Dement, 2011). Sleep is essential for children's development and well-being, and it allows children and their parents to restore energy for wakeful occupations. Appropriate sleep is paramount for optimal growth, development, and functioning and is an important part of a child's and family's life (Deshpande et al., 2022). Childhood sleep problems can disrupt family dynamics and lead to cognitive and behavioral issues in children, and early recognition can avert many of those issues (Deshpande et al., 2022). Healthy sleep includes several factors: quality, timing, regularity, and adequate duration (Paruthi et al., 2016). Sufficient sleep is associated with better health outcomes, including better attention, learning, emotional regulation, and physical and mental health. The ranges of "typical sleep" vary widely, which can be reassuring to parents and caregivers. See Table 12.1 for recommendations of typical sleep for children and situations that may impede sleep.

**Rest** refers to quiet and effortless actions that interrupt physical and mental energy (AOTA, 2020). According to the OTPF-4, rest includes "endeavors that restore energy and calm and renew interest in engagement" (AOTA, 2020, p. 46). Rest is important to calm and renew a child's interest and engagement and is important for maintaining one's energy and ability to attend to activities. Rest is an important part of one's day. Rest can include small pauses during activity to reflect, relax, and manage one's emotional state. For example, infants may show signs of frustration during feeding and require a "rest" from this activity. They may cry or become disengaged as a way to communicate their need for a change. Toddlers may require breaks when play activities become overwhelming or frustrating. Adolescents may want to learn how to take care of themselves through rest (such as a breathing technique, a walk outside, or listening to a favorite song). Taking time for rest breaks or pauses supports renewed energy to focus on daily tasks.

Occupational therapy practitioners are uniquely qualified to help children with sleep and rest as they are versed in addressing physiological, behavioral, sensory, and environmental factors associated with sleep and rest (Gronski, 2022). Occupational therapy practitioners in pediatric practice work routinely with children who are at risk of sleep issues such as autism spectrum disorder (ASD, Franklin et al., 2015). However, although a survey of 141 occupational therapists in pediatric practice found that many addressed sleep and rest with their clients, a majority reported feeling inadequate in their knowledge (Piller et al., 2020). To help children with sleep, it is important that occupational therapy practitioners possess basic knowledge of typical sleep across the lifespan.

## TYPICAL SLEEP PROCESS

The two primary processes that regulate sleep and wakefulness in humans are the circadian and homeostatic processes (El Shakankiry, 2011). Human beings have rhythms in their body that operate in 24-hour cycles referred to as **circadian rhythms**. A tiny "very precise internal timekeeping mechanism" (Pelayo & Dement, 2017, p. 85) or "biological clock" is located in the brain (suprachiasmatic nuclei, SCN), and its job is to "synchronize the body's biological rhythms with the earth's cycles of dawn and dusk" (Pelayo, 2020, p. 12). The most important function of the clock is to manage sleep and wakefulness. The time cue that has the strongest influence on the clock is light, but other social and environmental processes such as mealtimes, temperature, bedtime routines, and physical activity also affect the circadian rhythm (El Shakankiry, 2011).

The clock alerts the body and brain to release melatonin after dusk when it starts to get dark. This results in a cascade of events in other parts of the brain, which leads to one becoming sleepy.

**TABLE 12.1 Typical Amount of Sleep Needed at Different Ages and Possible Factors Impeding Sleep**

| Age | Amount of Sleep Needed | Naps | Factors to Consider When Child Has Sleep Problems |
|---|---|---|---|
| Newborn, 1–2 months (See Fig. 12.2) | 12–18 h<br>50–60 min REM-NREM cycle | Throughout day | No established sleep/wake cycle<br>Interrupted sleep related to feeding, comfort needs (diaper changes), medical procedures, sleep apnea alarms (if used), or too much sleep during the day<br>When asleep and put to bed, baby wakes up with change in position |
| 3–11 months (Fig. 12.8) | 12–18 h | Three or four times daily, 30 min–2 h | Usually, cannot sleep through the night without feedings until 6 months of age<br>70%–80% sleep through the night by 9 months<br>Separation anxiety interferes with sleep<br>Has not learned to self-soothe and is dependent on parents (needs to be drowsy or already asleep to be placed in crib)<br>May be insecure with attachment or always wants to engage with others |
| Toddler, 1–3 years (See Fig. 12.5) | 12–14 h | Once or twice daily (18 months once a day), 1–3 h | Fewer naps needed<br>Needs independence<br>Anxiety about going to sleep (may relate to separation anxiety, inability to self-soothe, imagination, fear of being alone, nightmares)<br>Difficulty with transitions<br>Gets out of bed independently |
| Preschoolers 3.1–4.11 years (See Fig. 12.6) | 11–13 h | Once daily | Bed-wetting<br>Nighttime fears or nightmares because of imagination developing (e.g., fear of being alone, the dark, tigers under the bed)<br>Peak age for sleepwalking and sleep terrors<br>Television watching too close to bedtime<br>Outgrown the need for naps and not sleepy when put to bed |
| School age, 5–10 years (See Figs. 12.3 and 12.7) | 10–11 h | 10%–30% still nap until 7 | Bed-wetting (typical until age 7)<br>Medical issues: Tonsils enlarged, facial profile is convex, has crossbite, reflux, or medical procedure (e.g., positioning, suction)<br>Unaware of social cues for calming down to go to sleep<br>Increased demands for schoolwork or other extracurricular activities<br>More interest in computers and the internet<br>Caffeine consumption or eating close to bedtime<br>Electronic use in the bedroom or too close to bedtime (e.g., computers, televisions, tablets, video games)<br>Erratic sleep schedule<br>Lack of understanding of the importance of healthy routines for sleep |
| Teens, 10.1–17 years (See Fig. 12.1) | 8.5–9.25 h | | Increased demands of school, work, social life, or other activities<br>Anxiety or emotional event during the day<br>Caffeine consumption or eating close to bedtime<br>Electronic use in the bedroom or too close to bedtime (e.g., computers, televisions, tablets, video games, smartphones)<br>Erratic sleep schedule especially weekend versus weekday nights<br>Internal clock of teens—like late nights and waking up later in the morning<br>Lack of understanding of importance for healthy routines for sleep |

Collated from: Mindell, J. & Owens, J. (2015). *Clinical guide to pediatric sleep: Diagnosis and intervention.* Wolters Kluwer; Suni, E (2023). Sleep Foundation. https://www.sleepfoundation.org/articles/sleep-hygiene and https://www.sleepfoundation.org/bedroom-environment

Melatonin itself does not make one sleepy or fall asleep. As sleep occurs throughout the night, and as the sun rises, the release of melatonin slows and eventually stops, which leads to wakefulness. The primary times when we are the sleepiest are in the middle of the night (a few hours after midnight) and late in the afternoon after lunch, all as dictated by the suprachiasmatic nuclei (SCN). However, people's circadian rhythms vary such that some people prefer to go to sleep early and wake early, while others do not get sleepy until later in the night and prefer to sleep later into the morning.

Throughout the lifespan, sleep changes in terms of hours required and patterns and also circadian rhythm. Newborns' circadian rhythm is not fully developed, so they can easily sleep whether it is day or night (El Shakankiry, 2011). Teenagers' circadian rhythms shift, causing them to get sleepy later at night and to want to sleep in later (See Fig. 12.1). Teenagers may physically start to look like adults in size and appearance, but their sleep needs in terms of hours are higher than adults (See Table 12.1). Older adults' (65+) circadian rhythms may shift such that they get sleepy earlier and wake earlier. Ideally, to optimize health, a goal should be to work in concert with one's circadian rhythm instead of against it (Pelayo, 2020).

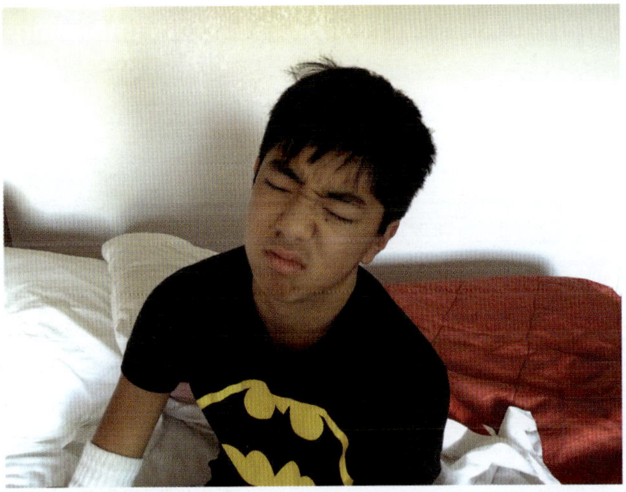

Fig. 12.1 This 14-year-old's circadian rhythm made waking up at 9:00 a.m. while on a family vacation an unhappy experience. He preferred staying up late and sleeping in later. (Photo courtesy of Jean Koketsu.)

## SLEEP STAGES

Studies of brain wave patterns via electroencephalograms show that sleep consists of several rounds of sleep cycles, with two major stages of sleep, non-rapid eye movement (NREM) and rapid eye movement (REM). Sleep stages follow a progression: N1, the transition from wakefulness to sleep; N2, true sleep, also referred to as light sleep; and N3 (slow wave sleep), referred to as deep sleep, when the brain and body recover. Within these stages, healthy young adults experience four to six cycles of NREM and REM sleep; each cycle lasts 90–120 minutes. REM is the phase when the brain is highly active, is associated with dreaming, memory consolidation, and learning, and is characterized by a paralysis of voluntary muscles (except the diaphragm and eyes) for protective reasons; adults spend about 20%–25% in REM sleep and 75%–80% in NREM sleep.

## TYPICAL DEVELOPMENT OF SLEEP

Sleep changes significantly throughout the lifespan (Pelayo & Dement, 2017). Unlike adults, who typically sleep through one large bout at night (approximately 7–9 hours), newborns and young infants sleep throughout the 24-hour day (See Fig. 12.2). Until infants are 3 months old, their sleep has only two distinct NREM ("quiet sleep") and REM ("active sleep") phases. Quiet sleep may include more rhythmic breathing and minimal movement, while active sleep may include more irregular breathing, twitches, facial expressions, and gross limb muscle movements but not the voluntary muscle paralysis seen later (El Shakankiry, 2011). Not until 3 months have elapsed does infant sleep resemble adult sleep with N1, N2, N3, and REM sleep (Pacheco, 2022). Unlike other age groups, newborns, and infants under 6 months cycle through the sleep stages in 50–60 minutes and enter sleep through REM and spend 50% each in REM and NREM sleep (El Shakankiry, 2011). Deep sleep in young children is also maximized in terms of quantity and quality, so it may be very difficult to wake a child when they are in N3 deep sleep (See Fig. 12.3). By 6 months of age, infants' sleep architecture resembles that of adults, and they experience longer consolidated sleep at night and sleep less during the day. By 4 years, children may not need a nap (El Shakankiry, 2011). See Fig. 12.4, which shows the changes in sleep patterns across the lifespan, and Figs. 12.5–12.7, illustrating the sleep habits of various ages of children. Box 12.1 summarizes the American Academy of Pediatrics (Moon et al., 2022) recommendations for infant sleep.

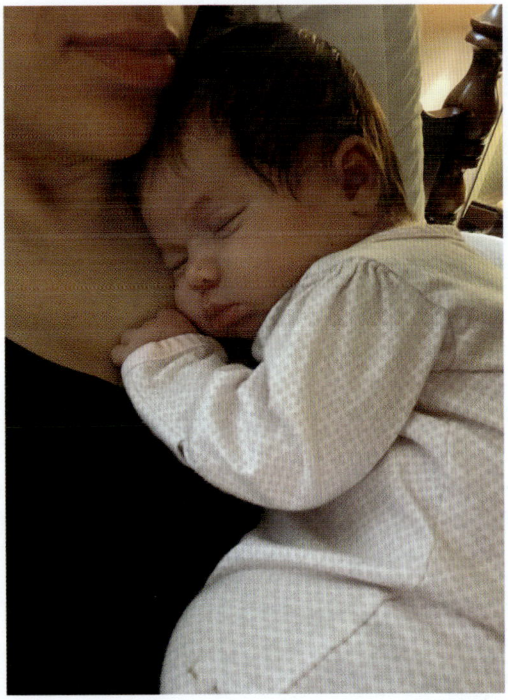

Fig. 12.2 Newborns' sleep differs from all other ages across the lifespan. This healthy two-week-old infant most likely entered sleep through REM sleep and cycled through REM and NREM sleep every 60 minutes and slept 12–18 hours a day. (Photo courtesy of Michelle Rodriguez.)

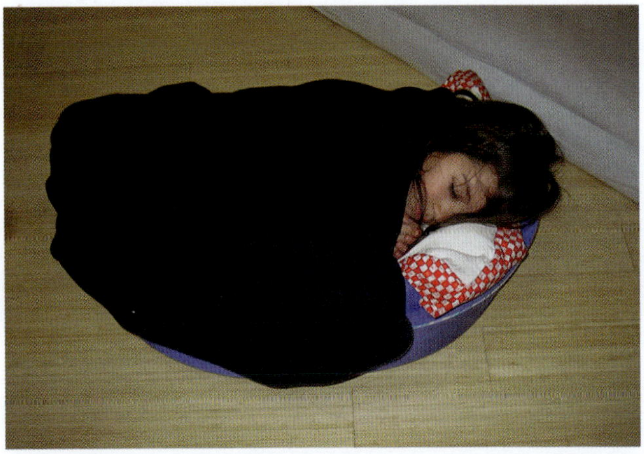

Fig. 12.3 Healthy young children spend more time in deep sleep and can fall asleep easily in less-than-optimal conditions like this 6-year-old who fell asleep while playing in the dog's bed. (Photo courtesy of Kirk Stromberg.)

## CONSEQUENCES OF POOR SLEEP

When inadequate sleep occurs, people experience shorter REM and NREM sleep, which interferes with memory, muscle repair, and hormone release. This may exacerbate an illness or its symptoms or cause changes in weight (Fatima et al., 2015; Souders et al., 2017). For example, babies who are more easily awakened have more episodes of apnea (stopped breathing) when they are sleep-deprived. Other symptoms of difficulty sleeping include blurred vision, fatigue, tiredness, sleepiness, change in appetite, sickness, difficulty learning, and difficulty managing stress. Studies show that sleep deprivation affects cognitive, attentive, and social skill development (Goldstein & Walker, 2014; Tso et al., 2019).

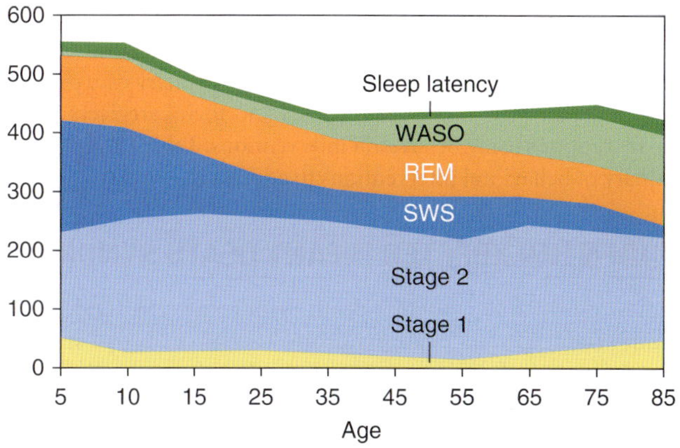


**Fig. 12.4** Sleep across the lifespan (ages 5–85 years). (From Koketsu, J. S. (2025). Sleep and rest. In H. M. Pendleton, & W. Schultz-Krohn (Eds.), *Pedretti's occupational therapy: Practice skills for physical dysfunction* (9th ed., p. 328). Elsevier. From Ohayon, M. M., Carskadon, M. A., Guilleminault, C., & Vitiello, M. V. (2004). Meta analysis of quantitative sleep parameters from childhood to old age in healthy individuals: Developing normative sleep values across the human lifespan. *Sleep, 27*(7), 1255–1273. https://doi.org/10.1093/sleep/27.7.1255.) Slow wave sleep (SWS) or deep sleep, wake after sleep onset (WASO), sleep latency (amount of time to fall asleep in minutes).

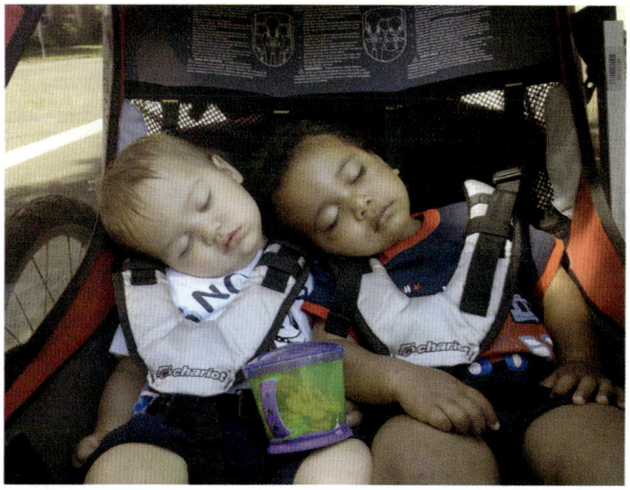

**Fig. 12.5** Healthy toddlers, such as these 15-month-old and 24-month-old children, sleep about 12–14 hours a day, including naps 1–2 times a day in 1–3-hour bouts. (Photo courtesy of Kirk Stromberg.)

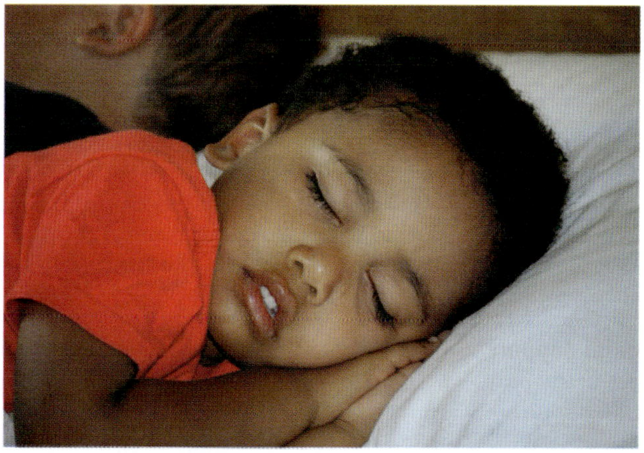

**Fig. 12.6** Three-year-olds sleep about 11–13 hours a day, including naps, and require one nap a day. (Photo courtesy of Kirk Stromberg.)

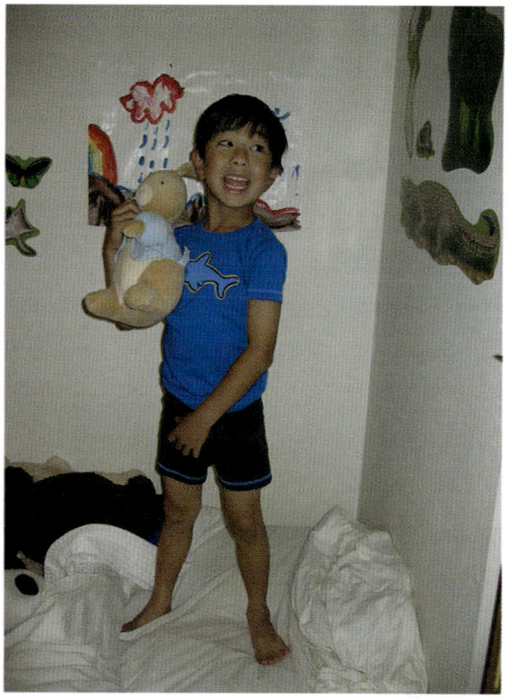

**Fig. 12.7** Healthy elementary school children are "the best sleepers in our society" (Pelayo, 2020, p. 51) as they tend to have consistent routines, fall asleep easily, and feel safe, comfortable, and loved. This 6-year-old sleeps 10 hours a night, takes daytime naps on occasion, looks forward to sleep, and energetically wakes up at 6:00 a.m. (Photo courtesy of Jean Koketsu.)

The prevalence of sleep problems in typical developing children is at least 25%, but it is up to 85% in children with neurodevelopmental disorders (Horwood et al., 2019; Maski & Owens, 2016). Children with diagnoses such as attention deficit hyperactivity disorder (ADHD), autism spectrum disorder (ASD), diabetes mellitus, or cerebral palsy often have sleep disturbances (Horwood et al., 2019; Macaulay et al., 2020; Miller et al., 2018; Papadopoulos et al., 2019). Chronic deprivation of sleep may result in a propensity for depression or substance use. This is particularly significant in adolescents; Lovato and Gradisar (2014) found that about 73% of adolescents who suffered from depression also experienced comorbid sleep problems. Sleep disturbance is also significantly associated with health-risk behaviors, leading to negative effects such as sports-related injuries, suicide attempts, dropping out of school, and difficulty maintaining social relationships (Lovato & Gradisar, 2014). Sleep problems are also significantly associated with excessive screen-time behaviors (Baiden et al., 2019; Guerrero et al., 2019). Engaging in an online game before bedtime may shorten sleep duration (Chan et al., 2022).

Parents and other household members may become sleep-deprived when a child has difficulty sleeping which may affect their ability to meet role expectations (at school, home, work, or in the community). Parents who are sleep-deprived are more likely to report stress, irritability, reduced concentration, increased sleepiness during the daytime, and impaired sleep quality at night (Levin & Scher, 2016; Martin et al., 2019). Therefore, when addressing sleep issues, occupational therapy practitioners examine and address the entire family's routine.

## COMMON SLEEP DISORDERS

Common sleep disorders in children are insomnia, obstructive sleep apnea, restless legs syndrome, parasomnias, and delayed sleep phase syndrome (Deshpande et al., 2022). Table 12.2 describes common sleep disorders in children. Table 12.3 further defines common

**BOX 12.1 American Academy of Pediatrics Recommendations for Infant Sleep**

**A Level Recommendations**

Place infants on their back to sleep for every sleep

Use a firm, flat, noninclined sleep surface to reduce the risk of suffocation or wedging/entrapment.

Feed infants human milk (like breastfeeding). Human milk is associated with a reduced risk of SIDS.

Share a room with an infant for at least the first 6 months. Infants should sleep in the parents' room, close to the parents' bed, but on a separate surface designed for infants.

Keep things out of the infant's sleep area, including soft objects, pillows, toys, quilts, comforters, mattress toppers, blankets, and nonfitted sheets, to reduce the risk suffocation, entrapment/wedging, and strangulation.

Offer the infant a pacifier at nap time and bedtime once they are breastfeeding well.

Avoid smoke, vaping, and nicotine exposure during pregnancy and after birth.

Avoid alcohol, marijuana, opioids, and illicit drug use during pregnancy and after birth.

Avoid letting an infant get too hot and keep their head and face uncovered during sleep.

Get regular medical care throughout pregnancy.

Immunize infants in accordance with guidelines from your healthcare provider per the American Academy of Pediatrics (AAP) and Centers for Disease Control (CDC).

Avoid heart, breathing, motion and other monitors to reduce the risk of SIDS.

Provide supervised, awake tummy time to facilitate development and to minimize the risk of positional plagiocephaly. Place the infant in tummy time while awake and supervised for short periods beginning soon after hospital discharge, increasing incrementally to at least 15–30 min total daily by age 7 weeks.

Physicians, nonphysician clinicians, hospital staff, and childcare providers should endorse and model safe infant sleep guidelines from the beginning of pregnancy.

Media and manufacturers should follow safe sleep guidelines in their messaging and advertising to promote safe sleep practices as the social norm.

Continue the NICHD "safe to sleep* campaign, focusing on ways to reduce the risk of all sleep-related deaths. Pediatricians and other maternal and child health providers can serve as key promoters of the campaign messages.

**B Level Recommendations**

Avoid products and devices that go against safe sleep guidance (especially those that claim to "prevent SIDS").

**C Level Recommendations**

Avoid swaddline once an infant starts to roll over (usually around 3 months of age). There is no evidence to recommend swaddling as a strategy to reduce the SIDS risk.

Continue research and surveillance on the risk factors, causes, and pathophysiological mechanisms of sleep-related deaths, with the ultimate goal of eliminating these deaths entirely.

Based on the strength-of-recommendation taxonomy Level A recommendations are based on consistent, good-quality patient-oriented evidence. Level B recommendations are based on inconsistent or limited-quality, patient-oriented evidence. Level C recommendations are based on consensus, usual practice, opinion, disease-oriented evidence, or case studies of diagnosis treatment, prevention, or screening. NICHD, Eunice Kennedy Shriver National Institute of Child Health and Human Development.

Adapted from Moon et al. (2022). Sleep-related infant deaths: updated 2022 recommendations for reducing infnat deaths in the sleep environment. *Pediatrics, 150*(1), e2022057990; Eunice Kennedy Shriver National Institute of Child Health and Human Development. (2022). *What does a safe sleep environment look like?* https://safetosleep.nichd.nih.gov.

parasomnias. Occupational therapy practitioners may be the first to notice features of sleep disorders and can refer clients to their healthcare providers. The practitioner can work with primary care providers and other team members to help clients and their caregivers address sleep disruptions using behavioral interventions. Table 12.4 provides a summary of behavioral interventions to address insomnia in children.

## SUDDEN UNEXPECTED INFANT DEATH SYNDROME

Sudden unexplained infant death syndrome (SUIDS), which includes sudden infant death syndrome (SIDS) is a broad spectrum of both explained and unexpected deaths of previously healthy infants under 1 year (Parks et al., 2021). In a review of 4929 SUIDS cases in the United States, 72% of deaths occurred in unsafe sleeping environments (Parks et al., 2021). Unsafe sleeping environments include those with soft surfaces or objects that can block an airway, those with shared sleeping with another person or a pet, and those where the infant's sleeping position can lead to airway blockage or entrapment. Children of color are disproportionately affected, with SUIDS rates in the United States which is highest for American Indian/ Alaska Natives, then Non-Hispanic, and Blacks (Parks et al., 2017).

## ENVIRONMENTAL AND PERSONAL FACTORS INFLUENCING SLEEP AND REST

### Environmental Factors

**Environmental factors** include the physical, social, and attitudinal atmospheres in which people live and engage in daily activities (AOTA, 2020). Occupational therapy practitioners examine the influence of environmental factors on a child's rest and sleep. See Case Example 12.1; Sarah for an illustration of occupational therapy addressing environmental factors.

**Physical.** The physical environment plays a key role in encouraging healthy rest and sleep. Physical factors include elements of the room where the infant or child rests and sleeps. Room temperature, light, sound, and smells can impact sleep. Other physical factors include products and technology such as sleeping surfaces, bedding, pillows, and availability and access to social media. Studies show that using technology before bedtime results in less sleep (AlShareef, 2022; Pillion et al., 2022). Furthermore, light from technology sources may even interrupt sleep. Setting up the physical environment to be a safe, calming, and comfortable space promotes sleep. Sleep areas should be comfortable temperatures for children. Fans, vents, or open windows may soothe children and provide a way to alert others of problems.

Providing a safe space without interruptions supports healthy sleep patterns. Generally, researchers recommend children and youth sleep in a dark room, although some children may benefit from a night-light or an open doorway. Calming sounds such as white noise help some children sleep. Some children benefit from soothing aromas, such as lavender. The occupational therapy practitioner collaborates with the child and family to determine aspects of space that may require modifications. For example, one child noted that they were afraid to sleep in their bed, as a doll was staring at them.

**Social Support and Relationships.** **Social and relational factors** refer to the people or animals that provide physical or emotional support, nurturing, protection, assistance, and connections to others (AOTA, 2020). Social support and relationships may affect sleep and rest. Children and youth benefit from predictable caring relationships with adults who protect them and nurture them. Establishing a calming and supportive bedtime routine benefits

TABLE 12.2 **Common Sleep Disorders in Children**

| Sleep Disorder (Prevalence) | Clinical Features | Diagnostic Criteria | Treatment Options[a] |
|---|---|---|---|
| Childhood insomnias (behavioral subtypes 10%–30%) | Sleep-onset association: children have trouble falling asleep without relying on a person or activity such as rocking or other environmental cues, which results in a significant delay or absence of sleep onset without caregiver involvement.<br>Limit-setting: parent or caregiver does not establish sleep routines, or limits are not consistently followed; mixed problems with associations and limit-setting | Diagnosis is clinical<br>Sleep-wake disturbances characterized by difficulties in initiating or maintaining sleep occurring at least 3 times per week for at least 3 months | Behavioral interventions (Table 12.4)<br>Hypnotic medications are not recommended |
| Obstructive sleep apnea (1%–5%; peaks between 2 and 8 years) | Recurrent episodes or partial or complete upper airway obstruction associated with arousals, awakenings, or oxygen desaturations<br>Obesity and tobacco smoke exposure are risk factors | Polysomnography<br>Home sleep apnea testing is not recommended | Adenotonsillectomy<br>Nasal continuous positive airway pressure for second-line treatment |
| Restless legs syndrome (2%–4%; more common in adolescents) | Unpleasant sensations in the legs that cause difficulty initiating and maintaining sleep. Daytime symptoms can happen with extended periods of inactivity or sitting. About one-fourth of patients with restless legs syndrome have attention-deficit/hyperactivity disorder symptoms, and up to one-third of those with attention-deficit/hyperactivity disorder have restless legs syndrome | Diagnosis is clinical and requires the following: (1) urge to move legs because of unpleasant or uncomfortable sensations. (2) sensations begin or worsen with rest ***or*** inactivity, tying down, or sitting. (3) temporary partial or complete relief with movement such as stretching or walking. (4) occurs mostly in the evening or night. (5) symptoms cause sleep disturbance or impairment of daytime functioning, and (6) symptoms need to be described in the child's words | Iron therapy of 3 mg per kg per day if ferritin levels <50 ng per mL (50 mcg per L)<br>Screen for and address triggers if identified as a cause or contributing factor (e.g., prolonged inactivity, sleep deprivation, diphenhydramine (Benadryl), selective serotonin reuptake inhibitors, metoclopramide (Reglan), caffeine, nicotine, alcohol. |
| Parasomnias (up to 50%) | During sleep-wake transitions, activities appear purposeful or automatic but the child has no meaningful interaction with the environment, child is difficult to arouse, appears contused, may quickly go back to sleep, and may have amnesia about the episode<br>Repetitive stereotypic behaviors and posturing indicate the need to investigate for nocturnal seizures | Diagnosis is clinical<br>Polysomnography is indicated if (1) the description is not typical or there has been an injury, (2) there is concern about nocturnal seizures or rapid eye movement sleep behavior disorder, or (3) there is concern about precipitating factors such as obstructive sleep apnea or periodic limb movement disorder (clustered neurologically mediated leg movements that disturb sleep) | Self-limiting; most resolve spontaneously by adolescence, education and reassurance, address sleep hygiene and stress; treat comorbid conditions such as gastroesophageal reflux, obstructive sleep apnea, and restless legs syndrome; take safety precautions refer for violent behavior or injury, or when there is no response to conservative treatment |
| Delayed sleep phase syndrome (7%–16%) | Sleep-onset and wake-up times are delayed | Diagnosis is clinical, with a sleep diary for 7–14 days showing a sleep period delayed by more than 2 hours for at least 3 months | Sleep-wake schedules with patient input<br>Avoid exposure to bright and blue light (e.g., electronic devices) before bedtime<br>Melatonin (0.3–5 mg) given about 1.5–6 5 hours before bedtime<br>Bright-light therapy in the first 1–2 hours after awakening |

[a]Note that the above treatment options are those recommended by physicians and primary care providers. Treatments such as provision of medications, supplements, procedures and continuous positive airway pressure devices are outside of the scope of occupational therapy.
From Deshpande, P, Salcedo, B., & Haq, C. (2022). Common sleep disorders in children. *American Family Physician, 105*(2), 170. From Carter et al. (2014). Recommendations for medications, supplements should be by the physician or primary care provider. Advanced training may be required for light therapy.

TABLE 12.3 **Differentiating Common Childhood Parasomnias**

| Parasomnia | Timing in Sleep Period | Sleep Stage | Amnesia | Out of Bed? | Behavior | Autonomic Nervous System |
|---|---|---|---|---|---|---|
| Confusional arousals | First half | Non- rapid eye movement | Yes | No | Confused appearance, eyes open or closed - attempts to wake child are unsuccessful and often resisted by the child | No |
| Nightmare | Last half | Rapid eye movement | Age-appropriate dream recall is present | No | Frightening dream resulting in a period of wakefulness | Absent to mild |
| Sleep terror | First half | Non- rapid eye movement | Yes | Yes | Child precipitously sits upright and screams; may jump out of bed and run blindly; child can become agitated or disoriented | High level of autonomic activation; tachycardia, mydriasis, sweating |
| Sleepwalking | First half | Non- rapid eye movement | Yes | Yes | Partial arousal from sleep with some ambulation young child may crawl out of bed' older child may be found asleep in a different location | No |

From Deshpande, P, Salcedo, B., & Haq, C. (2022). Common sleep disorders in children. *American Family Physician, 105*(2), 173.

TABLE 12.4 **Behavioral Interventions for Childhood Insomnias**

| Intervention | Method |
|---|---|
| Education | Parents or caregivers are educated on prevention and development of sleep problems; information about sleep hygiene. They receive education on sleep-wake routine, naps, and putting child to bed awake to promote self-soothing behaviors. |
| Graduated extinction | Modified extinction method to promote self-soothing behaviors by child, parents or caregivers. Briefly check on child on a fixed or progressive schedule; goal is the same as unmodified extinction. |
| Positive routines/faded bedtime/ response costs | **Positive routines:** Parents or caregivers develop a bedtime routine with a series of calming activities leading to sleep onset.<br>**Faded bedtime:** Bedtime is temporarily delayed to the natural sleep onset time, so child does not stay awake in bed; bedtime is then faded to an earlier time.<br>**Response cost:** Child is taken out of bed for scheduled periods if not able to fall asleep. |
| Scheduled awakenings | Parent or caregivers document the times of usual overnight awakenings; child is awakened before the anticipated awakening at night and then put to bed; number of awakenings is reduced over time. |
| Unmodified extinction (cry it out loud) | Parent or caregivers put child to bed at a designated bedtime; child is monitored for issues such as safety and illness but otherwise ignored for crying or screaming until morning. The objective is to reduce undesired behaviors by removing reinforcement from parental attention. |

From Deshpande, P, Salcedo, B., & Haq, C. (2022). Common sleep disorders in children. *American Family Physician, 105*(2), 171.

sleep patterns (Hoyniak et al., 2022). Allowing children and youth to feel emotionally supported and cared for promotes connection and supports sleep. Engaging children and youth in reflective, positive, and calming social activities before bedtime prepares them for sleep. High-intensity social activities before bedtime may excite children and make sleeping difficult.

**Attitudes.** *Attitudes* are defined as "observable evidence of customs, practices, ideologies, values, norms, factual beliefs, and religious beliefs held by people other than the client." (AOTA, 2020, p. 10). For example, some families and societies place importance on performance and achievement over restorative occupations. These attitudes may cause children and youth to feel pressure to succeed while ignoring the need to rest and sleep. Family routines may support or inhibit sleep and rest patterns. For example, busy working families may value time at the end of the day to catch up and enjoy time together. This pattern may support children and youth, allow them to feel family connections, and enhance rest and sleep. It may also cause families to stay up later and interfere with the child's sleep. Occupational therapy practitioners examine the attitudes and beliefs of families and support sleep and rest within the family system. Many different routines are successful. For example, some children sleep in the same room (or same bed) as their parents. For some children, room- or bed-sharing with an adult may promote "good sleep" (Hoyniak et al., 2022). The occupational therapy practitioner works with families to create a sleep-rest plan that meets the child's and family's values, routines, and needs.

**Systems and Policies.** Systems and policies can also affect rest and sleep. These include benefits, programs, and regulations that are designed to meet the needs of persons, groups, and populations (AOTA, 2020). For example, school policies regarding start times and bus schedules influence children's sleep patterns. Daylight savings time changes routines and affects sleep and wake hours. Systems, policies, and programs regarding healthcare coverage may influence activity choices and opportunities to support sleep and rest. For example, children may be afforded opportunities for specialized programs

### CASE EXAMPLE 12.1 SARAH, AN ADOLESCENT CHEERLEADER

Sarah is a 15-year-old high school student referred to outpatient occupational therapy after falling and hitting her head and breaking her right wrist during a cheerleading competition. She was diagnosed with a mild concussion and a radial wrist fracture, which required surgery. Usually an "A" student, since her fall, which was 2 months ago, Sarah has difficulty concentrating and organizing herself to complete her assignments. Headaches, sensitivity to lights, occasional dizziness along with wrist pain, weakness, and general fatigue, affect her ability to work on her computer or to write. Before the accident, Sarah had no difficulty falling asleep, did not wake up at night, and slept about 6 hours a night on school nights and 10 hours a night on weekends when there were no competitions.

Sarah states she is unable to sleep at night due to pain, concerns about school, and sadness that she may not be able to do cheerleading anymore. It can take her an hour to fall asleep, she wakes up 2–3 times a night, and has trouble falling back asleep. She must get on the bus at 6:30 a.m. to make it to school by 7:35 a.m. On Friday and Saturday nights, she stays up until 2:00 a.m. and sleeps until noon.

The occupational therapy practitioner completed an occupational therapy profile of sleep (Pierce & Summers, 2011) to collect information on Sarah's day and night routine, activities, and environment. The practitioner addressed Sarah's wrist pain issues that negatively affect her sleep. The practitioner educated Sarah and her parents on the importance of sleep, circadian rhythms, and how sleep changes across the lifespan. The occupational therapy practitioner provided the family with resources for establishing healthy sleep and rest patterns.

Together, the practitioner and Sarah created a plan to support her rest and sleep to prevent fatigue during the day and promote healing at night. Sarah decided she would take regular rest breaks (minimum every 30 minutes) while on her computer and devices. She would also stop using her computer and devices 1 hour before bedtime. They created a weekend and weekday schedule for wake and sleep times that was slightly different (but as congruent as possible so Sarah would remain on a healthy schedule). As part of her bedtime routine, Sarah added deep breathing exercises and gentle stretching to calm her mind and body without the expectation of falling asleep.

Sarah's sleep before her injuries was typical for a teenager, although she admitted she often sacrificed sleep and rest to get school assignments completed or socialize with friends (online). Given Sarah's recent head trauma, the occupational therapy practitioner referred Sarah to her primary care provider for further assessment of possible insomnia, mood, and cognitive issues and to determine the need for accommodations to her school schedule until full recovery from her injuries.

where they can be active during the day which promotes sleep and rest. They may receive programmatic support through school systems or healthcare providers to engage in psychological counseling to learn meditation strategies or coping techniques to better support emotional regulation, sleep, and rest. Occupational therapy practitioners understand the systems and policies that influence children's sleep and rest. They advocate for services and policies that support children and families.

**Culture.** Cultural values, beliefs, and practices influence bedtime routines, sleeping arrangements, physical activity, and psychological functioning (Jeon et al., 2021). Jeon and team (2021) looked at cross-cultural differences in child, parent, and environmental factors across 51 countries ($n = 19$) and found that children from Europe, North America, and Australasia were more likely to go to bed and wake up earlier and have longer nighttime sleep duration than children in Asia and the Middle East. Infants in Asia were more likely to have more frequent and longer regular naps than other countries. In America, to prevent SIDS, the American Academy of Pediatrics recommends that infants be placed supine on firm surfaces (See Fig. 12.8) and discourages bed-sharing. Stiffler et al. (2020) conducted a focus group with African American mothers of infants at least 6 months old to discuss sleep practices and experiences with providers. The mothers gave suggestions to providers regarding how to best educate them (See Box 12.2).

### Personal Factors

**Personal factors** are enduring features of a person that are internal to the person, not part of a health condition or status, and make up the person's background (AOTA, 2020). Personal factors include age, sexual orientation (preference and identity), gender identity, race and ethnicity, cultural identification and attitudes, social background, socioeconomic status (SES), upbringing and life experiences, behavioral patterns, psychological assets (temperament, character traits, coping styles), education, professional identity, lifestyle, and health condition and fitness status (AOTA, 2020). Activity level and SES influence sleep in children and adolescents (Sosso & Khoury, 2021). In both North America and Europe, children and teens from low socioeconomic backgrounds and those whose mothers have lower education levels report poorer or disrupted sleep. The Coordinated Health Care for Complex Kids project, which targets Medicaid-funded (lower SES) children, examined claims data from over 16,609 children ages 0–18 with chronic medical conditions (Adavadkar et al., 2022). They found that 14% of this population received a sleep disorder diagnosis, with the most frequent diagnosis being sleep-disordered breathing, then nocturnal enuresis and insomnia. The researchers suggest that sleep disorders are underdiagnosed in the most vulnerable, high-risk, and predominantly minority populations (Adavadkar et al., 2022). Although occupational therapy practitioners do not make assumptions about children's sleep based on SES alone, they examine the influence of both environmental and personal factors on rest and sleep. As Peloya (2020), a professor in sleep medicine states, "poor sleep has no age, social, or cultural boundaries" (p. 99).

## OCCUPATIONAL THERAPY INTERVENTIONS TO ADDRESS SLEEP AND REST

Occupational therapy practitioners must show respect and acknowledge family preferences when providing occupational therapy services. They listen to children and families and design client-centered interventions that are meaningful to the child and family. Understanding each family's unique situation and culture requires an openness and desire to learn from the families. This allows the occupational therapy practitioner to present materials and intervention activities that align with the child and family's routines, which are more likely to be followed.

Occupational therapy practitioners address sleep and rest challenges for children and adolescents through lifestyle modifications and the use of Cognitive Behavior Therapy for Insomnia (CBT-I) (Purdin et al., 2022), which requires advanced training. They also encourage children and teens to care for their assistive devices/equipment and to engage in sleep- and rest-promoting activities. They collaborate with children and their families to educate and train them to make needed changes and modifications to support consistent routines. They advocate for systems and policies to support children and their families (AOTA, 2020).

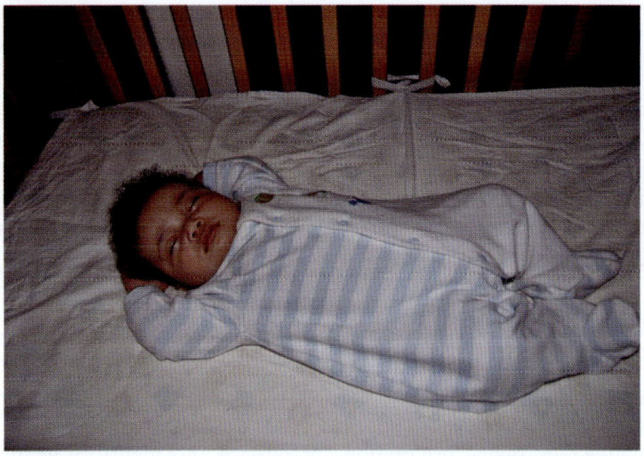

**Fig. 12.8** Per recommendations of the American Academy of Pediatrics (Moon, 2022), Table 12.4. This 5-month-old is sleeping on a firm, flat, noninclined surface, separately from the parents, with no pillows or bedding materials that pose an asphyxiation risk. (Photo courtesy of Kirk Stromberg.)

### BOX 12.2 Recommendations by African American Mothers for Infant Sleep Education (Stiffler et al., 2020)

- Do not just hand out pamphlets.
- Make sure that key family members are educated (e.g., father, grandparents, everyone).
- Emphasize the higher risk of African American infant mortality (twice the risk of SUIDS).
- Have a person who looks like them deliver the message (not a video).
- Tell stories of real people.
- Continue the education process throughout the first year of the baby's life (not just when the baby is delivered) (Stiffler et al., 2020).

## Lifestyle Modifications

### Sleep Hygiene: Bedtime Routines, Habits, and Environment.

**Sleep hygiene** is defined as modifiable lifestyle and environmental practices that promote sleep (Ellis & Allen, 2019). General sleep hygiene recommendations for all children include a consistent bedtime and wake-up time, a dark and quiet bedroom that is comfortably cool, minimal external noise, avoidance of excessive fluids before bedtime, avoidance of caffeine several hours before bedtime, avoidance of vigorous activity before bedtime, and satiated in terms of hungry (may provide a small snack before bedtime if hungry) (Deshpande et al., 2022). Deshpande and colleagues also added that children should learn to fall asleep alone. The Sleep Foundation recommends limiting screen use close to bedtime, getting adequate exercise, avoiding frightening or violent content, not sleeping with pets, and providing soothing smells in the bedroom (Pacheco, 2022).

***Bedtime Routines and Habits.*** Bedtime routines are created specifically for each child and family to support sleep. For example, initiating a bath close to bedtime with a child who does not like baths may have a negative alerting effect, which may lead to resistance to going to sleep. Another child may enjoy bath time and may become calm and drowsy afterward. Children with sensory processing disorders may find tooth brushing; face washing; texture, weight, or tightness of clothing or blankets; or donning and doffing orthotics as being aversive, which may affect the child's readiness to go to sleep at night or for naps. The Carson case example (Case Example 12.2) illustrates an occupational therapy intervention to support a child's bedtime routine.

### CASE EXAMPLE 12.2 CARSON

Carson is an active 5-year-old who was evaluated by an occupational therapist in an outpatient clinic. Carson's mother reported Carson has "high activity level" and adverse reactions to bathing and tooth brushing. The mother reports he has irregular sleep patterns and is not able to stay in bed or stay asleep for more than 2 or 3 hours at a time. Carson has difficulty getting to sleep (latency) and remaining asleep (night awakening). He does not have a regular bedtime. Because Carson continually gets out of bed and refuses to go to sleep, his mother brings Carson to bed with her to "keep an eye on him." Mom also revealed that she continually argues over the phone with Carson's father (regarding custody and support) after she puts Carson to bed.

#### Intervention Plan

The therapist used a variety of approaches to address Carson's activity level, his sensory modulation difficulties, and the lack of a consistent, calming bedtime routine. The practitioner educated both parents on the importance of daily routines (e.g., physical activity, consistent meal times) and sleep routines so Carson knows what to expect and is rested for the next day.

Together, they developed an after-school routine that included taking the dog for a short walk so Carson could get fresh air and physical activity. They decided to reduce food and drink consumption at nighttime. They created a checklist for Carson's bedtime routine after dinner that both parents agreed to follow.

Carson brushed his teeth after dinner since he became irritated during this activity. He was rewarded by playing a quiet board game of his choice. To prepare for sleep, his parents turned the television off, provided hugs for deep pressure, and he took a warm calming bath. The parents were instructed to provide firm pressure during the washing and drying-off process and when applying lotion. To give Carson control, his parents allowed Carson to pick a special soap (with smells that Carson liked), washcloths, and rhythmic songs (e.g., "This is the way we wash our face.").

His parents read him a bedtime story while Carson rested under heavy blankets. The heavy blankets provide deep pressure and proprioceptive input throughout the night. The parents added a small night light in the hallway and a white noise machine to comfort Carson for sleep. They moved his bed away from the vent that blew air directly on him. Carson received a sticker for staying in his own bed each night. His parents agreed that they would discuss parenting and custody issues during the day while Carson was at school instead of at nighttime when they both were tired.

Carson was also referred for a psychological assessment because he continued to experience difficulty at school (e.g., high activity level, anxiety, and difficulty paying attention). This assessment was also important because of the stress of the family going through a custody hearing. In addition, because Carson seemed to appear bored and unchallenged during the day and was not getting enough exercise or activity, his parents enrolled him in different camps during the summer months. These behavioral strategies, environmental changes, and changes in routine improved Carson's sleep patterns. The changes benefited Carson and his parents as they all felt more rested and supported.

*Much gratitude to Audrey Kane, PhD, OTR/L, Assistant Professor, Virginia Commonwealth University, Richmond, VA, who originally contributed the case study.*

Occupational therapists can help develop tailored routines for naps, rest, or bedtime for their clients. Mindell et al. (2015) considered that **bedtime routines** were the "activities that occur right before lights out" and found that the earlier the routines start in a child's life the better. Prokasky and colleagues' (2019) research on toddlers suggests that consistent bedtime routines between weeknights and weekends are important to optimize sleep See Box 12.3 for recommendations regarding routines for toddlers through school-aged children.

## BOX 12.3 Suggested Recommendations for Bedtime Routines

- To signal that bedtime is approaching and to relax and get ready for sleep, turn off the TV, and have the child pick up and put away toys.
- To empower children to develop confidence and overcome possible nighttime fears, make supportive positive statements to let them know they are safe.
- Ensure that the physical environment is safe for sleep by removing dangling cords from blinds, trip hazards, toys from beds. If a child tends to use the bathroom at night consider motion detector night lights.
- If a child is at risk of rolling out of bed, consider padded mats on the floor, lowered beds, or baby monitors. Caution should be used when recommending rails as there may be a risk of asphyxiation.
- Establish a quiet time before bedtime for reading, rocking together in a chair, singing quiet rhythmic songs, or giving the child a back rub or gentle massage (Pacheco, 2023).
- Use transition objects (e.g., special blanket, cuddle toy) reserved for nighttime to help develop between the item to segue into the bed and sleep (Franklin et al., 2015)
- Implement a screen curfew (Pacheco, 2023).
- Keep the routine and environment as consistent as possible. Use familiar objects and sequence of tasks (such as self-care, reading a bedtime story, and turning off the lights).
- Develop a routine for going back to sleep if the child wakes up during the night. The checks should be brief, with the purpose to let a child know they are safe and attended to while fostering a child's ability to self-soothe and sleep on their own. Caregivers may choose to wait a few minutes before responding to allow the child to fall asleep on their own (Pacheco, 2023).

***Environment.*** The location and sensory aspects of the sleep environment and the type of bedding and clothing may facilitate or hinder the quality of sleep. As children grow, they may need different firmness in a mattress or type of bed (e.g., from a crib to a youth bed [once a child is 35 in tall], or a longer bed for the teen who is now 6 ft 4 in, or 193 cm tall). The sleeping area needs to be quiet and away from activity. Bedrooms should be used for sleeping and not for other activities. The following suggestions relate to modifying the physical sleep environment, if needed (Hannan & Hiscock, 2015; Ho & Siu, 2018; Reynolds & Andelin, 2021; Suni, 2023).

- *Light*: Use a blackout curtain to keep the bedroom dark; use a nightlight if a child is afraid of the dark. Limit screen time as blue light emitted from LED-lit devices (e.g., smartphones, tablets, computers, and television screens) can delay circadian rhythms and cause the child to take a longer time to fall asleep. If needed, switch to red lights that do not suppress melatonin production.
- *Sound*: Keep the room quiet or use a white noise machine at low decibels if a child accepts the sound.
- *Temperature*: Keep the temperature consistent and determine if vents, windows, or fans that are near the bed are problematic or if the child may be too cold or hot.
- *Smell*: Determine if smells are alerting or calming in the room (e.g., kitchen smells, deodorant in a diaper pail, smell of sheets or clothing). Add calming and soothing smells, such as lavender, cinnamon, and baby powder.
- Consider the weight, texture, and visual attractiveness of clothing and bedding and the personal preference of the child. Use favorite pillows or stuffed animals in the bed to help children feel more secure (not for babies).
- Limit technology use before bedtime: set a curfew, make the bedroom or mattress a technology-free zone, use blue-light filters, or alter settings (e.g., night mode or dark mode).
- Secure outside doors or windows if sleepwalking or escaping from the home are issues. Alarms may be installed so that parents are alerted if children start to leave the sleep environment.

Modification of the physical environment may include simple changes to lighting, floor surface, amount and type of furniture or objects, and overall traffic pattern of the room or building. For some children, minimizing sensory stimuli and eliminating visual and auditory distractions may help.

***Positioning.*** Occupational therapists may change the position of the child and of the materials or activity when making recommendations for both engagement in wakeful and rest/sleep occupations. Occupational therapy practitioners examine body positions and promote regular positional changes for sleep for children who have mobility issues. Limitations in body functions such as strength, joint movement, motor control, and endurance can affect a child's ability to position themselves comfortably in bed during sleep, so caregivers may have to help to ensure the child is comfortable to optimize sleep. It is important to provide pressure relief via special bed surfaces or regular bed position changes during sleep to protect the skin from breakdown, particularly to areas of the body with bony prominences for children who have limitations in mobility. A comprehensive program including but not limited to regular skin checks, turning schedules, and pressure reduction surfaces for children who are hospitalized and on prolonged bed rest due to illness is particularly important (Simsic et al., 2019).

***Safety, Fear, and Sleep.*** Teaching children that they are safe in the dark is important so that they can sleep better (Pelayo, 2020). Pelayo (2020) recommends not using a child's sleeping space as punishment or for time-outs but rather allowing the sleep environment to be a safe and comfortable space for a child. Caregivers can acknowledge fears that children may have without reinforcing the fears or validating irrational fears (such as looking for monsters in the closet) (Pelayo, 2020). If a child's anxiety is strong and affects functioning, they should be referred to a primary care provider. Some children may respond to cognitive behavioral training to address their fears that interfere with sleep.

## Cognitive Behavioral Training for Insomnia

There is emerging evidence that cognitive behavioral training for insomnia (CBT-I) is effective for children and adolescents (Peersmann et al., 2021; Schlarb et al., 2018; Zachariae et al., 2016). The CBT-I protocols include psychoeducation, stimulus control, sleep restriction, relaxation, and cognitive restructuring. Research supports the use of these techniques online (such as with the i-sleep app) (Peersmann et al., 2021; Zachariae et al., 2016). This technique involves understanding the child or adolescent's thinking and promoting positive "self-talk" and self-soothing techniques. The occupational therapy practitioner may promote journaling, guided imagery, and slow deep breathing techniques (Eakman et al., 2022). They may support the child's bedtime routine by engaging the child in visualization and positive mantras. Throughout the process, practitioners empower the child or youth to create their own rest and sleep routines. They collaborate with children and youth to develop goals and identify rewards. They involve children in the established routine, discuss progress, and may engage in role-play activities. Occupational therapy practitioners using CBT-I benefit from advanced education on the protocols and techniques (Baglioni et al., 2022).

## Education and Training

Occupational therapy practitioners educate parents and caregivers about sleep and its connection to positive development as the first step of the intervention (Franklin et al., 2015). Educational programs about healthy sleep habits can benefit children and families (Russell et al., 2019; Wooster et al., 2015). Russell et al. (2019) found positive sleep results after providing a program to educate families of children 3 years old and younger from an Arizona Navajo Nation, diagnosed with a developmental disability. Wooster et al. (2015) reported evidence that an occupational-therapy-designed, parent-educational program for children with ASD regarding sleep preparation and participation was effective. Educating children and families about the benefits of sleep and rest requires practitioners to engage families and children in conversations to understand their routines, habits, patterns, and goals. Occupational therapy practitioners use this knowledge to design creative intervention plans that are meaningful to children and their families (Beisbier & Laverdure, 2020).

## Advocacy

Advocacy to support sleep and rest can occur at the person, group, and population level. For example, occupational therapy practitioners can ensure that an adolescent in an inpatient rehabilitation unit is not scheduled for a 7:00 a.m. occupational therapy session if the teen prefers to be sleeping. School-based therapists advocate for adjusted schedules to accommodate the sleep needs of their clients. At the societal level, efforts to protect the sleep of children and teens can occur in the form of research, policy, and political advocacy.

Research suggests that later school start times help adolescents get adequate sleep (Wahlstrom et al., 2014; Wheaton et al., 2016). Researchers reported significant improvements in sleep duration, school attendance, grades, and less tardiness and falling asleep in class, and fewer car crashes with later school start times (Wheaton et al., 2016). Wahlstrom et al. (2014) found that high school students whose schools started at 8:30 a.m. or later were less likely to report low mood or to use caffeine or substances such as alcohol, tobacco, and drugs and they achieved higher test scores on national achievement tests.

US schools have complex bureaucratic structures that maintain the status quo, making it difficult to change start times in high school (Wahlstrom et al., 2014). Changing school start times requires support from all interested parties and their inclusion in decision-making and planning committees (Fitzpatrick et al., 2021). The American Academy of Sleep Medicine supports delaying school start times for middle and high school students to 8:30 a.m. (Watson et al., 2017) and the elimination of Daylight Saving Time in the United States to a fixed, national year-round time (Rishi et al., 2020). Daylight savings time is not in alignment with the human circadian rhythm and can be detrimental to sleep, and it is another hotly debated issue (Watson, 2019). Occupational therapy practitioners advocate for changes in policies that support children and families.

## Caring for Assistive Devices/Equipment

As they mature, children learn to take care of their personal devices, such as hearing aids, glasses, contact lenses, orthotics, prosthetics, catheters, insulin pumps, glucose monitors, and/or a variety of pieces of assistive devices used for toileting, grooming, feeding, and dressing. Females need to learn to care for their menses needs at night to ensure proper hygiene. About 75%–90% of young women experience dysmenorrhea (period pain) during their reproductive life, so they need to learn to manage that as well (Armour et al., 2019). Many items used for self-care are part of bedtime and morning routines, such that children and caregivers may need to allow extra time to manage those items both before bed and upon awakening.

Adenotonsillectomy is the first-line treatment of obstructive sleep apnea in children while a nasal continuous positive airway pressure (CPAP) device is the second-line treatment if the outcome of surgery is not optimal or if the adenotonsillectomy is contraindicated (Deshpande et al., 2022). Management of the device requires appropriate donning and doffing of the device, maintaining and managing it before bed, and once the child wakes up.

Occupational therapy practitioners may assist children and families in understanding how to care for personal devices and integrate the management into the child's daily routine which may include rest and sleep routines. For example, as part of a child's sleep routine, they may create adaptations to support children who have fine motor skill challenges in managing their glasses, insulin, or catheters.

## Activities

Occupational therapy practitioners engage children and youth in activities to address routines for health. They use their skills in occupational analysis to evaluate the steps and tasks required for the child to be successful. As experts at grading and adapting activities along with viewing the whole perspective, occupational therapy practitioners create client-centered intervention plans. They carefully measure the outcomes of the plan and adjust the plan and recommendations throughout. When addressing sleep and rest, they collaborate with children and their families often and reinforce positive changes to support the child and family. Beisbier and Laverdure (2020) found strong evidence to support occupation and activity-based interventions to improve sleep quality and routines.

**Mindfulness Meditation, Yoga, and Progressive Muscle Relaxation.** Research shows the positive influence of physical activity (Beisbier & Laverdure, 2020), mindfulness meditation (Zaccari et al., 2022), yoga (Narasingharao et al., 2017), and progressive muscle relaxation (Franklin et al., 2015) on children's sleep and rest routines. Mindfulness meditation practices have been found to help people with sleep (Rusch et al., 2019; Shallcross et al., 2019). These practices have also been instituted in schools in the United States to help with stress. From 2012 to 2017 there was a rise in children aged 4–17 years using mindfulness or spiritual meditation in their life (National Center for Complementary and Integrative Health, 2022). One study applied mindfulness-oriented meditation (MOM) to help children with ADHD sleep and showed promising results (Zaccari et al., 2022). Twenty-five children with ADHD (7–11 years) underwent two programs three times per week for 8-weeks. Fifteen children received MOM training, while 10 children in the control group did not. Children who received MOM training showed significantly improved scores on sleep and behavioral measures than the controls.

Similarly, structured yoga sessions were found to be helpful when provided to children with ASD with parent involvement. Results showed improvement overall in sleep, gastrointestinal issues, and behaviors for the 32 children who received the intervention compared with the 32 controls (Narasingharao et al., 2017). Progressive muscle relaxation (systematic contraction and relaxation of muscles) before sleep and gentle massage may be incorporated into bedtime routines to help children with relaxation (Franklin et al., 2015).

**Integrating Rest Breaks Throughout Activities.** Occupational therapy practitioners understand the importance of rest throughout the day. Rest breaks allow children and youth to manage their emotions and responses so that they can reengage in activities as needed (AOTA, 2020). Rest allows children to relax and renew their energy. Essentially rest provides a break from activities to allow the body and mind to calm, refocus, and approach activities with a renewed interest. Rest may include stopping the activity altogether and taking a few breaths before returning. It may include sitting in a favorite spot and closing one's eyes briefly. Rest may also include replacing the activity with a more calming one (such as swinging or listening to one's favorite song). The occupational therapy practitioner often creates "rests" specific to the child and family. They identify rests that are acceptable to the situation. Sometimes, a rest break whereby children go outside for a walk or play provides renewed energy.

Children and youth may benefit from replacing cognitive activities with more physical activities (such as gym, dancing, and playing). For example, many preschool classroom schedules have scheduled rest periods for students throughout the day. Parents may schedule breaks (i.e., quiet time or naps) for children throughout the day. Occupational therapy practitioners may identify behaviors that signify a child's or youth's need for a rest. For example, children may experience frustration while playing. Instead of waiting for the child to become agitated, the practitioner provides a natural rest. Teaching parents and caregivers to observe the child's behaviors and integrate rests (which may take many forms) throughout the day often results in improved engagement in daily activities.

Adolescents may benefit from understanding the importance of rest throughout their day and identifying how they can incorporate breaks. For example, some adolescents take "technology breaks" to allow themselves a rest from social media influences. They may discover benefits in reflecting, relaxing outside, or reading a book.

## SUMMARY

Occupational therapy practitioners provide services to children and youth who are at risk of having sleep issues. They understand that children's sleep influences their growth and development. Sleep routines affect caregivers and household members. Sleep and rest are important restorative occupations.

1. Sleep and rest are important for memory, muscle, repair, and hormone release. Appropriate sleep is paramount for optimal growth, development, and functioning and is an important part of a child's and family's life (Deshpande et al., 2022). Childhood sleep problems can disrupt family dynamics and lead to cognitive and behavioral issues in children and adolescents, and early recognition can avert many of those issues (Deshpande et al., 2022).
2. Environmental and personal factors affect participation in sleep and rest as well as client factors (such as the child's cognitive, sensory, social, emotional, and physical strengths and challenges). Environmental factors include physical, social, and attitudinal characteristics. Personal factors include culture, social background, lifestyle, family routines, and structures. Occupational therapy practitioners consider these factors when creating intervention plans to address rest and sleep.
3. Infants require 12–18 hours of sleep (with frequent naps); toddlers 12–14 hours (with one or two naps); preschoolers 11–13 hours (one nap); school-age 10–11 hours (some children still nap); and teenagers 8.5–9.25 hours (no naps). Teens prefer staying up late and waking up later.
4. Occupational therapy practitioners address sleep and rest challenges for children and adolescents through the use of education, activities, therapeutic interventions (such as CBT-I), lifestyle modifications, and assistive devices and equipment (Purdin et al., 2022). They collaborate with children and their families to educate and train them to make needed changes and modifications to support consistent rest and sleep routines. They advocate for systems and policies to support children and their families (AOTA, 2020).

## REFERENCES


Adavadkar, P. A., Pappalardo, A. A., Glassgow, A. E., Zhang, C., Schwartz, A., Brooks, L. J., & Martin, M. A. (2022). Rates of diagnoses of sleep disorders in children with chronic medical conditions. *Journal of Clinical Sleep Medicine*, *18*(8), 2001–2007.

AlShareef, S. M. (2022). The impact of bedtime technology use on sleep quality and excessive daytime sleepiness in adults. *Sleep Science*, *15*(Spec. 2), 318.

American Occupational Therapy Association. (2020). Occupational therapy practice framework: Domain and process. *American Journal of Occupational Therapy*, *74*(Suppl. 2), 7412410010p1–7412410010p87.

Armour, M., Smith, C. A., Steel, K. A., & Macmillan, F. (2019). The effectiveness of self-care and lifestyle interventions in primary dysmenorrhea: A systematic review and meta-analysis. *BMC Complementary and Alternative Medicine*, *19*(22), 1–16.

Baglioni, C., Espie, C. A., Spiegelhalder, K., Gavriloff, D., & Riemann, D. (2022). Recommendation of the European Academy for Cognitive–Behavioural Therapy for Insomnia (CBT–I) for high quality training for health professionals. *Cognitive-Behavioural Therapy for Insomnia (CBT-I) Across the Life Span: Guidelines and Clinical Protocols for Health Professionals*, 243–250.

Baiden, P., Tadeo, S. K., & Peters, K. E. (2019). The association between excessive screen-time behaviors and insufficient sleep among adolescents: Findings from the 2017 youth risk behavior surveillance system. *Psychiatry Research*, *281*, 112586.

Beisbier, S., & Laverdure, P. (2020). Occupation- and activity-based interventions to improve performance of instrumental activities of daily living and rest and sleep for children and youth ages 5–21: A systematic review. *American Journal of Occupational Therapy*, *74*(2), 7402180040.

Carskadon, M. A., & Dement, W. C. (2011). Normal human sleep: An overview. In M. H. Kryger, T. Roth, & W. C. Dement (Eds.), *Principles and practice of sleep medicine* (5th ed.). Elsevier/Saunders.

Carter, K. A., Hathaway, N. E., & Lettieri, C. F. (2014). Common sleep disorders in children. *American Family Physician*, *89*(5), 368–377.

Chan, G., Huo, Y., Kelly, S., Leung, J., Tisdale, C., & Gullo, M. (2022). The impact of eSports and online video gaming on lifestyle behaviours in youth: A systematic review. *Computers in Human Behavior*, *126*, 106974.

Deshpande, P., Salcedo, B., & Haq, C. (2022). Common sleep disorders in children. *American Family Physician*, *105*(2), 168–176.

Eakman, A. M., Schmid, A. A., Rolle, N. R., Kinney, A. R., & Henry, K. L. (2022). Follow-up analyses from a wait-list controlled trial of occupational therapist–delivered cognitive–behavioral therapy for insomnia among veterans with chronic insomnia. *American Journal of Occupational Therapy*, *76*(2).

El Shakankiry, H. M. (2011). Sleep physiology and sleep disorders in childhood. *Nature and Science of Sleep*, *3*, 101–114.

Ellis, J. G., & Allen, S. F. (2019). Sleep hygiene and the prevention of chronic insomnia. In *Sleep and health* (pp. 137–145). Academic Press.

Eunice Kennedy Shriver National Institute of Child Health and Human Development. (2022). *What does a safe sleep environment look like?* https://safetosleep.nichd.nih.gov/reduce-risk/reduce.

Fatima, Y., Doi, S., & Mamun, A. (2015). Longitudinal impact of sleep on overweight and obesity in children and adolescents: A systematic review and bias–adjusted meta–analysis. *Obesity Reviews*, *16*(2), 137–149.

Fitzpatrick, J. M., Silva, G. E., & Vana, K. D. (2021). Perceived barriers and facilitating factors in implementing delayed school start times to improve adolescent sleep patterns. *Journal of School Health*, *91*(2), 94–101.

Franklin, J., Smith-Windsor, J., & Brown, C. (2015). In A. Green, & C. Brown (Eds.), *An occupational therapist's guide to sleep and sleep problems* (pp. 160–184). Jessica Kingsley Publishers.

Goldstein, A. N., & Walker, M. P. (2014). The role of sleep in emotional brain function. *Annual Review of Clinical Psychology, 10*, 679.

Gronski, M. (2022). Evidence connection—occupational therapy interventions to support sleep in children from birth to age 5 years. *American Journal of Occupational Therapy, 76*, 7605390010.

Guerrero, M. D., Barnes, J. D., Chaput, J. P., & Tremblay, M. S. (2019). Screen time and problem behaviors in children: Exploring the mediating role of sleep duration. *International Journal of Behavioral Nutrition and Physical Activity, 16*, 105.

Hannan, K., & Hiscock, H. (2015). Sleep problems in children. *Australian Family Physician, 44*(12), 880–884.

Ho, E. C. M., & Siu, A. M. H. (2018). Occupational therapy practice in sleep management: A review of conceptual models and research evidence. *Occupational Therapy International*. https://doi.org/10.1155/2018/8637498. 2018.

Horwood, L., Li, P., Mok, E., Shevell, M., & Constantin, E. (2019). A systematic review and meta-analysis of the prevalence of sleep problems in children with cerebral palsy: How do children with cerebral palsy differ from each other and from typically developing children? *Sleep Health, 5*(6), 555–571.

Hoyniak, C. P., Bates, J. E., Camacho, M. C., McQuillan, M. E., Whalen, D. J., Staples, A. D., Rudasill, K. M., & Deater-Deckard, K. (2022). The physical home environment and sleep: What matters most for sleep in early childhood. *Journal of Family Psychology, 36*(5), 757–769.

Jeon, M., Dimitriou, D., & Halstead, E. J. (2021). A systematic review on cross-cultural comparative studies of sleep in young populations: The roles of cultural factors. *International Journal of Environmental Research and Public Health, 18*(4), 2005.

Koketsu, J. S. (2025). Sleep and rest. In H. M. Pendleton, & W. Schultz-Krohn (Eds.), *Pedretti's occupational therapy: Practice skills for physical dysfunction* (9th ed.) (p. 328). Elsevier.

Levin, A., & Scher, A. (2016). Sleep problems in young children with autism spectrum disorders: A study of parenting stress, mothers' sleep–related cognitions, and bedtime behaviors. *CNS Neuroscience and Therapeutics, 22*(11), 921–927.

Lovato, N., & Gradisar, M. (2014). A meta-analysis and model of the relationship between sleep and depression in adolescents: Recommendations for future research and clinical practice. *Sleep Medicine Reviews, 18*(6), 521–529.

Macaulay, G. C., Boucher, S. E., Yogarajah, A., Galland, B. C., & Wheeler, B. J. (2020). Sleep and night-time caregiving in parents of children and adolescents with type 1 diabetes mellitus–A qualitative study. *Behavioral Sleep Medicine, 18*(5), 622–636.

Martin, C. A., Papadopoulos, N., Chellew, T., Rinehart, N. J., & Sciberras, E. (2019). Associations between parenting stress, parent mental health and child sleep problems for children with ADHD and ASD: Systematic review. *Research in Developmental Disabilities, 93*(2019), 103463.

Maski, K., & Owens, J. A. (2016). Insomnia, parasomnias, and narcolepsy in children: Clinical features, diagnosis, and management. *The Lancet Neurology, 15*(11), 1170–1181.

Miller, M. A., Kruisbrink, M., Wallace, J., Ji, C., & Cappuccio, F. P. (2018). Sleep duration and incidence of obesity in infants, children, and adolescents: A systematic review and meta-analysis of prospective studies. *Sleep, 41*(4), 1–19.

Mindell, J. A., Li, A. M., Sadeh, A., Kwon, R., & Goh, D. Y. (2015). Bedtime routines for young children: A dose-dependent association with sleep outcomes. *Sleep, 38*(5), 717–722.

Moon, R. Y., Carlin, R. F., & Hand, I. (2022). Sleep-Related infant deaths: Updated 2022 recommendations for reducing infant deaths in the sleep environment. *Pediatrics, 150*(1), e2022057990.

Narasingharao, K., Pradhan, B., & Navaneetham, J. (2017). Efficacy of structured yoga intervention for sleep, gastrointestinal and behaviour problems of ASD children: An exploratory study. *Journal of Clinical and Diagnostic Research: JCDR, 11*(3), VC01–VC06.

National Center for Complementary and Integrative Health. (June 2022). Meditation and mindfulness: What you need to know. Retrieved March 4, 2023, from https://www.nccih.nih.gov/health/meditation-and-mindfulness-what-you-need-to-know.

Ohayon, M. M., Carskadon, M. A., Giulleminault, C., & Vitiello, M. V. (2004). Meta analysis of quantitative sleep parameters from childhood to old age in healthy individuals: Developing normative sleep values across the human lifespan. *Sleep, 27*(7), 1255–1273. https://doi.org/10.1093/sleep/27.7.1255.

Pacheco, D. (2022). How your baby's sleep cycle differs from your own. Retrieved March 3, 2023 from *Sleep Foundation*. https://www.sleepfoundation.org/baby-sleep/baby-sleep-cycle#references-83522.

Pacheco, D. (2023). Sleep strategies for kids. https://www.sleepfoundation.org/children-and-sleep/sleep-strategies-kids.

Papadopoulos, N., Sciberras, E., Hiscock, H., Mulraney, M., McGillivray, J., & Rinehart, N. (2019). The efficacy of a brief behavioral sleep intervention in school-aged children with ADHD and comorbid autism spectrum disorder. *Journal of Attention Disorders, 23*(4), 341–350.

Parks, S. E., Erck Lambert, A. B., Hauck, F. R., Cottengim, C. R., Faulkner, M., & Shapiro-Mendoza, C. K. (2021). Explaining sudden unexpected infant deaths, 2011-2017. *Pediatrics, 147*(5), e2020035873.

Parks, S. E., Erck Lambert, A. B., & Shapiro-Mendoza, C. K. (2017). Racial and ethnic trends in sudden unexpected infant deaths: United States, 1995–2013. *Pediatrics, 139*(6), e20163844.

Paruthi, S., Brooks, L. J., D'Ambrosio, C., Hall, W. A., Kotagal, S., Lloyd, R. M., Malow, B. A., Maski, K., Nichols, C., Quan, S. F., Rosen, C. L., Troester, M. M., & Wise, M. S. (2016). Recommended amount of sleep for pediatric populations: A consensus statement of the American Academy of Sleep Medicine. *Journal of Clinical Sleep Medicine, 12*(6), 785–786.

Peersmann, S. H., van Straten, A., Kaspers, G. J., Thano, A., van den Bergh, E., Grootenhuis, M. A., & van Litsenburg, R. R. (2021). Does the guided online cognitive behavioral therapy for insomnia "i-Sleep youth" improve sleep of adolescents and young adults with insomnia after childhood cancer?(MICADO-study): Study protocol of a randomized controlled trial. *Trials, 22*(1), 1–11.

Pelayo, R., & Dement, W. (2017). *Dement's sleep & dreams* (2nd ed.). Rafael Pelayo and William Dement.

Pelayo, R. (2020). *How to sleep: The new science-based solutions for sleeping through the night*. Artisan Books.

Pierce, D., & Summers, K. (2011). Rest and sleep. In C. Brown, & V. C. Stoffel (Eds.), *Occupational therapy in mental health: A vision for participation* (pp. 736–757). F. A. Davis.

Piller, A., Torrez, E., Keenportz, M., Maki, K., Rudkoski, T., & Hawk, K. (2020). Pediatric sleep difficulties: How OTs address sleep as an occupation. *American Journal of Occupational Therapy, 75*(Suppl. 2), 7512505094p1.

Pillion, M., Gradisar, M., Bartel, K., Whittall, H., & Kahn, M. (2022). What's "app"-ning to adolescent sleep? Links between device, app use, and sleep outcomes. *Sleep Medicine, 100*, 174–182.

Prokasky, A., Fritz, M., Molfese, V. J., & Bates, J. E. (2019). Night-to-Night variability in the bedtime routine predicts sleep in toddlers. *Early Childhood Research Quarterly, 49*, 18–27.

Purdin, S., Selhorst, M., Rospert, S., Baker, V., & Tanner, K. (2022). Sleep interventions for children 0-18. *OT Practice, 27*(6), 37–40.

Reynolds, S., & Andelin, L. (2021). Sleep and screens: How technology can be used to improve sleep in children. *SIS Quarterly Practice Connections, 6*(4), 2–5.

Rishi, M. A., Ahmed, O., Barrantes Perez, J. H., Berneking, M., Dombrowsky, J., Flynn-Evans, E. E., Santiago, V., Sullivan, S. S., Upender, R., Yuen, K., Abbasi-Feinberg, F., Nisha Aurora, R., Carden, K. A., Kirsch, D. B., Kristo, D. A., Malhotra, R. K., Martin, J. L., Olson, E. J., Ramar, K., … Gurubhagavatula, I. (2020). Daylight saving time: An American Academy of Sleep Medicine position statement. *Journal of Clinical Sleep Medicine, 16*(10), 1781–1784.

Rusch, H. L., Rosario, M., Levison, L. M., Olivera, A., Livingston, W. S., Wu, T., & Gill, J. M. (2019). The effect of mindfulness meditation on sleep quality: A systematic review and meta-analysis of randomized controlled trials. *Annals of the New York Academy of Sciences, 1445*(1), 5–16.

Russell, M., Baldwin, C. M., Roberts, K., & Quan, S. F. (2019). Mixed method sleep intervention for Navajo caregivers and their children with developmental disabilities. *Sleep, 42*(Suppl. 1), A397.

Schlarb, A. A., Bihlmaier, I., Velten-Schurian, K., Poets, C. F., & Hautzinger, M. (2018). Short-and long-term effects of CBT-I in groups for school-age children suffering from chronic insomnia: The KiSS-program. *Behavioral Sleep Medicine, 16*(4), 380–397.

Shallcross, A. J., Visvanathan, P. D., Sperber, S. H., & Duberstein, Z. T. (2019). Waking up to the problem of sleep: Can mindfulness help? A review of theory and evidence for the effects of mindfulness for sleep. *Current Opinion in Psychology, 28*, 37–41.

Simsic, J. M., Dolan, K., Howitz, S., Peters, S., & Gajarski, R. (2019). Prevention of pressure ulcers in a pediatric cardiac intensive care unit. *Pediatric Quality & Safety, 4*(3), e162.

Sosso, F. E., & Khoury, T. (2021). Socioeconomic status and sleep disturbances among pediatric population: A continental systematic review of empirical research. *Sleep Science, 14*(3), 245–256.

Souders, M. C., Zavodny, S., Eriksen, W., Sinko, R., Connell, J., Kerns, C., Schaff, R., & Pinto-Martin, J. (2017). Sleep in children with autism spectrum disorder. *Current Psychiatry Reports, 19*(6), 1–17.

Stiffler, D., Matemachani, S. M., & Crane, L. (2020). Considerations in Safe to Sleep® messaging: Learning from African-American mothers. *Journal for Specialists in Pediatric Nursing, 25*(1), e12277.

Suni, E. (2023). Sleep Foundation. (2023). *Sleep Hygiene*. Retrieved March 3, 2023, from https://sleepfoundation.org/sleep-topics/sleep-hygiene.

Tester, N. J., & Foss, J. J. (2018). Sleep as an occupational need. *American Journal of Occupational Therapy, 72*(1), 7201347010p1–7201347010p4.

Tso, W., Chan, M., Ho, F. K., Rao, N., Li, A. M., Chan, K. L., Tiwari, A., Wong, I. C. K., Wing, Y. K., Van Voorhees, B., Li, S. L., Goh, W. H. S., & Ip, P. (2019). Early sleep deprivation and attention-deficit/hyperactivity disorder. *Pediatric Research, 85*(4), 449–455.

Wahlstrom, K., Dretzke, B., Gordon, M., Peterson, K., Edwards, K., & Gdula, J. (2014). *Examining the impact of later school start times on the health and academic performance of high school students: A multi-site study*. Center for Applied Research and Educational Improvement. University of Minnesota.

Watson, N. F., Martin, J. L., Wise, M. S., Carden, K. A., Kirsch, D. B., Kristo, D. A., Malhotra, R. K., Olson, E. J., Ramar, K., Rosen, I. M., Rowley, J. A., Weaver, T. E., & Chervin, R. D. (2017). Delaying middle school and high school start times promotes student health and performance: An American Academy of sleep medicine position statement. *Journal of Clinical Sleep Medicine, 13*(4), 623–625.

Watson, N. F. (2019). Time to show leadership on the daylight saving time debate. *Journal of Clinical Sleep Medicine, 15*(6), 815–817.

Wheaton, A. G., Chapman, D. P., & Croft, J. B. (2016). School start times, sleep, behavioral, health, and academic outcomes: A review of the literature. *Journal of School Health, 86*(5), 363–381.

Wooster, D., Gwin, H., Gwin, S., Hargis, L., Papania, J., Register, J., & Rood, K. (2015). Efficacy of sleep education for parents with children with autism spectrum disorder. *American Journal of Occupational Therapy, 69*(Suppl. 1), 6911515153p1.

Zaccari, V., Santonastaso, O., Mandolesi, L., De Crescenzo, F., Foti, F., Crescentini, C., Fabbro, F., Vicari, S., Curcio, G., & Menghini, D. (2022). Clinical application of mindfulness-oriented meditation in children with ADHD: A preliminary study on sleep and behavioral problems. *Psychology and Health, 37*(5), 563–579.

Zachariae, R., Lyby, M. S., Ritterband, L. M., & O'Toole, M. S. (2016). Efficacy of internet-delivered cognitive-behavioral therapy for insomnia–a systematic review and meta-analysis of randomized controlled trials. *Sleep Medicine Reviews, 30*, 1–10.

13

# Interventions to Address Activities of Daily Living

*Carole Ivey and Jayne Shepherd*

## GUIDING QUESTIONS

1. What factors influence children's performance and participation in ADLs?
2. How do occupational therapy practitioners address children's challenges in ADL participation?
3. What intervention approaches and strategies promote children's ADL performance and development?
4. How is collaboration with caregivers, parents, and children important for occupational therapy intervention to address ADLs?

## KEY TERMS

Activities of daily living (ADLs)
Activity demands
Environmental factors
Personal factors
Client factors
Social stories
Visual stories
Video modeling

## ACTIVITIES OF DAILY LIVING

Some of the earliest occupations that children engage in are activities of daily living (ADLs). According to the Occupational Therapy Practice Framework (fourth edition), ADLs are bathing and showering; toileting and toilet hygiene; dressing; eating and swallowing; feeding; functional mobility; personal hygiene and grooming; and sexual activity (American Occupational Therapy Association [AOTA], 2020). This chapter focuses on bathing and showering, toileting and toilet hygiene, dressing, and personal hygiene and grooming. Please see Chapters 11,12,19, 20 and 32 for the other ADLs and Chapter 8 for information about the developmental progression of these skills.

Young children often perform ADLs as co-occupations with their caregivers. The foundations for mastering ADLs begin in infancy and are refined throughout childhood and adolescence. Children develop habits and routines to perform ADLs with ease and independence leading to more time to engage in other occupations with their family, friends, and community. Culture, caregiver expectations, social and family routines, and the physical environment influence when children begin to bathe, dress, groom, and toilet themselves. Overall, society and families expect that as children age, they develop increasing levels of competence and self-reliance to meet their daily living needs. These expectations influence the ability to participate in other occupations, for instance, being toilet trained to go to school. ADLs also relate to a child's self-efficacy, social participation, belonging, and sense of autonomy (Costa et al., 2017). Children's performance in ADLs is a strong predictor of adult outcomes, including employment, quality of life, and socialization (Klinger et al., 2015). Performance in ADLs is complex and dynamically related to client factors, performance skills, performance patterns, and contexts, as well as the demands of the specific activity (AOTA, 2020).

### Client Factors, Performance Patterns, and Performance Skills

Client factors, performance patterns, and performance skills support or inhibit participation and performance in ADLs. Client factors refer to the child's capacities, characteristics, beliefs, body functions, and body structures (AOTA, 2020). The severity of the child's disability, symptoms, and health status is related to self-care function; specifically, when skills are less affected, functional skill performance increases, and the amount of caregiver assistance decreases (Kilincaslan et al., 2019; Phipps & Roberts, 2012; Zapata-Figueroa & Ortiz-Corredor, 2022). Children who are acutely ill or who have multiple disabilities that require numerous procedures throughout the day (e.g., tube feeding, tracheostomy care, bowel, and bladder care) may not have the time or energy to perform ADLs independently. This care may also affect their daily habits and routines. Children with multiple disabilities may be physically unable to do all or any part of ADLs, but they may partially participate in or direct others on how to care for them (See Case Example 13.1 and Fig. 13.1). Family beliefs, values, and attitudes about child-rearing, autonomy, and self-reliance influence how caregivers and children perceive and prioritize ADLs and therefore, must be considered for intervention planning.

### Environmental and Personal Factors

Environmental and personal factors influence engagement with, participation in, and performance of ADLs (AOTA, 2020). Occupational therapy practitioners must be aware of their own and others' cultural beliefs, customs, activity patterns, and expectations for ADLs. Cultural expectations of family, caregivers, and their social group may determine standards and expectations for ADLs. Personal factors, (e.g., unique features of person, such as age, gender identity, race, culture, beliefs, or socioeconomic status; AOTA, 2020), may influence the type and availability of tools, equipment, and materials that a child uses to perform ADLs (e.g., types of clothes; hair products; use of toilet, bidet, or outhouse; type of adaptations that are acceptable). Economic conditions, geographic location, and opportunities for education and employment determine the types of resources and supports available to families.

The initiation and completion of ADLs are also influenced by environmental factors (i.e., physical, support relationships, attitudinal

## CASE EXAMPLE 13.1 KARINA: PARTIAL PARTICIPATION

Four-year-old Karina is hospitalized every 2 months because of respiration complications related to a muscular disorder. Karina has an opinion about and preference for how her hair is styled, and she likes to wear barrettes, ribbons, jewelry, and pretend makeup. Karina has a tracheostomy, poor endurance, limited strength, and limited postural control to sit independently. Although sitting independently in bed to groom is limited by these client factors, with partial participation, Karina is still part of the activity. She can sit up and bend forward with physical support from the occupational therapy practitioner, reach and choose her barrettes, and with assistance, comb her hair. See Fig. 13.1.

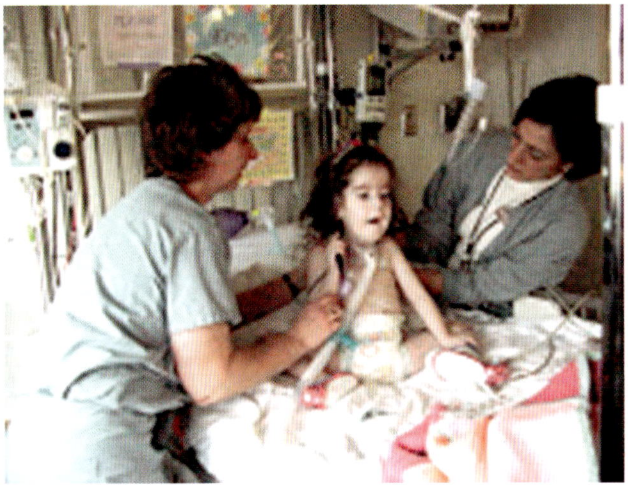

**Fig. 13.1** This child partially participates in hair combing and chooses her barrettes while therapists support her in her hospital bed.

surroundings, and available products/technology and systems; AOTA, 2020). Primary settings that children may experience include home, school, childcare, community, and work. The physical environment will likely be different across the places where the child completes ADLs. For instance, in the daycare setting, there may be a child-sized toilet, but at home, there may be an adult-sized toilet. The supports and relationships in an environment also shapes expectations for ADLs and will differ across settings. For example, the family may have the child use the toilet whenever they need it, while teachers may allow students to use the toilet at fixed times. The variation in the environments may confuse or be disorganizing to children with intellectual disabilities or autism but may be motivating to children without attention, sensory, or cognitive issues. The differing contextual components may result in differences in a child's participation and performance across settings.

### Activity Demands

The activity demands (i.e., aspects of activity needed to engage in it, such as importance to the child or caregiver, object properties, space and social demands, sequencing and timing of required action, and underlying body functions and structures) facilitate or inhibit the quality of performance during ADLs. Occupational analysis helps the occupational therapy practitioner understand the complexity and various components of the activity (Table 13.1). An occupational analysis of activity demands often are different in the clinic, compared with the home, school, or community. It is important to understand this and plan for carryover to different settings.

The objects used to perform ADLs may also help or hinder performance. Clothing items (e.g., clothes with snaps, hooks, and loop shoes), grooming items (e.g., toothbrush and size and design of toothpaste dispenser), or bathing items (e.g., type of soap, bathing mitt, or the feel of a towel) may motivate or distract the child. Objects or assistive devices need to be accepted by the child and family, fit the child and caregivers' skills, needs, and preferences, and meet the demands of the social, cultural, and physical environment.

## EVIDENCE-BASED INTERVENTIONS THAT SUPPORT PARTICIPATION AND PERFORMANCE IN ACTIVITIES OF DAILY LIVING

Current evidence indicates that the most effective interventions to support participation and performance in ADLs (1) are directly focused on ADLs, (2) incorporate client and caregiver training and education, (3) are performed in natural contexts, and (4) are developed and completed collaboratively with the child and caregivers. Occupational therapy practitioners address performance in ADLs by creating occupation-based intervention plans that include participation in the target ADL within the child's environment (and using familiar objects) and in collaboration with the child and family. They provide child and caregiver training to empower them to participate in desired activities. Please see Box 13.1 for reflective questions to guide the practitioner in considering family priorities for ADL interventions.

### Occupation-Based Interventions

Interventions that explicitly and directly address functional life skills training improve participation and performance in ADLs for children and youth (Gronski & Doherty, 2020; Laverdure & Beisbier, 2021; Novak & Honan, 2019). Interventions should be occupation-based and outcomes should be focused on occupation, rather than on client factors (Daud et al., 2016; Kreider et al., 2014). While this may sound obvious, many practitioners report an emphasis on performance skills and client factors (e.g., developing strength and movement) or the use of equipment or technologies due to reported challenges with implementing occupation-based interventions (Daud et al., 2016). However, interventions that focus on ADLs directly confer larger clinical gains than interventions focused on client factors or performance skills (Novak & Honan, 2019).

Directly working on ADLs allows the occupational therapy practitioner to observe supports and barriers to performance and initiate collaborative problem-solving with the child and caregivers on modifications for tasks, materials, environment. or the approach used. For instance, the practitioner may work to improve a child's dressing skills by offering the caregiver and child choices of various dressing strategies to use. Once the method is chosen, anticipatory problem-solving is used to help prepare for unexpected events in the environment. Selection or modification of materials, assistive technology, and adaptations to the task are all methods for improving a child's performance in ADLs (Table 13.2). Occupational therapy practitioners suggest methods to modify the demands of the activity, such as supportive positioning, or the use of adaptive aids such as button hooks, rings on zippers, one-handed shoe fasteners, or hook and loop closures during dressing.

Occupational therapy practitioners may attempt to establish or develop performance skills and patterns for ADLs using a developmental or restorative approach by using activities unrelated to ADLs. For instance, self-care skills require specific motor skills such as grasping, pinching, reaching, and calibrating. A practitioner may address those areas directly and give caregivers ideas for skill development. Developmental, restorative, or remedial approaches may be components of a comprehensive intervention plan but are most effective when they are tied explicitly and directly to structured practice of ADLs

**TABLE 13.1 Analysis and Interventions for Toileting**

| Area | Analysis | Intervention Ideas |
|---|---|---|
| Occupational analysis | Recognizes signal to go to the bathroom (visual or interoceptive sensation).<br>Goes to bathroom and closes door.<br>Pulls clothes down (only as much as needed).<br>Sits or stands at toilet<br>Urinates or defecates (or words child uses).<br>Gets toilet paper.<br>Wipes, then throws toilet paper in toilet.<br>Flushes once.<br>Pulls clothes up.<br>Washes and dries hands.<br>Throws away trash.<br>Leaves bathroom. | Visual schedule on bathroom wall.<br>Make tasks smaller or larger, depending on child's abilities (e.g., separate washing and drying of the hands).<br>Add task if child is omitting it or is having trouble (e.g., if child is smearing feces, use "wipe" as one of the steps).<br>Child uses too much toilet paper: (1) remove toilet paper roll and use tissues or pull off correct amount to be used and hand it to child; or (2) place a tape mark on the wall of how much paper to roll out.<br>Child does not sit: Use timer and instruct child to stay "seated" until timer rings; use potty that is close to the floor. |
| Client factors | Sensory function (toilet paper texture, smells, noise of flushing)<br>Interoception (bladder fullness, voluntary control, emptying bladder).<br>Physiologic readiness.<br>Strength, coordination, and endurance to manage clothing and fasteners.<br>Stability to stand at or sit on toilet. | Use habit training if no pattern is evident: go at the same times every day.<br>Use preparatory activities at other times to build strength and coordination for fasteners.<br>Support child's body (e.g., grab bars, foot support, ring reducer, potty chair on floor).<br>Change toilet paper or use different material, such as wet wipes or cloth.<br>Cover automatic flushers to reduce noise.<br>Consider smells and how to manage. |
| Environmental and personal factors | Cultural: family and societal expectations of toileting; words used; whether child uses a public bathroom and sits on the toilet seat; institutional practices (e.g., toileting in preschool, language used).<br>Size, temperature, sounds; set up; way to flush, height of toilet, adaptations (toilet seat or potty chair; grab bars or safety frame around toilet); faucets and other fixtures. | Dedicate a bathroom to toilet training, if possible.<br>Play soft music or toilet song.<br>Cueing and/or social story for bathroom behavior. For example, leave a space between yourself and someone else at a urinal; keep your pants up over your buttocks while urinating at a urinal; don't talk or look others in the eye while at the urinal; be quick and leave when you are finished; only you will touch your body while in the bathroom (unless catheterization training). |
| Performance skills (motor, process, social interaction) | Motor: Posture, mobility, coordination, and effort needed.<br>Process: Initiate, sequence, and terminate.<br>How child communicates the need to go to the bathroom (e.g., physically or by speaking).<br>Social interaction during toileting. | Consistent communication to indicate need to use the bathroom<br>Picture cues of entire sequence<br>Object cues or transitional object<br>Social story<br>Timer<br>Spoken cues<br>Positioning body on toilet<br>Physical, gestural cues<br>Bathroom etiquette/social expectations (touching, personal space, conversations) |
| Performance patterns | Recognizes typical routines in the family for eating and drinking.<br>Recognizes typical times and patterns for urination and defecation.<br>Uses habit training to go at a certain time of the day, every day.<br>Cleans up accidents without harsh reprimanding. | Limit or increase liquids.<br>Use wet-dry chart to determine typical times for toileting.<br>Use visual schedule for toileting steps (including wiping) and times, as well as times for drinking fluids.<br>Use same routine, habits, and rituals for toileting (e.g., particular times or when waking, before trips, after meals).<br>Urge family, school, and daycare center all to follow the same routine and collect data. |
| Activity demands | Placement of potty chair or toilet seat; height of toilet, flushing mechanism, toilet paper dispenser.<br>Space in bathroom, arrangement of items.<br>Door shut or closed; whether child announces it's time to go.<br>Steps to toileting, flushing after going potty; when to close door, get toilet paper or paper towel.<br>Public bathroom social expectations. | Change layout of objects or accessibility of environment.<br>Include "shut the door" as part of toileting sequence.<br>Discuss public bathroom expectations; have social story available to talk about them. |

Adapted from Wheeler, M. (2007). *Toilet training for individuals with autism and other Developmental disabilities* (2nd ed.). Future Horizons.

**BOX 13.1 Reflective Questions to Consider Child's and Family's Priorities**

The following reflective questions may help practitioners in considering how to understand the child's and family's priorities:

- What ADLs are useful and meaningful in current and future contexts?
- What are the preferences of the child and/or family?
- Are the activities age-appropriate?
- Is it realistic to expect the child to perform or master this task?
- Which alternative methods can the child use to perform the tasks?
- Does learning this task improve the child's health, safety, and social participation?
- Do cultural issues influence how tasks are taught?
- Can the task be taught, and practiced in a variety of environments?

in their natural contexts without assuming carry over of skills (e.g., if strength increases the child can pull up pants) (Gronski & Doherty, 2020; Laverdure & Beisbier, 2021; Novak & Honan, 2019).

## Education, Training, and Coaching

Evidence supports that families respond well to education and training (Novak & Honan, 2019) and that their intervention is as effective as therapist-delivered intervention with education and training (Baker et al., 2012). Therefore, home programs and self-management programs can be effective in improving participation and performance in ADLs (Laverdure & Beisbier, 2021; Novak & Honan, 2019). Caregiver education and training are consistent with family-centered philosophy, early intervention legislation, and client-centered practice. Client and caregiver education and training can improve participation and performance through increasing understanding of conditions and intervention

**TABLE 13.2 Typical Adaptation Principles Used With Children and Adolescents With Disabilities**

| Behavior or Disability | Adaptation Principles |
|---|---|
| Low vision or hearing (or both) | Use intact or residual senses.<br>Amplify sensory characteristics of objects (e.g., color, size, tactile and auditory features).<br>Give cues consistently to determine whether activity is beginning or ending.<br>Use tactile, verbal, visual, or object cues (e.g., hand child washcloth, use hand under hand cuing or say, "It's time to wash your face.").<br>Use gestures (e.g., point to arm that is put in sleeve first).<br>Decrease auditory and visual distractions. |
| Dislike of being touched (tactile overresponsivity) | Prepare child for touch by giving deep pressure and applying organized, rhythmic touch.<br>Give choices for tactile preferences (e.g., clothes, washcloths, brushes).<br>Let child perform touching on themself (e.g., use toothbrush or wash face or body).<br>Allow child to wear snug clothing (e.g., turtleneck) or loose clothing in accordance with their preference. |
| Inability to find clothes or understand top, front, or bottom | Amplify characteristics.<br>Reduce distracters (e.g., place only one utensil on countertop for grooming activity).<br>Use visual or gestural cues (e.g., mark medial border of shoes with "happy faces" to keep shoes on correct feet).<br>Use systematic scanning when searching for objects (e.g., clothes in closet). |
| Inability to sit up or maintain balance | Provide support externally (e.g., use positioning device on floor or chair, use walls for support).<br>Change position of child (e.g., have child sit to put on shoes or dress in side-lying position).<br>Change position of activity (e.g., keep grooming items together in a bucket on top of the sink). |
| Limited reach | Reduce amount of reach needed.<br>Change position of activity.<br>Lengthen handles (e.g., use long-handled bath sponge or reacher). |
| Difficulty grasping objects | Build up handles of objects with foam or wrapping tape (e.g., brushes, spoons).<br>Substitute assistive devices so that grasping is not necessary (e.g., use universal cuffs or straps).<br>Stabilize objects with other body parts (e.g., in teeth or between legs). |
| Weakness, with little endurance | Eliminate gravity (e.g., prop elbow or dress in side-lying position).<br>Use lightweight objects.<br>Use power equipment (e.g., a lift, to transfer to tub bench or toilet; an electric toothbrush, a stand to hold a hair dryer). |
| Difficulty controlling movement | Provide stable base of support (e.g., sit on floor with wide base, or sit on chair).<br>Eliminate need for fine control (e.g., use an enlarged zipper pull).<br>Use weighted devices to give proprioceptive feedback (e.g., weighted toothbrushes and cups).<br>Increase practice opportunities using the desired movement. |
| Poor memory; inability to remember sequences or directions | Establish and practice set routines and sequences.<br>Use partial participation, grading techniques, and backward and forward chaining.<br>Use visual cues (e.g., pictures, labels, checklists, color coding).<br>Substitute assistive technology (e.g., alarm on watch or timers).<br>Use verbal cues (e.g., "first, then second"; jingles, rhymes, songs).<br>Use real-life materials in the setting in which the occupation occurs. |
| Tendency to become easily frustrated; outbursts | Identify purpose of "problem behavior" (e.g., escape, avoid, attention, obtain, transition, or stimulate) by analyzing antecedents and consequences.<br>Limit exposure to context associated with misbehavior.<br>Use preferred tasks and give choices.<br>Reinforce, coach, and expand appropriate alternate behaviors.<br>Avoid personal assistance and coaching (use partial participation).<br>Use grading, prompting, fading prompts, and generalization. |

options, adherence, and decreasing caregiver stress (Gronski & Doherty, 2020; Laverdure & Beisbier, 2021; Novak & Honan, 2019). Education and training may help children perform ADLs in their natural environments and help teachers, caregivers, and children learn safety information, specific techniques, and coping strategies. To provide clear education and training, occupational therapy practitioners must consider the knowledge, skills, desired outcomes, learning capacity, literacy, learning preferences, and environmental contexts of children and caregivers, as well as the activity demands (Shepherd & Hanft, 2016). This requires asking the right questions. Questions to reflect (e.g., who, what, when, where), compare (how), and interpret (e.g., why did this work? What other issues may arise?) give practitioners the information to help coach the child and family. Shepherd and Hanft (2016) suggest observing, listening, responding, and planning collaboratively with the child and all caregivers involved in the task for the best outcome.

Occupational therapy practitioners use a variety of education, training, and coaching methods. Grading, forward and backward chaining, partial participation, and modeling can assist caregivers in teaching ADLs. Box 13.2 provides an overview of these training techniques. In addition, the occupational therapy practitioner may use visual aids, written instructions, infographics, audio, video, apps, and checklists to support the education and training. Two areas that tend to be a specific focus for education and training are positioning and safety.

**Education and Training on Positioning.** Occupational therapy practitioners consider the position of the child and the materials in relation to the activity. When possible, the practitioner uses the most typical position for the given activity, with the fewest restrictions or adaptations. Limitations with posture and movement often result in a lack of sufficient control to assume or maintain stable postures during ADLs and thus benefit from adaptive positioning. Adaptive positioning may include using alternate positions (e.g., sitting instead of standing), low-technology devices (e.g., lap boards, pillows, towel rolls), or high-technology devices (e.g., customized cushions, wheelchairs, braces or orthotics). If adaptive positioning is used, the occupational therapy practitioner needs to systematically determine whether the device supports or hinders performance. See Chapter 32 for more information on positioning.

Adaptive positioning may help compensate for physical limitations in body functions such as strength, joint movement, control, and endurance, as well as provide relief to skin areas and bony prominences. For example, dressing while sitting in a chair may eliminate balance or endurance limitations. Although it is common to dress infants while they are lying in the supine position, this position may increase extensor tone for those with neurologic impairment. Positioning the child prone across the knee of the caregiver (for infants and small children) or in a side lying position may decrease extensor and adductor tone, allowing for the range of motion needed for dressing (Fig.13.2A) and diapering (Fig. 13.2B).

**Education and Training on Safety.** Education and training of caregivers should include proper body mechanics to prevent injury. For instance, to lessen strain during bathing, an adult may sit on a stool beside the tub or kneel on a cushion. Lifting is done with the knees bent and the back straight, with the legs used for power. As children get older and heavier, a lift or an easily accessed shower stall arrangement may be necessary. Caregivers may need assistance in planning renovations that will assist the child in being independent and/or assist them in the future growth of the child.

### Providing Training in Natural Contexts

Explicit training on ADLs and structured practice in the natural context is effective for engagement and performance in ADLs (Laverdure & Beisbier, 2021). Practice in the natural context leads to better outcomes and aligns with legislative requirements that require children to receive services in their natural or least restrictive environment, such as in the home or classroom during daily life routines (Gronski & Doherty, 2020).

**BOX 13.2 Training Techniques to Teach Activities of Daily Living**

| Technique | Description | Example |
|---|---|---|
| Grading | Changing the degree of difficulty of the activity | • Providing pull-on pants so child does not have to manage a zipper<br>• Allowing child to eat "finger foods" for lunch or use a spork to stab fruits<br>• Setting out child's clothes so they do not have to find things |
| Forward chaining | Child completes the first step in the sequence and adds additional steps until the child completes all steps. | **Morning grooming:** Turn on the water, pick up the washcloth, rub soap on the cloth, wash face and hands, and turn off the water.<br>Child turns on the water, and the caregiver completes the remaining steps.<br>As the child progresses, the child turns on the water and picks up the washcloth, and the caregiver completes the rest of the sequence. |
| Backward chaining | Child completes the last step in the sequence (so is successful) and adds additional steps until they complete all steps. | **Brushing teeth:** Pick up the toothbrush, pick up toothpaste, squeeze toothpaste on the toothbrush, turn on the water, place toothbrush under water briefly, brush teeth, spit out toothpaste, repeat, turn off water, and return toothbrush to holder.<br>In this example, the caregiver completes all steps except the last—the child returns the toothbrush to the holder. As the child progresses, the caregiver initiates the activity, and the child turns off the water and returns the toothbrush to the holder. |
| Partial participation | Child engages in those aspects of occupation for which they are able. | • Child makes choices of what they want to wear, child pulls shirt over head and caregiver finishes the rest of dressing task.<br>• Child splashes hands in bath water; puts washcloth to body; caregiver washes child and dries them off. |
| Modeling | Practitioner demonstrates actions; shows child how to complete an action or uses video (video-modeling) of occupation. | • Demonstrating how to comb hair or put lotion on<br>• Showing a video to a child of how to tie shoes<br>• Providing simple 1 step directions with a demonstration of dressing. |

Grading, forward and backward chaining, partial participation, and modeling can assist caregivers in teaching ADLs. Box 13.2 provides an overview of these training techniques.

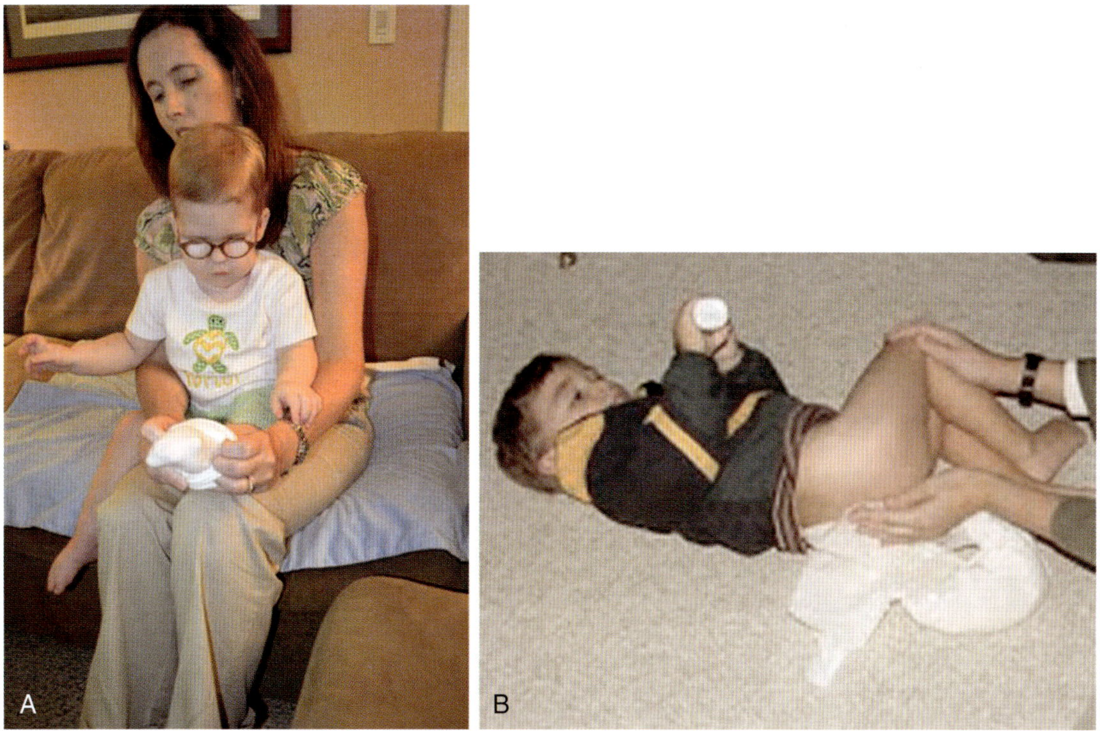


Fig. 13.2 (A) When dressing a child who is hypertonic, the caregiver should carefully flex the child's hips and knees before putting on socks and shoes. (B) The side-lying position may reduce stiffness and make diapering easier.

When children engage in daily activities, at the times and places where they naturally occur, they benefit from the natural cues and the occupation becomes part of the child's repertoire. They benefit from practicing activities in their own environments using their own materials, and the activity holds more meaning to them as it is part of their daily routine.

## Collaboration

Collaboration with the child and caregiver improves the child's participation and performance (King, 2017; Laverdure & Beisbier, 2021). King (2017) frames occupational therapy as a change process "where the client is the ultimate direct change agent—not the therapist" (p. 130). Collaboration with children and caregivers begins with the codevelopment of goals and intervention plans (Laverdure & Beisbier, 2021). This collaboration is essential for client-centered intervention. Building trust and rapport for client engagement, and for carryover of strategies into daily routines, results in increased effectiveness and efficiency in intervention (Costa et al., 2017).

Children about 5 years of cognitive age may contribute their views and priorities to the goal-setting process. Costa et al. (2017) found that children "clearly expressed their concerns and wishes related to their activity performance and to their participation in everyday life and chose very distinct, individual, and specific activity- and participation-oriented goals that were meaningful for them for occupational therapy intervention" (p. 1595). Occupational therapy practitioners embrace the child's and parent's (or caregiver's) goals. They collaborate with children and caregivers to understand the child's skills, priorities, preferences, and interaction styles when making decisions about the occupational therapy evaluation and intervention process.

Collaboration continues during intervention in which priorities about goals, equipment, methods, and other intervention approaches depend on client and caregiver preferences. Coaching and feedback during ADLs to support in-the-moment sharing of challenges and successes allows for collaborative problem-solving. Having clients or caregivers be responsible for monitoring their practice and performance has been shown to improve performance in ADLs (Laverdure & Beisbier, 2021).

## Visual Supports

Emerging evidence suggests that incorporating visual support and technology in ADLs is beneficial to improving performance. Visual supports are used to promote engagement in routines, support home programs, and provide additional cues to children. Occupational therapy practitioners may use visual support to address sequencing, timing, and pacing and as a reminder to complete the ADL. Visual supports (including schedules, modeling, and stories) are specific to the child and family and should be written in plain language with clear pictures. Occupational therapy practitioners collaborate with children and families and sometimes speech and language practitioners when designing visual supports. They may include visuals created with technology (such as apps). Visual supports (such as schedules, modeling, and stories) are effective in improving participation and performance in ADLs (Hong et al., 2016; Laverdure & Beisbier, 2021; Novak & Honan, 2019). The greatest gains have been reported in young children with intellectual disabilities and autism spectrum disorders (Akers et al., 2016; Aldi et al., 2016). Occupational therapy practitioners evaluate the need to continue the visual support over time as performance may return to baseline if the support is removed (Akers et al., 2016; Aldi et al., 2016).

**Visual Activity Schedules.** Visual activity schedules are an effective strategy to improve independence in ADLs and on-task behaviors, and to decrease challenging behaviors and caregiver prompts (Lequia et al., 2012; Spriggs et al., 2017). Visual activity schedules are a sequence of visual cues (e.g., objects, pictures, words) used to depict any sequence of an ADL task (e.g., schedule, occupational analysis) (Fig.13.3). They may include laminated pictures, handheld devices, albums, projections, rings with pictures, horizontal or vertical schedules, 3-ring binders, or pictures in an album. The occupational therapy practitioner creates a visual schedule that matches the child's preferences, cognition, and physical skills and is easy to use within the specific context and socially accepted (e.g., technology-based modality for an adolescent vs. a ring-binder).

**Video Modeling.** Video modeling is a well-researched technique used by a variety of professionals (Campbell et al., 2015; Hong et al., 2016; Piccin et al., 2017). In video modeling, a child learns a specific activity (e.g., dressing) by watching a video of someone doing the activity. There are different types of video modeling. In one form, a peer or an adult are filmed to provide the model. In video self-modeling, the child is filmed engaging in the activity. In point-of-view video modeling, the video images look like they would from the child's point of view when the child completes the task, showing the arms and hands of a model completing the activity (Fig. 13.4).

Video modeling promotes independence in ADLs and, when used with supported instruction, may enhance the learning and generalization of life skills (Campbell et al., 2015; Hong et al., 2016). It provides children with accurate and consistent examples of the desired behavior through a video presentation that is often motivating for children (Hong et al., 2016). A review of studies on video modeling suggests that custom-made videos resulted in better outcomes than commercially available videos (Piccin et al., 2017). Custom-made videos are personalized to the child's needs and preferences; and include voiceovers or written cues specific to the child to promote success (Aldi et al., 2016; Campbell et al., 2015; Hong et al., 2016; Piccin et al., 2017). Video modeling is more effective for elementary and adolescent children than for children under 5 years of age (Hong et al., 2016). Portable technology such as smartphones or tablets allows children to bring videos to different settings (Aldi et al., 2016; Campbell et al., 2015; Hong et al., 2016). Video modeling is most effective when the child uses it in the natural context (Campbell et al., 2015).

Video modeling should include an opportunity to practice the skills immediately following the video, with feedback, error correction, or prompting techniques to support children's learning in the moment before moving to the next step in the sequence. The occupational therapy practitioner uses video modeling to teach the child skills needed within the sequence (by stopping the video) until the child masters the task (Gardner & Wolfe, 2015). Once the child completes the task independently using video modeling, the practitioner engages the child in the practice of maintenance sessions to support the generalization and carryover of previously learned skills (Aldi et al., 2016; Campbell et al., 2015).

**Visual Stories.** Visual stories or social stories are social learning tools for a specific context, skill, achievement, or context created as a personalized illustration with text (Gray, 2015). The repetition of positive statements and personalization makes children more willing to follow the routine in a story and initiate the task themselves. Gray (2015) established criteria for creators of the stories to follow when using social stories to promote participation and performance. Gray (2015) recommends reading the story to the child daily and reading it before beginning the task. While visual stories are effective in improving social skills, the research evidence for improving ADL performance and participation is limited.

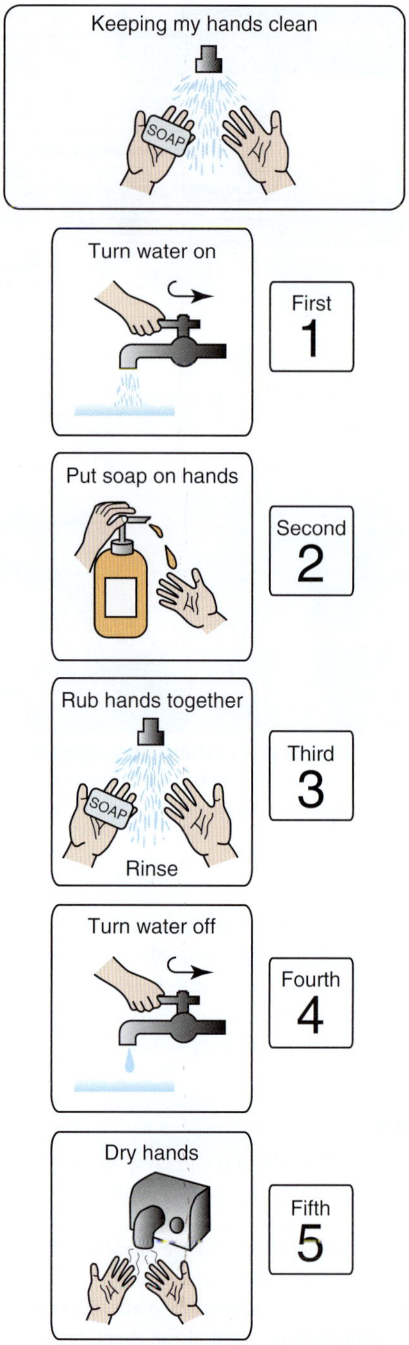


**Fig. 13.3** This simple picture sequence gives children the needed cues to wash their hands independently. (Courtesy Judith Schoonover, Loudoun County Public Schools, Virginia; Picture Communication Symbols from Mayer–Johnson, Solana Beach, CA.)

## ACTIVITIES OF DAILY LIVING—SPECIFIC INTERVENTION STRATEGIES AND APPROACHES

As described above, occupational therapy practitioners engage children in meaningful practice of whole ADLs within natural environments and using familiar objects. Evidence suggests supporting children's participation by adapting activities and expectations promotes self-determination and belongingness in the family. Practitioners use visual supports, coaching strategies, and child and parent training techniques to promote performance and participation in ADLs. The following are specific intervention strategies for dressing; bathing, and showering;

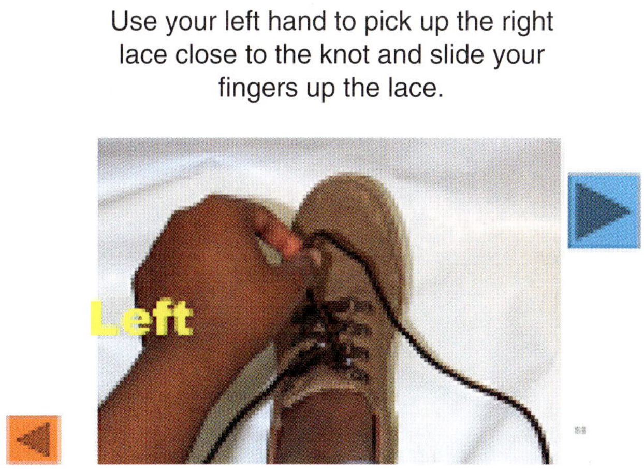


**Fig. 13.4** Point of view modeling to tie shoes. (Courtesy Laura Pal and Kelly Showalter, Virginia Commonwealth University.)

personal hygiene and grooming; and toileting, toilet hygiene, and bowel and bladder management.

## Dressing

Clothing is connected to social, cultural, and religious values and beliefs. Occupational therapy practitioners are respectful of children and their family's beliefs regarding dressing and clothing. They assure privacy and ask permission from parents and child to engage the child in dressing/undressing. Understanding the family's routines and expectations is essential to the occupational therapy process. For example, practitioners ask parents or caregivers for permission before changing an infant's diaper. They should not assume all parents are comfortable with others changing their child.

Children with tactile sensitivity (such as children with sensory processing challenges or children with autism) may find certain clothing uncomfortable. Occupational therapy practitioners may identify aspects of clothing (such as seams, tags, textures, and fabrics) that may be uncomfortable. They may suggest removing tags or purchasing tagless and seamless clothing. They may recommend using clothing made of soft cotton or other natural fabrics, like bamboo, rather than stiff or rough textured clothing (such as jeans or acrylic). Children may be sensitive to the smell of clothing requiring parents to use an odorless or mild-smelling laundry detergent. Children may be sensitive to colors. For example, children may describe feeling nauseous when wearing certain colors.

Occupational therapy practitioners consider how and where the clothing provides tactile input to the body. Clothing that tends to move or "bunch up" may be more irritating. Clothing that binds unevenly, like elastic waistbands, may also be irritating. Compression garments, like bike shorts or compression tees, can be helpful under clothing to provide uniform pressure if needed.

Sensory sensitivity to clothing affects home routines. Allowing children to pick out their own clothing may support daily dressing. Some children are so sensitive to clothing that they refuse to get dressed or even wear clothes. The occupational therapy practitioner analyzes the child's challenges with dressing to create an intervention plan, which may include making clothing changes (based on the child's preferences, strengths, and challenges), establishing home routines (to support sequencing, timing, and choice), and training children and families (on cognitive, motor, or social aspects) of dressing.

Children who have difficulty with motor skills may have challenges with dressing and managing clothing. Clothing fit, donning, and doffing requirements, and performance patterns (e.g., routines and habits) can influence the child's choice of clothing and their ability to dress independently. Most clothing is designed for individuals in a standing position. For those who spend long hours sitting (e.g., in a wheelchair), the sitting position causes pulling and straining on areas of the garment and a surplus of fabric in others. Alterations to the clothing can allow for more comfort in sitting. For example, designers who create adapted clothing may design pants that are higher in the back and lower in the front, or larger to give additional room in the hips and thighs (Fatima & Paul, 2015). Since pockets in the back may cause shearing or skin breakdown with prolonged sitting, they may place pockets on the top of the thigh or the side of the calf for easy access. Front and side seams can include hook and loop fasteners zippers, or loops to assist in donning (Fig. 13.5A–C). Similarly, clothing may be adapted or modified to promote ease of care when children require gastrostomy feedings, tracheostomy care, catheterization, or diapering. Caregivers can sew moisture-resistant fabric into the seat of pants, on collars, on attaching bibs, and on sleeve cuffs (if the child bites clothing) or can consider using stretch fabrics that dry quickly (Fatima & Paul, 2015). Many clothing adaptations are now available commercially. Manufactures are beginning to offer attractive fashionable clothing that meets functional requirements and conforms to the child's peer group standards and fashion trends.

Bras can be particularly challenging for individuals with sensory or motor limitations. Most bras include hook and eye closures, requiring coordinated fine motor use of both hands to hold and hook the bra together, either in the front or in the back. Front closures may be easier but still require significant bilateral dexterity. Some bras use snaps or magnetic closures. Pullover bras eliminate the manual dexterity required for the closures; however, they often require an adequate range of motion and strength to pull over the head and down to adjust the cups.

A variety of adaptive equipment is available to assist with dressing (such as long-handled shoehorns, reachers, and button hooks). The Bra Angel Dressing Aid (designed by an occupational therapist) helps a client put on a bra. The device is placed over the neck, hanging down to the chest, and holds one end of the straps in place so that the user can bring the other end together to fasten it.

## Bathing or Showering

Occupational therapy practitioners work with caregivers to support both client and caregiver comfort and safety with bathing and showering. Adaptive positioning or special equipment may provide support that helps the child feel safe and secure while bathing. Bath hammocks, support rings, bath seats, and shower benches hold the body fully and enable the caregiver to wash the child thoroughly (Fig. 13.6A). A light inconspicuous bath support offers design features well adapted to the needs of children with motor deficits (Fig. 13.6B). The front half of the support ring swings open for easy entry and then locks securely, holding the child at the chest to give trunk stability. Various types of bath seats and shower benches (Fig. 13.6C) are available to assist children in bathtub seating and transfers. For a child with severe motor limitations who lies supine in the tub in shallow water, a horseshoe-shaped inflatable bath collar (Fig. 13.6D) supports the neck and keeps the child's head above water. A bath stretcher is constructed like a cot and fits inside the bathtub at the rim or midtub level to minimize the caregiver's bending while transferring and bathing the child. Home modifications such as roll in shower stalls or built-in bath benches increase independence and/or protect the caregiver's back.

Caregivers and children's education about bathing safety helps prevent injury. Constant monitoring until the child demonstrates safety in the tub is necessary, even if using supported adaptive equipment. A study found that caregivers who believed their child was safe and well supported left the child unsupervised in the bathtub briefly, even

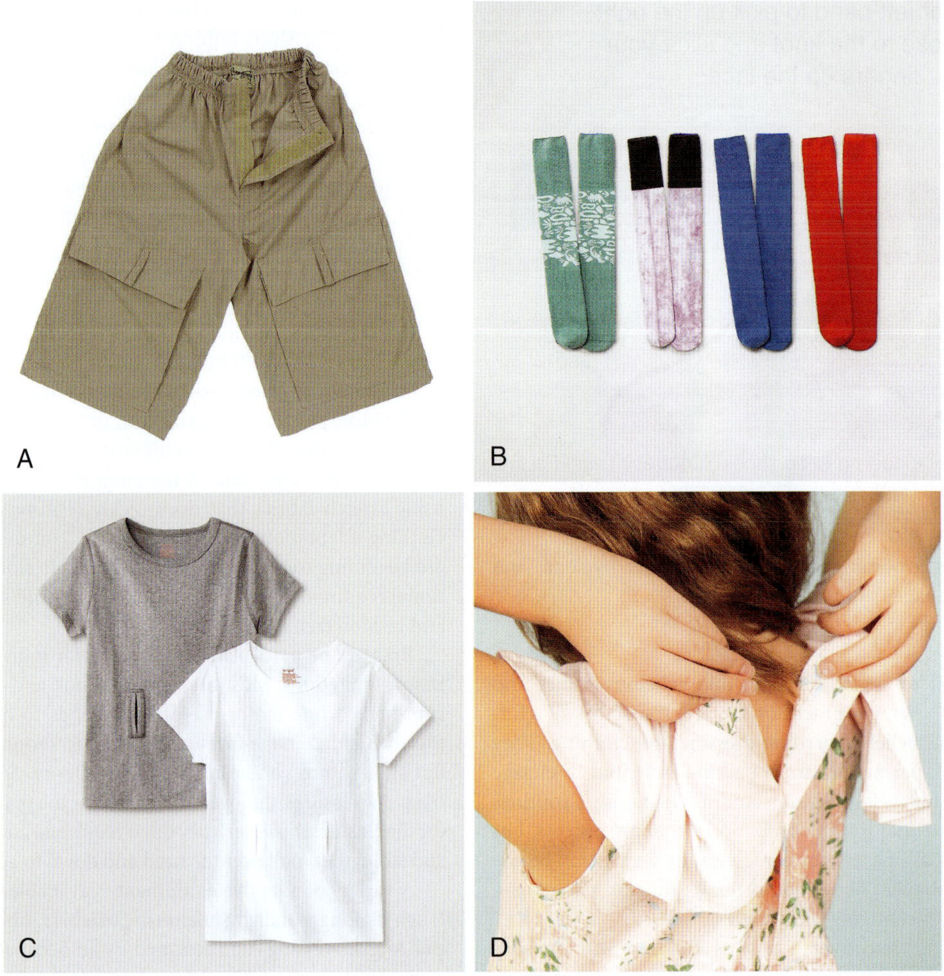


**Fig. 13.5** (A) Shorts with easy access, an elasticized waistband, and a Velcro fly with a finger loop allow children to manage clothing. From easy access clothing at https://easyaccessclothing.com/collections/clothing-for-disabled-children/products/childrens-cargo-shorts?variant=29503545081923). (B) Adaptive knee-high socks are soft, stretchy, with no-heel design. From Cat & Jack TM at https://www.target.com/c/kids-adaptive-clothing/sensory-friendly/-/N-1laueZ82xbj (C) Short sleeve undershirts with 0easy abdominal access, soft with no tags. From Cat & Jack at https://www.target.com/c/kids-adaptive-clothing/sensory-friendly/-/N–1laueZ82xbj). (D) Magnetic fasteners make it easy for children to put on and take off clothing. (From Magnetic Me clothing at: https://magneticme.com/products/2458_ainsl)

after indicating that they would never leave their child unattended (Snider-Riczker et al., 2005). Conversely, some caregivers do not teach independence in bathing because they worry that children may injure themselves if left alone. Following a safe routine for bathing, teaching the child what they are and are not allowed to do in the tub or shower, and grading the amount of assistance and monitoring helps develop independence. Nonslip bath mats beside and in the tub are essential for safety. Grab bars and their placement require careful thought and planning. A rubber cover for the bathtub faucet may prevent injury if the child touches it or slips and hits their head. Faucets should be marked (visually, or tactically for individuals who are blind) for temperature, and children can be directed to begin running their bath water by first putting on the cold water and then slowly adding hot water if they have adequate sensation.

The caregiver's positioning and handling are prime considerations when modifying the bathing of children. For example, children with neurological disorders may lose their balance when startled. Keeping the child's head and arms forward when lifting and lowering them into the tub prevents a reaction of full extension. The caregiver uses slow gentle movements with the child and provides simple verbal cues about the steps of bathing. Draining the tub and wrapping the child in a towel before lifting them from the tub allows the child to feel more secure.

Children who are hypersensitive to touch or temperature may avoid bathing and showers. Understanding the child's sensory needs and modifying techniques may help bathing become a more positive experience for the child and caregiver. Preparatory activities (e.g., deep pressure, visual support) before bathing may be helpful. The child may prefer a consistent routine, for instance insisting on always washing the back and extremities first, and then the stomach and face. Using rhythmic, organized, deep strokes for washing is often most accepted. Some caregivers and children find a hand-held shower with an eye guard hat useful to avoid getting soap in the eyes. Adjusting the water flow or temperature of the handheld shower and allowing the child to operate it gives the child more control over the direction and water pressure on their body. Alternately, using a cup with water may be a preferable way to rinse off than a shower spray. Wrapping the child in a tight towel after bathing and holding the child with deep pressure can help with the transition out of the tub.

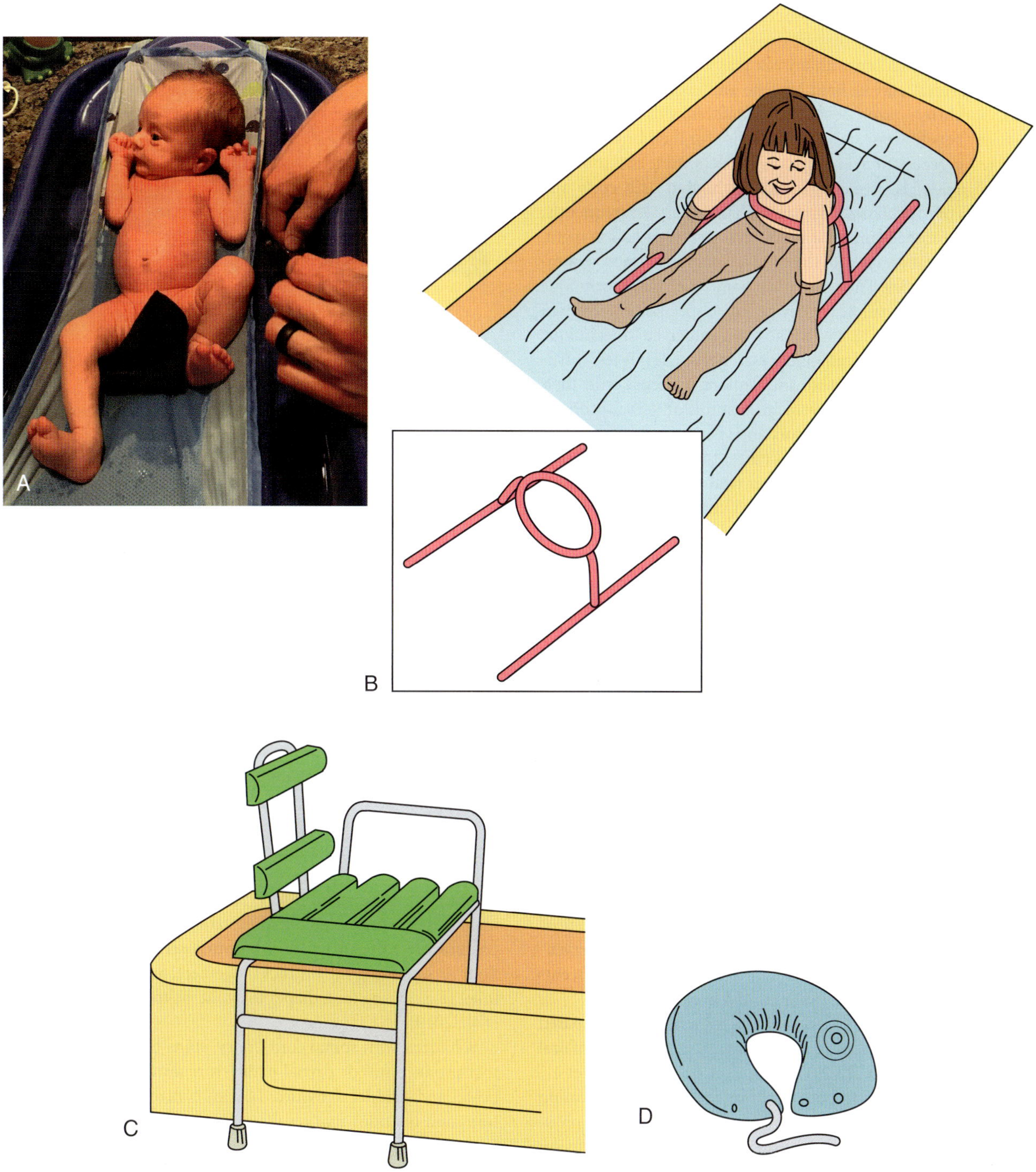


**Fig. 13.6** (A-D) adapted seating equipment for bathing. (A) The hammock chair is adjustable and equipped with oversized suction cups. (B) A trunk support ring is lightweight and compact and fits all bathtubs. (C) A shower bench aids seating and transfers. (D) An inflatable bath collar can be used when the child is in either the supine or the prone position.

Bathing may also be used therapeutically to improve body capabilities that interfere with independence. A warm bath may calm a distressed child, decrease muscle tonicity, and increase range of motion and independent movement. Caregivers may purposefully schedule bath times to promote relaxation before bedtime (Coutinho et al., 2016); or to help wake up a child before school. The occupational therapy practitioner needs to reinforce this positive behavior and work to understand the reasoning for the family's decisions.

## Personal Hygiene and Grooming

Personal hygiene and grooming are important to self-care, but also to health management, social participation, and work. An occupational therapy practitioner may collaborate with the client and caregivers to modify or adapt the environment, method, task, or tools used based on client factors and performance skills. For example, for brushing teeth, a small, soft brush is easier to move around in the mouth for younger children or children who have a tongue thrust or gag reflex. Children may accept a water flosser or battery-operated toothbrush rather than a standard toothbrush and it may be easier for children with limited dexterity to handle. Children with a weak grasp may use an enlarged handle or a universal cuff to hold hygiene and groom devices (e.g., washcloth, toothbrush, razor, deodorant). Children with limited range of motion may benefit from an extended device for their brush, comb, or hair pick. An occupational analysis helps determine the routines, methods, and materials used. For instance, children with curly and coiled hair types of African descent may wash their hair less frequently, use oils and wide toothed combs or picks, and wrap their hair at night. The practitioner collaborates with the child and family to teach grooming and hygiene activities. They may use a hand-over-hand technique to teach the child how to handle the devices when specificity is required (such as brushing teeth in Fig. 13.7). The hand-under-hand technique is effective for children with deaf blindness or autism as it is less intrusive and allows the child to initiate and explore materials with their hands. As the child learns the movement, gestures or verbal prompts may be needed (Fig. 13.8A–D). Auditory and visual cues may motivate a child to engage in the activity; for instance, toothbrushes that play music may motivate a child to brush their teeth or brush for longer. The practitioner works with the parent and child to develop a routine sequence and determine the supports needed (e.g., visual pictures, physical cues, verbal directions). As the child progresses, the caregiver provides fewer cues.

Personal hygiene and grooming activities can be particularly challenging for individuals with sensory sensitivities. Occupational therapy practitioners collaborate with the child and caregivers to educate them on the heightened sensory experiences in these activities and problem-solve alternatives. Allowing the child to select their materials, such as toothpaste flavor, hair products, soap, and deodorant, may help them manage their sensory experiences. Similarly, children should select their hair care, haircuts, and hair style.

With the onset of puberty, new self-maintenance activities emerge, including skin care, hair styling, hair removal, and application of cosmetics. It is important to collaborate with the client and caregivers to develop new routines and habits. Case Example 13.2 is an example of an adolescent who desires independence in grooming. Visual schedules and reminders (on phones or watches) may support routines. The occupational therapy practitioner uses approaches and evidence-based interventions discussed throughout this chapter to help children and adolescents learn how to complete these new grooming and hygiene tasks.

Children with disabilities have poorer oral hygiene when compared with their peers without disabilities, leading to a heightened risk of oral health problems (Joybell et al., 2015; Popple et al., 2016; Stein et al., 2012). Contributing factors to poor oral hygiene include medication effects, medical issues (e.g., gastric reflux), cognition, diet, and physical and sensory issues. Occupational therapy practitioners focus on prevention as management of dental disease in a dental clinic can be challenging for children with disabilities. They work with the child and caregivers to determine a plan of action and collaborate with other professionals, such as the dental clinician, to help them understand the relationship among sensory and motor issues, dental care, and dental health (Cermak et al., 2015; Kim et al., 2019; Kuhaneck & Chisholm, 2012).

## Toileting and Toilet Hygiene

Toileting is a complex activity requiring a thorough analysis of how activity demands, context, and the child's capabilities influence performance skills and patterns. Independence in toileting requires body functions (e.g., interoception, strength, range of motion), motor skills (e.g., postural stability, reach, bend, dexterity), and process skills (e.g., initiation, sequencing, memory of toileting steps). To begin to learn this task, a child must be physically (e.g., they have a pattern of urine and feces elimination) and psychologically ready. Caregivers also need to be ready to devote the time and effort needed to follow evidenced-based toilet training protocols (e.g., scheduled toileting sits and increasing fluid intake) (Gronski & Doherty, 2020). The occupational therapy practitioner considers cultural factors that may influence toileting. For example, some individuals use a bidet instead of toilet paper or require that only the left hand does wiping. While working with children and families on toileting routines, occupational therapy practitioners ask permission before touching a child while explaining what they are doing and why. In some cultures, it is inappropriate to work alone with someone of the opposite gender on ADLs that require visual inspection or touch of body parts (e.g., toileting, bathing, dressing) (Padela & Rodriguez del Pozo, 2011).

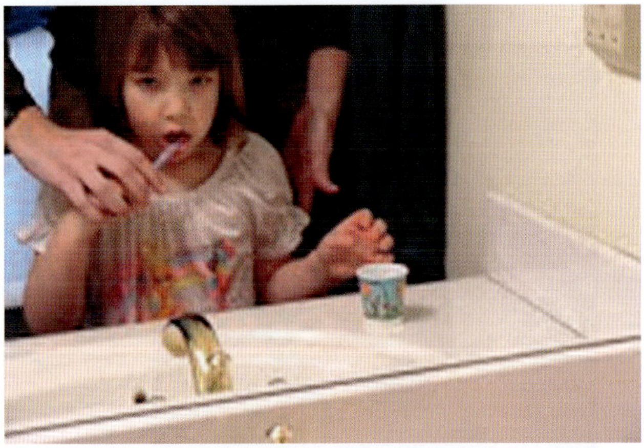

**Fig. 13.7** Brushing teeth with hand-over-hand assistance.

Occupational therapy practitioners examine and address factors that may impede progress in toileting independence. Beaudry-Bellefeuille et al. (2019) highlight the relationship between functional defecation issues and sensory reactivity and perception. Behaviors include defecation-related manifestations of pain, adapting a retentive posture (avoiding defecation by purposefully contracting the pelvic floor or squeezing the buttocks together), and avoiding the use of the toilet (e.g., asking for a diaper to avoid the toilet) (Beaudry-Bellefeuille et al., 2019).

Children with spinal cord injury, spina bifida, or other conditions that produce full or partial paralysis require special management for bowel and bladder activities. Loss of control over these bodily functions and the odor that results can cause embarrassment, reduce self-esteem, and limit social participation (Fischer et al., 2015). The type of bladder problem depends on the level and type of neurologic impairment. When the lesion is in the lumbar region or below, the reflex arc is no longer intact, and the bladder is flaccid (lower motor neuron bladder). When the lesion is above the level of bladder innervation, the result is an automatic bladder (upper motor neuron bladder). The child undertakes training programs to develop an automatic response for the upper motor neuron bladder. In children with a flaccid bladder, training will be ineffective because the bladder has insufficient tone and requires assistance in emptying.

The occupational therapy practitioner works with physicians and nurses to determine bladder training and management programs after medical testing and has collaborative discussions with children and their caregivers. Four main methods are used to manage urine: (1) condom catheterization (for use with a penis), (2) indwelling catheters, (3) intermittent catheterization (every 4–6 h), and (4) ileal conduits.

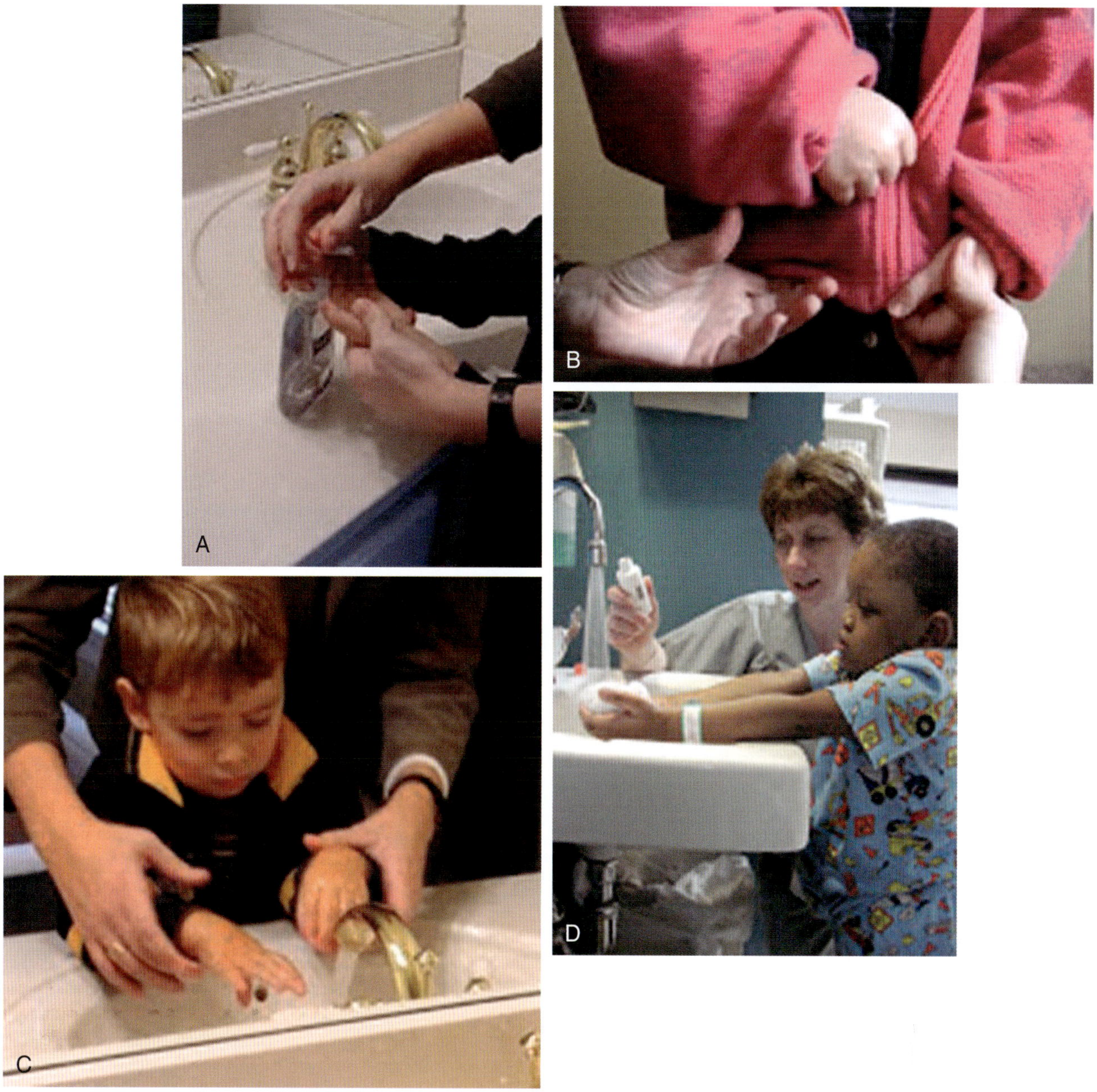


**Fig. 13.8** (A) Hand-over-hand approach is used to help children squirt soap onto their hands. (B) Two fingers are used to guide the zipping of the child's coat. (C) The occupational therapy practitioner shadows her hand over the top of the child's hands to cue hand movements for hand washing. (D) The practitioner verbally cues the child on how to wash their hands.

Children can learn to do their own intermittent catheterization as early as 6 years old if they have the performance skills (e.g., motivation, dexterity), visual perceptual skills, and learning supports.

Children with congenital or acquired neurologic disorders often undergo catheterization or bowel programs. Compared with the toileting practices of their peers, these additional bowel and bladder tasks require more time, established routines, and higher cognitive functions to plan, organize, and remember to perform the procedure (Tarazi et al., 2007). In addition, children may have difficulty in any of the following areas: maintaining a stable yet practical position; hand dexterity (praxis and speed); perceptual awareness; strength, range of motion, and stability; and accuracy in emptying collection devices. Children need memory, safety, and sensory awareness to complete many of these procedures. Although nurses often teach bowel and bladder control methods, the occupational therapy practitioner helps establish the necessary fine motor skills, adapts the context by providing assistive devices, positioning, environmental changes, or adapted methods, and/or establishes a routine that becomes habitual and easy for the child that helps prevent future infections or embarrassment.

A basic principle for success in bowel reeducation for individuals with neurologic disorders is to have a regular and consistent evacuation of the bowel. Bowel program timing is a matter of choice, but it requires a consistent schedule. In some cases, the child receives suppositories and a warm drink before evacuation. This stimulates the contraction and relaxation of muscle fibers in the walls of the intestine, moving the contents onward. Other techniques include digital

## CASE EXAMPLE 13.2 JOSIE: GROOMING INDEPENDENCE

Josie is a 12-year-old girl who demonstrates incoordination, poor memory, and limited judgment, but she wants to be independent in her grooming. Josie has worked on improving her coordination so that she can brush her hair or manipulate the grooming materials, but adaptation strategies are essential to increase her independence in grooming.

The occupational therapy practitioner recommends that Josie uses a brush with a built-up handle, rests her elbow on the table while brushing her hair to stabilize her ataxic movements, uses a checklist and visual model, and finds several simple hairstyles that Josie likes and can complete. They explore a variety of makeup that is easier to manipulate (https://glowsly.com/makeup-products/best-accessible-beauty-products/#tips), and together, they make decisions on how Josie applies it for a daily look. The practitioner provides directions on the application of makeup and lip gloss. Together, they create a grooming and makeup routine. Josie and her parents are educated about ways to incorporate grooming tasks into everyday routines by placing visual and natural cues in the environment, such as keeping the deodorant on the dresser. Leaving facial cleansing equipment out on the sink gives Josie a visual cue to use before applying makeup. These strategies allow Josie to engage in her grooming with minimal support.

stimulation, massage around the anal sphincter, and manual pressure on the abdomen. Occasionally, removal of the stool by hand or by a colostomy is recommended. As with an ileostomy, colostomy collection bags are emptied and cleaned regularly, and the child is taught to do this independently as soon as possible.

Closely associated with bowel and bladder care is perianal skin care. The skin is cleansed thoroughly to protect the tissue against the effects of contact with waste matter and eliminate odor. All children with decreased sensation are susceptible to decubitus ulcers, pressure sores that develop rapidly when blood vessels are compressed (e.g., around a bony prominence, such as the ischial tuberosity). Daily inspection of the buttocks with a long-handled mirror is needed.

Of all ADLs, toileting requires the most sensitive approach on the part of those who work with the child on a self-maintenance program. Children may purposely restrict their fluid intake at school to avoid the need for elimination. Unfortunately, limited fluid intake promotes infections, which increases the difficulty of regulating the bowel and bladder. Occupational therapy practitioners may work with families, teachers, nurses, and paraprofessionals to evaluate the social environment and find the best place, time, and routine for the child.

The bathroom is often the most inaccessible room, yet every person must have access to it. The floor space and object clearance may be insufficient to allow the child to turn a wheelchair for a toilet transfer. The location and height of the sink, faucets, towels, soap, and toilet paper may make them inaccessible to young children. In home and public bathrooms, the sensory aspects of the environment may overwhelm some children. Bathroom odors (e.g., air freshener, perfumed toilet paper or soap, stool odor) and auditory aspects (e.g., automatic flush toilets, defecating, hand dryers, fans; touch or coolness of the toilet seat or washing hands) may restrict participation for children who demonstrate heightened responses to sensory stimuli (Schaaf et al., 2011). Therefore, the bathroom's space, equipment, and objects may need to be adapted or modified. Review Table 13.1 for other toileting analyses and adaptations.

Numerous adaptations are available to assist the child in positioning and maintaining cleanliness after toileting. Occupational therapy practitioners may provide a variety of assistive devices for toileting. Some examples include: hand held urinals, catheters, leg bag clamps, long-handled mirrors, positioning devices to provide postural stability or hold the legs open, and universal cuffs with a catheter or digital stimulator attached. For children with good postural control but limited range of motion or grasp, simple and inexpensive aids include toilet paper tongs and toilet paper–holding devices. A combined bidet and toilet offer a means of total independence (Fig. 13.9). Various toilet seats or chairs and special cushions designed to prevent tissue trauma are available commercially.

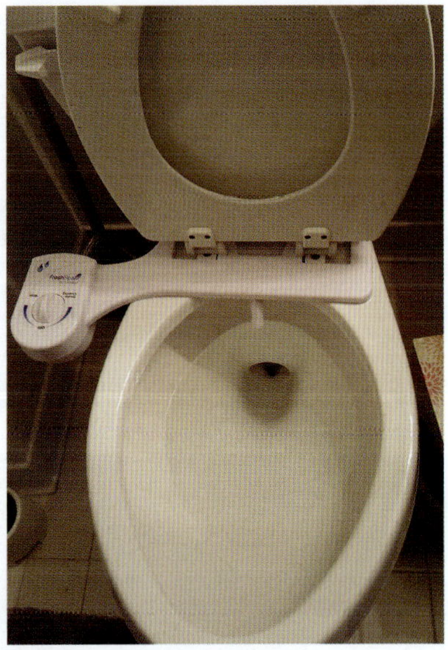

**Fig. 13.9** Electrically powered bidet makes it possible to clean the perianal area independently, without using hands or paper.

The type of clothing worn during toileting may hinder the child's independence or the caregiver's ability to promote independence. Tight stretch garments are often recommended to help with postural control or sensory needs, but these may result in problems with toileting independence or incontinence. For children who wear diapers, a full-length crotch opening with a zipper or hook and loop (e.g., Velcro) closure makes changes easier. When children are first learning toilet training, the use of elastic-waisted diapers that pull up and down gives them the opportunity to practice this part of the toileting sequence while protecting clothing from accidents. As children mature, they may be responsible for changing their own diapers or caring for their appliances and equipment.

When children sit on the toilet, they need postural security. When toilet seats are low enough that the feet rest firmly on the floor, the abdominal muscles that aid in defecation effectively fulfill their function. Reducer rings are used for small children to decrease the size of the toilet seat opening and thus improve sitting support and eliminate fears of falling into the toilet. A stepstool placed in front of the toilet helps small children get on and off and have foot support. Safety rails that attach to the toilet or wall assist with balance or provide lateral support. For the child who has outgrown small training potties, freestanding commodes may be useful when wheelchair access to the bathroom is impossible. Commodes that feature such modifications as adjustable legs, safety bars, angled legs for stability, lifts, and padded, upholstered, and adjustable backrests and head rests are often helpful to caregivers. Commodes are also available with seat reducer rings, seat belts, and adjustable footrests.

Toilet training is often challenging for families with young children, particularly children with disabilities. The most effective interventions included caregiver education and training and caregiver-implemented interventions focused on teaching "positive reinforcement and rewards for in-toilet elimination, scheduled toileting sits, increased fluid intake during training, and the exclusion of punitive or negative language" (Gronski & Doherty, 2020, p. 5).

## SUMMARY

This chapter presents a wide range of options for promoting participation and enhancing performance in ADLs. Occupational therapy practitioners collaborate with children, caregivers, and other professionals to support children's ADL performance. They create interventions that meet the child's unique needs and are consistent with their cultural and family routines and beliefs.

1. Children's performance and participation in ADLs is the result of the interaction among a variety of factors, including client factors (characteristics of the child that include their beliefs, capacities, body functions, and body structures); personal factors (unique features of the child, such as race, living situation, disability status, age); and environmental factors (physical, social, and attitudinal spaces). Occupational therapy practitioners consider the unique family situation and daily routines; the child's strengths and challenges; environmental resources; and the activity demands when creating intervention plans to address ADL performance.
2. Occupational therapy practitioners create intervention plans to address a child's participation in ADLs. They evaluate the child's motor, cognitive, sensory, and social-emotional skills and abilities in addition to the environment, and family culture. They collaborate with children and families to identify meaningful ADLs and identify intervention strategies to address the goals. Current evidence indicates that the most effective interventions to support participation and performance in ADLs are occupation-based (i.e., focused on ADLs), incorporate client and caregiver training and education, are performed in natural contexts, and involve collaboration with the child and caregivers.
3. Occupational therapy intervention approaches to address ADLs may include those to develop skills and abilities (i.e., rehabilitate or remediation), create habits and routines (i.e., education), compensate for performance challenges (i.e., adaptations or modifications), and advocate (i.e., provide additional opportunities). Emerging evidence suggests visual supports and technology are beneficial to improving performance in ADLs. They may provide assistive technology or make modifications to how tasks are completed or may address routines to support participation and performance in ADLs.
4. Occupational therapy practitioners collaborate with children and their caregivers to address ADL participation. The practitioner seeks to understand the child and their family's beliefs, routines, and priorities to create meaningful intervention plans that will make a difference in their daily activities.

## ACKNOWLEDGMENT

Thank you to Tara Weinstein, OTD, OTR/L for her contributions to this chapter.

## REFERENCES


Akers, J. S., Higbee, T. S., Pollard, J. S., Pellegrino, A. J., & Gerencser, K. R. (2016). An evaluation of photographic activity schedules to increase independent playground skills in young children with autism. *Journal of Applied Behavior Analysis, 49*(4), 954–959. https://doi.org/10.1002/jaba.327.

Aldi, C., Crigler, A., Kates-McElrath, K., Long, B., Smith, H., Rehak, K., & Wilkinson, L. (2016). Examining the effects of video modeling and prompts to teach activities of daily living skills. *Behavior Analysis in Practice, 9*, 384–388. https://doi.org/10.1007/s40617-016-0127-y.

American Occupational Therapy Association. (2020). Occupational therapy practice framework: Domain and process-fourth edition. *American Journal of Occupational Therapy, 74*(Suppl. 2),7412410010.

Baker, T., Haines, S., Yost, J., DiClaudio, S., Braun, C., & Holt, S. (2012). The role of family-centered therapy when used with physical or occupational therapy in children with congenital or acquired disorders. *Physical Therapy Reviews, 17*(1), 29–36. https://doi.org/10.1179/1743288X11Y.0000000049.

Beaudry-Bellefeuille, I., Lane, S. J., & Lane, A. E. (2019). Sensory integration concerns in children with functional defecation disorders: A scoping review. *American Journal of Occupational Therapy, 73*(3), p1–p13. https://doi.org/10.5014/ajot.2019.030387.

Campbell, J. E., Morgan, M., Barnett, V., & Spreat, S. (2015). Handheld devices and video modeling to enhance the learning of self-help skills in adolescents with autism spectrum disorder. *OTJR: Occupation, Participation and Health, 32*, 95–100. https://doi.org/10.1177/1539449215570040.

Cermak, S. A., Duker, S. L. I., Williams, M. E., Dawson, M. E., Lane, C. J., & Politico, J. C. (2015). Sensory adapted dental environments to enhance oral care for children with autism spectrum disorders: A randomized controlled pilot study. *Journal of Autism and Developmental Disorders, 45*, 2876–2888. https://doi.org/10.1007/s10803-015-2450-5.

Costa, U. M., Brauchle, G., & Kennedy-Behr, A. (2017). Collaborative goal setting with and for children as part of therapeutic intervention. *Disability & Rehabilitation, 39*, 1589–1600. https://doi.org/10.1080/09638288.2016.1202334.

Coutinho, K., Pacheco, S., Rodriques, B., & de Moraes, J. (2016). Body hygiene of children with encephalopathy: A creative-sensible method for relatives. *Online Brazilian Journal of Nursing, 15*, 443–453. https://doi.org/10.17665/1676-4285.20165533.

Daud, A. Z. C., Judd, J., Yan, M., & Barnett, F. (2016). Issue in applying occupation-based intervention in clinical practice: A delphi study. *Procedia: Social and Behavioral Sciences, 222*, 272–282. https://doi.org/10.1016/j.sbspro.2016.05.158.

Fatima, N., & Paul, S. (2015). Assessment of clothing needs of physically challenged children. *International Journal of Multidisciplinary Approach & Studies, 2*, 78–82.

Fischer, N., Church, P., Lyons, J., & McPherson, A. C. (2015). A qualitative exploration of the experiences of children with spina bifida and their parents around incontinence and social participation. *Child: Care, Health and Development, 41*, 954–962. https://doi.org/10.1111/cch.12257.

Gardner, S. J., & Wolfe, P. S. (2015). Teaching students with developmental disabilities daily living skills using point-of-view modeling plus video prompting with error correction. *Focus on Autism and Other Developmental Disabilities, 30*, 195–207. https://doi.org/10.1177/1088357614547810.

Gray, C. (2015). *The new social story book, revised and expanded* (15th ed.). Future Horizons.

Gronski, M., & Doherty, M. (2020). Interventions within the scope of occupational therapy practice to improve activities of daily living, rest, and sleep for children ages 0–5 years and their families: A systematic review. *American Journal of Occupational Therapy, 74*, 7402180010. https://doi.org/10.5014/ajot.2020.039545.

Hong, E. R., Ganz, J. B., Mason, R., Morin, K., Davis, J. L., Ninci, J., Neely, L. C., Boles, M. B., & Gilliland, W. D. (2016). The effects of video modeling in teaching functional living skills to persons with ASD: A meta-analysis of single-case studies. *Research in Developmental Disabilities*, *57*, 158–169. https://doi.org/10.1016/j.ridd.2016.07.001.

Joybell, C., Krishnan, R., & Kumar, S. (2015). Comparison of two brushing methods-Fone's vs. modified bass method in visually impaired children using the Audio Tactile Performance (ATP) technique. *Journal of Clinical and Diagnostic Research*, *9*, 19–22.

Kilincaslan, A., Kocas, S., Bozkurt, S., Kaya, I., Derin, S., & Aydin, R. (2019). Daily living skills in children with autism spectrum disorder and intellectual disability: A comparative study from Turkey. *Research in Developmental Disabilities*, *85*, 187–196. https://doi.org/10.1016/j.ridd.2018.12.005.

Kim, G., Carrico, C., Ivey, C., & Wunsch, P. B. (2019). Impact of sensory adapted dental environment on children with developmental disabilities. *Special Care in Dentistry*, *39*, 180–187. https://doi.org/10.1111/scd.12360.

King, G. (2017). The role of the therapist in therapeutic change: How knowledge from mental health can inform pediatric rehabilitation. *Physical & Occupational Therapy in Pediatrics*, *37*, 121–138. https://doi.org/10.1080/01942638.2016.1185508.

Klinger, L. G., Klinger, M. R., Mussey, J. L., Thomas, S. P., & Powell, P. S. (2015). Correlates of middle adult outcome: A follow-up study of children diagnosed with ASD from 1970–1999. In *International Society for Autism Research*. https://imfar.confex.com/imfar/2015/webprogram/Paper20033.html.

Kreider, C. M., Bendixen, R. M., Huang, Y. Y., & Lim, Y. (2014). Centennial Vision—review of occupational therapy intervention research in the practice area of children and youth 2009–2013. *American Journal of Occupational Therapy*, *68*, e61–e73. https://doi.org/10.5014/ajot.2014.011114.

Kuhaneck, H. M., & Chisholm, E. C. (2012). Improving dental visits for individuals with autism spectrum disorders through an understanding of sensory processing. *Special Care in Dentistry*, *32*(6), 229–233. https://doi.org/10.1111/j.1754-4505.2012.00283.x. PMID: 23095065.

Laverdure, P., & Beisbier, S. (2021). Occupation- and activity-based interventions to improve performance of activities of daily living, play, and leisure for children and youth ages 5 to 21: A systematic review. *American Journal of Occupational Therapy*, *75*, 7501205050. https://doi.org/10.5014/ajot.2021.039560.

Lequia, J., Machalicek, W., & Rispoli, M. J. (2012). Effects of activity schedules on challenging behavior exhibited in children with autism spectrum disorders: A systematic review. *Research in Autism Spectrum Disorders*, 6(1), 480–492. https://doi.org/10.1016/j.rasd.

Novak, I., & Honan, I. (2019). Effectiveness of paediatric occupational therapy for children with disabilities: A systematic review. *Australian Occupational Therapy Journal*, *66*, 258–273. https://doi.org/10.1111/1440-1630.12573.

Padela, A., & Rodriguez del Pozo, P. (2011). Muslim patients and cross-gender interactions in medicine: An Islamic bioethical perspective. *Journal of Medical Ethics*, *37*, 40–44. https://doi.org/10.1136/jme.2010.037614.

Phipps, S., & Roberts, P. (2012). Predicting the effects of cerebral palsy severity on self-care, mobility, and social function. *American Journal of Occupational Therapy*, *66*, 422–429. https://doi.org/10.5014/ajot.2012.003921.

Piccin, S., Crippa, A., Nobile, M., Hardan, A. Y., & Brambilla, P. (2017). Video modeling for the development of personal hygiene skills in youth with autism spectrum disorder. *Epidemiology and Psychiatric Sciences*, *27*, 127–132. https://doi.org/10.1017/S2045796017000610.

Popple, B., Wall, C., Flink, L., Powell, K., Discepolo, K., Keck, D., Mademtzi, M., Volkmar, F., & Shic, F. (2016). Brief report: Remotely delivered video modeling for improving oral hygiene in children with ASD: A pilot study. *Journal of Autism and Developmental Disabilities*, *46*, 2791–2796. https://doi.org/10.1007/s10803-016-2795-4.

Schaaf, R. C., Toth-Cohen, S., Johnson, S. L., Outten, G., & Benevides, T. W. (2011). The everyday routines of families of children with autism: Examining the impact of sensory processing difficulties on the family. *Autism*, *15*, 373–389. https://doi.org/10.1177/1362361310386505.

Shepherd, J., & Hanft, B. (2016). Teamwork verses the lone ranger. In B. Hanft, & J. Shepherd (Eds.), *Collaborating for student success: A guide for school-based occupational therapy* (2nd ed.) (pp. 107–146). AOTA Press.

Snider-Riczker, P., Ryan, S., Campbell, K., & Bortolussi, J. (2005). Adaptive seating for young children: Parents' perceptions of injury risk in the bathtub. *Technology and Disability*, *17*, 165–171.

Spriggs, A. D., Mims, P. J., van Dijk, W., & Knight, V. F. (2017). Examination of the evidence base for using visual activity schedules with students with intellectual disability. *The Journal of Special Education*, *51*, 14–26. https://doi.org/10.1177/0022466916658483.

Stein, L. I., Polido, J. C., & Cermak, S. A. (2012). Brief report—oral care and sensory concerns in autism. *American Journal of Occupational Therapy*, *66*, e73–e76. https://doi.org/10.5014/ajot.2012.004085.

Tarazi, R. A., Mahone, E. M., & Zabel, T. A. (2007). Self-care independence in children with neurological disorders: An interactional model of adaptive demands and executive dysfunction. *Rehabilitation Psychology*, *52*, 196–205. https://doi.org/10.1037/0090-5550.52.2.196.

Wheeler, M. (2007). *Toilet training for individuals with autism and other developmental disabilities* (2nd ed.). Future Horizons.

Zapata-Figueroa, V., & Ortiz-Corredor, F. (2022). Assessment of manual abilities using the box and block test in children with bilateral cerebral palsy. *Occupational Therapy International*, *2022*. :9980523. https://doi.org/10.1155/2022/9980523.

14

# Interventions for Instrumental Activities of Daily Living

*Theresa Carlson Carroll, Ashley Stoffel, and Vivian Villegas*

## GUIDING QUESTIONS

1. What are common types of instrumental activities of daily living (IADLs) that are expected of children and adolescents?
2. How do performance and participation in IADLs contribute to the positive skill development of children and adolescents?
3. What are common types of intervention approaches that an occupational therapy practitioner uses to improve children's IADL performance and participation?

## KEY TERMS

**Cognitive orientation to daily occupational performance (CO-OP)**
**Environmental factors**
**Instrumental activities of daily living**
**Learned helplessness**
**Natural environment**
**Occupational performance coaching**
**Person factors**
**Self-determination**
**Technology supports**
**Visual supports**

## DEFINING INSTRUMENTAL ACTIVITIES OF DAILY LIVING

According to the Occupational Therapy Practice Framework, fourth edition (OTPF-4) (AOTA, 2020), **instrumental activities of daily living (IADLs)** support daily life within the home and community and are generally considered to require more complex interactions than activities of daily living (ADLs). These activities include care of others, care of pets and animals, child rearing, communication management, driving and community mobility, financial management, home establishment and management (e.g., clothing care, cleaning), meal preparation and cleanup, religious and spiritual expression, safety and emergency maintenance, and shopping.

Children and youth who are referred to occupational therapy services often experience IADL performance and participation challenges. As part of interprofessional teams, occupational therapy practitioners have the expertise to partner with children, adolescents, and families in enabling IADL performance and participation as it contributes to positive skill development.

The authors define IADLs and discuss how children and youth learn to perform and participate in IADLs. They outline key factors that influence a child's or adolescent's IADL performance and participation and provide intervention approaches. Case vignettes illustrate intervention approaches that occupational therapy practitioners use to promote IADL performance and participation for children and youth.

## INFLUENCE OF CONTEXT ON INSTRUMENTAL ACTIVITIES OF DAILY LIVING PERFORMANCE AND PARTICIPATION

A complex host of factors can support or hinder a child's IADL performance and participation. Children and youth participate in IADLs in a variety of home, school, and community settings. For example, parents can encourage young children to participate in IADLs such as assisting with laundry and putting away clothing. Successful participation in this home management IADL can support the development of the child's motor, process, and social interaction skills (e.g., taking turns, motor planning to fold the laundry or match the clothing and engagement in social exchanges) and also promotes the child's self-efficacy and contributes to the child's feelings of confidence and pride in contributing to household tasks. Providing opportunities for children and youth to participate in IADLs can lead to skill development for future IADL performance and participation. The child's age, developmental skills, and family expectations are important considerations for IADL performance and participation. See Fig. 14.1A through D for illustrations of children's involvement in IADLs.

Context includes environmental and personal factors that impact participation in occupations (AOTA, 2020) and influence access to occupations and quality and satisfaction of performance (WHO, 2008). Personal factors that impact IADL performance and participation include those of the child, youth, and family members. Children and caregivers each have abilities and preferences that can influence a child's IADL performance and satisfaction with participation. Caregiver beliefs, expectations, and habits regarding IADLs can influence the child's performance and participation. For example, a caregiver might have certain expectations for their child's participation in home management or meal preparation and cleanup activities based on that caregiver's experiences growing up. Children of parents who provide encouragement and support for IADL participation are more likely to participate in these activities with other adults (Hammond & Carpendale, 2015). Some families may value play and engagement in extracurricular activities more than participation in household chores or meal preparation, while in other families it may be essential for children to participate in household maintenance tasks. Occupational

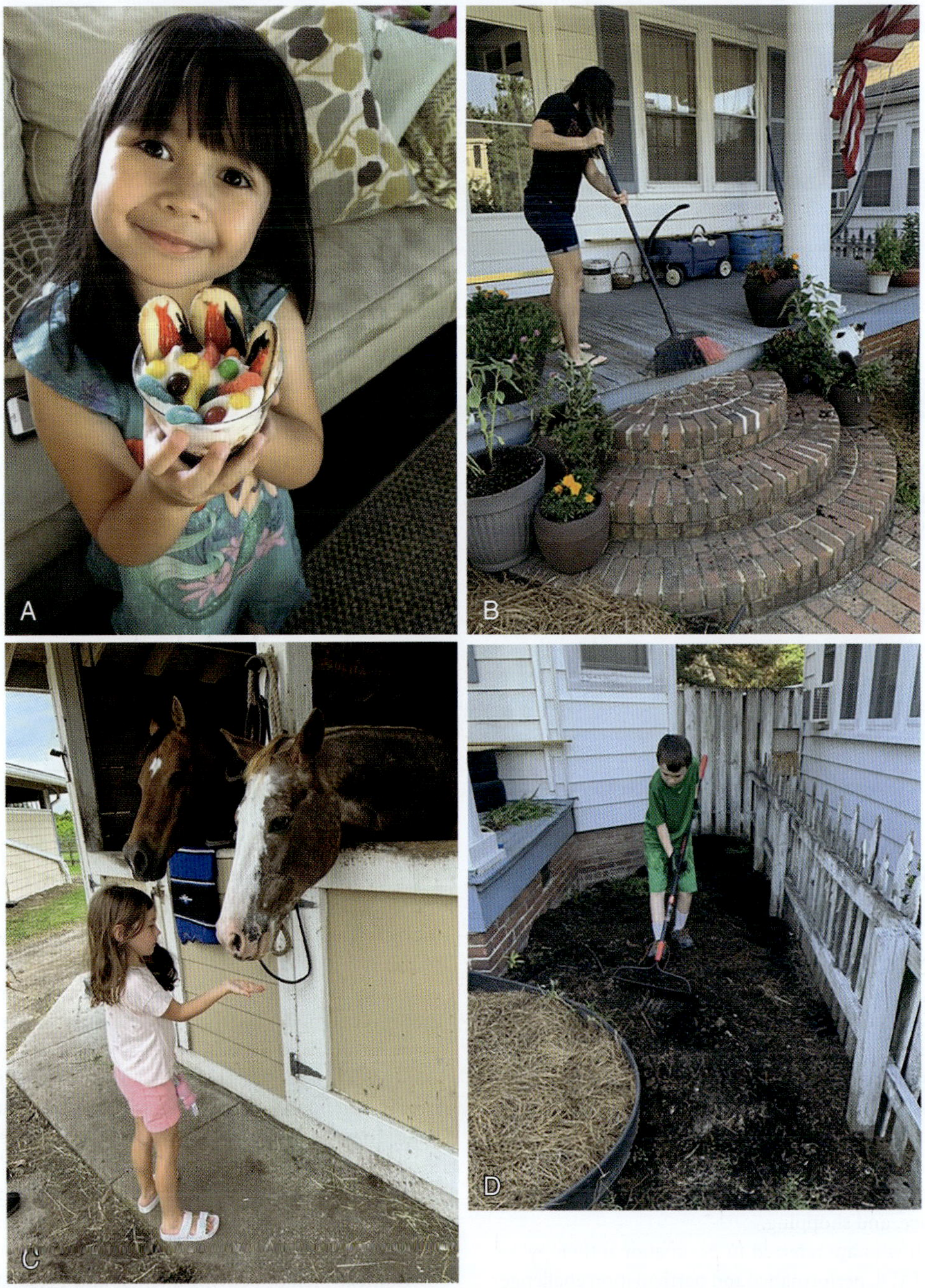

Fig. 14.1 (A–D) Children engage in tasks associated with IADLs. (A) This young girl enjoys making her own dessert (meal preparation). (B) This young girl helps manage the home by sweeping the porch. (C) This young girl feeds the horses as part of her IADLs. (D) A young boy attends to the yard work (home management).

therapy practitioners communicate with caregivers about their expectations and willingness to support IADL participation for their child or youth. In some cases, the practitioner may need to support the child or youth in advocating for their desire to be independent in an IADL activity if this is not congruent with family expectations.

The child's abilities also influence the IADLs that they are interested in and see as strengths, and their preferences may be influenced by the child's prior success with the IADL. While independent performance of some IADLs may not be expected until adolescence, even very young children demonstrate the ability to participate in IADLs. Increasing evidence (Berge et al., 2018; Davis et al., 2016; Hammond et al., 2017) supports the importance of addressing IADLs in young children to promote skill development, prosocial behaviors, and self-determination which are necessary for supporting a child's growth toward adulthood and independence (Angell et al., 2018; Dang et al., 2015; Shogren et al., 2015). Even young children demonstrate motivation to participate in IADL-related tasks, such as household chores, and children may be more motivated to participate in an actual task (e.g., washing dishes, setting the table) rather than imitating the task through play (Taggart et al., 2018). See Fig. 14.2A and B showing young children helping with chores. As children grow older, their opportunities to engage in IADLs increase and they become capable of greater independence. Participation and performance of IADLs are important, as they relate to outcomes in adolescence and adulthood. Research demonstrates that engagement in IADLs at younger ages is related to engagement and performance in adolescence and adulthood (Dang et al., 2015). As

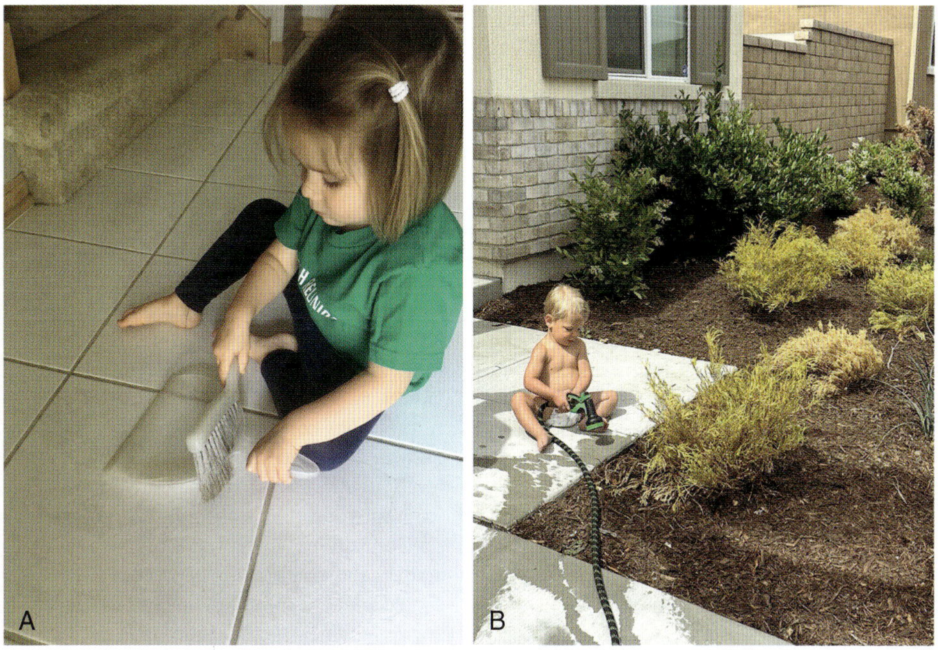

Fig. 14.2 Even young children can participate in IADLs, such as (A) sweeping the floor or (B) watering the lawn.

adolescents prepare to transition to adulthood, the ability to perform IADLs becomes important for independent living and work.

**Environmental factors** that influence IADL performance and participation include physical features (e.g., housing layout, physical items in the home), sensory features (e.g., noise and other stimuli), social relationships (e.g., supportive sibling), and attitudes of individuals who are present with and encourage the child (e.g., peer advocate) during IADL completion. Attitudes, systems, policies, and location can influence the occupation of IADLs. For example, in urban environments, parents may expect children and youth to demonstrate more independent community mobility such as walking in the community and using public transportation independently, than children and youth who live in suburban and rural environments. Children may need to be more independent with laundry and meal preparation if their parents work long hours or they might need to assist more with childcare of younger siblings.

## SELF-DETERMINATION

**Self-determination** is a "dispositional characteristic manifested as acting as the causal agent in one's life" (Shogren et al., 2015, p. 258). According to Causal Agency Theory, self-determined actions are volitional, self-directed, and linked to a belief that the individual can create change or achieve a goal (Shogren et al., 2015). Self-determination closely aligns with the domain and process of occupational therapy and develops from early childhood through adulthood. Component elements of self-determined action include making choices, expressing preferences, solving problems, making decisions, setting and attaining goals, self-managing and self-regulating action, self-advocating, and acquiring self-awareness and self-knowledge (Shogren et al., 2015). Many of these elements are key components of client-centered occupational therapy practice.

Foundations for self-determination begin in early childhood as children engage in activities at home, school, and in the community (Palmer et al., 2019). Young children can learn age-appropriate skills in problem-solving, choice-making, self-regulation, basic goal-setting, and decision-making. As children become older, they become able to demonstrate more complex self-determination skills. Self-determination plays a critical role in independent living outcomes into adulthood. Youth with disabilities who demonstrate greater self-determination skills in high school are more likely to be employed and engaged in the community as adults (Shogren et al., 2015).

Instrumental activities of daily living are closely related to self-determination. IADLs are complex and require component elements of self-determined actions such as decision-making, problem-solving, self-regulation, and self-evaluation. Children of all ages can develop self-determination through participation in IADL. In the home, preschool children assist with many household tasks such as putting away their toys, making their beds, putting away their clothes, helping set the table, and preparing cold snacks (Rodger, 2006). These tasks provide opportunities for self-regulation, problem-solving, and decision-making to develop. For example, a young child who participates in meal preparation with an adult may have the opportunity to make choices about the food prepared for the meal, collaborate to solve problems during the process, and self-evaluate the results of the prepared food. As youth develop self-determination skills, they are often able to engage in more complex IADLs. Adolescents may become more independent with community mobility, which provides them with increased opportunities to make decisions about where to spend their time, solve problems encountered while driving or using public transportation, and self-regulate emotions if they get lost.

IADLs are highly individualized and influenced by environment and culture, providing opportunities for choice and decision-making. For example, there are a variety of ways to maintain a home, and young adults who take on more home maintenance responsibilities will have opportunities to decide on home décor, cleaning routines, and standards for organization and cleanliness. Through engagement in IADL, youth can develop self-determination skills that may generalize to other aspects of their lives, improving their independent living outcomes as adults (McPherson et al., 2018). For example, grocery shopping is an IADL that could be used as an intervention to facilitate the performance of self-determined actions such as decision-making, self-regulation, problem-solving, and goal-setting. Fig.14.3 shows a child making her own decisions while shopping. Engagement in IADLs can be both a result of self-determined actions and a means for developing self-determination.

When options and opportunities for the development of self-determination and engagement in IADL are severely limited or absent there is an increased risk of **learned helplessness** (which refers to a person's disbelief that they have the skills and abilities to perform or make choices for themselves) (Filippello et al., 2015). Learned helplessness occurs when actions repeatedly fail to produce results or when individuals are not afforded the opportunity to make repeated attempts with specific activities or tasks. Many children and adolescents with disabilities have decisions made for them or have developed a habit of deferring to others (Gomez et al., 2015; Sparks & Cote, 2012). Children and adolescents with various disabling conditions often have limited opportunities to engage in IADLs that involve self-determination, such as shopping for their clothes or preparing their meals. Adolescents in foster care often lack knowledge and experience with independent living, especially safety and home and health maintenance (Olson et al., 2017; Radey et al., 2016). Children and adolescents with cognitive/behavioral disorders such as traumatic brain injury (TBI), intellectual disability (ID), and autism spectrum disorder (ASD) often lack opportunities to engage in household tasks and community activities such as shopping (Bedell et al., 2005; Bedell et al., 2013; Hodgetts & Park, 2016; Larson, 2010; Law et al., 2013; Murphy et al., 2011). For at least the past 10 years, research has consistently shown that youth with Autism Spectrum Disorder, intellectual disability, and multiple disabilities show lower levels of self-determination compared with students in other disability groups and their non-disabled peers (Qian et al., 2022).

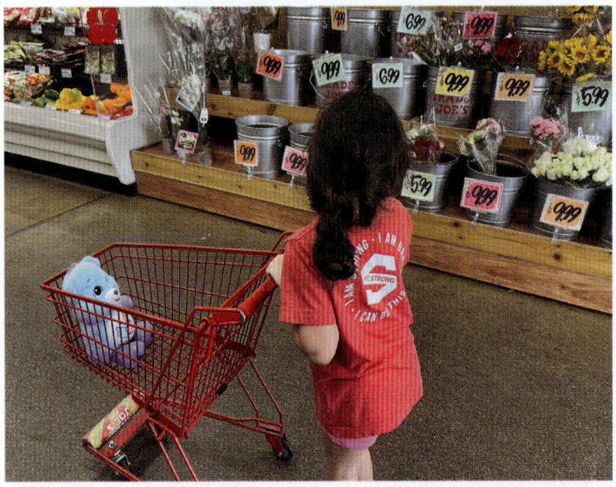

**Fig. 14.3** Engaging children in shopping provides opportunities to support decision-making and self-determination. This toddler is excited to pick out flowers and bring them home to decorate the house.

Occupational therapy practitioners are well suited to explore and address the relationship between IADL and self-determination and should advocate for expanding our role in this area. Occupational therapy practitioners should incorporate age-appropriate self-determination into their interventions with youth of all ages. See Fig. 14.4A and B show children engaged in activities to designed to promote self-determination. Providing opportunities for youth to make choices, coaching youth through problem-solving embedded in IADL, involving youth in goal setting, and designing interventions to foster self-regulation and self-awareness are all ways that occupational therapy practitioners can promote self-determination for youth. Evidence supports family involvement in interventions to support both self-determination and IADLs (Beisbier & Laverdure, 2020; Dean et al., 2021). Practitioners coach families on the importance of incorporating opportunities to develop self-determination into the family's environments and routines.

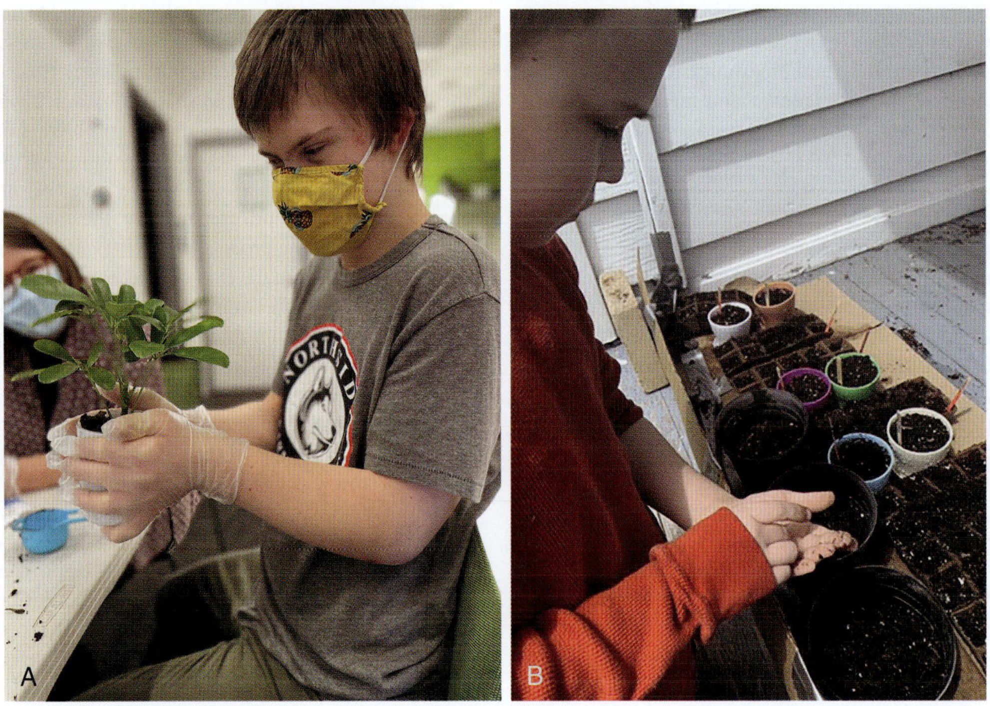



**Fig. 14.4** (A and B) Children learn to make choices and feel a sense of belonging, achievement, and self-determination while engaging in IADLs, such as gardening.

TABLE 14.1 **Occupational Therapy Intervention Approaches and Examples to Address IADLs**

| Intervention Approach (AOTA, 2020) | Example |
|---|---|
| Create, promote | • Create a vegetable "alien" as part of theme luncheon.<br>• Healthy cooking group to promote physical health of children and families at community center.<br>• Makeover your room (e.g., clean, decorate) in a new way.<br>• Plan to save money for something special (create a goal). |
| Establish, restore | • Use processing skills to sequence, time, and read directions to make a new recipe for breakfast.<br>• Improve a youth's grip strength after injury so they can effectively grasp utensils while cooking.<br>• Consult with a caregiver to establish a chore routine that supports caregiver's needs and provides opportunity for child to demonstrate responsibility and develop useful life skills.<br>• Engage children in pet care by establishing a schedule of tasks.<br>• Work on activity endurance by doing outside chores (e.g., raking lawn, picking up the yard, sweeping the porch) for 20 min a day. |
| Maintain | • Teach children to communicate to parents school tasks that they need to complete (and supplies they may need). Set up a system to have homework requirements each day.<br>• Instruct youth in using talk-to-text feature to maintain text and social media communication with peers after upper extremity injury.<br>• Enable families to maintain participation in religious activities by collaborating with them to identify strategies for autistic child's behavior during church service.<br>• Find inclusive community programs, such as parks, recreation centers, or spaces that are welcoming to all. |
| Modify | • Instruct adolescents how to use financial management app in lieu of balancing checkbook.<br>• Rearrange kitchen cabinets so that the materials needed for packing school lunches are accessible and organized for children.<br>• Put dog food in a smaller container so youth can pour food into dog bowl, rather than lifting the large bag. |
| Prevent | • Teach children and adolescents safety and emergency maintenance (as appropriate to their age).<br>• Practice basic safety and emergency preparedness.<br>• Create visual supports and provide instruction to youth with IDD on emergency procedures within the school environment (e.g., tornado drills, fire drills).<br>• Create an emergency kit. |

## INTERVENTION APPROACHES TO TARGET INSTRUMENTAL ACTIVITIES OF DAILY LIVING

IADLs can be a component of occupational therapy intervention as both a strategy for addressing underlying skills as well as an outcome of the intervention, meaning the performance of the IADL is the primary focus of the occupational therapy treatment. Occupational therapy practitioners may use a variety of intervention approaches that address IADLs or include IADLs as intervention activities. See Table 14.1 for a summary of intervention approaches from the OTPF-4 (AOTA, 2020) and sample IADL interventions for each approach.

Aligned with the AOTA's recommendations from the Choosing Wisely Initiative, OT practitioners should utilize purposeful, occupation-based interventions to enhance client motivation and outcomes (Gillen et al., 2019). Furthermore, research evidence supports the use of occupation and activity-based interventions to support occupational performance and participation in IADL for children and youth ages 5–21 (Beisbier & Laverdure, 2020; Laverdure et al., 2021). Interventions to address IADL for children and youth should be family-centered, delivered in the **natural environment** (i.e., the place and space that the child spends their time, such as home, school, community), when possible, individualized, and incorporated into the child's routines (Beisbier & Laverdure, 2020). Additionally, a study by McPherson et al. (2018) demonstrated the positive effects of a group IADL intervention for youth with disabilities. Following these evidence-based guidelines results in greater client motivation and better client outcomes.

Occupational therapy practitioners are not the only professionals who may address IADL skills for children and youth. However, occupational therapy practitioners can demonstrate distinct value by applying occupational therapy theory and practice models. They consider the interaction between the person, task, and environment to design meaningful and effective interventions. Some examples of intervention strategies that support occupational performance are described below.

### Occupational Performance Coaching

**Occupational Performance Coaching (OPC)** is a strengths-based approach that focuses on enabling children and parents to participate in occupations within the home and community (Graham et al., 2009). Dunn et al. (2017) identified four overall guiding principles of OPC:

1. Situation coaching in the client's everyday life;
2. Seek understanding by working collaboratively with others;
3. Foster the client's deep thinking about their own life; and
4. Explore resources with clients (Dunn et al., 2017).

While most often described as an intervention for young children and their caregivers, principles of occupational performance coaching may be applied to older children as well. Laverdure et al. (2021) identified caregiver coaching as an effective intervention for improving participation in household chores for children and youth. Occupational performance coaching and caregiver coaching strategies can improve engagement of various IADLs in the home, school, and community. Box 14.1 provides an example of the use of occupational performance coaching principles to address home management.

## BOX 14.1 Home Management

Mazy is a 3-year-old child with seizure disorder (controlled on medications) and developmental delays who lives with her 5-year-old sister and parents in a small apartment. While her parents realize that Mazy is only 3, they want to teach her to help around the house and follow a routine so they can enjoy time at home as well. Mazy's parents admit they have been reluctant to expect her to help at home and asked the occupational therapy practitioner for assistance.

The occupational therapy practitioner observed Mazy playing at home. When it was time to clean up her toys for dinner, Mazy became upset and threw the toys and kept playing. When her parents approached her, she said "no, I play." Mazy continued to play by herself and eventually went to the table to eat. She disrupted the family meal by demanding different foods and throwing things.

The occupational therapy practitioner used the guiding principles of Occupational Performance Coaching (OPC) (Dunn et al., 2017) to provide intervention to promote Mazy's participation in home management (routines and picking up toys).

| Guiding Principles OPC | Actions of Practitioner |
|---|---|
| Situation coaching in client's everyday life: | Provided simple strategies in real time. Focused on the main issues by setting firm but gentle limits and using clear verbal directions, "all done." practiced this with games and short wait times (to reinforce following directions in a way that Mazy could be successful). |
| Seek understanding by working collaboratively with family: | Showed parent strategies, asked them to try them (in real time), and asked for feedback (i.e., did they think they could follow through with it? What did they think of the strategies? What were their expectations). Asked them for suggestions of things that Mazy likes (for reinforcers). Each week provided time for them to reflect on the process and provide feedback to the practitioner. Adjusted strategies and techniques based on parent and family feedback. |
| Foster client's deep thinking about own life: | Reinforced parents' goals and the importance of Mazy being a member of the family. Supported family efforts and asked the sibling how she was doing. |
| Explore resources with client: | Provided tips and strategies each week. Together they found resources, such as using colorful bins for Mazy to drop all her toys in to make clean up faster. The therapist found an online support group of parents. She also provided information on the development of IADLs to show the parents the possible progression. |

### Visual Supports

**Visual supports** may include visual schedules, visual cues in the environment, and video modeling or prompting, such as the examples shown in Fig. 14.5A–C. Visual activity schedules have been found to improve the performance of life skills for children and adolescents with intellectual and developmental disabilities (Spriggs et al., 2017). Research evidence supports video modeling, an intervention that provides a video example of a task being performed to aid in teaching the task, for autistic individuals (Auld et al., 2022). Visual supports can be customized for a variety of IADL tasks and may be created using real life photos or icons. Box 14.2 provides an example of a visual schedule.

### Cognitive Orientation to Daily Occupational Performance to address Money Management

**Cognitive Orientation to Daily Occupational Performance (CO-OP)** is a client-centered, performance-based, problem-solving approach that enables skill acquisition through a process of guided discovery and strategy use (Polatajko & Mandich, 2005). See Chapter 26 for more information on the CO-OP approach. The CO-OP approach can be useful when clients identify the performance of an IADL as an intervention priority. The approach engages children in a process that includes "Goal, Plan, Do, Check," as shown in Fig. 14.6. CO-OP is likely an effective intervention for improving IADL task performance among adolescents with ASD (Weaver, 2015). Wilson and colleagues found that pairing CO-OP with concept mapping supported occupational engagement in IADL for youth with ASD and was motivating to the participants (Wilson et al., 2018). Box 14.3 provides an overview of a CO-OP intervention to address money management.

### Task and Environmental Modification

While addressing **person factors** (i.e., unique features of the person, such as age, race, ability status) and client factors (i.e., specific capacities, characteristics of beliefs, body functions and structures) (AOTA, 2020) such as strength or attention to task may result in improved participation in IADLs, modifying the IADL task(s) or the environmental context of the IADL may be equally, or more, effective. Context therapy, or therapy in which only the characteristics of the task and/or environment are addressed during intervention has been found to be equally effective as interventions in addressing personal factors for children with cerebral palsy (Darrah et al., 2011). Project TEAM, an intervention designed to teach youth with developmental disabilities to identify environmental barriers and supports to participation, generate solutions for barriers, and advocate for environmental changes that support participation, resulted in intervention participants achieving their participation goals and improving problem-solving and self-advocacy skills (Kramer et al., 2018). When addressing IADLs in intervention, modifying the way an IADL is completed, such as using a handheld vacuum for crumbs instead of sweeping the floor, or the environmental context of the IADL, such as rearranging kitchen cupboards so meal preparation materials are within reach, may be effective methods for improving IADL performance. Fig. 14.8A through C shows other ways to modify the task and environment to support children's engagement in meal preparation. Box 14.4 provides sample suggestions for task modifications.

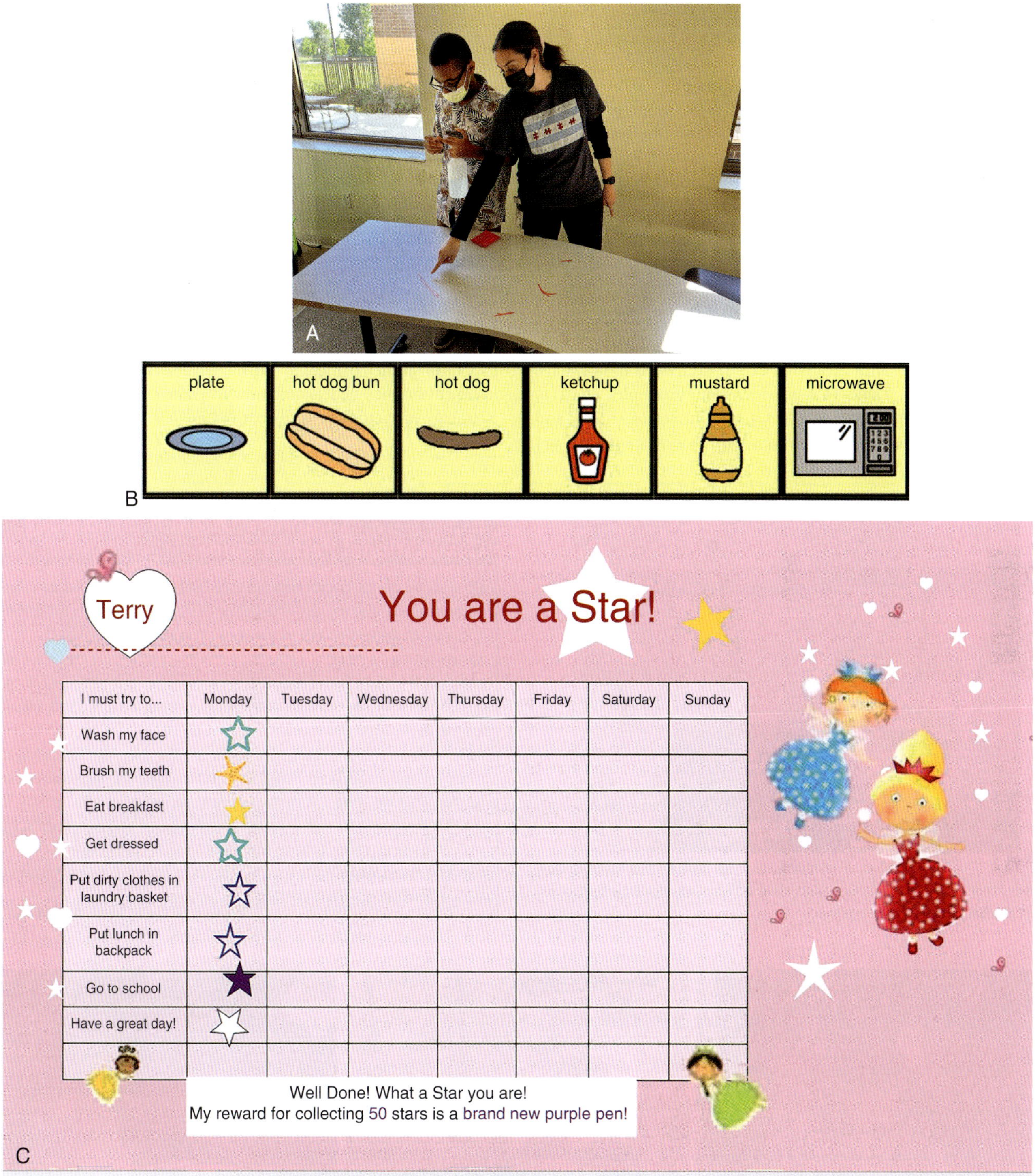
A
plate
hot dog bun
hot dog
ketchup
mustard
microwave
B
Terry
You are a Star!
I must try to...
Monday
Tuesday
Wednesday
Thursday
Friday
Saturday
Sunday
Wash my face
Brush my teeth
Eat breakfast
Get dressed
Put dirty clothes in laundry basket
Put lunch in backpack
Go to school
Have a great day!
Well Done! What a Star you are!
My reward for collecting 50 stars is a brand new purple pen!
C

**Fig. 14.5** (A) Visual environmental cues (such as the red tape on the table) can be useful when teaching children to complete tasks, such as cleaning marks on table. (B) Visual supports or schedules can be customized for a variety of IADL tasks and may be created using real-life photos or icons. (C) Visual schedules are best when tailored to the child.

> **BOX 14.2 Visual Supports**
>
> Visual schedules help children organize their routines, such as the morning schedule provided (See Fig. 14.5C). The child is more invested when they pick the design and select the reward for earning "stars." Parents can change the template weekly and the reward. It is important to have rewards that vary (for example, they should now always be food-related). Some children enjoy special time with their parents as a reward.

## Technology Supports

Technology is increasingly becoming a part of everyday life and can be an effective support for IADL participation. **Technology support refers** to the use of phones, laptops, computers, and other devices to support children and youth in participating in IADLs. Fig. 14.9 shows a teen using technology. For example, smartphones and other handheld devices can be used to provide reminders (e.g., a reminder to take medication or schedule a doctor's appointment) or to remember sequences or lists (e.g., grocery list, bus route). Mobile devices also are effective for video prompting during IADL tasks (e.g., meal preparation) for middle school students with intellectual disability (Shepley et al., 2018). Laverdure et al. (2021) identify technology-based interventions as being effective in improving participation in household chores for children and youth. Occupational therapy practitioners should consider using technology support in intervention, especially as technology advances and becomes more accessible for children and youth. Box 14.5 provides tips on using technology.

## ADDRESSING INSTRUMENTAL ACTIVITIES OF DAILY LIVING ACROSS PRACTICE SETTINGS

IADLs are a relevant intervention for children and adolescents across practice settings and, with creativity, can be addressed in hospitals, clinics, and schools. Table 14.2 provides some examples of IADL intervention across practice settings. Case Examples 14.1, 14.2, and 14.3 provide examples of IADL interventions. Evidence suggests that the best outcomes occur when IADLs can be addressed using occupation- and activity-based interventions within the natural environment, such as the home, grocery store, public transportation, or other community environment (Beisbier & Laverdure, 2020). However, when intervention cannot occur within the natural environment, occupational therapy practitioners can use strategies to increase the likelihood that skills will generalize, such as simulating the natural environment as much as possible, using materials that are familiar or the same as the child's materials and collaborating closely with the child's family member to identify strategies that will easily carry over at home or in the community. The purpose of IADLs may vary across settings. For example, in an inpatient setting, meal preparation may be an activity that motivates children to improve their strength after injury. In schools, adolescents preparing to graduate high school may have postsecondary goals to independently travel by public transportation so they can get to work independently. A toddler in early intervention may be learning how to gather the family's laundry as a strategy for getting proprioceptive and vestibular sensory input in the home.

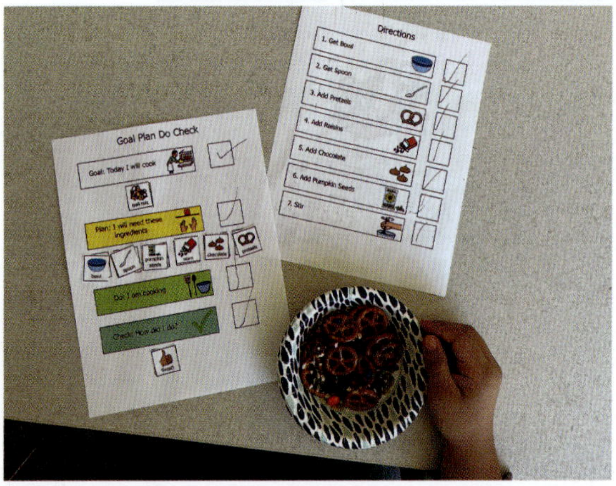

**Fig. 14.6** The child makes a pretzel snack as part of the intervention session using the CO-OP approach. The child uses strategies to organize his plan and sequence tasks.

### BOX 14.3 Cognitive Orientation to Daily Occupational Performance

Occupational therapy practitioners using the CO-OP approach involve the child in problem-solving, planning, and reflecting on their performance. This collaborative approach allows the child to learn the steps of the process (Goal, Plan, Do, Check) so they can internalize the process and use it in everyday life. For example, a teen may express a desire to eventually live on their own but have no experience managing their money. The occupational therapy practitioner and teen create a goal to learn to earn, budget, and spend money. They create goals (GOAL), identify strategies for making money (PLAN), earn money and spend it as budgeted (DO), and reflect on the process (Check). During the reflection phase, the child considers how his plan went and areas that were challenging, as well as areas of growth. The practitioner engages the teen in sessions to practice the skills necessary as they work through the process and they also discuss with his parents who support the teen's goals and reinforce the steps at home. See Chapter 26 for more details on the CO-OP model.

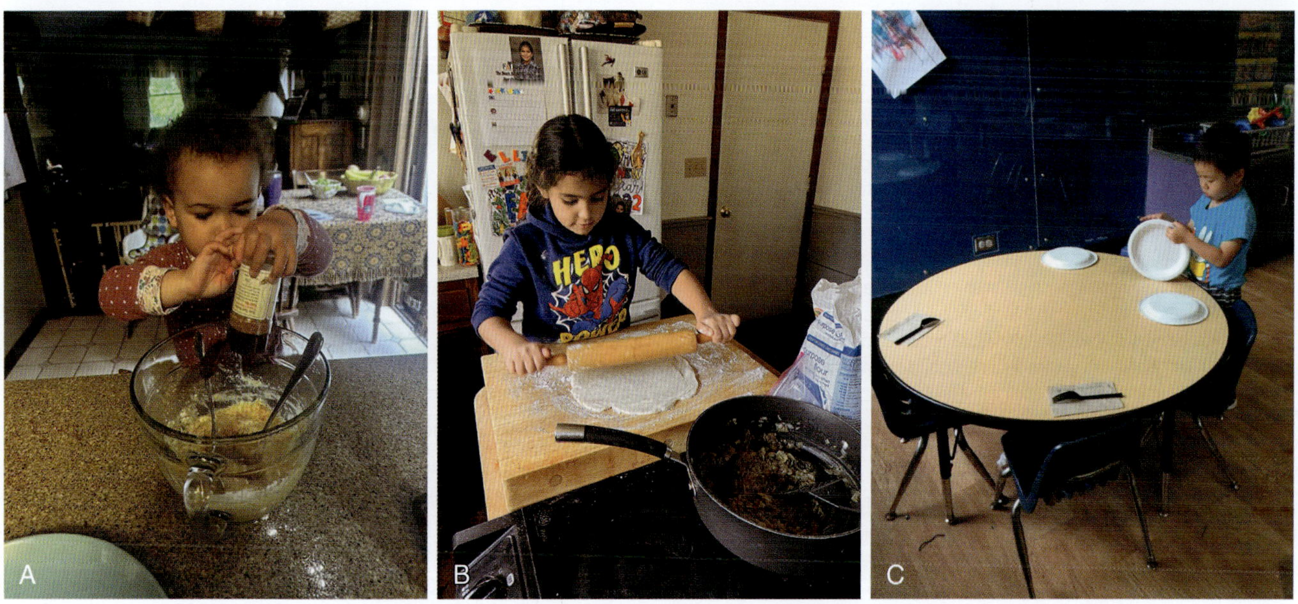


**Fig. 14.8** Meal preparation tasks can be adapted for young children. (A) Toddler pouring and stirring (items have been pre-measured). (B) Ellie rolling out the dough (standing on stool to be the correct height; dough is adjusted so it is easily rolled by young child) and (C) Child setting the table (items handed to child one item at a time).

## BOX 14.4 Task and Environmental Modifications

*Caring for pets* is an important IADL for many children and families (Fig. 14.7). Occupational therapy practitioners may create intervention plans to enable children and families to establish skills, routines, and knowledge to care for pets. The following is a brief analysis examining walking the family dog in the morning with possible task and environmental modifications.

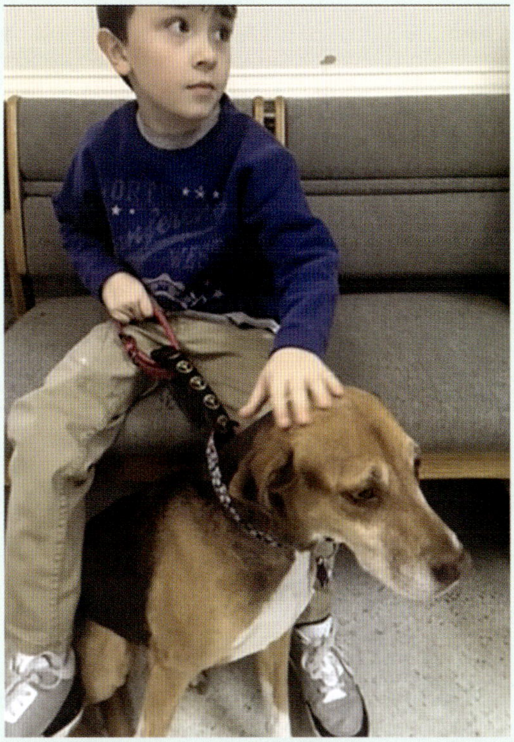

**Fig. 14.7** A young boy cares for his pet dog by taking the dog for walks daily.

**CARING FOR THE FAMILY DOG: TAKING REMY FOR A MORNING WALK**

| Steps | Task Modifications | Environment |
|---|---|---|
| Take the dog outside for a 20-minute walk in the morning. | Child can walk for 20 min holding small dog on leash (who is trained to stay close).<br>Child requires supervision to be outside with dog.<br>Child can problem-solve as situations may arise.<br>Child can walk dog for 10 min.<br>Child can watch dog outside (in fenced in yard) for 10 min. | Child is responsible and aware of safety situations to walk the dog on leash around the block by themself.<br>Child goes with parent (or older sibling) but is responsible for holding dog on leash.<br>Child stays with dog in the fenced- in backyard. |
| Pick up dog waste (i.e., poop). | Child can handle baggy by themselves.<br>Child can use an adapted 'scooper' with baggy that does not require as much fine motor coordination.<br>If the child is with someone, the child can hold baggy open, while other person scoops it in.<br>If a child is with someone, the child is not required to pick up waste, the other person will do that. Child can throw baggy away when they get home. | The environment requires scooping up dog waste.<br>The environment (i.e., home backyard) allows for some waste to be left unattended. |

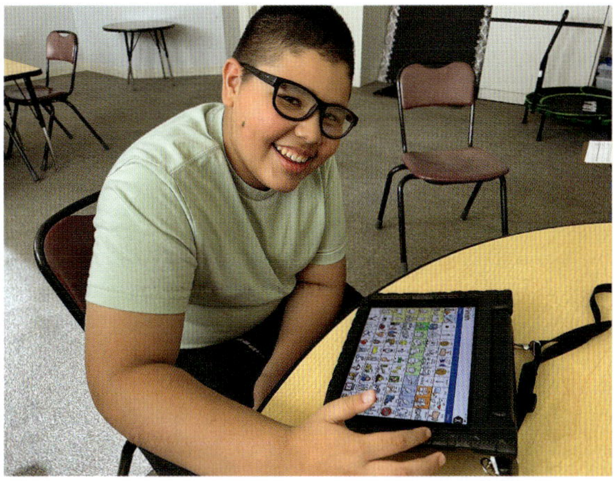

**Fig. 14.9** Technology can help teenagers participate in IADLs. This teen uses technology to engage in school and communicate with friends.

## BOX 14.5 Technology Tips

- Know child's and family's strengths, challenges, and needs.
- Do research.
  - Search a variety of sites and talk to users.
  - Collaborate with other professionals (e.g., speech-language therapists, physical therapists, educators).
- Try different applications. Keep track of uses.
  - Sesame Enable: Touch-free app that enables user to operate a smartphone with head movements.
  - Kurzweil 3000: Text to speech software.
  - Life360: Allows family to be aware of the child's whereabouts.
  - Find My Kids: GPS tracker that finds child's location (of phone) at any time.
  - Kidgy: Internet safety app which allows parents to monitor and block websites and track real-time location of children.
- Consider the child's motor, processing, and sensory strengths and challenges when recommending products.
- Collaborate with family and child.
  - Consider environmental support and barriers, including physical and human resources.
  - Finances: Keep it simple and affordable.
  - Consider the child's opinion of technology. (Does the child like it? Will they use it?)
  - Try out applications with the child before making recommendations.
- Follow-up to observe how technology helps the child engage in their daily activities. Make revisions as needed.

## TABLE 14.2 Examples of Intervention Activities and Strategies for Addressing IADLs Across Practice Settings

| Practice Setting | Example IADL Intervention Activities | Strategies |
|---|---|---|
| Early intervention | • Folding laundry.<br>• Putting items away where they belong (e.g., toys, utensils/plates, groceries).<br>• Simple food preparation for snacks and meals (encourage child to help sort, pour, stir). | • Interventions should be embedded into the family's everyday activities and routines.<br>• Use the family's materials instead of bringing in a toy bag.<br>• Have child prepare a special snack to share with family. |
| Schools | • Financial management - may be linked to math instruction or learning standards.<br>• Classroom jobs that relate to IADLs (e.g., wiping tables, putting classroom items away).<br>• Prepare lunch (e.g., make sandwich and select dessert and drink).<br>• Engage a child in community mobility (e.g., fieldtrips, community-based instruction).<br>• Engage child in planning how they will study or complete a classroom project. | • Goals should be related to the student's participation in educational activities.<br>• Occupational therapy practitioner supports individualized education plan (IEP) goals written by education team.<br>• Transition age students may have postsecondary goals on their IEP transition plan that relate to independent living or employment. |
| Outpatient | • Simple food preparation in clinic kitchen that they may carryover to home.<br>• Simulated financial management activities.<br>• Community mobility (e.g., safely crossing the street outside the clinic) or using the bus system.<br>• Engage children and youth in activities to encourage physical activity, such as care of pets, home maintenance. | • Involve family as much as possible.<br>• Promote generalization and transfer to natural settings.<br>• Have the family bring in materials that the child or youth uses as home (e.g., a favorite recipe and ingredients). |
| Hospital inpatient | • Simple meal preparation in hospital kitchen.<br>• Simple household chores in hospital simulated living environment.<br>• Care of pets (e.g., caring for therapy dogs visiting hospital).<br>• Encourage attending hospital chapel if they desire (spiritual expression). | • Transition back to natural settings (home, school).<br>• Promote generalization and transfer. |
| Community | • Assisting with shopping; child can have their own shopping list.<br>• Gardening at home or within the community (e.g., picking flowers, fruit).<br>• Community mobility (e.g., safely crossing streets, using public transportation).<br>• Planning to attend an event with money saved. | • Collaborate with client and caregiver to identify strategies that are likely to be used outside of therapy session. |

## CASE EXAMPLE 14.1 MEAL PREPARATION

Justine is a 14-year-old with hemiplegia referred to an outpatient clinic due to left upper extremity weakness and mild cognitive deficit. Justine typically neglects to use their left hand in everyday activities. Justine's occupational profile reveals that they are interested in cooking.

Justine's occupational therapy intervention plan included following a written recipe to make a mug cake in the outpatient clinic's kitchen as shown in Fig. 14.10. Justine worked with the occupational therapy practitioner to find a recipe online, wrote the recipe on a recipe card, and then made the recipe. While in the kitchen, Justine was required to use their left hand to hold the handle of the mug while stirring the contents with a spoon held in their right hand. Justine also had to use both hands to measure ingredients and wash dishes after cooking. Justine's occupational therapy practitioner provided structured prompting to support Justine's executive functioning skills while cooking.

Over the course of occupational therapy intervention, Justine compiled a collection of mug cake recipe cards that they were able to take home. The occupational therapy practitioner consulted with Justine's foster parent to ensure that they were comfortable with Justine using the microwave to cook mug cakes in the home. The occupational therapy practitioner also coached Justine's foster parent on how to best support Justine while they cook at home, and how the home kitchen could be arranged to best support their occupational performance.

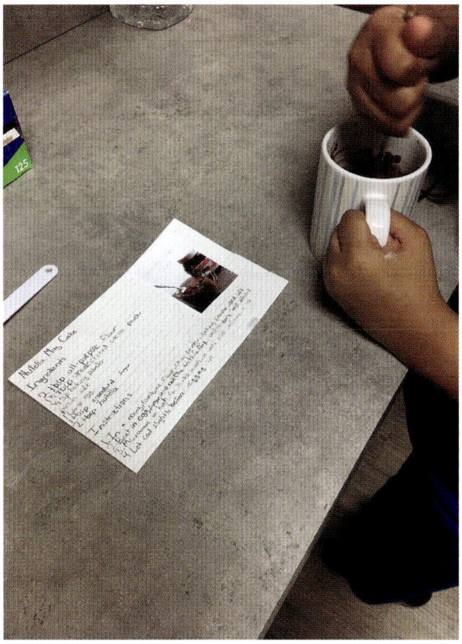

**Fig. 14.10** The occupational therapy practitioner engages the child in meal preparation activity to make a mug cake.

### CASE EXAMPLE 14.2 GROCERY SHOPPING

Matthew is a 17-year-old high school student with a goal to live independently after high school. Matthew has an Intellectual and Developmental Disability (IDD) and ambulates using crutches and lower limb prostheses as both of their legs were amputated as a young child due to a congenital lower limb deficiency. One of the postsecondary goals on Matthew's IEP transition plan is to independently shop for groceries, as this is related to Matthew's goal of living independently.

**Guided discovery strategies:** The occupational therapy practitioner used guided discovery strategies to help Matthew problem solve how to shop independently. With the support of the occupational therapy practitioner, Matthew determined that they could put both of his crutches in a standard grocery cart and use the cart as support while pushing it during the shopping trip. During an intervention session at the grocery store, the occupational therapy practitioner realized that Matthew was distracted by the many foods available in the store and attempted to make several impulsive purchases.

The occupational therapy practitioner worked with Matthew to create a shopping list and encouraged them to stick to the list to ensure they stayed within their budget for the trip. During the first few intervention sessions, the occupational therapy practitioner carried the grocery bags back to school on the city bus for Matthew. The occupational therapy practitioner used coaching strategies to help Matthew understand the importance of being able to perform all steps of grocery shopping independently.

The occupational therapy practitioner again used guided discovery techniques with Matthew, and Matthew identified that they could put the groceries in a backpack after shopping to independently transport them back to school or home on public transportation. The occupational therapy practitioner observed Matthew while they trialed this strategy, and coached Matthew on strategies for arranging the groceries in the backpack so they would not become damaged in transit (e.g., eggs on the top, heavy items on the bottom).

### CASE EXAMPLE 14.3 HOME MANAGEMENT (CLOTHING CARE)

Jamal, an autistic, nonspeaking, sixth-grade student, had an IEP goal of working independently for 15 minute on structured activities within the classroom. Jamal's classroom teacher consulted with the school occupational therapy practitioner to design some structured activities that were relevant to the real world. The occupational therapy practitioner suggested that one of the structured activities be folding washcloths.

**Task modification:** To help Jamal understand the task and complete the task independently, the occupational therapy practitioner colored the edges of the washcloths either blue or red (See Fig. 14.11). Jamal was instructed to match "blue to blue" and "red to red." Over time, Jamal mastered this task without the color cues and was able to meet their goal of working independently for 15 minutes.

At his annual IEP meeting, Jamal demonstrated his new washcloth folding skills to the educational team and his mother at the beginning of the meeting. His caregiver was in tears after this brief demonstration. They explained to the team, "I didn't know Jamal could do that. Jamal's brothers have chores at home, but I never thought that Jamal would be able to contribute to our family by doing chores. Now Jamal can do something to help our family and I'm just so grateful that they can be included in this way, like a typical kid. Jamal might not be excited to have chores, but this means so much to me."

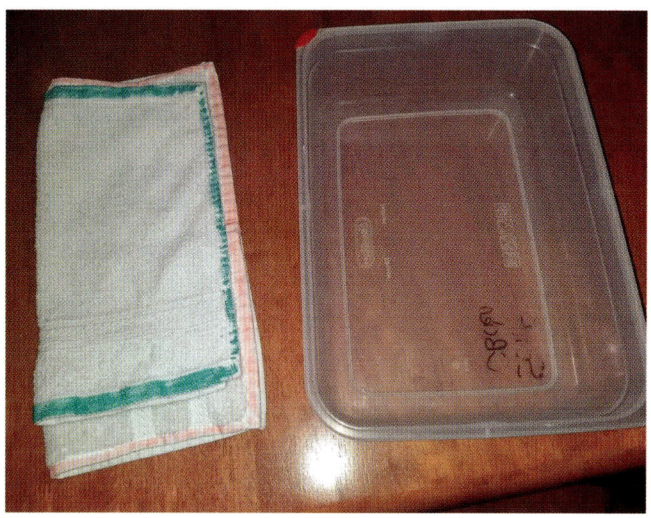

**Fig. 14.11** Towels with colored edges can help children fold them more easily.

## SUMMARY

Children and youth of all ages can benefit from meaningful participation in IADLs. Engagement in IADLs can lead to the development of self-determination skills (McPherson et al., 2018) and greater self-determination skills can lead to increased motivation to participate in IADL. Children and youth with disabilities and chronic conditions are less likely to demonstrate self-determination and less likely to be engaged in the community than their non-disabled peers, which provides an opportunity for occupational therapy practitioners to intervene and address this societal need.

Occupational therapy practitioners have the expertise to support their clients who are experiencing IADL performance and participation challenges. The occupational therapy process in addressing IADL involves

## SUMMARY—cont'd

using occupation-focused models to identify person, environment, and occupation factors. The occupational therapy practitioner can then use this information to analyze the client's abilities, IADL task demands, and environmental barriers and supports through a variety of evaluation methods, which can then guide the development of client goals and occupation-based, family-centered interventions delivered in the natural environment. Through this process, occupational therapy practitioners can assist clients in greater IADL performance and participation, which can then lead to more positive outcomes throughout childhood and into adulthood.

1. IADLs that develop during childhood and adolescence include care of others, care of pets and animals, child rearing, communication management, driving and community mobility, financial management, home establishment and management (e.g., clothing care, cleaning), meal preparation and cleanup, religious and spiritual expression, safety and emergency maintenance, and shopping.
2. Participation in IADLs and community activities prepares children and adolescents for work, vocational roles, and independent and interdependent community living.

   IADL participation also helps children develop feelings of competence and self-determination as they make choices and contribute to their family or community. Children and adolescents who demonstrate self-determined actions are more likely to report better quality of life and engage in social activities.
3. Performance and participation in independent or interdependent IADLs can be supported through family-centered, occupation-based, purposeful interventions delivered within the natural environment as much as possible where intervention is embedded into the child's already occurring routines.

## REFERENCES


American Occupational Therapy Association. (2020). Occupational therapy practice framework: Domain and process-fourth edition. *American Journal of occupational therapy*, *74*(Suppl. 2):7412410010. https://doi.org/10.5014/ajot.2020.74S2001.

Angell, A. M., Carroll, T. C., Bagatell, N., Chen, C., Kramer, J. M., Schwartz, A., Tallon, M., & Hammel, J. (2018). Understanding self-determination as a crucial component in promoting the distinct value of occupational therapy in post-secondary transition planning. *Journal of Occupational Therapy, Schools, & Early Intervention*, 1–15. https://doi.org/10.1080/19411243.2018.1496870.

Auld, C., Foley, K.-R., & Cashin, A. (2022). Daily living skills of autistic adolescents and young adults: A scoping review. *Australian Occupational Therapy Journal*, *69*(4), 456–474. https://doi.org/10.1111/1440-1630.12806.

Bedell, G., Coster, W., Law, M., Liljenquist, K., Kao, Y.-C., Teplicky, R., Anaby, D., & Khetani, M. A. (2013). Community participation, supports, and barriers of school-age children with and without disabilities. *Archives of Physical Medicine & Rehabilitation*, *94*(2), 315–323.

Bedell, G. M., Cohn, E. S., & Dumas, H. M. (2005). Exploring parents' use of strategies to promote social participation of school-aged children with acquired brain injury. *American Journal of Occupational Therapy*, *59*, 273–284.

Beisbier, S., & Laverdure, P. (2020). Occupation- and activity-based interventions to improve performance of instrumental activities of daily living and rest and sleep for children and youth ages 5–21: A systematic review. *American Journal of Occupational Therapy*, *74*, 7402180040. https://doi.org/10.5014/ajot.2020.039636.

Berge, J. M., Draxten, M., Trofholz, A., Hanson-Bradley, C., Justesen, K., & Slattengren, A. (2018). Similarities and differences between families who have frequent and infrequent family meals: A qualitative investigation of low-income and minority households. *Eating Behaviors*, *29*, 99–106. https://doi.org/10.1016/j.eatbeh.2018.02.007.

Dang, V. M., Colver, A., Dickinson, H. O., Marcelli, M., Michelsen, S. I., Parkes, J., Parkinson, K., Rapp, M., Arnaud, C., Nystrand, M., & Fauconnier, J. (2015). Predictors of participation of adolescents with cerebral palsy: A European multi-centre longitudinal study. *Research in Developmental Disabilities*, *36C*, 551–564. https://doi.org/10.1016/j.ridd.2014.10.043.

Darrah, J., Law, M. C., Pollock, N., Wilson, B., Russell, D. J., Walter, S. D., Rosenbaum, P., & Galuppi, B. (2011). Context therapy: A new intervention approach for children with cerebral palsy. *Developmental Medicine and Child Neurology*, *53*(7), 615–620. https://doi.org/10.1111/j.1469-8749.2011.03959.x.

Davis, J. N., Martinez, L. C., Spruijt-Metz, D., & Gatto, N. M. (2016). LA sprouts: A 12-week gardening, nutrition, and cooking randomized control trial improves determinants of dietary behaviors. *Journal of Nutrition Education and Behavior*, *48*(1), 2–11. https://doi.org/10.1016/j.jneb.2015.08.009.

Dean, E. E., Kirby, A. V., Hagiwara, M., Shogren, K. A., Ersan, D. T., & Brown, S. (2021). Family role in the development of self-determination for youth with intellectual and developmental disabilities: A scoping review. *Intellectual and Developmental Disabilities*, *59*(4), 315–334. https://doi.org/10.1352/1934-9556-59.4.315.

Dunn, W., Little, L. M., Pope, E., & Wallisch, A. (2017). Establishing fidelity of occupational performance coaching. *OTJR: Occupation, Participation and Health*, *38*(2), 96–104. https://doi.org/10.1177/1539449217724755.

Filippello, P., Sorrenti, L., Buzzai, C., & Costa, S. (2015). Perceived parental psychological control and learned helplessness: The role of school self-efficacy. *School Mental Health*, *7*, 298–310. https://doi.org/10.1007/s12310-015-9151-2.

Gillen, G., Hunter, E. G., Lieberman, D., & Stutzbach, M. (2019). The Association—AOTA's top 5 Choosing Wisely recommendations. *American Journal of Occupational Therapy*, *73*. :7302420010. https://doi.org/10.5014/ajot.2019.732001.

Gomez, R. J., Ryan, T. N., Norton, C. L., Jones, C., & Galan-Cisneros, P. (2015). Perceptions of learned helplessness among emerging adults aging out of foster care. *Child and Adolescent Social Work Journal*, *32*, 507–516.

Graham, F., Rodger, S., & Ziviani, J. (2009). Coaching parents to enable children's participation: An approach for working with parents and their children. *Australian Occupational Therapy Journal*, *56*(1), 16–23. https://doi.org/10.1111/j.1440-1630.2008.00736.x.

Hammond, S. I., Al-Jbouri, E., Edwards, V., & Feltham, L. E. (2017). Infant helping in the first year of life: Parents' recollection of infants' earliest prosocial behaviors. *Infant Behavior and Development*, *47*, 54–57. https://doi.org/10.1016/j.infbeh.2017.02.004.

Hammond, S. I., & Carpendale, J. I. M. (2015). Helping children help: The relation between maternal scaffolding and children's early help. *Social Development*, *24*(2), 367–383. https://doi.org/10.1111/sode.12104.

Hodgetts, S., & Park, E. (2016). Preparing for the future: A review of tools and strategies to support autonomous goal setting for children and youth with autism spectrum disorders. *Disability & Rehabilitation*, *39*, 535–543. https://doi.org/10.3109/09638288.2016.1161084.

Kramer, J. M., Hwang, I.-T., Helfrich, C. A., Samuel, P. S., Carrellas, A., & the YELL Lab Project TEAM Youth Research Collaborators. (2018). Evaluating the social validity of project TEAM: A problem-solving intervention to teach transition age youth with developmental disabilities to resolve environmental barriers. *International Journal of Disability, Development and Education*, *65*(1), 57–75. https://doi.org/10.1080/1034912X.2017.1346237.

Larson, L. (2010). Ever vigilant: Maternal support of participation in daily life for boys with autism. *Physical & Occupational Therapy in Pediatrics, 30*, 16–27. https://doi.org/10.3109/01942630903297227.

Laverdure, P., Nemec, E., Johnson, C., & Blake, T. (2021). Evaluating interventions that improve participation in chores in children and youth with disabilities: A systematic review. *Journal of Occupational Therapy, Schools, & Early Intervention, 14*(3), 257–273. https://doi.org/10.1080/19411243.2021.1875384.

Law, M., Anaby, D., Teplicky, R., Khetani, M., Coster, W., & Bedell, G. (2013). Participation in the home environment among children and youth with and without disabilities. *British Journal of Occupational Therapy, 76*(2), 58–66.

McPherson, A. C., Rudzik, A., Kingsnorth, S., King, G., Gorter, J. W., & Morrison, A. (2018). "Ready to take on the world": Experiences and understandings of independence after attending residential immersive life skills programs for youth with physical disabilities. *Developmental Neurorehabilitation, 21*(2), 73–82. https://doi.org/10.3109/17518423.2016.1141254.

Murphy, E., Clegg, J., & Almack, K. (2011). Constructing adulthood in discussions about the futures of young people with moderate-profound intellectual disabilities. *Journal of Applied Research in Intellectual Disabilities, 24*, 61–73.

Olson, A., Scherer, D. G., & Cohen, A. L. (2017). Decision-making skills of emerging adults aging out of foster care. *Children and Youth Services, 82*, 81–86.

Palmer, S. B., Fleming, K. K., Summers, J. A., Erwin, E. J., Maude, S. P., Brotherson, M. J., Stroup-Rentier, V., Haines, S. J., Zheng, Y. Z., Peck, N. F., & Wu, H. Y. (2019). Foundations for self-determination in early childhood: Preliminary preschool study. *Advances in Neurodevelopmental Disorders, 3*(2), 188–196. https://doi.org/10.1007/s41252-019-00106-0.

Polatajko, H. J., & Mandich, A. (2005). Cognitive orientation to daily occupational performance with children with developmental coordination disorder. In N. Katz (Ed.), *Cognition and occupation across the life span* (2nd ed.) (pp. 237–260). American Occupational Therapy Association Press.

Qian, X., Shogren, K., Odejimi, O. A., & Little, T. (2022). Differences in self-determination across disability categories: Findings from national longitudinal transition study 2012. *Journal of Disability Policy Studies, 32*(4), 245–256. https://doi.org/10.1177/1044207320964396.

Radey, M., Schelbe, L., McWey, L. M., Holtrop, K., & Canto, A. I. (2016). "It's really overwhelming": Parent and service provider perspectives of parents aging out of foster care. *Children and Youth Services Review, 67*, 1–10.

Rodger, S. (2006). I can do it: Developing, promoting, and managing children's self-care needs. In S. Rodger, & J. Ziviani (Eds.), *Occupational therapy with children* (pp. 200–221). Blackwell.

Shepley, C., Allday, R. A., & Shepley, S. B. (2018). Towards a meaningful analysis of behavior analyst preparation programs. *Behavior Analysis in Practice, 11*(1), 39–45.

Shogren, K. A., Wehmeyer, M. L., Palmer, S. B., Forber-Pratt, A., Little, T. J., & Lopez, S. (2015). Causal agency theory: Reconceptualizing a functional model of self-determination. *Education and Training in Autism and Developmental Disabilities, 50*(3), 251–263.

Sparks, S. C., & Cote, D. L. (2012). Teaching choice making to elementary students with mild to moderate disabilities. *Intervention in School and Clinic, 47*, 290–296.

Spriggs, A. D., Mims, P. M., van Dijk, W., & Knight, V. F. (2017). Examination of the evidence base for using visual activity schedules with students with intellectual disability. *The Journal of Special Education, 51*(1), 14–26. https://doi.org/10.1177/0022466916658483.

Taggart, J., Heise, M. J., & Lillard, A. S. (2018). The real thing: Preschoolers prefer actual activities to pretend ones. *Developmental Science, 21*(3):e12582. https://doi.org/10.1111/desc.12582.

Weaver, L. L. (2015). Effectiveness of work, activities of daily living, education, and sleep interventions for people with autism spectrum disorder: A systematic review. *American Journal of Occupational Therapy, 69*. :6905180020. https://doi.org/10.5014/ajot.2015.017962.

Wilson, J., Mandich, A., Magalhaes, L., & Gain, K. (2018). Concept mapping and the CO-OP approach with adolescents with autism spectrum disorder: Exploring participant experiences. *The Open Journal of Occupational Therapy, 6*(4). https://doi.org/10.15453/2168-6408.1455.

World Health Organization. (2008).

# 15

# Intervention for Education: Early Intervention Through Transition from High School

*Gloria Frolek Clark, Meira L. Orentlicher, and Yvonne Swinth*

## GUIDING QUESTIONS

1. What type of services do occupational therapy practitioners provide to children in educational systems?
2. How do policies support the continuum of services for children and youth?
3. What is the process to create an IEP or IFSP?
4. What best practice strategies are associated with improved outcomes and participation in postsecondary occupations?

## KEY TERMS

Early intervention
Ecological assessment
Individuals with Disabilities in Education Improvement Act (IDEA)
Individualized Education Program (IEP)
Individualized Family Service Plan (IFSP)
Multi-tiered System of Supports (MTSS)
Special education
Universal design
Universal Design for Learning (UDL)

## OVERVIEW OF OCCUPATIONAL THERAPY IN EDUCATION

Occupational therapy practitioners work with children and adolescents in homes, daycares, public schools, charter schools, private schools, and alternative schools. Public schools and early intervention are the most common work setting for occupational therapy practitioners; approximately 24% of occupational therapists and 20% of occupational therapy assistants, who are members of the American Occupational Therapy Association (AOTA), identified public school/early intervention as their primary work setting (AOTA, 2020a).

Occupational therapy practice within the public schools and most early intervention (EI) settings is guided by several federal laws, with a focus on development and preparation for learning and family services in EI and the occupation of education/learning for children ages 3–21 years. As students become adolescents, emphasis on transition and preparation for life beyond school is a key part of the educational program. If an occupational therapy practitioner works in a charter school or private school, their services may not be guided by federal education law, allowing more flexibility in how services are provided.

US public education policy is governed by the Elementary and Secondary Education Act of 1965 (Public Law 114-95), amended in 2015 and now called the Every Student Succeeds Act (ESSA, 2015). Within ESSA, occupational therapy practitioners are identified as specialized instructional support personnel (SISP), which promotes the value of practitioners working with all education stakeholders to enhance learning for all children.

The purpose of the latest reauthorization of the education law, the **Individuals with Disabilities in Education Improvement Act (IDEA** 2004; P.L. 108-446) for 3–21 years is "to ensure that all children with disabilities have available to them a free appropriate public education that emphasizes special education and related services designed to meet their unique needs and prepare them for further education, employment and independent living" (Section 300.1). IDEA specifies that students who receive special education and related services should be prepared for "further education, employment, and independent living" (§ 1401[d]). This explicit statement clarifies that **Individualized Education Program (IEP)** teams, parents, and students must consider adult outcomes as they plan students' school experiences and individualized education programs. The reauthorization added early intervening services (commonly referred to as "response to intervention") to address children who were at risk for learning and behavior needs; placed emphasis on the use of scientifically based practices, high-quality preservice training, and professional education; and the use and development of appropriate technology (including assistive technology). This reauthorization also included services for children birth to 3 years old for the purpose of providing comprehensive statewide EI services for children with disabilities and their families. New language ensured that EI services were based on scientifically based research, specific EI services were based on peer-reviewed research to the extent practicable, and that measurable results include preliteracy and language skills. States were given an option to continue EI services until a child enters kindergarten or elementary school to ensure smooth transitions.

### Emphasis on Access and Participation

School-based occupational therapy services have evolved from a clinical model (pull out and serve) to a focus on participation and educational performance (Frolek Clark & Polichino, 2020) across naturally occurring environments and settings, routines, and roles. Occupational therapy practitioners focus on ensuring children and youth can access and participate in the same settings and routines as their peers rather than "fixing" the person or increasing scores

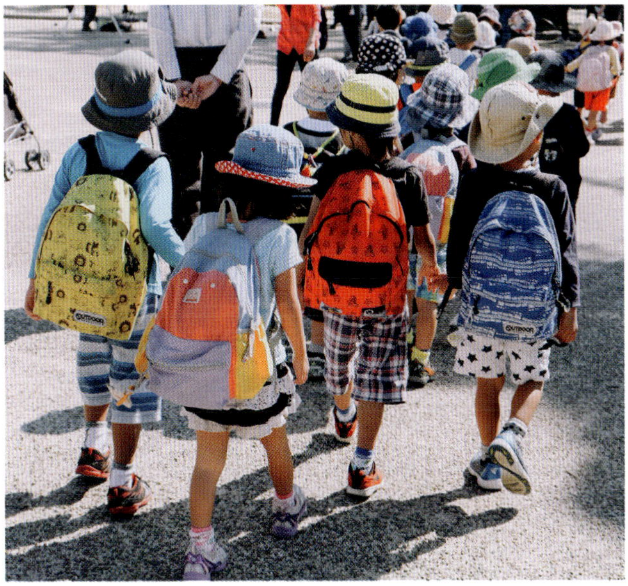

**Fig. 15.1** Occupational therapy practitioners in the schools focus on ensuring all children have access to participate in the same routines as their peers. (From www.unsplash.com)

on standardized tests (see Fig. 15.1). Under IDEA, services may be provided to the child, family, educational staff, or other colleagues in the natural environment for children birth to 3 years and least restrictive environment (LRE) for 3–21 years. Examples are provided in Table 15.1.

**TABLE 15.1 Examples of Occupational Performance Addressed in Early Intervention and Schools**

| Occupational Performance | Example Intervention Outcomes |
|---|---|
| Activities of daily living (basic and instrumental) | • Caregivers manage child's needs in the home or daycare (e.g., feeding, dressing, bathing, diapering).<br>• Takes care of self-care needs within school environment.<br>• Uses accommodations and modifications, including assistive technology to complete daily routines (e.g., taking the bus, managing school materials, eating lunch, playing with peers). |
| Education | • Attends to teacher, completes schoolwork, and able to listen, ask questions in class.<br>• Completes assignments on time.<br>• Uses seat adaptations and modifications to engage in academics.<br>• Uses strategies, such as text-to-speech software to complete written assignments.<br>• Exhibits communication skills to show knowledge.<br>• Preparing for transition out of high school to college, vocational school, or employment.<br>• Engages in reading, writing, and math work with accommodations or modifications. |
| Work | • Explores options, interests.<br>• Determines possible work options considering interests, skills, and aptitude.<br>• Engages in prevocational activities.<br>• Identifies work accommodations or adaptations to support success.<br>• Develops "soft skills" for employment. |
| Play/leisure | • Participates in activities with peers during recess.<br>• Uses equipment and toys to play.<br>• Engages in pretend play with others.<br>• Shows a playful attitude.<br>• Explores and creates during play.<br>• Tries out new activities.<br>• Negotiates with friends while engaged in fun activities. |
| Social participation | • Communicates with family, peers, and teachers.<br>• Establishes friendships.<br>• Reads and responds to social cues.<br>• Provides social cues to others.<br>• Engages in safe social activities.<br>• Learns to say no when needed.<br>• Develops one's own voice. |

## PROVIDING SERVICES ACROSS THE CONTINUUM

Occupational therapy practitioners believe "active engagement in occupation promotes, facilitates, supports, and maintains health and participation" (AOTA, 2020b, p. 5). Occupational therapy practitioners working in EI and schools provide a distinct value in services for children, families, and educational staff through their knowledge of the interplay between occupations and underlying components, the environment, and context, as well as the person's supports and challenges for access and participation in their daily life skills. Occupational therapy services are provided to enhance outcomes for children and their families through the following: (1) *systems* (e.g., services directed at administration or operation of federal, state, district, or local school); (2) *population and group* (e.g., services directed at people with common attributes); and (3) *individual* (e.g., child, including those involved in the care of the child). Practitioners consider approaches to intervention and types of occupational therapy interventions. Occupational therapy practitioners use frames of reference, theories, and practice models to guide intervention approaches to facilitate engagement in occupations (AOTA, 2020b). Table 15.2 provides examples of intervention approaches. Practitioners document their approaches on the intervention plan to achieve the child or family outcomes. See Chapter 9 regarding additional models of practice and frames of reference.

### Services to Support Systems

The complexity of addressing the diverse needs of today's students requires changes in how services have been traditionally provided. Services not only teach discrete skills to families or students, but also ensure that the context supports ongoing success. System supports are the "formal and informal initiatives, programs, and communications that occupational therapy practitioners and other education partners engage in together to address the education needs of an entire grade, school building, or population of students within a district, county, or state" (Hanft et al., 2016, p. 244). For young children, support may also be provided at the state level (e.g., statewide committees), community level (e.g., day care), or to groups of families to enhance child and family outcomes.

Partnership between professionals in the community and schools is essential. The World Health Organization (2012) recognizes that effective interprofessional collaboration leads to better outcomes for those receiving services. Thus, when an occupational therapy practitioner works with a team of interested parties to address the needs of a system, outcomes for all may improve.

**Early Intervention.** Occupational therapy practitioners may advocate for systems support as part of Early Intervention (EI) services

**TABLE 15.2 Occupational Therapy Intervention Approaches and Types Based on the OTPF-4 (AOTA, 2020)**

| Occupational Therapy Intervention Approaches | Description | Examples |
|---|---|---|
| Create, promote | Enriches a child's experiences, development, and environment. | Provide the family with a list of developmentally appropriate toys to promote the child's learning. |
| Establish, restore | Establish new skills or restore skills/abilities that are impaired. | Teach a child with Down syndrome how to feed themselves or dress.<br>Engage children with developmental delays in play activities to learn how to crawl, stand, or walk. |
| Maintain | Provide resources and support to preserve performance. | Create a feeding program for safe feeding for a child with severe/profound disability. |
| Modify (adaptation) | Change the context of the activity of the objects of the activity to support the child's performance in their environment. | Provide a visual schedule so youth can complete morning routines.<br>Provide a built-up handle toothbrush to allow child to grasp more effectively. |
| Prevent | Prevent the occurrence of barriers to occupational performance. | Provide antibullying training to school children so they feel comfortable and safe at school.<br>Engage children in activities to interact with others on the playground so all children feel included.<br>Advocate for inclusive spaces at school, home, and in the community. |
| **Types of Occupational Therapy Interventions** | | |
| Occupations and activities | Meaningful daily life events or parts of these events that meet therapeutic goals. | Engaging teens in prevocational training in the community.<br>Taking a nature walk to explore physical activity options for a healthy lifestyle. |
| Interventions to support occupations | Methods and tasks that prepare child to engage in desired activities. | Occupational therapy practitioner engages classroom in morning movement session, so they are ready for the day. |
| Education and training | Imparting knowledge and facilitating skills to improve performance. | Discussing reasons why a child may benefit from energy conservation strategies.<br>Demonstrating (and asking child to demonstrate back) how to use coping strategies to decrease anxiety. |
| Advocacy | Promoting occupational justice and empowering children to seek and obtain resources for their health and well-being. | Engaging a child in activities to ask teachers for assistance with learning.<br>Empowering teen to find resources (such as inclusive dance classes, adaptive sports programs), so they can engage in healthy activities. |
| Group interventions | Facilitate learning and skill development through groups. | Engaging in summer camps for children who have disabilities.<br>Group sessions to address bullying and friendships. |
| Virtual interventions | Use of technologies for service delivery | Providing online social skills group for teenagers with autism. |

by joining statewide interagency committees to discuss services for children birth to 3 years. Participating as part of an interagency committee helps all interested parties understand the distinct lens and role of occupational therapy, allowing the importance of focusing on the child's routine within the natural environment to be paramount within the discussion.

Occupational therapy practitioners may also participate in a committee to address implementing strategies and activities for recruitment and retention of early education service providers. This may include promoting preparation of EI providers, supporting children and families who have experienced developmental trauma, and addressing early needs of children on the spectrum to support occupational therapy providers that are qualified to work in EI and schools.

**Preschool and Schools.** The system's approach to services may include seeking membership on specific committees. For example, serving on a district literacy committee would allow an occupational therapy practitioner to help develop district-wide strategies to support the development of literacy with an emphasis on functional literacy (Frolek Clark, 2016; Grajo & Gutman, 2019) or participating on a playground committee to ensure playgrounds designs support social interactions among peers (see Fig. 15.2). As a member of the transportation committee, occupational therapy practitioners can ensure that the proper seating devices are available for children.

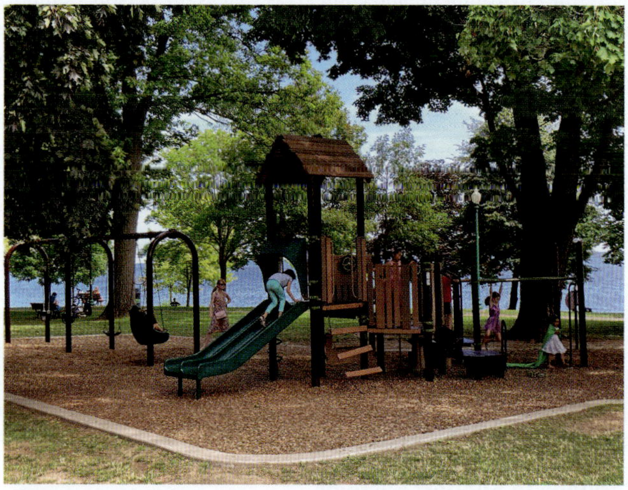

**Fig. 15.2** Occupational therapy practitioners serve on committees to help with playground modifications and adaptations so all children can participate. (From www.unsplash.com)

Another example is the collaboration between school districts and the local vocational rehabilitation agency (through Workforce Innovation and Opportunity Act) to ensure career and training services for youth.

## Services to Support Populations and Groups

Occupational therapy practitioners provide services in the home, community, and school to *populations* (e.g., people with common attributes such as students in general education) and *groups* (e.g., collections of individuals with shared characteristics or common purpose). The purpose of these services is to enhance the participation of children in their occupations and include working with families, educators, and others. The following section describes some examples of services provided for EI, preschools, and schools.

**Early Intervention.** EI services for populations are often provided as advocacy or education to people within the community. Examples include educating primary referral sources about EI services as part of Child Find or providing training to day care providers on child development. Some group activities are directed at the family, caregivers, and children. Examples may include including postpartum screenings for new mothers of infants referred to EI, providing developmental resources to parents and caregivers of young children who are in homeless shelters or foster care, or leading an EI play group.

**Preschool and Schools.** Occupational therapy practitioners (under early intervening or as SISP) engage in services with populations when they provide services under Tier 1 of Multi-tiered System of Supports (MTSS) with educational staff. Examples include professional development, assisting in the planning of universal screening tools, participating on the problem-solving team, or serving on school committees such as curriculum or playground committees (note: committee work can be at a system or a group level, depending upon the purpose of the committee).

Activities with groups may include working with the school on accessibility for all children with medical conditions, working with teams to identify prevocational training sites in the community for students with cognitive or physical impairments, and working with the early childhood special education teacher to set up centers to enhance literacy, motor, and self-regulation skills for children with special needs. Examples of group services in the classroom include co-instruction in the classroom, social skills training to a group of students with autism spectrum disorder, stress management, social-emotional learning, or literacy.

A strong leadership model of advocacy, including promotion and prevention, is often seen as occupational therapy practitioners expand their role to groups of children who are at risk. This may include being involved with the schools' positive behavior interventions and supports; school mental health; science, technology, engineering, and mathematics programs; literacy programs; UDL and assistive technology for diverse learners; and health promotion initiatives such as safe and healthy school, school bus and pedestrian safety, employee safety, healthy lifestyles, and nutrition (Bazyk, 2019; Candler, 2019; Frolek Clark & Bainter, 2019; Schoonover, 2019; Shrumpt, 2019). Every Moment Counts, developed by an occupational therapist, is a "multipronged mental health promotion initiative to help all children and youth be mentally healthy in order to succeed in school, at home, and in the community" (Every Moment Counts, 2022, Guiding Philosophy section). Guided by a public health framework and applied in the school setting, the emphasis is on embedding strategies throughout the school day to support the mental health of all students. See everymomentcounts.org for free resources regarding programming, such as Comfortable Cafeteria Program and Refreshing Recess.

## Services to Support the Individual

This section focuses on services to children in EI programs, general education, under Section 504, and special education.

**Early Intervention.** If states choose to participate in EI services, they must complete several requirements such as determining eligibility and identifying the lead agency. The service coordinator serves as the single point of contact for the EI team and provides the parent with resources and access to services through Part C and the community. The service coordinator may be any professional on the EI team (e.g., such as the occupational therapist).

***Identification and Referral.*** The EI program may receive a referral from multiple referral sources (e.g., parent, doctor, or daycare), which begins the 45-day timeline to conduct the process and complete the Individualized Family Service Plan (IFSP), which refers to the plan for services created in collaboration with the family.

***Intake and Family Assessment.*** The service coordinator is assigned and contacts the family to share information about the EI program, discuss their concerns about the child, and to schedule an initial visit if the family is interested. On the first visit, the family may request a screening (e.g., optional) or sign for evaluation and assessment of their child. The family assessment is optional. Part C process includes the families concerns, priorities, and resources for their child and the family.

***Child Evaluation and Assessment.*** The service coordinator requests medical information, as applicable. Some children are automatically eligible (based on the state's policy of diagnosed conditions). A multidisciplinary team (e.g., at least two professionals) conducts the evaluation and assessment, gathering information in all five required developmental areas: adaptive, cognitive, communication, physical (including hearing and vision), and social-emotional.

The occupational therapist may play one or two roles. These include participating in the multidisciplinary assessment to determine eligibility of the child or conducting an occupational therapy evaluation to determine the child's and family's strengths and need for occupational therapy services.

***Eligibility.*** Eligibility is defined by each state and must include conditions with a probability of resulting in developmental delay (children with these conditions are automatically eligible for EI services). Eligibility includes a rigorous definition of developmental disability typically defined between broad (e.g., at risk, 25% delay in one or more domains) or restrictive (e.g., 50% delay in one or more domains) range (Lucas, 2021). When an area of development is difficult to assess, the professionals can form an eligibility determination using qualitative and quantitative information to determine eligibility. This professional judgment should be based on data and is referred to as "informed clinical opinion" and can be used, for example, with adaptive skills (e.g., feeding), social-emotional (e.g., behavior, self-regulation), and physical skills (e.g., range of motion, muscle tone, strength, endurance).

***IFSP Development.*** If the child meets state eligibility, the IFSP team meets to review the child's evaluation and assessment, family assessment, and other information. Occupational therapy practitioners are actively involved with the development of the IFSP. Contents of the IFSP include the following: a child's present level of development (physical, cognitive, communication, social or emotional, adaptive) based on objective criteria; families' resources, priorities, and concerns; measurable results or outcomes for the child and family; specific EI services based on peer-reviewed research, to the extent practicable; natural environment where services will be provided, or a justification if held elsewhere; projected dates for beginning of services and length, duration, and frequency of services; identification of the service coordinator; and transition of a toddler from the program to appropriate services by age of 3 years.

Based on the individualized needs and family priorities and concerns, child and family outcomes are identified. Outcomes are typically written in the family voice and "describe the child's participation in naturally occurring routines and activities and promote skill development across multiple domains" (Lucas, 2021, p. 125). Outcomes are typically addressed by IFSP team members and are not discipline specific.

***Service Delivery.*** IDEA requires that EI services be provided in the natural environment (e.g., home, daycare, park). Supporting the child and family outcomes, the occupational therapist develops an intervention plan including occupation-based goals and interventions, intervention approaches, and delineation of services (if applicable) (AOTA, 2018). Approaches to interventions and types of occupational therapy interventions are also listed (see Table 15.2). In addition, occupational therapy practitioners working in EI services generally practice using the primary service provider model, where one professional (whose expertise matches the child's and family's needs) provides services in collaboration with the child, family, and IFSP team to achieve the desired outcomes. They frequently use a coaching approach to empower children and their families. When using a coaching model in occupational therapy, practitioners collaborate with family and children by listening to their feedback and carefully monitoring the child's progress. They provide strategies at the right level, so the child and family are successful but making progress toward their goals. Throughout the process, they listen to children and their families and adjust intervention based on feedback, progress, and professional reasoning. In all cases, evaluations should be conducted by occupational therapists before providing any child-specific intervention or strategies.

***Periodic or Annual Review.*** IDEA requires the IFSP plan to be reviewed at least annually. A periodic review must be held to with the family to determine progress towards the outcomes at least every 6 months (1436[b]).

***Transition.*** IDEA requires that a transition plan be developed for children on IFSP no less than 90 days and not more than 9 months before the child turns 3 years. Parents are an integral part of the child's transition and make decisions for their child (see Fig. 15.3). Options for a child may include the following: no additional services, transition to community activities or preschool program, or referral for a Part B evaluation to determine eligibility for special education and related services. Occupational therapists are actively involved with the transition by assisting parents in visiting programs being considered, sharing information with the transitioning partners, or educating parents on upcoming changes.

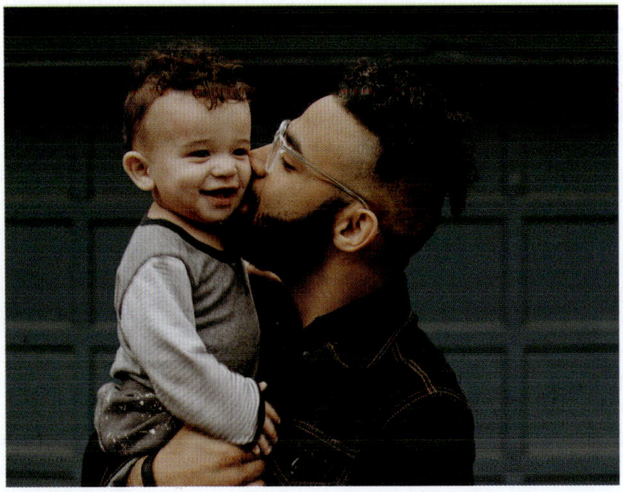

**Fig. 15.3** Early intervention focuses on the concerns, priorities, and resources of each family. The family is a core part of the team making service decisions impacting the child and family. (From www.unsplash.com)

***Discharge.*** The occupational therapist, as part of the IFSP team, should review the child's performance with the parent and plan to discharge when the family feels there is no longer a need, when child has met outcomes relating to occupational therapy services, or other reasons determined by the team.

**Preschool and Schools.** The continuum of educational services is typically described within a three-tiered MTSS model for kindergarten to grade 12 for all children in the general education curriculum to children eligible for special education. Many educators have also included preschool initiatives within this model.

***Multitiered Systems of Support.*** Many states use a **MTSS** to address the learning, social, and behavioral needs of all students. School districts are required to provide all students with high-quality instructional, behavioral, and social support in general education (Tier 1). If students in general education are struggling, they may be given additional practice or instruction in groups or individually (Tier 2). Students who do not demonstrate strong progress and continue to need extra resources and support may need specific one-to-one instruction and can be considered for evaluation to determine special education eligibility (Tier 3). Box 15.1 provides examples of interventions specific to each tier.

***Referral for Section 504.*** A child with a medical condition or suspected disability *impacting access and participation in school,* should be referred to their school district's Section 504 Committee. Section 504 provides the following: *accommodations* (e.g., does not change the test or assignments but provides changes including timing, formatting, scheduling, or setting); *modifications* (e.g., change to test or assignment that lowers or reduces what is measured or learned such as completing an alternative test), and *services* (e.g., some states provide related services such as occupational therapy services). Disability is broadly defined under Section 504 and the Americans with Disabilities Amendment Act (ADAA); a disability is "(1) A physical or mental impairment that substantially limits a major life activity; (2) A record of such impairment; or (3) being regarded as having such an impairment" (US DOE, 2012; para. 2). A major life activity includes "major bodily functions … and to include sleeping, standing, lifting, bending, reading, concentrating, thinking, communicating, and working" (Richards, 2021, p. 7). If a child appears to need specially designed instruction, a referral for evaluation for special education and related services under IDEA should be considered.

There is no formalized testing process. Determination for eligibility under Section 504 is made on a case-by-case basis using data from a variety of sources (e.g., parent information, health records, teacher report, student grades, occupational therapy evaluation).

### BOX 15.1 Occupational Therapy Intervention based on Multitiered Levels of Support

- **Tier 1.** Provide teachers with information about evidence-based curriculum for literacy or math. Provide suggestions for support for behaviors, physical activity, sensory, and motor skills for education. Provide teacher support and consultation on general classroom activities.
- **Tier 2.** Assist teachers in identifying activities to enhance targeted concern and set up data collection for decision-making. If allowed under state licensure, provide episodic (short-term) group or individual intervention to enhance performance in general education.
- **Tier 3.** Provide intensive activities to target concerns for specific students within the classroom. Provide individualized evaluation and intervention to target concerns if needed.

The occupational therapy evaluation process should obtain and interpret data necessary to understand the person's "health, well-being, and participation in life engagement in occupation" (AOTA, 2020b) and strengths and challenges within the education context and expectations from educational staff.

If the child is determined to meet eligibility, an individualized 504 plan is developed that outlines the accommodations, modifications, or services that will be provided by the school district. While the school district must notify the parents that a plan has been developed, there are no legal implications for timelines to implement the plan, parent participation in the development of the plan, format of the plan, or review of the plan (Jackson, 2019).

Some school districts provide accommodations under the Americans with Disabilities (ADA) Amendment Act of 2008. Title II of ADA prevents discrimination of individuals with disabilities by any state or local programs that receive federal funds. The definition of disability is similar within Title II ADA or Section 504.

***Referral for Full and Individual Initial Education Evaluation.*** A referral for a comprehensive individual education evaluation may be initiated by the parent, legal guardian, or member of the school team. After the parent or legal guardian has provided written consent for the evaluation, the team has approximately 60 calendar days (state timeline may vary) to complete the evaluation. Team members should understand appropriate and inappropriate referrals to occupational therapy.

***Evaluation to Determine if Child has an Educational Disability and Need for Special Education.*** The occupational therapy evaluation must provide valid and useful information to be used by the team in determining eligibility for special education and related services. The evaluation should be strengths based, person centered, and include a determination of all the occupations that are impacted (e.g., activities of daily living, instrumental activities of daily living, health management, rest and sleep, education, work, play, leisure, and social participation). This may be gathered through parent or teacher interview as part of the occupational profile. Contact with the family during the evaluation to understand the child and the family concerns should be considered essential to the process of data collection. Review of the records may also indicate the child's strengths and needs. Observation should also be included within the evaluation process to provide a deeper understanding of the impact of the environment, instruction and curriculum, and occupations upon the learner. For example, observing the child's social and physical interactions with equipment and peers on the playground may indicate strengths or challenges that must be addressed. Observing the child's work during classroom activities provides insight to their ability to access, participate, and complete tasks (see Fig. 15.4).

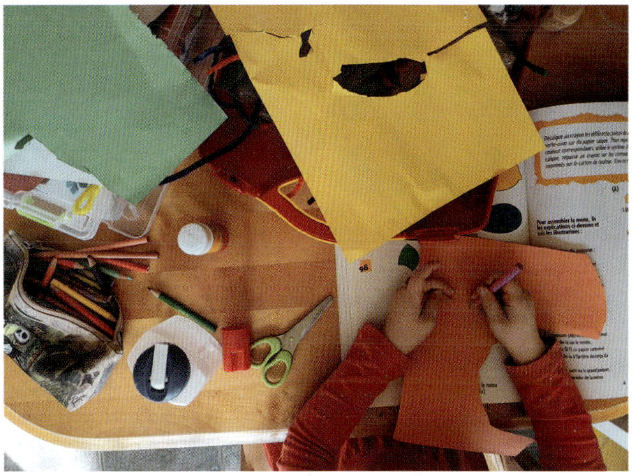

**Fig. 15.4** Observation in the student's daily routine offers insight into classroom expectations as well as peer performance. This provides information about the child's strengths and challenges relating to the task, environment, and performance. (From www.unsplash.com)

Assessment tools should be selected to provide accurate and unbiased information about the child's strengths and barriers to their educational program. See Appendix A for a list of assessment tools. Tools grounded in occupation assist in understanding engagement in occupation performance. Some states require specific results from an assessment tool for eligibility to occupational therapy services; however, IDEA does NOT require this and leaves the determination of related services to the IEP team after identification of student strengths, needs, and IEP goals.

The occupational therapist's professional report documents the evaluation process and recommendations. This includes a description about how the child's concern is impacting their participation in age-appropriate activities (e.g., choking on foods, hits peers if they come nearby) and their general education curriculum (e.g., unable to independently journal, does not complete work), what the child needs to learn (e.g., curriculum, needs to learn to feed self, to hold scissors and cut, to remove coat, to initiate and maintain positive interactions with peers); appropriate strategies to teach the child (e.g., verbal prompting, adding motivational strategies, use of special techniques); and accommodations, modification, and assistive technology needed for learning (e.g., quiet work area, peer role models, adaptive spoon, physical assistance from adult). The most important statement is how the expertise of an occupational therapy practitioner is needed (e.g., providing skill building activities, educating teacher, providing modifications). In some cases, only skill building requires ongoing services, while the others may be completed in a few sessions.

***Determine Eligibility.*** Eligibility for special education is based on two factors that must both be present. First, the child must have an educational disability (e.g., intellectual disability, orthopedic impairment), and second, the child must need special education and related services (1401[3][A]). **Special education** is defined as "specially designed instruction, at no cost to the parents, to meet the unique needs of the child with a disability" (1401[29]). Once a child is found to be eligible, the team determines the services based on the child's needs (e.g., they do not need to "qualify" for services once they are eligible for special education). Occupational therapy practitioners are often included in this process, or the team may use their report. IDEA considers the parent an essential part of the IEP team and provides parents specific rights to make decisions about their child's program.

***Development of an IEP.*** IDEA mandates attendees of the IEP meeting to include the parent, child (if appropriate), child's general education teacher, special education teacher, representative from the local educational agency, individual who can interpret evaluation results, and related service personnel (such as the occupational therapist) (300.321). The IEP process includes identifying the child's present levels of academic achievement and functional performance (e.g., impact of child's educational disability on participation in activities or general education curriculum); measurable goals based on strengths, needs, and concerns; description of how the child's progress will be measured and reported to families; special education, related services, and supplementary aids and services provided to or on behalf of the child; program modifications; any lack of participation with nondisabled peers in general education class or activities; accommodations necessary for performance on state and district-wide assessments; and beginning dates of services.

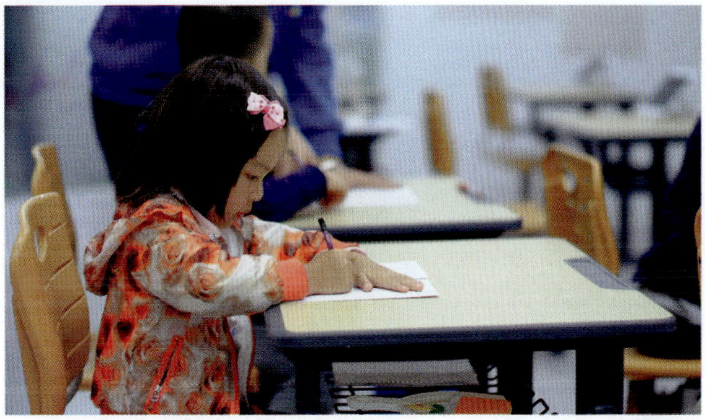

Fig. 15.5 Occupational therapy practitioners use co-instruction or co-teaching in the classroom with the teacher as a method to enhance learning for general and special education children. (From www.unsplash.com)

By age 16 years, the IEP must include "appropriate measurable post-secondary goals based upon age-appropriate transition assessments related to training, education, employment, and, where appropriate, independent living skills" (§ 1414[d][1][A][VIII]). Services from the local education agency or agencies outside the community must be listed on a transition plan and be provided to assist each student in meeting these goals. Postschool activities to be addressed during transition planning listed in the IDEA include postsecondary education, vocational education, integrated employment (including supported employment), continuing and adult education, adult services, independent living, and community participation.

***Service Delivery.*** Occupational therapy practitioners provide interventions to support physical, emotional, mental health, and social competence of students. The IDEA requires services to be provided in the LRE, or a statement justifying why the services cannot be provided there must be listed on the IEP. Table 15.2 identifies various approaches to intervention and types of interventions used by occupational therapy practitioners. These include preventing barriers to participation (e.g., supporting school-wide programs such as universal design for learning), providing modifications and accommodations in the environment and classroom activities, educating and training others to enhance the child's performance, co-instructing in the classroom, teaching students to advocate for their needs, and establishing skills and abilities. Fig. 15.5 shows a classroom where the occupational therapy practitioner and teacher co-instruct young children on handwriting skills.

Effective occupational therapy services to students are provided along a continuum of least to most restrictive and may include services on behalf of the student or directly with the student or groups of students. Frolek Clark and Hollenbeck (2019) provide the following descriptions of each service:

- *Services on behalf of the student.* The educator is present, but the child might not be. Services may include modifications and accommodations, education and training, consultation, and advocating.
- *Services directly with students.* The child and educator are both present. For example, services may include (a) groups in natural context and within regular routine such as co-instruction in the classroom, fine motor preschool groups, and (b) individualized intervention in the natural context and within regular routine such as dressing for recess, writing in a journal, and social skills coaching on the playground.
- *Services directly with the student.* The student is present, but the educator is not. Services provided in this way are the most restrictive because the child receives intervention outside of their natural routine and context. Examples may include services such as working on cutting in the hallway or skills in a "therapy" room.

***Annual Review/Re-evaluation.*** The IDEA requires the IEP team to review the IEP at least annually to determine if the child's goals are being achieved. Revisions may be made to the IEP with parent input (states have various procedures for IEP revisions). Parents are typically informed of the ongoing progress on the child's goals on a quarterly or trimester basis (e.g., typically following the district's report card schedule). Parents may request a meeting at any time to discuss progress or lack of progress.

The occupational therapy practitioner documents services provided to the child, progress toward the child's goals, and any recommendations for services. If the child is eligible, the team develops an IEP with new goals and services for the child.

Re-evaluation of the child must occur at least every 3 years (unless parents and schools agree that it is unnecessary) to determine if the child continues to have a disability and their educational needs (300.303). A re-evaluation may not occur more than once a year unless parents and schools agree. If new data are being collected, the family must be notified and provide written consent (e.g., the initial goal was to address eating, but the team has current concerns regarding organization, coping strategies, and visual perceptual skills).

***Transition by Age 16 Years.*** Although the IDEA requires transition planning to begin no later than age 16 years, research suggests that planning should begin earlier (Cimera et al., 2013) to increase employment after high school and to help the student earn higher wages. Occupational therapy researchers also propose preemployment and other transition preparation programs for students in middle school (Hollenbeck et al., 2015).

When conducting an assessment for students who are transitioning out of school settings, the occupational therapy practitioner identifies the child's abilities and access to potential resources. Some abilities that strength-based transition assessment can identify are self-determination skills, social skills, and positive character traits (Carter et al., 2015). Potential resources that a strength-based approach can identify include a student's access to social, economic, and cultural capital, as well as social networks, financial support, and cultural values. Creating a structure of future activities for students reduces their social isolation and segregation, provides opportunities for new friendships, develops the student's competence, and promotes respect for the student (Holburn & Vietze, 2002).

Best practices are associated with improved outcomes and predict participation in postsecondary occupations among students with disabilities. Although the emphasis is on long-term postschool outcomes, these practices should be used throughout the student's school career: (1) inclusion in general education, (2) paid and unpaid work experience while in high school, (3) employment preparation emphasizing career awareness, job-searching skills, and vocational training (4) family involvement, (5) parent high expectations, (6) self-care and independent living skills, (7) interagency collaboration, (8) self-advocacy and self-determination, (9) social skills, and (11) community integration (Haber et al., 2016; Kutscher & Tuckwiller, 2020; Mazzotti et al., 2015). Box 15.2 provides suggestions from best practices for positive postschool outcomes. More information about the laws connected to transition such the Workforce Innovation and Opportunity Act (WIOA, 2014), ADA Amendments Act (ADAA, 2008) can be found in the chapter activities online.

***Discharge.*** The occupational therapist, as part of the IEP team, reviews the child's performance and plan to discharge when the IEP team feels there is no longer a need, when child has met outcomes relating to occupational therapy services, or other reasons determined by the team.

**BOX 15.2 Best Practice Suggestions for Positive Post-School Outcomes**

- Begin the transition process early and discuss it with the child, family, and teachers. Provide opportunities for children, families, and team members to discuss resources, future goals, and opportunities for children. Focus on child's strengths, motivations, and desires. Be open minded and help the child and family see possibilities, opportunities, and resources to support the child's future.
- Inclusion in general education. Children benefit from participating in all aspects of life with typically developing peers, in schools, and in the community (AOTA, 2014, 2017). Occupational therapy practitioners may recommend modifications to increase physical access, accommodations to increase social participation, or strategies to improve the child's ability to meet the performance and behavioral expectations.
- Work experience. Match students with career readiness and employment preparation activities based on their age, individual needs, and goals (e.g., career exploration, job shadowing, job samplings). Occupational therapy practitioners help students develop "soft" skills, such as work completion, task accuracy, punctuality, social skills, and self-regulation that benefit them in the work setting. They can provide intervention to address specific skills for work and volunteer settings.
- Self-care and independent living skills. Functional skills such as cooking, appropriate dressing, reading the news, and computing sales tax can be integrated into academic content such as vocabulary, properties of elements in the periodic table, and mathematic computation (Chapman et al., 2019; Karl et al., 2013). Occupational therapy practitioners work with children to develop daily living skills.
- Self-advocacy and self-determination. Self-determination is defined as acting as a causal agent in one's life, that is, having the skills, opportunities, and supports to engage in goal-directed actions (Shogren et al., 2015). Occupational therapy practitioners promote self-determination by encouraging children to make choices, decide, problem solve, set goals and achieve them, plan, self-manage, and advocate for themselves (Burke et al., 2020; Mazzotti et al., 2021).
- Community integration. Community participation represents both physical presence and meaningful involvement in community events and organizations, leading to a network of personal relationships (Lee & Morningstar, 2019). To achieve community integration, it is important to teach functional skills along with how the student will get to the community site. Occupational therapy practitioners can encourage children to participate in community events with their peers.

Rather, the focus of intervention should include the child, environment, and the activities. For example, the occupational therapy practitioner observes the child in the classroom to determine how the environment influences their learning. Box 15.3 provides questions for occupational therapy practitioners to consider when observing children within their classroom environment.

**BOX 15.3 Potential Modifications for Classroom Environments**

- Removing distracting items to enhance attention
- Altering seating arrangements to promote child engagement with others
- Adding movement opportunities into the classroom routine, such as when it is time to line up
- Providing calming items or objects for a student who becomes easily frustrated
- Creating a quiet area of a room or an area for calming and relaxing experiences, such as a reading den, or small tent filled with pillows
- Reducing the noise level or providing methods to reduce a student's exposure, such as noise cancelling headphones
- Removing or rearranging room decoration to reduce visual stimulation
- Removing or dimming bothersome classroom lighting
- Altering the arrangement of desks to improve line of sight for a student to the teacher or the board
- Altering the physical setup or equipment to better allow navigation throughout the room and changes in body postures, such as sitting on a carpet versus sitting at a desk

## SETTING THE ENVIRONMENT AND TASKS FOR A CHILD'S SUCCESS

Occupational therapy practitioners focus their interventions on the child's ability to complete activities within the routine of the school day (e.g., access and participation). Removal of a child from the natural routine and environment for services should seldom occur. Rather, the focus of intervention should include the child, environment, and the activities. For example, the occupational therapy practitioner may determine the need to modify the environment or a task for a student in order to enhance their learning. They communicate respectfully and collaborate with the classroom teacher to establish appropriate and acceptable classroom changes. Box 15.3 provides ways in which occupational therapy practitioners may collaborate with a teacher to modify the classroom environment.

Working with the child or educator within the classroom allows the occupational therapy practitioner to observe the social, physical, and temporal aspects influencing the child's classroom participation so that they may identify and address the underlying reasons for the child's challenges. The ability to function and complete tasks in natural environments is also important for the transition to adult life. For example, young adults function in noisy and ever-changing work and community environments, such a noisy supermarket or a crowded bus. The student's ability to complete activities and routines should be evaluated in other environments, for example, transitioning from one classroom to another, navigating through crowded and noisy hallways, accessing lockers, eating lunch in the cafeteria, and using the restrooms. Knowledge regarding the influence of environmental and sensory stimuli on the student's occupational performance allows practitioners to create intervention that supports students' engagement in daily routines within their environments. Regardless of age, children and youth can benefit from environments that have been designed to support their ability to participate successfully.

### Ecological Assessment

**Ecological assessments** are used to evaluate the environment (e.g., physical, sensory, social features) for the child's learning, social interactions, or work experience. Occupational therapy practitioners understand the interplay between the person, environment, and the occupation (tasks) and are qualified to assess environments, such as the classroom, cafeteria, or community-based job site to identify student's strengths and needs in relation to the demands of the environment and to determine what resources and expectations the environment can provide (see Fig. 15.6). In addition to performing ecological assessments, occupational therapists are experts in modifying the environment and task demands to improve performance.

### Assistive Technology

Assistive technology plays an instrumental role in assisting children with disabilities in performing daily occupations and to participate more fully

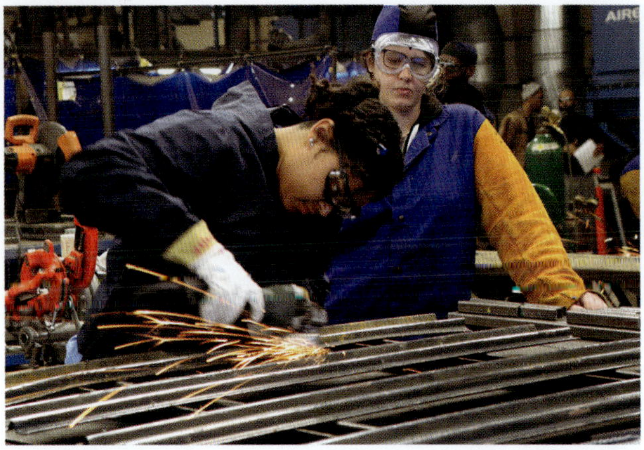

**Fig. 15.6** Ecological assessments allow occupational therapy practitioners to identify student needs during prevocational job experiences. Environmental or task modifications may allow the student to be more successful. (From www.unsplash.com)

in the community (e.g., functional mobility, communicating, reading, writing). See Chapter 34 for more on assistive technology. Assistive technology can mitigate the impact of sensory, cognitive, and/or physical challenges that cause functional limitations. Recent changes to learning environments include a wider implementation of blended or digital learning, providing new and practical options for students with disabilities to access the curriculum and receive content. Occupational therapy practitioners can assist in adapting and providing technology to facilitate students' access to their curriculum and environment.

## Universal Design for Learning

**Universal design** is referred to in The Tech Act (The Improving Access to Assistive Technology for Individuals with Disabilities Act of 2004; P. L. 108-364) as "a concept or philosophy for designing and delivering products and services that are useable by people with the widest possible range of functional capabilities, which include products and services that are directly accessible (without requiring assistive technologies) and products and services that are interoperable with assistive technologies" (29 USC 3002 [19]). Universal design principles have been applied to education to ensure that all learners can access and participate in meaningful and challenging learning opportunities.

**Universal Design for Learning (UDL)** reduces barriers for accessing instruction by providing appropriate accommodations and supports (Higher Education Opportunity Act, 2008, p. 20, USC 1002). Rather than solely focusing on the capabilities of the learners, UDL advocates for examining the environment in which students learn and their interactions with educational goals, materials, methods, and assessments. The learning environment includes the physical layout of the classroom, the way that the space is being used, environmental elements and sensitivities such as lighting, as well as the social interactions and other covert and overt behavioral expectations. Occupational therapy practitioners can help create learning environments that are positive, structured, and supportive for all students. For example, occupational therapy practitioners can recommend flexible and varied types of furniture and arrangements, areas for quiet individual work, visual schedules, activities to help students transition between classes and activities, and strategies for providing sensory-friendly environments and positive behavior supports.

**Not Just Classroom.** It is important to consider the impact of the environment on children's engagement in meaningful activities, tasks, and life roles during and after the transition from home to school and school to adult life. In addition to the classroom, occupational therapy practitioners advocate for a variety of environmental factors to promote a child's engagement. For example, students who use personal mobility aids (e.g., walkers, wheelchairs) require adequate space for maneuvering, as well as accessible buildings. Young children and families need quiet places in the community for their children with noise sensitivities. Occupational therapy practitioners provide consultation on the school and community level to increase access for all students.

## SUMMARY

Occupational therapy practitioners provide services in EI programs and schools directed at systems, populations, groups, and individuals. Their focus is on the child's access, participation, and progress in the natural environment (EI programs) and LRE (school programs). Evaluation and intervention emphasize the person's occupations (activities) within their environment. Collaboration with the family, educators, and community partners is critical to successful outcomes for the child.

1. Occupational therapy practitioners are involved in creating intervention plans to support the education of children. They provide direct services in homes (as in EI) and schools. They consult with team members (such as teachers) and address physical (e.g., motor, sensory), social-emotional, and behaviors (e.g., planning, attention) required for children to benefit from education. They examine the environment and suggest modifications of technology to support children.
2. Legislation (e.g., PL 94-142, IDEA 2004, No Child Left Behind, ESSA, Section 504, and the ADA) provides guidelines for the provision of services of children birth to 21 years of age. They provide details of funding sources, eligibility criteria, and intervention processes. Occupational therapy practitioners working with children and youth practicing in EI and school settings use the key concepts of each of these pieces of legislation/reauthorizations to support the occupational therapy intervention process.
3. The IFSP is created in collaboration with children (birth to 3 years) and their families for education plan as part of the EI process. As children transition to school settings, the team collaborates with families to create an IEP to support the child's progress in school settings. Each plan includes a description of the child's goals, services, and timelines for measuring progress.
4. The following strategies are associated with best practice in occupational therapy to facilitate children and youth's education and occupational participation: inclusion in general education; work experiences; engagement in self-care and independent living skills training; promotion of self-advocacy and self-determination; and opportunities for community integration.

## REFERENCES


American Occupational Therapy Association. (2020a). *2019 Workforce and salary survey*. Author. https://library.aota.org/AOTA-Workforce-Salary-Survey-2019/?_ga=2.2387888.1244685793.1662380027-26548289.1653474380.

American Occupational Therapy Association. (2020b). Occupational therapy practice framework: Domain and process-Fourth edition. *American Journal of Occupational Therapy, 74*(Suppl. 2),412410010p412410011–412410074. https://doi.org/10.5014/ajot.2020.74s2001.

American Occupational Therapy Association. (2018). Guidelines for documentation of occupational therapy. *American Journal of Occupational Therapy, 72*(Suppl. 2),721241001.

American Occupational Therapy Association. (2017). Guidelines for occupational therapy Services in early intervention and schools. *American Journal of Occupational Therapy, 71*(Suppl. 2),7112410010.

American Occupational Therapy Association. (2014). Occupational therapy's commitment to nondiscrimination and inclusion. *American Journal of Occupational Therapy, 68*(Suppl. 3), S23–S24. https://doi.org/10.5014/ajot.2014.686s05.

Americans with disabilities amendment Act of 2008, HR 3195 S. 3406 § 1–7 (ADAA, 2008).

Bazyk, S. (2019). Best practices in school mental health. In G. Frolek Clark, J. Rioux, & B. Chandler (Eds.), *Best practices for occupational therapy in schools* (2nd ed.) (pp. 153–160). AOTA Press.

Burke, K. M., Shogren, K. A., Antosh, A. A., LaPlante, T., & Masterson, L. H. (2020). Implementing the SDLMI with students with significant support needs during transition planning. *Career Development and Transition for Exceptional Individuals, 43*(2), 115–121. https://doi.org/10.1177/2165143419887858.

Candler, C. (2019). Best practices in school health and wellness. In G. Frolek Clark, J. Rioux, & B. Chandler (Eds.), *Best practices for occupational therapy in schools* (2nd ed.) (pp. 143–151). AOTA Press.

Carter, E. W., Boehm, T. L., Biggs, E. E., Annandale, N. H., Taylor, C. E., Loock, A. K., & Liu, R. Y. (2015). Known for my strengths: Positive traits of transition-age youth with intellectual disability and/or autism. *Research and Practice for Persons with Severe Disabilities, 40*(2), 101–119. https://doi.org/10.1177/1540796915592158.

Chapman, S. M., Ault, M. J., Spriggs, A. D., Bottge, B. A., & Shepley, S. B. (2019). Teaching algebra with functional application to students with moderate intellectual disability. *Education and Training in Autism and Developmental Disabilities, 54*(2), 161–174.

Cimera, R. E., Burgess, S., & Wiley, A. (2013). Does providing transition services early enable students with ASD to achieve better vocational outcomes as adults? *Research and Practice for Persons with Severe Disabilities, 38*(2), 88–93.

Every Moment Counts. (2022). *Every moment counts guiding philosophy, framework, and goals*. Retrieved from https://everymomentcounts.org/guiding-philosophy-goals/.

Every Student Succeeds Act, Pub. L. 114-95, 20 U.S.C. 6301 *et seq.* (ESSA, 2015).

Frolek Clark, G., & Bainter, S. (2019). Best practices in literacy and STEM skills to enhance participation at the district and building levels. In G. Frolek Clark, J. Rioux, & B. Chandler (Eds.), *Best practices for occupational therapy in schools* (2nd ed.) (pp. 135–141). AOTA Press.

Frolek Clark, G., & Hollenbeck, J. (2019). Best practices in school occupational therapy interventions to support participation. In G. Frolek Clark, J. Rioux, & B. Chandler (Eds.), *Best practices for occupational therapy in schools* (2nd ed.) (pp. 341–348). AOTA Press.

Frolek Clark, G., & Polichino, J. (2020). School occupational therapy: Staying focused on participation and educational performance. *Journal of Occupational Therapy, Schools, & Early Intervention, 14*, 19–26.

Frolek Clark, G. (2016). The occupations of literacy: Occupational therapy's role. *Journal of Occupational Therapy, Schools, & Early Intervention, 9*, 27–37.

Grajo, L., & Gutman, S. (2019). The role of occupational therapy in functional literacy. *Open Journal of Occupational Therapy, 7*(1).

Haber, M. G., Mazzotti, V. L., Mustian, A. L., Rowe, D. A., Bartholomew, A. L., Test, D. W., & Fowler, C. H. (2016). What works, when, for whom, and with whom. *Review of Educational Research, 86*(1), 123–162.

Hanft, B., Swinth, Y., & Shepherd, J. (2016). Initiating and sustaining system supports. In B. Hanft, & J. Shepherd (Eds.), *Collaborating for student success* (pp. 243–281). AOTA Press.

Higher Education Opportunity Act of 2008, Pub. L. 110-315, 122 STAT. 3078 (2008).

Holburn, S., & Vietze, P. M. (Eds.). (2002). *Person-centered planning: Research, practice, and future directions*. Paul H. Brookes.

Hollenbeck, J., Orentlicher, M., & Handley-More, D. (2015). Expanding roles, expanding impact: Supporting work readiness in middle school. *Early Intervention & School Special Interest Section Quarterly, 22*(3), 1–4.

Individuals with disabilities education improvement Act of 2004. P.L. 108-446, 20 U.S.C. § 1400 *et. seq.*

Jackson, L. (2019). Best practices in supporting students with a 504 plan. In G. Frolek Clark, J. Rioux, & B. Chandler (Eds.), *Best practices for occupational therapy in schools* (2nd ed.) (pp. 219–226). AOTA Press.

Karl, J., Collins, B. C., Hager, K. D., & Ault, M. J. (2013). Teaching core content embedded in a functional activity to students with moderate intellectual disability. *Education and Training in Autism and Developmental Disabilities, 48*, 363–378.

Kutscher, E. L., & Tuckwiller, E. D. (2020). A mixed methods study of K-12 influences on college participation for students with disabilities. *Career Development and Transition for Exceptional Individuals, 43*(2), 101–114. https://doi.org/10.1177/2165143420905104.

Lee, H., & Morningstar, M. E. (2019). Exploring predictors of community participation among young adults with severe disabilities. *Research and Practice for Persons with Severe Disabilities, 44*(3), 186–199.

Lucas, A. (2021). Understanding Part C: Early identification law and individualized family service plan (IFSP) process. In G. Frolek Clark, & S. Parks (Eds.), *Best practices for occupational therapy in early intervention* (2nd ed.) (pp. 119–128). AOTA Press.

Mazzotti, V. L., Rowe, D. A., Kwiatek, S., Voggt, A., Chang, W.-H., Fowler, C. H., Poppen, M., Sinclair, J., & Test, D. W. (2021). Secondary transition predictors of postschool success: An update to the research base. *Career Development and Transition for Exceptional Individuals, 44*(1), 47–64.

Mazzotti, V. L., Rowe, D. A., Sinclair, J., Poppen, M., Woods, W. E., & Shearer, M. L. (2015). Predictors of post-school success: A systematic review of NLTS2 secondary analyses. *Career Development and Transition for Exceptional Individuals, 39*, 196–215.

Richards, J. (2021). *The fundamentals of Section 504 eligibility*. https://www.504idea.org/wp-content/uploads/2021/03/2021-504-eligibility.pdf.

Schoonover, J. (2019). Best practices in universal design for learning. In G. Frolek Clark, J. E. Rioux, & B. E. Chandler (Eds.), *Best practices for occupational therapy in schools* (2nd ed.) (pp. 161–176). AOTA Press.

Shogren, K., Wehmeyer, M., Palmer, S., Rifenbark, G., & Little, T. (2015). Relationships between self-determination and postschool outcomes for youth with disabilities. *The Journal of Special Education, 48*(4), 256–267.

Shrumpt, S. (2019). Best practices in safe transportation. In G. Frolek Clark, J. Rioux, & B. Chandler (Eds.), *Best practices for occupational therapy in schools* (2nd ed.) (pp. 177–185). AOTA Press.

The Improving Access to Assistive Technology for Individuals with Disabilities Act of 2004, 108-364.

U.S. Department of Education. (2012). *Questions and answers on the ADA Amendments Act of 2008 for students with disabilities attending public elementary and secondary schools*. Retrieved from https://www2.ed.gov/about/offices/list/ocr/docs/dcl-504faq-201109.html.

Workforce Innovation and Opportunity Act, Pub. L. 113-128, 3101, *et. seq.* Cong. Rec. (2014) https://www.gpo.gov/fdsys/pkg/PLAW-113publ128/html/PLAW-113publ128.htm.

World Health Organization. (2012). *The world health report 2010: Health systems financing: The path to universal coverage*. Author.

16

# Play Intervention

*Helen Lynch and Alice Moore*

## GUIDING QUESTIONS

1. How is play defined from an occupational perspective?
2. What are play issues related to childhood development, social sciences, and anthropology?
3. What are the characteristics of play and its contribution to issues of mastery, identity, belonging, community connectedness, and participation?
4. What are different approaches in the continuum of play-based occupational therapy, and what are their benefits?

## KEY TERMS

Context
Context therapy
Form, function and meaning
Occupational justice
Play
Play as an occupation
Play as progress
Play deprivation
Playfulness
Universal Design for Play

> ***Quote:*** *"How do we discover who we are? How do we determine the character of the world in which we live? And how do we decide what we can do in the world so configured? We learn about ourselves and the world through acts of play." (Henricks, 2015, p. 1)*

This chapter aims to explore play in occupational therapy, which requires us to explore first, play as an occupation and its place in childhood. So, let's begin with a focus on situatedness: where is play in your life, in your community, and in your situated experience?[1] These questions are important because play is an occupation that is shaped by the sociocultural, spatial, historical, and political context within which it is conducted (Lynch, 2023). While it certainly has a universal dimension (i.e., play is a universal human behavior), that does not mean play is universally the same across cultures. So, taking an occupational perspective requires us to not only consider development but to also consider play from other lenses such as sociology and anthropology. Importantly, there is a multidimensional aspect to **play as an occupation** that is subjective, situated within specific contexts, and therefore requires a deeper insight into how it is shaped and influenced by the diverse environments in which it is enacted.

In moments of crises, we realize most visibly the fundamental place of play in children's lives. Children from war-torn countries seek to play to help make sense of their worlds, to express the meaning of things they are experiencing, and to solve emotional distress. In response, adults seek to provide play spaces in refugee centers, and play programs have a significant place in program provision in response to crises (see, for example, Chatterjee, 2017). During COVID-19 lockdowns, schools were closed in many countries, in addition to local playgrounds, and children were unable to play together in their communities. See Fig. 16.1. The impact of such restrictions soon became obvious at a societal level, and in some countries, it led to a government-level response, supported by the International Play Association who produced materials in various languages to support parents and carers to address play, due to its "significant therapeutic role in helping children recover a sense of normality and joy" (see https://ipaworld.org/resources/for-parents-and-carers-play-in-crisis/).

The importance of play is currently well acknowledged by adults in many countries who have developed new insights into its significance for children to thrive in childhood. Yet adults need a lot of help to truly understand play from a child's perspective. For example, think about play … think about your memories of play when you were young. Can you feel the moment, and can you figure out why it stays in your memory? Usually when we ask people to remember moments of play from their childhood, there is a lot of excitement and laughter in the discussions and shared experiences of what seems in hindsight quite simple events—often without the use of toys or what adults might consider play objects. It often involves the freedom of the outdoors and is away from adults, and it may or may not be with others. Yet play in occupational therapy is typically quite different from these kinds of memories: it is often adult led, involving manufactured toys and objects designed to support skill development. Indeed, when we explore the use of play in occupational therapy in countries from different continents including North America, Europe, and Asia, we see similar patterns in practice: play is most often used as a means to an end, to support skill development for other reasons (e.g., to develop fine motor skills), and practitioners often have had little training on play as an occupation (Lynch et al., 2017; Miller Kuhaneck et al., 2013; Moore & Lynch, 2018a; Yakup & Dahlan, 2022). Why is there such a chasm between what we know play to be and how we use play in practice?

[1]Note: situatedness is the concept related to knowing how your specific historical, cultural, and family experiences shape the way you interpret and respond to the world.

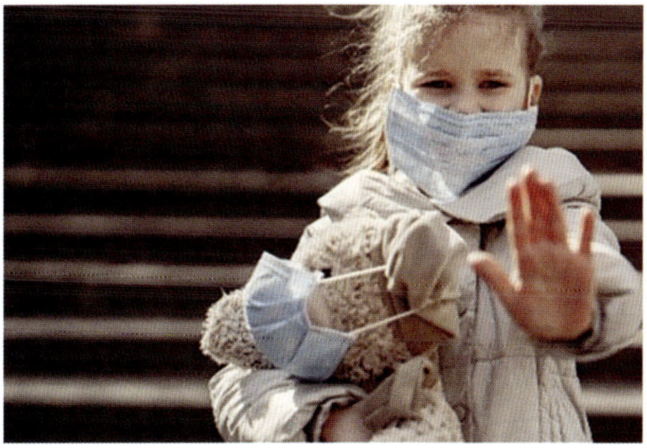

**Fig. 16.1** COVID-19 had an impact on children's play. (*Source*: Photo by Gustavo Fring, Pexels.)

This chapter seeks to address some of the problems occupational therapy practitioners face in addressing play. It aims to support occupational therapy practitioners to incorporate play in practice by providing deeper insights into play as an occupation, play theory, and evidence and, with this knowledge, how we can aim for more authentic evidence-informed play-based practice to truly address play as a goal and play as participation.

## WHAT IS PLAY? AN OCCUPATIONAL SCIENCE PERSPECTIVE

Play is accepted as a major area in a child's life, noted to be the primary occupation of childhood and the earliest occupation to develop (Adolfsson et al., 2010; Bundy, 1993; Lynch, 2012). So, it is essential that occupational therapy practitioners develop a strong knowledge of play theory, play as an occupation, and occupational development to develop evidence-informed practice.

The first place to start is usually to define a concept, so we ask what is play? Play is rather difficult to define as it has been the focus of intensive interdisciplinary research, resulting in multiple varied definitions due to these diverse perspectives. In addition, in the past in occupational therapy, it was often ignored or sometimes defined in a similar way to leisure (Bundy & Du Toit, 2023), but in the American Occupational Therapy Practice Framework, fourth edition (OTPF-4), play is established as a stand-alone occupation, where **play** is defined as follows: activities that are intrinsically motivated, internally controlled, and freely chosen and that may include suspension of reality (e.g., fantasy; Skard & Bundy, 2008), exploration, humor, risk-taking, contests, and celebrations (Eberle, 2014; Sutton-Smith, 1997). Play is a complex and multidimensional phenomenon that is shaped by sociocultural factors (American Occupational Therapy Association [AOTA], 2020, p. 34; Lynch et al., 2016).

Play is defined in relation to the child's level of control and the associated experience of the activity as being fun or joyful; i.e., it is determined by the player (Bundy, 1993). In this regard, play is clearly defined here as an occupation, as it is presented as a subjective experience that evolves through the process of playing. It is also transformative, as it includes elements of flexibility, spontaneity, and testing of ideas, as players engage in forming and reforming events and actions in ways they devise and control themselves (Henricks, 2008). Other key elements that characterize play include that it is more about the process rather than the outcome, that it is noncompulsory, and that it can take place "whenever and wherever opportunities arise" (Committee on the Rights of the Child [CRC], 2013). Fig. 16.2. Play may be viewed, experienced, or defined differently among cultures. See Box 16.1. A key aspect to play that practitioners need to understand is that play is how a child engages in the world, to learn, develop, and flourish, without needing to be taught. This is a crucial factor as adults often logically assume that if a child learns through play, then providing more intensified or structured play will enhance learning, but often this results in adults high-jacking play for other purposes, and play disappears (CRC, 2013). Because of this threat to play, many play advocates have taken a clear stance on differentiating play from leisure and recreation, which are less central to learning as children move into adolescents and adulthood. So, while play is often used interchangeably and synonymously with recreation, play is distinguishable from recreational activity: even though both are voluntary, play is directed by children themselves, as a subconscious driver of learning, whereas recreation commonly takes the forms of activities for relaxation, often in the form of sport and games directed by adults (CRC, 2013).

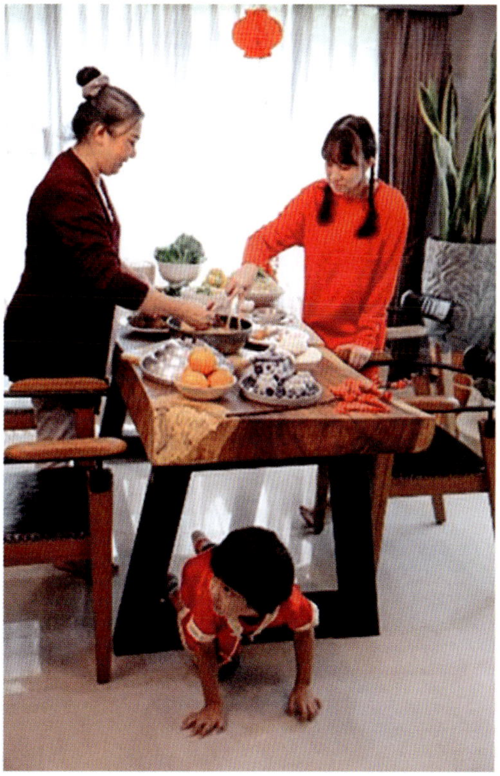

**Fig. 16.2** Children find places and spaces to play anywhere. (*Source*: Photo by Angela Roma, Pexels.)

### BOX 16.1 Cultural Definitions of Play

When we explore the meaning of play in different languages, we find that while it usually pertains to the child, it is not so clearly distinguishable from other concepts such as dallying, being playful, or amusement (Huizinga, 1950).

- Is there a word for play in your language?

See Huizinga's chapter on play concepts as expressed in language (1950) or a play on words by Bryan Boyle (https://www.p4play.eu/news/blog-posts/a-play-on-words-or-words-on-play/2021/10/22/).

Within the AOTA definition of play is the concept that is closely intertwined with play, i.e., the concept of playfulness. The definition of **playfulness** consists of the same three elements outlined above in play: intrinsic motivation, internal control, and freedom of constraints from reality (Bundy, 2011). Through decades of research on play and playfulness, Bundy and colleagues have progressed our knowledge of playfulness, which is considered to be a "disposition to engage in play" (Muys et al., 2006, p. 160). Playfulness as a disposition to play is expressed by children (and is also evident in adults), across the daily pattern of engagement in occupation, whether at mealtimes, while doing work/schoolwork, or indeed in play. In

**TABLE 16.1 Examples of Play Categories or Taxonomies and the Disciplinary Source**

| Categories or Taxomonies | Source | Disciplinary Focus | Age Group |
|---|---|---|---|
| Sensory-motor or exploratory play | Piaget (1962)<br>Hutt (1979) | Cognitive psychology<br>Behavioral psychology | Infancy<br>Preschool children aged 3–5 years |
| Object play | Rochat (1989, 1993), Rochat et al. (1999) | Developmental psychology | Infants aged 1 to 12 months |
| Physical activity play as it evolves (rhythmic stereotypies; exercise play; rough-and-tumble play) | Pellegrini and Smith (1998) | Educational psychology: Physical play taxonomy | Infancy to middle childhood |
| Risky play types (great height; high speed; dangerous tools; dangerous elements; rough-and-tumble; disappearing and getting lost) | Sandseter (2007) | Early childhood education: Risky play types | Preschool children aged 4–5 years |
| Social play as it evolves (unoccupied; onlooker; solitary; parallel; associative; cooperative) | Parten (1932) | Sociology: Social play taxonomy | Preschool children aged 2–5 years |
| Pretend play as it evolves (functional; constructive; pretend/dramatic; games with rules) | Smilansky (1968) | Cognitive psychology | Preschool children aged 3–5 years |
| Symbolic and imaginative play subcategories: Themes/play scripts; sequences of play actions; object substitution; social interaction; role-play; doll/teddy play | Stagnitti (2007) | Occupational therapy | Infants and preschoolers aged 18 months to 5 years |

this way, playfulness can be seen in many occupations other than play, as it is more about a person's approach or attitude toward the activity at hand.

In the study of occupational science, **form, function, meaning**, and **context** are central to understanding an occupation (Clark et al., 1991), and for play, this includes explaining the research on what children themselves say about play. The next sections outline these core considerations beginning with forms of play, so readers can consider the breadth of play as an occupation that has been identified and then onto meaning to centralize the subjective experiences of children from their own words and continuing with connecting function and context.

## FORMS OF PLAY

In occupational therapy, it is helpful to know the different forms or patterns of play (also known as a taxonomy), as this captures some ways to think about what children do when they play. Understanding the different types of play helps the occupational therapy practitioner better observe skills for occupational analysis. It is helpful to know firstly the disciplinary origins of the evidence as these influence what is prioritized in the research itself. For example, Piaget was a cognitive psychologist and valued play for what illuminates children's cognitive abilities in assimilation and accommodation or learning, which is an expression of the mental processes (Piaget, 1962). While many of the play forms that have been identified in research are drawn from psychology, not all of them are (see Table 16.1).

Play can be described in terms of the activity type or general patterns of behavior and can be categorized into various subtypes (e.g., social play or risky play). Indeed, Henricks described at least 12 forms of play types, including mastery play, construction play, and language play (Burghardt, 2011). Research has also identified how the type of play evolves in different phases of development as it becomes more complex. For example, Piaget identified the phases of play from sensorimotor/exploratory or practice play, from birth to 2 years, to preoperational/symbolic play from 2 to 7 years, and games with rules, from seven onward (Piaget, 1962). While it is helpful to identify the various types of play, children typically play in multiple ways in any one play event, so an integrated perspective of play is also required, where the phases and forms of play are considered concurrently.

These different play taxonomies can be applied universally in general, although it is acknowledged that these taxonomies were drawn primarily from research in Europe and North America (Trawick-Smith, 2010). It is therefore important to consider that there may be differences due to culture or disability within them. Play development is culturally situated and influenced and therefore can develop differently depending on the context. For example, in Trawick-Smith's (2010) study of children's play in Puerto Rico, he identified music play as a common form of play for these preschoolers, which reflected the dominance of music on their communities. In our occupational therapy community, Dender and Stagnitti (2015) completed a historical review of research on play in an Australian indigenous context, which resulted in them challenging the deterministic view that all children play in the same or similar ways: "it can be argued that play is situational, culturally contextual and socially constructed because play takes different forms in different cultures and some forms of play are discouraged or have a different emphasis in some cultural groups" (p. 3). In another example relating to disability, Barton (2010) analyzed studies of play in autistic children and found that their development of pretend play had its own pattern or trajectory that differed from typically developing children. Few studies have been conducted to repeat this approach to researching play taxonomies across other disability groups. Given that children of different types of disabilities often have unique play patterns, more research is needed to identify potential diversity across these common play types and sequences of development outlined in Table 16.1.

### Infant Play

For young children, and children with disabilities, exploratory and sensorimotor play dominates in the early years and begins with a focus on body play (Nagy, 2011). This phase of play moves into exploration of the world around the infant and is where the child explores what objects can do and what they can do with objects (e.g., moving from banging an object on the floor to banging two objects together as the infant learns to work both hands concurrently) as they learn to consciously control body movements and work toward mastery (Galloway & Thelen, 2004). Indeed, in more mature forms of play, this exploratory phase is often still evident as the child figures out how to play with the material world around them before engaging in more complex forms of play such as symbolic play or risky play. Early social play is evident with games such as peekaboo, common across the world, where the carer hides and then reappears to the infant (Lancy, 2007). These examples of infant play contain experiences that are based on cause-and-effect games or turn-taking. Typically, the child

**TABLE 16.2 Mapping Infant Space and Object Play (Lynch, 2012)**

| INFANT PLAY: CHARACTERISTICS OF PLAY WITH THE PHYSICAL ENVIRONMENT | | | |
|---|---|---|---|
| **STATIONARY PLAY** | | **MOBILE PLAY** | |
| **Body Space** | **Near Space** | **Middle Space** | **Home Space** |
| Body play: sitting play; floor play; reaching and crawling play; platform play; walking play | | | |
| Objects brought into the infant's space | | Infants move into the objects' space | |
| Baby toys/soft toys; objects in the home; sharing toys; "learning" toys and pretend play | | | |

expands their repertoire of play of skills in parallel to their emerging ability to move about the home setting (Karasik et al., 2011; Lynch, 2012), so it is impossible to separate out the object play aspect from the environmental affordances (Table 16.2). Overall, during this first phase of play, the infant engages in many forms of play that are evident in play events, including object play, early social play, and physical activity play.

### Preschooler Play

As the child develops further skills and abilities, from about 18 months to 6 years, their use of language influences their play, as it enables the child to explore ideas, use their imagination, and develop mental representations through pretend and symbolic play (Haight & Miller, 1993; Nicolich, 1977). This leads to an expanded ability to engage in pretend play as it evolves from using real objects or miniatures to represent the real object (e.g., a mobile phone or pretend phone) to using other objects as substitutes (Pellegrini & Bjorklund, 2004). It is a phase of play where the child is engaged in inner processes that are expressed externally in what they do (Stagnitti & Unsworth, 2000). Pretend play is closely embedded in social play also as the child engages in associative and cooperative play together with other children (Parten, 1932). Imitation and turn-taking with peers are more evident, as well as the capacity to use humor and mischievousness (Bergen, 2006). As noted earlier, some children with disabilities, such as those with autism, may develop social play in a different trajectory, with parallel play being an important aspect of their play for longer than other children (Kangas et al., 2012). Case Example 16.1 describes an occupational therapy intervention session to promote symbolic play.

**CASE EXAMPLE 16.1 PROMOTING PRETEND PLAY**

**Imagination and Playfulness**

Phoenix is a 5-year-old child with mildly delayed motor skills but very limited pretend play. Whenever the occupational therapist says, "Ok, now you be the fireman, and we can pretend to ..." Phoenix will respond, "I'm not a fireman, I am Phoenix." Attempts to use hose-shaped objects to pretend to spray water on pretend fires are unsuccessful. The occupational therapy practitioner's (Malik's) attempts at pretending with role-play are also unsuccessful until he brings in very realistic props. When Malik comes in with a firefighter's outfit and a plastic fire hat, Phoenix smiles and enthusiastically puts his outfit and hat on too. They build a firehouse out of red cardboard blocks and use a red ride-on toy as the fire truck. Malik encourages Phoenix to ride the fire truck to the fire (making siren noises for added effect). He rides to the sink area, where Phoenix can put out the "fire" (a picture of a fire drawn with washable red, orange, and yellow markers) using a plant sprayer with water. As the water sprays on the washable marker drawing of the fire, it washes away, and the fire is then out.

The practitioner then creates similar games such as this using realistic props for playing doctor and police officer. Over time, Malik can get Phoenix to pretend with fewer realistic props, then with fewer props, until eventually he can just role-play using his imagination and whatever materials happen to be on hand.

This case example illustrates how to promote pretend play in a therapy session. In this scenario, the practitioner directs a play session engaging the child in symbolic play. While Malik directs the session, he is mindful that the child should be in control if possible. Play should be spontaneous, free from rules, and internally motivated. Therefore, the practitioner gives Phoenix time and space to initiate ideas and contribute to the pretend games. Malik uses a playful approach throughout the session to model play for the child. This example illustrates engaging children in the occupation (play) to enhance their abilities at that occupation.

During this preschool phase, children are at the same time increasing their repertoire in physical activity play and risky play, which are significantly associated with aspects of exploratory play as the child seeks to explore the expanded environment, often outdoors, and to master challenges relating to intensified sensory experiences related to greater height and more speed in movement for example (Pellegrini, 2006; Sandseter, 2007). With the enhanced engagement in increasingly more diverse community settings, the preschooler becomes more connected to their local community, which enhances feelings of belonging, and they begin to take a more active role in social participation.

### Play in Middle Childhood

In school and community settings, as the child moves into middle childhood (6–12 years), this intensified physical play phase is further enhanced by peer play, where the influence on others is evident. For example, children can be seen showing their skills to each other or helping and encouraging their friends to try something challenging (Hinchion et al., 2021). During this middle childhood phase, physical activity play includes rough-and-tumble play and play fighting, which are thought to contribute to a child's ability to control their social and antisocial behavior, and it results in increased social competence (Brussoni et al., 2015). However, these opportunities are impacted by the cultural context, which may support or hinder these types of play, which can sometimes result in children seeking to play away from adult gaze more often (Lynch, 2023). It is at this stage that children's play preferences become strongly established, along with their growing sense of identity (Phelan & Kinsella, 2009, 2014). Typically, at this stage however, pretend play is becoming less evident, and children seek more opportunities to develop games together or role-play scenarios, while at home, more board games and online play in digital environments are used more often (Kuhaneck & O'Brien, 2022; Loudoun et al., 2022). By late middle childhood, as the child moves toward adolescence, play evolves into leisure and recreation and typically is more focused on collective social pursuits that move away from family toward peers and include activities such as sports, online gaming, and hanging-out activities (Bazyk, 2022).

## MEANING OF PLAY

When considering **play as an occupation**, the subjective **meaning** of play for an individual is regarded as one of the most important considerations (Kuhaneck & O'Brien, 2022). Kuhaneck and O'Brien (2022) recently asserted that "the meaning attributed to play may be as varied and unique as the individual players" (p. 58). Yet, for many years, adults considered childhood work (e.g., schooling) and play to be the same thing, until researchers began to explore ways to study the child's experience (Howard & McInnes, 2013a, 2013b). In their study of preschoolers in Wales, Howard and McInnes found that children could identify what they thought of play in school; it was most like play when there was no adult, when they could choose and control their play and choose the location for play, which was usually away from the classroom table (see Fig. 16.3).

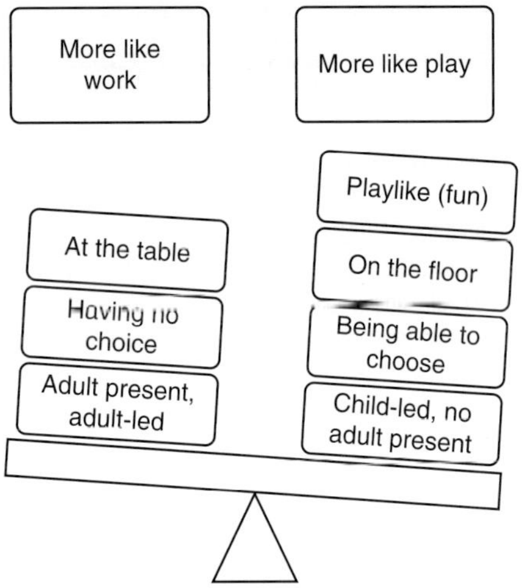


**Fig. 16.3** Work-play continuum at preschool from a child's perspective.

More recently, in a review of studies seeking to understand play from a child's perspective across 14 countries from five continents, Lynch found that this idea of play appears to be consistent across cultures (Lynch, 2023). So, play is understood by children to be different from work, and if it is play, it is something they choose and control for themselves. When we think of using play therefore in therapy, we can see that the children may not experience it as play at all.

Children have also said how play makes them feel, and this has become an important avenue for exploring well-being in children. The strong connection with well-being and happiness has led to researchers using happiness as a measure of quality of life and well-being in childhood (Moore & Lynch, 2018b). For example, in this occupational science study of children aged 6–8 years in Ireland, children identified that happiness is strongly related to play, because play means something that is fun and makes them feel good (Moore & Lynch, 2018b). In this study, it was evident how play was central to an enhanced feeling of belonging and connectedness to family and community. Furthermore, Howard and McInnes (2013a, 2013b) compared the well-being of children experiencing work-like or play-like practices in preschool, and those who engaged in play-like approaches scored higher on well-being. However, in studies of children with disabilities, community play events were not always associated with fun, as in their experience, places to play were not accessible, and therefore they were often excluded from play experiences with their friends (Prellwitz & Skär, 2007). The outcome for these children and families is that they do not feel like they belong in their communities, so inclusion in play is a vital component of belonging and well-being.

When children are asked more about play, they also provide more insight on what kind of play is valuable for them and why. For example, play is something that involves challenge (Miller & Kuhaneck, 2008) and some sense of achievement (Prellwitz & Skär, 2007) but should not be too hard or too easy (Norðdahl & Einarsdóttir, 2014). It is most fun when it involves some risk or excitement (Sandseter, 2009). As children grow older, studies have also highlighted that children seek valued play experiences that sometimes are not valued equally by adults, such as online gaming or more risk-taking in play (Glenn et al., 2012). So, although occupations are typically considered to be defined as socially sanctioned activities (Yerxa, 1990), this is not always the case when you consider the different and often conflicting views of adults and children in relation to play.

While there is evidently a universal experience associated with the meaning of play among children, this does not mean there are no cultural differences in their communities, however. Anthropological studies across cultures confirm play differences that are due to geographic factors such as indoor play being prioritized in colder climates (Lancy, 2007) or sociocultural factors such as play not being valued among adults in the culture (Bazyk et al., 2003) or work being prioritized for girls as they get older (CRC, 2013). Indeed, in a review of 186 ethnographies, Lancy (2007) found that infant-mother play is common across cultures in infancy but is quite rare in many cultures as the child ages. In addition, Munambah et al. (2022) found that male family members (fathers or grandfathers) are not free to play with their children in their culture in Zimbabwe, as children have to show their fathers respect. These cultural differences have significant implications for therapy practice as we may automatically assume that infant-mother/father/carer play is happening at home and beyond childhood, but this may not be how play occurs in a specific cultural context. Therefore, occupational therapy practitioners need to attune to the cultural values and attitudes toward play if they seek to address play authentically in practice (Lynch, 2023; Lynch et al., 2016).

To summarize, when children are asked about their play, they consistently highlight the importance of fun, pleasure, choice, and freedom (Alexander et al., 2014; Glenn et al., 2012; Moore & Lynch, 2018a). Researchers have identified that if these qualities identified by the children are absent, children no longer consider it play (Glenn et al., 2012). However, Kuhaneck and O'Brien (2022) recently reminded us that not all play is wonderful: play may be scary, cruel, dangerous, risky, sexualized, and not completely free. It can be about struggles for power and dominance, and it may not always be accessible and available for all (Kuhaneck & O'Brien, 2022).

## IDENTIFYING THE CONTRIBUTION PLAY MAKES TO CHILDHOOD: FUNCTION OF PLAY

Analysis of the distinctive forms or categories of play inevitably questions why this behavior is important (Lester & Russell, 2008). Historically, as the focus of play shifted from determining what play is to establishing what play is good for, scientific research established its beneficial effects (Wood & Chesworth, 2021). Indeed, the traditional emphasis from play studies has concentrated on the benefits that an individual might accrue from participating in play (Lester & Russell, 2010). Reviews of the research evidence conducted by the American Academy of Pediatrics identified the "critical importance of play in facilitating parent engagement; promoting safe, stable and nurturing relationships; encouraging the development of numerous competencies, including executive functioning skills; and improving life course trajectories" (Ginsburg, 2007; Milteer et al., 2012; Yogman et al., 2018). Moreover, in the International Play Association (IPA) Declaration (2014), play was deemed to be essential for children's physical and mental growth and for enhancing their ability to function in the culture and society in which they are born. Furthermore, Lester and Russell (2010) determined that play promotes creativity, imagination, self-confidence, self-efficacy, and physical, social, cognitive, and emotional strength and skills, and as a protective process, it can enhance adaptive capabilities and resilience.

In addition to these reviews, further research provides evidence on the wide-ranging benefits of play (e.g., Brussoni et al., 2015; Gleave & Cole-Hamilton, 2012; Tremblay et al., 2015; Whitebread et al., 2017). One dimension of the wide-ranging positive effects is the development of cognitive capacities (Nielsen, 2021). Interaction with other children through the practice of playing is also thought to be critically important for children's development of certain social skills essential for the ability to participate in social life (Nielsen, 2021). Moreover, a large body of evidence in the field of early childhood has established the importance of diverse forms of playing for early learning and development.

Historically, research in the field of occupational therapy has demonstrated the benefits of play for children's skill development (Rodger &

Ziviani, 1999; Stagnitti, 2004; Sturgess, 2003); indeed, occupational therapy practitioners often use play to support the skill development of children with disabilities (Parham, 2008; Rodger & Ziviani, 1999). Also, there is increasing recognition of the importance of play for learning-relevant processes such as self-regulation, meta-cognition, memory, attention, and problem-solving (Robson, 2010; Whitebread et al., 2017).

Additionally, there is increasing recognition of the importance of play from a public health perspective (Alexander et al., 2014; Vitale, 2011). Specifically, researchers have attributed a myriad of social, emotional, cognitive, and physical benefits that children can accrue from participating in outdoor play that is less supervised, less structured, more adventurous, and includes elements of challenge and risk (Brussoni et al., 2015; Gill, 2007; Sandseter, 2011). Moreover, numerous health benefits have been attributed to play that involves physical activity, such as enhanced efficacy of the immune, endocrine, and cardiovascular systems (Lubans et al., 2010), decreased body mass index (Ansari et al., 2015), and reduced depressive symptoms (Korczak et al., 2017).

Outdoor play is increasingly recognized as significant for children's development, health, and well-being (Loebach et al., 2021; Lynch et al., 2020; Tremblay et al., 2015). In particular, children's participation in outdoor play has been associated with positive effects on cardiorespiratory fitness (Schaefer et al., 2014) and cardiovascular and metabolic health biomarkers (Clements, 2004), alongside overall health (Alexander et al., 2014; Brussoni et al., 2012) and quality of life (Bento & Dias, 2017). Additionally, researchers have identified that when children play outside, they benefit from being exposed to sunlight, natural elements, and open air, all of which relate to a stronger immune system, bone development, as well as physical activity (Bilton, 2010; Dyment & Bell, 2008).

Furthermore, research in the field of neuroscience has associated play in childhood with brain development and functioning (Loebach & Cox, 2020). For example, neuroscience studies have demonstrated that when children play, all areas of the brain "light up," leading to adaptive and prosocial changes at each of the molecular, cellular, and behavioral levels, reinforcing that play activities can simultaneously foster development and learning across all domains—physical, social, cognitive, and emotional (Brown, 2009; Yogman et al., 2018). Emerging from these insights, Loebach and Cox (2020) recently asserted that "we should guard against an approach to play which creates artificial silos between developmental domains, associating certain types of play with a single area of development, but rather understanding play as activities which integrate development across domains" (p. 2). It is perhaps not surprising then that the impact of play is considered cumulative and iterative; indeed, researchers have asserted that skills and knowledge that children accrue from participating in play nurture both short- and long-term developmental benefits (Athey, 2018; Brown, 2009).

## CONTEXT OF PLAY

Context is defined as the environmental and personal factors specific to each person/group/population that influence engagement and participation in occupations (AOTA, 2020). Occupations (in this case, play) occur in contexts and are influenced by the transaction between each element: the person, their contexts, and the occupation. Therefore, context must always be considered when looking at play (AOTA, 2020). The terms context and environment are often used interchangeably in the literature; however, according to the OTPF-4, context includes consideration for environmental factors and personal factors (AOTA, 2020). For this section, we focus specifically on environmental factors, and we consider the environment as a determinant of occupation (Hocking, 2021).

Early descriptions of the environment in occupational science focused on its sociocultural characteristics (Hocking, 2021), whereby environments were considered to include conventions guiding behavior, expectations about successful performance, and "psychological, social, cultural, and spiritual demands" (Yerxa, 1990, p. 7). Building on these initial ideas, AOTA expanded on environmental factors to include consideration for the physical (i.e., natural and built environment, including products and technology), social, attitudinal, familial, and political surroundings (i.e., services, systems, and policies) that influence people's lives (AOTA, 2020). Play is known to be highly susceptible to all these environmental factors and can be impacted by the actions or inactions of adults (Casey, 2017).

In relation to the political environment for play, the right to play was established as one of the 41 rights of the child, known as articles (United Nations Convention on the Rights of the Child [UNCRC], 1989). It is important to note that this right to play is for children and does not apply to adults. Article 31, as the right to play, values and protects children's play irrespective of its development and social imperatives (Lester & Russell, 2008). Even so, the child's right to play "is one of the least-known, least-understood and least-recognized rights of childhood and is therefore currently one of the most consistently ignored, undervalued and violated around the world" (IPA, 2010, p. 3). Moreover, many children experience inequity in play opportunities and participation (CRC, 2013). Furthermore, the United States remains one of the only countries that has not ratified the UNCRC, which means that rather than being viewed as a right, play can be seen as a privilege that is granted to certain groups of children and denied to others (Souto-Manning, 2017).

To inform policy, the CRC outlines how play environments need to be considered to realize the child's right to play and determined that certain optimal environmental conditions need to be assured if children are to realize their Article 31 rights (see Box 16.2; CRC, 2013). They also identified several factors that are impacting upon children's ability to access, use, and be included in spaces for play (CRC, 2013). These include unsafe and hazardous environments, resistance to children's use of public spaces balancing risk and safety, lack of access to nature, pressure for educational achievement, overly structured and programmed schedules, and lack of investment, for example (CRC, 2013).

In relation to the physical environment, the provision of space for play in the built environment takes many forms, including, for example, parks, playgrounds, school playgrounds, public open spaces, streets, and green spaces (IPA, 2016). The International Play Association (2016) further identified that although some of these spaces are perceived and valued as "natural" and others are planned, designed, and managed, they can serve the same purpose. However, listing spaces where children's play takes place does not adequately reflect the range of places in which children (by choice or necessity) play; these spaces may include spaces temporarily claimed by children, spaces disregarded by adults or authorities, and the spaces between buildings and settlements, such as streets (IPA, 2016). So, playgrounds are not the only community places for play that need to be explored when working with children and when aiming to enhance play participation in their communities. See Fig. 16.4 showing the influence of geography and climate on play.

When the sociocultural environment for play is explored, many attitudinal and sociocultural factors have been identified showing how play is changing internationally. Indeed, there is considerable evidence emerging that documents how children's play, particularly in outdoor environments, has dramatically declined across the past several generations particularly in the Global North (Dodd et al., 2021; Gray, 2011; Lee et al., 2021; Loebach et al., 2021; Tremblay et al., 2015). Several ongoing societal shifts have been identified as contributing factors, including neighborhood social and environmental conditions, children's safety and parental concerns, lifestyle changes, and changing social norms around children's independent mobility (Brussoni et al., 2012; Loebach et al., 2021; Singer et al., 2009; Tremblay et al., 2015).

**BOX 16.2 Factors for an Optimum Play Environment**

Children and youth have a spontaneous urge to play and participate in recreational activities and will seek out opportunities to do so. The following factors should be available to support children's play, based on Article 31 (CRC, 2013).

- Accessible play environments that support their play and recreation, which include freedom from stress, social exclusion, prejudice, or discrimination.
- The play environment should be secure from social harm and violence and sufficiently free from pollution, traffic, and other hazards that impede free and safer movement.
- Availability for rest and leisure time, as well as space that is free from adult control and management.
- Space to play outdoors in diverse and challenging physical environments, with access to supportive adults, when necessary.
- Opportunities to experience, interact with, and play in natural environments and the animal world.
- Opportunities to invest in their own space and time to create and transform their world, using their imagination and languages.
- Opportunities to explore and understand the cultural and artistic heritage of their community and participate, create, and shape it.
- Opportunities to participate with other children in games, sports, and other recreational activities, supported, where necessary, by trained facilitators or coaches.
- Recognition by parents, teachers, and society of the value and legitimacy of the rights provided for in Article 31 (CRC, 2013).

Modified from Committee on the Rights of the Child [CRC]. (2013). *General comment No. 17 on the right of the child to rest, leisure, play, recreational activities, cultural life, and the arts*, pp. 10–11 https://www.refworld.org/docid/51ef9bcc4.html.

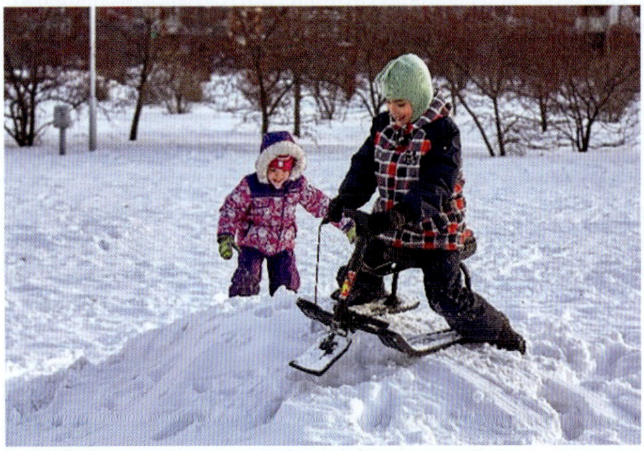

**Fig. 16.4** Geography and climate influence play. Children enjoy playing in the snow. (*Source*: Photo by Bulat Khamitov, Pexels.)

Consequently, researchers have coined numerous terms to document this decline in play opportunities, such as **play deprivation** (Bundy et al., 2011) and "poverty of experience" (Welsh Government, 2014). Moreover, the CRC (2013) identified that certain groups of children are at increased risk of fewer opportunities to participate in play (often referred to as "at risk of play deprivation" in the literature). These groups include children with disabilities, girls, children living in poverty, children in institutions, children from indigenous and minority communities, as well as children in situations of conflict and humanitarian and natural disasters. And while decreased opportunities apply to many children, it is potentially amplified for children with disabilities because of additional factors including attitudinal, physical, and social barriers resulting in reduced opportunities to benefit from participating in play compared with other children (Anaby et al., 2014).

However, most countries around the world have ratified the UNCRC, where ratification means that state parties (i.e., governments) commit to undertaking all appropriate legislative, administrative, and other measures for the full realization of provisions of the UNCRC, and thus, they can be held accountable for violations of the rights it contains. Therefore, to provide for the child's right to play requires governments to value play as important for its own sake, as outlined in Article 31. This suggests a shift from viewing play solely for instrumental purposes, that is, nonplay skill development, to appreciating the intrinsic, or autotelic, value of play (Lester & Russell, 2010). While not the only profession concerned with the right to play, occupational therapy provides a unique perspective on play as an occupation. In this way, play is valued for its intrinsic, or autotelic, value and not only for the using to learn other skills (Lynch & Moore, 2016).

## THEORIES OF PLAY: PLAY RHETORIC AND MOVING BEYOND PLAY AS DEVELOPMENT

Now that we have explored some of the foundational characteristics of play as an occupation, it is also important to situate these in relation to the bigger theories of what play means in human beings. For over 100 years, this topic has been the concern of many theorists and philosophers, from education and psychology, and animal behaviorists (or ethologists) among others (Henricks, 2008). From our knowledge of animal behavior, we know that play is a common behavior in juvenile animals and not just juvenile humans (Burghardt, 2005). Such play behavior appears to be dominant in youth and then fades as animals mature. In a similar manner, humans appear to grow out of play in many ways and engage in more mature behavior often called leisure or recreation, with a similar inner motivation and internal control (or playfulness) but with more focus on outcome (Bundy & Du Toit, 2023).

Play theories may be divided into classical and modern theories of play (Mellou, 1994; Parham, 2008). Classical play theories (e.g., surplus energy theory, recreation or relaxation theory, pre-exercise theory, and recapitulation theory) emerged in the 19th century and attempted to explain the existence and purpose of play (Mellou, 1994). Classical theories were developed by opinion or observation of children, and most of these theories indicated some future benefit with reference to survival (Kuhaneck & O'Brien, 2022). Modern play theories (e.g., arousal modulation theories, psychodynamic theories, cognitive development theories, play as socialization, and metacommunicative theory) emerged after 1920 and tried to explain the role of play in child development (Mellou, 1994). Modern theorists have subsequently developed more complex insights into play and consequently have expanded on play theories.

In 1997, an eminent scholar of play, Brian Sutton-Smith, undertook a review and synthesis of hundreds of play studies to seek some synthesis and proposed they could be aligned with seven categories (or rhetoric of play) that dominated the diverse literature (Sutton-Smith, 1997). Of these, the one that seems to relate most closely to occupational therapy is "play as progress." **Play as progress** refers to play primarily as it relates to child development. This means that play is primarily valued for its contribution to skill development, while undervaluing any inherent fun or well-being aspects. The danger of adopting or prioritizing this rhetoric is that we are at risk of high-jacking play for other means (i.e., only using play as a medium in therapy to achieve progress in skill development). This, it is argued, has given rise to the development of "instrumentalized" "good" and "correct" forms of play, which subsequently questions the essence of play (Gleave & Cole-Hamilton, 2012). Although play is primarily described in the literature as something that belongs to children, an occupation that they are intrinsically motivated to participate in, placing adults in control of children's play to instrumentalize it for other reasons results in the children no longer being the rightful owners of play. Indeed, Parham (2008) suggests we need to take care in how we approach play in occupational therapy, especially if we only consider a play-as-progress approach, and to consider instead a further rhetoric of "play as health" (Parham, 2008, p. 18).

However, there is also a more recent rhetoric to consider. Since 1997, much work has been done to examine play from a social science perspective and most significantly from a child's rights perspective, as noted earlier (e.g., Lester & Russell, 2010; Woolley, 2013). Both perspectives view play as an occupation that is inherently fundamental to the now of childhood and not about a future child. That means play is important in and of itself and not for some future benefit in adulthood. This aligns closely with an occupational science approach, where doing, being, and belonging are already valued, alongside becoming (Wilcock & Hocking, 2015). For occupational therapy practitioners, including this perspective on play in the now of childhood, which talks of play for the sake of play (and not for something else such as fine motor skill development), expands our potential to address play provision as an issue of social and occupational justice (AOTA, 2008; Lynch et al., 2018; Lynch & Moore, 2018).

## PLAY IN OCCUPATIONAL THERAPY

From our overview of play so far, it is clear how central it is in childhood, fundamental for development, health, and well-being, as well as enabling children to enact culture, while strengthening meaning and belonging in their communities. It is important to begin by asking occupational therapy practitioners why they are interested in play, where does play fit within their service, or where is the potential to focus on play within their practice.

Many practitioners report barriers to implementing play-based practice. They identify challenges from micro to macro levels, including poor knowledge of play theory or value, no training on play-based interventions, no autonomy in introducing play alongside other service provision priorities, and no insurance or funding approval to address play (Lynch et al., 2017; Miller Kuhaneck et al., 2013; Moore & Lynch, 2018a; Yakup & Dahlan, 2022). Yet, evidence consistently shows that children with disabilities are most frequently excluded from play compared with other groups of children and in most need of support for play participation (Adolfsson et al., 2010; Lynch & Moore, 2018; Prellwitz & Skär, 2016). Reassuringly however, practitioners are aware of this injustice, and there is evidence that they value play and consider it a fundamentally important occupation.

Following the occupational therapy commitment to person-environment-occupation models, play in occupational therapy needs to consider each of these three elements. Person-environment fit theories are built on three hypotheses (Van Vianen, 2018). First, the fit between a person and the environment is a better predictor of outcomes than person or environment factors only (Spitzer et al., 2022). Second, the greatest outcomes are likely when the characteristics of the person and the environment are well suited (Spitzer et al., 2022). Third, positive outcomes are lessened when the fit between a person and the environment does not occur; this can be the result of too little or too much of an attribute, for example (Spitzer et al., 2022). With reference to play and play spaces, person applies to the player, environment relates to play spaces, playthings, and play mates, as well as the sociocultural context of the home and community, while occupation refers to play (Kuhaneck & Metz, 2022). Together, the theories suggest that the fit between a child's characteristics and the play environment is significantly important when predicting play in play spaces (Spitzer et al., 2022). Examining this fit must be part of a comprehensive evaluation of play, as described in Chapter 9.

## PLAY-CENTERED OCCUPATIONAL THERAPY PRACTICE: CONTINUUM OF PLAY PROVISION

Play in occupational therapy has been influenced significantly by the play as progress rhetoric that was described earlier (Sutton-Smith, 1997), whereby there is a commonly accepted idea that play is primarily a means to support development. In doing so, occupational therapy practitioners have adopted many complimentary approaches such as play therapy to implement play-based interventions (Brown & Lynch, 2023). However, practitioners need to differentiate play therapy from play-based therapy: play therapy is an approach that requires further training and utilizes play to support children who deal with trauma, or stress, and usually play itself is not the goal. The primary focus is to examine the place of play in occupational therapy when play is the goal.

Historically in many countries, play-based occupational therapy approaches have been implemented using well-known concepts such as the zone of proximal development (Vygotsky, 1978). In Vygotsky's work, he proposes that the child is best helped when a caring adult knows the child's level of ability and can provide appropriate assistance to progress their play. However, as we have seen, this can result in an activity that is not actually play, when you consider the definition of play. It is often not controlled or informed by the child's play needs or process oriented. So, how do practitioners address play in therapy intervention so that play itself is the goal, i.e., that therapy is play-centered? They begin by analyzing the role they need to take on in delivering play intervention. This role analysis can be helped by considering play intervention as a continuum from work to play-like work, to work-like play, and finally to play as an occupation as illustrated in Fig. 16.5 (Lynch, 2016; Ray-Kaeser & Lynch, 2017).

The work-play continuum builds on the consensus in play research that adult-child play activities map across the play, playfulness, and work continuum (Wood, 2007; Zosh et al., 2018) and that practitioners need to be able to work fluidly across these approaches to be most effective. The following paragraphs describe these work-play roles beginning with (1) work, then (2) directed and guided play, and finally (3) play as an occupation.

### Work/Nonplay

Occupational therapy practitioners who take on a work role typically focus on a nonplayful approach to teach skills, for example using an acquisitional frame of reference or behavioral approach, using repetition and practice (Kramer & Hinojosa, 2010). The practitioner draws from knowledge of task analysis and task modification to support the child's learning, using techniques such as prompting, modeling, or reinforcement of behavior. While the goal might be to enhance play, the focus in the therapy session is teaching a specific skill such as turn-taking or practicing with miniature toys to teach symbolic play skills (Luckett et al., 2007), and the practitioner may not be working in a playful manner. Specifically, the therapy intervention is not play based, as play is not the focus in the therapy session (Fisher, 2013). Instead, the target skill is practiced, usually in an adult-led structured way and may also involve an award system.

In their review of 47 behavioral interventions to improve play skills in children with autism, Luckett et al. (2007) found that the interventions typically aimed at addressing "appropriate play" rather than respecting the play styles of the children and often focused on reducing stereotyped

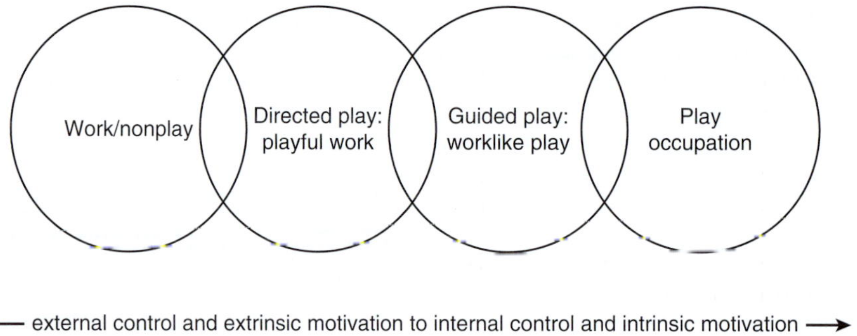


**Fig. 16.5** Play-centered occupational therapy roles: the work-play continuum. (From Lynch, H. (2023). Perspectives on the meaning of play: International, cultural and individual contexts. In H. Kuhaneck & S. Spitzer (Eds.), *Making play just right: Unleashing the power of play in occupational therapy* (2nd ed., pp. 399–430). Jones & Bartlett Learning; and Ray-Kaeser, S., & Lynch, H. (2017). Occupational therapy perspective on play for the sake of play. In S. Besio, D. Bulgarelli, & V. Stancheva-Popkostadinova (Eds.), *Play development in children with disabilities* (pp. 155–165). De Gruyter)

behaviors. While many of the studies reported changes in behavior following intervention, the extent to which it was generalized into a change in spontaneous play in natural environments after intervention was less clear. Interestingly, in a review of interventions for children with autism particularly targeting functional and symbolic play with toys, researchers found that the most effective studies included three core elements: modeling, prompting with reinforcement, and with some element of choice for the child in a natural learning setting (Lang et al., 2009). Yet, when typical children's play is explored in relation to activities that involve toys and play materials, researchers found that using a work role can override the child's drive to explore and discover for themselves, which are fundamental attributes for play and learning (Bonawitz et al., 2011). It is therefore important to carefully weigh any evidence for adult-led teaching and structured approaches, as they apply to specific populations, when play is the focus or goal of therapy.

## Directed Play/Guided Play

In directed or guided play, play is the focus in the therapy session as well as the goal, so it is considered a play-based intervention (Fisher, 2013). In play-based occupational therapy, the occupational therapy practitioner adopts a playful approach and targets play-based work occupations (Brown & Lynch, 2023). When the practitioner adopts a directed play or guided play role, they are playful and work to develop an atmosphere of play in the therapy session but guide the therapy session with a focus on a play skill or activity (Spitzer, 2022). This playful approach uses nonverbal and verbal communication to communicate playfulness, to build rapport, and to share control for the therapy session. Spitzer (2022) notes that this approach takes time to develop and requires practitioners learn to play and understand their own play styles as well as the sociocultural contexts of the children to ensure the intervention is authentic to their family values and community contexts. In play-based approaches, the practitioner draws from their knowledge of child development and uses play as the medium of learning either explicitly (Wilkes-Gillan, Bundy, Cordier, Lincoln, et al., 2016) or implicitly (Schaaf et al., 2013). In Wilkes-Gillan, Bundy, Cordier, Lincoln, et al. (2016) and Wilkes-Gillan, Bundy, Cordier, and Lincoln (2016) play-based intervention for children with ADHD, the practitioner explicitly models play behaviors for the child during child-led play sessions, whereas in Schaaf et al.'s (2013) play-based sensory integration intervention, play is the means through which the child leads the therapy session guided by the occupational therapy practitioner, who responds to the child's inner drive and scaffolds their engagement in self-selected sensory-motor play activities without modeling or coaching. Case Example 16.2 illustrates an occupational therapy intervention session using directed or guided play.

Guided play is effective in supporting learning, due to key factors relating to the context for learning: that the child learns best when they are actively involved and engaged and when the task is meaningful and the environment allows social interaction (Zosh et al., 2018). Interestingly, in Luckett et al.'s (2007) review of evidence of behavioral approaches to enhancing play in children with autism, the most effective studies were those that were not solely behavioral in their approach but also involved elements of guided play or scaffolded peer-supported play. See Fig. 16.6.

**Evidence for Play-Based Interventions Using Directed or Guided Play.** In recent years, researchers have examined the evidence for play-based therapy interventions. Commonly, the recognition of complexity in trying to do this is acknowledged due to the multiple philosophies involved. Consequently, the authors propose that there is a need to examine interventions using several factors, such as (1) identifying the role of play within the intervention, (2) the underpinning philosophy (e.g., behaviorist or developmental), and (3) the role of the practitioner (e.g., one-to-one intervention, group facilitation, parent feedback) (Gibson et al., 2021). It may also be important to include the nature of the child's play style as it relates to their diagnosis as this may influence how the child responds to play interventions also. Two examples of play based interventions that come from a developmental perspective and are implemented by occupational therapy practitioners will be presented to illuminate this approach to examining play interventions: for children with autism and for children with ADHD.

Several studies reviewed evidence for play-based interventions for children with autism (Gibson et al., 2021; Jung & Sainato, 2013; Kent et al., 2020; Kuhaneck et al., 2020; Lang et al., 2009). Children with autism often face challenges in forming relationships with others, and this is often associated with their different play styles in childhood, when friendships typically form. Therefore, many efforts have gone into developing interventions to enhance their abilities in social play, mostly in relation to typical development (Gibson et al., 2021; Jung & Sainato, 2013). One study specifically examined interventions for play for children with autism that have potential application in occupational therapy (Kuhaneck et al., 2020). Kuhaneck et al. found 20 studies that related to potential occupational therapy practice and identified that the most consistent and effective approach used was imitation of the child as they play, which was used in conjunction with other strategies such as modeling.

Kent et al. (2020) examined the strength of evidence for social play skills interventions from an randomized control trial (RCT) perspective in their

## CASE EXAMPLE 16.2 PLAY-BASED INTERVENTION USING GUIDED OR DIRECTED PLAY

### Sarah and Her Magic Beads

Sarah is a 2.5-year-old girl with mild spastic diplegia. She is playful, talkative, and extremely imaginative. A former premature infant, her primary motor impairment is independent ambulation, and despite the ability to walk, she is generally fearful of taking more than a few steps. Her favorite activity in occupational therapy is to play dress-up and direct everyone in the play theme of the day. Costumes are always involved for both Sarah and her occupational therapy practitioner, as are long strings of colorful beads. Most of the time, she crawls around in costume with her beads dragging along the therapy mats, or she walks holding the practitioner's hand. As a means of improving Sarah's confidence with walking, and to decrease her reliance on others, the practitioner begins using a string of Sarah's beads to gradually wean her from holding hands. First, the practitioner simply holds the beads in her palm as she holds Sarah's hand. Next, the clinician has Sarah help her hold the beads between their clasped hands. Then, the occupational therapy practitioner begins to lengthen the beads from a ball in the palms to a single strand of bead, one end held by Sarah and one by the practitioner. As Sarah's confidence grows, the practitioner gradually lengthens the bead fully out between them—a distance of about 18 inches—and then she eventually lets go of the bead chain completely! Sarah keeps walking with a big smile on her face, waving at the occupational therapy practitioner.

This case example illustrates the use of play to address intervention goals. Play is the focus of the therapy session and the goal (that Sarah can engage in play as she wishes), while the practitioner also guides the therapy session to focus on play skills (of mobility). The practitioner uses a playful approach and models play and play skills to engage in the session and scaffolds the activity so that Sarah can participate.

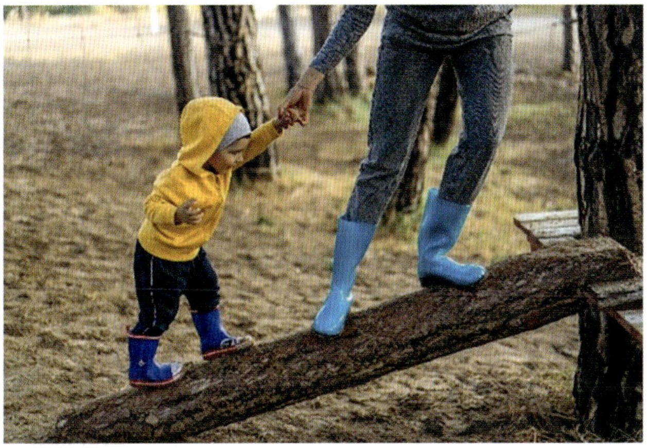

**Fig. 16.6** Scaffolding the activity so the child is successful is an example of guided play. The adult offers the toddler a hand, so the child can balance as they move along the slope in the playground. (*Source*: Photo by Oleksandr Pidvalnyi, Pexels.)

review. Of the 19 studies they identified, all used an outcome to measure impact on play. The meta-analysis identified that the strongest evidence so far is for interventions that focus on the individual child, rather than on groupwork, or on peers and parents, and for interventions that consist of combinations of approaches such as coaching and video modeling within the context of naturally occurring play opportunities. The duration and frequency of intervention sessions to achieve these outcomes were daily or twice a week for 30 minutes to 1 hour, over 6 to 12 weeks (Kent et al., 2020). However, across these 19 studies, the ability to determine whether the social play skills were generalized to other environments was not possible and has been flagged as an area for further study.

Finally, Gibson et al. (2021) review of 388 studies reported no play-based social play intervention that used a strengths-based approach, so none took into account the child's own play style and preferences. In summary, common to many of these reviews is the acceptance that while play skills can be taught for children with ASD in structured settings, there is a need to ensure that interventions are designed that build on the child's own interests to support free play with peers in natural settings as this is where children form friendships and social connections.

Similar to autism, children with ADHD experience significant difficulties in social play and forming friendships, and researchers have examined play-based occupational therapy interventions for this group of children (Barnes et al., 2017; Cordier et al., 2009; Cornell et al., 2018; Wilkes-Gillan, Bundy, Cordier, & Lincoln, 2016; Wilkes-Gillan, Bundy, Cordier, Lincoln, et al., 2016). Informed by the key characteristics of playfulness and play, Cordier, Wilkes-Gillan, Bundy, Cordier, Lincoln, et al. (2016) and Wilkes-Gillan, Bundy, Cordier, and Lincoln (2016) were able to identify which aspects of playfulness are likely to be impacted by the symptoms of ADHD and consequently to determine key objectives for intervention, namely "(1) to capture children's intrinsic motivation through the natural context of play, (2) facilitating the development of interpersonal empathy, (3) including a regular typically-developing playmate, for friendship development and (4) involving parents, to assist skill generalisation, and (5) therapist [practitioner] modeling to promote cooperative play between the two children" (p. 3). The intervention involved seven, weekly 1-h sessions over 10 weeks and included play in a clinic playroom where the children are filmed playing, and the practitioner models desired social play, based on preparation work with parents beforehand to gain insight into the child's play. The clinic session is accompanied by homework and training elements for the family. The results of this RCT show effectiveness for this approach to addressing social peer play for children with ADHD aged from 5 to 11 years. In these examples for children with ADHD, similar ingredients for successful outcomes are evident, when compared with the studies of interventions for children with autism, which include the use of multiple strategies to support learning, including modeling and video, while the importance of strengths-based, child-led play, with a focus on the play needs for a natural context, is promoted as the way forward.

## Play as an Occupation

When the occupational therapy practitioner's role is to address play as an occupation, guided play is not the main approach. Instead, the practitioner uses an occupation-focused approach and primarily works to provide space and time to play (CRC, 2013), so that the child's intrinsic motivation, internal control, and freedom of choice are supported. This requires the practitioner to consider how the environment supports or constrains the child's participation in play and identify modifications or accommodations to the environment to maximize play participation. See Case Example 16.3 for an example of how to engage children in play as an occupation. Recently, this approach has been termed a context therapy approach (Anaby et al., 2014; Darrah et al., 2011; Gibson et al., 2021; Law et al., 2011), which necessitates "a shift from individual, treatment focus of the profession to one which takes a population, advocacy perspective" (Hitch et al., 2012, p. 382). The practitioner may find that indirect therapy using consultative approaches and advocacy skills are the primary modes of intervention, along with universal or targeted approaches such as those involving environmental adaptations (Bundy et al., 2011; Hutton et al., 2016; Moore & Lynch, 2015). Although the evidence for context therapy approaches is only emerging, there are many examples of how addressing the environmental barriers can enhance play.

**Evidence for Interventions for Play as an Occupation.** Because children participate in play in home, school, and community environments, occupational therapy practitioners target these environments to improve the opportunities for play. Moore and Lynch (2015) proposed that practitioners can do this effectively by broadening their approach to include targeted and universal interventions that include other children and the broader community (Moore & Lynch, 2015).

Occupational therapy practitioners address play in the community through involvement in universal approaches with community based playgroups, which have been identified as effective for developing community belonging, as well as enhancing playfulness among families (Armstrong et al., 2019; Fabrizi & Hubbell, 2017). In home environments, occupational therapy practitioners work in a targeted way with parents and caregivers to determine family choices and preferences for play that reflect a family perspective rather than just focusing on the child (Coughlan & Lynch, 2011; Graham et al., 2015; Sterman et al., 2016). Additionally, occupational therapy practitioners work within educational settings to introduce new universal play-related activities on the playground for all children (Bundy et al., 2009, 2011, 2015, 2017; Sterman, Naughton, et al., 2020; Sterman, Villeneuve, et al., 2020) and to assess and/or modify the setting to make it more play friendly (Blake et al., 2018; Fahy et al., 2021; O'Connor et al., 2021).

Furthermore, in community contexts, significant attention has, in recent years, been directed toward the use of universal design to enhance inclusive design for public playgrounds (Moore & Lynch, 2018a; Perry et al., 2018; Prellwitz & Lynch, 2018; Sterman et al., 2016; Sterman, Villeneuve, et al., 2020). Occupational therapy practitioners may focus on the design of public spaces and showing how they can contribute their knowledge on play as an occupation in implementing universal design solutions to enable play (Moore et al., 2022a, 2022b, 2022c, 2023). Recently, Moore (2023) identified that occupational therapy practitioners can advance the conversation on how to apply universal design in public playgrounds as they possess unique knowledge on play as well as the transactional relationship between people, environments, and occupations. Specifically, Moore (2023) proposed a novel framework, **Universal Design for Play**, to communicate how the discourse on universal design may be expanded to include play as a central concern when designing built environments. This example illustrates how occupational therapy practitioners can provide interventions to impact individuals, communities, and populations.

Finally, occupational therapy practitioners providing direct interventions can support accommodations to remove barriers to play. For example, early provision of wheelchairs for children under 12 years who had mobility problems enhanced their play and their ability to participate in play with friends (Rousseau-Harrison & Rochette, 2012).

## TOYS

Toys are an important ingredient of play, and indeed, any object can become a toy if a child chooses to play with it (Kuhaneck & O'Brien, 2022; Ray-Kaeser et al., 2018). Anthropologists have found evidence of toys dating back for centuries and across continents (Lynch, 2023). Typically, such toys represented the culture within where they were found and often consisted of miniature versions of what adults use in daily routines for cooking or hunting (Chick, 2015).

In many countries, toys are now manufactured and given to children as gifts or to support learning and development (Edwards, 2000). Toys are designed to entice children to play, and a variety of characteristics are known to influence their use, usefulness, and/or desirability such as availability, materials and type, realism, novelty, control, and complexity (Kuhaneck & O'Brien, 2022). In selecting toys for play-based interventions, occupational therapy practitioners also need to consider core factors such as age appropriateness of the toy, the category of toy, and the child's age (Ray-Kaeser et al., 2018; Richards et al., 2020). In relation to addressing play, Ray-Kaeser et al. (2018) assert that well-chosen toys, when used in a suitable environment, in a playful context, with play partners, have the best chance to allow children to play for the sake of play. To articulate what was meant, they established a list of considerations/questions to consider when selecting toys, as summarized in Box 16.3.

### CASE EXAMPLE 16.3 PLAY AS AN OCCUPATION

**Arts and Crafts as Play**

Rachel is a 9-year-old child in the third grade. Rachel has been diagnosed with generalized anxiety disorder, bipolar disorder, and attention deficit disorder. Her home environment is unstable, and child protective services is involved with the family, who struggles financially. Rachel lives with her mother (who has depression, substance abuse, and bipolar disorder) and brother (who was recently incarcerated because of substance abuse). Rachel enjoys arts and crafts and likes to be involved in after-school activities. She can be pleasant and talkative to adults but seems to stand on the sidelines with peers and has episodes in which she gets very angry with peers when waiting her turn. Rachel exhibits good gross and fine motor skills. However, she sometimes completes schoolwork quickly and shows poor attention to details. She is struggling in the classroom.

The occupational therapist completed the Child Occupational Self-Assessment with Rachel where she reported she was "not very good" at socializing with peers. However, Rachel said this was not important to her. After further conversation, Rachel admitted she would like to have some friends at school. The therapist designed interventions to help Rachel learn to play with peers and express her frustration in an appropriate fashion. The therapist modeled play behaviors, engaged Rachel in individual sessions with arts and crafts, and later invited peers to join. Rachel began to share objects with peers once she realized these items would also be available to her. She began to interact with peers and complete arts and crafts projects together. The occupational therapist focused sessions on increasing Rachel's belief in her own abilities (self-competency) to increase her ability to play with peers.

Through play with crafts, Rachel experienced an outlet to be creative, and she expressed pride with her products. Engaging in craft sessions (play) provided Rachel with space to laugh, engage, and make her own decisions. While the goal of the occupation therapy intervention was for Rachel to develop a sense of belonging, spending time playing supported her emotional needs. This case illustrates the use of play both as the occupation and method to support Rachel's goals (of making friends).

### Toy Design

Another important consideration for universal design of toys is that the more universal design features a toy has, the more likely it can be used by a broad range of children, including children with disabilities (Ray-Kaeser et al., 2018). Using a toy analysis checklist for usability is recommended. The Toys and Games Usability Evaluation Tool was developed to assist with designing, selecting, and adapting toys to the needs of children with hearing, visual, or motor difficulties and is available free of charge (https://www.tuet.eu).

Spitzer (2022) asserted that if toys and environments do not represent the children and do not include what is important in a positive manner, then children may experience stigma about culture, gender, disability, or other factors. Therefore, it is essential that inclusive play spaces provide a diversity of play objects with toys that are representative of the children who will be playing with them, without biased divisions (Spitzer, 2022). As such, it is important to consider the appropriateness of specialized toys and whether

## BOX 16.3 Considerations When Selecting Toys for Children

**General considerations as they relate to the toy:**

- For what age group or developmental level is the toy or activity appropriate?
- Is the toy typically associated with gender or culture (e.g., dolls, trucks, toys for cooking)?
- What is the cost of the toy?
- What are the requirements (e.g., physical, space, time) to play with the toy?
- Are there any safety precautions (i.e., potential for physical harm, allergic reaction, or psychological distress)?
- Is the toy flexible?
- Does the toy require a peer to engage with the child?

**Specific considerations as they relate to the toy:**

- **Motor requirements**, such as position, posture, mobility, range of movements, dexterity, bilateral hand use, coordination, motor planning, strength, and endurance. What is the level of motor skills required?
- **Sensory requirements**, such as sensory input and feedback and sensory discrimination. What are the sensory properties of the toy?
- **Cognitive requirements**, including attention span, concentration, memory, planning, problem-solving, level of arousal, judgment, understanding, and learning. Does the toy require creativity or curiosity?
- **Perceptual requirements**, such as matching by size, color, shape, or quantity, distinguishing left from right, figure-ground perception, depth perception, or visual-perceptual-motor integration. Is the toy visually pleasing to the child?
- **Social-emotional and psychological aspects,** for example structured or unstructured toys, creativity and expression, motivation, interaction, cooperation, sharing, turn-taking, choice, control, and challenge. Can the child play with the toy by themselves?

**Considerations as they relate to the child:**

- What toys does the child consider fun and enjoyable?
- Will the child be able to use the toy?
- What ways might the child use the toy?
- Does the toy provide any challenge to the child? Does the toy provide any interest to the child?
- With whom does the child like to play?
- What is the preferable play context for the child?
- Does the child have time for play?
- What games or toys are available for the child to play with?
- Can the toy be used in creative ways?
- Are there differences in the child's level of performance, such as persistence, attention, coordination, mobility, communication, well-being, or enjoyment with different kinds of toys, play partners, or play context?

Adapted from Ray-Kaeser, S., Chatelain, S., Kindler, V., & Schneider, E. (2018). The evaluation of play from occupational therapy and psychology perspectives. In S. Besio, D. Bulgarelli, & V. Stancheva-Popkostadinova (Eds.), *Evaluation of children's play: Tools and methods* (pp. 75–77). De Gruyter. https://doi.org/10.1515/9783110610604.

## BOX 16.4 Principles for Selecting Inclusive Toys for Children

Finding inclusive toys for children to play with promotes play. The following principles can guide adults when selecting toys for children.

1. Toys and games that are accessible, flexible, and adjustable.
2. Toys and games that offer multiple means of play promote the child's interest and experiences.
3. Toys and games that appeal to children with different abilities, encouraging exploration and discovery.
4. Toys and games that offer easy ways to use them successfully.
5. The overall structure and pieces of the toy or game should feature useable shapes, dimensions, and weights: stable, big, light, and allowing it to be grasped in different ways.
6. Toys and games that can be used in different positions or be disassembled in modules to adjust them to the child.
7. Toys and games that promote interactive actions and stimulate multisensory and multimodal experiences.
8. Toys and games that have multiple sensory effects, such as sounds, lights, pictures, movements, vibrations, scents, textures, and colors.
9. Toys and games that include adjustable features for sound, height, and level of difficulty to adapt to individual users.
10. Toys and games that offer written and/or audible messages to adapt to individual user capabilities.
11. Toys and games that have a quick and simple means of activation and do not require many steps to begin play.
12. The toy and game components as well as buttons, switches, etc., should be easy to connect, to press, to turn on, fit in, or grasp.
13. The activation buttons, knobs, or connectors of the toy or game should be highlighted and differentiated from the background.
14. The toy and game material should be washable.

Adapted from Ray-Kaeser, S., Chatelain, S., Kindler, V., & Schneider, E. (2018). The evaluation of play from occupational therapy and psychology perspectives. In S. Besio, D. Bulgarelli, & V. Stancheva-Popkostadinova (Eds.), *Evaluation of children's play: Tools and methods* (pp. 71–71). De Gruyter. https://doi.org/10.1515/9783110610604.

these are necessary and appropriate; this will vary depending on children's needs and preferences. Box 16.4 describes principles of inclusive toys.

## RECOMMENDATIONS AND GUIDANCE FOR THE FUTURE

Play is one of the core occupations of childhood. Play leaders such as Bundy (1993), Florey (1981), and Parham (1996) recommend the occupational therapy profession embrace play as a legitimate practice area and validate its importance through research. Furthermore, AOTA (2008) acknowledged the importance of play in its Societal Statement on Play.

Occupational therapy practitioners support, enhance, and defend children's right to play as individuals and as members of their families, peer groups, and communities by promoting recognition of play's crucial role in children's development, health, and well-being; establishing and restoring children's skills needed to engage in play; adapting play materials, objects, and environments to facilitate optimal play experiences; and advocating for safe, inclusive play environments that are accessible to all.

Further guidance is available for play recommendations in relation to specific groups of children (Table 16.3). For children with intellectual impairments, developmental delays, and learning disabilities, Arbesman et al. (2013) recommend that occupational therapy practitioners promote positive mental health outcomes through activity-based interventions including social skills programming as well as play. For children with specific learning difficulty, Esmaili et al. (2019) recommend that occupational therapy practitioners consider group therapy-led peer play activities including practice play, symbolic play, and games with rules to improve executive function skills and behavior regulation. For children and young people with or at risk of mental health concerns, Cahill and Beisbier (2020) recommend that occupational therapy practitioners match the desired therapy outcome with appropriate play-based interventions.

**TABLE 16.3 Play Strategies to Address Characteristics Associated With Childhood Conditions**

| Condition | Characteristics | Play Strategies |
|---|---|---|
| Attention deficit disorder | • Short attention span<br>• Easily distracted<br>• Enjoys novelty<br>• Impulsive behaviors | • Identify play preferences<br>• Explore strategies for making friendships<br>• Provide opportunities to play outdoors<br>• Engage child in high impact play events (such as trampolining, jumping rope, wheelbarrow racing, crawling)<br>• Encourage activities that can be achieved in short timespan |
| Autism | • Likes repetitive behaviors<br>• Needs routines for successful engagement<br>• Enjoys objects and natural elements in environment<br>• Needs help to understand humor, jokes, or nonverbal communication | • Identify play preferences<br>• Explore strategies for making friendships<br>• Provide outdoor experiences for play that allow freedom to self-control play choices<br>• Use social stories when introducing new playgrounds or places for play |
| Visual and hearing impairment | • Needs time to orient and understand the physical layout and opportunities in the play environment | • Identify play preferences<br>• Explore strategies for making friendships<br>• Provide structured play opportunities with enhanced multisensory characteristics<br>• Support risk-taking at the just-right level |
| Developmental coordination disorder/ dyspraxia | • Difficulty with coordination and balance<br>• May prefer activities that do not involve a lot of manipulation<br>• Enjoys games or activities they can control themselves, which are not competitive<br>• Able to problem solve and figure things out | • Identify play preferences<br>• Explore strategies for making friendships<br>• Encourage more varied and intense outdoor play and large body movements<br>• Play games that require problem-solving<br>• Engage child in planning activities |

Promoting play in communities is an emerging area of practice and is less developed or less evident as a scope of practice in occupational therapy. Occupational therapy practitioners are well positioned to address children's play rights and take seriously the need to increase their understanding of how environments, particularly public playgrounds, support or prevent participation in play and contribute to the **occupational justice** agenda of creating the context for the realization of Article 31 (Lynch et al., 2020; Moore & Lynch, 2015; Sterman et al., 2016). Indeed, Hitch et al. (2012) asserted that "if as a profession we are committed to equity and diversity and the health and wellbeing of communities and the individuals within them, we need to ensure that we have the understanding, skills and expertise to ensure that built environments are not a barrier to people's ability to participate in their everyday occupations and roles" (p. 382). Moore (2023) provides ideas about how to progress this work in designing inclusive play spaces, with the emerging UD for Play model. This is based on the knowledge that occupational therapy practitioners have something unique to offer in terms of environmental design given their knowledge on play and the transactional relationship between people, environments, and occupations. As such, it is essential that occupational therapy practitioners adopt not only conventional ways of working but also nonconventional ways of working to address play needs at the individual level as well as community and policy levels through engagement in social and political action (Lynch, 2023; Moore, 2023; Moore & Lynch, 2015).

## SUMMARY

Since the work of Reilly, occupational therapy practitioners have more carefully considered their practices in relation to play (Bundy, 1993; Florey, 1981; Kuhaneck & O'Brien, 2022; Parham, 1996), which has resulted in the promotion of new practices (Kuhaneck et al., 2010; Kuhaneck & Spitzer, 2023) as well as new models and ideas about the way in which play is used in therapy (Moore, 2023; Ray-Kacser & Lynch, 2017). By committing to developing one's knowledge beyond play development theories, occupational therapy practitioners are seeing and discovering that play is a core area of concern and study in occupational therapy research and practice. Practitioners who are committed to occupational justice can extend their knowledge toward the child's right to play and continue to provide play interventions as solutions that address not only the play needs of the child but also of their family and communities.

1. Play is defined in relation to the child's level of control and the associated experience of the activity as being fun or joyful (i.e., as determined by the player) (Bundy, 1993). In this regard, play is clearly an occupation, as it is a subjective experience that evolves through the process of playing. It is also transformative, as it includes elements of flexibility, spontaneity, and testing of ideas, as players engage in forming and reforming events and actions in ways they devise and control themselves (Henricks, 2008). Other key elements that characterize play include that it is more about the process rather than the outcome, that it is noncompulsory, and that it can take place "whenever and wherever opportunities arise" (CRC, 2013).
2. Children learn cognitive, motor, social, and developmental skills through play. They learn to negotiate and engage with others while learning how to move, experience, and engage with toys and the environment. They learn cultural expectations and develop an approach or attitude toward play (i.e., playfulness) that may be used later in life to flexibly solve problems and engage with others.
3. Children's play begins as they explore their bodies and the environment. They learn to communicate, move, interact, and manipulate objects through play. They develop competence and mastery in their skills and abilities, which leads to a sense of identity (e.g., this is who I am, my preferences, talents, and abilities). As children

and youth participate in play, they develop a sense of belonging and connectedness with others.

4. Occupational therapy practitioners may use play as the tool to target skills. For example, they may work on fine motor skills during a play activity. They also may address play as an occupation, whereby the goal of the occupational intervention sessions is to facilitate activity (or play) that is spontaneous, intrinsically motivated, internally controlled, and free from rules. They may use directed play or guided play.

## REFERENCES


Adolfsson, M., Simeonsson, R., Lee, A., & Ellingsen, K. (2010). Major life areas: Play and education. In A. Majnemer (Ed.), *Measures for children with developmental disabilities: An ICF-CY approach* (pp. 404–415). Mac Keith Press.

Alexander, S. A., Frohlich, K. L., & Fusco, C. (2014). Playing for health? Revisiting health promotion to examine the emerging public health position on children's play. *Health Promotion International, 29*(1), 155–164.

American Occupational Therapy Association. (2008). AOTA's societal statement on play. *American Journal of Occupational Therapy, 62*(6), 707–708.

American Occupational Therapy Association. (2020). Occupational therapy practice framework: Domain and process (4th ed.). *American Journal of Occupational Therapy, 74*(Suppl. 2) 7412410010p1–7412410010p87.

Anaby, D., Law, M., Coster, W., Bedell, G., Khetani, M., Avery, L., & Teplicky, R. (2014). The mediating role of the environment in explaining participation of children and youth with and without disabilities across home, school, and community. *Archives of Physical Medicine and Rehabilitation, 95*(5), 908–917.

Ansari, A., Pettit, K., & Gershoff, E. (2015). Combating obesity in head start: Outdoor play and change in children's BMI. *Journal of Developmental and Behavioral Pediatrics: Journal of Developmental and Behavioral Pediatrics, 36*(0), 605.

Arbesman, M., Bazyk, S., & Nochajski, S. M. (2013). Systematic review of occupational therapy and mental health promotion, prevention, and intervention for children and youth. *American Journal of Occupational Therapy, 67*, e120–e130. https://doi.org/10.5014/ajot.2013.008359.

Armstrong, J., Paskal, K., Elliott, C., Wray, J., Davidson, E., Mizen, J., & Girdler, S. (2019). What makes playgroups therapeutic? A scoping review to identify the active ingredients of therapeutic and supported playgroups. *Scandinavian Journal of Occupational Therapy, 26*(2), 81–102.

Athey, I. (2018). Contributions of play to development. In *Children's play* (pp. 8–28). Routledge.

Barnes, G., Wilkes-Gillan, S., Bundy, A., & Cordier, R. (2017). The social play, social skills and parent–child relationships of children with ADHD 12 months following a RCT of a play-based intervention. *Australian Journal of Occupational Therapy, 64*, 457–465.

Barton, E. (2010). Development of a taxonomy of pretend play for children with disabilities. *Infants and Young Children, 23*(4), 247–261.

Bazyk, S. (2022). Creative play and leisure for adolescents. In H. Kuhaneck, & S. Spitzer (Eds.), *Making play just right: Unleashing the power of play in occupational therapy* (2nd ed.) (pp. 347–376). Jones and Bartlett Learning.

Bazyk, S., Stalnaker, D., Llerena, M., Ekelman, B., & Bazyk, J. (2003). Play in Mayan children. *American Journal of Occupational Therapy, 57*(3), 273–283.

Bento, G., & Dias, G. (2017). The importance of outdoor play for young children's healthy development. *Porto Biomedical Journal, 2*(5), 157–160.

Bergen, D. (2006). Play as a context for humor development. In D. Fromberg, & D. Bergen (Eds.), *Play from birth to twelve: Contexts, perspectives and meanings* (2 ed.) (pp. 141–156). Routledge.

Bilton, H. (2010). *Outdoor learning in the early years: Management and innovation.* Routledge.

Blake, A., Sexton, J., Lynch, H., Moore, A., & Coughlan, M. (2018). An exploration of the outdoor play experiences of preschool children with autism spectrum disorder in an Irish preschool setting. *Today's Children are Tomorrow's Parents: An Interdisciplinary Journal, 47*, 100–116.

Bonawitz, E., Shafto, P., Gweon, H., Goodman, N., Spelke, E., & Schulz, L. (2011). The double-edged sword of pedagogy: Instruction limits spontaneous exploration and discovery. *Cognition, 120*(3), 322–330.

Brown, S. L. (2009). *Play: How it shapes the brain, opens the imagination, and invigorates the soul.* Penguin.

Brown, T., & Lynch, H. (2023). Children's play–work occupation continuum: Play-based occupational therapy, play therapy and playwork. *Canadian Journal of Occupational Therapy, 90*(3), 249–256. https://doi.org/10.1177/00084174221130165.

Brussoni, M., Gibbons, R., Gray, C., Ishikawa, T., Sandseter, E. B. H., Beinenstock, A., & Tremblay, M. (2015). What is the relationship between risky outdoor play and health in children? A systematic review. *International Journal of Environmental Research and Public Health, 12*(6), 6423–6454.

Brussoni, M., Olsen, L. L., Pike, I., & Sleet, D. A. (2012). Risky play and children's safety: Balancing priorities for optimal child development. *International Journal of Environmental Research and Public Health, 9*(9), 3134–3148.

Bundy, A. (1993). Assessment of play and leisure: Delineation of the problem. *American Journal of Occupational Therapy, 47*, 217–222.

Bundy, A. (2011). Children: Analysing the occupation of play. In L. Mackenzie, & G. O'Toole (Eds.), *Occupational analysis in practice* (pp. 133–146). Wiley-Blackwell.

Bundy, A., & Du Toit, S. (2023). Chapter 47: Play and leisure. In B. Schell, & G. Gillen (Eds.), *Willard and Spackman's Occupational Therapy* (14 ed.) (pp. 793–818). Wolters Kluwer.

Bundy, A., Naughton, G., Tranter, P., Wyver, S., Baur, L., Schiller, W., … Brentnall, J. (2011). The Sydney playground project: Popping the bubblewrap - unleashing the power of play: A cluster randomised controlled trial of a primary school playground-based intervention aiming to increase children's physical activity and social skills. *BMC Public Health, 11*(680), 1–9.

Bundy, A., Waugh, K., & Brentnall, J. (2009). Developing assessments that account for the role of the environment: An example using the test of playfulness and test of environmental supportiveness. *OTJR: Occupation, Participation and Health, 29*(3), 135–143.

Bundy, A. C., Wyver, S., Beetham, K. S., Ragen, J., Naughton, G., Tranter, P., Norman, R., Villeneuve, M., Spencer, G., Honey, A., Simpson, J., Baur, L., & Sterman, J. (2015). The Sydney playground project-levelling the playing field: A cluster trial of a primary school-based intervention aiming to promote manageable risk-taking in children with disability. *BMC Public Health, 15*(1), 1125–1130.

Burghardt, G. (2005). *The genesis of animal play: Testing the limits.* MIT Press.

Burghardt, G. (2011). Defining and recognising play. In A. Pellegrini (Ed.), *The Oxford handbook of the development of play* (pp. 9–37). Oxford Library of Psychology.

Cahill, S. M., & Beisbier, S. (2020). Occupational therapy practice guidelines for children and youth ages 5-21 years. *American Journal of Occupational Therapy, 74*(4), 1–47.

Casey, T. (2017). Outdoor play and learning in the landscape of children's rights. In T. Waller, E. Arlemalm-Hagser, E. B. H. Sandseter, L. Lee-Hammond, K. Lekies, & S. Wyver (Eds.), *The SAGE handbook of outdoor play and learning* (pp. 362–377). Sage.

Chatterjee, S. (2017). *Access to play for children in situations of crisis: Synthesis of research in six countries.* International Play Association. http://ipaworld.org/wp-content/uploads/2020/04/IPA-APC-Research-Synthesis-Reportsinglepg.pdf.

Chick, G. (2015). Anthropology and the study of play. In J. Johnson, S. Eberle, T. Henricks, & D. Kuschner (Eds.), *The handbook of the study of play* (pp. 71–84). Lanham: Rowman and Littlefield.

Clark, F. A., Parham, D., Carlson, M. E., Frank, G., Jackson, J., Pierce, D., Wolfe, R. J., & Zemke, R. (1991). Occupational science: Academic innovation in the service of occupational therapy's future. *American Journal of Occupational Therapy, 45*(4), 300–310.

Clements, R. (2004). An investigation of the status of outdoor play. *Contemporary Issues in Early Childhood, 5*(1), 68–80.

Committee on the Rights of the Child. (2013). *General comment No. 17 on the right of the child to rest, leisure, play, recreational activities, cultural life and the arts.* https://www.refworld.org/docid/51ef9bcc4.html.

Cordier, R., Bundy, A., Hocking, C., & Einfeld, S. (2009). A model for play-based intervention for children with ADHD. *Australian Occupational Therapy Journal, 56*, 332–340.

Cornell, H. R., Lin, T. T., & Anderson, J. A. (2018). A systematic review of play-based interventions for students with ADHD: Implications for school-based occupational therapists. *Journal of Occupational Therapy, Schools, and Early Intervention, 11*(2), 192–211.

Coughlan, M., & Lynch, H. (2011). Parents as environmental managers: The Irish home as a play space for toddlers. *Irish Journal of Occupational Therapy, 39*(1), 34–41.

Darrah, J., Law, M., Pollock, N., Wilson, B., Russell, D., Walter, S., Rosenbaurm, P., & Galupp, B. (2011). Context therapy: A new intervention approach for children with cerebral palsy. *Developmental Medicine and Child Neurology, 53*(7), 615–620.

Dender, A. M., & Stagnitti, K. (2015). Children's play in the Australian Indigenous context: The need for a contemporary view. *International Journal of Play, 4*(1), 3–16.

Dodd, H. F., FitzGibbon, L., Watson, B. E., & Nesbit, R. J. (2021). Children's play and independent mobility in 2020: Results from the British Children's Play Survey. *International Journal of Environmental Research and Public Health, 18*(8), 4334. https://doi.org/10.3390/ijerph18084334.

Dyment, J. E., & Bell, A. C. (2008). Grounds for movement: Green school grounds as sites for promoting physical activity. *Health Education Research, 23*(6), 952–962.

Eberle, S. (2014). The elements of play: Towards a philosophy and a definition of play. *American Journal of Play, 6*(2), 214–233.

Edwards, C. (2000). Children's play in cross-cultural perspective: A new look at the six cultures study. *Cross-Cultural Research, 34*, 318–338.

Esmaili, S. K., Mehraban, A. H., Shafaroodi, N., Yazdani, F., Masoumi, T., & Zarei, M. (2019). Participation in peer-play activities among children with specific learning disability: A randomized controlled trial. *American Journal of Occupational Therapy, 73*(2) 7302205110p1–7302205110p9. PMID: 30915972.

Fabrizi, S., & Hubbell, K. (2017). The role of occupational therapy in promoting playfulness, parent competence, and social participation in early childhood playgroups: A pretest posttest design. *Journal of Occupational Therapy, Schools, and Early Intervention, 10*(4), 346–365.

Fahy, S., Delicate, N., & Lynch, H. (2021). Now, being, occupational: Outdoor play and children with autism. *Journal of Occupational Science, 28*(1), 114–132.

Fisher, A. (2013). Occupation-centred, occupation-based, occupation-focused: Same, same or different. *Scandanavian Journal of Occupational Therapy, 20*, 162–173.

Florey, L. L. (1981). Studies of play: Implications for growth, development, and for clinical practice. *American Journal of Occupational Therapy, 35*(8), 519–524.

Galloway, J., & Thelen, E. (2004). Feet first: Object exploration in young infants. *Infant Behavior and Development, 27*, 107–112.

Gibson, J., Pritchard, E., & de Lemos, C. (2021). Play-based interventions to support social and communication development in autistic children aged 2-8 years: A scoping review. *Autism & Developmental Language Impairments, 6*, 1–30. https://doi.org/10.1177/23969415211015840.

Gill, T. (2007). *No fear: Growing up in a risk averse society.* Caloustie Gulbenkian Foundation.

Ginsburg, K. R., & Committee on Communications, & Committee on Psychosocial Aspects of Child and Family Health. (2007). The importance of play in promoting healthy child development and maintaining strong parent-child bonds. *Pediatrics, 119*(1), 182–191.

Gleave, J., & Cole-Hamilton, I. (2012). *A world without play: A literature review* (Play England).

Glenn, N., Knight, C., Holt, N., & Spence, J. (2012). Meanings of play among children. *Childhood, 20*, 185–199. https://doi.org/10.1177/0907568212454751.

Graham, N. E., Truman, J., & Hoigate, H. (2015). Parents' understanding of play for children with cerebral palsy. *American Journal of Occupational Therapy, 69*(3), 1–9.

Gray, P. (2011). The decline of play and the rise of psychopathology in children and adolescent. *American Journal of Play, 3*(4), 443–463.

Haight, W., & Miller, P. (1993). *Pretending at home: Early development in a sociocultural context.* State University of New York Press.

Henricks, T. S. (2015). Play as experience. *American Journal of Play, 8*(1), 18–49.

Henricks, T. (2008). The nature of play: An overview. *American Journal of Play, 1*(2), 157–180.

Hinchion, S., McAuliffe, E., & Lynch, H. (2021). Fraught with frights or full of fun: Perspectives of risky play among six-to-eight year olds. *European Early Childhood Education Research Journal, 29*(4), 696–714.

Hitch, D., Larkin, H., Watchorn, V., & Ang, S. (2012). Community mobility in the context of universal design: Inter-professional collaboration and education. *Australian Occupational Therapy Journal, 59*(5), 375–383.

Hocking, C. (2021). Occupation in context: A reflection on environmental influences on human doing. *Journal of Occupational Science, 28*(2), 221–234.

Howard, J., & McInnes, H. (2013a). Playfulness. In J. Howard, & H. McInnes (Eds.), *The essence of play: A practice companion for professionals working with children and young people* (pp. 39–48). Taylor and Francis Group.

Howard, J., & McInnes, K. (2013b). The impact of children's perception of an activity as play rather than not play on emotional well-being. *Child Health and Development, 39*(5), 737–742.

Huizinga, J. (1950). *Homo Ludens: A study of the play element in culture.* Beacon Press.

Hutt, C. (1979). Exploration and play. In B. Sutton-Smith (Ed.), *Play and learning* (pp. 175–194) Gardner.

Hutton, E., Tuppeny, S., & Hasselbusch, A. (2016). Making a case for universal and targeted children's occupational therapy in the United Kingdom. *British Journal of Occupational Therapy, 79*(7), 450–453.

International Play Association. (2010). *IPA global consultations on children's right to play: Summary report* (Author).

International Play Association. (2014). *Declaration on the importance of play* (Author).

International Play Association. (2016). *Children's right to play and the environment: A discussion paper prepared by the IPA for the UN committee on the rights of the child day of general discussion 2016* (Author).

Jung, S., & Sainato, D. M. (2013). Teaching play skills to young children with autism. *Journal of Intellectual and Developmental Disability, 38*(1), 74–90.

Kangas, S., Maatta, K., & Uusiautti, S. (2012). Alone and in a group: Ethnographic research on autistic children's play. *International Journal of Play, 1*(1), 37–50.

Karasik, L., Tamis-LeMonda, C., & Adolf, K. (2011). Transition from crawling to walking and infants' actions with objects and people. *Child Development, 82*(4), 1199–1209.

Kent, C., Cordier, R., Joosten, A., Wilkes-Gillan, S., Bundy, A., & Speyer, R. (2020). A systematic review and meta-analysis of interventions to improve play skills in children with autism specturm disorder. *Review Journal of Autism and Developmental Disorders, 7*, 91–118.

Korczak, D. J., Madigan, S., & Colasanto, M. (2017). Children's physical activity and depression: A meta-analysis. *Pediatrics, 139*(4) e20162266.

Kramer, P., & Hinojosa, J. (2010). *Frames of reference for pediatric occupational therapy* (3rd ed.). Wolters Kluwer Health/Lippincott Williams and Wilkins.

Kuhaneck, H., & Metz, A. (2022). Informal play assessment and activity analysis. In H. Kuhaneck, & S. Spitzer (Eds.), *Making play just right: Unleashing the power of play in occupational therapy* (2nd ed.) (pp. 109–140). Jones and Bartlett Learning.

Kuhaneck, H., & O'Brien, K. (2022). Answering the big questions about play. In H. Kuhaneck, & S. Spitzer (Eds.), *Making play just right: Unleashing the power of play in occupational therapy* (2nd ed.) (pp. 1–54). Jones and Bartlett Learning.

Kuhaneck, H., Spitzer, S., & Bodison, S. (2020). A systematic review of interventions to improve the occupation of play in children with autism. *OTJR: Occupation, Participation and Health*, *40*(2), 83–98.

Kuhaneck, H., Spitzer, S., & Miller, E. (2010). *Activity analysis, creativity, and playfulness in pediatric occupational therapy: Making play just right*. Jones and Bartlett Learning.

Kuhaneck, H., & Sptizer, S. (Eds.). (2023). *Making play just right: Unleasing the power of play in occupational therapy* (2nd ed.) Jones and Bartlett Learning.

Lancy, D. (2007). Accounting for variability in mother-child play. *American Anthropologist*, *109*, 273–284.

Lang, R., O'Reilly, M., Rispoli, M., Shogren, K., Machalicek, W., Sigafoos, J., & Regester, A. (2009). Review of interventions to increase functional and symbolic play in children with autism. *Education and Training in Developmental Disabilities*, *44*(4), 481–492.

Law, M., Darrah, J., Pollock, N., Wilson, B., Russell, D., Walter, S., Rosenbuam, P., & Galuppi, B. (2011). Focus on function: A cluster, randomized controlled trial comparing child-versus context-focused intervention for young children with cerebral palsy. *Developmental Medicine and Child Neurology*, *53*, 621–629.

Lee, E.-Y., Bains, A., Hunter, S., Ament, A., Brazo-Sayavera, J., Carson, V., Hakimi, S., Huang, W. Y., Janssen, I., & Lee, M. (2021). Systematic review of the correlates of outdoor play and time among children aged 3-12 years. *International Journal of Behavioral Nutrition and Physical Activity*, *18*(1), 1–46.

Lester, S., & Russell, W. (2008). *Play for a change: Play, policy and practice: A review of contemporary perspectives*. National Children's Bureau.

Lester, S., & Russell, W. (2010). Children's right to play: An examination of the importance of play in the lives of children worldwide. *Working Papers in Early Childhood Development, No. 57* ERIC.

Loebach, J., & Cox, A. (2020). Tool for observing play outdoors (TOPO): A new typology for capturing children's play behaviors in outdoor environments. *International Journal of Environmental Research and Public Health*, *17*(15), 5611.

Loebach, J., Sanches, M., Jaffe, J., & Elton-Marshall, T. (2021). Paving the way for outdoor play: Examining socio-environmental barriers to community-based outdoor play. *International Journal of Environmental Research and Public Health*, *18*(7), 3617.

Loudoun, F., Boyle, B., & Larsson-Lund, M. (2022). Children's experiences of play in digital spaces: A scoping review. *PLoS One*, *17*(8) e0272630.

Lubans, D. R., Morgan, P. J., Cliff, D. P., Barnett, L. M., & Okely, A. D. (2010). Fundamental movement skills in children and adolescents. *Sports Medicine*, *40*(12), 1019–1035.

Luckett, T., Bundy, A., & Roberts, J. (2007). Do behavioural approaches teach children with autism to play or are they pretending? *Autism*, *11*(4), 365–388.

Lynch, H. (2012). *Infant places, spaces and objects: Exploring the physical in learning environments for infants under two [Unpublished PhD thesis]*. Dublin Institute of Technology.

Lynch, H. (2023). Perspectives on the meaning of play: International, cultural and individual contexts. In H. Kuhaneck, & S. Spitzer (Eds.), *Making play just right: Unleashing the power of play in occupational therapy* (2nd ed.) (pp. 399–430). Jones and Bartlett Learning.

Lynch, H., Hayes, N., & Ryan, S. (2016). Exploring socio-cultural influences that impact on infant play occupations in Irish home environments. *Journal of Occupational Science*, *23*(3), 352–369.

Lynch, H., & Moore, A. (2016). Play as an occupation in occupational therapy. *British Journal of Occupational Therapy*, *79*(9), 519–520.

Lynch, H., & Moore, A. (2018). What barriers to play do children with disabilities face? In P. Encarnação, S. Ray-Kaeser, & N. Bianquin (Eds.), *Guidelines for supporting children with disabilities' play. Methodologies, tools, and contexts* (pp. 27–40). De Gruyter.

Lynch, H., Moore, A., Edwards, C., & Horgan, L. (2020). Advancing play participation for all: The challenge of addressing play diversity and inclusion in community parks and playgrounds. *British Journal of Occupational Therapy*, *83*(2), 107–117.

Lynch, H., Moore, A., & Prellwitz, M. (2018). From policy to play provision: Universal design and the challenge of inclusive play. *Children, Youth, and Environments*, *28*(2), 12–34.

Lynch, H., Prellwitz, M., Schulze, C., & Moore, A. (2017). The state of play in children's occupational therapy: A comparison between Ireland, Sweden and Switzerland. *British Journal of Occupational Therapy*, *81*(1), 42–50.

Mellou, E. (1994). Play theories: A contemporary review. *Early Child Development and Care*, *102*(1), 91–100.

Miller, E., & Kuhaneck, H. (2008). Children's perceptions of play experiences and play preferences: A qualitative study. *American Journal of Occupational Therapy*, *62*(4), 407–415.

Miller Kuhaneck, H., Tanta, K., Coombs, A., & Pannone, H. (2013). A survey of pediatric occupational therapists' use of play. *Journal of Occupational Therapy, Schools, & Early Intervention*, *6*, 213–227.

Milteer, R. M., Ginsburg, K. R., & Mulligan, D. A. (2012). The importance of play in promoting healthy child development and maintaining strong parent-child bond: Focus on children in poverty. *Pediatrics*, *129*(1), e204–e213.

Moore, A., Boyle, B., & Lynch, H. (2022a). Designing public playgrounds for inclusion: A scoping review of grey literature guidelines for universal design. *Children's Geographies*, *21*(3), 422–441.

Moore, A., Boyle, B., & Lynch, H. (2023). Designing for inclusion in public playgrounds: A scoping review of definitions, and utilization of universal design. *Disability and Rehabilitation: Assistive Technology*, *18*(8), 1453–1465. https://doi.org/10.1080/17483107.2021.2022788. Epub 2022 Feb 9. PMID: 35138989.

Moore, A., & Lynch, H. (2015). Accessibility and usability of playground environments for children under 12: A scoping review. *Scandanavian Journal of Occupational Therapy*, *22*(5), 331–344.

Moore, A., & Lynch, H. (2018a). Play and play occupation: A survey of paediatric occupational therapy practice in Ireland. *Irish Journal of Occupational Therapy*, *46*(1), 59–72. https://doi.org/10.1108/IJOT-08-2017-0022.

Moore, A., & Lynch, H. (2018b). Understanding a child's conceptualisation of well-being through an exploration of happiness: The centrality of play, people and place. *Journal of Occupational Science*, *25*(1), 124–141. https://doi.org/10.1080/14427591.2017.1377105.

Moore, A., Lynch, H., & Boyle, B. (2022b). A national study of playground professionals universal design implementation practices. *Landscape Research*, *47*(5), 611–627.

Moore, A., Lynch, H., & Boyle, B. (2022c). Can universal design support outdoor play, social participation, and inclusion in public playgrounds? A scoping review. *Disability & Rehabilitation*, *44*(13), 3304–3325. https://doi.org/10.1080/09638288.2020.1858353.

Munambah, N., Ramugondo, E., & Cordier, R. (2022). Play of children living with HIV/AIDS in a low-resourced setting: Perspectives of caregivers. *British Journal of Occupational Therapy*, *85*(4), 292–300.

Muys, V., Rodger, S., & Bundy, A. C. (2006). Assessment of playfulness in children with autistic disorder: A comparison of the children's playfulness scale and the test of playfulness. *OTJR: Occupational Therapy Journal of Research*, *26*(4), 159–170. https://doi.org/10.1177/153944920602600406.

Nagy, E. (2011). The newborn infant: A missing stage in developmental psychology. *Infant and Child Development*, *20*, 3–19.

Nicolich, L. (1977). Beyond sensorimotor intelligence: An assessment of symbolic maturity through analysis of pretend play. *Merrill-Palmer Quarterly*, *23*(2), 89–99.

Nielsen, L. (2021). Don't downplay "play": Reasons why health systems should protect childhood play. *Journal of Medicine and Philosophy: A Forum for Bioethics and Philosophy of Medicine*, *46*(5), 586–604.

Norðdahl, K., & Einarsdóttir, J. (2014). Children's views and preferences regarding their outdoor environment. *Journal of Adventure Education and Outdoor Learning*, *15*(2), 152–167. https://doi.org/10.1080/14729679.2014.896746.

O'Connor, D., Lynch, H., & Boyle, B. (2021). A qualitative study of child participation in decision-making: Exploring rights-based approaches in pediatric occupational therapy. *PLoS One*, *16*(12) e0260975.

Parham, L. D. (1996). Perspectives on play. In R. Zemke, & F. Clark (Eds.), *Occupational science: The evolving discipline* (pp. 71–80). Philadelphia, PA: F. A. Davis.

Parham, L. D. (2008). Play and occupational therapy. In L. D. Parham, & L. Fazio (Eds.), *Play in occupational therapy for children* (2 ed.) (pp. 219–249). Mosby Elsevier.

Parten, M. (1932). Social participation among preschool children. *Journal of Abnormal Child Psychology, 27*(3), 243–269.

Pellegrini, A. (2006). Rough-and-tumble play from childhood through adolescence. In D. Fromberg, & D. Bergen (Eds.), *Play from birth to twelve: Contexts, perspecitves and meanings* (2 ed.) (pp. 111–118). Routledge.

Pellegrini, A., & Bjorklund, D. (2004). The ontogeny and phylogeny of children's object and fantasy play. *Human Nature, 15*(1), 23–43.

Pellegrini, A., & Smith, P. (1998). Physical activity play: The nature and function of a neglected aspect of play. *Child Development, 69*(3), 577–598.

Perry, M. A., Devan, H., Fitzgerald, H., Han, K., Liu, L. T., & Rouse, J. (2018). Accessibility and usability of parks and playgrounds. *Disability Health Journal, 11*(2), 221–229. https://doi.org/10.1016/j.dhjo.2017.08.011. Epub 2017 Sep 8. PMID: 28918095.

Phelan, S., & Kinsella, E. A. (2009). Occupational identity: Engaging socio–cultural perspectives. *Journal of Occupational Science, 16*(2), 85–91.

Phelan, S. K., & Kinsella, E. A. (2014). Occupation and identity: Perspectives of children with disabilities and their parents. *Journal of Occupational Science, 21*(3), 334–356.

Piaget, J. (1962). *Play, dreams and imitation in childhood.* W. W. Norton.

Prellwitz, M., & Lynch, H. (2018). Universal design for social inclusion: Playgrounds for all. In M. Twomey, & C. Carroll (Eds.), *Seen and heard: Exploring participation, engagement and voice for children with disabilities* (pp. 267–296). Oxford: Peter Lang.

Prellwitz, M., & Skär, L. (2007). Usability of playgrounds for children with different abilities. *Occupational Therapy International, 14*(3), 144–155.

Prellwitz, M., & Skär, L. (2016). Are playgrounds a case of occupational injustice? Experiences of parents of children with disabiliites. *Children, Youth, and Environments, 26*(2), 28–42.

Ray-Kaeser, S., Chatelain, S., Kindler, V., & Schneider, E. (2018). The evaluation of play from occupational therapy and psychology perspectives. In S. Besio, D. Bulgarelli, & V. Stancheva-Popkostadinova (Eds.), *Evaluation of children's play: Tools and methods* (pp. 19–57). De Gruyter. https://doi.org/10.1515/9783110610604.

Ray-Kaeser, S., & Lynch, H. (2017). Occupational therapy perspective on play for the sake of play. In S. Besio, D. Bulgarelli, & V. Stancheva-Popkostadinova (Eds.), *Play development in children with disabilities* (pp. 155–165). De Gruyter.

Richards, M. N., Putnick, D. L., Suwalsky, J. T. D., Bornstein, M. H., Phillips, K. H., & Hurley, J. (2020). *Age determination guidelines: Relating consumer product characteristics to the skills, play behaviors, and interests of children.* National Institute of Child Health and Human Development and U.S. Consumer Product Safety Commission. https://www.cpsc.gov/s3fs-public/Age-Determination-Guidelines-Relating-Consumer-Product-to-Characteristics-Skills-Play-Behavior-Intersts-to-Children-January-2020.pdf.

Robson, S. (2010). Self-regulation and metacognition in young children's self-initiated play and reflective dialogue. *International Journal of Early Years Education, 18*(3), 227–241.

Rochat, P. (1989). Object manipulation and exploration in 2-5-month-old infants. *Developmental Psychology, 25*(6), 871–884.

Rochat, P. (1993). Hand-mouth coordination in the newborn: Morphology, determinants, and early development of a basic act. *Advances in Psychology, 97*, 265–288.

Rochat, P., Goubet, N., & Senders, S. (1999). To reach or not to reach? Perception of body effectivities by young babies. *Infant and Child Development, 8*(3), 129–148.

Rodger, S., & Ziviani, J. (1999). Play-based occupational therapy. *International Journal of Disability, Development and Education, 46*(3), 337–365.

Rousseau-Harrison, K., & Rochette, A. (2012). Impacts of wheelchair acquisition on children from a person-occupation-environment interactional perspective. *Disability and Rehabilitation: Assistive Technology, 8*(1), 1–10.

Sandseter, E. B. H. (2007). Risky play among four-and five-year-old children in preschool. In *Vision into practice: Making quality a reality in the lives of young children* (pp. 248–256). Dublin Castle, Ireland.

Sandseter, E. (2009). Children's expressions of exhilaration and fear in risky play. *Contemporary Issues in Early Childhood, 10*(2), 92–106.

Sandseter, E. B. H. (2011). Children's risky play in early childhood education and care. *ChildLinks. Children's Risky Play, 3*, 2–6.

Schaaf, R., Benevides, T., Mailloux, Z., Faller, P., Hunt, J., & van Hooydonk, E. (2013). An intervention for sensory difficulties in children with autism: A randomised control trial. *Journal of Autism and Developmental Disorders, 44*(7), 1493–1506.

Schaefer, L., Plotnikoff, R. C., Majumdar, S. R., Mollard, R., Woo, M., Sadman, R., Rinaldi, R. L., Boulé, N., Torrance, B., Ball, G. D., et al. (2014). Outdoor time is associated with physical activity, sedentary time, and cardiorespiratory fitness in youth. *The Journal of Pediatrics, 165*(3), 516–521.

Singer, D., Singer, J., Dagostino, H., & DeLong, R. (2009). Childrens' pastimes and play in sixteen nations: Is free play declining? *American Journal of Play, 1*, 283–312.

Skard, G., & Bundy, A. (2008). Test of playfulness. In L. D. Parham, & L. Fazio (Eds.), *Play in occupational therapy for children* (pp. 71–93). Mosby Elsevier.

Smilansky, S. (1968). *The effects of sociodramatic play on disadvantaged preschool children.* Wiley.

Souto-Manning, M. (2017). Is play a privilege or a right? And what's our responsibility? On the role of play for equity in early childhood education. *Early Child Development and Care, 187*(5–6), 785–787.

Spitzer, S. (2022). Being playful: Therapeutic use of self in pediatric occupational therapy. In H. Kuhaneck, & S. Spitzer (Eds.), *Making play just right: Unleashing the power of play in occupational therapy* (2nd ed.) (pp. 157–196). Jones & Bartlett Learning.

Spitzer, S. L., Metz, A. E., & Kuhaneck, H. M. (2022). Playful play spaces. In H. Kuhaneck, & S. L. Spitzer (Eds.), *Making play just right: Activity analysis, creativity and playfulness in pediatric occupational therapy* (pp. 241–268). Jones and Bartlett Learning.

Stagnitti, K. (2004). Occupational performance in pretend play: Implications for practice. In M. Mollineux (Ed.), *Occupation for occupational therapists* (pp. 103–121). Blackwell Science.

Stagnitti, K. (2007). *Child-initiated pretend play assessment (ChIPPA) manual and kit.* Co-ordinates Publications.

Stagnitti, K., & Unsworth, C. (2000). The importance of pretend play in child development: An occupational therapy perspective. *British Journal of Occupational Therapy, 63*(3), 121–127.

Sterman, J., Naughton, G. A., Bundy, A. C., Froude, E., & Villeneuve, M. A. (2020). Is play a choice? Application of the capabilities approach to children with disabilities on the school playground. *International Journal of Inclusive Education, 24*(6), 579–596.

Sterman, J., Naughton, G., Froude, E., Villeneuve, M., Beetham, K. S., Wyver, S., & Bundy, A. C. (2016). Outdoor play decisions by caregivers of children with disabilities: A systematic review of qualitative studies. *Journal of Developmental and Physical Disabilities, 28*(6), 931–957.

Sterman, J., Villeneuve, M., Spencer, G., Wyyer, S., Beetham, K. S., Naughton, G., Trnater, P., Ragen, J., & Bundy, A. C. (2020). Creating play opportunities on the school playground: Educator experiences of the Sydney playground project. *Australian Occupational Therapy Journal, 67*, 62–73.

Sturgess, J. (2003). A model describing play as a child-chosen activity—is this still valid in contemporary Australia? *Australian Occupational Therapy Journal, 50*, 104–108. https://doi.org/10.1046/j.1440-1630.2003.00362.x.

Sutton-Smith, B. (1997). *The ambiguity of play.* Harvard University Press.

Trawick-Smith, J. (2010). Drawing back the lens on play: A frame analysis of young children's play in Puerto Rico. *Early Education & Development, 21*(4), 536–567.

Tremblay, M., Gray, C., Babcock, S., Barnes, J., Bradsheet, C., Carr, D., … Brussoni, M. (2015). Position statement on active outdoor play. *Environmental Research and Public Health, 12*, 6475–6505.

United Nations. (1989). *Convention on the rights of the child.* United Nations High Commissioner for Human Rights. https://treaties.un.org/pages/ViewDetails.aspx?src=IND&mtdsg_no=IV-11&chapter=4&lang=en.

Van Vianen, A. E. (2018). Person–environment fit: A review of its basic tenets. *Annual Review of Organizational Psychology and Organizational Behavior, 5*, 75–101.

Vitale, A. (2011). Children's play: A tool for public health interventions. *International Journal of Pediatric Obesity, 6*(S2), 57–59.

Vygotsky, L. (1978). *Mind in society: The development of higher psychological processes.* Cambridge University Press.

Welsh Government. (2014). *Wales-a play friendly country statutory guidance document.* wales-a-play-friendly-country.pdf (gov.wales).

Whitebread, D., Neale, D., Jensen, H., Liu, C., Solis, S. L., Hopkins, E., … Zosh, J. (2017). *The role of play in children's development: A review of the evidence.* Billund, Denmark: LEGO Foundation.

Wilcock, A., & Hocking, C. (2015). *An occupational perspective of health* (3rd ed.). Slack.

Wilkes-Gillan, S., Bundy, A., Cordier, R., & Lincoln, M. (2016). Child outcomes of a pilot parent-delivered intervention for improving the social play skills of children with ADHD and their playmates. *Developmental Neurorehabilitation, 19*, 238–245.

Wilkes-Gillan, S., Bundy, A., Cordier, R., Lincoln, M., & Chen, Y. (2016). A randomised controlled trial of a play-based intervention to improve the social play skills of children with attention deficit hyperactivity disorder (ADGD). *PLoS One, 11*(8), 1–22.

Wood, E. (2007). New directions in play: Consensus or collision? *Education 3–13, 35*(4), 309–320.

Wood, E., & Chesworth, L. (2021). Framing and defining play in early childhood. In L. Arnott, & K. Wall (Eds.), *Research through play: Participatory methods in early childhood* (pp. 3–18). Sage.

Woolley, H. (2013). Now being social: The barrier of designing outdoor play spaces for disabled Children. *Children and Society, 27*, 448–458.

Yakup, K. A., & Dahlan, A. (2022). The Malaysian occupational therapist perspective on the use of play in children with disabilities. *Malaysian Journal of Medicine and Health Sciences, 18*(8), 322–332.

Yerxa, E. J. (1990). An introduction to occupational science, a foundation for occupational therapy in the 21st Century. *Occupational Therapy in Health Care, 6*(4), 1–17.

Yogman, M., Garner, A., Hutchinson, J., Hirsh-Pasek, K., Golinkoff, R. M., Baum, R.… , & and Committee on Psychosocial Aspects of Child and Family Health. (2018). The power of play: A pediatric role in enhancing development in young children. *Pediatrics, 142*(3) e20182058.

Zosh, J., Hirsh-Pasek, K., Hopkins, E., Jensen, H., Liu, C., Neale, D., … Whitebread, D. (2018). Accessing the inaccessible: Redefining play as a spectrum. *Frontiers in Psychology, 9*, 1–12.

17

# Promoting Leisure Participation

*Susan Bazyk*

*It is widely claimed that positive leisure pursuits contribute to the development of self-fulfilled and mentally healthy young people (Passmore & French, 2001, p. 68).*

## GUIDING QUESTIONS

1. What are the personal and interpersonal benefits associated with structured leisure participation in children and youth?
2. How does the quality (context, breadth, and density) of leisure participation influence positive outcomes?
3. How do you identify children and youth at risk of leisure deprivation?
4. How can occupational therapy practitioners promote leisure participation within a multitiered public health framework at the universal, targeted, and intensive levels?
5. What environment-focused, coaching, and strength-based methods promote leisure participation?
6. What individual, group, and whole-school occupational therapy strategies promote leisure participation in children and youth with and without disabilities and/or mental health challenges?

## KEY TERMS

Activity analysis
Active leisure
Coaching
Context therapy
Environment-focused intervention
Flow
Passive leisure
Structured leisure
Unstructured leisure
Personal development
Identity work
Social skills

Core to occupational therapy is the belief that what we do impacts how we feel and function. Thus, a major aim of occupational therapy practitioners is to help people participate in and enjoy a range of occupations, including leisure, to promote health and well-being (American Occupational Therapy Association [AOTA], 2020a; Wilcock & Hocking, 2015). Through occupations, we define who we are, where we have been, and where we are going. When people learn to enjoy complex occupations that provide challenges corresponding to their skills, they are more likely to develop innate abilities, experience positive self-esteem, and be happier overall (Csikszentmihalyi, 1993). The focus of this chapter is on occupational therapy practitioners' role in promoting healthy leisure participation in *all* children and youth with and without disabilities and/or mental health challenges.

Leisure is discussed from a multitiered, public health perspective (Bazyk, 2011a). The emphasis is on addressing the leisure participation needs of children and youth at individual, targeted, and universal levels. The author describes the application of the occupational therapy process in promoting leisure participation in diverse schools, clinics, and communities. Practice examples highlight occupational therapy's role in embracing occupational justice—that all youth have a right to explore and engage in a range of meaningful and health-promoting leisure occupations.

## LEISURE PARTICIPATION DURING THE DEVELOPING YEARS

Exposure to a range of opportunities beyond merely family and school helps expand the social world of children and youth and fosters psychosocial autonomy from parents (Passmore & French, 2001). Freely chosen leisure activities are important for the development of autonomy during childhood and adolescence (Pavlova & Silbereisen, 2015). Children and youth take an active role in shaping their interests by selecting and repeating activities based on the quality of the experience (Delle Fave & Bassi, 2000). Having access to diverse leisure opportunities that are both socially desirable and enjoyable is critical to identity development. Structure, active involvement, breadth, and amount of leisure as well as the role of context are critical factors that occupational therapy practitioners must address.

### Defining and Categorizing Leisure

Leisure is defined as freely chosen, intrinsically motivated, and enjoyable activities pursued during discretionary time that provide a sense of personal meaning (Passmore, 2003; Zhang et al., 2014). Given opportunities to explore a variety of leisure activities, youth gradually develop personal preferences for specific kinds of activities (Passmore & French, 2001). One's leisure interests reveal what makes a person unique (Zhang et al., 2014). A variety of terms are used in the literature outside of occupational therapy to describe leisure participation, such as structured leisure activities, organized out-of-school activities, and extracurricular activities (Bazyk, 2011a). For this chapter, leisure activities refer to all these variations.

Leisure activities are commonly categorized based on the amount of structure and effort. **Structured leisure** activities are associated with regular participation schedules, direction by one or more adults, rule-guided interaction, skill development, and performance that requires sustained active attention and the provision of feedback (e.g., school or community-sponsored clubs, athletics, theater, dance). Higher social complexity involving peer cooperation, support from family members, and guidance from adult role models is also associated with structured leisure activities (Eccles et al., 2003; Mahoney & Stattin, 2000). In contrast, **unstructured leisure** is generally spontaneous, occurs without formal rules and adult direction, and includes few opportunities for skill development (e.g., watching television, listening to music, and hanging out with friends). Based on the amount of effort required, leisure can be described as either active or passive (Nishino & Larson, 2003). **Active leisure** involves some challenge, combining effort and enjoyment, and opportunities for learning a skill (e.g., playing an instrument, learning a sport). **Passive leisure** includes nonchallenging activities for pleasure, relaxation, coping with stress, or filling free time.

## Benefits of Structured Leisure Participation

The contribution of leisure participation to physical and mental health, quality of life, and better life outcomes is well documented (Brajsa-Zganec et al., 2011; Mahoney et al., 2005; Trainor et al., 2010). Research has consistently confirmed a positive relationship between participation in *structured leisure* and positive youth development which emphasizes building assets that enable youth to grow and flourish throughout life (Fredricks & Eccles, 2006; Larson, 2000; Leversen et al., 2012). The quality of the leisure experience is also an important consideration. Csikszentmihalyi and Larson (1984) found that the most intrinsically rewarding leisure occupations were highly structured and organized, had rules, and required the development and use of skills. These types of activities were also found to promote **flow** – a state of consciousness characterized by deep concentration and absorption associated with identity formation and optimal experience (Csikszentmihalyi & Larson, 1984). Research using youth inventories of participation and focus groups yield similar findings—that participation in structured leisure is associated with both personal and interpersonal development (Mahoney et al., 2005; Trainor et al., 2010).

**Personal Development.** Several areas of **personal development** have been identified as benefitting from participation in structured leisure (Hansen et al., 2003; Trainor et al., 2010). First, participation in leisure fosters **identity work** (i.e., work on establishing one's values, beliefs, and sense of self, including style, lifestyle, interests, and routines). Exposure to and participation in a variety of leisure activities allows a young person to explore, express, and refine one's identity and passion (Zhang et al., 2014). Youth assess their talents, interests, values, and place in the social world. Choices communicate to oneself and others that "this is who I am" or "what I am meant to do" and are based on the person's expectations for successful performance and enjoyment of the activity (Barber et al., 2005, p. 188). Second, organized activities have been viewed as providing a context for the development of *initiative* (Larson, 2000). Initiative reflects the self-motivation needed to devote effort over time to achieve a challenging goal—a core quality youth need to transition to adulthood and future work (Wilson et al., 2010). Three elements of initiative include intrinsic motivation (wanting to do the activity), concerted engagement, and commitment over time (Larson, 2000). Third, structured activities are associated with greater skill development (e.g., athletics, artistic, homemaking) (Wilson et al., 2010), higher academic achievement (Passmore, 2003), and the development of beginning work skills (Dworkin et al., 2003; Mahoney & Stattin, 2000). Finally, participation in structured leisure is associated with greater degrees of subjective well-being and positive mental health (Leversen et al., 2012). Several emotional competencies have been associated with participation in structured leisure including managing feelings, controlling impulses, increasing self-esteem, and reducing stress (Mahoney et al., 2005; Trainor et al., 2010). In terms of positive mental health, Csikszentmihalyi (1993) found that when people learn to enjoy complex occupations that provide challenges corresponding to their skills, they are more likely to develop innate abilities, experience positive self-esteem, and be happier overall.

**Interpersonal Development.** Participation in structured leisure activities fosters *interpersonal development* by expanding the social world of youth and requiring a higher level of interpersonal skills than in unstructured activities. First, participation in shared structured leisure provides an important context for the development of *new peer friendships* with youth who have similar interests. Many structured leisure pursuits provide opportunities for youth to interact with peers outside their typical network, such as youth representing different ages, racial and ethnic backgrounds, and socio-economic status (Trainor et al., 2010). Second, youth activities provide opportunities to develop a variety of **social skills** including working effectively with others, giving and receiving feedback, and learning how to interact appropriately across settings (Hansen et al., 2003; Mahoney et al., 2005). Third, leisure participation brings about *close connections to adults with social capital*, such as coaches, artists, dancers, musicians, and other valued community members. These adults offer special skills and knowledge to youth and provide a sense of belonging to a network of people valued in the community. Close relationships with adults with social capital may provide long-term sources of emotional support and social networking (e.g., access to information about future jobs or colleges).

**Preparation for Future Work.** According to Passmore (2003), participation in leisure provides a positive training ground for future work. Many structured leisure pursuits require specific knowledge, concentration, task commitment, persistence, and teamwork—all critical for success at work. These abilities are typically encouraged and modeled by adult supervisors. The actual structure of leisure activities imposes organization on youth time helping in the development of time management and health-promoting habits for independent living (maintaining a balance among work, rest, and leisure). Involvement in positive structured extracurricular activities has important implications regarding a young person's perceptions of and investment in their future (Bazyk, 2005).

## Challenges Associated With Unstructured and Passive Leisure

Outcomes associated with unstructured and passive forms of leisure are mixed. Some leisure scientists contend that certain types of unstructured leisure (e.g., attending concerts, hiking, and going out to dinner) contribute to positive adolescent development (Caldwell & Faulk, 2013). Such activities are chosen for enjoyment and personal interests and may occur in isolation or within a group without adult supervision. However, other studies consistently link engagement in unstructured or passive leisure (e.g., hanging out with peers, watching TV, playing video games) with poor academic performance, antisocial behaviors, and becoming young offenders (Farnworth, 1999). The social context of unstructured leisure is different in that adult supervision is typically lacking, allowing for greater opportunities to engage in risky behaviors (drinking, unsupervised sex, drugs) (Mahoney & Stattin, 2000). Furthermore, less time spent in structured activities is associated with less time with positive adult role models and subsequently an increased risk of developing maladaptive attitudes about school and the future in general (Sharp et al., 2015). Passive forms of leisure generally lack complexity, provide little or no challenge, and require limited skills, which may result in boredom.

**Boredom.** Boredom is a subjective experience of feeling that there is nothing meaningful to do and that time is passing slowly (Spaeth et al., 2015). Feelings of dissatisfaction, stress, and annoyance may accompany boredom. During these times, the person may experience a sense of bodily tension and restlessness (fidgeting, sighing, yawning) from an underaroused nervous system. Boredom may occur when families, schools, and communities do not offer a range of developmentally appropriate leisure opportunities and contexts for children and youth. As a result, boredom may lead a person to seek stimulation from any activity (even illegal) that is interesting or challenging to reach an optimal level of arousal (Farnworth, 1999).

Recently, in the United States, boredom rates in adolescents have been rising, with up to 20% of teens reporting feeling bored (Martz et al., 2018; Weybright et al., 2020). As boredom has been linked to poorer quality of life, mental health concerns, delinquency, and a variety of risky behaviors in teenagers, occupational therapy practitioners working with adolescents should be attuned to its indications (Biolcati et al., 2018; Schwartze et al., 2021). Additionally, although boredom is often associated with deprivation, it is frequently reported even in those with affluence and significant opportunities. Because of this, newer research and models of boredom distinguish between chronic boredom and situational boredom and more thoroughly consider the impact of attention and executive function in relation to boredom (Danckert & Merrifield, 2018; Hunter & Eastwood, 2018; Raffaelli et al., 2018; Tam et al., 2021). It may be that boredom is an outcome of negative attitudes coupled with limited attentional capacities (Martin et al., 2012), suggesting avenues of interventions that could be provided in occupational therapy such as mindfulness (Martin, 2009; Martin et al., 2012) in addition to attending to access to meaningful leisure experiences.

## Qualities Associated With Healthy Leisure Participation

Both exposure to a range of potential leisure occupations and the availability of resources to support engagement are critical factors linked with the likelihood that youth will develop and maintain healthy leisure interests. Furthermore, simply participating in structured leisure may not always result in positive outcomes—the context, breadth, and density are also important considerations.

**Context.** It is important that occupational therapy practitioners consider the physical, social, and emotional aspects of where leisure is occurring. Eight key features of the leisure context are associated with positive leisure participation and include physical and psychological safety, appropriate structure, supportive relationships, opportunities for belonging, positive social norms, support for efficacy and mattering, opportunities for skill building, and integration of family, school, and community efforts (Mahoney et al., 2005). Although many organized leisure activities incorporate several of these features, occupational therapy practitioners can screen and advocate for such features in youth programming.

**Breadth.** Although benefits are consistently associated with participation in structured versus unstructured leisure activities, involvement in a greater breadth of activities has also been advocated. A study of rural adolescents found that those who participated in the most structured and unstructured activities did better in terms of grades, school attachment, and future educational expectations (Sharp et al., 2015). Those with a lower breadth of participation showed poorer outcomes. These findings are important to consider since youth in rural and lower socioeconomic status (SES) settings report limited options for organized activities compared with suburban youth. Occupational therapy practitioners should encourage participation in a variety of activities (both structured and unstructured) to help youth explore interests, skills, and personal characteristics across settings (Sharp et al., 2015).

**Density.** In terms of leisure, density means frequency of participation. In a study of leisure participation in Norwegian adolescents, Leversen et al. (2012) found a strong relationship between the amount of leisure participation and life satisfaction suggesting that density is important in addition to the variation of activities. Leisure activities engaged in frequently over time provide opportunities for skill development, allowing adolescents to feel that they are good at something (Leversen et al., 2012). Developing new skills, forming new behaviors, and building relationships takes time.

## Barriers and Constraints to Leisure Participation

To experience the benefits of leisure, youth must participate. The home, school, and community environments may either support or undermine youth's engagement in complex activities that they can enjoy. Both exposure to potential leisure occupations and the availability of resources to support engagement are critical factors influencing the likelihood that youth will develop and maintain healthy leisure interests (Mahoney et al., 2005). Resources such as parks, organized sports, other community programs, and competent adults to oversee the activities are essential. If only mindless or aggressive opportunities for action are available, youth will miss the opportunity to seek out and experience health-promoting challenges (Bazyk & Bazyk, 2009). Occupational therapy practitioners need to be aware of the multiple factors that may limit the availability of and access to healthy leisure activities, such as systemic racism, cultural bias, or gender-related issues (AOTA, 2020b). It is important to recognize how these factors might limit leisure participation and advocate minimizing disparities affecting marginalized groups. For example, practitioners need to become aware of and support community-driven initiatives aimed at providing healthy recreation, sports, and after-school activities in low-income environments.

**Youth with Disabilities and/or Mental Health Challenges.** Despite the importance of leisure and its positive impact on health outcomes, participation in community-based leisure is significantly restricted among youth with various types of disabilities compared with nondisabled peers (Bedell et al., 2013; Law et al., 2015; Powrie et al., 2020). Those with more significant functional impairment report lower levels of participation in leisure activities (Schreuer et al., 2014). A North American study found that 37% of youth with disabilities never took part in organized physical activities compared with only 10% among nondisabled peers (Bedell et al., 2013). Researchers found that youth with physical disabilities tend to participate more in informal, unstructured activities alone at home and less in structured community-based leisure (Law et al., 2006). Youth experiencing depression and peer rejection are at higher risk for leisure deprivation and may benefit from services aimed at fostering meaningful leisure participation and peer-related social skills (Spaeth et al., 2015).

**Financial and Transportation Limitations.** Low-income urban and rural youth generally have less opportunity to engage in structured leisure because of limited finances and/or transportation (Bazyk, 2011d). An important predictor of structured leisure participation is financial capital. Youth from families with higher socioeconomic status (SES) have greater financial capacity to pursue a larger range of leisure activities (Bazyk, 2011d; Farnworth, 1999). Most structured leisure activities (organized sports, dance lessons, and Scouts) require some sort of transportation and a participation fee. Many activities also require expensive equipment or specialized clothing.

## PROMOTING LEISURE PARTICIPATION WITHIN A MULTITIERED FRAMEWORK IN OCCUPATIONAL THERAPY

Given the developmental, mental, and physical health benefits of participation in a range of leisure occupations, occupational therapy practitioners need to address the leisure needs of *all* children and youth—those with and without disabilities and/or mental health challenges. A multitiered, public health framework has been described (Bazyk, 2011b) and applied by practitioners to address the mental health needs of children and youth. This framework has been effective in helping practitioners articulate and advocate for occupational therapy's distinct value in mental health promotion, prevention, and intervention (Bazyk et al., 2015) and has also been applied to promote leisure participation (Bazyk, 2011a).

A multitiered framework is compatible with the *Occupational Therapy Practice Framework: Domain and Process (OTPF-4)* (AOTA, 2020a) which broadly describes occupational therapy's contribution to promoting the health and participation of clients including persons, groups, and populations through engagement in occupations. Given this broad framework, it is timely for occupational therapy practitioners to reframe how they address leisure to include promotion and prevention in addition to a traditional focus on intervention for those with limitations due to disability, illness, injury, or poverty. Such a shift in thinking requires practitioners to reflect on who they serve and where, followed by a strategic conceptualization of what services might entail (Bazyk, 2011a, 2019). To address the leisure needs of *all* adolescents, the following sections provide descriptions of occupational therapy services at the universal, targeted, and individualized levels with practice examples representing diverse settings (school, clinic, and community). Although occupational therapy's emphasis varies depending on context, all efforts share a common belief in the positive relationship between participation in meaningful leisure and health (Bazyk, 2011b). The following sections describe key intervention approaches to facilitate leisure participation at the universal, targeted, and individualized levels of service provision.

### Intervention Approaches Used to Promote Leisure Participation

Based on current literature on leisure, an overall goal for occupational therapy practitioners is to foster leisure exploration and participation in a variety of structured activities within natural contexts. The following intervention approaches guide efforts to promote successful and enjoyable leisure participation.

**Use of an Ecological Model.** An ecological model, focusing on the relationship among the person, occupation, and environment (PEO), has been widely supported in occupational therapy (Law et al., 1996). Just as factors within the person may support or impede occupational performance, the environment can have a positive or negative influence. A core skill for all occupational therapy practitioners is **activity analysis** – the ability to analyze the relationship among the person, environment, and occupation and determine the factors needed for successful participation. When the activity-environment demands are greater than the person's abilities, adaptation of the environment or the activity may be provided to foster successful participation (Bazyk, 2011a).

Environmental barriers and social support have been linked to limited participation in leisure activities among youth with disabilities (Anaby et al., 2016). Despite the impact of environmental factors on participation, therapy has traditionally focused on improving performance component functioning (Anaby et al., 2016; Law et al., 2015). In contrast, with **environment-focused interventions**, the occupational therapy practitioner, youth, and family collaborate to remove environmental barriers, provide the necessary supports (e.g., physical, social, activity-based), and build on strengths to enhance successful participation (Anaby et al., 2016; Law & Darrah, 2014). Similarly, **context therapy** (Darrah et al., 2011) focusses on modifying environmental conditions and activity demands to foster leisure participation. For example, to decrease the activity demands of independent performance during a dance class, a peer buddy (e.g., a child with higher skills and positive social interaction) may dance alongside a child with autism to provide the needed environmental supports (e.g., verbal, and physical prompts) for successful participation.

**Leisure Coaching.** Environment-focused intervention may also involve a **coaching** element (Graham et al., 2009) where the occupational therapy practitioner coaches the young person and parent on identifying and implementing effective strategies to improve leisure participation (Anaby et al., 2016). There is evidence that implementing coaching among youth with physical disabilities is effective (Law et al., 2015). In a 12-week occupational therapy intervention involving environmental modifications and coaching with six adolescents with disabilities, Anaby et al. (2016) found clinically significant improvements in occupational performance. Contemporary approaches emphasize the importance of targeting modifiable factors within real-life environments rather than focusing solely on "fixing a deficit" to foster leisure participation.

**Focus on Strengths.** "Disability has long been defined and described in the language of deficits" (Carter et al., 2015, p. 101). An overemphasis on the remediation of deficits for youth with disabilities may have important limitations, particularly related to transition to adulthood. Participating in the community and developing relationships are heavily dependent on personal strengths. All young people possess a unique combination of strengths, struggles, interests, personality traits, and passions. In a mixed-method study of youth and young adults with intellectual disability and/or autism, Carter et al. (2015) found that that youth who participated in a higher number of community based after-school activities had more personal and interpersonal strengths. Assisting adolescents to develop leisure interests and activities that enhance and showcase their strengths may provide a relevant context within which youth develop and deepen strengths over time (Carter et al., 2015).

**Embed Playfulness.** When promoting leisure, it is important for the occupational therapy practitioners to embed playful interactions to communicate "having fun" together (Proyer et al., 2018). Playfulness can be used to diffuse tension and to move beyond resistance to participate. For example, one teenage female refused to participate in a mock TV production during an after-school leisure group by stating, "that's stupid." The skilled practitioner quickly quipped in a joking manner, "I'll tell you what, why don't you do the activity and afterward, you can tell me how much you hated it." This made the teen laugh. She participated in the activity and told the practitioner afterward how much she loved it and that she wanted to do it again. Playfulness can be powerful in building relationships between practitioners and youth, increasing motivation and the possibility of having fun together. It is also important to recognize and encourage a young person's playfulness by explicitly pointing it out as an important character strength to both the young person and parents. For example, "Joey has a great sense of humor. He makes us all laugh which adds to our fun and wanting to spend time together!"

### Occupational Therapy Strategies for Promoting Leisure Participation Within a Tiered Framework

A multitiered, public health framework supports a change in thinking from an individually focused deficit driven model of occupational therapy intervention to a whole population strength-based approach. The three major tiers of service can be depicted in a pyramid (see Fig. 17.1) and include *Tier 1 universal leisure promotion* (for all), *Tier 2 targeted prevention* (for those at-risk of limited leisure), and *Tier 3 individualized* (for those with leisure deficits). Universal leisure *promotion* emphasizes competence enhancement as well as environmental modifications to support leisure participation for all children and youth with and without limitations. Targeted *prevention* efforts focus on reducing the occurrence of leisure deficits in youth at-risk (e.g., those with disabilities, social challenges, limited finances) by providing targeted services. *Individualized intervention* focuses on leisure coaching with the young person and family to foster successful leisure participation for those with leisure deficits (Bazyk, 2011b). The occupational therapy process in addressing leisure within a multitiered framework follows a traditional process of evaluation, intervention, and targeting outcomes (AOTA, 2020a). It is important to remember that "client" is defined broadly and includes the young person, parents and family, peer groups, school community, clinic setting, and community (Bazyk, 2011c).

In the following sections, information specific to the occupational therapy process focusing on leisure participation is presented for each of the three tiers of service provision along with examples of occupational therapy implementation and outcomes. Although these are presented separately, there is often overlap in actual practice. A summary description of tiered occupational therapy services for promoting leisure participation is provided in Table 17.1. Occupational therapy examples

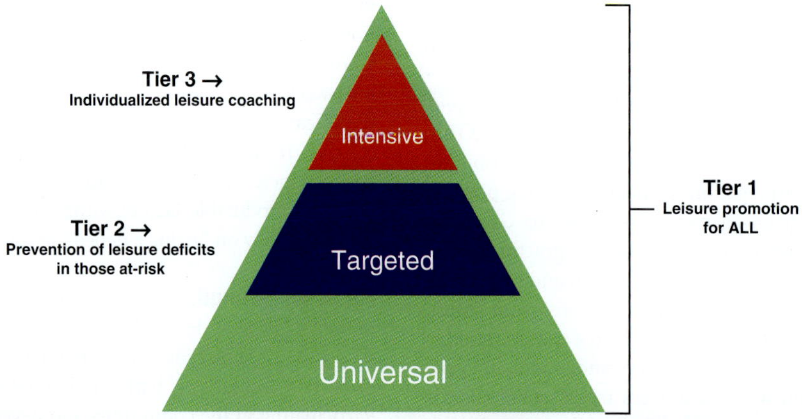


**Fig. 17.1** Tiered public health framework for addressing leisure in occupational therapy.

**TABLE 17.1 Description of a Tiered Services for Promoting Leisure Participation in Children and Youth**

| Focus of OT Services | Who Served? | Occupational Therapy Strategies |
|---|---|---|
| Tier 3 Individualized<br>Individualized OT Leisure Coaching | Youth with identified limitations in leisure participation | • Include leisure participation as a part of every OT evaluation. Begin with open-ended questions such as "What do you do for fun after school and on weekends?" Identify leisure strengths, limitations, and barriers to participation. Interview parents to learn about their daughter/son's leisure experiences, opportunities, and interests.<br>• Educate youth, parents, and school personnel about OT's role in promoting leisure participation.<br>• Use individual OT Leisure Coaching strategies over time to strategically foster structured leisure participation in one or more activities. |
| Tier 2 Targeted<br>OT Leisure Groups | Youth at risk of leisure deprivation | • Tune into youth who might be at risk of limited leisure participation such as those with challenges related to disabilities, mental health issues, sensory processing disorders, and/or obesity. Screen for leisure deficits.<br>• In addition to providing Tier 1 strategies, small group interventions targeting those at-risk during recess or after school focusing on exposure and participation in a variety of leisure activities. Unless exposed to leisure activities, youth will not discover interests and talents. Consider including peers with established leisure skills to lead various group activities. Youth often learn best from peer role models. |
| Tier 1 Universal<br>School-wide Leisure Promotion | All youth with and without disabilities and/or mental health challenges | • Explore local, state, and national resources focusing on inclusive community-based leisure.<br>• Educate youth, families, and school providers about the mental and physical health benefits of structured leisure participation and advocate for participation in a variety of activities (arts, music, theater, sports, clubs).<br>• Implement Every Moment Counts' *Refreshing Recess* program to promote participation in healthy play and leisure for all students.<br>• Help develop school-wide inclusive leisure activities such as The Sparkle Effect inclusive cheerleading or inclusive drama clubs.<br>• Develop and share a handout highlighting the benefits of structured leisure participation and a list of school and community-sponsored options. |

of addressing the leisure needs of adolescents are derived from *Every Moment Counts' Making Leisure Matter* initiative. Background information and a summary of this initiative can be found in Box 17.1.

**Tier 3: Individualized Intervention.** Following a comprehensive evaluation as described in Chapter 9, occupational therapy services at this level focus on helping youth with disabilities and/or mental health challenges who have little or no leisure participation to explore and participate in meaningful and healthy hobbies and interests. Tier 3 individualized intervention involves a variety of strategies, as described above, including an ecological PEO analysis, environment-focused services, embedding playfulness, strength-based strategies, and leisure coaching. Specific to youth with physical disabilities, the Pathways and Resources for Engagement and Participation (PREP) intervention has been effective in improving performance in meaningful community-based activities (Anaby et al., 2016, 2018; Law et al., 2015). This 12-week client-centered intervention focuses on enhancing participation by focusing on strengths, removing environmental barriers, and coaching youth and parents. The five steps guiding intervention are (1) making goals; (2) mapping out a plan; (3) making it happen; (4) measuring process and outcomes; and (5) moving forward (Law et al., 2016). In an interrupted time series design study involving 28 adolescents with physical disabilities, the PREP intervention resulted in statistically significant improvements in leisure participation (Anaby et al., 2018). A similar 6-step occupational therapy (OT) leisure coaching process has been developed as a part of *Every Moment Counts'* Making Leisure Matter initiative (refer to Box 17.2). Tier 3 OT Leisure Coaching success stories can be found in Table 17.2. Fig. 17.2 depicts a young boy with developmental and mental health challenges successfully participating in adaptive soccer with the support of his occupational therapy practitioner.

## BOX 17.1 Every Moment Counts' Making Leisure Matter Initiative

The occupational therapy examples shared throughout this chapter of promoting leisure participation are derived from work completed as a part of *Every Moment Counts (EMC).* Originally funded by the Ohio Department of Education (2012–15), *EMC* is a multipronged mental health promotion initiative developed to help all children and youth become mentally healthy to succeed in school, at home, and in the community (Bazyk, 2019; Bazyk et al., 2015). This initiative emphasizes mental health promotion, inclusion of children with disabilities and/or mental health challenges in school and community settings, integrating occupational therapy services in natural settings throughout the day (classroom, recess, cafeteria, and after school), and collaborating with all relevant stakeholders to enhance their ability to be mental health promoters (refer to www.everymomentcounts.org).

*Making Leisure Matter (MLM)* is one of EMC's initiatives that was originally developed as an exploratory research study (2014–16). A convenience sample of 20 occupational therapists and occupational therapy assistants committed to working together for 2 years to strategically foster leisure participation in youth with disabilities and/or mental health challenges who were identified as engaging in few or no leisure occupations. Practitioners worked in a variety of schools, private practice outpatient, and community-based settings. The focus of the first year (Phase 1) involved Tier 3 Individualized OT Leisure Coaching. Findings from the first year resulted in expanding the leisure coaching to address the needs of youth at Tiers 1 and 2 during Phase 2. Implementation and outcomes at each phase are summarized below.

### Making Leisure Matter, Phase 1 Implementation and Outcomes

Occupational therapy practitioners involved in this initiative selected youth (ages 8–20 years) on their caseloads that they knew had little or no leisure participation. Youth with a variety of diagnoses were represented including Down syndrome, ADHD, spina bifida, sensory processing disorder, autism, anxiety, serious emotional disturbance, and depression. After learning about the benefits and barriers associated with structured leisure participation (Anaby et al., 2016; Graham et al., 2009) during an orientation session, the practitioners used several strategies (coaching, strength-based, environmental modifications) over time to promote participation in one or more community or school-based leisure occupations. Data collection involved the practitioners writing monthly reflections of what they did with the young person during each meeting, outcomes, and personal reflections. At the end of the first year, practitioners reflected on the entire process noting successes, barriers, and challenges. Each participant summarized what they felt were essential elements of the OT Leisure Coaching process (refer to Box 17.2).

Outcome: Participation in one or more structured leisure activities on a routine basis (minimum of once per week) over an extended period (minimum of 2 months) was the targeted outcome. Nineteen of the 20 youths successfully participated in one or more structured leisure activities within three to 9 months of OT Leisure Coaching. A range of leisure activities was chosen based on the young person's interests, family resources, and community availability (e.g., pottery, crocheting, bird watching, adapted football, running, softball, theater, horticulture, and cooking). It is important to note that a variety of interest inventories were used as a part of the OT Leisure Coaching process to educate and expose the young person to possible leisure pursuits. Practitioners noted that both adolescents and parents were often unaware of the wide variety of possibilities. Once an interest was sparked, the practitioner and young person explored community options using online resources with parent input.

*Occupational spin-off:* In some cases, the occupational therapy practitioner noted that 'success bred further success." Parents were excited to observe their child's successful participation in the community and the associated benefits of expressed joy, new friends, expanded skills, and independence. An occupational spin-off was noted, which represents the notion that success and enjoyment experienced during a new leisure occupation lead to further leisure exploration (Rebeiro & Cook, 1999). Parents were observed as feeling more confident in their ability to find leisure activities in the community and in the belief that their child could be successful in a community-sponsored activity. OT leisure coaching not only helps youth expand their leisure interests but also helps parents develop the skills and confidence needed to search for options and complete the registration process.

### Making Leisure Matter, Phase 2 Implementation and Outcomes

During Phase 2 of the *Making Leisure Matter* initiative, practitioners expanded services to include Tier 1 and 2 strategies for promoting leisure participation at the universal and targeted levels in school and community settings. Tuning into youth at risk of leisure deprivation, practitioners providing after-school outpatient clinic services realized that they were not effectively promoting leisure participation. Given practitioners' ability to facilitate occupation-based groups, several practitioners developed and implemented groups to foster both social-emotional learning and leisure participation. Practitioners identified leisure needs at the universal, whole-school, and community levels. Creative ways to promote leisure at school such as the development of Special Olympics and walking and running clubs occurred. Other practitioners brought community leisure organizations into the school or offered leisure groups at local recreation centers. The longer occupational therapy practitioners were involved in the *Making Leisure Matters* initiative, the more their services expanded to the universal and targeted levels. Specific success stories are described in Table 17.2.

From Bazyk, S. (2022). 'Making Leisure Matter.' Every Moment Counts. https://everymomentcounts.org/making-leisure-matter/

## BOX 17.2 Making Leisure Matter's Occupational Therapy Leisure Coaching Process

**Every Moment Counts' OT Leisure Coaching**

**Vision Statement:** All children and youth have a right to participate in and enjoy healthy hobbies and interests in inclusive school and community settings.

***Why Occupational Therapy?***

Occupational therapy practitioners (OTPs) are skilled in being able to analyze the social, emotional, physical, and sensory aspects involved in doing an activity to make the modifications needed for successful participation. Using a collaborative coaching approach, OTPs provide the support and adaptations needed for successful participation (e.g., enhance needed skills; adapt entry into the activity; modify the activity; educate the activity director; etc.).

***About OT Leisure Coaching***

The focus of OT Leisure Coaching is to help *all* children and youth explore, select, and participate in extracurricular leisure activities to develop enjoyable hobbies and interests. OT Leisure Coaching can be provided either *individually* with a youth and family, within a *small group* context, or at a *school-wide level*. The occupational therapy practitioner serves as an:

- *Educator*, sharing information about the health benefits of participation in enjoyable hobbies and interests with children/youth, families, and school personnel;
- *Facilitator* of the change process, by working collaboratively with youth to help them explore and participate in enjoyable leisure activities; and
- *Advocate* inclusive leisure participation by promoting involvement in integrated school and community-sponsored extracurricular activities.

**OT leisure coaching** combines the use of emotional support and encouragement, information exchange, and a structured process of planning for and participating in chosen activities. The OTP serves as a facilitator of the change process:

- *Emotional Support and encouragement* are provided to build trust and help the youth and family explore and pursue leisure participation. OTP uses listening, empathy, reframing abilities, guidance, and encouragement.
- *Information exchange* between the OT, youth, and family. OT shares information about the health benefits of leisure participation. The child/youth shares information about potential leisure interests. Family shares information about available resources (financial, transportation, time, etc.) and values related to leisure participation.
- *Structured process* involving identifying interests, exploring options, and planning for and engaging in leisure activities (see OT Leisure Coaching process). This process often involves activity analysis, problem-solving, and scaffolding the experience; advocating for the child/youth/family; and therapeutic use of self to enable successful participation.

***OT Leisure Coaching Process: Six Steps to Success***

1. **Start the conversation about the importance of leisure**—Meet with children/youths and parents and educate them about the health benefits of participation in meaningful hobbies and interests during out-of-school time. Obtain parental buy-in and support. Begin to develop a trusting relationship.
2. **Interest Inventory: Spark an interest**—Complete an interest inventory with child/youth; provide education about a variety of creative arts, sports, and nature-based activities; help child/youth prioritize a list of interests; share with caregivers.
3. **Explore school or community-sponsored options**—Explore options for participation using the Internet based on the family resources; engage the child/youth and family in this process as much as possible. Know your community and venues for inclusive participation!
4. **Make a match and a plan**—Discuss school and/or community-sponsored options for participation with the child/youth and caregivers; plan for registration and entry into the activity. Contact the program instructor/coach (if necessary) to discuss relevant information regarding the child/youth's strengths. And needs related to accommodations and successful participation.
5. **Just do it! Child/youth participates in the activity.** Occupational therapy (OT) coaching provided to foster success—only as much as needed (e.g., adapting entry into the activity, modifying the environment, coaching and support to instructor/coach, etc.).
6. **Occupational reflection and future plans**—Following participation, talk with the child/youth and caregivers (separately) about the experience—Explore likes? Dislikes? Foster ongoing exploration and participation in a variety of healthy hobbies and interests.

**Developed for Every Moment Counts by:** Bazyk, S., Weiss, D., Negrey, J., Llerena, M., Thompson-Repas, K., LaGuardia, T., Michaud, P., & Kennedy, M. (2015). *Making Leisure Matter.*

Bazyk, S. (2022). '*Making Leisure Matter*'. Every Moment Counts. https://everymomentcounts.org/making-leisure-matter/

## TABLE 17.2 Occupational Therapy Success Stories of Individual, Targeted, and Universal Leisure Promotion

| Client, Setting, and OTP | Evaluation; Identifying a Need | Intervention | Leisure Outcomes |
|---|---|---|---|
| **Tier 3: Individual OT Leisure Coaching** | | | |
| **Kelson** (14 y.o., diagnosed with autism, anxiety, severe emotional disturbance, optic nerve hypoplasia)<br>**Setting:** Prentiss Autism Center, Positive Education Program, Cleveland, OH<br>**OT:** David Weiss, OTR/L | • Kelson lives with his mother, Sonia, on the second floor of a two-family home.<br>• He is very social and enjoys being helpful but struggles with aggressive and violent behavior causing his mother to call 911.<br>• He enjoys art activities, and his mother has a card table with art supplies set up at home.<br>• He doesn't have any extracurricular activities.<br>• Kelson likes to watch football and indicated he would like to play football. Sonia said she would like him to be a part of a team with positive male role models. | • David found a local adaptive football league and helped Sonia access and fill out the registration materials. This was an important part of leisure coaching because Sonia did not know how to find an appropriate football program to meet Kelson's needs. Because of her concerns, David provided the support and encouragement she needed to complete the registration process.<br>• David attended the first couple of sessions to share strategies with the coach for helping Kelson regulate behavior, communicate needs, and participate successfully. Sonia felt that David's input was significant in ensuring Kelson's transition and success in a new activity. | • Kelson participated in the entire 3-month weekly adaptive football program.<br>• Sonia was happy to see Kelson successfully participate and enjoy being a part of a football team. This experience increased her confidence in Kelson's ability to participate in a community-sponsored activity. Since then, he has participated in an adapted soccer program.<br>• In a short videotaped interview, Sonia stated that playing football has helped him be more focused and patient in working toward a goal and that he looks forward to football and it makes him happy.<br>• View the video at https://everymomentcounts.org/view.php?nav_id=192 |

## TABLE 17.2 Occupational Therapy Success Stories of Individual, Targeted, and Universal Leisure Promotion—cont'd

| Client, Setting, and OTP | Evaluation; Identifying a Need | Intervention | Leisure Outcomes |
|---|---|---|---|
| **Alex** (16 y.o., diagnosed with autism and severe anxiety)<br>**Setting:** Home-schooled, Cleveland, OH<br>**Family:** Single-parent household (father) and twin brother without a disability<br>**OT:** Paula Michaud, MEd, OTR/L | • Paula met with the father privately to discuss Alex's interests, strengths, and challenges; the father expressed a family interest in music and theater and significant challenges in taking Alex anywhere outside of the home due to his anxiety<br>• Paula completed the Sensory Profile and a leisure inventory with Alex; he identified music and theater as interests; he indicated that he wanted to be in a play like his twin brother | • Paula worked with Alex on self-regulation related to his anxiety using the "bucket filler" analogy and teaching self-regulation strategies<br>• Paula explored adapted theater programs and found a local one at a small college<br>• Peer coaching was used to help Alex participate in theater practice and the production of a Mary Poppins play | • Alex successfully participated in the *Mary Poppins* performance with the assistance of a peer mentor<br>• This success led to him participating in a general education high school theater performance the following year |
| **Shelly** (13 y.o, diagnosed with spina bifida and Type 1 diabetes)<br>**Setting:** Solon School District, OH<br>**OT:** Julie Brizes, MEd, OTR/L | • Started the discussion of leisure participation & possible new interests<br>• Shelley wanted to have something "portable" to do when she went to her brothers' sports events<br>• She had an IEP objective to be able to complete a multistep fine motor activity<br>• Shelly admired Julie's scarf which led to a conversation about crocheting | • Shelly indicated an interest in learning how to crochet<br>• Julie taught her how to crochet and make a scarf<br>• Julie taught Shelly the basic stitches and spent 5–10 minutes per OT session working on the scarf | • Shelly finished crocheting the scarf over the summer<br>• She explored high school clubs and decided to join the knitting/crocheting club |
| **Tier 2: Targeted OT Leisure Groups** | | | |
| **CLINIC**<br>**Cleveland Clinic Outpatient Therapy**, Westlake, OH<br>**OT:** Jenny Negray, MOT, OTR/L | • Typically provide 1:1 therapy 1 hour per week<br>• Provide therapy after school for children and youth with a wide variety of disabilities<br>• Many clients demonstrate challenges with making friends and participating in community-based leisure<br>• Parents report difficulties in finding leisure activities<br>• A large number of youths have comorbid anxiety and depression | • Developed their first OT-led leisure group in 2014, Game Break Group, focusing on learning how to play games and friendship skills. Targeted youths on their caseloads identify as having few or no friends and limited out-of-school leisure.<br>• Following this group's success, the OTPs developed and implemented a variety of occupation-based groups to foster exploration and participation: Green Thumbs Up Group, Artists Group, Mindful Movements Group, PPursuits Leisure Group | • Group participants enjoy the groups, leaving with new leisure interests and friends. One participant carried her UNO deck with her to school and was observed initiating a card game with a peer. One parent indicated that her daughter began having play dates with other children in the group.<br>• Hospital administration supported the continuation and expansion of the groups based on positive outcomes.<br>• Video vignette of Game Break Group - https://everymomentcounts.org/view.php?nav_id=193 |
| **RECREATION CENTER**<br>**The KIDnections Groups, LLC** (occupation-based groups provided for youth with and without disabilities at a recreation center)<br>North Olmsted, OH<br>**OT:** Maria Llerena, OTR/L | • Recognized that youth with disabilities often have limited leisure participation, especially in inclusive community settings.<br>• The local recreation facility did not have any classes that did not target and included youth with disabilities.<br>• Youth on Maria's caseload needed leisure groups facilitated by professionals knowledgeable and skilled in modifying the activity and/or environment to foster successful participation and who knew how to promote positive behavior and social interaction. | • Collaborated with a speech therapist and ABA therapist to develop a business, The KIDnections Groups, LLC, to meet a real community need.<br>• Met with and obtained buy-in from the director of a local recreation center to offer leisure groups targeting youth with autism and other disabilities and peers without disabilities.<br>• The groups are advertised on The KIDnections Group website where parents can register and pay for participation. Website: http://www.thekidnectionsgroup.com.<br>• They began by offering cooking groups for youth with autism and based on demand have expanded what they offer to a variety of groups and adapted parties.<br>• The groups foster leisure exploration, skill development, and social connections. Youths attend the groups without parents present. | • The recreation center is fully accessible for youth with disabilities.<br>• The KIDnections Group is provided as a therapeutic, social, and recreational service.<br>• Classes expand based on youth and parent input and include cooking, packing a brown lunch, planning your own party and meals, games, Lego groups, and arts and crafts.<br>• Participants make friends with youth from their community and feel like they "belong" in a recreation center setting.<br>• Skills learned include cooking and food safety, clean up, following directions, serving others, reading recipes, using kitchen tools, and teamwork. |

*Continued*

**TABLE 17.2 Occupational Therapy Success Stories of Individual, Targeted, and Universal Leisure Promotion—cont'd**

| Client, Setting, and OTP | Evaluation; Identifying a Need | Intervention | Leisure Outcomes |
|---|---|---|---|
| **Tier 1: Universal Leisure Promotion for ALL** | | | |
| Cleveland Metropolitan School District, Cleveland, OH<br>**OT:** Eileen Dixon, MS, OTR/L | • Students are primarily from low-income families<br>• Limited finances and transportation prevent exploration of a range of leisure activities<br>• School personnel and families are unaware of the health benefits of structured leisure participation | • Eileen completed a Leisure Environmental Scan of activities in her school's immediate area that are low-cost or free and that can be accessed by bus or on foot. | • Eileen made a poster and handout depicting the location and contact information for a variety of family-based leisure activities.<br>• The poster and handouts were made available to the school community in the school's entrance area. |
| Achievement Centers for children autism school, Westlake, OH<br>**OT:** Maria Llerena, OTR/L | • Students with autism receive education in self-contained classrooms.<br>• Many students engage in little to no out-of-school leisure and have few friends outside of school.<br>• Families are hesitant to try something new and are unsure whether programs will accept youth with autism and know how to support participation. They don't feel connected to the community.<br>• If youth don't have opportunities to be exposed to a variety of activities, they will not discover hidden interests and talents. | • Maria met with families and students to explore their interests.<br>• Maria searched the community for recreational activities and programs that welcome students with special needs and compiled a list of resources to give to families.<br>• Students with significant communication and behavior challenges often need to participate in adapted sports, dance, and art classes that were found in the community.<br>• Maria contacted several agencies and programs to provide background information about the need for inclusive participation and to invite them to provide an introductory, 1-day class presentation and demonstration. She set up some presentations that were given to the students as a part of the academic curriculum. | • The outside agency visits were a "hit." Students were engaged and excited to share information with parents.<br>• The following organizations provided class presentations and demonstrations:<br>  ◦ power Martial arts Academy<br>  ◦ Beck center for the arts<br>  ◦ Lake Erie Nature and science center<br>  ◦ St. Ignatius High School Juggling Group<br>  ◦ North pointe Ballet<br>• Beck center for the arts' 1-day class led to an 8-week theater class with a final production of *The Wizard of Oz.* All students participated in dance rehearsals, making props for the set, posters for advertising, managing audiovisuals, and performing for families and the school staff.<br>• Students with disabilities have amazing talents and interests that are discovered and developed if there are opportunities to participate.<br>• Programs are available, but families need help in finding them. |

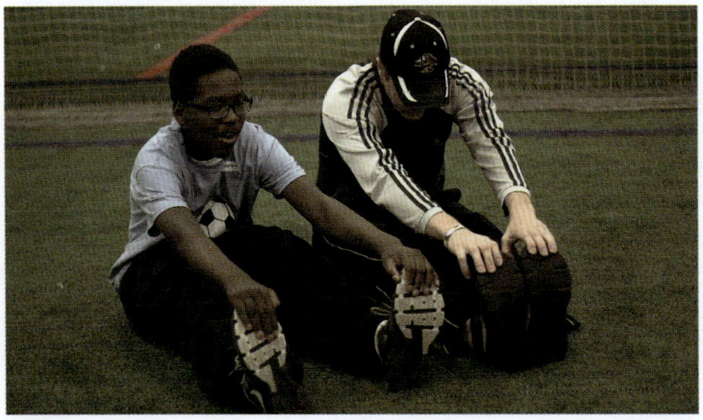

**Fig. 17.2** A young boy with developmental and mental health challenges successfully participates in adaptive soccer with the support of his occupational therapy practitioner.

**Tier 2: Targeted Leisure Groups for Youth at Risk of Leisure Deprivation.** Tier 2 services are developed and implemented with youth at risk of limited leisure participation such as children with disabilities and/or mental health challenges who may struggle with social interaction and friendship, anxiety and/or depression, and being bullied (Bazyk, 2011c). Young people experiencing obesity may struggle with self-esteem issues as well as physical challenges (Bazyk & Winne, 2013). Additionally, specific efforts to promote leisure participation with youth at risk due to restricted access and availability (e.g., low-income urban contexts or rural areas) may be provided (Bazyk & Bazyk, 2009). Targeted services emphasize both the prevention of the negative effects of leisure deprivation (e.g., boredom, participation in risky unstructured activities) as well as the promotion of a variety of healthy and meaningful leisure interests (Bazyk, 2011c).

Occupation-based groups focusing on leisure exploration can be an important strategy for fostering leisure interests in youth at risk of limited participation. There is strong evidence to support occupation-based social skills groups targeting leisure to enhance youth's social participation and mental health (Arbesman et al., 2013). All occupational therapy practitioners obtain entry-level skills and experience in developing and facilitating occupation-based groups (Olson, 2011). By "doing" together, occupation-based groups help participants work together cooperatively, experience group cohesion, and build friendships (Bazyk & Bazyk, 2009). At the same time, youth are exposed to novel activities giving them opportunities to try out something new, identify hidden strengths, and develop new leisure interests.

Traditional occupational therapy in clinic and school settings tends to focus on individual, one-to-one service delivery. This type of service provision may be less effective in helping youth develop important social skills and friendships. While the primary goal of these groups is to expose youth to a variety of occupations to foster the development of leisure interests, practitioners need to make the case that such groups can address occupational performance goals (e.g., fine motor, sensory processing, social, and emotional).

***Making the Case for Occupational Therapy Leisure Groups in Schools.*** For practitioners in school settings, it's critical to be aware of and to educate others on how the Individuals with Disabilities Education Act (IDEA) (Pub. L. 108–446) supports services that promote play and leisure in natural contexts throughout the day. First, IDEA mandates that schools must provide nonacademic and extracurricular services and activities in the manner necessary to afford students with disabilities an equal opportunity for participation in those services and activities (See Section 300. Nonacademic Services). These services and activities may include athletics, recreational activities, special interest clubs, and recess activities. Second, schools must ensure that each student with a disability participates with nondisabled peers in the extracurricular services and activities to the maximum extent possible (least restrictive environment). Further, supplementary aids and services deemed necessary by the IEP team need to be provided to help students participate in nonacademic settings.

Based on IDEA's mandate, occupational therapy practitioners need to talk about the importance of leisure participation with students, families, and school personnel and advocate for services that promote leisure participation during recess and after school. For example, small groups that integrate both students with and without disabilities can be offered during recess to enhance play, leisure, and social participation. Such recess groups, despite occurring over a short amount of time, can be effective in exposing youth to games (e.g., card games, board games, four square) or simple crafts (e.g., making friendship bracelets), building friendships, and reducing bullying.

An occupational therapy practitioner in a suburban school indicated that it is important to "look for the open doors" to provide needed services. At two separate IEP meetings, concerns about students' struggles with anxiety, making friends, and being bullied were discussed. Based on this awareness and the principal's support, the practitioner developed a group called "Friendship and Activity Detectives," which was offered 1 day per week for 8 weeks during recess targeting students who struggled, as well as nondisabled peer mentors. The groups focused on playing games, leisure exploration, friendship promotion, and social and emotional learning. Because the groups were so successful in helping the students have fun and make friends, the principal supported continued implementation. In another example, an occupational therapy practitioner developed an after-school game club, initially targeting youth with disabilities. She was aware that several high school students on her caseload had few friends and nothing to do after school. With principal support, space was provided for the teens to meet and play games, hang out, and enjoy a snack under the supervision of the occupational therapy practitioner. Soon, the club attracted teens without disabilities and has grown to be an inclusive club for students with and without disabilities to play games, have fun, and make friends. See Fig. 17.3.

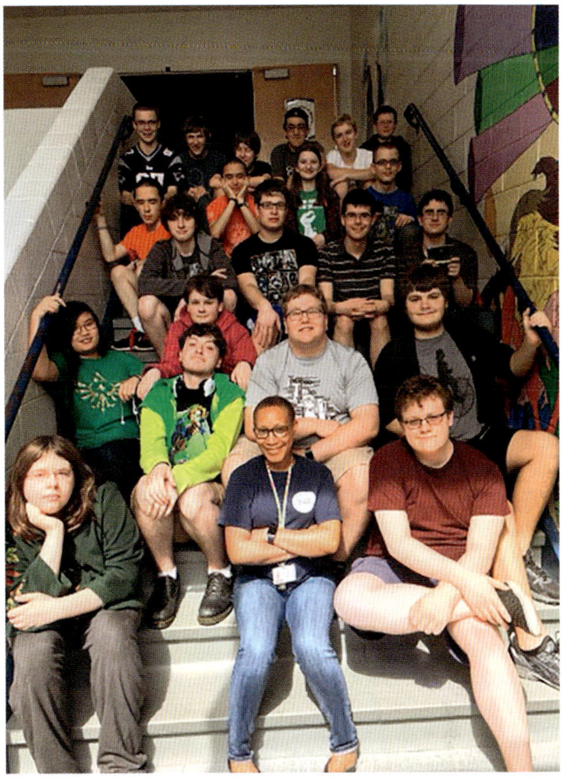

**Fig. 17.3** Teens enjoy participating in after-school leisure. The teens meet and play games, have snacks, socialize, and have fun after school.

***Making the Case for Occupational Therapy Leisure Groups in After-School Clinic Settings.*** Youth with disabilities and/or mental health challenges receiving outpatient services are often seen during the after-school hours. Providing individual services focusing on performance component functioning (e.g., fine motor skills, sensory processing, social skills) may limit opportunities to explore leisure activities within a social context. Given that youth with disabilities are at greater risk of leisure deprivation and being bullied (Bazyk, 2011d), developing and providing occupation-based groups is an important service delivery option for outpatient clinic settings. Participation in groups provides opportunities to develop friendships. Having high-quality friendships, or at least one best friend, can help prevent youth from being a victim of bullying (Bazyk, 2011d). Offering a range of leisure groups to expose youth to a variety of structured leisure (games, art, horticulture) can also provide opportunities to address performance goals such as fine motor skills, self-regulation, and sensory processing. Refer to Table 17.2 for a success story of Tier 2 leisure groups in a clinical setting. Fig. 17.4 depicts children with disabilities participating in an after-school game-playing group with occupational therapy practitioners.

***Making the Case for Occupational Therapy Leisure Groups in the Community.*** Community-based groups offered in natural settings such as recreation centers can foster participation in leisure. Recreation centers often offer a variety of classes for children and youth that require registration and class fees for participation. Refer to Table 17.2 for an example of OT leisure groups offered in a recreation center.

Occupation-based groups can also be embedded in after-school youth programs. Payment for services is possible if parents can obtain insurance coverage or pay out of pocket. This is not always feasible, especially in low-income urban contexts. Community-based after-school programs almost always lack the finances needed to provide occupational therapy services. Low-income urban youth are at risk of occupational deprivation in leisure due to a lack of family and financial resources. One way to meet the structured leisure and social and emotional needs of this population is through university-led occupational therapy service-learning programs. Refer to Box 17.3 for details

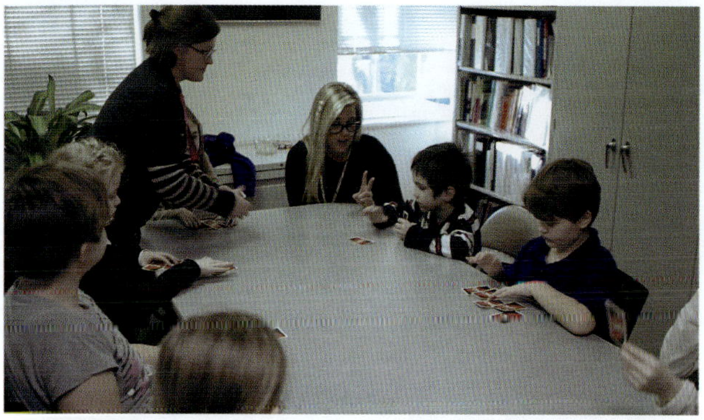

**Fig. 17.4** Children with disabilities participate in after-school games and activities with occupational therapy practitioners and students. They explore and engage in a variety of leisure activities.

about preventive leisure groups for low-income youth. Fig. 17.5 A and B demonstrates occupational therapy students facilitating occupation-based groups with low-income urban youth in an after-school setting.

**Tier 1: Universal School and Community-Based Leisure Promotion.** It is important that parents and school personnel learn about the multiple benefits of structured leisure for their children—that participation in self-selected structured leisure provides positive opportunities for fostering health, identity work, and life skill development. Given occupational therapy practitioners' scope of practice in the areas of play, leisure, and social participation combined with skills in analyzing the person, environment, and occupation, they provide services at the universal level. This is feasible in school settings given that IDEA mandates that students with disabilities receive services in the least restrictive environment to the maximum extent possible

## BOX 17.3 Tier 2 Preventive Occupational Therapy Leisure Groups With Low-Income Urban Youth

### HOPE Groups: Healthy Occupations for Positive Emotions (Bazyk, 2006)

The Occupational Therapy Groups for HOPE (Healthy Occupations for Positive Emotions), embedded in an after-school program in Cleveland, Ohio, were developed to address the occupation-based, social-emotional, and interaction needs of low-income urban youth.

**The HOPE Group Curriculum:** The integration of knowledge about group process, meaningful occupation, social and emotional learning (SEL), mental health literacy, and positive behavioral interventions and supports (PBS) provided the foundation for the 8-week HOPE groups. Under the supervision of the project director (S. Bazyk), two graduate occupational therapy students (OT) from Cleveland State University co-plan and facilitate the weekly groups, with 6–10 youth ages 6–14 years. Each Fall semester since 2004, approximately 60–80 children participate in the groups. The groups promote.

- ***Participation in Meaningful Leisure Occupation:*** Based on the risk of occupational deprivation in low-income urban youth, the HOPE groups expose youth to a variety of structured leisure occupations. Examples include games, drumming, horticulture, and arts and crafts. Activities are selected by occupational therapy students based on input from the youth to expose them to new activities and the development of new hobbies and interests.
- ***Social and Emotional Learning (SEL) Activities:*** SEL activities are embedded into each of the groups and focus on the development of social competencies (e.g., understanding the relationship among feelings, thoughts, and behaviors; empathy), friendship skills, conflict resolution skills, and anger management skills. The social-emotional aspects of the group session help youth recognize their emotions, think about their feelings and how they should act, and regulate their behavior based on thoughtful decision-making. The social-emotional learning curriculum *and* strategies for teaching appropriate ways to express anger are adapted from *Volcano in My Tummy: Helping Children to Handle Anger* (Whitehouse & Pudney, 1996).
- ***Group Process:*** Research suggests that children who demonstrate personal or social difficulties benefit more from small groups that provide a supportive environment and an opportunity to develop positive relationships with caring adults than those who receive individual interventions. Through "doing together," the HOPE groups foster peer interaction and teamwork leading to a sense of group cohesion.
- ***Positive Behavioral Interventions and Supports (PBIS):*** PBIS promotes the use of proactive strategies to prevent problem behavior by altering a situation before problems escalate, and to concurrently teach appropriate alternatives. Examples of strategies embedded during the HOPE groups included clearly communicating group rules and creating a warm and positive group environment.
- ***Mental Health Literacy:*** Youth learn about positive mental health (feeling good, doing well, coping with challenges) and strategies for managing stress. By participating in various leisure activities, they learn first-hand the relationship between enjoyable occupations and feeling good emotionally.

### Organization of the Group Sessions

Group sessions are structured into three segments: conversation time, project activity, and closure. *Conversation time* focuses on introducing the social-emotional theme for the session, setting the emotional tone, and promoting group cohesion. The *occupation-based project activity* is considered the "heart" of the group because it exposes the children to activities that may develop into long-term interests and allows them to practice the social-emotional skills introduced during conversation time. Examples of projects and activities include making greeting cards using rubber stamping, crocheting scarves, creating papier-mâché masks, and doing yoga. The project activities focus on exposing children to a variety of structured leisure occupations to broaden their repertoire of interests and promote the development of hobbies. *Closure* involves revisiting the SEL theme and occupational reflection—an opportunity to think about the influence of activity on emotional and physical health.

### Research Outcomes

- **Meaning of participation from youth's perspective: Becoming Hooked on Doing.** A phenomenology study, using a combination of in-depth interviews and participant observations, explored the meaning of group participation from the youth's perspective. Findings revealed that the youth perceive the groups to be *fun* (occupational meaning) because of engagement in novel and challenging projects and talking about feelings within a supportive group context (occupational form). Participation in creative leisure occupations that allow for choice transforms mood—youth experience happiness and forget their problems (occupational function). The children enjoy the projects and activities and express wanting to do more. Children are often heard saying "What are we going to do today?" or "I wish you could come every day." They become hooked on doing and experience firsthand the power of occupation—that participating in creative occupations fosters positive feelings. In addition, as the weeks pass, the youth begin to interact as a cohesive group—sharing materials and praising each other's accomplishments. Youth also indicated that they enjoy being able to talk about their feelings (Bazyk & Bazyk, 2009).
- **Meaning of participation from the OT students' perspective: Becoming and OT.** Reflective journals and focus groups were used to explore how OT students made sense of their experience of planning and facilitating the HOPE groups. Qualitative data analysis resulted in six major themes reflecting the process of professional growth over the 8 weeks. Professional reasoning progressed from mechanical procedural reasoning to flexible forms of conditioning reasoning. Findings emphasize the critical role of active participation in real-life contexts in learning how to become an OT and address the needs of youth deprived of leisure exploration (Bazyk et al., 2010).

(34 C.F.R. § 300.114(A) (2) (i)). Whenever possible, occupational therapy practitioners need to integrate services in natural contexts throughout the day (both academic and nonacademic) as opposed to providing individual therapy in isolated settings (Cahill & Bazyk, 2020). For example, an occupational therapy practitioner implementing a universal, school-wide program might embed accommodations and supports for students with disabilities to ensure successful and enjoyable participation (Mohler et al., 2014). When integrating services, practitioners have opportunities to observe how students on their caseload participate in play and leisure during recess, for example, and tune into students who demonstrate limited participation or who are at-risk but not on their caseloads. As such, integrated services maximize the impact of occupational therapy, allowing practitioners to address the leisure needs of more students and educate teachers and other school providers about occupational therapy's full scope of practice (Cahill & Bazyk, 2020).

In terms of evaluation and intervention at the universal level, practitioners focus on opportunities for quality play and leisure during recess and extracurricular after school activities. Recess is a critical time of the day to promote active play, friendship, teamwork, and inclusion of students with disabilities and/or mental health challenges. Due to the unstructured nature of recess combined with supervisors who are often unprepared to foster positive play and social interaction among large groups of students, there are often higher incidents of bullying and behavior challenges. Embedding occupational therapy services during recess can contribute to the promotion of enjoyable participation in healthy play and leisure activities for all students. Refer to Box 17.4 to learn

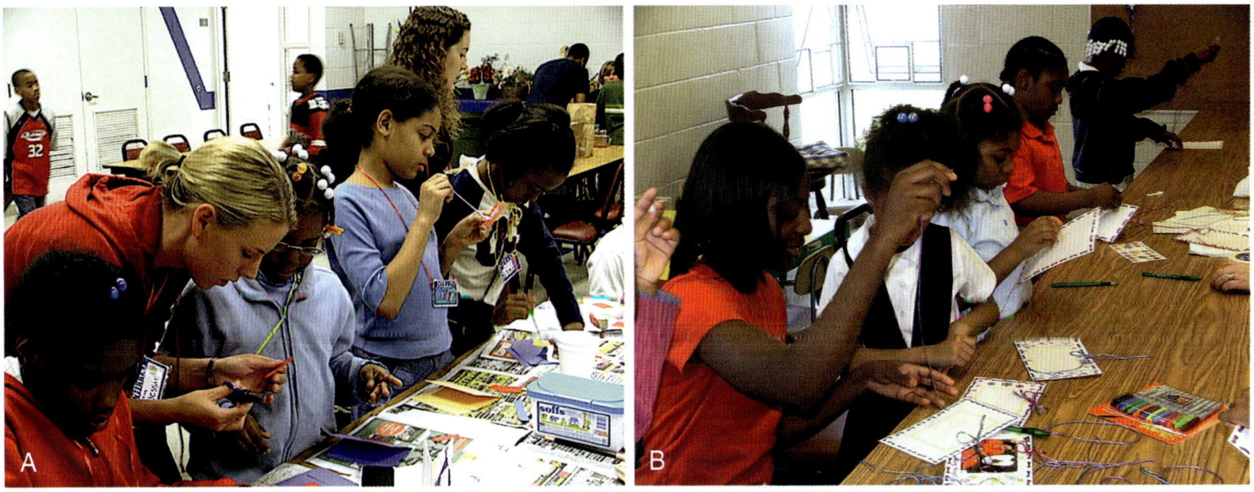

Fig. 17.5 (A) Occupational therapy students facilitate leisure groups with low-income urban youth in an after-school program. (B) They provide opportunities for children to experience leisure, develop interests, and develop a sense of identity.

## BOX 17.4 Tier 1, Universal Recess Program: Refreshing Recess

As a part of *Every Moment Counts*, this program is embedded during recess to create a positive recess experience so that all students can enjoy active play and socialization with friends. The goal is to provide the recess supervisors and students with the necessary knowledge, skills, and resources needed to sustain a positive recess environment. Specifically, the program was designed to support school personnel during recess and to give them strategies for fostering friendships, engaging children in a variety of play activities, resolving conflicts, promoting positive behavior, and creating opportunities for inclusion of all students. Any structured activities that are provided are strictly optional, so students may choose whether they would like to participate.

The evaluation consists of observing recess and completing a *Recess Environmental Scan* (refer to https://s3.us-east-2.amazonaws.com/s3.everymomentcounts.com/wp-content/uploads/2021/03/01192600/RR_EnvironmentalAnalysis_FINAL_fillable_3-1-21.pdf). During the observation, the occupational therapy practitioner tunes into the occupations of play and leisure as well as the physical, social, and emotional contexts. Do children and youth engage in enjoyable and healthy forms of play and leisure? Are there students who struggle to fit in? Do recess supervisors interact with students in positive ways and encourage a variety of play activities? Strengths and challenges specific to the recess experience help shape the implementation of the *Refreshing Recess* program.

***What does the program involve?*** This is a 6-week, 1 day/week program embedded into recess that involves a combination of:

- **Educating** recess supervisors, school administrators, teachers, and students about how to create a positive recess experience for all students by offering a variety of activity ideas and embedding strategies for promoting positive behaviors and social interactions during recess using a variety of methods such as an orientation session, newsletters, talking points, posters, and bookmarks.
- **Embedding weekly activities** 1 day per week for 6 weeks by an occupational therapy practitioner to encourage children to engage in active play, develop new interests, form friendships, interact positively with peers, include others, and decrease bullying.
- **Occupational therapy coaching** with recess supervisors to model positive social interaction with students, help problem-solve behavioral challenges, suggest a variety of enjoyable recess activities, and create opportunities for inclusion of all students with and without disabilities.

**Weekly themes!** Each week has a theme along with a suggested activity.

*Continued*

## BOX 17.4 Tier 1, Universal Recess Program: Refreshing Recess—cont'd

Week #1: Kickoff: Let's get started! Orientation: How to refresh recess. Students receive the *Refreshing Recess* bookmark. The occupational therapy practitioner provides an orientation to recess supervisors and explores challenges and needs.

Week #2: Let's make friends and have fun together. Students participate in a friendship scavenger hunt or game that fosters teamwork. Supervisors learn about fostering friendships.

Week #3: Let's play and work together. Students create something together with a variety of art materials. Supervisors learn about teamwork and conflict resolution.

Week #4: Let's get fit and get along. Students engage in Fitness Trail. Supervisors learn about positive behavioral interventions and supports (PBIS).

Week #5: Let's respect differences and include everybody. Students engage in Magic Tag. Supervisors learn how to promote inclusion.

Week #6: Let's make sure everyone has fun. Students engage in the Untying Knots game. Supervisors learn about bully prevention.

**Program outcomes:** Preliminary findings from survey data indicate that the Refreshing Recess program resulted in statistically significant changes in students perceiving outdoor recess to be fun, being engaged in active play, the number of games that adults promote; and looking forward to recess. By the end of the program, recess supervisors reported positive changes in the following areas: feeling adequately trained to supervise recess; having the necessary supports to promote play; knowing how to interact socially with students; and knowing how to successfully resolve conflict.

Information on how to implement this program with downloadable materials such as posters, newsletters, and lesson plans are available online: Mohler, R., Kerns, S., & Bazyk, S. (2014). *Refreshing recess.* https://everymomentcounts.org/refreshing-recess/

about *Refreshing Recess,* a universal occupational therapy recess program.

Developing an awareness of the school and community's extracurricular activities is also important so that the occupational therapy practitioner can foster exploration and participation for students receiving IEP services as well as those at risk. Being knowledgeable about local, state, and national resources focusing on inclusive recreation and leisure helps broaden practitioners' awareness of opportunities for participation. This knowledge is useful for actively advocating for inclusive participation—another important aspect of the occupational therapy practitioner's role within a school. For example, the occupational therapy practitioner can complete a leisure environmental scan of school and community-based activities and compile them in a handout to share with students and parents. When families have limited financial and transportation means, the practitioner can target and share low-cost activities that can be accessed by bus or on foot. An occupational therapy practitioner can also promote whole-school strategies targeting leisure participation (see Box 17.4 for examples). Fig. 17.6 depicts two teens with Down syndrome successfully participating in an inclusive local dance studio.

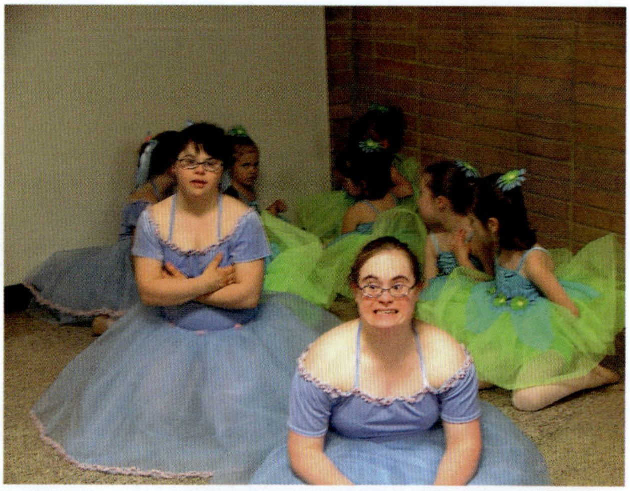

**Fig. 17.6** Two teens with Down syndrome successfully participate in an inclusive local dance studio. They express themselves in dance with others and gain a sense of self-efficacy while supporting their health and well-being.

## SUMMARY

Leisure participation helps promote skill development, health, and positive life outcomes for children and youth. With a commitment to occupational justice, occupational therapy practitioners are guided by the belief that all youth have a right to participate in and enjoy meaningful and health-promoting leisure despite barriers such as disabilities or poverty. This chapter provides information and examples of how occupational therapy practitioners promote leisure participation within a tiered public health framework. Occupational therapy leisure scenarios provide examples of individual leisure coaching, leisure groups for those at-risk, and whole-school initiatives that advocate for and result in inclusive leisure participation for all children and youth.

1. Participation in leisure contributes to physical and mental health, quality of life, and better life outcomes (Brajsa-Zganec et al., 2011; Mahoney et al., 2005; Trainor et al., 2010). Leisure participation promotes flow (i.e., a state of consciousness characterized by deep concentration and absorption associated with identity formation and optimal experience (Csikszentmihalyi & Larson, 1984). Engaging in organized leisure activities supports children and youth in developing initiative, self-motivation, and skills, as well as positive self-esteem and mental health.
2. Context (i.e., the physical, social, and emotional aspects) affect the benefit of leisure. Children and youth benefit from engaging in leisure activities that provide positive social norms, physical and psychological safety, support for meaningful opportunities for belonging, supportive relationships, and integration into the family, school, and community (Mahoney et al., 2005). Involvement in a variety of activities (i.e., breadth) that occur frequently over time (i.e., density) promotes relationships, connectedness, and the development of physical, social, and emotional skills.
3. Children and youth from lower socioeconomic communities or families may have fewer opportunities to participate in leisure activities. Furthermore, children with physical, mental health, or behavioral challenges may have difficulty finding leisure activities that are suited to them. Occupational therapy practitioners need to be aware of the multiple factors that may limit the availability of and access to healthy leisure activities, such as systemic racism, cultural bias, or gender-related issues (AOTA, 2020b).
4. Occupational therapy practitioners may address the needs of all children and youth by creating programming to foster leisure exploration and participation in the natural context for individuals, groups, and populations (such as the community). Programs such

as Every Moment Counts use a strength-based approach, embedding playfulness and positive opportunities for all children and youth. Occupational therapy practitioners use coaching methods to support leisure activities within the child's natural environment (such as home, school, and community.

5. Occupational therapy practitioners target leisure participation by finding opportunities to increase access and availability; exploring community options; creating new opportunities; educating others on the benefits; and integrating students with and without disabilities into programming (such as recess groups). They address barriers to leisure participation that may involve helping the child develop skills or a sense of competence to engage.
6. Occupational therapy practitioners promote leisure participation in children and youth with and without disabilities on the individual, group, and population levels. They may create programs to provide children and youth with positive experiences, such as social groups, task groups, interests groups, and intramural sports or physical activity groups. They may design groups to address timely topics, such as bullying, coping strategies, reading groups, or cooking groups (i.e., healthy eating). Occupational therapy practitioners may work with individuals to explore and engage in leisure activities, develop skills and abilities to engage in desired leisure, and help create routines to engage in leisure.

## REFERENCES


American Occupational Therapy Association. (2020b). Occupational therapy practice framework: Domain and process (4th ed.). *American Journal of Occupational Therapy*, *74*(Suppl. 2).

American Occupational Therapy Association. (2020a). *AOTA's guide to acknowledging the impact of discrimination, stigma, and implicit bias on provision of services.* Retrieved from https://www.aota.org/~/media/Corporate/Files/Practice/Guide-Acknowledging-Impact-Discrimination-Stigma-Implicit-Bias.pdf.

Anaby, D. R., Law, M. C., Majnemer, A., & Feldman, D. (2016). Opening doors to participation of youth with physical disabilities: An intervention study. *Canadian Journal of Occupational Therapy*, *83*(2), 83–90.

Anaby, D. R., Law, M., Feldman, D., Majnemer, A., & Avery, L. (2018). The effectiveness of the Pathways and Resources for Engagement and Participation (PREP) intervention: Improving participation of adolescents with physical disabilities. *Developmental Medicine and Child Neurology*, *60*(5), 513–519.

Arbesman, M., Bazyk, S., & Nochajski, S. M. (2013). Systematic review of occupational therapy and mental health promotion, prevention, and intervention for children and youth. *American Journal of Occupational Therapy*, *67*, e120–e130.

Barber, B. L., Stone, M. R., Hunt, J. E., & Eccles, J. S. (2005). Benefits of activity participation: The roles of identify affirmation and peer group norm sharing. In J. L. Mahoney, R. W. Larson, & J. S. Eccles (Eds.), *Organized activities as contexts of development: Extracurricular activities, after-school and community programs* (pp. 185–210). Lawrence Erlbaum.

Bazyk, S., & Bazyk, J. (2009). The meaning of occupational therapy groups for low-income youth: A phenomenological study. *American Journal of Occupational Therapy*, *6*, 69–80.

Bazyk, S. (2006). Creating occupation-based social skills groups in after-school care. *Occupational Therapy Practice*, *11*, 13–18.

Bazyk, S., Demirjian, L., LaGuardia, T., Thompson-Repas, K., Conway, C., & Michaud, P. (2015). Building capacity of occupational therapy practitioners to address the mental health needs of children and youth: Mixed methods study of knowledge translation. *American Journal of Occupational Therapy*, *69*, 6906180060p1–6906180060p10.

Bazyk, S. (2011d). Enduring challenges and situational stressors during the school years: Risk reduction and competence enhancement. In S. Bazyk (Ed.), *Mental health promotion, prevention, and intervention with children and youth: A guiding framework for occupational therapy* (pp. 119–139). AOTA Press.

Bazyk, S. (2005). Exploring the development of meaningful work for children and youth in Western contexts. *Work: A Journal of Prevention, Assessment, & Rehabilitation*, *24*, 11–20.

Bazyk, S., Gordon, R., Haines, J., Percociante, M., & Glorioso, M. (2010). Service learning: The process of doing and becoming an occupational therapist. *Occupational Therapy in Health Care*, *24*(2), 171–187.

Bazyk, S. (2022). *'Making Leisure Matter'*. Every Moment Counts. https://everymomentcounts.org/making-leisure-matter/.

Bazyk, S. (2019). Mental health promotion, prevention and intervention in schools: A guiding framework for occupational therapy. In C. Brown, & V. Stoffel (Eds.), *Occupational therapy in mental health: A vision for participation* (pp. 809–837). F. A. Davis.

Bazyk, S. (2011a). *Mental health promotion, prevention, and intervention with children and youth: A guiding framework for occupational therapy*. AOTA Press.

Bazyk, S. (2011c). Occupational therapy process: A public health approach to promoting mental health in children and youth. In S. Bazyk (Ed.), *Mental health promotion, prevention, and intervention with children and youth: A guiding framework for occupational therapy* (pp. 21–44). AOTA Press.

Bazyk, S. (2011b). Promotion of positive mental health in children and youth: A guiding framework for occupational therapy. In S. Bazyk (Ed.), *Mental health promotion, prevention, and intervention with children and youth: A guiding framework for occupational therapy* (pp. 3–20). AOTA Press.

Bazyk, S., & Winne, R. (2013). A multi-tiered approach to addressing the mental health issues surrounding obesity in children and youth. *Occupational Therapy in Health Care*, *27*(2), 84–98.

Bedell, G., Coster, W., Law, M., Liljenquist, K., Kao, Y. C., Teplicky, R., & Khetani, M. A. (2013). Community participation, supports, and barriers of school-age children with and without disabilities. *Archives of Physical Medicine and Rehabilitation*, *94*(2), 315–323.

Biolcati, R., Mancini, G., & Trombini, E. (2018). Proneness to boredom and risk behaviors during adolescents' free time. *Psychological Reports*, *121*(2), 303–323.

Brajsa-Zganec, A., Merkas, M., & Sverko, I. (2011). Quality of life and leisure activities: How do leisure activities contribute to subjective well-being? *Social Indicators Research*, *102*(1), 81–91.

Cahill, S., & Bazyk, S. (2020). School based occupational therapy. In J. O'Brien, & H. Kuhaneck (Eds.), *Case-Smith's occupational therapy for children* (8th ed.) (pp. 627–658). Elsevier.

Caldwell, L., & Faulk, M. (2013). Adolescent leisure from a developmental and prevention perspective. In T. Freire (Ed.), *Positive leisure science: From subjective experience to social contexts* (pp. 41–60). Springer.

Carter, E. W., Boehm, T. L., Biggs, E. E., Annandale, N. H., Taylor, C. E., Loock, A. K., & Liu, R. Y. (2015). Known for my strengths: Positive traits of transition-age youth with intellectual disability and/or Autism. *Research and Practice for Persons with Severe Disabilities*, *40*(2), 101–119.

Csikszentmihalyi, M. (1993). Activity and happiness: Towards a science of occupation. *Occupational Science: Australia*, *1*(1), 38–42.

Csikszentmihalyi, M., & Larson, R. (1984). *Being adolescent: Conflict and growth in the teenage years*. Basic. 9780465006458 (ISBN10: 0465006450).

Danckert, J., & Merrifield, C. (2018). Boredom, sustained attention and the default mode network. *Experimental Brain Research*, *236*, 2507–2518.

Darrah, J., Law, M. C., Pollock, N., Wilson, B., Russell, D. J., Walter, S. D., & Galuppi, B. (2011). Context therapy: A new intervention approach for children with cerebral palsy. *Developmental Medicine and Child Neurology*, *53*, 615–620.

Delle Fave, A., & Bassi, M. (2000). The quality of experience in adolescents' daily lives: Developmental perspectives. *Genetic, Social, and General Psychology Monographs*, *126*(3), 347–367.

Dworkin, J. B., Larson, R., & Hansen, D. (2003). Adolescents' accounts of growth experiences in youth activities. *Journal of Youth and Adolescence*, *32*, 17–26.

Eccles, J. S., Barber, B. L., Stone, M., & Hunt, J. (2003). Extracurricular activities and adolescent development. *Journal of Social Issues, 59*, 865–889.

Farnworth, L. (1999). Time use and leisure occupations of young offenders. *American Journal of Occupational Therapy, 54*(3), 315–325.

Fredricks, J. A., & Eccles, J. S. (2006). Is extracurricular participation associated with beneficial outcomes? Concurrent and longitudinal relations. *Developmental Psychology, 42*(4), 698–713.

Graham, F., Rodger, S., & Ziviani, J. (2009). Coaching parents to enable children's participation: An approach for working with parents and their children. *Australian Occupational Therapy Journal, 56*(1), 16–23.

Hansen, D., Larson, R., & Dworkin, J. B. (2003). What adolescents learn in organized youth activities: A survey of self-reported developmental experiences. *Journal of Research on Adolescence, 13*(1), 25–55.

Hunter, A., & Eastwood, J. D. (2018). Does state boredom cause failures of attention? Examining the relations between trait boredom, state boredom, and sustained attention. *Experimental Brain Research, 236*, 2483–2492.

Individuals with Disabilities Education Improvement Act of 2004, Pub. L. 108–446, 20 U.S.C. §§ 1400–1482.

Larson, R. W. (2000). Toward a psychology of positive youth development. *American Psychologist, 55*, 170–183.

Law, M., Anaby, D., Teplicky, R., & Turner, L. (2016). Pathways and resources for engagement and participation (PREP): A practice model for occupational therapists [Internet]. https://www.canchild.ca/en/shop/25-prep.

Law, M., Anaby, D., Imms, C., Teplicky, R., & Turner, L. (2015). Improving the participation of youth with physical disabilities in community activities: An interrupted time series design. *Australian Occupational Therapy Journal, 62*(2), 105–115.

Law, M., Cooper, B., Strong, S., Stewart, D., Rigby, P., & Letts, L. (1996). The Person-Environment-Occupation Model: A transactive approach to occupational performance. *Canadian Journal of Occupational Therapy, 63*(1), 9–23.

Law, M., & Darrah, J. (2014). Emerging therapy approaches: An emphasis on function. *Journal of Child Neurology, 29*, 1101–1107.

Law, M., King, G., King, S., Kertoy, M., Hurley, P., Rosenbaum, P., et al. (2006). Patterns of participation in recreational and leisure activities among children with complex physical disabilities. *Developmental Medicine and Child Neurology, 48*(5), 337–342.

Leversen, I., Danielsen, A. G., Birkeland, M. S., & Oddrun, S. (2012). Basic psychological need satisfaction in leisure activities and adolescents' life satisfaction. *Journal of Youth and Adolescence, 41*, 1588–1599.

Mahoney, J. L., Larson, R. W., & Eccles, J. S. (2005). Organized activities as developmental contexts for children and adolescents. In J. L. Mahoney, R. W. Larson, & J. S. Eccles (Eds.), *Organized activities as contexts of development: Extracurricular activities, after-school and community programs* (pp. 3–22). Lawrence Erlbaum.

Mahoney, J. L., & Stattin, H. (2000). Leisure activities and adolescent antisocial behavior: The role of structure and social context. *Journal of Adolescence, 23*(2), 113–127.

Martin, M. (2009). Boredom as an important area of inquiry for occupational therapists. *British Journal of Occupational Therapy, 72*(1), 40–42.

Martin, M., Sadlo, G., & Stew, G. (2012). Rethinking occupational deprivation and boredom. *Journal of Occupational Science, 19*(1), 54–61.

Martz, M. E., Schulenberg, J. E., Patrick, M. E., & Kloska, D. D. (2018). "I am so bored!": Prevalence rates and sociodemographic and contextual correlates of high boredom among American adolescents. *Youth & Society, 50*(5), 688–710.

Mohler, R., Kerns, S., & Bazyk, S. (2014). *Refreshing recess*. Retrieved from https://everymomentcounts.org/refreshing-recess/.

Nishino, H. J., & Larson, R. (2003). Japanese adolescents' free time: *Juku, Bukatsu*, and government efforts to create more meaningful leisure. *New Directions for Child and Adolescent Development, 99*, 23–35.

Olson, L. (2011). Development and implementation of groups to foster social participation and mental health. In S. Bazyk (Ed.), *Mental health promotion, prevention, and intervention with children and youth: A guiding framework for occupational therapy* (pp. 95–115). AOTA Press.

Passmore, A., & French, D. (2001). Development and administration of a measure to assess adolescents' participation in leisure activities. *Adolescence, 36*, 67–75.

Passmore, A. (2003). The occupation of leisure: Three typologies and their influence on mental health in adolescents. *OTJR: Occupation, Participation and Health, 23*, 76–83.

Pavlova, M. K., & Silbereisen, R. K. (2015). Leisure activities choices among adolescents. In J. Wright (Ed.), *International encyclopedia of the social & behavioral sciences* (2nd ed.) (pp. 830–837). Elsevier.

Powrie, B., Copley, J., Turpin, M., Ziviani, J., & Kolehmainen, N. (2020). The meaning of leisure to children and young people with significant physical disabilities: Implications for optimizing participation. *British Journal of Occupational Therapy, 83*(2), 67–77.

Proyer, R. T., Gander, F., Bertenshaw, E. J., & Brauer, K. (2018). The positive relationships of playfulness with indicators of health, activity, and physical fitness. *Frontiers in Psychology, 9*, 1–16.

Raffaelli, Q., Mills, C., & Christoff, K. (2018). The knowns and unknowns of boredom: A review of the literature. *Experimental Brain Research, 236*, 2451–2462.

Rebeiro, K. L., & Cook, J. V. (1999). Opportunity, not prescription: An exploratory study of the experience of occupational engagement. *Canadian Journal of Occupational Therapy, 66*, 176–187.

Schreuer, N., Sachs, D., & Rosenblum, S. (2014). Participation in leisure activities: Differences between children with and without physical disabilities. *Research in Developmental Disabilities, 35*(1), 223–233.

Schwartze, M. M., Frenzel, A. C., Goetz, T., Pekrun, R., Reck, C., Marx, A. K., & Fiedler, D. (2021). Boredom makes me sick: Adolescents' boredom trajectories and their health-related quality of life. *International Journal of Environmental Research and Public Health, 18*(12), 6308.

Sharp, E. H., Tucker, C. J., Baril, M. E., Van Gundy, K. T., & Rebellon, C. J. (2015). Breadth of participation in organized and unstructured leisure activities over time and rural adolescents' functioning. *Journal of Youth & Adolescents, 44*, 62–76.

Spaeth, M., Weichold, K., & Silbereisen, R. K. (2015). The development of leisure boredom in early adolescence: Predictors and longitudinal associations with delinquency and depression. *Developmental Psychology, 51*(10), 1380–1394.

Tam, K. Y., Van Tilburg, W. A., Chan, C. S., Igou, E. R., & Lau, H. (2021). Attention drifting in and out: The boredom feedback model. *Personality and Social Psychology Review, 25*(3), 251–272.

Trainor, S., Delfabbro, P., Anderson, S., & Winefield, A. (2010). Leisure activities and adolescent well-being. *Journal of Adolescence, 33*(1), 173–186.

Weybright, E. H., Schulenberg, J., & Caldwell, L. L. (2020). More bored today than yesterday? National trends in adolescent boredom from 2008 to 2017. *Journal of Adolescent Health, 66*(3), 360–365.

Whitehouse, E., & Pudney, W. (1996). *A volcano in my tummy*. New Society Publishers.

Wilcock, A. A., & Hocking, C. (2015). *An occupational perspective of health*. Slack.

Wilson, D. M., Gottfredson, D. C., Cross, A. B., Rorie, M., & Connell, N. (2010). Youth development in after-school leisure activities. *The Journal of Early Adolescence, 30*(5), 668–690.

Zhang, S., Shi, R., Liu, X., & Miao, D. (2014). Passion for leisure activity, presence of meaning, and search for meaning: The mediating role of emotion. *Social Indicators Research, 115*(3), 1123–1135.


## FURTHER READING


Bundy, A. (1993). Assessment of play and leisure: Delineation of the problem. *American Journal of Occupational Therapy, 47*(3), 217–222.

Carter, E. W. (2018). Supporting the social lives of secondary students with severe disabilities: Considerations for effective intervention. *Journal of Emotional and Behavioral Disorders, 26*(1), 52–61.

Henry, A. (2008). Assessment of play and leisure in children and adolescents. In L. D. Parham, & L. S. Fazio (Eds.), *Play in occupational therapy for children* (2nd ed.) (pp. 95–193). Mosby, Inc.

Takata, N. (1974). Play as prescription. In M. Reilly (Ed.), *Play as exploratory learning* (pp. 209–246). Sage Publications.

# 18

# Social Participation and Community Integration

*Karen Ratcliff and Claudia List Hilton*

## GUIDING QUESTIONS

1. What comprises social participation?
2. How does social participation relate to community integration?
3. What are the important outcomes of social participation and community integration?
4. What intervention strategies can occupational therapy practitioners use to promote social participation and community integration?

## KEY TERMS

Community integration
Goal attainment scaling
Identity development
Self-advocacy
Self-determinism
Social coaching
Social participation

## AN INTRODUCTION TO SOCIAL PARTICIPATION AND COMMUNITY INTEGRATION

Social participation, the involvement in everyday life situations with others (WHO, 2007), is essential to human development and contributes to physical, mental, and emotional well-being (Piškur et al., 2014; Sylvestre et al., 2013). **Social participation** is defined in the Occupational Therapy Practice Framework (4th ed.; AOTA, 2020, p. 83) as follows:

> *"the interweaving of occupations to support desired engagement in community and family activities as well as those involving peers and friends (Schell & Gillen, 2019a, p. 711); involvement in a subset of activities that involve social situations with others (Bedell, 2012); and in activities that support social interdependence (Magasi & Hammel, 2004,)"*

Qualitative studies with adolescents, experts, and parents have described the importance of context to social participation, the distinction between active and passive participation, and the importance of feeling one belongs (Bärwalde et al., 2023; Hoffman et al., 2023). A recent scoping review found that the majority of papers defining social participation focused on involvement in activities that provided social interactions in the community, and that as a group, the papers discussed the who, what, where, and why of social participation. Therefore, the authors suggested a new definition of social participation that included all of those elements. Although this definition was created from a review of papers that focused on elderly populations, the definition is fitting for children and youth as well. These authors suggest that social participation is "a person's involvement in activities providing interactions with others in community life and in important shared spaces, evolving according to available time and resources, and based on the societal context and what individuals want and is meaningful to them" (Levasseur et al., 2022, p. 8).

**Community integration** is an overlapping concept that refers to an individual moving toward becoming independent and taking on typical adult roles in the community. Community integration means the individual will not be steered into settings away from typical community life such as day treatment centers, sheltered workshops, and the like. Community integration requires more than performance in activities of daily living or other skills, but it includes the acceptance of others, life satisfaction, and autonomy with decision-making. Therefore, although there are similarities between social participation and community integration, they are distinct concepts. A recent model of community integration, built from a review of the literature, proposes that it encompasses the following six attributes: independence, a place to live, social connection, occupational performance, adjustment, and a sense of belonging (Shaikh et al., 2019). Community integration means being part of the community and not merely existing in or residing in a community (Bond et al., 2004).

One can view social participation and community integration as an outcome of the interaction or fit between a person and their environment, the result of the interplay between barriers to them, and supports for both. Alternatively, one can consider the outcomes of social participation and community integration, where they are the agent of change for other traits, characteristics, and abilities, such as self-determination, mental health and well-being, quality of life, and life satisfaction. This chapter will consider both and then provide a discussion of the ways in which occupational therapy practitioners can support and promote social participation and community integration through our interventions.

### Barriers to Social Participation and Community Integration

Potential barriers to social participation include the physical or built environment, attitudes, policies, and specific child or adolescent characteristics. Methods to intervene to improve or manage many of these barriers are provided below. Box 18.1 provides examples of how different environmental factors influence social participation.

**Physical Environment.** Physical environments may hinder social participation when structures limit access, and many structural

## BOX 18.1 Environmental Factors and Social Participation based on the International Classification of Functioning, Disability, and Health (WHO, 2007)

**Products and Technology:** Natural or synthetic products or systems of products, equipment, and technology in an individual's immediate environment that are gathered, created, produced, or manufactured.

- Augmentative communication devices can be used to share ideas with other students in a class activity.
- Smartphone apps can be used to help individuals remember the steps of a game or organize their social time.

**Natural and Human-Made Changes to the Environment:** Animate and inanimate elements of the natural or physical environment and components of that environment that have been modified by people.

- Weather, such as extreme temperatures, may affect the ability of individuals with chronic medical conditions to move about their community.
- Universal design, such as curb cuts and well-lit signage, can provide access for a broad range of individuals in a community—for example, parents who push strollers, persons who use a wheelchair, or an older adult who may have an unsteady gait.

**Support and Relationships:** Physical or emotional support, nurturing, protection, assistance, and relationships provided by people or animals to other persons in their homes, places of work, schools, at play, or in other aspects of their daily activities.

- A service dog may help a teenager with ASD feel more comfortable in a new social setting, such as a community dance.
- An encouraging teacher assists a student with a disability with his college application, providing additional postsecondary opportunities for the student.

**Attitudes:** Observable consequences of customs, practices, ideologies, values, norms, factual beliefs, and religious beliefs.

- A coach may think that it is not safe for a youth with a disability to play sports. The coach requires a teenager to obtain extensive medical documentation before allowing him or her to join the team.
- An occupational therapist works under the assumption that skills are best developed during engagement in meaningful occupations, rather than in contrived situations. Instead of pretending to plan a route using the bus, the occupational therapist rides the bus with a young adult to practice going to a new job site.

**Services, Systems, and Policies:** Services that provide benefits, structured programs, and operations in various sectors of society designed to meet the needs of individuals. This may include systems that exert administrative control and organizational mechanisms and are established by governments at the local, regional, national, and international levels or by other recognized authorities, and policies constituted by rules, regulations, conventions, and standards established by governments at the local, regional, national, and international levels or by other recognized authorities.

- The Americans with Disabilities Act ensures that persons with disabilities can access businesses in their community such as movie theaters, recreational centers and pools, and restaurants.
- A local center for independent living provides access to personal care attendants. Having assistance to get ready in the morning allows a young adult to move out of his or her parents' house into an apartment with a roommate.

barriers exist that lead to social isolation of individuals with disabilities (Eisenberg et al., 2020; Macdonald et al., 2018). Fig. 18.1 shows children in a classroom setting that supports their learning but may not be accessible to all children. Children and youth who have physical, sensory, cognitive, or emotional challenges may require physical modifications to enable them to participate in varied activities. Physical barriers to social participation include the physical layout of spaces, such as the presence of stairs and other structural features that limit mobility, or limited modifications in the community such as curb cuts and accessible sidewalks (Eisenberg et al., 2020; Hemmingson & Borell, 2002; Pivik et al., 2002). Camps, playgrounds, amusement parks, swimming facilities, and water parks, for example, all may be difficult to access for children and teens with mobility impairments (Burns & Graefe, 2007; Koontz et al., 2021; Moore & Lynch, 2015). The physical environment may be uncomfortable and crowded and not allow adequate room for children to engage. Inaccessibility, unsuitable equipment or devices, limited availability of space, and limited access to adaptive aids or technology all interfere with children's social participation (Anaby et al., 2016; Elfassy et al., 2020; Wenger et al., 2021).

Inadequate transportation is a major barrier to social and community participation and integration (Anaby et al., 2016; Crabtree, 2017; Sze & Christensen, 2017; Verdonschot et al., 2009; Wasfi et al., 2017). Lack of proper transportation, particularly in school-related endeavors such as field trips, limits the social participation of children with disabilities (Dudgeon et al., 1997; Mancini & Coster, 2004). Inaccessible public transportation can make full community integration quite difficult for some as it can hinder housing, employment, and social possibilities (Bezyak et al., 2017; Crabtree, 2017; Koontz et al., 2021).

Lack of adequate space can lead to misperceptions among peers, putting the child with a disability at a social disadvantage. One youth described the uncomfortableness of going into the classroom in their wheelchair and seeing all the desks attached to chairs and not knowing what to do, yet not wanting to cause a commotion (Forber-Pratt et al., 2021).

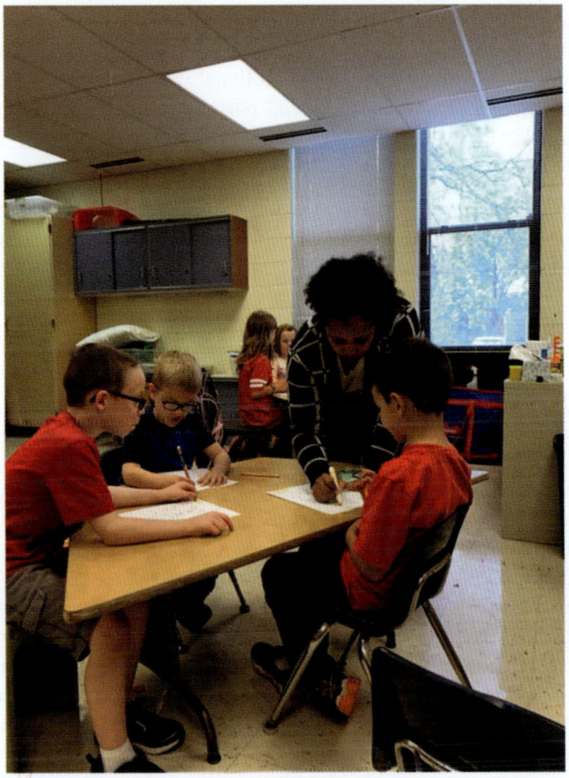

**Fig. 18.1** Physical spaces may not be accessible to all children. This classroom group may not be accessible to children who require wheelchairs or for children who have sensory challenges.

Another explained "A few teachers took me aside and went through things with me. But we had to work in the canteen, there was nowhere else. Classmates were astonished at me—spending time with a teacher!

If they knew what [we] were talking about, they'd know I needed the extra help" (Shevlin et al., 2002, p. 164).

**Attitudes.** The attitudes of others often interfere with social participation. For example, adults who overestimate or underestimate the needs of an individual youth with a disability may restrict choices and opportunities for participation. Similarly, attitudes of others may lead to social limitations because of misunderstandings. For example, a teacher may single out a child, informing the class that the child will not be able to engage in the activity because of their motor challenges, or believe a child is not trying hard enough and therefore push the child too far in front of their peers. Just having adults nearby can reduce social engagement with peers (Carter & Pesko, 2008; Diez, 2010; Kramer et al., 2012; Verdonschot et al., 2009).

Attitudes of others may also push families to limit their excursions into the community. Stigma "is the unwanted shadow of a person, produced when society disdains certain human differences, retaining its ancient Greek meaning as a mark or branding on the body made with a sharp instrument ....it has also come to connote a flawed psychological or physical state. Stigmatized people are often seen as incompetent, blamed for their suffering, and socially marginalized in ways that we might now consider ableist" (Grinker, 2020, p. S55). The impact of stigma on social participation has been reported in many studies of families of children with disabilities (Green, 2003; Kinnear et al., 2016; Lalvani, 2015; Mitter et al., 2019; Scior et al., 2020). For example, families of children with autism often reduce their levels of social participation because of the attitudes of others (Smith et al., 2023; Zuckerman et al., 2018).

**Policies.** A lack of services and services that are not tailored to the youth's needs and interests are barriers to participation (Kramer et al., 2012). Services are driven by policy. Policies either create structures and opportunities for inclusion in social activities or limit or hinder them. In the United States and many Westernized countries, since the 1960s, policies have granted greater access to education and employment for individuals with disabilities. However, there remain enormous gaps between those with and without disabilities in relation to adequate housing, employment, and access to public transportation, public spaces, and community activities (Anaby et al., 2016; Bascom & Christensen, 2017; Bedell et al., 2013; Bezyak et al., 2020; Hardman & Dawson, 2008; Kapsalis et al., 2022; Kirchner et al., 2008; Stienstra, 2018).

**Child Characteristics.** Children's feelings of competence play a role in their willingness to participate in social activities (Duffey et al., 2021; Maciver et al., 2019; Steinhardt et al., 2021). Children and youth may feel anxious, afraid of being perceived differently than peers, or concerned that they do not have the abilities to "fit in" and make friends. They may have experienced negative situations such as not being included, having others bully them, or being left alone (Lindsay & McPherson, 2012). Many understand the experience of stigma and seek to avoid discomfort, or they may struggle with understanding whether or not they have a disability and how they fit in (Ali et al., 2012; Jones et al., 2015; Mazumder & Thompson-Hodgetts, 2019; Mueller, 2019). These issues can further result in social isolation.

**Family Characteristics.** Family socioeconomic status (SES) and level of education may interfere with social participation of youth with disabilities. For early adolescents with cerebral palsy, lower levels of parent education (which may be associated with lower income) were associated with lower scores of social functioning (Voorman et al., 2010). Shattuck et al. (2011) found that autistic youth, ages 13–17 years, with family incomes higher than $75,000 were more likely to be involved in extracurricular activities, have friends, and be invited to activities compared with youth with autism spectrum disorder (ASD) with family incomes lower than $50,000. Youth with ASD ages 18–21 years were four times more likely to be employed or enrolled in postsecondary education if their families were above the poverty level during early adolescence (ages 13–16 years; Liptak et al., 2011).

## Supports for Social Participation

Having considered some of the many factors that are barriers to social participation, how might these barriers be removed or mitigated? Many policies and strategies foster social participation for children with disabilities.

**Policy Supports.** Policies may create structures that facilitate the inclusion and participation of youth with disabilities. Legislation such as the Individuals with Disabilities Education Act guarantees youth with disabilities the right to be educated next to their general education peers in the least restrictive environment. Although this policy does not guarantee social participation, it encourages practices that may lead to increased social participation (Lüddeckens, 2021). This includes regulations such as inclusion in the standard curriculum next to students without disabilities. Similarly, the US Department of Education (2013) called for educational systems to provide equal opportunities for youth with disabilities to participate in sports. Participating in school sports opens opportunities for youth with disabilities to interact with peers and belong to a group.

The United Nations Convention on the Rights of the Child stated that all children, including children with disabilities, are entitled to be involved in matters and decisions concerning them (Bearman et al., 2005; Cavet & Sloper, 2004; Garth & Aroni, 2003; Lansdown & Karkara, 2006; Sloper & Lightfoot, 2003; Tisdall & Davis, 2004). These policies encourage federal and state governments, international nonprofit organizations, and other groups to develop practices that systematically include youth with disabilities in society.

**Opportunities and Outcomes.** Several factors have been shown to consistently improve social participation such as providing children and adolescents with the opportunity to choose the activities they find interesting, motivating, and comforting (Steinhardt et al., 2021; Vänskä et al., 2020). Service and support systems that provide opportunities for young people to make choices and that involve youth in organizational decision-making support social participation (Verdonschot et al., 2009).

Youth with disabilities appreciate the opportunity to engage socially and to interact with others who experience similar daily life challenges; they can acquire new skills and insights when exposed to others who have resolved similar challenges (Joseph Rowntree Foundation, 2003; Kotzer & Margalit, 2007; Lopes et al., 2019; Powers et al., 2007; Valnes et al., 2003). Socially connecting with other youth with disabilities was identified as fundamental to the identity development of adolescents with disabilities (Forber-Pratt et al., 2021). Connecting with others who have disabilities helps youth identify and appreciate valuable aspects of their disabilities. For example, youth attending a disability-only summer camp indicated that camp participation facilitated personal and group identity formation (Goodwin & Staples, 2005). Camp provided them with opportunities to spend time with other youth who had disabilities, to manage their time and schedules without assistance from their parents, and to explore a range of new activities in a safe and supportive environment. After these experiences, they expressed positive changes in feelings about their disabilities, identities, and possibilities for the future. Although equal access and inclusion with all peers are important for young people with disabilities, experiences within the disability community are essential for the development of a positive disability identity (Gill, 1997).

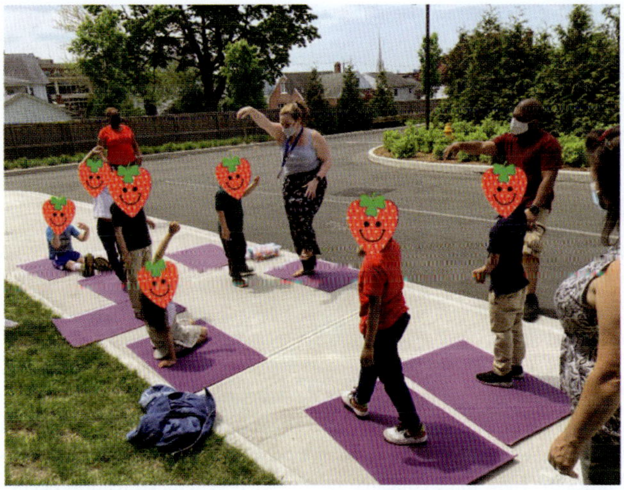

**Fig. 18.2** Occupational therapy practitioners lead a group of youth in outdoor games.

Children and youth who have the opportunity for social participation and inclusion benefit in multiple ways. First, they may gain skills in self-determination and learn strategies for self-advocacy, and second, they are better able to develop their identity, a critical aspect of adolescent development. Third, they learn valuable life lessons and skills. Finally, they may experience belonging, an important outcome for families of children with disabilities. Fig. 18.2 shows a group of youth who are participating in an outdoor game.

**Self-Determination and Self-Advocacy.** As adolescents participate in social activities, they develop autonomy and self-determination skills to make plans and decisions to create their futures (Kingsnorth et al., 2019). **Self-determination** refers to a person's sense that they have choice (autonomy) and a say in their actions (mastery), which promotes satisfaction and relatedness (feelings of closeness) leading to well-being (Ryan & Deci, 2000). Autonomy refers to having a sense of choice, initiative, and endorsement of one's activities. Competency represents a sense of mastery over one's capacity to act in the environment. Relatedness denotes feelings of closeness and connectedness to significant others. As young children make choices, indicate preferences, problem solve, plan, and initiate, they make sense of the world around them to ultimately produce feelings of competence, confidence, and empowerment (Erwin & Brown, 2003).

Children and youth need opportunities to develop skills, make choices, and establish their goals. Children very early in life can make choices through motor movements, eye gaze, or nonattention (Palmer, 2011). The skills of self-determination continue to evolve over time. For example, as children choose new activities, they must work on developing new skills, adjusting to performance challenges, and persevering. As they work toward goals, they develop feelings of competence and develop new coping strategies. They may have to learn self-advocacy to get their needs met. They may find skills that are difficult for them to complete. They may have to ask for accommodation to meet the demands. Children with disabilities will likely have to speak up and advocate for themselves if the environment does not support their participation. **Self-advocacy** is knowledge of self, knowledge of rights, being able to communicate effectively, and leadership that involves moving from advocating for self to advocating for all (Test et al., 2005). Social participation provides opportunities to practice both skills and allows them to grow and develop over time. Fig. 18.3A and B shows children engaged in activities to promote decision making and self-determination.

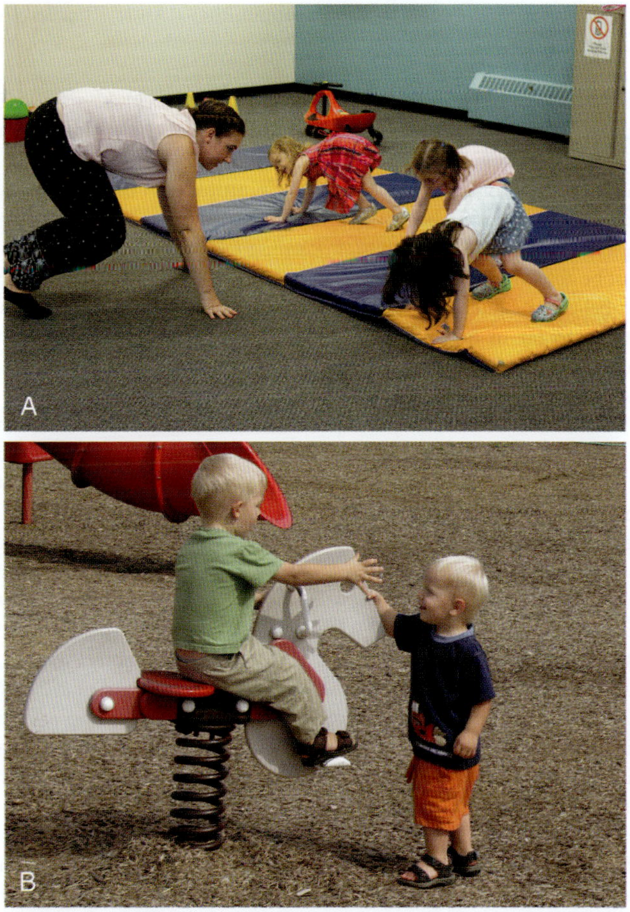


**Fig. 18.3** Children develop skills of self determination as they learn to make choices in early childhood through group play and social activities, both (A) with adult supervision, or (B) independently.

**Identity.** Social participation is important for identity development (Hansen et al., 2003), especially in adolescence (Erikson, 1968). **Identity development** includes defining who one is, what one values, and which directions to pursue in life. It is a dynamic and individualized process that begins in childhood, evolves during adolescence, and continues in one's career, social, and leisure choices (Meeus et al., 1999). Trying new things and challenging oneself lead to identity development. Trying new things allows children and adolescents to discover how new activities suit their developing identity. New activities may require youth to use or develop different skills. Thus, participation in new activities provides young children a chance to explore their abilities and furthers the development of their identities (i.e., their unique style, approach to situations, strengths, and challenges).

**Skills and Competence.** Social participation is essential to development (Hoehne et al., 2020; Piškur et al., 2014; Wang et al., 2009). Social participation leads to feelings of self-efficacy and competence, which allow children to understand their skills and abilities. Through social participation, children and youth develop friendships, express autonomy, make choices, and identify preferences and interests (Sylvestre et al., 2013). As children socially engage, they also learn cultural expectations and societal norms (Samanci et al., 2018), gain a sense of self, and experience feelings of success (Hoehne et al., 2020). They develop communication, negotiation, planning, coping strategies, self-regulation (e.g., flexibility and self-advocacy), self-esteem, and resiliency as they engage with others (Nario-Redmond et al., 2013; Rutter, 1990; Sezici et al., 2017).

**Belonging and Friendship.** As children engage socially, they experience feelings of connectedness (Hoehne et al., 2020). Parents reported that one of their main hopes for their children is that they "fit in" and be included socially at school and in the community (Cohn et al., 2000). They cited the need for their children to learn behaviors to conform to the settings and to fully interact and form meaningful relationships with siblings, same-aged peers, and other children. Social participation allows children and youth to connect and relate to other people in a variety of situations (Fig. 18.4A and B). As children and adolescents become competent in social interaction skills, they use the skills to engage in friendships, education, work, community life, religion and citizenship, recreation, and leisure. Successful social participation in a range of interests leads to a rich and fulfilling life.

Social participation often results in friendships. Friendships are defined as reciprocal, mutual, co-constructed relationships that have a sense of equality at their core (Bagwell & Schmidt, 2011). Children develop skills of friendship such as sharing and engaging in prosocial behaviors as early as the first 2 years of life (Vandell & Mueller, 1980). In preschool, children with friends exhibit more prosocial behaviors and are more likely to be accepted and less likely to be rejected and bullied by peers (Howes, 1988; Sebanc, 2003; Vaughn et al., 2001). In middle childhood (ages 3–12), children become more competent and confident and more selective when choosing their friends (Bagwell & Schmidt, 2011). As they develop self-awareness, communication, and understanding of the thoughts and feelings of others, their social skills increase, and they improve their emotional control, which allows them to "fit in" and belong to groups and start to create interpersonal relationships. Adolescent friendships become more complex, intimate, and significant to one's psychological adjustment (Buhrmester, 1996; Hartup, 1996; Rubin et al., 2005; Selfhout et al., 2009). They evolve from early needs for companionship to needs for reciprocity, intimacy, self-disclosure, and emotional support. Friendships cannot develop without social interaction and social participation in the community.

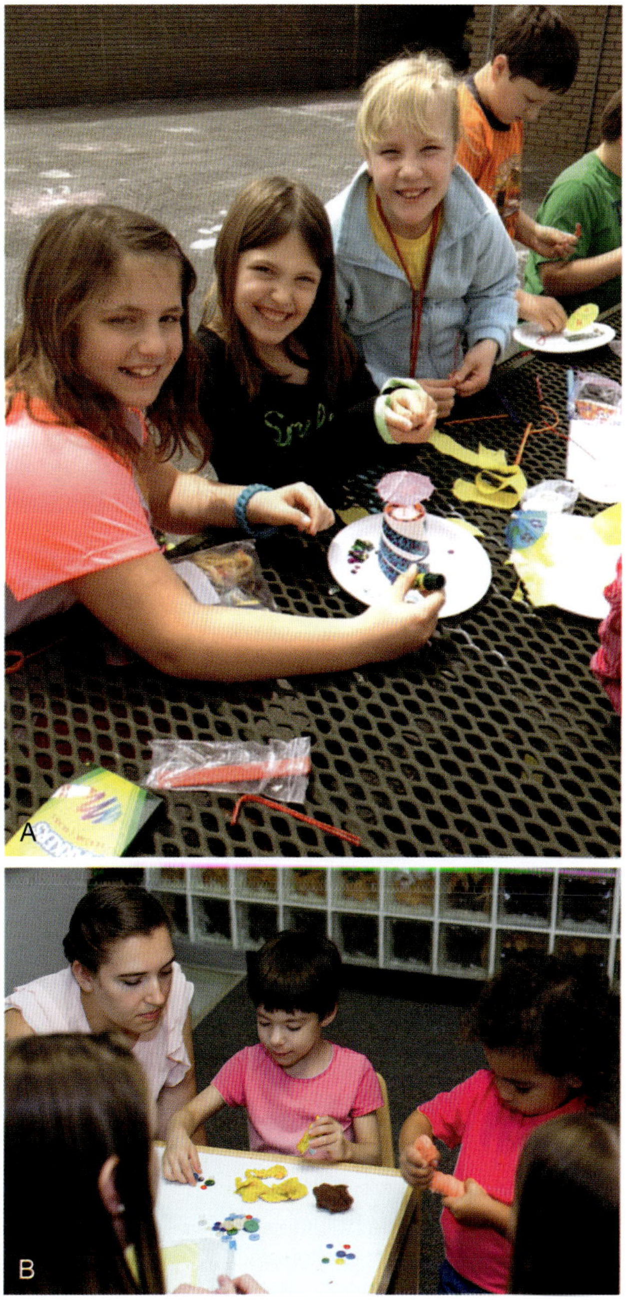

Fig. 18.4 (A) These young girls enjoy spending time with friends as they engage in craft activities. (B) The occupational therapy practitioner promotes social interaction and belonging as children to play together, in the group.

## SOCIAL PARTICIPATION IN YOUTH WITH DISABILITIES

Although social participation has been described as incredibly important for development and adult outcomes, youth with disabilities often lack social participation experiences (Kingsnorth et al., 2019) or have negative experiences (Anaby et al., 2016; Vänskä et al., 2020), leaving them unprepared for the transition from adolescence to adulthood. They experience systems (such as school settings) that lack disability representation, do not foster a disability community, and do not represent people with disabilities (Mueller, 2021).

Youth with disabilities have fewer opportunities to participate in social activities in home, school, and community environments (Anaby et al., 2016; Arakelyan et al., 2020; Chien & Lin, 2021; Jeong, 2020; Simpson et al., 2019; Steinhardt et al., 2021; Walker & Berthelsen, 2007). Youth with different disabilities experience a varying amount of social contact and social participation experiences (Shattuck et al., 2011). Of adolescents ages 13–17 years with autism, 43% reported never seeing friends, compared with 15.7% of youth with intellectual disabilities. In a study of adolescent telephone communication, 47.7% with intellectual disabilities reported getting calls from friends once a week, while only 9.6% with autism reported getting calls as frequently (Shattuck et al., 2011). High school students with disabilities receiving special education services in public schools often remain socially isolated because of the possibility of disability-related stigma or other barriers to friendship opportunities, such as the presence of adult paraprofessionals and limited inclusion in nonacademic school activities (Kramer et al., 2012). Research studies found disparities in the social participation of youth with and without disabilities in recreation and leisure activities (Askari et al., 2015; Ratcliff et al., 2018). In one study that included youth with autism and intellectual disabilities, 16%–23% belonged to a sports team, and 7%–10% belonged to a performing group (Shattuck et al., 2011). Therefore, children and youth with disabilities often require assistance or intervention to engage fully with peers and in the community with their families and friends.

Youth with disabilities have lower rates of enrollment and completion of postsecondary education compared with their peers without disabilities (Newman et al., 2011). They often experience social isolation, reduced social participation, and higher unemployment rates. Youth with disabilities also report low levels of civic engagement; only 35% of autistic youth and 33% of youth with intellectual disabilities ages 13–17 years completed volunteer or community service (Shattuck et al., 2011) compared with youth without disabilities (Howlin et al., 2013; Sattoe et al., 2014).

Persons with and without disabilities also differ in religious participation; 50% of adults with disabilities attend religious services regularly compared with 57% of adults without disabilities (Kessler Foundation, 2010). Only about 27% of youth with autism or intellectual disability reported that they belonged to a religious youth group (Shattuck et al., 2011), but belonging to a community of faith and incorporating those values into everyday life is important for persons with disabilities (Carter, 2013).

Occupational therapy practitioners can identify physical and social religious environments that are more likely to facilitate the inclusion and social participation of youth with disabilities and their families.

**TABLE 18.1 Examples of Goals for Social Participation**

| Area of Social Participation | Examples of Goals |
|---|---|
| Environment | • Client will identify a modification that would allow for participation in art class.<br>• Client will identify one strategy to participate in swimming lessons without getting upset and leaving the lessons.<br>• Client will use one resource to enable participation in choir at school. |
| Self-determination | • Client will choose one activity they would like to participate in during session.<br>• Client will identify one leisure activity to explore.<br>• Client will be able to participate in circle time for the duration of circle time. |
| Self-advocacy | • Client will express an identified need to a teacher to facilitate participation in the classroom setting.<br>• Student will identify a self-need for which they might need accommodations or modifications.<br>• Client will make a request to advocate for a need to the teacher or educational staff when an opportunity arises. |
| Social engagement | • Client will initiate a conversation with peer in the classroom every day.<br>• Client will engage in a reciprocal interaction during recess with a peer.<br>• Student will engage in a game with a peer by taking turns until the game is completed. |

Occupational therapy practitioners can support children and youth with disabilities and their families in their quest for social participation and should consider including social participation goals as they are planning for intervention.

## GOALS FOR SOCIAL PARTICIPATION

Occupational therapy intervention to enhance social participation may focus on social skills (the underlying requirements needed to improve one's abilities), or it may focus on social engagement (opportunities for child or adolescent to engage in social events). The goals of the intervention clearly outline the focus of occupational therapy intervention. See Table 18.1 for examples of social participation goals. **Goal attainment scaling (GAS)** (GAS; Kiresuk et al., 1994) can be a useful tool to identify and measure progress toward individualized goals, such as social participation goals. For example, GAS was used to measure friendship skills (King et al., 2020) and physical activity (Willis et al., 2018). GAS is a flexible means to measure changes based on client-centered goals and changes. Table 18.2 provides examples of GAS for social participation. See Chapter 10 for more information on GAS.

## OCCUPATIONAL THERAPY INTERVENTIONS FOR SOCIAL PARTICIPATION

Occupational therapy practitioners can assist families in generating opportunities for social participation through a variety of methods and in a variety of settings. These strategies can be categorized into removing barriers, providing supports, teaching skills, and fostering peer relationships and friendships.

### Removing Barriers

Accessible and useable spaces encourage participation. Objects, such as accessibility devices also support social participation (Maciver et al., 2019). For example, playgrounds can be designed to be physically accessible to children and family members as well as accessible to children and families with sensory challenges (e.g., enlarged print, Braille directions, tactile variety) and to support varied levels of cognition (e.g., provide equipment that easy to engage with or direction in multiple languages). Occupational therapy practitioners examine the environment and create intervention plans to address identified barriers to social participation for children and youth. Studies illustrate the impact of these environmental factors on the social participation of children and adolescents with disabilities (Anaby et al., 2013; Kramer et al., 2012).

Attitudes may be present as invisible barriers. Occupational therapy practitioners look for attitudinal barriers and address them as needed to support children's social participation. Maciver et al.'s (2019) systematic review revealed that competent, knowledgeable, and facilitative adults formed environments conducive to social participation by

**TABLE 18.2 Goals Attainment Scaling of Social Participation Goals**

| Goal | −2 | −1 | 0 | 1 | 2 |
|---|---|---|---|---|---|
| Increase social participation during lunch | Eat lunch in a small room with a peer 5 days in a row without leaving. | Eat lunch in the cafeteria at a smaller, separated table with a peer 5 days in a row without leaving. | Eat lunch in the cafeteria 1 day/week without leaving. | Eat lunch in the cafeteria 3 times a week without leaving. | Eat lunch in the cafeteria for an entire week without leaving. |
| Increase social participation at community art program | Attend art class, observe, and remain in the class. | Participate in art class by engaging in the activity for the day. | Participate in art class and respond to social questions. | Participate in art class and initiate a conversation with a peer. | Participate in art class and ask a peer if you can join them and converse with them. |

creating positive roles and attitudes. Wenger et al. (2021) found that there were invisible barriers on the playground that both children with disabilities and without experienced. The study recounts the experience of two children with disabilities sitting at the entrance of the slide when a nondisabled child was too uncomfortable to approach the children and say they wanted to go down the slide. The researchers suggest that there remained some barrier preventing successful interaction between the two groups (children with and without disability) despite having a space designed for inclusion and accessibility. They concluded that just because a space is designed to be inclusive does not mean that it is inclusive because of the invisible barriers (Wenger et al., 2021). See Case Example 18.1 on creating an inclusive environment for social participation in a preschool classroom.

## CASE EXAMPLE 18.1 AN INCLUSIVE PRESCHOOL ENVIRONMENT

Marissa is a 3-year-old that attends a preschool program for half a day. She has spastic quadriplegia. She is unable to sit upright without the support of adaptive equipment and has limited upper extremity control. Every morning her class has circle time sitting on the carpet where they learn about the days of the week, months of the year, weather, and the theme of the week. Marissa is unable to sit on the floor with her peers and her wheelchair puts her at a level much higher than her peers. The occupational therapist (OT) and physical therapist worked together to get her appropriate seating on the floor with her classmates. To help Marissa communicate, the OT and speech therapist found a switch that allows you to record a message and change the message to allow her to participate in the classroom activities. They identified the best placement for Marissa to access the switch. Marissa's teacher incorporates activities that she can participate in either using her switch or within the available movement that she has. Everyone wants to sit by Marissa because her teacher tried to include her in the activities that occur during circle time. With these environmental accommodations, Marissa can participate in circle time with her classmates at a level that offers her success and fosters relationships with her peers.

## Providing Supports and Adapting Activities

Steinhardt et al. (2021) suggested finding ways for children to shift their roles in the activity that allows for successful participation to facilitate participation. Occupational therapy practitioners adapt social activities to fit the capabilities of the child and enable the child to participate (Fig. 18.5). This may involve providing physical or emotional support, emotional strategies, or communication devices or ensuring the child understands the expectations for the activity (Vänskä et al., 2020).

Occupational therapy practitioners offer supports through education. Arakelyan et al. (2019) suggest that providing information to parents about community programs supports social participation. Occupational therapy practitioners provide families and children with resources (local community programs, national programs, and resources) to promote access to programming for social participation. Table 18.3 lists some community programs in the United States providing social participation opportunities for families of children with disabilities.

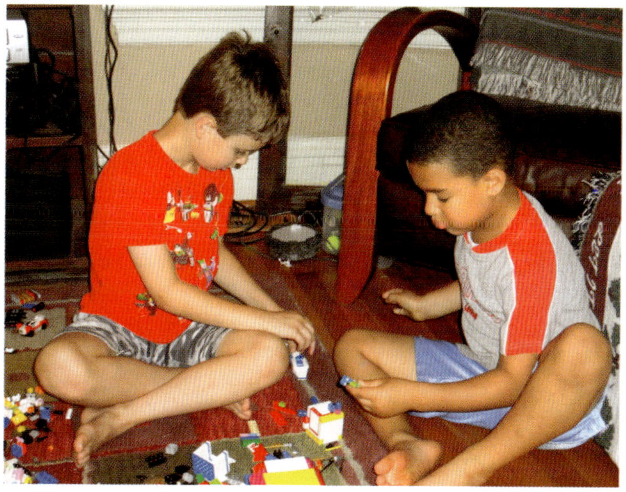

Fig. 18.5 Some children who may not be ready for social skills groups can benefit from the less threatening structure of a dyad. (Photo by Cheryl Klohr.)

## Teaching Specific Skills

Occupational therapy practitioners are skilled at examining the child's factors (i.e., skills, abilities, including motor, sensory, cognitive, feelings, emotions, interests, communication) that may interfere with social participations (Jeong, 2020; Steinhardt et al., 2021). They may provide intervention to address the specific factors such as engaging children in play activities to address turn taking and sharing. They may role play to prepare the child for behavioral expectations of the situation (for example, how to enter a party and start a conversation). They may address the child's physical abilities (e.g., assure the setting is accessible prior to the event). Fig. 18.6A and B shows children learning social interaction skills through play.

Occupational therapy practitioners may teach skills to children explicitly (Hengen & Weaver, 2018). Cook (2020) used a therapeutic theater intervention that taught self-advocacy skills through characters advocating for their needs to individuals with disabilities between the ages of 13–27 and found a statistically significant change in the assertiveness scores of the participants. Shogren et al. (2018) implemented interventions to improve self-determination using a *Self-Determined Learning Model* of instruction and *Whose Future Is It* curriculum and measured outcomes using GAS and a measure of self-determination. Students that received intervention improved in self-determination and met their goals. Findings indicate that teaching self-advocacy and self-determination are effective and result in improved outcomes. Occupational therapy practitioners promote self-determination during intervention sessions as they encourage children to make decisions, problem solve, and flexibly learn to address challenges.

Adolescents may need support as they begin to explore vocational interests. Developing the skills to participate in vocational planning and programming is important to develop the skills of holding a job and the self-direction to complete those tasks. Parents, occupational therapy practitioners, and teachers can help develop these skills in children. See Box 18.2 on developing self-determination skills and Case Example 18.2.

**Group Interventions.** Occupational therapy practitioners may design social skills intervention groups based on the interests of the members and focus on skill development as the children work together. The leaders (e.g., occupational therapy practitioners) or other participants (if possible) describe and demonstrate the social skills required for the group session. All members engage in the group together. They might work on social skills such as introducing themselves, giving compliments, or starting a conversation within the context of participation in activities and occupations within a social group. Members may have different social skill goals. For example, a play group may target goals related to turn taking, emotional regulation, communication, and decision-making. The practitioner can engage children in the social group to address each

TABLE 18.3 **Community Organizations for Social Participation Programs in the United States**

| Community Organization | Location | Services Provided |
|---|---|---|
| Pacer Center Champions for Children with Disabilities | 8161 Normandale Blvd. Minneapolis, MN 55437-1044<br>(952) 838-9000, (800) 537-2237<br>PACER@PACER.org PACER.org | Pacer provides many programs and opportunities for education including:<br>• Resources for children's mental health<br>• Bullying resources<br>• Resources and training for dispute resolution<br>• Early childhood information<br>• Social events for high school teens with and without disabilities<br>• Grandparent to grandparent program<br>• Health information<br>• Housing project<br>• International activities<br>• Family engagement<br>• Multicultural services<br>• Transitional services<br>• Puppet program<br>• School behavioral supports<br>• Technology center<br>• Special education information<br>• Information on working with culturally diverse families |
| Christina Sullivan Foundation | 4116 avenue N1/2 room 106<br>Galveston, Texas 77550<br>Mailing address:<br>P.O. BOX 504<br>Galveston, Texas<br>77553-0504<br>Galveston: (409) 209-0581<br>info@christinasullivanfoundation.org | • Christina Sullivan Foundation offers:<br>• Summer camps<br>• Adaptive and inclusive sports<br>• Tennis program<br>• Inclusion and acceptance programs in schools<br>• Resource center |
| Triangle, Inc. | Headquarters, Triangle, Inc.<br>450 Broadway<br>Malden, MA 02148<br>Phone (781) 322-0400<br>Fax (781) 322-0410 | • Community-based day services and supported employment<br>• Prism program<br>• Residential services<br>• Workforce development and career services<br>• IMPACT Boston & impact: Ability<br>• Empowering People for Inclusive Communities<br>• Clinical supports<br>• Testing centers |
| Little League Challenger | https://www.littleleague.org/play-little-league/challenger/ | • Website provides information about playing baseball for children with intellectual disability<br>• Locates team nearest you<br>• Provides information |
| Adaptive Sports Center | Kelsey Wright Building<br>19 Emmons road<br>Mt. Crested Butte, CO 81225<br>(970) 349-2296<br>https://www.adaptivesports.org/ | • Camp for teenage burn survivors |
| New Horizons Unlimited | New Horizons Unlimited Inc.<br>811 East Wisconsin Avenue, Suite 937<br>Milwaukee, WI 53202<br>https://www.new-horizons.org/ | • Provides resources for individuals with disabilities to find programs, adaptive technology, advocacy, education, employment, and much more |
| Easter Seals | https://www.easterseals.com/ | • Offers programs, services, and information in the areas of enriching education, enhancing health, expanding employment, and elevating community<br>• Many resources and opportunities for inclusive activities |
| United Cerebral Palsy | https://ucp.org/ | • Resources on the website for individuals with cerebral palsy |
| Friendship Circle | https://www.friendshipcircle.com/ | • Resources and programming to promote friendships |

## BOX 18.2 Promoting Self-Determination Skills

Occupational therapy practitioners promote children's self-determination to empower children to make choices based on their own feelings (autonomy) and to act in accordance to their desires, which promotes satisfaction, relatedness, and well-being. Children develop self-determination, confidence, and a sense of self by engaging in all aspects of the intervention. Specifically, they:

- create their own goals;
- identify the focus (goal[s]) for each session;
- identify rules of behavior for the session;
- make choices about the content of activities;
- choose snacks;
- choose rewards for goal attainment;
- engage in challenging activities;
- reflect upon their successes and times when they struggled;
- problem solve to "figure things out"
- explore alternative ways of doing;
- observe and engage with others (adults and other children).

## CASE EXAMPLE 18.2 SELF-DETERMINATION

Self-determination theory was used to develop a school-based physical activity program in a school with children of low socioeconomic status (Shannon et al., 2018). The intervention group of students was given physical activity choices and participatory learning about fitness and health that were not given to the control group. They also received positive constructive feedback during their daily mile walk and engaged in weekly discussion sessions with the teachers in which they could give feedback to make changes to the program. The students in the intervention group spent more time in moderate to vigorous activity levels than the control group, suggesting that actions to support self-determination (e.g., providing choice and opportunities to provide feedback) improved the healthy activity levels of the students.

member's separate goals. The practitioner ends each session with a group reflection or conclusion, whereby peers may provide each other feedback.

Social cognitive groups can also work on developing specific skills such as self-advocacy (Cook, 2020), friendships (King et al., 2022), and social skills (Cheung et al., 2021). These groups occur in two phases: acquisition and performance. During acquisition, the child observes the behavior of others and the consequences and remembers the observations. During the performance phase the child engages in the behavior, based on their perception of the situation and the consequences. Social interactions provide opportunities for a child to serve as a role model for others while simultaneously acquiring new behaviors or attitudes through imitation of others (O'Handley et al., 2015; Post et al., 2014). Peer mentorship, support, and modeling are effective in helping youth with disabilities develop their identity for successful transition to adulthood (Beresford, 2004; Britner et al., 2006; Cavet & Sloper, 2004; Field & Hoffman, 2002).

**Social Coaching.** Skills may also be developed through social coaching. Social coaching is an interactive process that promotes the caregiver's ability to support a child's participation in everyday experiences and interactions across settings by developing new skills, refining existing abilities, and gaining a deeper understanding of their actions (Rush & Shelden, 2005). Social coaching uses reflections and questioning of behaviors about what a child is doing (Fig. 18.7 A and B). It often involves videotaping and reviewing footage to help the child have a clearer idea of the behaviors.

Social coaching has been used successfully with college-aged individuals with attention deficit hyperactivity disorder (Swartz et al., 2005; Zwart & Kallemeyn, 2001) and adolescents between the ages of 14–22 with traumatic brain injury (Wade et al., 2018). Social coaching focuses on the trigger or antecedent that prompts the child to act in a certain way. It can also be used to empower children to organize and execute their responsibilities, both in academia and in everyday life. Parents can be taught coaching to help their child participate socially (Anaby et al., 2016; Hoehne et al., 2020; King et al., 2020). Social coaching can be used by occupational therapy practitioners working with parents or directly with children to increase the child's ability to interact with others and participate in social activities (Gregson et al., 2017).

**Peer-Mediated Intervention.** Occupational therapy practitioners may choose to use peer-mediated interventions to target specific social skills. Peer-mediated intervention partners children with disabilities and typically developing peers to promote behavioral changes in the children with disabilities (Odom, 2019; Roeyers, 1996). Peer-mediated intervention is based on the following premises:

- Peers can be as good as or even more effective than adults at promoting skills.
- The contexts created by peers are closer to the natural environments where children must function.
- The abundance of peers creates natural opportunities for youth to learn from multiple examples.
- The natural variability of peers' methods creates many opportunities for children to learn under "loose" training conditions, which is widely believed to facilitate generalized outcomes (Strain et al., 1996).

Peer-mediated approaches show that autistic children become more responsive to social interactions when peer support is present (Barry et al., 2003; Kamps et al., 1997). However, evidence for peer-mediated interventions was mixed for autistic children and adolescents since the gains achieved were not generalized to other contexts (Tanner et al., 2015). Recommendations for increasing success included choosing the peer wisely, controlling the interaction, looking at the activity context, working on generalization, and having specific goals in mind (Odom, 2019). Case Example 18.3 describes how a peer-mediated intervention helped one young man, Dylan, develop social relationships with other high school students.

## Fostering Relationships

Occupational therapy practitioners create opportunities for children to engage with peers by preparing the children, exploring a variety of social activities so the child is empowered to choose, and by coaching children through the process so they can succeed. Occupational therapists can create participation-based friendship interventions to help youth achieve their goals (King et al., 2020). Programs that foster relationships through matching or mentoring are often the only opportunities for youth with and without disabilities to interact. Such programs may be avenues for those without disabilities to begin to better understand that youth with disabilities have interests, feelings, and experiences like all teenagers (Carter et al., 2005; Carter & Hughes, 2005). Sometimes these programs can lead to meaningful and long-lasting friendships, as in the story of Joshua and Stephanie in Case Example 18.4. The youth in a study of 24 middle and high school adolescents with disabilities identified friendships with other youth with disabilities as vehicles for making deeper friendships because they had similar lived experiences and helped them to feel like they were not so different from others (Forber-Pratt et al., 2021). They found nondisabled peers understood fewer aspects of their lives. Finding opportunities for children

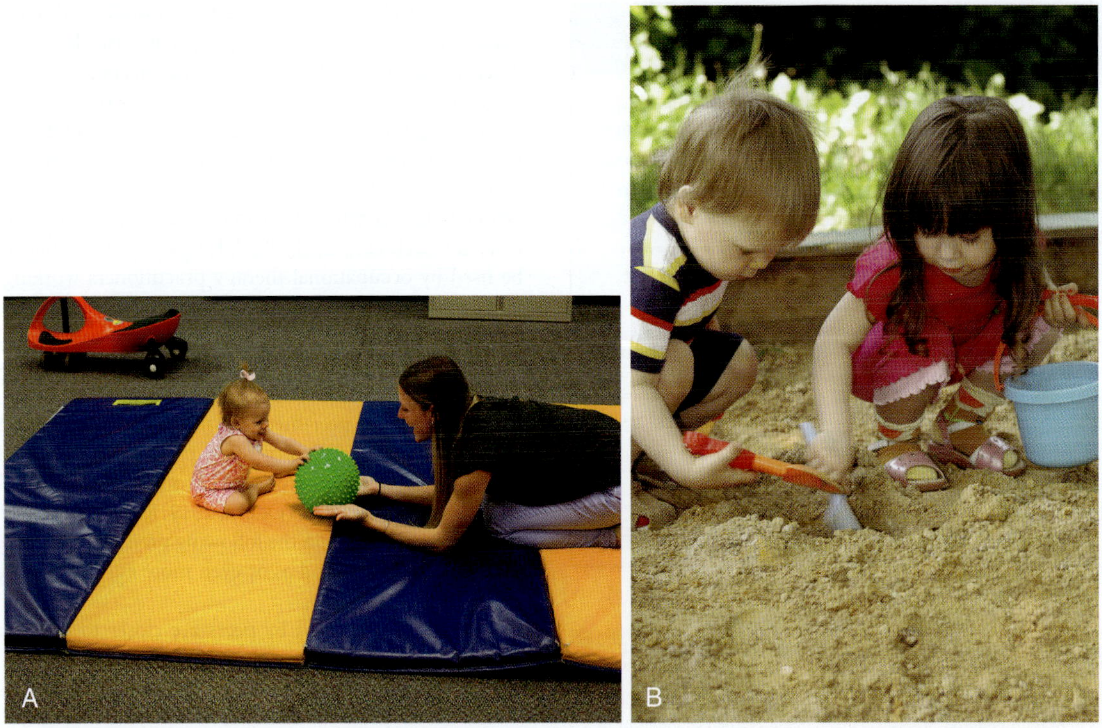

**Fig. 18.6** (A) Occupational therapy practitioners promote social interactions during play. (B) Children learn social interaction skills (such as negotiation, timing, sharing, responding to cues, giving cues) while playing together.

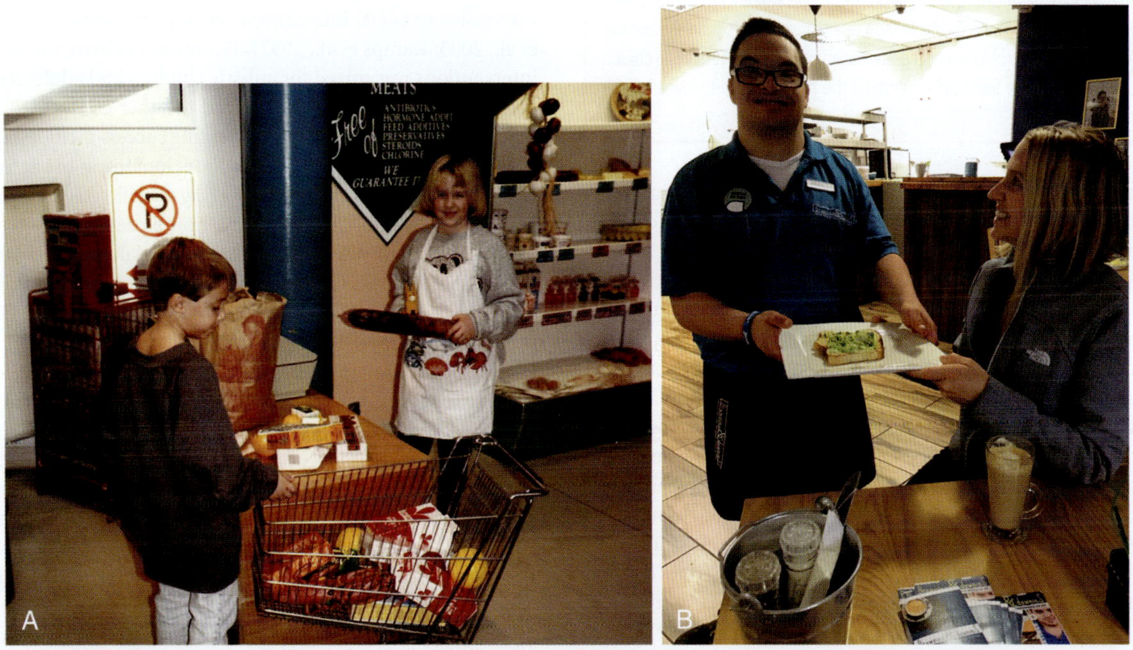

**Fig. 18.7** The occupational therapy practitioner uses social coaching to promote the child's social participation. (A) Shopping theme can give children an opportunity to role play social situations in the community. (B) This young man practices social skills in a cafeteria setting as the occupational therapist provides coaching. ((A) Photo by Claudia Hilton. (B) Photo by Claudia Hilton.)

and adolescents to socially connect with peers who have similar experiences is important to the development of friendships. Many adolescents in the study found opportunities for friendships in adaptive sports teams (Forber-Pratt et al., 2021). Youth may also be able to foster connections and friendships through their use of technology and social media, although they may need support, training, or adaptations to become independent in the use of specific devices (Björquist & Tryggvason, 2022).

### CASE EXAMPLE 18.3 PEER SUPPORT INTERVENTION: DYLAN

Like many other seniors at his high school, Dylan is a fan of stock car racing and enjoys listening to country music. Dylan also has autism. He communicates using sign language or a program on his iPad through which he can select or spell out words. Although he spends most of his school day in a special education classroom, he attends a general education environmental science class every morning.

At first, Dylan had fairly limited participation in his environmental science class. He sat toward the back of the room next to Ms. Collins, an individually assigned paraprofessional. Ms. Collins worked to create activities for Dylan that were related to class content and could be completed successfully (e.g., word searches, matching worksheets). With help from Ms. Collins, Dylan completed these worksheets as his classmates participated in lectures, engaged in class discussions, and completed other individual and group assignments. Dylan's classmates were never unkind to him, but they hardly ever talked to him. Dylan did not complain about the class, but as soon as he finished a worksheet, he looked at Ms. Collins and pointed to his wrist—his way of asking her if he could return to the special education classroom.

Ms. Collins took steps to establish a peer support arrangement in Dylan's class. First, she identified peers who might be willing to participate. On a day when Dylan was absent, she spoke with the class about the purpose of peer support and how this might be a fun opportunity to work with Dylan and get to know him better. She was pleasantly surprised by the number of students who expressed interest and she decided to initially involve three students—Chris, Alisha, and Sarah—as Dylan's peer supports.

Next, Ms. Collins held a brief orientation session with the peers to tell them more about Dylan and discuss how they might help support and interact with him during class. When she shared how Dylan liked stock car racing and listening to popular country music artists, Ms. Collins explained that Dylan used his iPad and some sign language to communicate. She showed the peers the various signs Dylan uses most often and demonstrated how to program new words or phrases into Dylan's iPad. Ms. Collins then showed the peers a support plan she created for Dylan. She explained that the plan offered a starting point for the peers to interact with Dylan and support him during various class activities, but she also encouraged the students to come up with their own ideas for how Dylan could become more actively involved in the class. Excited, Sarah asked if they could all begin working together with Dylan the next day.

Over the next few months, Chris, Alisha, and Sarah found creative ways to interact with Dylan. They introduced Dylan to other students, and soon many others were greeting Dylan in the hallways and in class. Alisha noticed Dylan's iPad did not include the vocabulary used in discussions during environmental science class, so she asked Ms. Collins if it would be okay to help Dylan program in new words. Ms. Collins worked with the teacher to get a list of key words each week, so Alisha could help Dylan program with these words on a regular basis. Knowing Dylan has access to content-related words on his device, Dylan's teacher began to call on him to answer questions for the very first time. Sarah helped Dylan find a correct response on his iPad, and Chris started prompting Dylan to raise his hand in class to share answers. Before long, Dylan volunteered to answer questions on his own and was noticeably excited when he knew the right answer.

Involvement in community, service, and religious organizations may contribute to an adolescent's identity development. Community organizations (such as charities, clubs, and professional organizations), service opportunities (such as local shelters, organizations), and religious settings provide youth with opportunities to engage in social activities outside their families and schools. For example, youth may find a sense of belonging and social connectedness through religious communities as they explore or deepen their spiritual beliefs. They may become involved in cultural organizations or local civic life. As adolescents become aware of problems in their communities and approach voting age, they may become involved in advocating for local or national legislation and policies that reflect their expanding belief systems. A national survey of adults in the United States found that persons with and without disabilities are equally likely to vote in national elections (Kessler Foundation, 2010).

Participating in community service is beneficial to young adults; for example, youth who participate in volunteer service are more likely to have higher grades and graduate from college (Davila & Mora, 2007; Scales et al., 2000). Providing service-learning opportunities in middle school and high school is associated with reduced disciplinary referrals

### CASE EXAMPLE 18.4 THE FRIENDSHIP OF STEPHANIE AND JOSHUA: DEFINING FRIENDSHIP ON THEIR OWN TERMS

Stephanie and Joshua are sophomores at a suburban public high school. Stephanie is an outgoing young woman with an easygoing nature who does not have a disability. Joshua is an outgoing young man with a playful nature who has Menkes syndrome. He is very expressive with his facial features and watches everything going on around him, constantly looking to interact with people who are close by. He uses a wheelchair, does not speak words, and needs support with most daily tasks because his one consistent movement is to reach out with his left hand. The two have been friends since they met as reading partners in an inclusive fifth grade classroom. Since then, Stephanie followed the general education curriculum in classes with her peers, while Joshua received special education services in a separate, self-contained class.

One day, Stephanie knelt to the right of Joshua's wheelchair, and he reached across his body with his left hand toward her head. He flashed a wry grin, looking as if he knew exactly what he was doing when he tugged at her hair. She said, "Hey! Josh!" She pulled her hair out of his hand and stood back up. He laughed, and she shook her head with a friendly and feigned look of exasperation. She smiled at him, and he straightened up with excitement in his wheelchair. They held hands for a moment before leaving.

Joshua displayed intentionality using one of the few movements that he can control to interact playfully with Stephanie. He demonstrated a type of slapstick humor that represents a complex form of nonspoken communication and helped form their connection. Whenever either one of them entered a room, they immediately scanned it to find the other and share a smile. They consistently expressed enjoyment to be together.

Stephanie struggled to describe her friendship with Joshua in any way other than with the immediate connection she felt with him.

> We just kind of clicked and I felt comfortable with him from the start. Being with him is a lot of fun. He's always smiling, and we just really get along. I can't imagine not seeing him.... We just click, and it doesn't matter what either of us can do. We just have a close relationship. It shouldn't be compared to others. It's just our relationship.

Later, to define friendship generally, she returned to the metaphor of clicking:

> Oh, wow. Just having a bond. You can't explain it. You can't explain why you click, but you just do. You just mesh together with someone.

Joshua does not have a way to communicate by speaking words or selecting or typing words and letters. Stephanie stated that she knows what Joshua likes from spending so much time together and reading his facial expressions and reactions:

> I know Joshua and I are such good friends because of all the time we spend together. Both of us know a lot about the other. Joshua is really good at sensing what kind of mood I'm in. I know he enjoys seeing me from his expression when I get there, happy, and when I leave, sad. I'd say for any friendship to become a great one you need to spend a lot of time with the friend. I'd say that any good friendship evolves from spending as much time together as possible.

### CASE EXAMPLE 18.5 EPIC SERVICE WARRIORS: "DISCOVER GREATNESS THROUGH SERVICE"

EPIC Service Warriors is a community service and education program for youth with disabilities between the ages of 16 and 23. By creating the change they want to see in the world, the Service Warriors learn more about local communities and develop practical skills that will help them develop as leaders and pursue future goals. This program also flips the switch on assumptions of many community members by changing the position of power; instead of being served, youth with disabilities serve others.

Each month, the Service Warriors engage in a day of service such as a clean-up of a local park or school, making food at homeless shelters and food kitchens, and wrapping toys for a toy drive. Often, the Service Warriors partner with other service and community organizations for the day of service. Partnering not only increases manpower for the service day but also increases the other organizations' awareness of the capacity of youth with disabilities and demonstrates how service organizations can become more inclusive (Fig. 18.8).

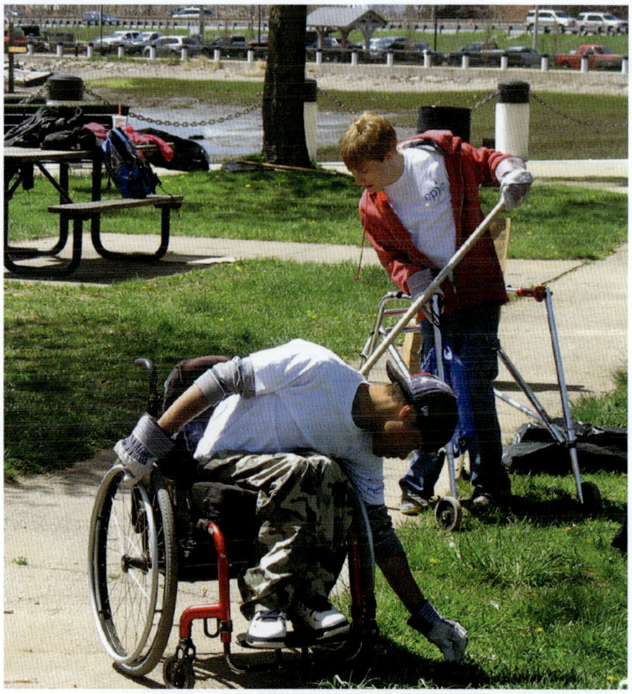

**Fig. 18.8** EPIC Service Warriors clean up their community.

(Potts et al., 2001). Providing opportunities to engage in community service for youth with disabilities is one avenue for increasing their social networks and can support successful transition to adulthood. This is a potential area to address in occupational therapy intervention because research findings show that only one in six adults with disabilities has participated in a group or organized activity that advocates for the rights of people with disabilities (Kessler Foundation, 2010). Innovative programs such as Empowering People for Inclusive Communities (EPIC) Service Warriors (Case Example 18.5) can provide unique opportunities for youth with disabilities to build social networks and serve their community.

## EVIDENCE FOR OCCUPATIONAL THERAPY SOCIAL PARTICIPATION INTERVENTIONS

Although much of the research on social participation has been completed with elderly populations, a recent review of occupational therapy interventions for social participation in youth found strong evidence to support the use of sports interventions and lesser evidence for the use of yoga (Cahill et al., 2020). Coupled with an understanding of the relationship between recreation and leisure and quality of life (Billstedt et al., 2011) and skill development (Bedell et al., 2013) provides support for occupation-based approaches that foster social participation.

A systematic review by Adair et al. (2015) indicated that interventions with multiple approaches are effective, but those targeting the participation level (occupation-centered models) versus the body function or activity level are more successful. In a study examining intervention that targeted changing the environment and coaching parents, adolescents who participated met their participation goals and improved participation scores, and parents had higher satisfaction (Anaby et al., 2018). Another study of physical participation after a family-centered, goal-directed intervention at a community health center found that physical participation was positively affected (Willis et al., 2018).

## SUMMARY

Infants, children, and youth engage in social interactions with others as they develop cognitive, motor, emotional, and communication skills. Through social participation, children and youth develop friendships, express autonomy, make choices, identify preferences and interests, and establish a sense of who they are (i.e., identity). Occupational therapy practitioners facilitate social participation by promoting self-determination, self-advocacy, social skill development, and social participation in the natural environment. They use behavioral, social, and skills training techniques such as behavioral modification, social cognitive groups, social coaching, peer mediation, and skills training. They provide children and youth with access to social participation opportunities at the child's level within the child's community. Occupational therapy practitioners provide parent education of opportunities and resources to promote social participation for children with and without disabilities.

1. Social participation includes activities that involve relationships with others and includes social interactions and social skills that are required during home, school, work, and community events (such as leisure, recreation, sports). Social participation includes all the daily interactions in which children and adolescents engage.
2. Community integration allows children and youth to engage in a variety of social events and opportunities based on their interests, which develops a sense of belonging attributing to quality of life.
3. Children and adolescents develop a sense of themselves (identity) through interactions with family and others. As children and teens interact and relate, they learn about their own strengths and challenges and develop a sense of who they are, what they value and find interesting, and what they believe.
4. Occupational therapy practitioners can create intervention to address social participation, self-determination, self-advocacy, social skills training, and occupation-based groups to allow children and teens to learn and practice skills in a safe setting. They may design inclusive programs in the community and advocate for resources to enable children and youth access to community events.

## REFERENCES


Adair, B., Ullenhag, A., Keen, D., Granlund, M., & Imms, C. (2015). The effect of interventions aimed at improving participation outcomes for children with disabilities: A systematic review. *Developmental Medicine and Child Neurology*, *57*(12), 1093–1104. https://doi.org/10.1111/dmcn.12809.

Ali, A., Hassiotis, A., Strydom, A., & King, M. (2012). Self-stigma in people with intellectual disabilities and courtesy stigma in family carers: A systematic review. *Research in Developmental Disabilities*, *33*(6), 2122–2140.

American Occupational Therapy Association. (2020). Occupational therapy practice framework: Domain and process-fourth edision. *American Journal of Occupational Therapy*, *74*(Suppl. 2). https://doi.org/10.5014/ajot.2020.74S2001.

Anaby, D., Hand, C., Bradley, L., DiRezze, B., Forhan, M., DiGiacomo, A., & Law, M. (2013). The effect of the environment on participation of children and youth with disabilities: A scoping review. *Disability & Rehabilitation*, *35*(19), 1589–1598. https://doi.org/10.3109/09638288.2012.748840.

Anaby, D. R., Law, M. C., Majnemer, A., & Feldman, D. (2016). Opening doors to participation of youth with physical disabilities: An intervention study. *Canadian Journal of Occupational Therapy. Revue Canadienne d'Ergotherapie*.

Anaby, D. R., Law, M., Feldman, D., Majnemer, A., & Avery, L. (2018). The effectiveness of the pathways and resources for engagement and participation (PREP) intervention: Improving participation of adolescents with physical disabilities. *Developmental Medicine and Child Neurology*, *60*(5), 513–519. https://doi.org/10.1111/dmcn.13682.

Arakelyan, S., Maciver, D., Rush, R., O'Hare, A., & Forsyth, K. (2019). Family factors associated with participation of children with disabilities: A systematic review. *Developmental Medicine and Child Neurology*, *61*(5), 514–522. https://doi.org/10.1111/dmcn.14133.

Arakelyan, S., Maciver, D., Rush, R., O'Hare, A., & Forsyth, K. (2020). Community-based participation of children with and without disabilities. *Developmental Medicine and Child Neurology*, *62*(4), 445–453. https://doi.org/10.1111/dmcn.14402.

Askari, S., Anaby, D., Bergthorson, M., Majnemer, A., Elsabbagh, M., & Zwaigenbaum, L. (2015). Participation of children and youth with autism spectrum disorder: A scoping review. *Journal of Autism and Developmental Disorders*, *2*, 103–114. https://doi.org/10.1007/s40489-014-0040-7.

Bärwalde, T., Hoffmann, L., Fink, A., Völlm, C., Martin, O., Bernard, M., & Richter, M. (2023). The adolescent concept of social participation—a qualitative study on the concept of social participation from adolescents with and without physical disabilities. *Qualitative Health Research*, *33*(3), 143–153.

Bagwell, C. L., & Schmidt, M. E. (2011). *Friendships in childhood and adolescence*. New York: Guilford Press.

Barry, T., Klinger, L., Lee, J., Palardy, N., Gilmore, T., & Bodin, S. (2003). Examining the effectiveness of an outpatient clinic-based social skills group for high-functioning children with autism. *Journal of Autism and Developmental Disorders*, *33*(6), 685–701. https://doi.org/10.1023/b:jadd.0000006004.86556.e0.

Bascom, G. W., & Christensen, K. M. (2017). The impacts of limited transportation access on persons with disabilities' social participation. *Journal of Transport & Health*, *7*, 227–234.

Bearman, M., Bowes, G., & Jolly, B. (2005). Looking for the child's perspective. *Medical Education*, *39*, 757–759. https://doi.org/10.1111/j.1365--2929.2005.02253.x.

Bedell, G., Coster, W., Law, M., Liljenquist, K., Kao, Y. C., Teplicky, R., Anaby, D., & Khetani, M. A. (2013). Community participation, supports, and barriers of school-age children with and without disabilities. *Archives of Physical Medicine and Rehabilitation*, *94*(2), 315–323. https://doi.org/10.1016/j.apmr.2012.09.024.

Bedell, G. M. (2012). Measurement of social participation. In V. Anderson, & M. H. Beauchamp (Eds.), *Developmental social neuroscience and childhood brain insult: Theory and practice* (pp. 184–206). NewYork: Guilford Press.

Beresford, B. (2004). On the road to nowhere? Young disabled people and transition. *Child: Care, Health and Development*, *30*(6), 581–587. https://doi.org/10.1111/j.1365-2214.2004.00469.x.

Bezyak, J. L., Sabella, S. A., & Gattis, R. H. (2017). Public transportation: An investigation of barriers for people with disabilities. *Journal of Disability Policy Studies*, *28*(1), 52–60. https://doi.org/10.1177/1044207317702070.

Bezyak, J. L., Sabella, S., Hammel, J., McDonald, K., Jones, R. A., & Barton, D. (2020). Community participation and public transportation barriers experienced by people with disabilities. *Disability & Rehabilitation*, *42*(23), 3275–3283.

Billstedt, E., Gillberg, I. C., & Gillberg, C. (2011). Aspects of quality of life in adults diagnosed with autism in childhood. *Autism*, *15*(1), 7–20. https://doi.org/10.1177/1362361309346066.

Björquist, E., & Tryggvason, N. (2022). When you are not here, I cannot do what I want on the tablet–The use of ICT to promote social participation of young people with intellectual disabilities. *Journal of Intellectual Disabilities*.

Bond, G. R., Salyers, M. P., Rollins, A. L., Rapp, C. A., & Zipple, A. M. (2004). How evidence-based practices contribute to community integration. *Community Mental Health Journal*, *40*, 569–588.

Britner, P. A., Balcazar, F. E., Blechman, E. A., Blinn-Pile, L., & Larose, S. (2006). Mentoring special youth populations. *Journal of Community Psychology*, *34*(6), 747–763. https://doi.org/10.1002/jcop.20127.

Buhrmester, D. (1996). Need fulfillment, interpersonal competence, and the developmental contexts of early adolescent friendship. In W. M. Bukowski, A. F. Newcomb, & W. W. Hartup (Eds.), *The company they keep: Friendships in childhood and adolescence* (pp. 346–365). Cambridge University Press.

Burns, R., & Graefe, A. (2007). Constraints to outdoor recreation: Exploring the effects of disabilities on perceptions and participation. *Journal of Leisure Research*, *39*, 156–181.

Cahill, S. M., Egan, B. E., & Seber, J. (2020). Activity-and occupation-based interventions to support mental health, positive behavior, and social participation for children and youth: A systematic review. *American Journal of Occupational Therapy*, *74*(2), 7402180020p1–7402180020p28.

Carter, E. W., Cushing, L. S., & Clark, N. M. (2005). Effects of peer support interventions on students' access to the general curriculum and social interactions. *Research and Practice for Persons with Severe Disabilities*, *30*, 15–25.

Carter, E. W., & Hughes, C. (2005). Increasing social interaction among adolescents with intellectual disabilities and their general education peers: Effective interventions. *Research and Practice for Persons with Severe Disabilities*, *30*(4), 179–193.

Carter, E. W., & Pesko, M. J. (2008). Social validity of peer interaction intervention strategies in high school classrooms: Effectiveness, feasibility, and actual use. *Exceptionality*, *16*, 156–173. https://doi.org/10.1080/09362830802198427.

Carter, E. W. (2013). Supporting inclusion and flourishing in the religious and spiritual lives of people with intellectual and developmental disabilities. *Inclusion*, *1*(1), 64–75. https://doi.org/10.1352/2326-6988-1.1.064.

Cavet, J., & Sloper, P. (2004). Participation of disabled children in individual decisions about their lives and in public decisions about service development. *Children & Society*, *18*, 278–290. https://doi.org/10.1002/chi.803.

Cheung, P. P. P., Brown, T., Yu, M., & Siu, A. M. H. (2021). The effectiveness of a school-based social cognitive intervention on the social participation of Chinese children with autism. *Journal of Autism and Developmental Disorders*, *51*, 1894–1908. https://doi.org/10.1007/s10803-020-04683-1.

Chien, C. W., & Lin, C. Y. (2021). Community participation of school-age children: Who is at risk of restricted participation? *Physical & Occupational Therapy in Pediatrics*, *41*(5), 447–463. https://doi.org/10.1080/01942638.2021.1900489.

Cohn, E., Miller, L. J., & Tickle-Degnen, L. (2000). Parental hopes for therapy outcomes: Children with sensory modulation disorders. *American Journal of Occupational Therapy*, *54*(1), 36–42. https://doi.org/10.5014/ajot.54.1.36.

Cook, A. G. (2020). Using an inclusive therapeutic theatre production to teach self-advocacy skills in young people with disabilities. *The Arts in Psychotherapy*, *71*, 101715. https://doi.org/10.1016/j.aip.2020.101715.

Crabtree, J. (2017). The importance of public transportation to community mobility and participation. *OT Practice*, *22*(3), 1–8.

Davila, A., & Mora, M. (2007). *Civic engagement and high school academic progress: An analysis using NELS data*. University of Maryland School of Public Policy, Center for Information and Research on Civic Learning and Engagement (CIRCLE).

Diez, A. M. (2010). School memories of young people with disabilities: An analysis of barriers and aids to inclusion. *Disability & Society, 25*(2), 163–175. https://doi.org/10.1080/09687590903534346.

Dudgeon, B. J., Massagli, T. L., & Ross, B. W. (1997). Educational participation of children with spinal cord injury. *American Journal of Occupational Therapy, 51*, 553–561. https://doi.org/10.5014/ajot.51.7.553.

Duffey, K., Barbosa, A., Whiting, S., Mendes, R., Yordi Aguirre, I., Tcymbal, A., Abu-Omar, K., Gelius, P., & Breda, J. (2021). Barriers and facilitators of physical activity participation in adolescent girls: A systematic review of systematic reviews. *Frontiers in Public Health, 9*. :743935. https://doi.org/10.3389/fpubh.2021.743935.

Eisenberg, Y., Heider, A., Gould, R., & Jones, R. (2020). Are communities in the United States planning for pedestrians with disabilities? Findings from systematic evaluation of local government barrier removal plans. *Cities, 102*. https://doi.org/10.1016/j.cities.2020.102720.

Elfassy, C., Cachecho, S., Snider, L., & Dahan-Oliel, N. (2020). Participation among children with arthrogryposis multiplex congenita: A scoping review. *Physical & Occupational Therapy in Pediatrics, 40*(6), 610–636. https://doi.org/10.1080/01942638.2020.1754319.

Erikson, E. H. (1968). *Identity, youth, and crisis*. Norton.

Erwin, E., & Brown, F. (2003). From theory to practice: A contextual framework for understanding self-determination in early-childhood environments. *Infants & Young Children, 16*(1), 77–87.

Field, S., & Hoffman, A. (2002). Preparing youth to exercise self-determination: Quality indicators of school environments that promote the acquisition of knowledge, skills, and beliefs related to self-determination. *Journal of Disability Policy Studies, 13*(2), 114–119.

Forber-Pratt, A. J., Minotti, B. J., Burdick, C. E., Kate Brown, M., & Hanebutt, R. A. (2021). Exploring disability identity with adolescents. *Rehabilitation Psychology, 66*(4), 550–564. https://doi.org/10.1037/rep0000411.

Garth, B., & Aroni, R. (2003). "I value what you have to say": Seeking the perspective of children with a disability, not just their parents. *Disability & Society, 18*(5), 561–576. https://doi.org/10.1080/0968759032000097825.

Gill, C. J. (1997). Four types of integration in disability identity development. *Journal of Vocational Rehabilitation, 9*, 39–46. https://psycnet.apa.org/doi/10.1016/S1052-2263(97)00020-2.

Goodwin, D. L., & Staples, K. (2005). The meaning of summer camp experiences to youths with disabilities. *Adapted Physical Activity Quarterly, 22*, 159–178. https://doi.org/10.1123/apaq.22.2.160.

Green, S. E. (2003). "What do you mean 'what's wrong with her?'": Stigma and the lives of families of children with disabilities. *Social Science & Medicine, 57*(8), 1361–1374.

Gregson, K. D., Tu, K. M., Erath, S. A., & Pettit, G. S. (2017). Parental social coaching promotes adolescent peer acceptance across the middle school transition. *Journal of Family Psychology, 31*(6), 668–678. https://doi.org/10.1037/fam0000314.

Grinker, R. R. (2020). Autism,"stigma," disability: A shifting historical terrain. *Current Anthropology, 61*(S21), S55–S67.

Hansen, D. M., Larson, R. W., & Dworkin, J. B. (2003). What adolescents learn in organized youth activities: A survey of self-reported developmental experiences. *Journal of Research on Adolescence, 13*(1), 25–55. https://doi.org/10.1111/1532-7795.1301006.

Hardman, M. L., & Dawson, S. (2008). The impact of federal public policy on curriculum and instruction for students with disabilities in the general classroom. *Preventing School Failure: Alternative Education for Children and Youth, 52*(2), 5–11.

Hartup, W. W. (1996). The company they keep: Friendships and their developmental significance. *Child Development, 67*(1), 1–13.

Hemmingson, H., & Borell, L. (2002). Environmental barriers in mainstream schools. *Child: Care, Health and Development, 28*, 57–63. https://doi.org/10.1046/j.1365-2214.2002.00240.x.

Hengen, S., & Weaver, A. D. (2018). Post-secondary student with disabilities: Increasing self-advocacy through educational plan participation. *School Psychologist, 72*(2), 7–18. https://escholarship.org/uc/item/1h35r6zr.

Hoehne, C., Baranski, B., Benmohammed, L., Bienstock, L., Menezes, N., Margolese, N., & Anaby, D. (2020). Changes in overall participation profile of youth with physical disabilities following the PREP Intervention. *International Journal of Environmental Research and Public Health, 17*(11), 3990. https://doi.org/10.3390/ijerph17113990.

Hoffmann, L., Völlm, C., Bernard, M., Fink, A., Richter, M., & Dawal, B. (2023). What does social participation mean? A qualitative study exploring the concept of participation from the perspectives of experts and parents. *BMJ Open, 13*(7):e072684. https://doi.org/10.1136/bmjopen-2023-072684.

Howes, C. (1988). Peer interaction of young children. *Monographs of the Society for Research in Child Development, 53*(1). https://doi.org/10.2307/1166062.

Howlin, P., Moss, P., Savage, S., & Rutter, M. (2013). Social outcomes in mid- to later adulthood among individuals diagnosed with autism and average nonverbal IQ as children. *Journal of the American Academy of Child & Adolescent Psychiatry, 52*(6):572–81.e1. https://doi.org/10.1016/j.jaac.2013.02.017.

Jeong, Y. (2020). Participation, supports, and barriers of Korean children and youth with and without disabilities in the school environment. *Disability & Rehabilitation, 42*(12), 1667–1674. https://doi.org/10.1080/09638288.2019.1567836.

Jones, J. L., Gallus, K. L., Viering, K. L., & Oseland, L. M. (2015). 'Are you by chance on the spectrum?'Adolescents with autism spectrum disorder making sense of their diagnoses. *Disability & Society, 30*(10), 1490–1504.

Joseph Rowntree Foundation. (2003). *An evaluation of a young disabled people's peer mentoring/support project*. Joseph Rowntree Foundation.

Kamps, D. M., Potucek, J., Lopez, A. G., Kravits, T., & Kemmerer, K. (1997). The use of peer networks across multiple settings to improve social interaction for students with autism. *Journal of Behavioral Education, 7*(3), 335–357. https://doi.org/10.1023/A:1022879607019.

Kapsalis, E., Jaeger, N., & Hale, J. (2022). Disabled-by-design: Effects of inaccessible urban public spaces on users of mobility assistive devices–a systematic review. *Disability and Rehabilitation: Assistive Technology*, 1–19.

Kessler Foundation/National Organization on Disability. (2010). The 2010 survey of Americans with disabilities. http://www.kesslerfoundation.org/.

King, G., Keenan, S., McDougall, C., & Oake, M. (2020). Investigating a participation-based friendship intervention for youth with disabilities: Effects on goal attainment, social self-efficacy, and engagement. *Physical & Occupational Therapy in Pediatrics, 40*(2), 152–167. https://doi.org/10.1080/01942638.2019.1646376.

King, G., Smart, E., Bowman, L., & Pinto, M. (2022). Social participation interventions targeting relational outcomes for young people with physical and developmental disabilities: An umbrella review and narrative synthesis. *Disability & Rehabilitation*, 1–14.

Kingsnorth, S., Rudzik, A., King, G., & McPherson, A. C. (2019). Residential immersive life skills programs for youth with disabilities: A case study of youth developmental trajectories of personal growth and caregiver perspectives. *BMC Pediatrics, 19*(1), 413. https://doi.org/10.1186/s12887-019-1793-z.

Kinnear, S. H., Link, B. G., Ballan, M. S., & Fischbach, R. L. (2016). Understanding the experience of stigma for parents of children with autism spectrum disorder and the role stigma plays in families' lives. *Journal of Autism and Developmental Disorders, 46*, 942–953.

Kirchner, C. E., Gerber, E. G., & Smith, B. C. (2008). Designed to deter: Community barriers to physical activity for people with visual or motor impairments. *American Journal of Preventive Medicine, 34*(4), 349–352.

Kiresuk, T. J., Smith, A., & Cardillo, J. E. (1994). *Goal attainment scaling: Application, theory and measurement*. Erlbaum.

Koontz, A. M., Bass, S. R., & Kulich, H. R. (2021). Accessibility facilitators and barriers affecting independent wheelchair transfers in the community. *Disability and Rehabilitation: Assistive Technology, 16*(7), 741–748.

Kotzer, E., & Margalit, M. (2007). Perception of competence: Risk and protective predictors following an e-self-advocacy intervention for adolescents with learning disabilities. *European Journal of Special Needs Education, 22*(4), 443–457. https://doi.org/10.1080/08856250701650060.

Kramer, J. M., Olsen, S., Mermelstein, M., Balcells, A., & Liljenquist, K. (2012). Youth with disabilities' perspectives of the environment and participation: A qualitative meta-synthesis. *Child: Care, Health and Development, 38*(6), 763–777. https://doi.org/10.1111/j.1365-2214.2012.01365.x.

Lüddeckens, J. (2021). Approaches to inclusion and social participation in school for adolescents with autism spectrum conditions (ASC)—a systematic research review. *Review Journal of Autism and Developmental Disorders*, *8*, 37–50.

Lalvani, P. (2015). Disability, stigma and otherness: Perspectives of parents and teachers. *International Journal of Disability, Development and Education*, *62*(4), 379–393.

Lansdown, G., & Karkara, R. (2006). Children's right to express views and have them taken seriously. *Lancet*, *367*, 690–692. https://doi.org/10.1016/S0140-6736(06)68268-8.

Levasseur, M., Lussier-Therrien, M., Biron, M. L., Raymond, É., Castonguay, J., Naud, D., & Tremblay, L. (2022). Scoping study of definitions of social participation: Update and co-construction of an interdisciplinary consensual definition. *Age and Ageing*, *51*(2):afab215.

Lindsay, S., & McPherson, A. C. (2012). Experiences of social exclusion and bullying at school among children and youth with cerebral palsy. *Disability & Rehabilitation*, *34*(2), 101–109.

Liptak, G. S., Kennedy, J. A., & Dosa, N. P. (2011). Social participation in a nationally representative sample of older youth and young adults with autism. *Journal of Developmental and Behavioral Pediatrics*, *32*, 277–283. https://doi.org/10.1097/DBP.0b013e31820b49fc.

Lopes, P. B., Shikako-Thomas, K., Cardoso, R., & Simões Matsukura, T. (2019). Social participation: The perspectives of adolescents with cerebral palsy and their mothers. *International Journal of Developmental Disabilities*, *67*(4), 263–272. https://doi.org/10.1080/20473869.2019.1623596.

Macdonald, S. J., Deacon, L., Nixon, J., Akintola, A., Gillingham, A., Kent, J., & Highmore, L. (2018). The invisible enemy': Disability, loneliness and isolation. *Disability & Society*, *33*(7), 1138–1159.

Maciver, D., Rutherford, M., Arakelyan, S., Kramer, J. M., Richmond, J., Todorova, L., Romero-Ayuso, D., Nakamura-Thomas, H., Ten Velden, M., Finlayson, I., O'Hare, A., & Forsyth, K. (2019). Participation of children with disabilities in school: A realist systematic review of psychosocial and environmental factors. *PLoS One*, *14*(1):e0210511. https://doi.org/10.1371/journal.pone.0210511.

Magasi, S., & Hammel, J. (2004). Social support and social network mobilization in African American woman who have experienced strokes. *Disability Studies Quarterly*, *24*(4). https://doi.org/10.18061/dsq.v24i4.878.

Mancini, M., & Coster, W. (2004). Functional predictors of school participation by children with disabilities. *Occupational Therapy International*, *11*(1), 12–25. https://doi.org/10.1002/oti.194.

Mazumder, R., & Thompson-Hodgetts, S. (2019). Stigmatization of children and adolescents with autism spectrum disorders and their families: A scoping study. *Review Journal of Autism and Developmental Disorders*, *6*, 96–107.

Meeus, W., Iedema, J., Helsen, M., & Vollenbergh, W. (1999). Patterns of adolescent identity development: Review of literature and longitudinal analysis. *Developmental Review*, *19*, 419–461. https://doi.org/10.1006/drev.1999.0483.

Mitter, N., Ali, A., & Scior, K. (2019). Stigma experienced by families of individuals with intellectual disabilities and autism: A systematic review. *Research in Developmental Disabilities*, *89*, 10–21.

Moore, A., & Lynch, H. (2015). Accessibility and usability of playground environments for children under 12: A scoping review. *Scandinavian Journal of Occupational Therapy*, *22*(5), 331–344.

Mueller, C. (2019). Adolescent understandings of disability labels and social stigma in school. *International Journal of Qualitative Studies in Education*, *32*(3), 263–281.

Mueller, C. O. (2021). "I didn't know people with disabilities could grow up to be adults": Disability history, curriculum, and identity in special education. *Teacher Education and Special Education*, *44*(3), 189–205. https://doi.org/10.1177/0888406421996069.

Nario-Redmond, M. R., Noel, J. G., & Fern, E. (2013). Redefining disability, re-imagining the self: Disability identification predicts self-esteem and strategic responses to stigma. *Self and Identity*, *12*, 468–488. https://doi.org/10.1080/15298868.2012.681118.

Newman, L., Wagner, M., Knokey, A.-M., Marder, C., Nagle, K., Shaver, D., Wei, X., with Cameto, R., Contreras, E., Ferguson, K., Greene, S., & Schwarting, M. (2011). *The Post-high school outcomes of young adults with disabilities up to 8 years after high school. A report from the national longitudinal transition study-2 (NLTS2) (NCSER 2011-3005)*. SRI International.

O'Handley, R. D., Radley, K. C., & Whipple, H. M. (2015). The relative effects of social stories and video modeling toward increasing eye contact of adolescents with autism spectrum disorder. *Research in Autism Spectrum Disorders*, *11*, 101–111. https://doi.org/10.1016/j.rasd.2014.12.009.

Odom, S. L. (2019). Peer-based interventions for children and youth with autism spectrum disorder: History and effects. *School Psychology Review*, *48*(2), 170–176. https://doi.org/10.17105/SPR-2019-0019.V48-2.

Palmer, S. B. (2011). Self-determination - a life-span perspective. *Focus on Exceptional Children*, *42*(6), 1–16.

Piškur, B., Daniëls, R., Jongmans, M. J., Ketelaar, M., Smeets, R. J., Norton, M., & Beurskens, A. J. (2014). Participation and social participation: Are they distinct concepts? *Clinical Rehabilitation*, *28*(3), 211 220. https://doi.org/10.1177/0269215513499029.

Pivik, J., McComas, J., & LaFlamme, M. (2002). Barriers and facilitators to inclusive education. *Exceptional Children*, *69*(1), 97–107.

Post, M., Haymes, L., Storey, K., Loughrey, T., & Campbell, C. (2014). Understanding stalking behaviors by individuals with autism spectrum disorders and recommended prevention strategies for school settings. *Journal of Autism and Developmental Disorders*, *44*(11), 2698–2706. https://doi.org/10.1007/s10803-012-1712-8.

Potts, S., Kirkham, M., Monsour, F., Grinde, J., & Planner, M. (2001). *Sustaining service learning in Wisconsin: What principals, teachers, and students say about service-learning*. Department of Public Instruction.

Powers, L. E., Garner, T., Valnes, B., Squire, P., Turner, A., Couture, T., & Dertinger, R. (2007). Building a successful adult life: Findings from youth-directed research. *Exceptionality*, *15*(1), 45–56. https://doi.org/10.1080/09362830709336925.

Ratcliff, K., Hong, I., & Hilton, C. L. (2018). Leisure participation patterns for school age youth with autism spectrum disorders: Findings from the 2016 national survey of children's health. *Journal of Autism and Developmental Disorders*, *48*(11), 3783–3793. https://doi.org/10.1007/s10803-018-3643-5.

Roeyers, H. (1996). The influence of nonhandicapped peers on the social interactions of children with a pervasive developmental disorder. *Journal of Autism and Developmental Disorders*, *26*, 303–320. https://doi.org/10.1007/BF02172476.

Rubin, K. H., Coplan, R. J., Chen, X., Buskirk, A. A., & Wojslawowicz, J. C. (2005). Peer relationships in childhood. In M. H. Bornstein, & M. E. Lamb (Eds.), *Developmental science: An advanced textbook* (pp. 269–512). Psychology Press.

Rush, D. D., & Shelden, M. L. (2005). Evidence-based definition of coaching practices. *CASE in Point: Insights into Early Childhood and Family Support Practices*, *1*(6), 1–6.

Rutter, M. (1990). Psychosocial resilience and protective mechanisms. In J. Rolf, A. S Masten, D. Cicchetti, K. H Nüchterlein, & S. Weintraub (Eds.), *Risk and protective factors in the development of psychopathology* (pp. 181–214). Cambridge University Press.

Ryan, R., & Deci, E. (2000). Self-determination theory and the facilitation of intrinsic motivation, social development, and well-being. *American Psychologist*, *55*(1), 68–78. https://doi.org/10.1037//0003-066x.55.1.68.

Samanci, O., Ocakci, E., & Secer, I. (2018). Developing scale for determining the sSocial participation skills for children and analyzing its psychometric characteristics. *International Education Studies*, *11*(6), 92. https://doi.org/10.5539/ies.v11n6p92.

Sattoe, J. N., Hilberink, S. R., van Staa, A., & Bal, R. (2014). Lagging behind or not? Four distinctive social participation patterns among young adults with chronic conditions. *The Journal of Adolescent*, *54*(4), 397–403. https://doi.org/10.1016/j.jadohealth.2013.09.017.

Scales, P. C., Blyth, D. A., Berkas, T. H., & Kielsmeier, J. C. (2000). The effects of service-learning on middle school students' social responsibility and academic success. *The Journal of Early Adolescence*, *20*(3), 332–358. https://doi.org/10.1177/0272431600020003004.

Schell, B.A.B, & Gillen, G. (2019a). Introduction to evaluation, intervention, and outcomes for occupations. In Schell B.A.B. & Gillen G. (Eds.), *Willard and Spackman's occupational therapy* (p. 711). Wolters Kluwer.

Scior, K., Hamid, A., Hastings, R., Werner, S., Belton, C., Laniyan, A., … Kett, M. (2020). Intellectual disability stigma and initiatives to challenge it and promote inclusion around the globe. *Journal of Policy and Practice in Intellectual Disabilities*, *17*(2), 165–175.

Sebanc, A. M. (2003). The friendship features of preschool children: Links with prosocial behavior and aggression. *Journal of Occupational and Organizational Psychology*, *12*(2), 249–268. https://psycnet.apa.org/doi/10.1111/1467-9507.00232.

Selfhout, M. H., Branje, S. J., & Meeus, W. H. (2009). Developmental trajectories of perceived friendship intimacy, constructive problem solving, and depression from early to late adolescence. *Journal of Abnormal Child Psychology*, *36*, 471–485. https://doi.org/10.1007/s10802-008-9273-1.

Sezici, E., Ocakci, A. F., & Kadioglu, H. (2017). Use of play therapy in nursing process: A prospective randomized controlled study. *Journal of Nursing Scholarship*, *49*(2), 162–169. https://doi.org/10.1111/jnu.12277.

Shaikh, N. M., Kersten, P., Siegert, R. J., & Theadom, A. (2019). Developing a comprehensive framework of community integration for people with acquired brain injury: A conceptual analysis. *Disability & Rehabilitation*, *41*(14), 1615–1631.

Shannon, S., Brennan, D., Hanna, D., Younger, Z., Hassan, J., & Breslin, G. (2018). The effect of school-based intervention on physical activity and well-being: A non-randomized controlled trial with children of low socio-economic status. *Sports Medicine-Open*, *4*(1), 16. https://doi.org/10.1186/s40798-018-0129-0.

Shattuck, P. T., Orsmond, G. I., Wagner, M., & Cooper, B. P. (2011). Participation in social activities among adolescents with an autism spectrum disorder. *PLoS One*, *6*(11):e27176. https://doi.org/10.1371/journal.pone.0027176.

Shevlin, M., Kenny, M., & McNeela, E. (2002). Curriculum access for pupils with disabilities: An Irish experience. *Disability & Society*, *17*(2), 159–169. https://doi.org/10.1080/09687590120122314.

Shogren, K. A., Burke, K. M., Anderson, M. H., Antosh, A. A., Wehmeyer, M. L., LaPlante, T., & Shaw, L. A. (2018). Evaluating the differential impact of interventions to promote self-determination and goal attainment for transition-age youth with intellectual disability. *Research and Practice for Persons with Severe Disabilities*, *43*(3), 165–180. https://doi.org/10.1177/1540796918779775.

Simpson, K., Adams, D., Bruck, S., & Keen, D. (2019). Investigating the participation of children on the autism spectrum across home, school, and community: A longitudinal study. *Child: Care, Health and Development*, *45*, 681–687. https://doi.org/10.1111/cch.12679.

Sloper, P., & Lightfoot, J. (2003). Involving disabled and chronically ill children and young people in health service development. *Child: Care, Health and Development*, *29*(1), 15–20. https://doi.org/10.1046/j.1365--2214.2003.00315.x.

Smith, J., Halliwell, N., Laurent, A., Tsotsoros, J., Harris, K., & DeGrace, B. (2023). Social participation experiences of families raising a young child with autism spectrum disorder: Implications for mental health and well-being. *American Journal of Occupational Therapy*, *77*(2):7702185090.

Steinhardt, F., Ullenhag, A., Jahnsen, R., & Dolva, A. S. (2021). Perceived facilitators and barriers for participation in leisure activities in children with disabilities: Perspectives of children, parents and professionals. *Scandinavian Journal of Occupational Therapy*, *28*(2), 121–135. https://doi.org/10.1080/11038128.2019.1703037.

Stienstra, D. (2018). Canadian disability policies in a world of inequalities. *Societies*, *8*(2), 36.

Strain, P. S., Kohler, F. W., & Goldstein, H. (1996). Learning experiences: An alternative program: Peer-mediated interventions for young children with autism. In E. D. Hibbs, & P. S. Jensen (Eds.), *Psychosocial treatments for child and adolescent disorders: Empirically based strategies for clinical practice* (pp. 573–587). American Psychological Association.

Swartz, S. L., Prevatt, F., & Proctor, B. E. (2005). A coaching intervention for college students with attention deficit/hyperactivity disorder. *Psychology in the Schools*, *43*, 647–656. https://doi.org/10.1002/pits.20101.

Sylvestre, A., Nadeau, L., Charron, L., Larose, N., & Lepage, C. (2013). Social participation by children with developmental coordination disorder compared to their peers. *Disability & Rehabilitation*, *35*(21), 1814–1820. https://doi.org/10.3109/09638288.2012.756943.

Sze, N. N., & Christensen, K. M. (2017). Access to urban transportation system for individuals with disabilities. *IATSS Research*, *41*(2), 66–73.

Tanner, K., Hand, B. N., O'Toole, G., & Lane, A. E. (2015). Effectiveness of interventions to improve social participation, play, leisure, and restricted and repetitive behaviors in people with autism spectrum disorder: A systematic review. *American Journal of Occupational Therapy*, *69*, p1–p12. https://doi.org/10.5014/ajot.2015.017806.

Test, D. W., Fowler, C. H., Wood, W. M., Brewer, D. M., & Eddy, S. (2005). A conceptual framework of self-advocacy for students with disabilities. *Remedial and Special Education*, *26*(1), 43–54.

Tisdall, E. K. M., & Davis, J. (2004). Making a difference? Bringing children's and young people's views into policy-making. *Children & Society*, *18*, 131–142. https://doi.org/10.1002/chi.816.

Vänskä, N., Sipari, S., & Haataja, L. (2020). What makes participation meaningful? Using photo-elicitation to interview children with disabilities. *Physical & Occupational Therapy in Pediatrics*, *40*(6), 595–609. https://doi.org/10.1080/01942638.2020.1736234.

Valnes, B., et al. (2003). Future directions agenda for youth with disabilities. In *National Youth Leadership Network*.

Vandell, D., & Mueller, E. C. (1980). Peer play and friendships during the first two years. In H. C. Foot, A. J. Chapman, & J. R. Smith (Eds.), *Friendships and social relationships in children* (pp. 181–208). John Wiley.

Vaughn, B., Colvin, T. N., Azria, M. R., Caya, L., & Krzysik, L. (2001). Dyadic analyses of friendship in a sample of preschool-age children attending Head Start: Correspondence between measures and implications for social competence. *Child Development*, *72*(3), 862–878. https://www.jstor.org/stable/1132460.

Verdonschot, M. M., de Witte, L. P., Reichrath, E., Buntinx, W. H., & Curfs, L. M. (2009). Impact of environmental factors on community participation of persons with an intellectual disability: A systematic review. *Journal of Intellectual Disability Research: Journal of Intellectual Disability Research*, *53*(1), 54–64. https://doi.org/10.1111/j.1365-2788.2008.01128.x.

Voorman, J., et al. (2010). Social functioning and communication in children with cerebral palsy: Association with disease characteristics and personal and environmental factors. *Developmental Medicine and Child Neurology*, *52*, 441–447. https://doi.org/10.1111/j.1469-8749.2009.03399.x.

Wade, S. L., Bedell, G., King, J. A., Jacquin, M., Turkstra, L. S., Haarbauer-Krupa, J., Johnson, J., Salloum, R., & Narad, M. E. (2018). Social participation and navigation (SPAN) program for adolescents with acquired brain injury: Pilot findings. *Rehabilitation Psychology*, *63*(3), 327–337. https://doi.org/10.1037/rep0000187.

Walker, S., & Berthelsen, D. (2007). The social participation of young children with developmental disabilities in inclusive early childhood programs. *Electronic Journal for Inclusive Education*, *2*(3).

Wang, T. N., Tseng, M. H., Wilson, B. N., & Hu, F. C. (2009). Functional performance of children with developmental coordination disorder at home and at school. *Developmental Medicine and Child Neurology*, *51*(10), 817–825. https://doi.org/10.1111/j.1469-8749.2009.03271.x.

Wasfi, R., Steinmetz-Wood, M., & Levinson, D. (2017). Measuring the transportation needs of people with developmental disabilities: A means to social inclusion. *Disability and Health Journal*, *10*(2), 356–360.

Wenger, I., Schulze, C., Lundström, U., & Prellwitz, M. (2021). Children's perceptions of playing on inclusive playgrounds: A qualitative study. *Scandinavian Journal of Occupational Therapy*, *28*(2), 136–146. https://doi.org/10.1080/11038128.2020.1810768.

Willis, C., Nyquist, A., Jahnsen, R., Elliott, C., & Ullenhag, A. (2018). Enabling physical activity participation for children and youth with disabilities following a goal-directed, family-centered intervention. *Research in Developmental Disabilities*, *77*, 30–39. https://doi.org/10.1016/j.ridd.2018.03.010.

World Health Organization. (2007). *International classification of functioning, disability and health: Children and youth version*. Author.

Zuckerman, K. E., Lindly, O. J., Reyes, N. M., Chavez, A. F., Cobian, M., Macias, K., … Smith, K. A. (2018). Parent perceptions of community autism spectrum disorder stigma: Measure validation and associations in a multi-site sample. *Journal of Autism and Developmental Disorders*, *48*, 3199–3209.

Zwart, L. M., & Kallemeyn, L. M. (2001). Peer-based coaching for college students with ADHD and learning disabilities. *Journal of Postsecondary Education and Disability*, *15*(1), 1–15.

19

# Sexuality

*Elizabeth Koss Schmidt and Jenn Soros*

## GUIDING QUESTIONS

1. What is the role of occupational therapy in sexuality?
2. What are the constructs addressed in the Occupational Therapy Sexual Assessment Framework (OTSAF), and how can occupational therapy practitioners use this framework to guide their practice?
3. What specific intervention approaches do occupational therapy practitioners use to support youth to ensure safe participation in meaningful tasks associated with sexual occupations?

## KEY TERMS

Gender identity
Family planning
Intimacy
Intimate partner relationships
Occupational Therapy Sexual Assessment Framework
Personal safety skills
Sexual activity
Sexual scripts
Sexual education
Sexual expression
Sexual health
Sexual interest
Sexual knowledge
Sexual orientation
Sexual response
Sexual self-view

## THE ROLE OF OCCUPATIONAL THERAPY: INTIMATE PARTNER RELATIONSHIPS AND SEXUAL ACTIVITY

Occupational therapy practitioners advocate for equality and equal access to occupations, which is a principle that is essential for human rights (Wilcock & Hocking, 2015; World Federation of Occupational Therapists, 2019). Every individual has the right to education to provide them with the highest standard of health and well-being (UNESCO, 2021). Sexual health is a basic component of a person's overall health and is essential to well-being (Amjadi et al., 2017; UNESCO, 2021). Occupational therapy practitioners have expertise in understanding and analyzing the effects of client factors, performance skills, and the context to promote participation and performance in occupations related to sexuality and intimacy (Walker, 2020). While occupational therapy practitioners possess the skills needed to address sexuality, many are uncomfortable addressing the topic in practice (Mc Grath & Sakellariou, 2016; Soros & Reese, 2021), especially with young people. Increasing knowledge surrounding sexuality can increase occupational therapy practitioners' competency and comfort level in addressing this critical area of development for their clients.

Within the Occupational Therapy Practice Framework: Domain and Process fourth edition (OTPF-4), **intimate partner relationships** are included under the occupation of social participation and are defined as "engaging in activities to initiate and maintain a close relationship, including giving and receiving affection and interacting in desired roles; intimate partners may or may not engage in sexual activity" (American Occupational Therapy Association, 2020, p. 34). **Sexual activity** is considered an activity of daily living and is defined as "engaging in the broad possibilities for sexual expression and experiences with self or others (e.g., hugging, kissing, foreplay, masturbation, oral sex, intercourse)" (American Occupational Therapy Association, 2020, p. 30). Both intimate partner relationships and sexual activity fall within the scope of practice of occupational therapy practitioners.

Walker et al. (2020) developed the **Occupational Therapy Sexual Assessment Framework (OTSAF)** to be consistent with the OTPF-4 but expanded in scope and detail. The OTSAF includes the constructs of sexual knowledge, sexual activity, sexual interest, sexual response, sexual self-view, sexual expression, intimacy, sexual health, and family planning (Walker et al., 2020). Constructs that are considered occupations include sexual activity (ADL), family planning and sexual expression (IADLs), intimacy (social participation), and sexual health (health management) (American Occupational Therapy Association, 2020; Walker, 2020). Constructs that fall into the category of client factors are sexual knowledge and sexual self-view (values, beliefs, spirituality) and sexual interest and sexual response (body functions) (American Occupational Therapy Association, 2020; Walker, 2020). Occupational therapy practitioners also consider other client factors, including body structures and other domains, environmental and personal factors, and performance skills and patterns when working with children and young people (American Occupational Therapy Association, 2020; Walker, 2020). As explored in the following sections, the OTSAF can be applied to pediatric populations to help guide occupational therapy practice.

### Sexual Knowledge and Personal Safety

**Sexual knowledge** is what someone knows, understands, believes, and values about sexual activity (Walker et al., 2020). All individuals need to have knowledge regarding personal safety skills. Sexuality education should start at an early age for children to learn critical concepts, make informed decisions, and to develop critical thinking skills regarding topics related to sexual health and wellness (UNESCO, 2021). When children and young people have knowledge deficits regarding personal safety, they have an increased risk for sexual abuse and sexual victimization (Dewinter et al., 2020; Miller et al., 2017). **Personal safety skills** include knowledge about one's physical development, appropriate and inappropriate touch, and responding to inappropriate touch (Miller et al., 2017). Children and young people develop **sexual scripts**, which are perceptions, beliefs, and social and cultural norms about how to act in sexual and intimate situations (Gagnon & Simon, 2011; Vintor & Ribner, 2021). Often children and young people with disabilities rely on caregivers or others for their basic activities of daily living (Cella et al., 2010; Czapla & Otrebski, 2018; Kahn & Halpern, 2018; Kattari, 2014; Wiegerink et al., 2011). As a result, children and young people with disabilities may develop altered sexual scripts where boundaries and privacy may not be as clearly defined (Gagnon & Simon, 2011; Vintor & Ribner, 2021). Occupational therapy practitioners need to ensure that sexual education is inclusive for all people to develop personal safety skills regarding sexuality and intimacy.

People with other disabilities, including, but not limited to, those with intellectual disabilities, may have cognitive challenges and challenges with executive function that impact their sexual knowledge. Specifically, people with cognitive challenges may have increased difficulty acquiring and maintaining sexual health education content necessary to make safe decisions associated with sexual occupations and/or understanding rules associated with boundaries needed for healthy relationships or difficulty (Davis et al., 2016; McLay et al., 2015; DiGioia, n.d.; Wiegerink et al., 2010).

Comprehensive **sexual education** is vital for the health and wellbeing of all youth, including youth with disabilities. However, youth with disabilities are less likely to receive comprehensive sexual education (Barnard-Brak et al., 2014; Holmes et al., 2022; McDaniels & Fleming, 2018; Stoffelen et al., 2017) and for those who do receive education, it is unclear whether that content was adequate or accessible to each individual (Penwell Barnet & Maticka-Tyndale, 2015). Thus, it is unsurprising that research demonstrates limited knowledge of sexuality topics for youth with disabilities compared to those without disabilities (McDaniels & Fleming, 2018; Wiegierink et al., 2011). An exploratory study of the knowledge of personal safety skills among children with developmental disabilities demonstrated that children had difficulty distinguishing between appropriate and inappropriate touch and to whom to report concerns regarding inappropriate touch (Miller et al., 2017). The paucity of accessible sexual education available for children and young people with disabilities has also been identified as a concern in the transition stage from secondary education to adulthood (McDaniels & Fleming, 2018). Occupational therapy practitioners should advocate for the inclusion of sexual education in individualized education plans or health plans (Couwenhoven, 2007; D'Amico & Cahill, 2015).

## Sexual Activity

*Sexual activity* is a person's ability to engage in behaviors and actions such as hugging, kissing, foreplay, masturbation, oral sex, anal sex, vaginal sex, and using sexual devices, alone or with another person (Walker et al., 2020). People have the right to participate in desired sexual acts, accounting for consent and current laws regarding sexual activity, and to enjoy and feel satisfaction and pleasure from participating in sexual activity (Richardson, 2000). In addition, people have the right to bodily autonomy, control, and safety, including the right not to participate in sexual activity (Richardson, 2000).

Occupational therapy practitioners consider a young person's values, beliefs, and spirituality surrounding sexual activity to ensure that therapy is client centered. Several factors may affect a young person's participation in sexual activity. Young people with disabilities have sexual wants and needs but often face challenges in meeting their needs (Czapla & Otrebski, 2018; Sakellariou & Simo Algado, 2006; Vaughn et al., 2014; Wiegerink et al., 2011). Masturbation is an important topic for many young people, and young people with disabilities want masturbation to be easier (Morales et al., 2016b). Young people with disabilities often have their first partnered sexual experience later than their nondisabled peers (Czapla & Otrebski, 2018; Retznik et al., 2017). Young people may not participate in sexual activity because they fear their family or friends will not approve (Cella et al., 2010). Their religious or moral views also affect how and if they participate in sexual activity, including masturbation or sexual activity with a partner (Cella et al., 2010; Morales et al., 2016).

Additionally, certain conditions may cause increased fatigue and pain before, during, or after sexual activities that may impact participation (Mohammed, 2017; Wigerink et al., 2011). People with other developmental conditions that impact their physical abilities may experience issues with balance, positioning, spasticity, range of motion, and dexterity that are important in engaging in certain sexual activities (Wiegerink et al., 2011). For example, if someone has balance and core stability challenges, they may have increased challenges maintaining certain positions during sexual activities. Alternatively, suppose someone with a penis wants to put on a condom but lacks the dexterity and fine motor skills. In that case, this can impact their ability to independently participate in this task associated with intimacy and sexual activity. Lastly, people with physical disabilities may have specific questions about their abilities to safely participate in sexual activities and/or conceive (Manoj & Suja, 2017; Wiegerink et al., 2011).

## Sexual Interest

Occupational therapy practitioners must recognize that young people may be interested in sexual activity and must help them advocate for their sexual interests. **Sexual interest** is a person's physiological drive, motivation, or desire to participate in sexual activities (Walker et al., 2020). Often parents and school personnel may not take children and young people with developmental disabilities seriously when they express age-appropriate behaviors regarding sexuality, such as wanting to go on a date (Krantz et al., 2016).

## Sexual Response

**Sexual response** is the body's physical response associated with sexual activity (Walker et al., 2020). Sexual response may include arousal; erection of the nipples, clitoris, or penis; lubrication; ejaculation; or orgasm (Walker et al., 2020). Chronic illness and physical disabilities can disrupt sexual response, including negatively impacting libido, arousal, orgasm, or resolution (e.g., the process of returning to your normal vitals after engaging in sexual activities) (Hughes, 2000; Mohammed, 2017). In addition, medications may affect participation in sexual activities as medication may affect sexual drive or interest in sexual activities (Weinfurt et al., 2015). Occupational therapy practitioners should be aware of how different factors affect sexual response to discuss concerns with the family, child, and healthcare team.

## Sexual Self-View

A person's **sexual self-view** is how they perceive themselves as a sexual being and includes sexual identity, gender identity, sexual self-esteem, and body image (Walker et al., 2020). Often there is a denial of the existence of sexuality for children and young people with developmental disabilities, and they are often seen as not having a sexual identity by people within their lives (e.g., parents, caregivers, teachers, healthcare providers) and by society (Manor-Binyamini & Schreiber-Divon, 2019; Morales et al., 2016a; Sakellariou & Simo Algado, 2006; Sellwood et al., 2017; Vaughn et al., 2014; Wiegerink et al., 2011). As a result, young people with developmental disabilities may have their sexuality defined as abnormal, and it may be seen as deviant, instead of a typical part of development (Manor-Binyamini & Schreiber-Divon, 2019). How a young person's social environment, including doctors, partners, and society, views their disability may have both a positive and a negative effect on their self-esteem (Cella et al., 2010; Kattari, 2014; Morales et al., 2016b; Sakellariou & Simo Algado, 2006; Sellwood et al., 2017; Vaughn et al., 2014; Weinfurt et al., 2015). Some young people may view their disability as a part of their identity but may also feel defined by their disability when it comes to sexual activity (Kattari, 2014). Further, upper and lower limb differences, amputations, and other conditions that impact the physical configuration of one's body are associated with body image dissatisfaction, which in turn can negatively impact a person's satisfaction in relationships, sexual activities, and intimacy (Connell et al., 2014; Hawkins et al., 2009; Hughes, 2000; Mohammed, 2017). Despite the stigma surrounding young people with disabilities' sexual identity, many young people want to minimize others' perception of them as different and embrace their own sexual identity (Manor-Binyamini & Schreiber-Divon, 2019) (Fig. 19.1).

**Sexual Orientation.** Part of a young person's sexual identity includes their sexual orientation. **Sexual orientation** is a person's sexual and emotional attraction to another person (American Psychological Association, 2015). There are many sexual orientations that a person may identify with (see Box 19.1). One's sexual identity may foster a person's identity within the lesbian, gay, bisexual, transgender, queer, intersex, and asexual (LGBTQIA+) community (Bedard et al., 2010; Bernert et al., 2012; Richardson, 2000; Stadnyk et al., 2010; Walker, 2020; Walker et al., 2020). For young people that identify as LGBTQIA+, occupational therapy practitioners can provide education and support regarding self-advocacy skills, such as choosing to disclose their sexual orientation to others, such as friends, family, or teachers.

Often, young people with disabilities are more likely to be a part of the LGBTQIA+ community than the general population (Bernert et al., 2012; Kahn & Halpern, 2018; Lewis et al., 2021). While sexual identity can help to foster a person's sense of community, there are some challenges that people with disabilities face regarding their sexual identity. For example, people with disabilities may not feel visible within the LGBTQIA+ community. They may have the unique experience of having to "come out" twice (i.e., disclose their LGBTQIA+ identity as well as their disability identity) (Dewinter et al., 2020). Occupational therapy practitioners can assist young people in advocating for themselves both with their sexual identity and their disability identity.

**Gender Identity.** Gender identity is a separate concept from biologic sex. A person's biologic sex is based on sex chromosomes, internal reproductive organs, and external genitalia, including male, female, and intersex (American Psychological Association & National Association of School Psychologists, 2015). Gender is a social construct and can be separated into gender identity, social gender, and gender congruence (Gender Spectrum, 2019). **Gender identity** is how people define their gender based on who they are and an understanding of their sense of self (Gender Spectrum, 2019; Porta et al., 2020). Gender identities typically fall into the categories of binary, such as a man or a woman, nonbinary, those who have an identity that is not exclusively man or woman and may include terms such as ***genderqueer*** or ***genderfluid*** or ***ungendered***, and those that do not identify with a gender and may include terms such as ***agender*** and ***genderless*** (Gender Spectrum, 2019; Walsh et al., 2018). People whose gender identity is the same as their biologic sex assigned at birth are ***cisgender*** (Walsh et al., 2018). ***Transgender*** describes people whose gender identity is not the same as their sex assigned at birth (American Psychological Association, 2015). ***Social gender*** is how a person presents themselves to the world

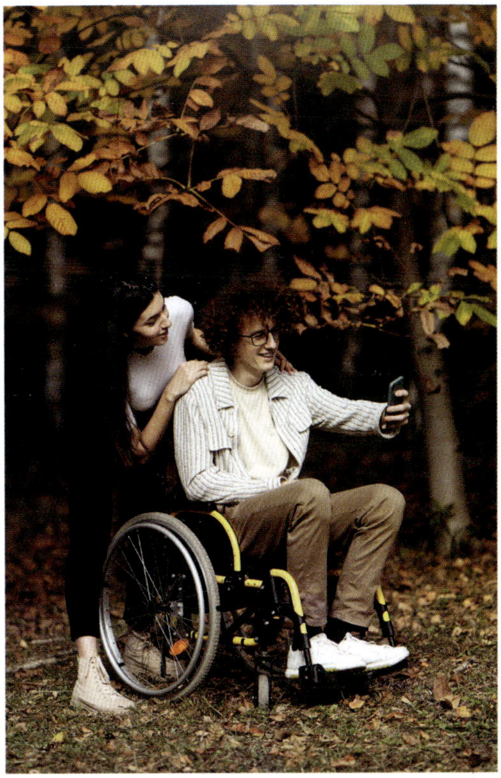

**Fig. 19.1** Young people may desire to establish intimate relationships and embrace their sexual identity. These teens spend time alone together to get to know each other better (Istock photo).

### BOX 19.1 Sexual Orientations

- Asexual: people who do not experience sexual attraction or have limited interest in sexual activity (American Psychological Association, 2015).
- Bisexual: people who are sexually attracted to more than one sex or gender (American Psychological Association, 2017).
- Gay: men who are sexually attracted to other men (American Psychological Association, 2015).
- Lesbian: women who are attracted to other women (American Psychological Association, 2015).
- Pansexual: attraction to a person regardless of their gender identity (American Psychological Association, 2022).
- Queer: an umbrella term used to describe a person's sexual orientation, gender identity, or gender expression that may not fit into societal norms. Queer has historically been used as a derogatory term; however, many people choose to use this term to describe their sexual identity. Many young people use the term queer to avoid gender binaries (American Psychological Association, 2015).
- Straight: people attracted to members of another gender (American Psychological Association, 2022).

(Gender Spectrum, 2019). A person may express their gender through various other occupations, such as dressing, grooming, hygiene, social participation, and play. Social gender is also influenced by how society, culture, and the community perceive and interact with gender concepts, such as gender roles and expectations (Gender Spectrum, 2019). ***Gender congruence*** is when a person feels a connection with their gender (Gender Spectrum, 2019). The connection with a person's gender may include feeling comfortable in one's own body; identifying one's gender based on whom they feel they are; expressing one's gender through clothing, interests, or activities; and being viewed by others as one sees themselves (Gender Spectrum, 2019).

When working with children and youth, it is essential to use inclusive language. American Occupational Therapy Association (AOTA) provides resources on diversity, equity, and inclusive language to use within the context of occupational therapy practice (AOTA, n.d.). Inclusive language can help develop and create the therapeutic relationship between occupational therapy practitioner and client by demonstrating respect for all people, and it is important to use inclusive language regarding a person's sexual self-view and all aspects of their identity.

## Sexual Expression

**Sexual expression** is how a person expresses themselves as a sexual being through behavior, mannerisms, preferences, appearance, pronouns, and daily routines, actions, and roles (Walker et al., 2020). Sexual expression may affect a variety of other occupations, including activities of daily living (ADLs) (dressing, toileting, bathing, dressing, and personal hygiene and grooming), instrumental activities of daily living (IADLs) (meal preparation, religious and spiritual expression, shopping, safety, and communication management), health management (copartners) (with health care system, medication management, physical activity, and personal care device management, which includes sexual devices), play/leisure, and social participation (community, family, friendships, peer groups, and initiate partners) (American Occupational Therapy Association, 2020). Occupational therapy practitioners must consider all occupations that may affect sexual expression to support children and young people to be their authentic selves.

Some children and young people who identify as transgender, genderqueer, agender, nonbinary, or gender diverse may seek to find congruence with their gender identity, a process known as ***transitioning*** (Gender Spectrum, 2019). Young people can transition in many ways, including social, hormonal, surgical, and legal (Gender Spectrum, 2019). Many aspects of transition include various occupations, which fall under the scope of practice for occupational therapy. During social transition, a person may change their social identifiers such as their clothing (dressing), hairstyle (grooming), and other aspects of their identity, including gender identity and pronouns (American Occupational Therapy Association, 2020; Gender Spectrum, 2019). With hormonal transition, people use medical approaches such as hormone therapy (medication management) to promote their physical, mental, and emotional alignment with their gender identity (American Occupational Therapy Association, 2020; Gender Spectrum, 2019). Surgical transition includes adding, removing, or modifying gender-related traits (Gender Spectrum, 2019). Recovery from surgical procedures may affect other occupations that occupational therapy practitioners may need to be involved in to enhance participation during the healing process. Youth may also benefit from a consultation with occupational therapy for wound management after surgical procedures. Finally, legal transition is changing a person's identification documents, such as their birth certificate, driver's license, or passport to reflect their gender identity (Gender Spectrum, 2019). Occupational therapy practitioners can use intervention methods related to self-advocacy to support young people during their legal transition.

## Intimacy

**Intimacy** relates to a person's ability to initiate and maintain close relationships and to give and receive affection (American Occupational Therapy Association, 2020; Walker et al., 2020). Children and young people encounter many types of relationships throughout their youth including family, friend, peer, professional, and intimate relationships (Bi et al., 2016; Soros & Reese, 2021). Family relationships include the interaction between the parent/caregiver and the child, between siblings, and relationships with other family members such as grandparents, aunts, uncles, and cousins (Bi et al., 2016; Soros & Reese, 2021). Friendships and peer relationships include relationships between all genders and platonic ones (Bi et al., 2016; Soros & Reese, 2021). Professional relationships include the relationships between teachers and students, the child or young person, and their healthcare provider (Soros & Reese, 2021). Children and young people who have high-quality interpersonal relationships have high overall levels of self-esteem (Bi et al., 2016).

People with attention, intellectual, or behavioral disabilities, among others, may have challenges with social and relational skills that impact their participation in sexual occupations, such as identifying potential partners, dating, establishing healthy boundaries, and maintaining intimate relationships (DiGioia, n.d.). Specifically, youth and young adults with language deficits, difficulties understanding social cues or nonverbal communication, or difficulty engaging in conversations may have fewer or reduced quality of relationships than desired (DiGioia, n.d.). Additionally, those with disabilities may have difficulty understanding subtle rules within social interactions, especially in intimate partnerships (Koller, 2000). However, people with disabilities express the same interests in social relationships, including intimate partnerships (Rushbrooke et al., 2014).

Children and young people need to be aware of the different types of relationships and what the social expectations may be within those relationships. For example, it may be acceptable to hug your family member, but it may not be acceptable to hug your teacher or healthcare provider (Fig. 19.2). Occupational therapy practitioners educate children and young people about the different types of relationships

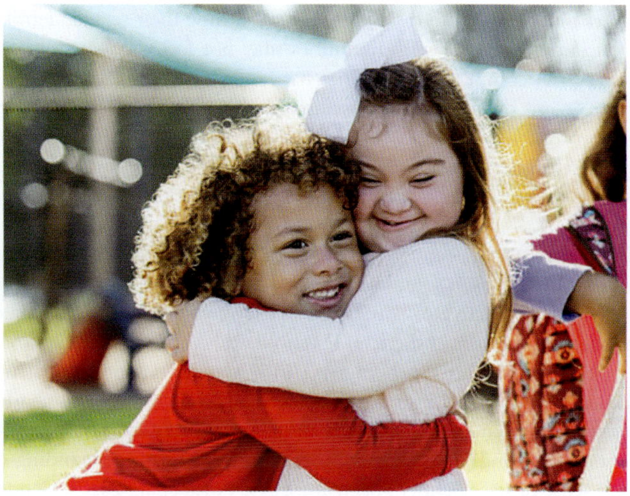

**Fig. 19.2** Young children may express themselves freely by hugging friends and family. They may need assistance learning to not hug strangers (Istock photo).

and model appropriate interactions during professional relationships. They also work with young people to develop the skills needed to engage in dating, including selecting a potential partner, asking someone out on a date, dealing with possible rejection, and maintaining intimate relationships.

## Sexual Health

Sexual health has been defined by the World Health Organization as "...a state of physical, emotional, mental and social well-being in relation to sexuality; it is not merely the absence of disease, dysfunction or infirmity. Sexual health requires a positive and respectful approach to sexuality and sexual relationships, as well as the possibility of having pleasurable and safe sexual experiences, free of coercion, discrimination and violence. For sexual health to be attained and maintained, the sexual rights of all persons must be respected, protected and fulfilled" (WHO, 2006). Included in sexual health is a person's ability to develop, manage, and maintain strategies and practices for safe sex, and the use of protection (Walker et al., 2020). Frequently parents and caregivers seek guidance from healthcare providers regarding their child or young person's sexual health related to menstruation, sexual behavior, and safety (Powell et al., 2020). Caregivers or parents need to be present when providing sexual health education (Powell et al., 2020). Including caregivers and parents during healthcare visits as part of patient and family-centered care has the potential to increase health care literacy regarding sexual health for children and young people. There are instances in which family members may be asked to leave the room during interventions to provide privacy related to sexual health topics. Occupational therapy practitioners use clinical judgment as to when to include caregivers and parents and when to provide interventions that respect the person's privacy.

As a part of typical development, infants and children rely on their parents or caregivers to manage their sexual health. However, as they get older and more independent, they may begin to assume more responsibility for their sexual health. To safely manage one's sexual health, they need access to comprehensive sexual health information. Comprehensive sexual education includes, at a minimum, anatomy and physiology, puberty and adolescent development, sexual self-view, pregnancy and reproduction, family planning, sexually transmitted infections, sexual health, healthy relationships, and personal safety (Schmidt, Brown, & Darragh, 2020; Koller, 2000) topics and should be culturally responsive and trauma informed (Campbell et al., 2020; Dewinter et al., 2020). Further, youth and young adults with various disabilities may need information specific to how their disability may impact their participation in intimate partnerships and sexual activities (Dewinter et al., 2020; Heller et al., 2016).

Menstruation management is an important activity of daily living for young people that have uteruses. Occupational therapy practitioners use their expertise in the area of activity analysis and contextual demands to support menstruation management and hygiene (Walker, 2020). For example, occupational therapy practitioners may help a young person with sensory sensitivities select the most comfortable menstrual product (e.g., disposable pads, reusable pads, tampons, menstrual cups, menstrual underwear, etc.) (see Fig. 19.3) based on their personal needs (Larson et al., 2021). Occupational therapy practitioners can also assist health management surrounding menstruation by developing methods to track a young person's menstrual cycle as well as developing strategies to manage medication related to a young person's menstrual cycle (Fig. 19.4). Strategies may include technology such as period tracking apps or written schedules to assist with menstruation management.

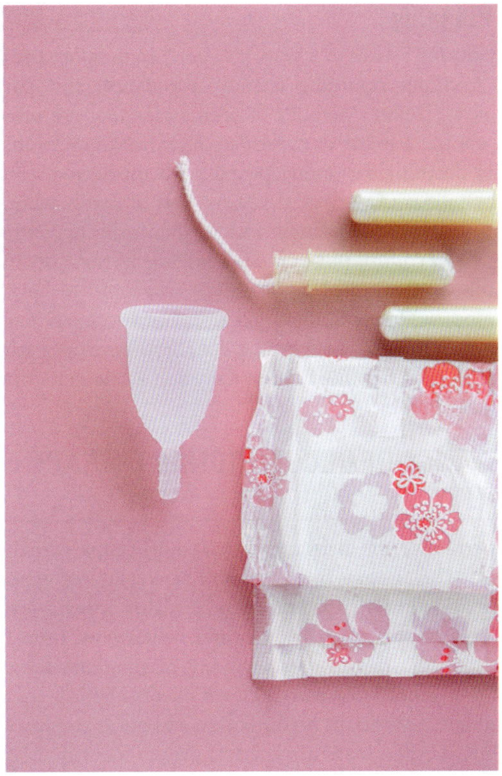

**Fig. 19.3** A variety of supplies are available for menstrual care, such as those illustrated in this picture. Occupational therapy practitioners may work with children and families to explain their options and provide some assistance.

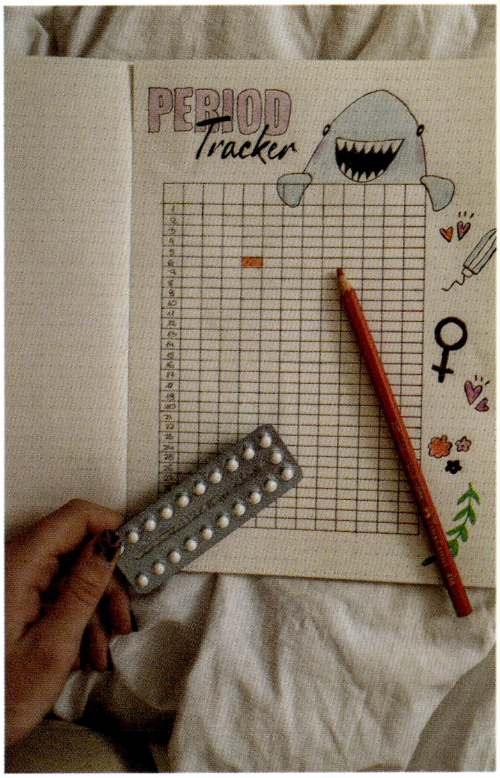


**Fig. 19.4** Occupational therapy practitioners often advise that children use schedules such as this one pictured to manage their medications related to their menstrual cycle.

### Family Planning

**Family planning** relates to a person's ability to develop, manage, and maintain routines regarding fertility, pregnancy, and parenthood (Walker et al., 2020). Methods of family planning are often a very personal choice. Parents or caregivers often make decisions regarding family planning for young people with intellectual or developmental disabilities (Powell et al., 2020). Part of family planning may include medication management with various forms of contraception, including birth control pills. Often family members assist in administering contraceptive medication to young people; to help increase independence with medication management, occupational therapy practitioners may work with young people to develop a schedule to remember to take their medication daily and at the same time of day (Roden et al., 2020).

## IMPORTANCE OF OCCUPATIONAL THERAPY FOR SEXUALITY

As described above, the societal view that young people with disabilities are not sexual beings puts them at risk of having limited opportunities for participation in varied aspects of the sexuality or sexual expression. Cultural concerns, personal values, and beliefs have been found to affect what healthcare providers, including occupational therapy practitioners, are comfortable working with clients about (e.g., difficulty navigating questions about masturbation and pornography) (Schmidt et al., 2021). Discrimination related to gender identity, LGBTQIA+, and ableism may limit occupational choices. In addition, many gender-based assumptions in society imply that certain occupations are more appropriate for specific genders, including sexual activity (Hammell, 2020). Often there are more opportunities, resources, and benefits for cis-gender and straight people (Hammell, 2020). Occupational therapy practitioners must advocate for their clients, including children and young people, and provide high-quality services regarding sexuality to promote equality and access to the full range of human occupation. They support children's identities by accepting, educating, and advocating that all children be included and treated fairly (see Fig.19.5).

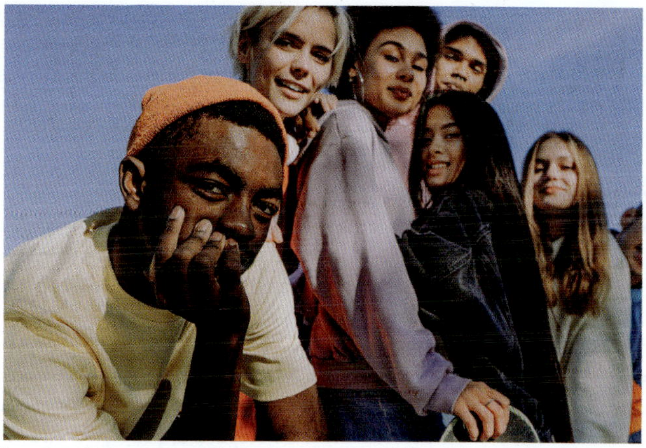

**Fig. 19.5** Children benefit from support from professionals, family, and friends as they develop their sexual identity and establish intimacy. This group of friends supports each other's identity (Istock photo).

## OCCUPATIONAL THERAPY INTERVENTIONS ADDRESSING SEXUALITY

Occupational therapy practitioners play a vital role in supporting youth by intervening to support clients' interdependence or independence in ADLs, which can impact their participation in occupations related to expression of sexuality. For example, occupational therapy practitioners address bowel and bladder management, which may include information about the importance of this management prior to engaging in sexual activities. Similarly, those addressing IADLs, such as meal preparation or financial management, can connect those skills to skills needed for dating (e.g., preparing a meal for a partner or budgeting for a date). Occupational therapy practitioners can also support their clients by advocating for and educating parents, caregivers, educators, and other healthcare providers. They also provide direct interventions, such as sexual education, social skills training, and through the promotion of sexual self-advocacy, adaptive equipment, or sensory interventions.

### Sexual Education

A variety of approaches have been identified as evidence-based interventions for providing sexual education to young people with disabilities, primarily surrounding the use of a Universal Design for Learning approach (Grove et al., 2018; Roden et al., 2020). Occupational therapy practitioners should individualize the content provided so

### CASE EXAMPLE 19.1 JALEN

Jalen is an 18-year-old teenager with intellectual disability, who is receiving services in a school-based setting for goals focused on vocational fit and training for his transition from secondary education. Specifically, Jalen's occupational therapy practitioner is working on career exploration, skill-building associated with specific careers that are identified as meaningful, time management, and social skill development.

Jalen demonstrates challenges with understanding different types of relationships (e.g., family, friend, teacher, peer) and healthy boundaries but is very interested in finding a girlfriend to ask to the senior prom. Jalen's parents are in support of him identifying a partner and having a date for prom, but they want to ensure he understands boundaries, consent, sexual health, and family planning first. Currently, Jalen does not have access to sexual education since it is only provided in the freshman regular education physical education classes at his school district. Jalen's occupational therapist understands how important and beneficial comprehensive sexual education is, so they educate administrators at the district who agree that the occupational therapist can provide school-based comprehensive sexual education within special education and use an opt-out approach for obtaining caregiver consent.

The occupational therapist partners with the health educator to provide accessible sexual health information, including a wide range of comprehensive sexual health topics, such as anatomy and physiology, puberty and development, sexually transmitted infections, family planning, sexual health management, sexual identity, and disability-specific information utilizing a culturally responsive and trauma-informed approach. After completing a sexual health information assessment with the class, they identify a need to define various sexual activities to aide in sexual self-advocacy and in understanding other sexual health topics. Therefore, the therapist tailors the program to include clear, concise definitions of sexual activities, including the use of other terms utilized commonly among peers or in media. The therapist also learns that many students want to learn more about relationships. The therapist and health educator team up to provide a "prom ready" after school group on relationships, respecting people's choices, and communication. They include information and fun games to illustrate concepts.

The therapist tailors the individual intervention plan within each session to meet Jalen's needs. They commonly utilize videos, visuals, and infographics to help him understand various sexual health-related topics. Additionally, the therapist uses videos, models and role-playing activities to facilitate Jalen's understanding, recognition, and ability to flirt or to ask someone on a date. The therapist shares the information with Jalen's parents.

that it is tailored to the needs of the person they are working with (McDaniels & Fleming, 2018; Schmidt, Robek, et al., 2020; Mackin et al., 2016; Roden et al., 2020; Krantz et al., 2016). See Case Example 19.1 Jalen.

There are a variety of evidence-based strategies that practitioners can utilize to support the understanding and retention of sexual health knowledge. They may provide concrete and specific examples using graphics, visuals, videos, social stories, and role-playing activities (Koller, 2000; Krantz et al., 2016; McDaniels & Fleming, 2018; Schaafsma et al., 2015; Schmidt, Brown, & Darragh, 2020; Schmidt, Robek, et al., 2020; Tarnai & Wolfe, 2008). Additionally, there is some evidence suggesting that technology may be a useful resource for youth when learning about sexuality topics, specifically ones that people can engage with the displays and allow for individualization of content (Mackin et al., 2016) or that utilize games (Persch et al., 2022; Gontijo et al., 2016).

Some occupational therapy practitioners may choose to organize and run sexual education courses for groups or classes of people with disabilities. This may be more common in school- or community-based settings. Occupational therapy practitioners who provide complete comprehensive sexual health education programs may develop their own or choose to use one of the few programs currently available on the market. The advisory group of the Sexual Health Equity for Individuals with Intellectual and Developmental Disabilities (SHEIDD) has reviewed seven curricula that offer a variety of educational materials to teach people with intellectual and developmental disabilities about sexual health topics. SHEIDD has reviewed the strengths and areas where these curricula could improve and published them for people considering utilizing a predeveloped program for youth with intellectual and developmental disabilities specifically (SHEIDD, n.d.). Similarly, the Massachusetts Department of Public Health and the Massachusetts Department of Developmental Services have developed and published a healthy relationship, sexuality, and disability resource guide that provides information about a variety of curricula available to support sexual education for people with disabilities (Massachusetts Department of Public Health, 2014). Respect Ability also has published a list of sexual education resources that include resources for parents and practitioners, as well as resources for comprehensive sexual education and other topics such as hygiene and self-care, masturbation, puberty and body changes, and exploitation that practitioners may review and consider utilizing resources from (Respect Ability, n.d.). Oak Hill provides an educational program for teenagers with intellectual disabilities related to safety and sexual health, called Positive Choices. This program is available online at https://relationshipandsexuality.oakhillct.org/positive-choices/.

## Caregiver Education

Occupational therapy practitioners can encourage caregivers to utilize open communication, humor, and natural opportunities to promote discussion about sexual health topics (e.g., television or movies that demonstrate healthy or unhealthy boundaries, consent, sexual activities, etc.) (Schmidt, Robek, et al., 2020) and educate them about how to respond to questions their child asks about sexual health topics. This includes reminding them not to jump to conclusions about what their child is asking, keeping responses brief, clear, and concise, and checking their child's understanding after they have answered (Planned Parenthood, n.d.). Parent support groups or education programs are often useful and necessary tools to support the accessibility of sexual education for youth with disabilities (Schmidt, Robek, et al., 2020). Occupational therapy practitioners may identify specific programs available for parents, share handouts with a summary of what they have been working on in their sessions with ideas

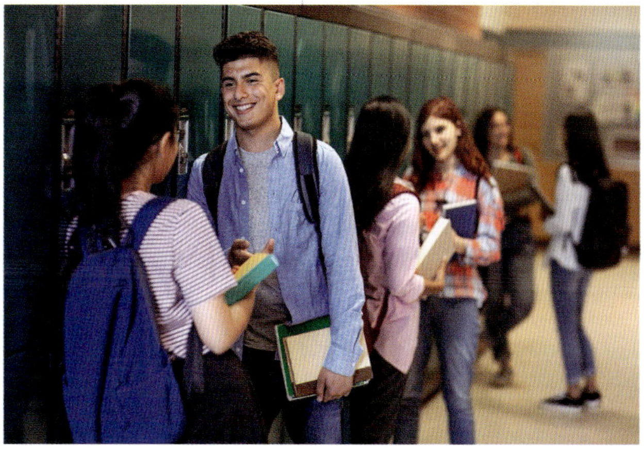

**Fig. 19.6** Youth may benefit from social skills training and support to establish their sexual identity and develop relationships with others. Training may include experiential "practice homework," such as observed as teens engage in conversations in the hallway. The training includes reflecting on the experience at the next session (Istock photo).

for parents to address those same skills at home to promote generalization, or suggest parent support groups (Schmidt, Robek, et al., 2020). There are freely available resources online that practitioners can utilize to help educate parents on the importance of addressing sexual health education with their youth with disabilities, including resources available in English and Spanish (Center for Parent Information and Resources, 2022).

## Social Skills Training

There are a variety of sexual education programs that include education on social skills specific to developing healthy and safe relationships, boundaries, and dating. For example, the "Boyfriends & Girlfriends: A Guide to Dating for People with Disabilities" (Couwenhoven, 2015) can guide teens and adults with intellectual and developmental disabilities on the "do's and don'ts" of dating. These programs utilize evidence-based strategies, such as videos, visuals, and role-playing, to generalize skills. For example, there is the Relationships Decoded curriculum that is freely available for practitioners to utilize with their clients and that offers a combination of education, videos, and visuals that support understanding boundaries, using assertive communication, understanding attraction, identifying sexual abuse, establishing healthy relationships, and handling emotions while dating (Relationships Decoded, 2020) (see Fig. 19.6). Additionally, practitioners may utilize social stories to model boundaries, respect others' boundaries, or even ask someone on a date (see Case Example 19.2 Samara). Practitioners can assist clients in understanding online safety and dating etiquette to create their online dating profiles and connect with potential partners safely. They may also provide videos on establishing boundaries or flirting with improving their safety and successful connection to partners (e.g., https://www.youtube.com/c/amazeorg/videos).

## Behavioral Interventions

Since some people with disabilities experience social and cognitive challenges, coupled with the limited accessibility of sexual health information, some people with disabilities may engage in sexual behaviors considered culturally inappropriate or illegal (e.g., public masturbation, stalking, touching without consent, etc.) (Stokes et al., 2007). Involvement in these behaviors can influence successful social participation in friendships and intimate relationships and present legal and safety concerns. Behavioral interventions are a common

## CASE EXAMPLE 19.2 SAMARA

Samara is a 14-year-old autistic girl who lives with her mother, grandmother, and three younger brothers. Samara has been receiving outpatient occupational therapy services related to her sensory processing, self-regulation, education, and self-help skills. Recently Samara's mother informed the occupational therapist that she has noticed that Samara has been masturbating more. She used to masturbate in her room, but recently she has begun to masturbate in the living room when watching TV with the rest of her family. Samara's mother is concerned about her masturbating in front of her brothers and is asking for help.

During the interview, the therapist asked Samara's mother for information about what time of day she is masturbating. Her mother stated that she primarily is masturbating in the evening before she gets ready for bed. Her mother also informed the therapist that she does not wash her hands after she is done masturbating. This is problematic when she is menstruating as Samara will get menstrual blood on the furniture, doors, and walls in the house. The therapist asked Samara's mother what she uses to clean herself after toileting. Samara's mother states that she uses a lota pot, a small vessel that is used to pour water over the genitals for cleansing and does not use toilet paper.

After gathering the information from Samara's mother, and using information from her previous occupational therapy evaluation, the therapist created a social story (see Fig. 19.8). Social stories are meant to describe situations and clarify social expectations (see https://vkc.vumc.org/assets/files/tipsheets/socialstoriestips.pdf for how to write a social story). This social story affirmed that masturbation was OK to do but explained that it was something to be done alone, without others watching, in her bedroom with the door closed. It was also important that the social story included information about cleaning up once done masturbating. The therapist made sure to include information about Samara's family's culture and use of the lota pot so that the social story was meaningful and individualized for Samara.

During the next occupational therapy session, the therapist had Samara write her name on the book, and they read the book together. The therapist asked Samara questions about the social story to check for clarification of the information. The therapist asked Samara "where in your house should you touch yourself?" Samara replied, "in my room." After evaluating and confirming that Samara understood the social story, the therapist instructed Samara to put her social story in a safe place in her room. The therapist also provided additional copies to the family, which could be used in other areas of the house.

The therapist followed up with the family a week later. Samara's mother stated that she has seen a reduction in Samara's masturbation in the common areas within the house. During times when she does attempt to masturbate in the common areas, Samara's mother handed her a copy of the social story to read, without bringing attention to her masturbation in front of her brothers. Samara would read the social story to herself and would then go into her bedroom, close the door, and finish masturbating, away from the rest of the family. Samara told the therapist that she likes her social story. Samara's mother was very happy with the outcome of the social story and told the therapist that Samara was independently cleaning up when she finished masturbating as well. The therapist continued to monitor Samara's masturbation and to adapt or modify the social story as needed until Samara mastered her goal.

evidence-based approach for eliminating or reducing these behaviors (Davis et al., 2016; McLay et al., 2015; Schaafsma et al., 2015; Schmidt, Brown, & Darragh, 2020). However, behavioral interventions have also been identified as a maladaptive approach to socialize people with disabilities to fit into an ableist society instead of celebrating differences between people (Gardner, 2017). Therefore, occupational therapy practitioners should utilize behavioral interventions only when focused on meaningful occupations for the client and to support their safety or the safety of others. See Chapter 25 for more information on behavioral approaches.

### Sexual Self-Advocacy

Self-advocacy and self-determination skills are critical for children and young people with disabilities so that they are able to use assertive communication, ask for what they need or want, establish healthy boundaries, and ask for help or report concerns that arise (Krantz et al., 2016). Sexual self-advocacy includes understanding one's choices, speaking up, and getting information, healthy relationships, and respect (Friedman et al., 2014). Access to sexual health information is critical as is a good understanding of sexual health information, including laws surrounding consent (Friedman et al., 2014).

Practitioners providing sexual education may focus on developing self-advocacy and self-determination skills related to sexual health information and topics, for example encouraging people to take charge of their reproductive healthcare, asking questions and making interdependent decisions as necessary, or empowering them to establish boundaries within relationships. Additionally, self-advocacy and self-determination skills are useful for promoting positive social participation and meaningful engagement with the client. In instances where we are not concerned about their safety or the safety of others (therefore, warranting a behavioral approach to eliminate or prevent certain inappropriate sexual behaviors), occupational therapy practitioners can educate people with a variety of disabilities about the unique attributes they bring to a relationship and help empower them to meet and date intimate partners confidently.

The inclusion of educational resources for clients from other people with disabilities may also help promote self-advocacy skills. For example, Vilissa Thompson's article "Take Me As I Am: Dating and Disability Etiquette" includes recommendations to embrace yourself as you are, embrace your disability, and not try to change to conform to others' expectations when trying to meet partners (Thompson, n.d.). Further, there is evidence suggesting that the inclusion of peer educators for sexual education or other interventions to support participation in sexual occupations is effective in empowering clients (Campbell et al., 2020; Frawley & O'Shea, 2019; Rothman et al., 2022).

### Adaptive Equipment

Occupational therapy practitioners may include adapted equipment to facilitate participation in sexual activities with and without partners. This may still be appropriate for practitioners working with children and young people with disabilities in pediatric settings depending on the individual's age, their guardianship status, their caregiver's consent or agreement to provide education on adapted equipment, and/or the specific state, facility, organization, and/or institution. Occupational therapy practitioners utilize their clinical reasoning skills and elicit appropriate consent before providing direct interventions to promote participation in sexual activities for youth. Occupational therapy practitioners who have appropriate permissions and are focused on adapted equipment education for youth consider the physical limitations of the individual, the occupational performance deficits impacting their participation in the specific sexual occupation, and various adapted equipment, sex toys, or devices that may help that individual participate in the identified meaningful sexual occupation. Practitioners should employ culturally responsive recommendations and take care not to assume one's sexual identity or how someone may want to participate in sexual activities by taking the time to ask questions and

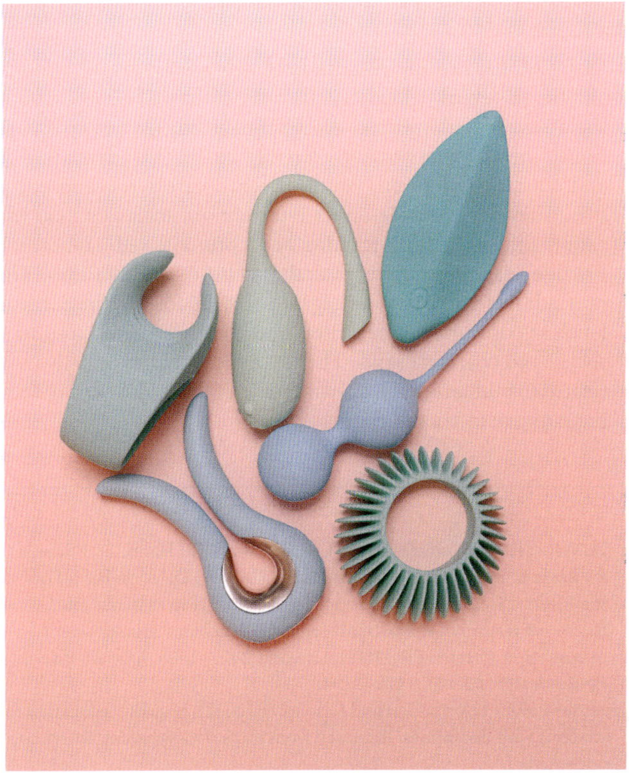

**Fig. 19.7** Occupational therapy practitioners may suggest adapted equipment or sex toys/devices, such as vibrators pictured here, to support client's engagement in partnered activities.

understand what the activity looks like for the individual. A variety of adapted equipment or sex toys/devices available on the market are suggested for people with physical disabilities engaging in partnered activities, such as slings, cushions, strap-ons, rings, and many others (Sportsheets, n.d.). For example, vibrators come in various shapes and sizes (see Fig. 19.7). Occupational therapy practitioners can use activity analysis skills to determine the best vibrator to promote independence with sexual activity. Additionally, practitioners may suggest various positions to facilitate participation in these meaningful occupations.

## Sensory Interventions

Youth with disabilities are more likely to experience sensory differences or dysregulation that impact their sexual occupations, such as engagement in intimate relationships and/or sexual activities alone and with partners. These sensory differences are often due to a mismatch between one's personal sensory needs and social context (Penwell Barnett & Maticka-Tyndale, 2015). Autistic people, in particular, have identified challenges with sensory overload in dating scenarios or negative sensory experiences associated with sexual activities (Penwell Barnett & Maticka-Tyndale, 2015). These experiences are reported to be emotionally upsetting and/or physically painful for people, in addition to negatively impacting their participation in sexual occupations (Penwell Barnett & Maticka-Tyndale, 2015). Occupational therapy practitioners can utilize their knowledge of assessment and intervention to address sensory differences that are impacting one's participation in meaningful occupations, including sexual activity (see Chapters 27 and 28).

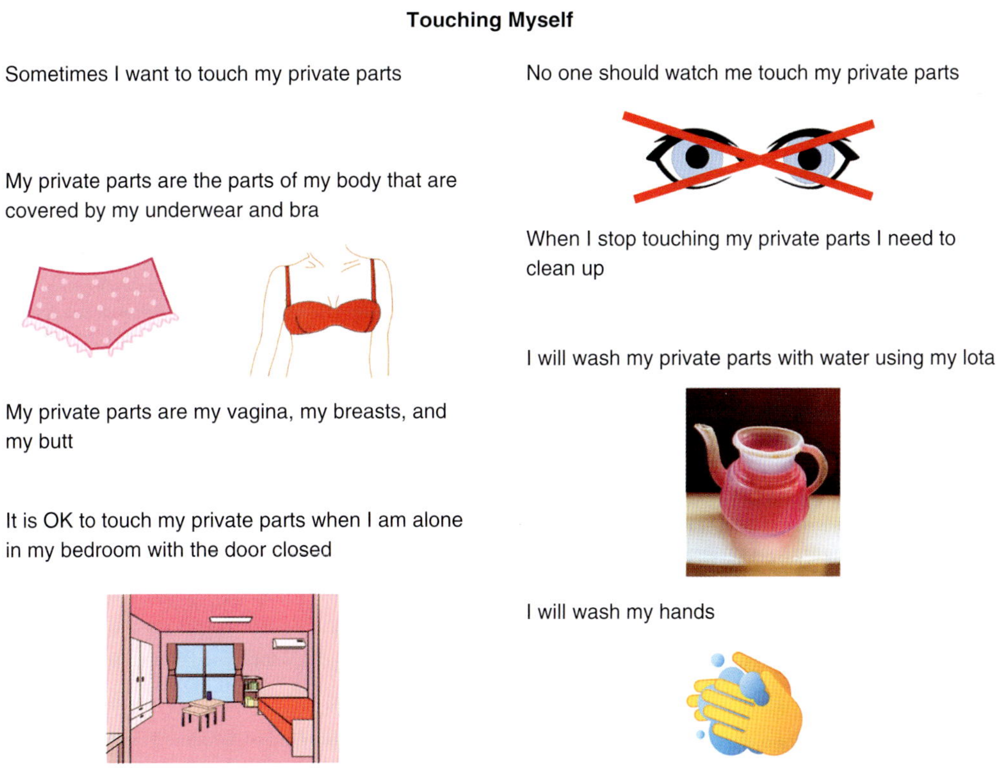


**Fig. 19.8** Practitioners may help children develop skills by using social stories, such as this one pictured.

## SUMMARY

Human sexuality is a normal part of life for our clients, no matter their disability, and access to the range of behaviors and activities that provide expression of sexuality is within the scope of occupational therapy. Occupational therapy practitioners should therefore advocate for and provide culturally responsive and trauma-informed interventions to support engagement and expression of sexuality for their clients with disabilities.

1. The OTSAF includes the following constructs: sexual activity, sexual interest, sexual response, sexual self-view, sexual expression, intimacy, sexual health, and family planning (Walker et al., 2020).
2. Occupational therapy practitioners can provide direct intervention individually and within groups using sexual education, caregiver education, social skills training, behavioral strategies, sensory strategies, and/or adaptive equipment.
3. Occupational therapy practitioners view young people with disabilities as sexual beings that are entitled to make choices about their sexual and intimate occupational engagement. Occupational therapy practitioners support clients by advocating for and educating children, youth, parents, caregivers, and educators. They may provide direct intervention, such as sexual education and social skills training or to promote self-advocacy, or provide adaptive equipment and/or sensory interventions. They may address barriers to engagement by addressing motor skills (such as positioning, fine motor, or endurance), communication, social, and cognitive skills. They support activities of daily living related to human sexuality such as when following health routines regarding menstruation.

## REFERENCES


American Occupational Therapy Association. (2020). Occupational therapy practice framework: Domain and process-fourth edition. *American Journal of Occupational Therapy*, *74*(Suppl. l._2). https://doi.org/10.5014/ajot.2020.74S2001.

American Psychological Association and National Association of School Psychologists. (2015). Resolution on gender and sexual orientation diversity in children and adolescents in schools. http://www.apa.org/about/policy/orientation-diversity.aspx.

American Psychological Association. (2015). Key terms and concepts in understanding gender diversity and sexual orientation among students: Informational guide. https://www.apa.org/pi/lgbt/programs/safe-supportive/lgbt/key-terms.pdf.

American Psychological Association. (2022). Sexual orientation. https://apastyle.apa.org/style-grammar-guidelines/bias-free-language/sexual-orientation#:~:text=Terms%20for%20sexual%20orientation&text=However%2C%20someone%20who%20identifies%20as,or%20delineated%20by%20gender%20identity.

American Psychological Association. (2017). Understanding bisexuality. https://www.apa.org/pi/lgbt/resources/bisexual#:~:text=The%20term%20%E2%80%9Cbisexual%E2%80%9D%20is%20used,than%20one%20sex%20or%20gender.

American Occupational Therapy Association. DEI word bank. https://www.aota.org/practice/practice-essentials/dei/dei-toolkit-word-bank.

Amjadi, M. A., Simbar, M., Hosseini, S. A., & Zayeri, F. (2017). The sexual health needs of women with spinal cord injury: A qualitative study. *Sexuality and Disability*, *35*(3), 313–330. https://doi.org/10.1007/s11195-017-9495-7.

Barnard-Brak, L., Schmidt, M., Chesnut, S., Wei, T., & Richman, D. (2014). Predictors of access to sex education for children with intellectual disabilities in public schools. *Intellectual and Developmental Disabilities*, *52*(2), 85–97. https://doi.org/10.1352/1934-9556-52.2.85.

Bedard, C., Zhang, H., & Zucker, K. J. (2010). Gender identity and sexual orientation in people with developmental disabilities. *Sexuality and Disability*, *28*(3), 165–175. https://doi.org/10.1007/s11195-010-9155-7.

Bernert, D. J., Ding, K., & Hoban, M. T. (2012). Sexual and substance use behaviors of college students with disabilities. *American Journal of Health Behavior*, *36*(4), 459–471. https://doi.org/10.5993/AJHB.36.4.3.

Bi, Y., Ma, L., Yuan, F., & Zhang, B. (2016). Self-esteem, perceived stress, and gender during adolescence: Interactive links to different types of interpersonal relationships. *Journal of Psychology*, *150*(1), 36–57. https://doi.org/10.1080/00223980.2014.996512.

Campbell, M., Löfgren-Mårtenson, C., & Martino, A. S. (2020). Cripping sex education. *Sex Education*, *20*(4), 361–365. https://doi.org/10.1080/14681811.2020.1749470.

Cella, D., Riley, W., Stone, A., Rothrock, N., Reeve, B., Yount, S., Amtmann, D., Bode, R., Buysse, D. J., Choi, S. W., Cook, K. F., DeVellis, R., DeWalt, D., Fries, J. F., Gershon, R., Hahn, E., Pilkonis, P., Revicki, D., Rose, M., Weinfurt, K., Hays, R. D., & on behalf of the PROMIS Cooperative Group. (2010). Initial item banks and first wave testing of the patient–reported outcomes measurement information system (PROMIS) network: 2005–2008. *Journal of Clinical Epidemiology*, *63*(11), 1179–1194.

Center for Parent Information and Resources. (2022). Sexuality education for students with disabilities. Retrieved from https://www.parentcenterhub.org/sexed/.

Connell, K. M., Coates, R., & Wood, F. M. (2014). Sexuality following trauma injury: A literature review. *Burns & Trauma*, *2*. https://doi.org/10.4103/2321-3868.130189. 20020061.

Couwenhoven, T. (2007). *Teaching children with Down syndrome about their bodies, boundaries, and sexuality*. Woodbine House.

Couwenhoven, T. (2015). *Boyfriends & girlfriends: A guide to dating for people with disabilities*. Woodbine House.

Czapla, K., & Otrebski, W. (2018). Differences in sexual behavior of teenagers and young adults with cerebral palsy: The role of sexual needs and sexual esteem. *Sexuality and Disability*, *36*(1), 33–46. https://doi.org/10.1007/s11195-017-9512-x.

D'Amico, M., & Cahill, S. M. (2015). Addressing sexuality with individuals with developmental disabilities and their families across the lifespan. *Special Interest Section Quarterly*, *38*(1), 1093–7196.

Davis, T. N., Machalicek, W., Scalzo, R., Kobylecky, A., Campbell, V., Pinkelman, S., Chan, J. M., & Sigafoos, J. (2016). A review and treatment selection model for individuals with developmental disabilities who engage in inappropriate sexual behavior. *Behavior Analysis in Practice*, *9*, 389–402. https://doi.org/10.1007/s40617-015-0062-3.

Dewinter, J., van der Miesen, A. I. R., & Graham Holmes, L. (2020). INSAR special interest group report: Stakeholder perspectives on priorities for future research on autism, sexuality, and intimate relationships. *Autism Research*, *00*, 1–10. https://doi.org/10.1002/aur.2340.

DiGioia, M.K. Taking a special education approach. Retrieved from https://www.uua.org/files/pdf/o/owl_specialed.pdf.

Frawley, P., & O'Shea, A. (2019). "Nothing about us without us": Sex education by and for people with intellectual disability in Australia. *Sex Education*. https://doi.org/10.1080/14681811.2019.1668759.

Friedman, C., Arnold, C. K., Owen, A. L., & Sandman, L. (2014). "Remember our voices are our tools": Sexual self-advocacy as defined by people with intellectual and developmental disabilities. *Sexuality and Disability*, *32*, 515–532. https://doi.org/10.1007/s11195-014-9377-1.

Gagnon, J. H., & Simon, W. (2011). *Sexual conduct: The social sources of human sexuality* (2nd ed.). Aldine Transaction.

Gardner, F. (2017). First-hand perspectives on behavioral interventions for autistic people and people with other developmental disabilities. https://autisticadvocacy.org/wp-content/uploads/2017/05/Behavioral-Interventions-Report-Final.pdf.

Gender Spectrum. (2019). Understanding gender. https://genderspectrum.org/articles/understanding-gender.

Gontijo, D. T., de Sena e Vasconcelos, A. C., Monteiro, R. J. S., Facundes, V. L. D., de Fátima Cordeiro Trajano, M., & de Lima, L. S. (2016). Occupational therapy and sexual and reproductive health promotion in adolescence: A case study. *Occupational Therapy International*, *23*(1), 19–28

Grove, L., Morrison-Beedy, D., & Kirby, R. (2018). The birds, bees, and special needs:Making evidence-based sex education accessible for adolescents with intellectual disability. *Sexuality and Disability*, *36*, 313–329. https://doi.org/10.1007/s11195-018-9547-7.

Hammell, K. W. (December 2020). Making choices from the choices we have: The contextual embeddedness of occupational choice. *Canadian Journal of Occupational Therapy*, *87*(5), 400–411. https://doi.org/10.1177/0008417420965741.

Hawkins, Y., Ussher, J., Gilbert, E., Perz, J., Sandoval, M., & Sundquist, K. (2009). Changes in sexuality and intimacy after the diagnosis and treatment of cancer: The experience of partners in a sexual relationship with a person with cancer. *Cancer Nursing*, *32*, 271–280.

Heller, M., et al. (2016). Sexuality and relationships in young people with spina bifida and their partners. *Journal of Adolescent Health*, *59*, 182–188. https://doi.org/10.1016/j.jadhhealth.2016.03.037.

Holmes, L. G., Rast, J. E., Roux, A. M., & Rothman, E. (2022). Reproductive health and substance use education for autistic youth. *Pediatrics*, *149*(s4) e20200493437T.

Hughes, M. (2000). Sexuality and the cancer survivor: A silent coexistence. *Cancer Nursing*, *23*(6), 477–482.

Kahn, N. F., & Halpern, C. T. (2018). Experiences of vaginal, oral, and anal sex from adolescence to early adulthood in populations with physical disabilities. *Journal of Adolescent Health*, *62*(3), 294–302. https://doi.org/10.1016/j.jadohealth.2017.08.003.

Kattari, S. K. (2014). Sexual experiences of adults with physical disabilities: Negotiating with sexual partners. *Sexuality and Disability*, *32*(4), 499–513. https://doi.org/10.1007/s11195014-9379-2.

Koller, R. (2000). Sexuality and adolescents with autism. *Sexuality and Disability*, *18*(2), 125–135.

Krantz, G., Tolan, V., Pontarelli, K., & Cahill, S. M. (2016). What do adolescents with developmental disabilities learn about sexuality and dating? A potential role for occupational therapy. *The Open Journal of Occupational Therapy*, *4*(2). https://doi.org/10.15453/2168-6408.1208.

Larson, S. K., Nielsen, S., Hemberger, K., & Klug, M. G. (2021). Addressing puberty challenges for adolescents with autism spectrum disorder: A survey of occupational therapy practice trends. *American Journal of Occupational Therapy*, *75*. https://doi.org/10.5014/ajot.2021.040105.7503180020.

Lewis, L. F., Ward, C., Jarvis, N., & Cawley, E. (2021). Straight sex is complicated enough!": The lived experiences of autistics who are gay, lesbian, bisexual, asexual, or other sexual orientations. *Journal of Autism and Developmental Disorders*, *51*(7), 2324–2337. https://doi.org/10.1007/s10803-020-04696-w.

Mackin, M. L., Loew, N., Gonzalez, A., Tykol, H., & Christensen, T. (2016). Parent perceptions of sexual education needs for their children with autism. *Journal of Pediatric Nursing*, *31*(6), 608–618.

Manoj, M. P., & Suja, M. K. (2017). Sexuality and reproductive health in young people with disability: A systematic review of issues and challenges. *Sexuality and Disability*, *35*, 507–516. https://doi.org/10.1007/s11195-017-9505-9.

Manor-Binyamini, I., & Schreiber-Divon, M. (2019). Parental perceptions of the sexuality of adolescents with intellectual disabilities. In *Sexuality and Disability*. https://doi.org/10.1007/s11195-019-09586-3..

Massachusetts Department of Public Health and Bureau of Community Health and Prevention. (2014). Healthy relationships, sexuality and disability: Resource guide 2014 edition. Retrieved from https://www.mass.gov/doc/healthy-relationships-sexuality-and-disability-resource-guide-0/download.

Mc Grath, M., & Sakellariou, D. (2016). Why has so little progress been made in the practice of occupational therapy in relation to sexuality? *American Journal of Occupational Therapy*, *70*(1). https://doi.org/10.5014/ajot.2016.017707. 7001360010pp.7001360011–7001360015.

McDaniels, B. W., & Fleming, A. R. (2018). Sexual health education: A missing piece in transition services for youth with intellectual and developmental disabilities? *Journal of Rehabilitation*, *84*(3), 28–38.

McLay, L., Carnett, A., Tyler-Merrick, G., & vans er Meer, L. (2015). A systematic review of interventions for inappropriate sexual behavior of children and adolescents with developmental disabilities. *Journal of Autism and Developmental Disorders*, *2*, 357–373. https://doi.org/10.1007/s40489-015-0058-5.

Miller, H. L., Pavlik, K. M., Kim, M. A., & Rogers, K. C. (2017). An exploratory study of the knowledge of personal safety skills among children with developmental disabilities and their parents. *Journal of Applied Research in Intellectual Disabilities*, *30*(2), 290–300. https://doi.org/10.1111/jar.12239.

Mohammed, A. (2017). Addressing sexuality in occupational therapy. *OT Practice*, *22*(9).

Morales, E., Gauthier, V., Edwards, G., & Courtois, F. (2016a). Masturbation practices of men and women with upper limb motor disabilities. *Sexuality and Disability*, *34*(4), 417–431. https://doi.org/10.1007/s11195-016-9445-9.

Morales, E., Gauthier, V., Edwards, G., & Courtois, F. (2016b). Women with disabilities' perceptions of sexuality, sexual abuse and masturbation. *Sexuality and Disability*, *34*(3), 303–314. https://doi.org/10.1007/s11195-016-9440-1.

Penwell Barnett, J., & Maticka-Tyndale, E. (2015). Qualitative exploration of sexual experiences among adults on the autism spectrum: Implications for sex education. *Perspectives on Sexual and Reproductive Health*, *47*(4), 171–179. https://doi.org/10.1363/47e5715.

Persch, A., Parsons, C., Anderson, S., & Schmidt, E. (2022). Transition technologies that support employment, community mobility, and interpersonal skills in autism and intellectual disabilities. *SIS Quarterly Practice Connections*, *7*(3).

Planned Parenthood, (n.d.). Tips for Talking: When should I start talking with my kid about sex and relationships? Retrieved from https://www.plannedparenthood.org/learn/parents/tips-talking.

Porta, C. M., Gower, A. L., Brown, C., Wood, B., & Eisenberg, M. E. (2020) Perceptions of sexual orientation and gender identity minority adolescents about labels. *Western Journal of Nursing Research*, *42*(2), 81–89. https://doi.org/10.1177/0193945919838618.

Powell, R. M., Parish, S. L., Mitra, M., & Rosenthal, E. (2020). Role of family caregivers regarding sexual and reproductive health for women and girls with intellectual disability: A scoping review. *Journal of Intellectual Disability Research*, *64*(2), 131–157. https://doi.org/10.1111/jir.12706.

Relationships Decoded. (2020). Relationships decoded: Social-sexual education for people with developmental disabilities. Retrieved from https://relationshipsdecoded.com/.

Respect Ability: Fighting stigmas, advancing opportunities. Sexual education resources. Retrieved from https://www.respectability.org/resources/sexual-education-resources/.

Retznik, L., Wienholz, S., Seidel, A., Pantenburg, B., Conrad, I., Michel, M., & Riedel-Heller, S. G. (2017). Relationship status: Single? Young adults with visual, hearing, or physical disability and their experiences with partnership and sexuality. *Sexuality and Disability*, *35*(4), 415–432. https://doi.org/10.1007/s11195-017-9497-5.

Richardson, D. (2000). Constructing sexual citizenship: Theorizing sexual rights. *Critical Social Policy*, *20*(1), 105–135.

Roden, R. C., Schmidt, E. K., & Holland-Hall, C. (2020). Sexual health education for adolescents and young adults with intellectual and developmental disabilities: Recommendations for accessible sexual and reproductive health information. *The Lancet*, *4*, 699–708.

Rothman, E. F., et al. (2022). Healthy relationships on the autism spectrum (hearts): A feasibility test of an online class co-designed and co-taught with autistic people. *Autism*, *26*(3), 690–702. https://doi.org/10.1177/13623613211069421.

Rushbrooke, E., Murray, C., & Townsend, S. (2014). The experiences of intimate relationships by people with intellectual disabilities: A qualitative study. *Journal of Applied Research in Intellectual Disabilities*, *27*, 531–541.

Sakellariou, D., & Simo Algado, S. (2006). Sex and disability: A case of occupational injustice. *British Journal of Occupational Therapy*, *69*(2), 69–76.

Schaafsma, D., Kok, G., Stoffelen, J. M. T., & Curfs, L. M. G. (2015). Identifying effective methods for teaching sex education to individuals with intellectual disabilities: A systematic review. *The Journal of Sex Research, 52*(4), 412–432.

Schmidt, E. K., Beining, A., Hand, B. N., Havercamp, S., & Darragh, A. (2021). Healthcare providers' role in providing sexual and reproductive health information to people with intellectual and developmental disabilities: A qualitative study. *Journal of Applied Research in Intellectual Disabilities*, 1–9.

Schmidt, E. K., Brown, C., & Darragh, A. (2020). Scoping review of sexual health educaiton interventions for adolescents and young adults with intellectual or developmental disabilities. *Sexuality and Disability, 38*, 439–453. https://doi.org/10.1007/s11195-019-09593-4.

Schmidt, E. K., Robek, N., Dougherty, M., Hand, B. N., Havercamp, S., Sommerich, C., Weaver, L., & Darrah, A. (2020). Recommendations to improve accessibility of sexuality education for individuals with intellectual or developmental disabilities: A qualitative study. *American Journal of Sexuality Education*. https://doi.org/10.1080/15546128.2020.1860177.

Sellwood, D., Raghavendra, P., & Jewell, P. (2017). Sexuality and intimacy for people with congenital physical and communication disabilities: Barriers and facilitators: A systematic review. *Sexuality and Disability, 35*(2), 227–244. https://doi.org/10.1007/s11195-017-9474-z.

Sexual Health Equity for Individuals with Intellectual/Developmental Disabilities, Multnomah County. (n.d.). SHEIDD* Review of sexual health education curricula designed for people with disabilities. Retrieved from https://www.ohsu.edu/sites/default/files/2019-08/Review%20of%20Sexual%20Health%20Education%20Curricula%20Designed%20for%20People%20with%20Disabilities%208.2019.pdf.

Soros, J., & Reese, K. (2021). Developing healthy relationships in youth: What is occupational therapy's role? *OT Now, 23*(2), 18–21.

Sportsheets (n.d.). Best sex toys and sexual positioning devices for people with disabilities. Retrieved from https://www.sportsheets.com/pages/best-sex-toys-sexual-positioning-devices-people-with-disabilities-slp.

Stadnyk, R., Townsend, E., & Wilcock, A. (2010). Occupational justice. In C. H. Christiansen, & E. A. Townsend (Eds.), *Introduction to occupation: The art and science of living* (2nd ed.) (pp. 329–358). Pearson Education.

Stoffelen, J. M. T., Herps, M. A., Buntinx, W. H. E., Schaafsma, D., Kok, G., & Curfs, L. M. G. (2017). Sexuality and individual support plans for people with intellectual disabilities. *Journal of Intellectual Disability Research, 61*(12), 1117–1129.

Stokes, M., Newton, N., & Kaur, A. (2007). Stalking, and social and romantic functioning among adolescents and adults with autism spectrum disorder. *Journal of Autism and Developmental Disorders, 37*, 1969–1980.

Tarnai, B., & Wolfe, P. S. (2008). Social Stories for sexuality education for persons with autism/pervasive developmental disorder. *Sexuality and Disability, 26*, 29–36. https://doi.org/10.1007/s11195-007-9067-3.

Thompson, V.K.. Take me as I am: Dating and disability etiquette. Retrieved from https://www.easterseals.com/thrive/take-me-as-i-am-disability.html.

UNESCO, United Nations Children's Fund. (2021). Joint united nations programme on HIV/AIDS, united nations population fund, world health organization, & united nations entity for gender equality and the empowerment of women. In *The journey towards comprehensive sexuality education: Global status report*.

Vaughn, M., Silver, K., Murphy, S., Ashbaugh, R., & Hoffman, A. (2014). Women with disabilities discuss sexuality in San Francisco focus groups. *Sexuality and Disability, 33*(1), 19–46. https://doi.org/10.1007/s11195-014-9389-x.

Vintor, S., & Ribner, D. (2021). Sexual scripts for individuals with intellectual/developmental disabilities. *Journal of Education & Social Policy, 8*(2), 70–79.

Walker, B. A. (2020). *Occupational performance inventory of sexuality and intimacy*. University of Indianapolis. https://uindy.edu/health-sciences/ot/opisi.

Walker, B. A., Otte, K., LeMond, K., Hess, P., & Kaizer, K. (2020). Development of the occupational performance inventory of sexuality and intimacy (OPISI): Phase one. *The Open Journal of Occupational Therapy, 8*(2), 1–18. https://doi.org/10.15453/2168-6408.1694.

Walsh, R. J., Krabbendam, L., Dewinter, J., & Begeer, S. (2018). Brief report: Gender identity differences in autistic adults: Associations with perceptual and socio-cognitive profiles. *Journal of Autism and Developmental Disorders, 48*(12), 4070–4078. https://doi.org/10.1007/s10803-018-3702-y.

Weinfurt, K. P., Lin, L., Bruner, D. W., Cyranowski, J. M., Dombeck, C. B., Hahn, E. A., Jeffery, D. D., Luecht, R. M., Magasi, S., Porter, L. S., Reese, J. B., Reeve, B. B., Shelby, R. A., Smith, A. W., Willse, J. T., & Flynn, K. E. (September 2015). Development and initial validation of the PROMIS((R)) sexual function and satisfaction measures version 2.0. *The Journal of Sexual Medicine, 12*(9), 1961–1974. https://doi.org/10.1111/jsm.12966.

WHO. (2006). *Defining sexual health: Report of a technical consultation on sexual health, 28–31 January 2002*. Geneva. Available from: https://www3.paho.org/hq/dmdocuments/2009/defining_sexual_health.pdf.

Wiegerink, D., Roebroeck, M., Bender, J., Stam, H., Cohen-Kettenis, P., & Transition Research Group South West, N. (2011). Sexuality of young adults with cerebral palsy: Experienced limitations and needs. *Sexuality and Disability, 29*(2), 119–128. https://doi.org/10.1007/s11195-010-9180-6.

Wiegerink, D. J., Stam, H. J., Gorter, J. W., Cohen-Kettenis, P. T., Roebroeck, M. E., & Netherlands, T. R. G. S. (2010). Development of romantic relationships and sexual activity in young adults with cerebral palsy: A longitudinal study. *Archives of Physical Medicine and Rehabilitation, 91*(9), 1423–1428.

Wilcock, A., & Hocking, C. (2015). *An occupational perspective of health* (3rd ed.). Slack Incorporated.

World Federation of Occupational Therapists. (2019). *Occupational therapy and human rights*.

20

# Driving and Community Mobility

*Melissa Missy Bell*

## GUIDING QUESTIONS

1. What is the importance of driving and community mobility for teens and young adults?
2. What are the dangers of driving and community mobility for teens and young adults?
3. What occupational therapy interventions address driving and community mobility?

## KEY TERMS

CarFit
Community mobility
Driving
Driver readiness
Driver rehabilitation specialist (DRS)
Generalist
Graduated driver licensing (GDL)
OT-FIRST

## DRIVING AND COMMUNITY MOBILITY

During adolescence, learning to drive and getting somewhere alone are considered valuable accomplishments in mobility independence. Learning to drive is considered a cultural rite of passage for teens and young adults, and most Americans believe the ability to drive is a right rather than a privilege. However, driving remains the most dangerous occupation of a young person's lifetime (CDC, 2022a). **Community mobility** refers to getting from one place to another regardless of the mode, with driving the preferred transit method in the United States (Scott & Tulloch, 2021). Community mobility includes using public or private transportation such as driving, walking, bicycling, or accessing and riding in buses, taxi cabs, ride shares, or other transportation systems (AOTA, 2020, p. 31). This chapter provides an overview of essential information for consideration when addressing driving and community mobility with youth. The author describes risk factors, cultural trends, and disparities that young people may face as barriers to community mobility and driving and provides an overview of potential challenges as related to specific conditions. The author outlines occupational therapy's role in driving and community mobility and presents creative solutions to address challenges. Case examples are provided in addition to practical resources, applications, and specific information to support occupational therapy practice.

### The Importance of Driving and Community Mobility

**Driving** and community mobility build social capital and provide greater accessibility to people, services, resources, work, and hobbies (Menzes, 2016; Monahan, 2009, 2012). The occupations of driving and community mobility affirm one's developing sense of identity, independence, freedom, and social connectedness throughout the lifespan (Monahan, 2012). Teens and young adults with disabilities face multiple barriers accessing the community for services that are necessary for health, development, and overall well-being (Stewart et al., 2014). In pediatric rehabilitation, there is limited attention on driving and community mobility and a lack of support services for teens transitioning into adulthood (NICHD, 2021). Occupational therapy practitioners play a key role in addressing driving and community mobility needs for children and youth (AOTA, 2016).

### Dangers of Driving and Community Mobility for Adolescents

According to the latest teen driving statistics, motor vehicle collisions remain the leading cause of teen deaths and disabilities (CDC, 2022a). Teen drivers (ages 16–19) are three times more likely to be involved in a crash than all other age groups (IHS, 2023a). In 2019, 4356 people were killed in young driver crashes. Of these fatalities, 1603 were young drivers, 880 were passengers of young drivers, and the remaining 1873 victims were occupants of the other vehicles involved (NHTSA, 2021). Male drivers aged 16–18, teenagers driving with teen passengers, and newly licensed teens are at high risk for being involved in car accidents (NHTSA, 2021). Males are more likely to engage in risky driving practices; females are more likely to be distracted by phones (IIHS, 2023b). Males are more likely to have severe automobile crashes; females are more likely to be killed or injured (IIHS, 2023b).

The concern for novice drivers, especially those with potentially invisible differences or undiagnosed conditions, cannot be ignored, since many new driver incidents are due to immature executive functions and inexperience (CDC 2022b; Monohan, 2012; Walshe et al., 2017). Teen driver crashes often involve driver error, lack of safety belt use, excessive speed, reckless driving, single-vehicle crashes, nighttime fatal crashes, increased risk with every additional passenger, distractions, alcohol, and drugs (NHTSA, 2021). Crash rates among young drivers are attributed to inexperience, risk-taking behaviors, peer pressure, and failure to notice or manage hazards (CDC, 2022b).

Insufficient sleep also contributes to driving accidents. The Center for Disease Control and Prevention identified that fewer than 30% of high school students get the recommended amount of daily sleep (Wheaton et al., 2016). The research shows a correlation between sleep hygiene, or fatigue, and other driving concerns such as texting while driving, failure to buckle, and driving under the influence (Wheaton et al., 2016). Young drivers (ages 15–25) are involved in over half of drowsy driving crashes annually (American Academy of Pediatrics, 2014).

Driving is not the only mode of transit with safety concerns for youth. In 2019, over 6000 pedestrians and nearly 1000 bicyclists were killed by drivers, and about 125,000 pedestrians and bikers were injured by drivers. Pedestrians comprise 17% of crash deaths, and bicyclists make up an additional 2% (IIHS/HLDI, 2023c).

## Cultural Trends and Disparities

There has been a declining driving interest and delayed licensure acquisition in young persons over the past 3 decades (Schoettle & Sivak, 2014). The trend for delayed permit and license acquisition has risen the most among urban-city youth and those living in poorer communities (Bush, 2016). Young people without a driver's license tend to have less education, lower median income, and higher unemployment than their peers who drive (Bush, 2016). Most students delaying licensure said they did not have a car but could get around fine without driving (Bush, 2016). Others stated cost as the main reason as related to vehicle expenses, gas prices, and driver education. Some adolescents gave reasons such as lack of interest or nervousness, not having time to get around to it, or having a medical issue. In summary, the reasons adolescents are not getting driving licenses are multifaceted, but the young driver culture is changing (Bush, 2016; Delbosc & Currie, 2013; Schoettle & Sivak, 2014).

Cultural dynamics such as expanding transportation options, affordable housing challenges, growing mental health concerns, and other factors contribute to the decline in licensure acquisition (Bush, 2016). During the Covid-19 pandemic, facility closures and other related factors made it difficult for many teens to obtain a driver's permit or license, causing many teens to postpone driving goals (Bell & Johns, 2022). Anxiety, depression, sleep and fatigue, suicidal thoughts, and the use of drugs and alcohol which all rose during this same time frame are important considerations for driving safety, (Center for Promise, 2020; NAMI, 2022).

Another possible contributor to delayed teen licensure is the implementation of **graduated driver licensing (GDL)** laws. GDL laws vary by state and include requirements for driver education, supervised driving hours, and other driving rules for safety and prevention. They are designed to prevent and reduce accidents by giving novice young drivers the chance to gain experience and improve their driving skills over time in lower-risk environments. GDL restrictions loosen in each state over certain ages, so teens may wait longer to avoid strict driving requirements (and practice less). This is especially concerning for new drivers with medical limitations who may benefit from more supervised driving training.

## Disability-Related Challenges for Driving and Community Mobility

Teens and young adults with physical differences such as spinal cord injury, hemiplegia, limb loss, or orthopedic conditions have mobility or transportation challenges that are often evident early on. These individuals typically postpone driving, rely on alternate modes of transportation, or get referred to specialists for support (Bell, 2022). The most common pediatric population with driving safety needs include those with neurodevelopmental disorders. Neurodevelopmental disorders may go undetected and fall in the category referred to as invisible disabilities, which potentially results in driving risks that are not identified before the teen gets behind the wheel (Morris-Rosendahl & Crocq, 2020). Examples of invisible disabilities include attention deficit/hyperactivity disorder (ADHD), autism (ASD), language or communication disorders, intellectual disability, and dyspraxia (which typically come with co-morbidities).

Occupational therapy practitioners evaluate children with a variety of conditions that can affect driving ability. It helps to gather general information pertaining to disability-related concerns for driving to guide and enhance the occupational therapy process. Occupational therapy practitioners identify children with potential risks, address foundations in fitness to drive, and provide necessary education or referrals before the teen begins to drive. This section describes how common disabilities (see Chapter 5 for more information) may influence driving and community mobility. This information may guide important conversations about potential driving risks that may facilitate further assessment, readiness intervention, planning, and/or professional referral. Occupational therapy practitioners consider the progression, symptoms of the condition, medication, along with motor, processing, and social-emotional skills to create intervention that is specific to each child's unique strengths and challenges.

**Attention Deficit Hyperactivity Disorder.** Biederman (2023) states, "Within the first month of driving, teens with ADHD are 62% more likely to be involved in an automobile crash. Over the first 4 years of having a license, drivers with ADHD are 37% more likely to get into a crash, twice as likely to drive while intoxicated, and 150% more likely to receive alcohol, drug, or moving violations" (Cited in Curry et al., 2019, paragraph 2). They may show difficulty with information processing, visual scanning, speed regulation, lane maintenance, and reacting to stimuli (Classen, Monahan, Brown, & Hernandez, 2013; Classen, Monahan, & Wang, 2013). Children with ADHD have trouble with sustaining attention, identifying road signs, recognizing danger hazards, and regulating impulsive behaviors. They may be prescribed medications that must be carefully monitored as they can both enhance and impair driver performance (Menzes, 2016).

**Autism.** Approximately one in three teens with autism spectrum disorder will become licensed drivers by age 21, which is lower than their peers (83.5%) (Curry et al., 2017). Autistic individuals experience social, sensory, motor, cognitive, and adaptive demands in public transportation and community environments. They report anxiety, sensory overload, and problems with attention (Silvi & Scott-Parker, 2018). The learn-to-drive process takes longer and can be more challenging for autistic teens. Children with autism need more practice and repetition, and tasks may have to be modified or adapted for each child (Monahan et al., 2019; Wilson et al., 2018). Teens with co-occurring symptoms may be at greater risk for driving accidents (Classen, Monahan, & Wang, 2013; Monahan et al., 2013). Drivers with autism are three times more likely to crash while making left or U-turns (Curry et al., 2021). They have difficulty with hazard detection (Sheppard et al., 2017), social and communicative skills (Lindsay, 2017), and adaptations to routines (Cox et al., 2012) while on the road or behind the wheel.

These challenges may cause teens with autism to avoid driving or be involved in accidents of unsafe situations. These same challenges may interfere with the teens' ability to navigate their community using public transportation. Myers et al. (2021) interviewed specialized driving instructors who provided behind the wheel training to autistic adolescents. Participants noted that children with autism present with different physical, social, and emotional challenges requiring instructors to view each child individually. They noted that autistic adolescents require practice and a longer time to apply skills in novel situations (due to mental inflexibility) (Myers et al., 2021). They reported the following instructional strategies that included scaffolding skills, repetition and continual practice, repetition of phrases or mnemonics, commentary driving, coaching and correction, calling out other drivers' social cues to help students make sense and interpret behaviors, provide instruction, and not treat the students like a neurotypical teen but use creativity and flexibility to teach (Myers et al., 2021).

**Anxiety and Mood Disorders.** Teen and young adult driver referrals for anxiety and mood disorders are on the rise (Bell, 2022). Approximately 52% of the young adult population (including ages 18–21) experience mild anxiety with driving, and 16% experience moderate to severe anxiety (Taylor et al., 2020). Anxiety may cause functional performance deficits that lead teens to reduce time driving or avoid driving completely due to a fear of driving (Taylor et al., 2020). Anxiety that interferes with an adolescent's driving community mobility independence reduces perceived quality of life (Stephens et al., 2020). Therefore, occupational therapy practitioners may address strategies to manage anxiety during driving and community mobility situations.

**Visual Impairment.** Most states have minimum visual acuity requirements such as 20/40 distance vision for daytime driving, 20/60 distance acuity for nighttime driving, absence of double vision, and continuous, uninterrupted field of view. In several states, individuals with visual deficits may earn a restricted driver's license using a bioptic telescope, if driving is a supported by a vision doctor and the user is properly trained (Wang et al., 2020). Driving restrictions may be enforced per state laws, medical board guidelines, or for additional safety.

Youth with visual impairments may require technologic support for community mobility, such as for reading signs, following directions, using public transportation, identifying locations, and moving within the community. For example, they may require directions in Braille, mobility devices, or technology to provide verbal directions. Many communities have orientation and mobility specialists to train children and adolescents to navigate their community. Occupational therapy practitioners may work with mobility specialists to reinforce concepts in practice.

**Language and Hearing Impairment.** Fewer individuals with a language impairment obtain a driver's license (Durkin et al., 2016). Learners need instruction in their preferred language or otherwise face barriers. Teens who have language impairments may have difficulty understanding or communicating with others in the community (or with peace officers). Hearing-impaired youth are often approached with questions or concerns about their driving capabilities (Feldman, 2022). However, there are new technologies available that emit visual warnings of sirens, and vehicle safety features such as cameras, collision warnings, or braking assist support safe driving. Drivers who are deaf often have better peripheral vision than others (Codina, Buckley, et al., 2011 and b; Feldman, 2022).

**Developmental Coordination Disorder/Dyspraxia.** Individuals with developmental coordination disorder (DCD), also known as "dyspraxia," have difficulties with sensory-perceptual functions, learning new motor tasks, and coordinating and timing movements, which are all important for driving. They may have difficulty perceiving distance (e.g., curb, parking, passing cars) and spaces between vehicles. They may have difficulty estimating speed and distance for driving. Children with DCD exhibit slower reaction time, steering errors, visual-motor integration challenges, and inconsistent gaze or perception (De Oliveira & Wann, 2012). These challenges influence consistency of driving. Children with dyspraxia may benefit from DriveSafety simulator training offered by The Dyspraxia Foundation and DriveSafety Team (Dyspraxia and Driving, 2018).

Children with dyspraxia may also have challenges moving quickly on public transportation, attending to signs, and motor planning through busy or unpredictable crowds. They may have difficulty with other modes of transportation, such as bicycle riding, due to motor challenges with coordination and timing.

**Spina Bifida/Hydrocephalus and Cerebral Palsy.** Spina bifida and hydrocephalus are neurological conditions which may include disruptions in movement, executive function, information processing, and visual deficits (Monahan et al., 2019). Children with neurological disorders such as spina bifida or cerebral palsy may experience challenges with motor skills (such as fine and gross motor coordination), timing and sequencing movements, reaction time, visual discrimination, multitasking, problem-solving, and attention. These challenges make learning to drive complex and place them at risk for motor vehicle accidents (Monahan et al., 2019). Children with neurologic challenges may require physical modifications (such as specialized vans, wheelchair, walkers, or canes) to navigate their community. They may have difficulty figuring out a map or bus schedule and understanding the concept of time. Children who face barriers in resources such as time, funding sources, transportation, and caregiver support may not successfully reach their desired community mobility or driving goals, which limits their access to housing, school, work, and social opportunities (Bell, 2022).

**Traumatic Brain Injury.** Traumatic brain injury (TBI) is the leading cause of acquired dysfunction in childhood (Thurman, 2016), which may result in deficits in executive function, emotional stability, consciousness, and motor skills (Barco et al., 2012). Distractibility, insight, awareness, judgment, information processing, and potential secondary complications of TBI (seizures, impaired sleep, or visual disturbance) interfere with community mobility and driving. Even a minor head injury or concussion can impair driving decisions (e.g., awareness, spatial awareness, timing, speed, location). Additionally, youth who return to driving without physician clearance or re-assessment of driving fitness put themselves and others at risk (Schmidt et al., 2017). Case example 20.1 provides an example of an occupational therapy approach to address driving and community mobility with a young man following a TBI.

## OCCUPATIONAL THERAPY'S ROLE IN DRIVING AND COMMUNITY MOBILITY

The American Occupational Therapy Association (AOTA) affirms the role occupational therapy practitioners hold in addressing driving and community mobility (AOTA, 2016). Driving and community mobility are instrumental activities of daily living (IADLs) and necessary occupations for general health and well-being (AOTA, 2020). Occupational therapy practitioners working in pediatric practice serve children and youth and address community mobility, independence, and safety as necessary life skills. Many children and youth exit occupational therapy services as a preteen, missing out on interventions that would support them in driving and community mobility. Occupational practitioners working in school systems address access to education and do not consistently address transportation-related concerns (Bell, 2022).

Occupational therapy practitioners educate various stakeholders about the importance of addressing driving and community mobility readiness skills during the teenage years and may offer expanded services, such as mobile service clinics, life skills training, and transportation assistance programs. Collaborative partnerships with traditional driver education schools, driver rehabilitation facilities, public transportation systems, and pediatrician offices improve educational outreach. If driving is not an appropriate goal, the occupational therapy practitioner working with children and adolescents may address safety and independence in community mobility and life skills. They remain current on driving standards of practice by reviewing documents such as the Novice Teen Driver Education and Training Administrative Standards, (2023) and AOTA documents on driving and mobility (AOTA, 2016).

## CASE EXAMPLE 20.1 TRAUMATIC BRAIN INJURY

The occupational therapy practitioner working in an in-patient hospital setting receives a referral for an 18-year-old-male with a TBI due to a motor vehicle collision after 2:00 a.m. on a Friday night. He presents with double vision, headaches, frequent pain, and impaired executive functions. A family member reports that the client plans to drive to all his appointments and wants to work for a food delivery or ride-share service. He has partial custody of an infant daughter.

After evaluating the client's readiness to drive, the therapist notes that the client is missing foundational skills (e.g., endurance, sitting balance, attention, judgment, problem-solving, awareness of space, timing, and reaction time) and is not ready to drive. The occupational therapist identifies multiple safety concerns and informs the client that he will need medical clearance to drive by his physician per state laws. They discuss ride options to get the patient to and from all appointments safely and review the support the patient will need upon discharge to safely care for his infant daughter. The therapist makes a referral to a vision doctor due to his double vision, which must be resolved per state restrictions, before it is possible for him to drive.

The discharge plan includes a referral for OT driver rehabilitation (CDRS) assessment and intervention to address driving readiness and skill acquisition for driving. Social work is involved in supporting the client's ability to care for his daughter. The client is reminded that he must notify the state's medical advisory board if he chooses to drive.

## Levels of Specialty: Community Mobility and Driving

All occupational therapy practitioners are qualified to address community mobility, which requires the ability to examine the child's strengths and challenges, environment, and the specific occupation. They use professional reasoning to consider the child's goals, safety, environmental barriers, and supports and carefully design a plan (with input from parents or caregivers) to promote community mobility. While no advanced specialization exists for community mobility, practitioners may seek additional training in conducting evaluations and specific focus areas (such as travel training, paratransit systems, and pedestrian safety) (AOTA, 2016).

There are several levels of specialty certification for interventionists who wish to specialize in driving, which are summarized in Table 20.1. Pediatric and school-based occupational therapy practitioners may be classified as driving and community mobility generalists. **Generalists** address driving and community mobility within the goal of promoting occupational participation. They address performance skills, make referrals, and make recommendations for alternate driving or community mobility (AOTA, 2016). They address underlying capacities (e.g., strength, seating, positioning, scanning, problem-solving) that influence driving. They provide interventions to remediate or adapt performance (AOTA, 2016). They can determine those clients at risk for compromised driving, and they are aware of state regulations regarding minimum criteria for safe driving (AOTA, 2016). Generalist practitioners do not make changes to vehicles or perform behind the wheel assessments or instruction. Case Example 20.2 illustrates the role of the generalist.

The occupational therapy practitioner can become a **driver rehabilitation specialist (DRS)** who is credentialed through the AOTA Board and Specialty Certificate program, certified through the Association for Driver Rehabilitation Specialists (ADED), or trained from other educational platforms (AOTA, 2016). Driver rehabilitation specialists can administer driver evaluations, help determine a person's fitness-to-drive, offer driver education and training, suggest modifications or adaptive equipment for driving, and provide both low- and high-technology equipment if qualified to do so (Lane et al., 2014). Occupational therapy practitioners who are certified Driver Rehabilitation Specialists (DRSs) receive advanced training and may also conduct "on-road" evaluations after meeting state requirements (see Case Example 20.3).

Occupational therapy assistants and occupational therapists have different roles in driver rehabilitation. The occupational therapist is responsible for the evaluation and interpretation of data. Occupational therapy assistants may administer individual assessments and contribute to the evaluation. Both can implement an intervention plan, including on-road training (if they meet qualifications and state guidelines).

## Assessment

Occupational therapists use principles of task analysis to evaluate and assess a child's ability to participate in community mobility (see Chapter 9). They evaluate the child's strengths and challenges including motor, processing, and social-emotional skills along with the environmental supports and barriers to create an intervention plan to address the child's mobility within the community. Occupational therapy assistants contribute to the evaluation process and conduct interventions.

Assessment of driving requires advanced education and training. Occupational therapy practitioners who are trained and licensed as Driver Rehabilitation Specialists (DRSs) and as driver instructors can complete comprehensive driver evaluation, which includes a clinical assessment of the teen's risk factors and readiness to drive and evaluation of the child's performance in the car. The occupational therapy practitioner (who is also a DRS) working with youth collects data from assessments, clinical observations, and professional reasoning to evaluate the youth's readiness to drive and to create an intervention plan. The assessment process is ongoing until the point where the teen completes the driving road test and obtains their driver's license. Often, training goes beyond earning a license and supports safety and functional driving skills. (See Chapter 9 for more on the assessment of driving.)

**TABLE 20.1 Level of Specialty, Training, and Roles**

| Level of Specialty | Training | Role and Services provided |
|---|---|---|
| Generalist | • Part of ACOTE-approved occupational therapy and occupational therapy assistant educational programs | • Promote occupational engagement in community mobility and driving.<br>• Assess performance skills.<br>• Identify performance deficits.<br>• Provide skilled interventions to remediate or adapt performance.<br>• Determine clients at risk for compromised driving.<br>• Refer to specialist as needed.<br>• Determine fit between community mobility task demands and ability of client. |
| Driver rehabilitation specialist (DRS) | • Advanced education and training through AOTA, ADED, or other driver rehabilitation education providers | • Plans, develops, coordinates, or implements driving rehabilitation services for individuals with disabilities.<br>• Works with people of all ages and abilities, exploring alternative transportation solutions.<br>• Performs evaluations to determine client's ability to safely engage in community mobility and driving. |
| Certified driver rehabilitation specialist (CDRS) | • Advanced education and training<br>• Meets education and experiential requirements and successfully completes certification examination provided by the Association for Driver Rehabilitation Specialists (ADED) | • Administer comprehensive driving or community mobility evaluations.<br>• Recommend continued, modified, or cessation of driving or community travel.<br>• Suggest appropriate modifications or adaptive equipment for driving or community travel.<br>• Provide retraining or specialized education for safe and effective travel through the community using the appropriate mode of transportation. |

American Occupational Therapy Association. (2016). Driving and community mobility. *American Journal of Occupational Therapy*, *70*(Suppl. 2), 7012410050. http://doi.org/10.5014/ajot.2016.706S04

### CASE EXAMPLE 20.2 THE ROLE OF THE GENERALIST

An occupational therapist working in home health receives a referral for a 17-year-old female who is recovering from traumatic injuries due to being struck by a driver while crossing the street. The accident was determined to be the result of negligent safety awareness by both the driver and the young girl. The client's prior medical history includes mild cerebral palsy and intellectual and developmental delays.

The child and family goals include establishing safe functional mobility for independence. The patient states, to everyone's surprise, that one goal she has is to learn to drive. The mother wonders about her daughter's potential for driving but thinks driver training may help her understand the danger of driving and motivate her to engage in therapy to improve her overall health and well-being.

The therapist evaluates the client's current level of functioning, given her injuries from the accident. The client is exhibiting many challenges related to her new injuries, which can be addressed to prepare the client for driving training. They discuss areas of concern and create goals to address foundation skills for driving with attention as well as on safe community mobility (e.g., taking the bus, riding her bike, walking on city paths). The therapist reminds the patient that she will still need to take a driver's education course and get a permit for training and informs her about adaptive driving equipment and programs. At that point, the client should be referred to a certified driving rehabilitation specialist.

### CASE EXAMPLE 20.3 REFERRALS TO DRIVING SPECIALISTS

Anna, a school-based occupational therapy practitioner, worked with a teenager who expressed concern that she could not drive or access community events because she had no mode of transportation. After discussing the issue in a team meeting with the teen and her family, Anna identified that the teen had adequate motor skills but lacked safety awareness, attention to details, and judgment. The family was receptive to the teen accessing public transportation and even driving, although they could not afford driver education and did not think their child would qualify, since she has trouble learning.

Anna referred the student and family to the state's vocational rehabilitation services and to a local occupational therapist who was a certified driving rehabilitation specialist (OT-CDRS) who can address the specific goal of driving (which falls outside of the school services scope). The OT-CDRS assesses potential to drive and completes necessary driver training as she is a licensed instructor in her state and offers guidance to the student and family for safe parent-taught driver education and a local driver school who can also help training. The vocational rehabilitation counselor offers support for student employment training opportunities as well as financial assistance for transportation and driver rehabilitation training services.

The school-based practitioner offered to set up an information station at an upcoming school fair for parent education and advertise a driving and community mobility readiness skills boot camp for the summer break. The occupational therapy practitioners (Anna and the OT-CDRS) discussed the possibility of offering a private-pay community-based service of helping teach teens how to use public and private transit options if this is something that health insurance plans or vocational rehabilitation services will not cover or reimburse.

## Interventions to Address Driving and Community Mobility

Occupational therapy practitioners collaborate with children, families, and other professionals to create intervention plans to address driving and community mobility. Each intervention plan is specifically designed to address the child's unique strengths and challenges and considers the child's culture, resources, and environment. For example, a child who lives in a busy city may use public transportation to access activities, whereas another child may need to learn to drive. Occupational therapy practitioners integrate knowledge from multiple sources to create a client-centered intervention plan. The plan often includes education, provision, and training in the use of technology and developing skills. Occupational therapy practitioners may create new programs, establish, maintain, or restore skills, modify, adapt for an individual's driving and community mobility needs or provide programming to prevent loss of driving and community mobility (AOTA, 2020).

**Education.** Client education on driving and community mobility often begins before services for driving are initiated during the initial referral process. Children are taught early to be aware of their surroundings, stay close to parents, look both ways before crossing the street, and wear their seat belts in the car. Children with disabilities may need practice, adaptations, or skill development to follow these socially accepted and safe ways of engaging in community events. They may require adaptive equipment for mobility and communication. Occupational therapy practitioners can educate children and family on safety (such as car seats, positioning, and awareness) and resources to support community mobility (such as public transportation, accessible programs, and technology).

Occupational therapy practitioners may educate students and parents on the permit process, graduated driving learning requirements, and state regulations. Students and parents may need assistance understanding rules, filling out forms, obtaining or interpreting information, and accessing services (Bell, 2022). Adolescents with disabilities and their families also need to be informed about liability and risks pertaining to driving. Some states have additional restrictions or medical advisory board guidelines.

Occupational therapy practitioners educate families on the role of a traditional driver education school and a driver rehabilitation facility. Families may need information regarding health insurance provider coverage or resources for financial assistance related to driving.

Practitioners provide education to support safe driving by emphasizing the importance of eliminating electronic distractions, specifically use of a cell phone while driving (Unni et al., 2017). Distracted driving, primarily related to cell phone use, even when the driver is not holding phone (i.e., handsfree), interferes with safe driving. Unni et al. (2017) created an anti-texting while driving campaign at 32 different high schools, resulting in a significant reduction in texting while driving. The occupational therapist can play a key role in such a program through analysis of when an adolescent is most likely to engage in texting behavior and providing suggestions to avoid this behavior. The profession of occupational therapy addresses issues not only at the individual level but also at the group and population level. Fostering safety campaigns to avoid texting while driving is an important role for an occupational therapist.

In addition to supporting youth regarding driving, occupational therapy practitioners educate teens on community mobility options. They explore resources within the community and provide opportunities for the child to practice safe mobility. For example, a youth may be able to use public transportation to attend events in the community. Occupational therapy intervention matches the adolescent's current skills with education on available resources.

Adolescents may benefit from instruction in the use of public transportation. Children may need education to understand money (costs) and the process (e.g., how to secure a bus or subway pass). Some communities have substantial support for community mobility such as wheelchair accessible buses and trains, where other communities may have extremely limited or potentially no form of public transportation. The practitioner may educate youth in advocating for accessible transportation to school events (as part of their Individualized Education Program). Together, they may find other sources of transportation (such as an adapted bike) or places that are more accessible. They may practice taking public transportation and review safety within the community (see Fig. 20.1).

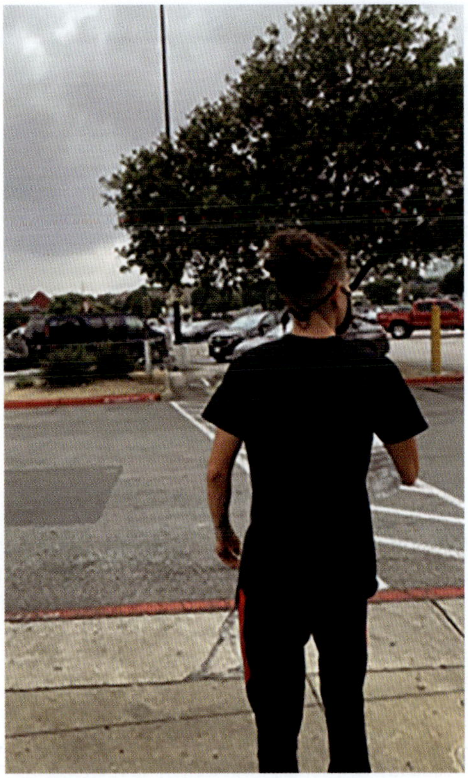

**Fig. 20.1** Safely crossing the street is an important skill for community mobility.

**Technology and Training.** Families and young people with access to the internet, computer devices, smart phones, and tablets benefit by using technology related to driving and community mobility. Table 20.2 provides apps and webpages that offer information and downloadable resources about young driver safety. Occupational therapy practitioners can assist in providing access, interpretation, and education to youth in need of technologic support.

For many American families and teenagers, new vehicles and supportive safety features are out of reach, while for others, simply having a car is too expensive. Some families may be able to afford new vehicles with advanced driver assistance systems and in-vehicle information systems and may be tempted to buy an autonomous (aka "self-driving") vehicle. Technologic advances in motor vehicle design have perceived benefits and can potentially enhance driver performance, but they come with high costs. Vehicle technology cannot replace the need for a knowledgeable, attentive driver with good safety awareness, insight, and maturity. Autonomous vehicles are not an appropriate accommodation or safer alternative for young drivers with disabilities (Monahan & Classen, 2019).

**TABLE 20.2 Web-Based Resources for Young Driver Readiness Training and Caregiver Support**

| **Auto Coach®** | Drive tracker and lesson planner for teaching teen drivers the rules of the road from the Shepard Center (which can be used with those with cognitive and physical differences) |
|---|---|
| **Drive Focus®** | Interactive video training from the Driver Rehabilitative Institute that targets noticing and prioritizing of critical information on the roadway as well as reaction time and accuracy |
| **DriveitHOME®** | A National Safety Council resource with pointers to help parents coach soon-to-be drivers as well as teens with a new permit or license |
| **Driving Skills for life** | A free online academy from Ford GM/The Governor's Highway Association and training tour that reviews safety related to vehicle technology and other modes of transportation |
| **Teen Driving Plan** | An interactive practice guide from the center for injury research and prevention at Children's Hospital of Philadelphia allowing parents to effectively supervise/guide training |

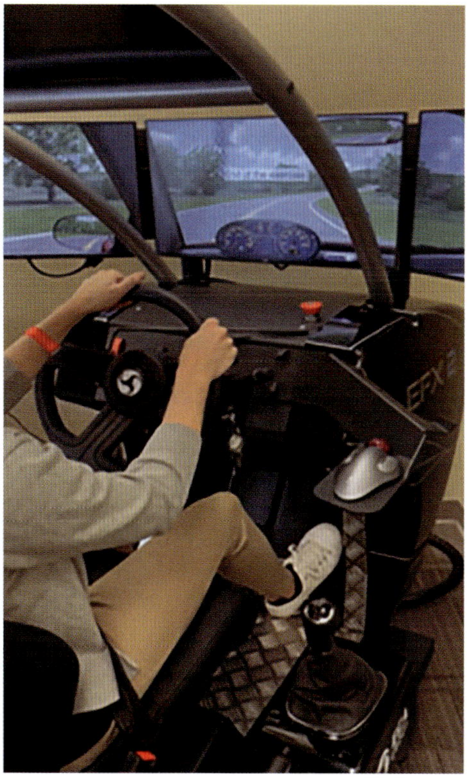

**Fig. 20.2** This teen practices driving using a driving simulator, which provides them a safe, controlled, and distraction-free environment to learn.

The advent of driving simulators has offered a new modality for intervention, most often found and used in research-based or driver education school settings (see Fig. 20.2 for an example of a driving simulator). The use of simulators with young adults with disabilities is limited (Classen, Monahan, & Wang, 2013; Monahan et al., 2013). The benefits of using a driving simulator with young people include perceived safety of a controlled environment, opportunity for repeated learning of a new task or experience, potential client enjoyment (less anxiety), and the ability for customization (Bell, 2022). Concerns with using a simulator include cost, space, time or maintenance requirements, and concern that the simulator can be perceived as play by users or does not represent the same functional reality that in-car training offers (Bell, 2022).

Adolescents with disabilities learning to drive may require assistive technology and vehicle modifications for driving. A variety of options exist that range from basic (e.g., seat cushion, steering wheel grip), low technology (e.g., seat cushion, steering wheel knobs, pedal extensions), to high technology (e.g., wheelchair van, ramp, left-foot accelerator, hand controls, cross-over turn signal notification). Basic technology is available to the public and often part of options. Fig. 20.3A–C show examples of adapted driving equipment.

CarFit (CarFit, 2023), a free national collaboration between the AOTA, American Auto Association, and American Association of Retired Persons, provides education, awareness, training, and resources regarding driving and community mobility. Occupational therapy practitioners can learn about additional devices to accommodate for drivers' needs, such as seat cushions, a leg lifter, extended handles, and button mirrors. While CarFit is designed for mature drivers (over age 65), a modified approach can be used with young drivers.

**Addressing Readiness Skills.** Teens with disabilities require support for driving and community mobility (Monahan, 2012). To drive and/or use other transportation options safely and independently, teens and young adults need to become proficient in multiple readiness skills (Monahan & Classen, 2019). Driver readiness skills include motor actions required to engage in driving, such as gripping a steering wheel, sitting upright, applying pressure to pedals, and turning one's head; cognitive actions, such as paying attention, sequencing, knowing road signage, understanding driving instruments, following a map, remembering a location, making judgments, and safety awareness; and social-emotional readiness, such as remaining calm, problem-solving, managing one's sensory reactions, attending, flexibility in situations, and communicating as needed. See Fig. 20.4 for an example of engaging a teen in activities to promote driving readiness. It is important to notice how the teen moves, sees, thinks, feels, and takes on general responsibilities (Menzes, 2016)

Occupational therapy practitioners examine young people's strengths and challenges regarding driving and may intervene at the driving readiness level before referring the teen to an in-vehicle program. They may address factors that interfere with youth engaging in community mobility activities, such as safety, planning, mobility, awareness, self-regulation, sensory processing, and judgment, flexibility, managing one's emotions, and communication. See Table 20.3 for intervention suggestions for readiness.

Occupational therapy practitioners use a variety of practice models and frames of reference to address readiness skills and factors that interfere with a young person's driving and community mobility. For example, they may use a biomechanical approach to address muscle strength challenges or use coaching strategies from a motor control approach to teach a teen to coordinate movements

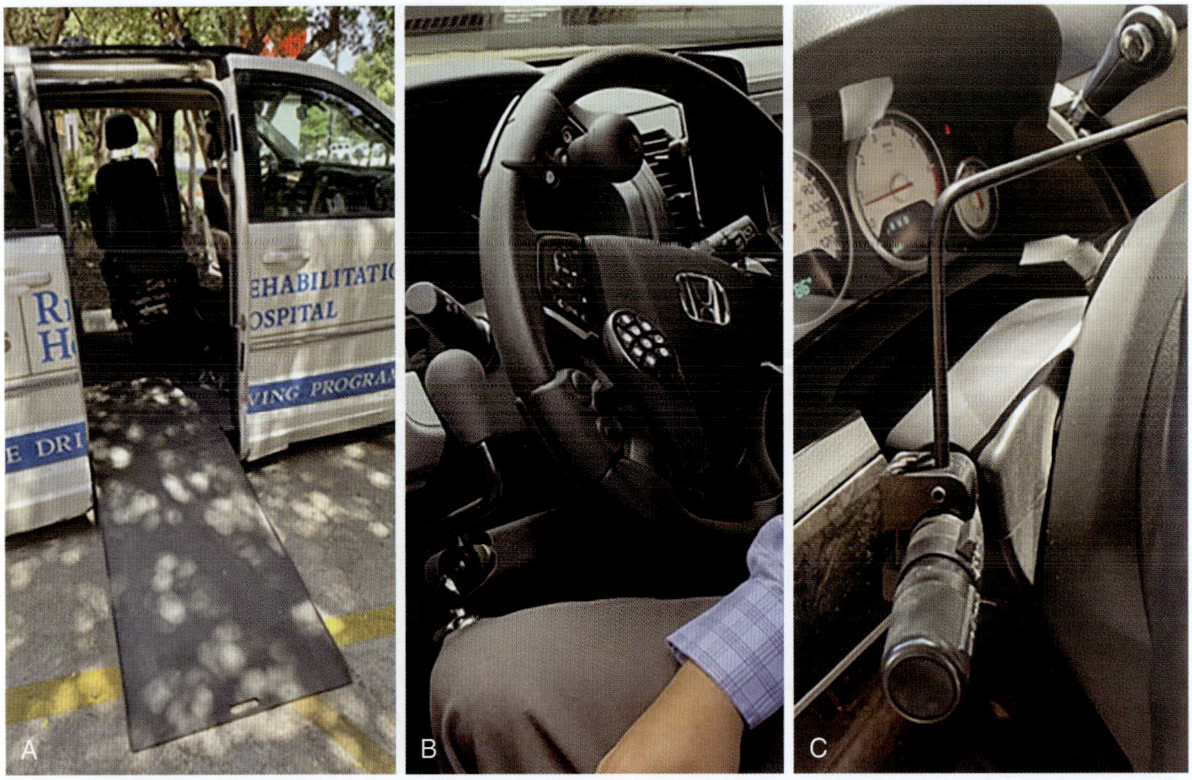

**Fig. 20.3** (A) Teens who require wheelchairs for mobility may learn to access an adapted van using a lowered floor, powered ramp and 6-way swivel seat (which could also be removed if safe and necessary). (B) A left-side hand control/spinner knob option (2 grasp options shown here) allows adolescents who have limited use of their right upper extremity to steer. (C) A cross-over extended turn signal adapter allows drivers to use their right hand for signaling.

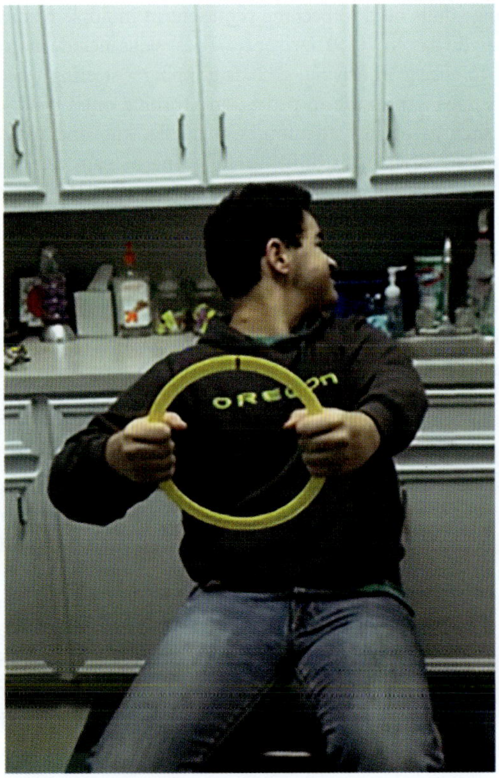

**Fig. 20.4** This teen practices basic bilateral motor and movement tasks associated with driving in the OT clinic setting.

for driving. They may use principles from sensory approaches to address self-regulation challenges and cognitive-behavioral strategies to promote engagement. They may use a behavioral approach to reinforce safety practices. See Chapter 9 for more on these approaches. Occupational therapy practitioners use these approaches within driving programs to promote learning and motor skills acquisition. See Table 20.4 for examples of different approaches to addressing driving readiness skills and activities that might be incorporated.

**Programs to Address Driving and Community Mobility for Adolescents.** A program called OT-FIRST was created by Bell (2019, 2020, 2022) to address driving and community mobility in teens and young adults from the OT perspective. Therapists can learn how to expand upon driving-related practice models developed for older adults, specifically OT-DRIVE (Davis & Dickerson, 2017) and MODEM (Hunt & Slater, 2012). The OT-FIRST methodology provides extensive educational programming, new screening tools, and a new evidence-based criterion-referenced assessment tool for driver readiness. OT-FIRST outlines the process for current best practice in addressing driving and community mobility readiness needs in young novice drivers. Occupational therapy practitioners using OT-FIRST methods address critical driving and mobility areas listed in Box 20.1. See online learning site for OT-FIRST materials and examples.

The OT-FIRST method follows a five-step framework (modified from Monahan & Classen, 2019) to address community mobility and driving. Occupational therapy practitioners use the steps within

**TABLE 20.3 Helpful Hints for Occupational Therapy Practitioners Addressing Readiness for Driving and Community Mobility**

| Category | Hints |
|---|---|
| Client-centered tasks | Identify, tap into, and use client-stated motivators to guide intervention for optimal gains. |
| Functional activities | Use simulated or modified tasks for safety; work toward doing real life tasks/settings. |
| Activity analysis | Identify skills required to complete the activity to assess suitability to client or intervention. |
| Chaining techniques | Break down the task into pieces and provide/remove support in areas needed for success. |
| Sensory strategies | Consider how children may respond to sensory aspects of activity. Provide sensory experiences that maintain optimal state of arousal for ideal performance. |
| Social and life skills | Build effective social interaction and self-care abilities for safety and independence within the community. |
| Modeling | Provide examples through demonstration (often beneficial if peer driven) or visual aides. Demonstrate using the actual objects (e.g., the actual bus schedule). |
| Facilitation and rest | Optimize performance with preparatory or guided inputs and rest breaks throughout a task, when necessary. |
| Motor timing tasks | Strength, stability, separation, and refined, graded, coordinated, timely responses aide driving. Provide clients with opportunities to practice motor tasks in a relaxed setting, using actual objects if possible. |
| Develop visual skills | Build rapid noticing, filtering, prioritizing, scanning, searching, judging, and differentiating to support client's skills for driving and community mobility. |
| Repetition of tasks | Repeating tasks (the same way, similar ways, new ways) encourages learning/generalization. |
| Monitoring resources | Track progress with notes, attendance logs, journals, video recordings, and goal attainment scales. Engage children in the reflective process to promote learning. |
| Life skills training | Improving life skills supports safety, independence, and well-being for mobility IADLs. Provide children with choices throughout. |
| Event preparedness | Collaborate with children on a plan for emergencies to develop their skills for dealing with unexpected events. |
| Checklists | Break multistep processes and critical information into manageable memorable pieces. Do this with the child to teach them ways to manage daily activities. |
| Task demonstration | Demonstrate a task or task components in a way that the learner can translate effectively. |
| Passenger level | Provide opportunities for learning and training in vehicles safely as an active passenger. |
| Commentary training | Instructor commentary teaches, while student commentary helps develop and assess skill level. |
| Multisensory methods | Utilize visual, auditory, tactile-kinesthetic, and combined strategies that support learning styles. |
| Fixed-route plans | Preplan routes that are mostly predictable, offering challenges suitable to client skill level. |
| Skilled observations | Examine the driver and driver settings and assist instructor processes for supports/barriers. |
| Self-management | Ensure students are rested, properly nourished, medicated, and otherwise supported as needed. |
| Driving agreement | Set clear rules and expectations to encourage responsibility and accountability for all actions. |
| Accommodations | Supports may include modification, restrictions, adaptive methods, and equipment training. |

Modified from Bell, M. (2022). *OT-FIRST method training manual for the OT practitioner*. Safe Driving Rehab, LLC.

the domain of occupational therapy practice and following ethical standards:

1. Examine youth-related client factors and performance skills pertaining to driving and community mobility risk assumptions or outcomes.
2. Identify appropriate, evidence-based occupational therapy assessments for the young person within the setting.
3. Address prerequisite skills (i.e., readiness) to support client goals (student and family).
4. Apply occupational therapy practice models, frames of reference, and approaches specific for each child to address driving and community mobility.
5. Refer to physicians, occupational therapy DRSs, and qualified driving instructors, and seek more training/support when necessary.

## ETHICAL CONSIDERATIONS IN DRIVING AND COMMUNITY MOBILITY

Occupational therapy practitioners addressing driving and community mobility follow the AOTA (2020) code of ethics. They also have an ethical responsibility to (1) warn clients and family of the potential anger of impaired performance and (2) recognize factors that compromise performance as public health safety risks (AOTA, 2016; Slater et al., 2014). Practitioners working with driving and community mobility must be aware and follow state laws and regulations regarding reporting obligations, driving processes, and professional responsibilities.

Berndt et al. (2022) conducted semistructured interviews and a focus group of experienced driver-trained occupational therapists.

**TABLE 20.4 Approaches to Address Readiness Skills for Driving and Community Mobility**

| Approach | Sample Approach with Driving and Community Mobility |
|---|---|
| Acquisitional | Facilitate higher level adaptive responses through passenger-level commentary and demonstration tasks for safety. |
| Biomechanical | Engage child in therapeutic programming and activities to improve strength and endurance for wheelchair transfers to and from driver's seat using family/client vehicle for transportation. |
| Cognitive behavioral | Promote problem-solving for person w/SCI returning to driving after major MVA and injury-related anxiety and use strategies (such as goal setting and working through challenges) to support performance. |
| Developmental | Address global developmental delays and learning issues with a teen wanting to get a job and live more independently by scaffolding tasks so that the child is successful over time. |
| Dunn's sensory processing model | Promote self-regulation strategies with a young adult with autism learning to use the city bus to go to his favorite store and purchase a small item. |
| Lifestyle performance model | Train child in their own community setting using similar vehicle and community routes to meet essential need (school, work, errands, or hobbies). |
| Motor skill acquisition | Train basics of steering/braking in open, empty parking lot (straightaways and at low speed) to a novice driver with a disability before adding turns or signal use. |
| Occupational adaptation | Teaches a driver how to drive using an adapted vehicle. Student chooses meaningful places they would like to drive to at a low-traffic time of day. |
| Visual perception | Address stationary functional visual abilities related to noticing and remembering critical information prior to advancing to motion-based tasks. |

Modified from Bell, M. (2022). *OT-FIRST method training for the OT practitioner.*

**BOX 20.1 Driving and Mobility Areas of Concern (Based on OT-FIRST)**

1. Visual motor and spatial integration
2. Functional vision (beyond acuity)
3. Cognitive perceptual integration
4. Bilateral motor integration
5. Executive functions and praxis
6. Task analysis and problem-solving
7. Knowing the "rules of the road"
8. Applying rules and generalizing abilities under stress
9. Insight into risk and liability
10. Guidance for treatment planning, referrals, and on-road assessments (Bell, 2022).

The themes were analyzed according to professional reasoning. Three subthemes emerged within ethical reasoning: (1) balance of safety vs. client independence, (2) objectivity (measuring driving performance), and (3) advocacy (supporting clients' interest to return to driving) (Berndt et al., 2022). The findings suggest that occupational therapy practitioners working in driving and community mobility examine processes to understand their responsibilities (along with state laws) when considering whether an adolescent is safe to drive or engage in community mobility. Practitioners have an obligation to identify resources that support client independence while assuring public safety as well. They may have to advocate for services for clients and assist families and adolescents in finding resources that allow them to participate in community events. Practitioners are responsible for using objective, evidence-based assessments to base decisions while weighing knowledge of youth and environmental factors.

## SUMMARY

Development of driving and community mobility skills are essential areas to address with children and youth. These IADLs allow children to engage in community events, provide independence, and promote life satisfaction. Children with disabilities may face barriers with these occupations and often need additional support. Occupational therapy practitioners identify affordances and barriers to engagement in community mobility and driving early and create intervention plans to address readiness skills, educate children on safety, and engage young children in activities in community activities. Addressing community mobility early (and as appropriate with the child's abilities and age) prepares them for future independence and driving.

1. Driving and community mobility build social capital and provide greater accessibility to people, services, resources, work, and hobbies (Menzes, 2016; Monahan, 2009, 2012). The occupations of driving and community mobility affirm one's developing sense of identity, independence, freedom, and social connectedness throughout the lifespan (Monahan, 2012).
2. Driving and community mobility can also be dangerous. Motor vehicle collisions remain the leading cause of teen deaths and disabilities (CDC, 2022a). Teen drivers (ages 16–19) are three times more likely to be involved in a crash than all other age groups (IHS, 2023a). Teen driver crashes often involve driver error, lack of safety belt use, excessive speed, reckless driving, single-vehicle crashes, nighttime fatal crashes, increased risk with every additional passenger, distractions, alcohol, and drugs (NHTSA, 2021). Crash rates among young drivers are attributed to inexperience, risk-taking behaviors, peer pressure, and failure to notice or manage hazards (CDC, 2022b). Insufficient sleep also contributes to driving accidents. Driving is not the only mode of transit with safety concerns for youth. In 2019, over 6000 pedestrians and nearly 1000 bicyclists were killed by drivers, and about 125,000 pedestrians and bikers were injured by drivers. Pedestrians comprise 17% of crash deaths, and bicyclists make up an additional 2% (IIHS/HLDI, 2023c).

3. Occupational therapy practitioners collaborate with children, families, and other professionals to create intervention plans to address driving and community mobility. Each intervention plan is specifically designed to address the child's unique strengths and challenges and considers the child's culture, resources, and environment. Occupational therapy practitioners integrate knowledge from multiple sources to create a client-centered intervention plan. The plan often includes education, provision, and training in the use of technology and developing skills. Occupational therapy practitioners may create new programs, establish or restore skills, maintain, modify, or adapt (or prevent) (AOTA, 2020).

## ACKNOWLEDGMENTS

This author acknowledges Dr. Miriam Monahan and Dr. Sherrilene Classen at The University of Florida, Dr. Angela Blackwell, Dr. Steven Gerardi, Destinee Logan, Tiffany Pham, Shelby Reed, and Celeste Johns at The University of St. Augustine, and Jennifer Perez Del Rio at St.David's Medical Center for important contributions to this chapter and sends gratitude to fellow exemplars in the field who are addressing community mobility safety and independence through research, education, advocacy, and innovation.

## REFERENCES

American Academy of Pediatrics. (2014). *Policy statement: School start times for adolescents*. www.pediatrics.org/cgi/doi/10.1542/peds.2014-1687.

American Occupational Therapy Association. (2020). Occupational therapy practice framework: Domain and process-fourth edition. *American Journal of Occupational Therapy*, *74*(Suppl. 2), 7412410010. https://doi.org/10.5014/ajot.2020.74S2001.

American Occupational Therapy Association. (2016). Driving and community mobility. *American Journal of Occupational Therapy*, *70*(Suppl. 2), 7012410050. https://doi.org/10.5014/ajot.2016.706S04.

Barco, P., Stav, W., Arnold, R., & Carr, D. (2012). Cognition: A vital component to driving and community mobility. In M. J. McGuire, & E. Schold Davis (Eds.), *Driving and community mobility: Occupational therapy strategies across the lifespan* (pp. 157–171). AOTA Press.

Bell, M. (2020). Applying the OT-DRIVE framework to serve young drivers: Perspectives from a pediatric focused driver rehabilitation specialist (Parts 1 &2). *ADED's NewsBrake*, *44*(2 &3), 10–11.

Bell, M. (2019). *Functional applications of the OT-DRIVE model with potential young driver needs and pediatric OTs*. https://safedrivingrehab.com/docs/Fuctional%20Applications%20of%20OTDRIVE.pdf.

Bell, M., & Johns, C. (2022). Feasibility study: Implementing the OT-FIRST methods and clinical observations measurement tool with young, novice drivers. Poster presentation available from: www.safedrivingrehab.com/ot-first/.

Bell, M. (2022). *OT-FIRST method training for the OT practitioner*.

Berndt, A., Hutchinson, C., Tepper, D., & George, S. (2022). Professional reasoning of occupational therapy driver rehabilitation interventions. *Australian Occupational Therapy Journal*, *69*, 436–446.

Biederman, J. (2023). Driving with ADHD: Pumping the brakes on vehicle safety risks. In *ADDitude*. https://www.additudemag.com/adhd-driving-risks-research-safety/.

Bush, E. (2016). Teens delay getting licenses – and their driving is worse. In *The Seattle Times*. http://www.seattletimes.com/seattle-news/transportation/young-drivers-wait-to-get-licenses-with-dangerous-consequences/.

CarFit. (2023). https://car-fit.org/.

Center for Promise. (2020). *The state of young people during Covid-19*. America's Promise Alliance. https://www.americaspromise.org/sites/default/files/d8/YouthDuringCOVID_FINAL%20%281%29.pdf.

Centers for Disease Control and Prevention. (2022a). *Get the facts: TBI data*. https://www.cdc.gov/traumaticbraininjury/data/index.html.

Centers for Disease Control and Prevention. (2022b). *Teen drivers and passengers: Get the facts*. https://www.cdc.gov/transportationsafety/teen_drivers/teendrivers_factsheet.html.

Classen, S., Monahan, M., Brown, K. E., & Hernandez, S. (2013a). Driving indicators in teens with attention deficit hyperactivity and/or autism spectrum disorder. *Canadian Journal of Occupational Therapy*, *80*(5), 274–283. https://doi.org/10.1177/0008417413501072.

Classen, S., Monahan, M., & Wang, Y. (2013b). Driving characteristics of teens with attention deficit hyperactivity and autism spectrum disorder. *American Journal of Occupational Therapy*, *67*(6), 664–673. https://doi.org/10.5014/ajot.2013.008821.

Codina, C., Pascalis, O., Mody, C., Toomey, P., Rose, J., Gummer, L., et al. (2011b). Visual advantage in deaf adults linked to retinal changes. *PLoS One*, *6*(6), e20417. https://doi.org/10.1371/journal.pone.0020417.

Codina, C., Buckley, D., Port, M., & Pascalis, O. (2011a). Deaf and hearing children: A comparison of peripheral vision development. *Developmental Science*, *14*(4), 725–737. https://doi.org/10.1111/j.1467--7687.2010.01017.x.

Cox, N. B., Reeve, R. E., Cox, S. M., & Cox, D. J. (2012). Brief report: Driving and young adults with ASD: Parents' experiences. *Journal of Autism and Developmental Disorders*, *42*, 2257–2262. https://doi.org/10.1007/s10803-012-1470-7.

Curry, A. E., Metzger, K. B., Carey, M. E., Sartin, E. B., Huang, P., & Yerys, B. E. (2021). Comparison of motor vehicle crashes, traffic violations, and license suspensions between autistic and non-autistic adolescent and young adult drivers. *Journal of the American Academy of Child & Adolescent Psychiatry*, *60*(7), 913–923. https://doi.org/10.1016/j.jaac.2021.01.001.

Curry, A. E., Pfeiffer, M. R., & Elliott, M. R. (2017). Compliance with and enforcement of graduated driver licensing restrictions. *American Journal of Preventive Medicine*, *52*(1), 47–54. https://doi.org/10.1016/j.amepre.2016.08.024.

Curry, A. E., Yerys, B. E., Metzger, K. B., Carey, M. E., & Power, T. J. (2019). Traffic crashes, violations, and suspensions among young drivers with ADHD. *Pediatrics*, *143*(6), e20182305. https://doi.org/10.1542/peds.2018-2305.

Davis, E. S., & Dickerson, A. (2017). OT-DRIVE: Integrating the IADL of driving and community mobility into routine practice. *OT Practice*, *22*(13), 8–14.

De Oliveira, R. F., & Wann, J. P. (2012). Driving skills of young adults with developmental coordination disorder: Maintaining control and avoiding hazards. *Human Movement Science*, *31*(3), 721–729. https://doi.org/10.1016/j.humov.2011.06.010.

Delbosc, A., & Currie, G. (2013). Causes of youth licensing decline: A synthesis of evidence. *Transport Reviews*, *33*(3), 271–290. https://doi.org/10.1080/01441647.2013.801929

Durkin, K., Toseeb, U., Pickles, A., Botting, N., & Conti-Ramsden, G. (2016). Learning to drive in young adults with language impairment. *Transportation Research Part F: Traffic Psychology and Behaviour*, *42*, 195–204. https://doi.org/10.1016/j.trf.2016.07.015.

Dyspraxia and Driving. (2018). In *DriveSafety*. https://drivesafety.com/driving-with-dyspraxia-2/.

Feldman, J. (2022). *Yes—the deaf (and those with hearing loss) are allowed to drive and do so as safely as hearing drivers*. https://www.enddd.org/end-distracted-driving/enddd-blog/yes-deaf-are-allowed-to-drive/.

Hunt, L. A., & Slater, D. (2012). Occupational therapy's ethical obligation to address driving and community mobility. In M. J. Maguire, & E. Schold Davis (Eds.), *Driving and community mobility: Occupational therapy strategies across the lifespan* (pp. 101–113). AOTA Press.

Insurance Institute for Highway Safety and Highway Loss Data Institute. (2023a). *Fatality facts 2019: Teenagers*. https://www.iihs.org/topics/fatality-statistics/detail/teenagers.

Insurance Institute for Highway Safety and Highway Loss Data Institute. (2023b). *Fatality facts 2022: Males & females*. https://www.iihs.org/topics/fatality-statistics/detail/males-and-females.

Insurance Institute for Highway Safety and Highway Loss Data Institute. (2023c). *Pedestrians and bicyclists*. https://www.iihs.org/topics/pedestrians-and-bicyclists.

Lane, A., Green, E., Dickerson, A., Davis, E. S., Rolland, B., & Stohler, J. T. (2014). Driver rehabilitation programs: Defining program models, services, and expertise. *Occupational Therapy in Health Care, 28*(2), 177–187.

Lindsay, S. (2017). Systematic review of factors affecting driving and motor vehicle transportation among people with autism spectrum disorder. *Disability & Rehabilitation, 39*(9), 837–846. https://doi.org/10.3109/09638288.2016.1161849.

Menzes, M. (2016). *Driving readiness for teens program outreach & therapist training*. Extra Credit! LLC.

Monahan, M. (2012). Assessing, treating, and preparing youth with special needs for driving and community mobility. In T. J. Maguire, & E. Schold Davis (Eds.), *Driving and community mobility: Occupational therapy strategies across the lifespan* (pp. 383–410). AOTA Press.

Monahan, M., & Classen, S. (2019). Best practices in driver's education to enhance participation. In G. Frolek-Clark, J. E. Rioux, & B. Chandler (Eds.), *Best practices for occupational therapy in schools* (pp. 437–445). AOTA Press.

Monahan, M., Classen, S., & Helsel, P. (2013). Pre-driving evaluation of a teen with attention deficit disorder and autism spectrum disorder. *Canadian Journal of Occupational Therapy, 80*(1), 35–41. https://doi.org/10.1177/0008417412474221.

Monahan, M. (2009). Driving assessment and training techniques: Addressing the needs of students with cognitive and social limitations behind the wheel. [AOTA CD or Online Format Course]. In *American Occupational Therapy Association.*

Morris-Rosendahl, D. J., & Crocq, M. A. (2020). Neurodevelopmental disorders-the history and future of a diagnostic concept. *Dialogues in Clinical Neuroscience, 22*(1), 65–72. https://doi.org/10.31887/DCNS.2020.22.1/macrocq.

Myers, R. K., Carey, M. E., Bonsu, J. M., Yerys, B. E., Mollen, C. J., & Curry, A. E. (2021). Behind the wheel: Specialized driving instructors' experiences and strategies for teaching autistic adolescents to drive. *American Journal of Occupational Therapy, 75*:7503180110. https://doi.org/10.501/ajot.2021.043406.

National Alliance on Mental Health NAMI. (2022). *Mental health by the numbers*. https://www.nami.org/mhstats.

National Highway Traffic Safety Administration. NHTSA. (2021). *Traffic safety facts: 2019 data, young drivers*. https://crashstats.nhtsa.dot.gov/Api/Public/ViewPublication/813130.

National Institute of Child Health and Human Development NICHD. (2021). *Theme 4: Improving child and adolescent health and the transition to adulthood*. http://www.nichd.nih.gov/about/org/strategicplan/researchthemes/theme4.

Novice Teen Driver Education and Training Administrative Standards NTDETAS. (2023). https://anstse.info/wp-content/uploads/2023/05/NTDETAS-May-2023-Edition-.pdf.

Schmidt, J. D., Hoffman, N. L., Ranchet, M., Miller, S., Tomporowski, P. D., Akinwuntan, A. E., & Devos, H. (2017). Driving after concussion: Is it safe to drive after symptoms resolve? *Journal of Neurotrauma, 34*, 1571–1578. https://doi.org/10.1089/neu.2016.4668.

Schoettle, B., & Sivak, M. (2014). The reasons for the recent decline in young driver licensing in the United States. *Traffic Injury Prevention, 15*(1), 6–9. https://doi.org/10.1080/15389588.2013.839993.

Scott, T. L., & Tulloch, K. (2021). Is community mobility contingent upon driving? Attitudes toward and intentions to use alternative modes of transportation according to a mixed-age sample. *Journal of Transport & Health, 20*. https://doi.org/10.1016/j.jth.2020.100974.

Sheppard, E., van Loon, E., Underwood, G., & Ropar, D. (2017). Attentional differences in a driving hazard perception task in adults with autism spectrum disorders. *Journal of Autism and Developmental Disorders, 47*(2), 405–414. https://doi.org/10.1007/s10803-016-2965-4.

Silvi, C., & Scott-Parker, B. (2018). Understanding the driving and licensing experiences of youth with autism. *Transportation Research Part F: Traffic Psychology and Behaviour, 58*, 769–781. https://doi.org/10.1016/j.trf.2018.04.021.

Slater, D. Y., National Highway Traffic Safety Administration, & American Occupational Therapy Association (2014). Consensus statements on occupational therapy ethics related to driving. *Occupational Therapy in Health Care, 28*(2), 163–168. https://doi.org/10.3109/07380577.2014.903356.

Stephens, A. N., Collette, B., Hidalgo-Munoz, A., Fort, A., Evennou, M., & Jallais, C. (2020). The impacts of anxiety over driving on self-reported driving avoidance, work performance and quality of life. *Journal of Transport & Health, 19*(1). https://doi.org/10.1016/j.jth.2020.100929.

Stewart, D., Law, M., Young, N. L., Forhan, M., Healy, H., Burke-Gaffney, J., & Freeman, M. (2014). Complexities during transitions to adulthood for youth with disabilities: Person-environment interactions. *Disability & Rehabilitation, 36*(23), 1998–2004. https://doi.org/10.3109/09638288.2014.885994.

Taylor, J. E., Sullman, M. J. M., & Stephens, A. N. (2020). Measuring anxiety-related avoidance with the driving and riding avoidance scale (DRAS). *European Journal of Psychological Assessment, 36*(1), 114–122. https://doi.org/10.1027/1015-5759/a000502.

Thurman, D. J. (2016). The epidemiology of traumatic brain injury in children and youths: A review of research since 1990. *Journal of Child Neurology, 31*, 20–27. https://doi.org/10.1177/0883073814544363.

Unni, P., Estrada, C. M., Chung, D. H., Riley, E. B., Worsley Hynd, L., & Stinson, N. (2017). A multiyear assessment of a hospital-school program to promote teen motor vehicle safety. *Journal of Trauma and Acute Care Surgery, 83*(2), 289–295. https://doi.org/10.1097/TA.0000000000001521.

Walshe, E. A., Ward McIntosh, C., Romer, D., & Winston, F. K. (2017). Executive function capacities, negative driving behavior and crashes in young drivers. *International Journal of Environmental Research and Public Health, 14*(11), 1314. https://doi.org/10.3390/ijerph14111314.

Wang, S., Moharrer, M., Baliutaviciute, V., Dougherty, B. E., Cybis, W., Bowers, A. R., & Luo, G. (2020). Bioptic telescope use in naturalistic driving by people with visual impairment. *Translational Vision Science & Technology, 9*(4). https://doi.org/10.1167/tvst.9.4.11.

Wheaton, A. G., Olsen, E. O., Miller, G. F., & Croft, J. B. (2016). *Sleep duration and injury related risk behaviors among high school students – United States, 2007–2013*. Centers or Disease Control and Prevention. http://www.cdc.gov/mmwr/volumes/65/wr/mm6513a1.htm.

Wilson, N. J., Lee, H. C., Vaz, S., Vindin, P., & Cordier, R. (2018). Scoping review of the driving behaviour of and driver training programs for people on the autism spectrum. *Behavioural Neurology, 2018*. https://doi.org/10.1155/2018/6842306.

21

# Treatment for Work Skills and Employment

*Andrew Persch and Beth Pfeiffer*

## GUIDING QUESTIONS

1. Who are some of the team members involved in transition planning?
2. How do self-direction, self-determination, and self-advocacy skills promote transition planning?
3. What laws support transition planning for children with disabilities?
4. What are the variety of transition options for children and youth?
5. How does Project SEARCH support employment for youth?

## KEY TERMS

Collaborative interdisciplinary and interagency teams
Customized employment
Individuals with Disabilities Education Improvement Act (IDEA)
Preemployment transition services (Pre-ETS)
Project SEARCH
Reasonable accommodations
Self-advocacy
Self-determination
Supported employment
Transition planning
Workforce Innovation and Opportunities Act (WIOA)
Vocational rehabilitation (VR) services

## OCCUPATIONAL THERAPY AND THE CONTEXT OF TRANSITION TO EMPLOYMENT

Employment has a significant impact on economic self-sufficiency, health, and overall quality of life (Berkman, 2014; Datson et al., 2012), making it an important focus of occupational therapy interventions. Unfortunately, people with disabilities have lower rates of competitive employment and lower pay than similar aged peers (Newman et al., 2011; Wehman, 2013), and people with developmental disabilities often experience greater disparities in employment compared to peers with other types of disabilities (Erickson et al., 2018). Occupational therapy practitioners can serve in a variety of roles and settings to support preemployment and employment skills for transition-age youth and young adults. Occupational therapy provides a unique and important role in the transition team to provide person-centered and environmentally focused interventions that improve employment outcomes and quality of life for transition-age youth. The evidence-based practices discussed within this chapter arise both from the profession of occupational therapy and from partners in special education, vocational rehabilitation (VR), and behavioral health.

There are many laws that codify the legal rights and support access to employment for individuals with disabilities (Table 21.1). These laws impact the service delivery models, funding, and types of services. The Individuals with Disabilities Education Act (IDEA) requires that children and youth with disabilities have access to publicly funded, individualized education including school-to-adult life transition services. This includes competitive employment (including supported employment); postsecondary education, vocational education, and continuing and adult education; and independent living and community participation. The occupational therapy practitioner offers skilled assessment and intervention strategies that are relevant to these targets.

The most recently amended version of IDEA (P.L. 108–446) states that transition-related planning must begin for students with disabilities when they are 16 years old or earlier based on individual student needs (§614[d][1][A][i][VII]). Beginning at age 16 (age 14 or 15 in some states), IDEA requires that a student's Individualized Education Plan (IEP) include measurable transition goals and needed services. Transition goals must be based on the results of age-appropriate assessments and relate to postsecondary priorities in the areas of education, employment, and community living. An occupational therapy practitioner may encourage students and families to advocate for this process to begin earlier when they feel that the extra time for transition planning and services is warranted. This is often justified with students who will not pursue postsecondary education, but rather for whom participation in community employment and independent living will be the primary indicators of successful transition to adulthood. Students receiving transition-related planning and services may graduate or complete high school around the age of 18 with their peers who do not have disabilities. Others may continue to receive school-funded education and transition services through the age of 21, though some states provide these services for longer. For example, Michigan provides special education until age 26. Because the legal requirement for special education and transition services ends upon high school graduation, some individuals may choose to delay graduation so that they continue to receive special education and transition services. High school exit decisions (before age 22) are based on individual student needs and goals as determined by the transition team. The occupational therapy practitioner can counsel the student, family, and IEP team about the value of delaying high school exit. In most cases the level of resources and services available through special education will exceed those available through adult service providers.

**TABLE 21.1 Laws and Regulations to Support Employment for People With Disabilities**

| Law/Regulation | Impact on Employment |
|---|---|
| Individuals with Disabilities Education Improvement Act of 2004 (IDEA) (PL 108–446) | Guarantees all children a free and appropriate public education including a federal mandate for comprehensive school-to-adult life transition services starting at the age of 16 years old or earlier based on the individual student needs. |
| Common Core State Standards | National curricula guide in English language arts (ELA) and mathematics that defines the knowledge and skills all students should master by the end of each grade level, so students are ready for college and career (Council of Chief State School Officers, 2013). These were developed in response to the increasing number of high school graduates who were not prepared for the rigor of college or the requirements of the workplace (Common Core State Standards Initiative, 2018). |
| Section 504 of the Rehabilitation Act (as amended in 1998 by PL 93–516) | The first civil rights law prohibiting discrimination based on disability by any program or agency that receives federal funding. Subparts of the law prohibit discrimination in employment, building and program accessibility, schooling (preschool through secondary education), and postsecondary education (colleges, universities, community colleges, vocational programs). Transition services may include reasonable accommodations under Section 504 of the Rehabilitation Act. |
| Americans with Disabilities Act (ADA) of 1990 (amended in 2008; PL 110–325) | ADA is a civil rights law that focuses on accessibility and nondiscrimination that extends protections beyond those programs and services that receive federal funding. The law also establishes clear accessibility standards for new building construction and public facilities. |
| Workforce Innovation and Opportunity Act (WIOA) of 2014 (implemented in 2016) | WIOA requires that state vocational rehabilitation agencies partner with students, their families, and school districts to encourage community-based employment as the desired high school graduation outcome (Fabian et al., 2016). This has altered the way that high school transition plans are written to better prepare a student with a disability for life after high school. |
| Home and Community Based Services (HCBS) | Home and Community Based Services (HCBS) final settings rule (Administration for Community Living, 2024) determines how Medicaid funds can be spent to support individuals with disabilities during the day. Medicaid will no longer pay for services provided in segregated settings (such as sheltered workshops) starting in 2022. The intention of the HCBS rule is twofold. First and foremost is the overriding principle that people with disabilities have the right to access and be fully integrated in their local community. The second intention is to raise expectations of how and where individuals with disabilities live, work, play, and participate. |

IDEA defines *transition services* as a coordinated set of activities for a child with a disability that:

(A) is designed to be within a results-oriented process, that is focused on improving the academic and functional achievement of the child with a disability to facilitate the child's movement from school to post-school activities, including postsecondary education, vocational education, integrated employment (including supported employment), continuing and adult education, adult services, independent living, or community participation;

(B) is based on the individual child's needs, taking into account the child's strengths, preferences, and interests; and

(C) includes instruction, related services, community experiences, the development of employment and other post-school adult living objectives, and, when appropriate, acquisition of daily living skills and functional vocational evaluation (§602[26]).

Post-school VR services support youth that have graduated or exited the educational system. These services are provided through mechanisms such as state and federally funded VR agencies and Medicaid Home and Community Based Services (HCBS; Medicaid.gov, 2022). VR agency titles vary by state and may also include phrases like rehabilitation services, disability employment, and adult career and education. Occupational therapy practitioners are too often under- or unrepresented on transition teams supporting school-to-work transitions (Abbott & Provident, 2017) and within VR services, although the unique training and approaches used by practitioners are potentially some of the most important (Rosner et al., 2020) in supporting successful employment outcomes for transition-age youth.

The *Workforce Innovation and Opportunity Act* (WIOA) of 2014 (implemented in 2016) altered the way that high school transition plans are written to better prepare a student with a disability for life after high school. The WIOA requires that state VR agencies partner with students, their families, and school districts to encourage community-based employment as the desired high school graduation outcome (Fabian et al., 2016). This significant change affects the students, their family, and the way that schools and state VR agencies deliver transition services. Previously, many students had transition plans with a goal for the student to attend a sheltered workshop or other segregated setting upon high school graduation. State departments of VR typically left the provision of services to the department of developmental disabilities and considered most of these individuals as unemployable. The WIOA made this practice illegal and requires that VR agencies offer community-based employment services to students with disabilities while they are still in high school. VR departments are now required to integrate into the school system, attend employment planning meetings, and pay for services that the student needs to discover their employment interests and develop employment skills. Specifically, WIOA requires that each state spends at least 15% of the federal VR funds it receives on preemployment transition services (Pre-ETS) for either students with disabilities (14–21) or youth with disabilities (14–24). Students are those who are in school with access to a free and appropriate education until the age of 22. Youths are those who graduate with a high school diploma or certificate.

Occupational therapy practitioners have a unique skill set that makes them qualified to provide Pre-ETS. In the assessment and treatment process, occupational therapy practitioners consider both the environment and individual client factors when implementing Pre-ETS and employment transition services (ETS) for transition-age youth. Table 21.2 includes the required Pre-ETS, exemplar applications, and links to the websites that contain these resources. All five types of Pre-ETS are within occupational therapy's scope of practice. In addition, occupational therapy practitioners have a long history of providing training in social skill development, independent living skills, and self-advocacy. WIOA provides an opportunity for occupational therapy practitioners to offer services in the community.

**TABLE 21.2 Required Preemployment Training Services**

| Pre-ETS | Exemplar Applications | Website |
|---|---|---|
| **Job exploration counseling** | | |
| | *Provide curricular options to the transition team and implement them* | |
| | • Explore-work.com | https://explore-work.com |
| | • T-Folio | https://www.cctstfolio.com |
| | • Transition Tennessee | https://transitiontn.org |
| | *Assess vocational interests using visual and video-based tools* | |
| | • Pictorial Interest Inventory (PII) | https://www.questar.org/wp-content/uploads/2017/08/pictorial-interest-inventory.pdf |
| | • Vocational Preference Inventory (VPI) | http://career.iresearchnet.com/career-assessment/vocational-preference-inventory-vpi/ |
| | • Career Cluster Survey | https://careerwise.minnstate.edu/careers/clusterSurvey |
| | • Photo Career Quiz | https://www.truity.com/test/photo-career-quiz |
| | *Explore careers* | |
| | • O*NET online | https://www.onetonline.org |
| | • Careeronestop.org | https://www.careeronestop.org |
| | • Workforce GPS | https://www.workforcegps.org |
| | • Khan Academy life skills career videos | https://www.khanacademy.org/college-careers-more/career-content |
| **Work-based learning experiences** | | |
| | • Job shadowing<br>• Career mentorship<br>• Informational interviews<br>• Workplace tours/field trips<br>• Paid internships<br>• Volunteering and unpaid internships, such as practicum, service-learning, simulated work, student-led enterprises | http://www.wintac.org/topic-areas/pre-employment-transition-services/overview/work-based-learning-experiences#JS |
| **Access to postsecondary education** | | |
| | • College and Career Competency Framework | https://www.cccframework.org |
| | • Increasing postsecondary opportunities and success for students and youth with disabilities | https://sites.ed.gov/idea/files/increasing-postsecondary-opportunities-and-success-09-17-2019.pdf |
| | • Think College | https://thinkcollege.net |
| **Workplace readiness training (with an emphasis on social skills and independent living at home and in the community)** | | |
| | • Social and interpersonal skills | https://transitionta.org/topics/pre-ets/workplace-readiness-training/#Chapter 24 |
| | • Independent living skills | Chapters 13 and 14<br>Also: https://transitionta.org/effective-practices/predictor/?id=self-care-independent-living-skills |
| | • Habits of work | https://nextsteps-nh.org/wp-content/uploads/2020/11/Habits-of-Work-Full-Curriculum-2012.pdf |
| | • Workplace readiness skills training checklist | http://wintac-s3.s3-us-west-2.amazonaws.com/topic-areas/ta01-pre-ets/checklist-WPRT-20-0806.pdf |
| **Instruction in self-advocacy** | | |
| | • Me! Lessons for teaching self-awareness and self-advocacy | https://www.ou.edu/education/zarrow/resources/curriculum<br>https://transitiontn.org/curriculum/me-lessons-for-teaching-self-awareness-and-self-advocacy/ |
| | • Project TEAM | https://yell.ot.phhp.ufl.edu/ |
| | • Self-advocacy and the transition to college | https://nextsteps-nh.org/wp-content/uploads/Self-advocacy-and-the-Transition-to-College-12-13-2011.pdf |
| | • Self-advocacy strategy | https://edgeenterprisesinc.com/product/self-advocacy-strategy-enhancing-student-motivation-and-self-determination/ |
| | • My journey of self discovery | https://www.crisoregon.org/cms/lib/OR01928264/Centricity/Domain/45/Documents/A-My-Journey-of-Self-Discovery.pdf |
| | • Instruction in self advocacy | https://transitionta.org/topics/pre-ets/self-advocacy/ |

*Continued*

**TABLE 21.2 Required Preemployment Training Services—cont'd**

| Pre-ETS | Exemplar Applications | Website |
|---|---|---|
| | • ChoiceMaker self-determination transition curriculum | https://www.ou.edu/education/zarrow/resources/curriculum |
| | • Whose future is it anyway? | https://www.ou.edu/education/zarrow/resources/curriculum |
| | • Transition guide – self-determination | https://www.imdetermined.org/tool/transition-guide-self-determination/ |
| | • Self-determined learning model of instruction | https://selfdetermination.ku.edu/wp-content/uploads/2019/05/Teachers-Guide-2019-Updated-Logos.pdf |
| | • Person-centered planning | https://transitionta.org/effective-practices/pd-person-centered-planning/ |
| | • Peer mentoring | https://www.pathwaysrtc.pdx.edu/model-my-life-tay |

Content on Pre-ETS is adapted from federally funded resources provided by the National Technical Assistance Center on Transition (NTACT) and the former Workforce Innovation Technical Assistance Center (WINTAC).

**TABLE 21.3 Examples of Person and Environment Employment Occupational Therapy Interventions for Transition-Aged Youth**

| Person-Focused Occupational Therapy Interventions | Environmentally Focused Occupational Therapy Interventions |
|---|---|
| Breaking down the job task into smaller chunks and providing structure or tools for learning (scaffolding the task) | Identifying and supporting the implementation of needed accommodations and modifications of job tasks for successful job performance |
| Role modeling and role-plays to learn interpersonal components of obtaining and maintaining a job (i.e., interviewing, interacting with coworkers, supervisors, and customers) | Adapting the physical environment as needed to ensure accessibility (i.e., modifying desk and seating ergonomics) and optimize employment outcomes (i.e., reducing distraction) |
| Teaching how to navigate job listing sites to identify employment opportunities and providing guidance to complete applications | Reducing sensory stimuli in the environment (i.e., moving desk to a quiet area of the office, using standing lights versus overhead lighting) to increase attention and focus to job responsibilities |
| Supporting problem-solving and providing feedback for learning new job tasks and technology | Educating and consulting with employers to identify strengths and potential accommodations for employees with disabilities |

## EMPLOYMENT AS AN OCCUPATION

Work is identified as one of the nine occupations within the domain of occupational therapy practice (American Occupational Therapy Association, AOTA, 2020). This establishes employment interventions as a part of the "profession's purview and an area in which its members have an established body of knowledge and expertise" (AOTA, 2020, p. 4). There are many occupational theories that conceptualize the relationship between the person, environment, and performance in an occupation that are applicable to the provision of transition to employment services (Goodman et al., 2020; Ivzori et al., 2020; Waisman-Nitzan et al., 2020). Intervention activities focus on strengthening the unique personal assets of each youth, capitalizing on their environmental resources, addressing their personal limitations and environmental challenges, and securing resources to enable successful employment outcomes.

The dual focus on personal and environmental factors is unique to occupational therapy. Table 21.3 provides examples of person- and environment-focused employment interventions for youth with disabilities. Despite overwhelming evidence that physical and social environmental barriers impede the success of obtaining and maintaining employment for people with disabilities (Pfeiffer et al., 2018; Scott et al., 2015; Walsh et al., 2014), most interventions place a heavy emphasis solely on person-level skill building. In contrast, occupational therapy practitioners personalize intervention components based on systematic assessments of both person- and environment-level barriers and facilitators to employment.

When evaluating person-level skills, occupational therapists often focus on performance skills (AOTA, 2020) that are needed for obtaining and/or maintaining employment. Although these can vary greatly based on the job itself, there are some skills that are needed across a variety of jobs. Employment skills are often classified into soft and hard job skills (United Disabilities Services Foundation, 2020). Soft job skills (Table 21.4) define how you work and involve interpersonal skills. These skills are important across all types of jobs and work environments (Fig. 21.1A–D). Occupational therapy practitioners can provide interventions to help people with soft skills such as time management, teamwork, problem-solving, and nonverbal communication.

Hard job skills are those that are specific to the job you are hired to perform. These are skills that are often taught in a step-by-step manner. The training in task analysis received by occupational therapy practitioners is helpful for breaking down whole job tasks into more easily learned portions or sequences for determining effective methods to teach them. Additionally, Occupational therapy-specific training in task analysis is helpful in being able to break down the job task and identify effective methods to teach the task. Additionally, occupational therapy practitioners can identify beneficial accommodations and assistive technology to support job skill performance. These types of interventions address the environmental components of the task.

Environmental factors include the physical, social, and attitudinal aspects of the job/work (AOTA, 2020). These factors can serve as a facilitator or barrier to successful employment. For example, a work environment that does not have an accessible physical workspace for someone who uses a wheelchair to mobilize is considered a barrier, whereas providing a quiet office space for someone who is easily distracted by sensory stimuli in the environment is a facilitator (Fig. 21.2). The attitudes of supervisors and peers toward disability can serve as a powerful facilitator or barrier within the work environment. In

**TABLE 21.4 Soft Skills Necessary for Any Job**

| Social/Interpersonal Skills | Independent Living Skills | Other Skills |
|---|---|---|
| • Communication | • Hygiene | • Financial literacy |
| • Positive attitude | • Time management | • Orientation and mobility |
| • Teamwork | • Healthy lifestyle | • Job-seeking skills |
| • Problem-solving | • Using a cell phone | • Understanding expectations |
| • Talking and writing | • Using transportation | |
| • Cooperation | • Money management | |
| • Active listening | • Meal preparation | |
| • Decision-making | • Community participation | |
| • Conflict resolution | • Safety | |
| • Body language | • Friendships | |
| • Empathy | • Dressing | |
| • Professionalism | • Behavior | |
| • Manners | | |
| • Supporting others | | |
| • Respectfulness | | |

Content on required Pre-ETS is adapted from federally funded resources provided by the National Technical Assistance Center on Transition (NTACT) and the former Workforce Innovation Technical Assistance Center (WINTAC).

addition to direct employment services provided to support the person, consultative services including environmental adaptations and education for employers can reduce environmental barriers and facilitate successful employment outcomes. Occupational therapy practitioners can assess the resources, attitudes, and opportunities for the person to determine if it is a high-functioning or low-functioning work environment (Patten, 2022). A high-functioning environment has numerous factors that facilitate successful employment outcomes, whereas a low-functioning environment has barriers that negatively impact these outcomes as a result of a poor person-environment fit. A primary role of occupational therapy practitioners in Pre-ETS is to identify the fit between the person's strengths and the environment of the job, as demonstrated in Case Example 21.1. This starts with a comprehensive occupational therapy evaluation as described in Chapter 9.

A wide range of other occupations of concern to occupational therapy practitioners, may serve as barriers or facilitators to successful employment outcomes (AOTA, 2020). These include the following.

- instrumental activities of daily living (e.g., driving and community mobility; see Chapter 14 & 20)
- activities of daily living (e.g., hygiene and grooming; see Chapter 13)
- health maintenance (e.g., medication and personal device management)
- social participation (e.g., engaging in social interactions with peers and other community members; see Chapter 24)
- rest and sleep (e.g., sleep preparation and participation; see Chapter 12)

For example, a lack of sleep can contribute to poor skill performance related to fatigue, whereas the inability to navigate use of transportation can influence the ability to get to a job site (Fig. 21.3) These must be considered in Pre-ETS, especially when there is an impact on employment outcomes for the youth.

## WORK SKILLS AND EMPLOYMENT: OCCUPATIONAL THERAPY APPROACHES AND INTERVENTIONS

As members of IEP and transition planning teams, occupational therapy practitioners are well positioned to implement evidence-based practices that are linked to positive postsecondary employment outcomes (Mazzotti et al., 2021). These approaches range from simple strategies designed to improve skills, knowledge, or access to community-based experiences to fully developed and tested transition programs or curricula that emphasize employment-related skills (Rosner et al., 2020). These interventions do not necessarily mention occupational therapy or include occupational therapy in their designs, but they fall within the profession's scope as defined within the Occupational Therapy Practice Framework: Domain and Process (4th ed.; AOTA, 2020). As such, the strategies included here are appropriate for occupational therapy intervention and represent the best evidence available in work skills and employment support.

### Collaborative Interdisciplinary and Interagency Teamwork

Outcome-oriented, student-centered planning and services based on collaborative interdisciplinary teamwork are at the center of high-quality transition services (Wehman, 2013). For transition-age students, this teamwork is accomplished by the IEP or transition team. As students with disabilities approach graduation from high school, all IEP planning and services must converge around the student's postsecondary goals and activities (Kohler & Field, 2003). When representatives from nonschool agencies join the student, family members, teachers, and related service personnel on the transition team, the interdisciplinary team becomes an interagency team. Congress, when crafting IDEA, did not intend for schools to have sole responsibility for transition processes and outcomes. Interagency linkages became a part of IDEA in 1990, indicating the expectation for shared responsibility across local education agencies and adult or community programs. Establishing interagency linkages, while challenging, can be an important benefit to students with disabilities who are preparing to exit the public education system (Stodden et al., 2004).

Upon graduation or completion of public education programs, a student's IDEA-based entitlement to school-sponsored educational, vocational, and other services ends. In the place of one lead agency (the school system), several service agencies such as the state VR agency, the state departments of mental health and developmental disabilities, state brain injury programs, postsecondary education, or training programs become responsible for providing services to individuals who qualify. Individuals who are no longer eligible for the school's transition-focused special education or related services become responsible for identifying where to obtain the ongoing services they

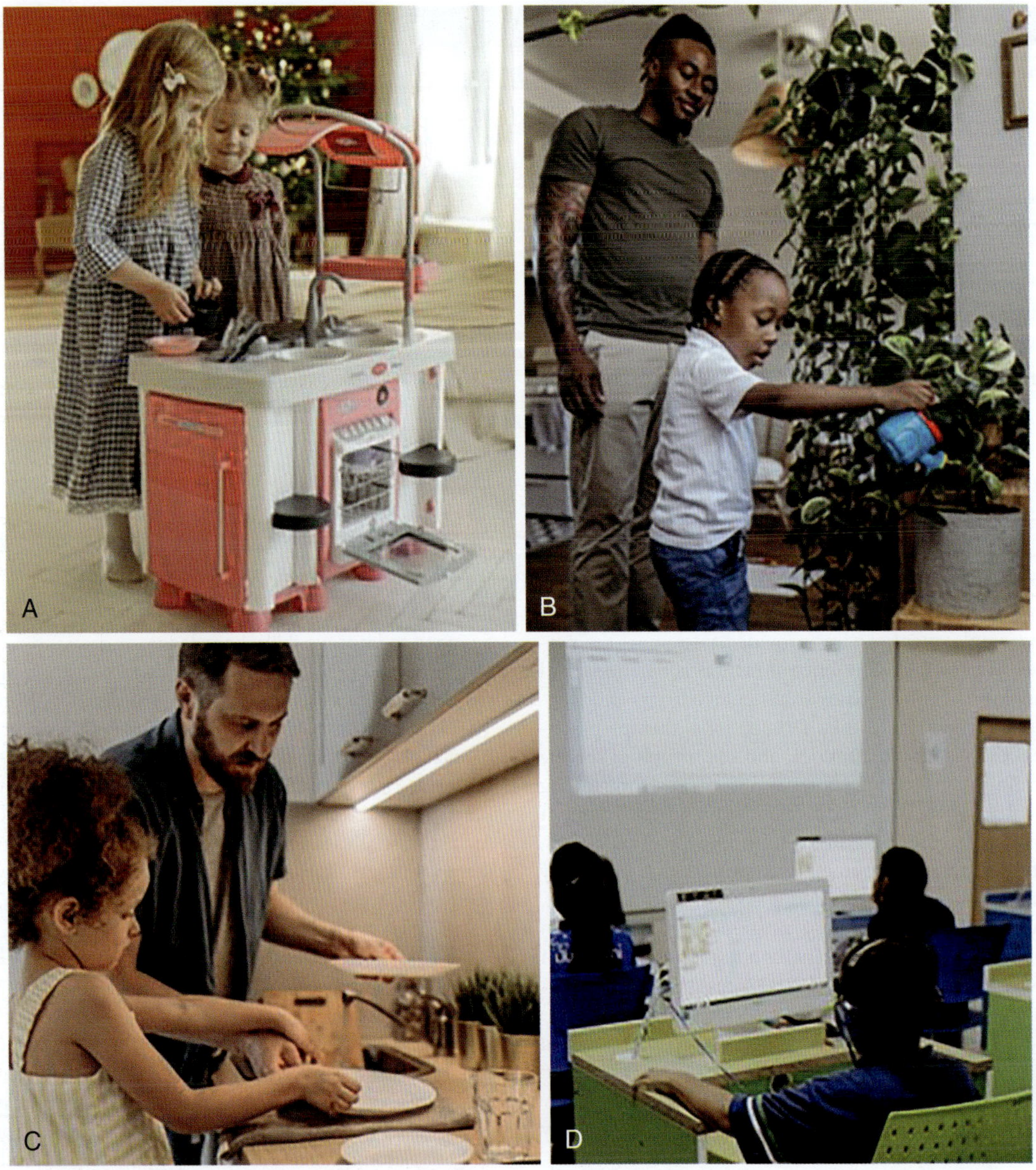

**Fig. 21.1** Childhood occupations provide opportunities for early development of employment-related soft skills. (A) Playing with kitchen toys. (B) Engaging in daily chores by watering houseplants. (C) Washing the dishes. (D) Learning to use computers for school. ((A) Polesie toys. (2018). *Photo of Kids Playing With Kitchen Plastic Toy* [Photograph]. Pexels. https://www.pexels.com/photo/photo-of-kids-playing-with-kitchen-plastic-toy-4484887/. (B) Mizuno K. (2022). *Daughter Watering Houseplants with Father* [Photograph]. Pexels. https://www.pexels.com/photo/daughter-watering-houseplants-with-father-12788487/. (C) Danilyuk, P. (2021). *Man in Blue Polo Washing the Dishes* [Photograph]. Pexels. https://www.pexels.com/photo/man-in-blue-polo-washing-the-dishes-8763141/. (D) Lach, R. (2021). *Students Using Computers* [Photograph]. Pexels. https://www.pexels.com/photo/students-using-computers-10638082/)

need and for demonstrating their eligibility to receive those services. Interagency responsibilities and linkages should be clearly stated in IEP documents developed by the transition team. Failure to initiate and formalize these connections during high school can result in the student missing opportunities to receive important services, coping with delays in receiving services, and potentially losing skills and motivation because of these delays and missed opportunities. The importance of strong interagency linkages cannot be overstated.

For transition-age students, collaboration is viewed as an effective way for a team to come together to help them plan for and achieve desired transition outcomes in the areas of postsecondary education, community living and recreation, and employment. Collaborative teams share a sense of purpose with shared responsibility for student outcomes (Hanft & Shepherd, 2016; Povenmire-Kirk et al., 2015). An effective transition team is not simply a collection of individuals, each with a different set of skills. Collaboration should be evident during the planning of individualized transition services and documented in the student's IEP and is essential given the variety of interdisciplinary team members representing the school's and community's interests. This type of planning is often termed person-centered and involves a group of individuals who know the student well and who have come together to engage in a positive, facilitated discussion focused on the

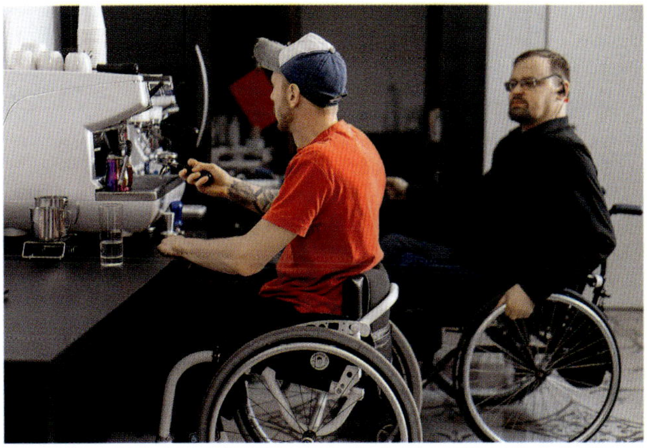

Fig. 21.2 A work environment that is accessible and spacious facilitates the ability for individuals who need wheelchairs to be able to work. (Source: Nilov, M. (2021). *People in Wheelchair Working in a Coffee Shop* [Photograph]. Pexels. https://www.pexels.com/photo/people-in-wheelchair-working-in-a-coffee-shop-7698023/)

## CASE EXAMPLE 21.1 ADDRESSING PERSON AND ENVIRONMENTAL FACTORS

Danny is a 21-year-old autistic young man who recently transitioned out of high school. He receives postsecondary VR services through HCBS waivers that include occupational therapy (Table 21.1). His most recent occupational therapy evaluation identified that stimulating environments are perceived as overwhelming and distracting for Danny. Strengths were identified in his attention to detail and his knowledge about different types of cars. He identified his long-term transition goals as obtaining a job that can support him to live on his own in the future and enjoy his interest in cars, although he did not want to learn to drive at that time. Danny was not interested in attending further schooling after high school.

**Occupational therapy intervention:** Occupational therapy focused on both person-centered and environmentally focused interventions based on Danny's self-identified goals using the Canadian Occupational Performance Measure (Table 21.5). Person-centered goals included developing the skills needed to obtain a job and identifying types of jobs that align with his interests and strengths. Danny worked with his occupational therapist to learn person-centered skills such as how to develop a resume, complete an interview, and interact with coworkers. They also focused on other work readiness skills (Table 21.4) such as learning how to use public transportation needed to get to a job and independent living skills such as health maintenance (e.g., scheduling health appointments, medicine organization and management), financial management (e.g., paying bills, budgeting), and home tasks (e.g., cleaning, doing laundry). Danny participated in a work-based internship program where he explored different types of jobs in the community based on his identified interests. Occupational therapy and other service providers supported his performance in these settings. The occupational therapist collaborated with Danny to identify environmental adaptations and accommodations based on the physical environment. This included wearing noise-attenuating headphones in loud and stimulating workspaces when not interacting with others or moving his workspace to a quieter area when possible. When job tasks involved multiple steps, an app on Danny's phone was used to provide a visual list of the steps needed to complete more complex tasks. The occupational therapist also collaborated with the job site supervisors and coworkers to reduce any attitudinal or social environmental barriers. In collaboration with his occupational therapist, Danny identified environmental barriers in each job setting and problem solved strategies to ensure the right person-environment fit for a high-performance environment. At the end of the program, Danny was offered a job at one of his preferred internship sites.

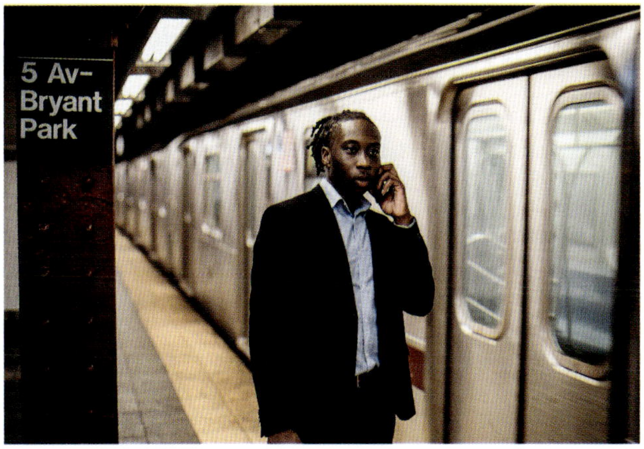


Fig. 21.3 The ability to navigate public transportation allows greater access to possible employment opportunities.

student's future. Emerging from this discussion is a comprehensive understanding of the student's unique strengths and interests, effective supports and accommodations, and potential resources and opportunities that can be incorporated into the student's transition services. Collaborative, group-oriented planning processes have been shown to be an effective approach to student evaluation and transition planning (Holburn & Vietze, 2002).

## Mental Health Interventions

Obtaining and maintaining employment is a challenge for those living with serious mental illness. There is strong evidence for cognitive interventions and the Individual Placement and Supports (IPS) model to improve employment skills and outcomes among those with severe mental illness (Noyes et al., 2018). Like Pre-ETS, soft skills, assessment, and collaborative strategies, IPS and cognitive interventions fall squarely within the occupational therapy scope of practice. Readers are encouraged to see the systematic review completed by Noyes et al., 2018), which provides an excellent summary on the substantial evidence in this area and a comprehensive list of references.

## Fostering Student Involvement in Transition Planning

IDEA requires that youth with disabilities be invited to IEP meetings when postsecondary goals are considered; however, actual participation of students with disabilities remains limited. Although almost half of students with disabilities provided at least some input at their most recent IEP meeting, only about 10%–20% took leadership roles at the meeting (Wagner et al., 2012). This limited participation is concerning because a student's ability to self-direct the IEP meeting and demonstrate self-advocacy for the transition planning process strongly relates to positive postsecondary outcomes (Clavenna-Deane & Coates, 2022; McConnell et al., 2012; Wehman, 2013).

The transition planning process is optimized by the inclusion of tools that enhance a student's ability to lead IEP meetings and make choices about postsecondary life. An occupational therapy practitioner who uses these tools contributes rigorous data to the transition planning process. At the same time, use of these instruments may help a student increase their awareness of personal strengths, needs, goals, and priorities. In many cases, direct instruction is required to teach individuals with disabilities to become aware of strengths and needs and to advocate for services. Over the past two decades, professionals, researchers, and other key stakeholders have developed several intervention techniques designed to improve a student's ability to participate in the IEP meeting and transition planning process (Alsaeed et al., 2023; Burke et al., 2020; Wehmeyer & Shogren, 2013). Several formal,

### TABLE 21.5 Self-Advocacy Strategy Steps Based on I PLAN Mnemonic

| Steps | Description |
|---|---|
| I | *Inventory* completed by students listing their strengths, weaknesses, learning needs, goals, and choices to prepare them for their upcoming IEP conference. |
| P | *Present* your inventory involves identifying appropriate time for the individual to share information during the conference, speaking clearly and completely, and referring to inventory as needed. |
| L | *Listen and respond* addresses being an active listener and responding to statements made by others in a positive manner. |
| A | *Ask questions* focuses on asking appropriate questions to gather needed information. |
| N | *Name your goals* to communicate goals and ideas on actions to be taken. |

Content is adapted from federally funded resources provided by the National Technical Assistance Center on Transition (NTACT).

evidence-based curricula exist for just this purpose. Occupational therapy practitioners interested in facilitating student participation in the transition planning process can incorporate these existing resources into their practice (see Table 21.2).

## Self-Advocacy Interventions

**Self-advocacy** refers to one's ability to communicate effectively and negotiate with others regarding rights and responsibilities. Self-advocacy is best viewed as a component of self-determination. Self-advocacy is of interest to many of the partners in the transition process. Here, we highlight three intervention approaches: (1) the Self-Advocacy Strategy (SAS), (2) ME! Lessons, and (3) Project TEAM. These are evidence based and suitable for use by occupational therapy practitioners supporting transition to employment. See Table 21.2 for links to these programs.

The SAS is an evidence-based practice designed to prepare youth to participate in IEP and transition planning meetings. The program consists of five steps that are built around the mnemonic "I PLAN" (Table 21.5). To date, the SAS program has been used to do the following: (1) improve student organization before IEP meetings (Cease-Cook et al., 2013); (2) identify goals before and during the IEP meeting (Lancaster et al., 2002; Van Reusen & Bos, 1994; Van Reusen et al., 1989); and (3) increase student verbal contributions and participation during the IEP meeting (Van Reusen & Bos, 1994; Lancaster et al., 2002; Hammer, 2004; Test & Neale, 2004; Cease-Cook et al., 2013). The skills emphasized by the SAS become increasingly important for adolescents as they encounter novel environments in adult life. For example, youth in need of reasonable accommodations (Box 21.1) will need to request, suggest, and negotiate these with their supervisor and/or employer's human resources department.

Similar to SAS, ME! Lessons is an evidence-based curriculum composed of modules designed to improve self-awareness and self-advocacy skills among youth (Cantley et al., 2010). Lesson plans and materials are designed for use with youth during the high school years and are aligned with Common Core State Standards (CCSS, 2018). Users of ME! Lessons are encouraged to modify the lessons to meet individual student and teacher needs. Units 8, 9, and 10 are especially relevant to employment and include content on disclosing one's disability, advocating for accommodations, and practice with performance evaluations and improvement plans (Table 21.6).

### BOX 21.1 Examples of Reasonable Accommodations for Employment Under the Americans With Disabilities Act

- Communications in writing such as email, using computers, mailboxes, bulletin boards, posters, and public addresses.
- Accessible training and in-service including sign language interpreters and written materials in alternative formats (e.g., PDF, large print, braille, audio).
- Restructuring of job tasks, functions, and the distribution of functions throughout the day.
- Flexible use of leave (e.g., sick, PTO, unpaid). For example, for medical treatment, recuperation, or rest, obtaining repairs to equipment and assistive devices, avoiding adverse environmental conditions, training a service dog, and/or to learning to use braille or sign language.
- Modified or part-time schedules, especially under the Family Medical Leave Act.
- Modified workplace policies such as permission to eat or drink at one's workplace, store medications (e.g., insulin), use phones or tablets to support performance, and modify attendance requirements.
- Environmental modifications that reduce sensory stimuli (e.g., changes in lighting, workstation relocation to a quieter area) and use of other tools (e.g., sunglasses, noise-attenuating headphones) that do not interfere with essential job functions (Case Example 21.1).
- Reassignment within the organization to an open position that better fits individual abilities.
- Provide reserved parking, aids, or services to improve access, including accessibility in the work area.

The "Project Teens making Environmental and Activity Modifications" (TEAM) program is a self-advocacy intervention for transition-age youth that emphasizes problem-solving (Kramer, 2015). Within this group-based intervention, participants identify environmental supports and barriers to participation, generate suggestions for modifications, and request reasonable accommodations. Project TEAM is grounded in evidence-based approaches including (1) cognitive-behavioral therapy, (2) Universal Design for Learning, (3) peer and social learning, and (4) experiential learning. A growing body of evidence on the Project TEAM intervention demonstrates that participants increased problem-solving, self-determination, and goal attainment (Kramer et al., 2017, 2018, 2019).

## Self-Determination Interventions

Self-determined students (1) demonstrate self-awareness and self-advocacy; (2) make choices and decisions; (3) problem-solve when issues arise; and (4) achieve self-identified goals. Beyond the self-advocacy interventions mentioned above, there are extensive self-determination curricula developed and tested by special educators. Here, we highlight three approaches that are especially well supported by research: (1) ChoiceMaker Self-Determination Curriculum and the Self-Directed IEP, (2) Whose Future Is It Anyway? and (3) the Self-Determined Learning Model of Instruction. See Table 21.2 for links to these programs.

**Choice Maker Program and Self-Directed IEP.** The ChoiceMaker program (Martin & Marshall, 1995, 1996) is designed to teach middle and secondary students skills needed for school and adult life and includes an additional evidence-based practice, the Self-Directed IEP (Allen et al., 2001; Martin et al., 2006). The ChoiceMaker curriculum consists of three complementary strands: (1) choosing goals, (2) communicating goals though Self-Directed IEP meetings, and (3) taking

TABLE 21.6 ***ME! Lessons*** **Content Focused on Employment**

| Unit 8: Advocating for My Needs After High School | Unit 9: Developing My Resources | Unit 10: Putting It All Together |
|---|---|---|
| • Disclosing disability<br>• Legal/illegal interview questions<br>• Responding to questions about disabilities<br>• Responding to inappropriate questions about disabilities | • Complete a summary of performance that describes impacts of disability, strengths, accommodations, and goals.<br>• Work with parents to complete the "YOU! Scale" that describes understanding and expectations. | • Work with student to complete the "ME! Scale," which reflects self-awareness and ability to self-advocate.<br>• Compare parent and student responses and identify discrepancies.<br>• Identify areas for continued improvement. |

TABLE 21.7 **Self-Directed Individualized Education Plan (IEP)**

| Lesson Number | Topic |
|---|---|
| 1 | Begin meeting by stating purpose |
| 2 | Introduce everyone |
| 3 | Review past goals and performance |
| 4 | Ask for others' feedback |
| 5 | State your school and transition goals |
| 6 | Ask questions |
| 7 | Deal with differences of opinion |
| 8 | State the support you'll need |
| 9 | Summarize your goals |
| 10 | Close meeting |
| 11 | Work on IEP goals all year |

action to attain goals. ChoiceMaker materials within the context of functional academic coursework and/or with students who are engaged in vocational activities such as work study, volunteering, on-the-job training, and paid work.

The Self-Directed IEP (Martin et al., 2006) is included within the ChoiceMaker curriculum, but it also stands on its own as an evidence-based practice. Lessons are provided in a multimedia format that includes an instructor's manual, student workbook, and two videos. The content is organized in 11 lessons (Table 21.7) and may be taught in 6–10 sessions. The developers of the Self-Determined IEP and the ChoiceMaker Curriculum suggest providing this instruction in a resource room, study skills class, or other settings. Occupational therapy practitioners working with special education teams may use these materials to teach middle and high school aged students to manage their own IEP.

**Whose Future Is It Anyway?.** Whose Future is it Anyway? is a 36-session transition-planning curriculum focused on individualized student needs, interests to build self-management, problem-solving, and goal-based decision-making skills (National Technical Assistance Center on Transition [NTACT], 2022). The program may be implemented in middle school for students with intellectual, learning, and/or developmental disabilities and is based on the following values: (1) students who engage in planning their transition will be more active in their planned education occupations, (2) students of all abilities are capable of education, and (3) giving children a voice may allow them to feel more likely to participate in future activities (NTACT, 2022). According to Lee et al. (2011), students that participated in Whose Future is it Anyway? program reported more confidence with transition planning, more determination in school, and higher self-efficacy with educational decisions. Occupational therapy practitioners working in schools and outpatient settings may use the free and accessible materials and handouts for Whose Future is it Anyway?

**Self-Determined Learning Model of Instruction.** The *Self-Determined Learning Model of Instruction (SDLMI)* is an evidence-based model that is oriented on self-direction and self-regulation for middle and high school students with and without disabilities. Occupational therapy practitioners can utilize this framework for their students to enhance self-determination through goal planning (National Technical Assistance Center on Transition, 2022b). The three phases of SDLMI include setting the goal, taking action, and adjusting as needed based on individual needs, environmental factors, and abilities (Wehmeyer & Shogren, 2013). SDLMI may be useful for occupational therapy practitioners aiming to focus on improving specific problem-solving and goal-oriented self-determination skills in inclusive academic classrooms.

## Early, Paid Work Experience

Among the many examples where occupation is used as both means (i.e., intervention) and ends (i.e., outcome), perhaps none is more relevant than work. Work is one of the most fundamental human occupations. Identity, self-worth, health, socioeconomic status, and quality of life (QoL) are strongly linked to one's ability to work independently and earn a living wage (Corcoran, 2004; Kober & Eggleton, 2005; Miller & Dishon, 2006). Beyond the functional and economic implications, work also provides a social-cognitive structure through which humans interact with and experience the world (Datson et al., 2012). Engagement in meaningful work enables development of social networks and self-efficacy, provides a sense of belonging and security, and contributes to overall health and QoL (Fig. 21.4). Occupational therapy practitioners employing a holistic approach are ideally situated to optimize the virtuous cycle of employment, health, and well-being.

Student engagement in paid work before their exit from high school is strongly associated with postsecondary employment (Newman et al., 2011) and is associated with the benefits described in the previous paragraph. Even for students who plan to pursue postsecondary education, the ability to maintain employment is considered a critical life skill that cannot be delayed until all formal education is complete (McConnell et al., 2012). Although postsecondary students secure paid work using a variety of strategies (Bolles, 2011), students who have disabilities may lack the skills needed to effectively access or use conventional job search strategies. For these students, supported employment provides an important evidence-based alternative (Mazzotti et al., 2016; Poppen et al., 2017; Test et al., 2009). In supported employment, youth and adults receive on-the-job training and ongoing supports provided by a job coach to acquire and sustain employment in community businesses and organizations.

When an individual with disability struggles to find or maintain employment through supported employment, the transition team may consider customized employment. An alternative approach, customized employment "is a process for individualizing the employment relationship between a job seeker or an employee and an employer in

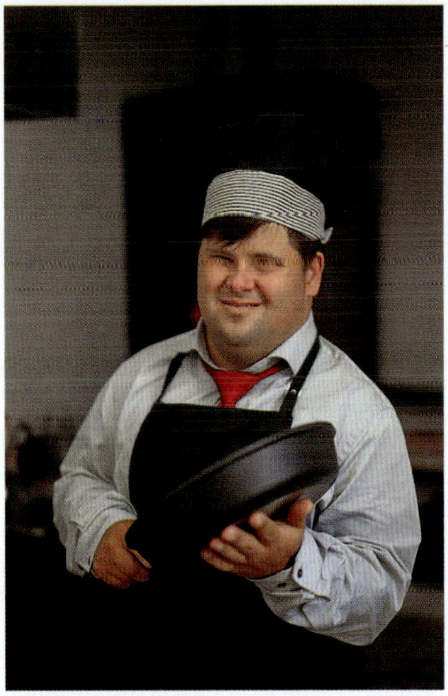

Fig. 21.4 Engagement in work that one finds enjoyable and meaningful provides a sense of belonging and security, and contributes to overall health and quality of life. This man was able to find employment in a restaurant, a job he enjoys.

**BOX 21.2 Vocational Choices for Transition-Age Youth and Young Adults**

- Internships to prepare for employment
- Work study
- Supported employment
- Customized employment
- Self-employment
- Day program or sheltered workshop
- Community rehabilitation program
- Competitive employment and business models

ways that meet the needs of both" (Inge, 2005, p. 1; Wehman & Brooke, 2013, p. 331). In this model, an employment specialist works with the client (i.e., individual with a disability) and prospective employers in the community to match the individual strengths and needs of the job seeker with the needs of the business. Oftentimes, this requires negotiating the rearranging or combining of job tasks into a job that is customized for the individual with a disability.

A review of the transition literature (McConnell et al., 2012) identified several work-related behaviors and experiences that relate to successful postsecondary employment outcomes. Participation in work study programs, vocational education classes, job internships, and mentoring experiences are all known to increase the likelihood of obtaining full-time employment after high school (Box 21.2). When students are given opportunities to practice self-management skills such as timeliness, orderliness, and cleanliness, they are more likely to succeed in the working world. Students who learn to express their desire for work, who actively pursue work, and who obtain work during the high school years are likely to matriculate into postsecondary education and/or employment after transition. Occupational therapy practitioners working with transition teams can help facilitate positive outcomes by ensuring that postsecondary goals and services target these factors.

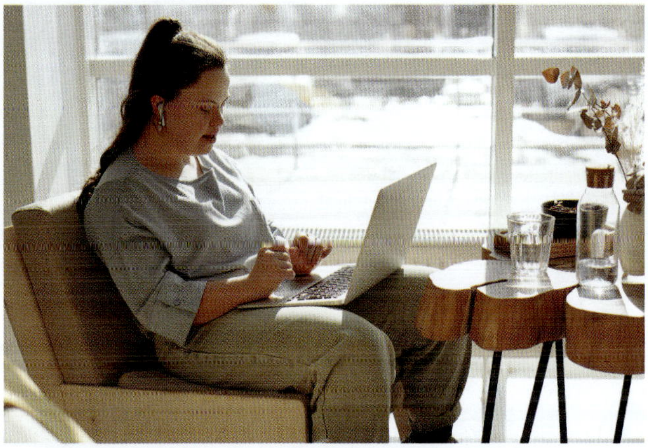

Fig. 21.5 Being able to use a computer is an important skill for many jobs. (Booth, C. (2020). *Girl Sitting on a Couch Using a Laptop* [Photograph]. Pexels. https://www.pexels.com/photo/girl-sitting-on-a-couch-using-a-laptop-4058219/)

## Technology Skills for Employment

Technology holds potential to assist students with disabilities as they transition into adulthood. The work of Wehman et al. (2015) demonstrates that youth with computer skills attain competitive employment at higher rates than those without (Fig. 21.5). Adolescents and young adults are avid users and consumers of technology and are "digital natives" who have been raised and educated with technology (Prensky, 2001). Wheelchairs, alternative and augmentative communication devices, environmental control units, and adaptive equipment can all help improve a person's ability to navigate and participate in life. While these supports can certainly increase independence, they may also make an individual appear disabled and different from their typical peers. New technologies and platforms allow students to use this assistive technology without separating them from their peers.

Concepts of Universal Design for Learning and accessibility mandates make commercially available technology useful in supporting students in transition (Case Example 21.2). Smart phones, tablets, and computers have accessible features that many consumers have found to improve efficiency and productivity. Additional applications (apps) or programs can be added to customize a device to the individual's unique needs.

Students have smartphones and tablet computers options from which they can choose. The operating system, size of the device, and technologic capabilities all dictate the device's functionality. Box 21.3 provides a brief overview of questions for practitioners to consider when they make technology recommendations for smartphone or tablet computer options (Cleary & Persch, 2013).

An advantage that tablets and smartphones have over other assistive technology is that students who use this technology are using the same technology that their typical peers use, so these devices can become tools of inclusion. These devices are also useful in supporting students as they transition into competitive employment. Business is ever increasing its reliance on information technology and adopting "paperless workplaces." In the past, a teacher or job coach may have photographed job tasks and assembled them into a three-ring paper binder that described how to perform a particular job. With smartphones and tablet computers, the bulky binders can be replaced by a tablet or smartphone with a series of photos or a video checklist to help support a student in employment (Gentry et al., 2012). Other

## CASE EXAMPLE 21.2

Carrie is a 16-year-old young woman with spina bifida who receives occupational therapy services in high school to support her transition. Occupational therapy service is focused on Pre-ETS provided through IDEA to support her transition to employment after high school. Carrie mobilizes with a cane or walker for short distances and uses a manual wheelchair when navigating longer distances. Her recent re-evaluation focused on the skills and abilities Carrie needs to be a healthy, independent, and productive adult using the Life Skills Inventory. Carrie and her occupational therapist also discussed her long-term goals. Carrie decided that she would like to live in her own apartment and have a job working with animals or children.

**Occupational therapy intervention:** Together, they developed a plan to help her reach her goals. For the occupational therapist, this plan also involved connecting Carrie and her family to programs that will support her as an adult with a disability. Occupational therapy helped Carrie learn self-determination skills necessary for making her own decisions and becoming more independent in her daily routines. Together, they identify assistive technology and environmental adaptations that will support independence. For example, Carrie's occupational therapist taught her how to use her smartphone to communicate with friends and family, set reminders, and use a navigation system when traveling by herself in the community. They also identified accessible forms of transportation and potential adaptations to work environments to ensure access when mobilizing with a wheelchair. A major aspect of Carrie's transition planning involved discovering her vocational interests, developing sustainable employment skills, and utilizing supports that facilitate successful employment in the community. Carrie enrolled in Project SEARCH, which provides opportunities for real-life work experience combined with training in employability and independent living skills. With this experience, Carrie can obtain employment as a veterinary technician at a local animal hospital. Carrie is learning independent living skills during occupational therapy so that she can eventually move to her own apartment and support herself financially. Occupational therapy services during this critical transition in her life can help Carrie become a healthy and productive adult.

## BOX 21.3 Smartphone and Tablet Computer Options: Which Device to Choose?

### What Operating System Should I Use?

- Android (Google) is often the least expensive device.
- iOS (Apple) has the most apps available to purchase.
- Windows (Microsoft Office) functions most like a typical computer operating system.

### What Hardware Capability Do I Need?

- Amount of storage: devices with greater storage are more expensive.
- Wi-Fi capability: will the student have access to a public Wi-Fi network (open or closed) to be able to access the device's full capability?
- Data network capability: will the student need the device in areas where there is no access to a public Wi-Fi network, and does a separate data plan need to be purchased?

### What Size of Device Would Be Best?

- Would the use of a smartphone and a tablet cause confusion?
- Does the device need to be small enough to be kept in a pocket?
- Does the device need to be large to allow for reduced visual or fine motor capability?
- Can the user manage a smart watch?

### What Built-in Accessibility Features Will the Student Need?

- Does the device offer text-to-speech?
- Does the device offer speech-to-text?
- Does the device offer options for those with low vision?
- Does the device have accessible options for individuals with physical limitations?

### What Apps Should Be Purchased to Make the Most out of the Device?

- What is the cost, and is it a one-time cost?
- Does the app require access to the internet to function properly?
- Does the app have an interface, so it can be used on a variety of devices?

examples of how this technology can support employment include the following.

1. Remote job coaching. A job coach can make a video call to an employee to check on how work is progressing, and the student can show the quality of their work remotely (Holm & Raina, 2012).
2. Telehealth. An occupational therapist can be brought in via video call (depending on state licensure requirements) to assess a task and help a student and job coach make adaptations to get the job done (Cason & Richmond, 2013). This approach is particularly beneficial in certain scenarios (e.g., when distance is a travel barrier, cramped workspaces, or workers who are uncomfortable drawing attention to themselves).
3. Video modeling applications can support a student as they move and learn to accomplish one task to the next on the job (Bennett et al., 2013; Hayes et al., 2015). Seaman et al. (2018) demonstrated the efficacy of paraprofessional-implemented video prompting to teach employment skills to youth with autism.
4. Emotional support applications can be customized to allow students to center and calm themselves during stressful situations (Blood et al., 2011).

Those looking to teach computer literacy and technology skills directly may want to consider EnvisionIT (EIT), a free career-readiness curriculum designed for middle and high school students. EIT is a digital, evidence-based curriculum (Izzo et al., 2010; Lombardi et al., 2017), appropriate both for students with and without disabilities, and focused on literacy and career skills. Lessons are aligned with learning standards in (1) information technology literacy, (2) English language arts, (3) college and career readiness, (4) financial literacy, and (5) career technical areas. The curriculum is in the public domain and freely available (https://transitiontn.org/curriculum/envision-it-curriculum/). Users may adapt the materials to suit individual needs (The Ohio State University Nisonger Center).

## The Project SEARCH Internship Model

Project SEARCH (https://projectsearch.us) is a 1-year transition to community employment program that combines on-site internships, job coaching, and an employment skills curriculum (Datson et al., 2012; Wehman et al., 2013). During their last year of public education (i.e., IDEA eligibility), students complete unpaid internships embedded within a host business (e.g., a Project SEARCH site). Students work approximately 20 hours per week with the support of a special education teacher and employment specialist (aka job coach) and complete a functional employment skills curriculum. Over the course of the academic year, student interns progress through a series of internships, typically two or three. Students build their resume, learn to utilize public transportation or drive, and practice job-searching strategies with the goal of interviewing for and obtaining a paid position at the end of the Project SEARCH year. Many Project SEARCH sites are in healthcare and hospitality settings with the emphasis on finding jobs that are well suited for an individual's unique talents (Fig. 21.6).

Cincinnati Children's Hospital developed the first Project SEARCH site in 1996. More than 25 years later, the model has been extended

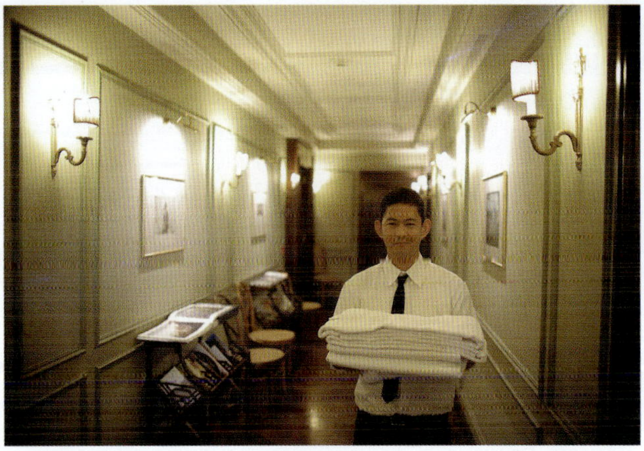

**Fig. 21.6** Many of the Project SEARCH sites are in healthcare or hospitality. (Piacquadio, A. (2017). *Man Holding White Linen Ad White Towel* [Photograph]. Pexels. https://www.pexels.com/photo/man-holding-white-linen-ad-white-towel-3770099/)

to approximately 700 Project SEARCH sites throughout the United States, Europe, and the Middle East (Project SEARCH, 2022).

Project SEARCH is made possible through innovative collaboration between transition partners. The public schools commit to provide a special educator to work with student internship on-site. That is, the special educator is embedded within the host business and not within a high school. This is usually sustainable for schools when 8–12 students participate in the program each year. A local "host" business provides a meeting space (i.e., classroom) and a variety of potential internships that students may pursue during the year. Additional funding comes from state VR agencies and departments of developmental disabilities. These resources are used to pay for the employment specialist, who also works on-site with student interns.

Research suggests that a history of participation in internships improves employment outcomes (Mazzotti et al., 2021). Internships may be chosen to suit an individual's skills or may be chosen to give an individual the opportunity to learn or develop new skills. The Vocational Fit Assessment (http://www.vocfit.com) was developed, in part, to inform selection of internship and job opportunities (Persch et al., 2015) and help transition teams identify priorities for intervention. Once the internship is selected, the job coach learns the job from the employer and instructs the student in how to complete the job. As the student's ability grows, the job coaching fades until the student is independent in completing the job.

A stated goal for this program is that 90% of Project SEARCH graduates become employed at the end of the program, and each year many sites achieve 90%–100% employment. Overall, the model achieves 60%–70% employment across all sites. This is a remarkable achievement, roughly double the national average for the population of transition-age youth.

Project SEARCH has partnered with occupational therapists, Drs. Dennis Cleary and Andrew Persch, for more than a decade. Cleary and Persch recognized the substantial opportunity for occupational therapy practitioners to support youth in transition to employment by collaborating with Project SEARCH sites. For example, occupational therapy practitioners working in the public schools may offer to consult or provide direct service under the IDEA to student interns participating in the program. Similarly, occupational therapy faculty and students may connect with sites to provide pro bono services that benefit both Project SEARCH interns and academic occupational therapy programs. Occupational therapy students can provide holistic assessments of person abilities and job demands, assist teams in goal setting, develop interventions (such as those in this chapter), modify work environments, and advocate for reasonable accommodations. Occupational therapy practitioners interested in working with Project SEARCH should visit https://projectsearch.us/.

## SUMMARY

Occupational therapy practitioners support work and employment skills across the lifespan. This work occurs in schools, clinics, and communities when occupational therapy practitioners provide a range of essential services that promote positive postsecondary employment outcomes for transition-age youth with disabilities. Occupational therapy practitioners understand the value of the occupation of work in fostering a person's sense of productivity, self-esteem, and self-determination; they also understand the societal barriers to employment that exist for many transition-age youth with disabilities. As such, they consider both environmental and individual client factors when providing preemployment transition services, offering a distinct perspective in the transition planning process.

Occupational therapy practitioners have unique training and expertise that make them well suited to use assessment tools and implement interventions and supports that meet the needs of transition-age youth during transition to employment. Using person-centered and environmentally focused interventions, occupational therapy practitioners can help facilitate successful transition to postsecondary employment for transition-age youth.

1. Transition planning requires the collaboration of multiple parties, including the student, family, teachers, related services personnel including occupational therapy practitioners, and community service providers. The plan includes clear goals and services that target participation in early work-based experiences and development of appropriate work-related behaviors.
2. Self-direction in the transition planning process is related to positive postsecondary outcomes for transition-age youth. Occupational therapy practitioners can facilitate development of self-determination and self-advocacy skills through various methods, including existing, evidence-based assessment tools and curricula.
3. Many laws require access to employment services for individuals with disabilities, including the IDEA and the WIOA. These laws impact service delivery models, funding mechanisms, and types of services provided to transition-age youth.
4. Vocational choices for transition-age youth include internships, work study, supported employment, customized employment, competitive employment and business models, community rehabilitation programs, and day programs or sheltered workshops. These options vary in their level of environmental support, community integration, and financial compensation. Occupational therapy practitioners should consider the needs and preferences of the student and family when recommending the least restrictive working environment.
5. Project SEARCH is a 1-year transition to community employment program for transition-age youth during their final year of IDEA eligibility (i.e., last year enrolled in public education). This internship model includes two to three on-site unpaid internships, job coaching, and employment skills curriculum. Project SEARCH aims to prepare student interns for full-time competitive employment in the community.

## REFERENCES


Abbott, B., & Provident, I. (2017). Changing occupational therapists' knowledge of their role in secondary transition planning. *Journal of Occupational Therapy, Schools, & Early Intervention*, *9*, 382–396. https://doi.org/10.1080/19411243.2016.1227760.

ADA Amendments Act of 2008, Pub. L. 110–325, 122 Stat. 3553–3559.

Administration for Community Living. HCBS settings rule. Retrieved on September 29, 2024. https://acl.gov/programs/hcbs-settings-rule#:~:text=The%20Home%20and%20Community%20Based,quality%20of%20Medicaid%2Dfunded%20HCBS.

Allen, S., Smith, A., Test, D. W., Flowers, C., & Wood, W. M. (2001). The effects of Self-Directed IEP on student participation in IEP meetings. *Career Development for Exceptional Individuals*, *24*, 107–120.

Alsaeed, A., Mansouri, M. C., Shogren, K. A., Raley, S. K., Kurth, J. A., Leatherman, E. M., & Lockman Turner, E. (2023). A systematic review of interventions to promote self-determination for students with extensive support needs. *Research and Practice for Persons with Severe Disabilities*, *48*(1), 3–24.

American Occupational Therapy Association. (2020). Occupational therapy practice framework: Domain and process (4th ed.). *American Journal of Occupational Therapy*, *74*(Suppl. 2), 7412410010. https://doi.org/10.5014/ajot.2020.74S2001.

Bennett, K. D., Gutierrez, A., & Honsberger, T. (2013). A comparison of video prompting with and without voice-over narration on the clerical skills of adolescents with autism. *Research in Autism Spectrum Disorders*, *7*(10), 1273–1281. https://doi.org/10.1016/j.rasd.2013.07.013.

Berkman, L. F. (2014). Commentary: The hidden and not so hidden benefits of work: Identity, income and interaction. *International Journal of Epidemiology*, *43*, 1517–1519. https://doi.org/10.1093/ije/dyu110.

Blood, E., Johnson, J. W., Ridenour, L., Simmons, K., & Crouch, S. (2011). Using an iPod Touch to teach social and self-management skills to an elementary student with emotional/behavioral disorders. *Education & Treatment of Children*, *34*(3), 299–321.

Bolles, R. N. (2011). *What color is your parachute? A practical manual for job-hunters and career-changers*. Ten Speed Press.

Burke, K. M., Raley, S. K., Shogren, K. A., Hagiwara, M., Mumbardó-Adam, C., Uyanik, H., & Behrens, S. (2020). A meta-analysis of interventions to promote self-determination for students with disabilities. *Remedial and Special Education*, *41*(3), 176–188.

Cantley, P., Little, K., & Martin, J. E. (2010). *ME! Lessons for teaching self-awareness and self-advocacy*. Retrieved from http://www.ou.edu/content/education/centers-and-partnerships/zarrow/trasition-education-materials/me-lessons-for-teaching-self-awareness-and-self-advocacy.html.

Cason, J., & Richmond, T. (2013). Telehealth opportunities in occupational therapy. In E. Kumar, & S. Cohn (Eds.), *Telerehabilitation* (pp. 139–162). Springer.

Cease-Cook, J., Test, D. W., & Scroggins, L. S. (2013). Effects of the CD-ROM version of the "Self-Advocacy Strategy" on quality of contributions in IEP meetings of high school students with intellectual disability. *Education and Training in Autism and Developmental*, *42*(2), 258–268. https://www.jstor.org/stable/23880644.

Clavenna-Deane, B. A., & Coates, W. R. (2022). High school experiences that support post-school success: What can We learn? *Career Development and Transition for Exceptional Individuals*, *45*(4), 176–186.

Cleary, D. S., & Persch, A. C. (April 2013). *iPads and iTechnology: Is it more engaging, efficient, and effective than traditional occupational therapy interventions in our schools?*. Retrieved from otwithanipad.blogspot.com.

Common Core State Standards Initiative. (2018). *In the states*. Retrieved from http://www.corestandards.org/standards-in-your-state/.

Corcoran, M. A. (2004). Work, occupation, and occupational therapy. *American Journal of Occupational Therapy*, *58*(4).

Council of Chief State School Officers. (April 2013). *Interstate Teacher Assessment and Support Consortium InTASC Model Core Teaching Standards and Learning Progressions for Teachers 1.0: A Resource for Ongoing Teacher Development*. Washington, DC: Author.

Datson, M., Riehle, J. E., & Rutkowski, S. (2012). *High school transition that works: Lessons learned from Project Search*. Paul H. Brookes.

Erickson, W., Lee, C., & von Schrader, S. (2018). *2016 Disability status report: United States*. Cornell University, Yang-Tan Institute on Employment and Disability.

Fabian, E., Simonsen, M., Deschamps, A., Shengli, D., & Luecking, D. M. (2016). Service system collaboration in transition: An empirical exploration of its effects on rehabilitation outcomes for students with disabilities. *Journal of Rehabilitation*, *82*(3), 3–10.

Gentry, T., Lau, S., Molinelli, A., Fallen, A., & Kriner, R. (2012). The apple iPod touch as a vocational support aid for adults with autism: Three case studies. *Journal of Vocational Rehabilitation*, *37*(2), 75–85.

Goodman, D., Caldwell, A., Bodnar, D., & Stover, A. (2020). Employable: Transition program to improve employment outcomes for students with disabilities-Needs assessment & current constraints. *Journal of Occupational Therapy, Schools, & Early Intervention*, *13*(2), 197–218.

Hammer, M. R. (2004). Using the self-advocacy strategy to increase student participation in IEP conferences. *Intervention in School and Clinic*, *39*(5), 295–380. https://doi.org/10.1177/10534512040390050601.

Hanft, B. E., & Shepherd, J. (Eds.). (2016). *Collaborating for student success: A guide for school-based occupational therapy* (2nd ed.) AOTA Press.

Hayes, G. R., Custodio, V. E., Haimson, O. L., Nguyen, K., Ringland, K. E., Ulgado, R. R., & Weiner, R. (2015). Mobile video modeling for employment interviews for individuals with autism. *Journal of Vocational Rehabilitation*, *43*(3), 275–287. https://doi.org/10.3233/JVR-150775.

Holburn, S., & Vietze, P. M. (2002). *Person-centered planning: Research, practice, and future directions*. Brookes.

Holm, M. B., & Raina, K. D. (2012). Emerging technologies for caregivers of a person with a disability. In R. Talley, & J. Crews (Eds.), *Multiple dimensions of caregiving and disability* (pp. 185–208). Springer.

Individuals With Disabilities Education Improvement Act of 2004, Pub. L. 108–446, 20 U.S.C. §§ 1400–1482.

Ivzori, Y., Sachs, D., Reiter, S., & Schreuer, N. (2020). Transition to employment program (SUPER) for youth at risk: A conceptual and practical model. *International Journal of Environmental Research and Public Health*, *17*(11), 3904

Izzo, M. V., Yurick, A., Nagaraja, H. N., & Novak, J. A. (2010). Effects of a 21st-century curriculum on students' information technology and transition skills. *Career Development for Exceptional Individuals*, *33*(2), 95–105. https://doi.org/10.1177/0885728810369348.

Kober, R., & Eggleton, I. R. C. (2005). The effect of different types of employment on quality of life. *Journal of Intellectual Disability Research*, *49*(10), 756–760.

Kohler, P. D., & Field, S. (2003). Transition-focused education: Foundation for the future. *The Journal of Special Education*, *37*(3), 174–183.

Kramer. (2015). Identifying and evaluating the therapeutic strategies used during a manualized self-advocacy intervention for transition-age youth. *OTJR*, *35*(1), 23–33. https://doi.org/10.1177/1539449214564146.

Kramer, J., Helfrich, C., Levin, M., Hwang, I., Samuel, P. S., Carrellas, A., Schwartz, A. E., Goeva, A., & Kolaczyk, E. D. (2018). Initial evaluation of the effects of an environmental–focused problem–solving intervention for transition–age young people with developmental disabilities: Project TEAM. *Developmental Medicine and Child Neurology*, *60*(8), 801–809. https://doi.org/10.1111/dmcn.13715.

Kramer, J., Helfrich, C., Schwartz, A., Samuel, P., Kolaczyk, E., & Goeva, A. (2019). Outcomes of an environmental-focused, problem-solving intervention for transition-age youth: Project TEAM. *American Journal of Occupational Therapy*, *73*(4_Suppl 1), 7311515321. https://doi.org/10.5014/ajot.2019.73S1-RP101C.

Kramer, J., Ryan, C. T., Moore, R. R., & Schwartz, A. A. (2017). Feasibility of electronic peer mentoring for transition-age youth and young adults with intellectual and developmental disabilities: Project TEAM (Teens making Environment and Activity Modifications). *Journal of Applied Research in Intellectual Disabilities*, *31*(1), e118–e129. https://doi.org/10.1111/jar.12346.

Lancaster, P. E., Schumaker, J. B., & Deshler, D. D. (2002). The development and validation of an interactive hypermedia program for teaching a self-advocacy strategy to students with disabilities. *Learning Disability Quarterly*, *25*(4), 277–302. https://doi.org/10.2307/1511358.

Lee, Y., Wehmeyer, M. L., Palmer, S. B., Williams-Diehm, K., Davies, D. K., & Stock, S. E. (2011). The effect of student-directed transition planning with a computer-based reading support program on the self-determination of students with disabilities. *The Journal of Special Education, 45*(2), 104–117. https://doi.org/10.1177/0022466909358916.

Lombardi, A. R., Izzo, M. V., Rifenbark, G. G., Murray, A., Buck, A., Monahan, J., & Gelbar, N. (2017). The impact of an online transition curriculum on secondary student reading: A multilevel examination. *Career Development and Transition for Exceptional Individuals, 40*(1), 15–24. https://doi.org/10.1177/2165143416681287.

Martin, J. E., & Marshall, L. H. (1995). Choice Maker: A comprehensive self-determination transition program. *Intervention in School and Clinic, 30*, 147–156

Martin, J. E., Van Dycke, J. L., Christensen, W. R., Greene, B. A., Gardner, J. E., & Lovett, D. L. (2006). Increasing student participation in their transition IEP meetings: Establishing the Self-Directed IEP as an evidenced-based practice. *Exceptional Children, 72*, 299–316.

Martin, J., & Marshall, L. (1996). Choice Maker: Infusing self determination instruction into the IEP and transition process. In D. J. Sands, & M. Wehmeyer (Eds.), *Self-determination across the lifespan: Independence and choice for people with disabilities* (pp. 215–236). Paul Brooks Publishing Co.

Mazzotti, V. L., Rowe, D. A., Kwiatek, S., Voggt, A., Chang, W.-H., Fowler, C. H., Poppen, M., Sinclair, J., & Test, D. W. (2021). Secondary transition predictors of postschool success: An update to the research base. *Career Development and Transition for Exceptional Individuals, 44*(1), 47–64. https://doi.org/10.1177/2165143420959793.

Mazzotti, V., Rowe, D., Sinclair, J., Poppen, M., Woods, W., & Shearer, M. (2016). Predictors of post-school success: A systematic review of NLTS2 secondary analysis. *Career Development and Transition for Exceptional Individuals, 39*(4), 196–215.

McConnell, Martin, J. E., Juan, C. Y., Hennessey, M. N., Terry, R. A., El-Kazimi, N. A., Pannells, T. C., & Willis, D. M. (2012). Identifying nonacademic behaviors associated with post-school employment and education. *Career Development and Transition for Exceptional Individuals, 36*(3), 174–187. https://doi.org/10.1177/2165143412468147.

Medicaid.gov. (2022). *Medicaid home and community based services.* Retrieved from https://www.medicaid.gov/medicaid/home-community-based-services/index.html.

Miller, A., & Dishon, S. (2006). Health-related quality of life in multiple sclerosis: The impact of disability, gender, and employment status. *Quality of Life Research, 15*(2), 259–271.

National Technical Assistance Center on Transition. (2022). http://transitionta.org/wp-content/uploads/docs/Whose-Future-Is-It-Anyway.pdf.

National Technical Assistance Center on Transition. (2022b). https://transitionta.org/wp-content/uploads/docs/PD_SDLMI-Self-Determination_Final.pdf.

Newman, L., et al. (2011). *The post-high school outcomes of young adults with disabilities up to 8 years after high school: A report from the national longitudinal transition study-2 (NLTS2)*. National Center for Special Education Research.

Noyes, S., Sokolow, H., & Arbesman, M. (2018). Evidence for occupational therapy intervention with employment and education for adults with serious mental illness: A systematic review. *American Journal of Occupational Therapy, 72*, 7205190010. https://doi.org/10.5014/ajot.2018.033068.

Patten, K. K. (2022). Finding our strengths: Recognizing professional bias and interrogating systems. *American Journal of Occupational Therapy, 76*(6), 7606150010.

Persch, A. C., Gugiu, P. C., Onate, J. A., & Cleary, D. S. (2015). Development and psychometric evaluation of the vocational fit assessment (VFA). *American Journal of Occupational Therapy, 69*(6):6906180080p1–6906180080p8. https://doi.org/10.5014/ajot.2015.019455.

Pfeiffer, B., Brusilovskiy, E., Davidson, A., & Persch, A. (2018). Impact of person-environment fit on job satisfaction for working adults with autism spectrum disorders. *Journal of Vocational Rehabilitation, 48*, 49–57.

Poppen, M., Linstrom, L., Unruh, D., Khurana, A., & Bullis, M. (2017). Preparing youth with disabilities for employment: An analysis of vocational rehabilitation case service data. *Journal of Vocational Rehabilitation, 46*, 209–224.

Povenmire-Kirk, T., Diegelmann, K., Crump, K., Schnorr, C., Test, D., Flowers, C., et al. (2015). Implementing CIRCLES: A new model for interagency collaboration in transition planning. *Journal of Vocational Rehabilitation, 42*, 51–65.

Prensky, M. (2001). Digital natives, digital immigrants part 1. *On the Horizon, 9*(5), 1–6.

Project SEARCH. (2022). Who we are. Retrieved from https://projectsearch.us/who-we-are/.

Rosner, T., Grasso, A., Scott Cole, L., Villalobos, A., & Mulcahey, M. J. (2020). Scoping review of school-to-work transition for youth with intellectual disabilities: A practice gap. *American Journal of Occupational Therapy, 74*, 7402205020. https://doi.org/10.5014/ajot.2020.035220.

Scott, M., Falkmer, M., Girdler, S., & Falkmer, T. (2015). View- points on factors for successful employment for adults with Autism Spectrum Disorder. *PLoS One, 10*(10), e0139281.

Seaman, Cannella-Malone, H. I., Brock, M. E., & Dueker, S. A. (2018). Efficacy of paraprofessional-implemented video prompting to teach vocational skills to students with Autism Spectrum Disorder. *Career Development and Transition for Exceptional Individuals, 41*(2), 68–76. https://doi.org/10.1177/2165143417708191.

Stodden, R. A., Brown, S. E., Galloway, L. M., Mrazek, S., & Noy, L. (2004). *Essential tools: Interagency transition team development and facilitation.* University of Minnesota, Institute on Community Integration, National Center on Secondary Education and Transition.

Test, D. W., Mazzotti, V. L., Mustian, A. L., Fowler, C. H., Kortering, L., & Kohler, P. (2009). Evidence-based secondary transition predictors for improving postschool outcomes for students with disabilities. *Career Development for Exceptional Individuals, 32*(3), 160–181.

Test, D. W., & Neale, M. (2004). Using the self-advocacy strategy to increase middle graders' IEP participation. *Journal of Behavioral Education, 13*(2), 135–145. https://doi.org/10.1023/B:JOBE.0000023660.21195.c2.

United Disabilities Services Foundation. (2020). *Top soft and hard job skills for adults with disabilities.* Retrieved from https://udservices.org/job-skills-adults-with-disabilities/.

Van Reusen, A. K., & Bos, C. S. (1994). Facilitating student participation in individualized education programs through motivation strategy instruction. *Exceptional Children, 60*(5), 466–475. https://doi.org/10.1177/001440299406000510.

Van Reusen, A. K., Deshler, D. D., & Schumaker, J. B. (1989). Effects of a student participation strategy in facilitating the involvement of adolescents with learning disabilities in individualized education program planning process. *Learning Disabilities, 1*(2), 23–34.

Wagner, Newman, L., Cameto, R., Javitz, H., & Valdes, K. (2012). A national picture of parent and youth participation in IEP and transition planning meetings. *Journal of Disability Policy Studies, 23*(3), 140–155. https://doi.org/10.1177/1044207311425384.

Waisman-Nitzan, M., Schreuer, N., & Gal, E. (2020). Person, environment, and occupation characteristics: What predicts work performance of employees with autism? *Research in Autism Spectrum Disorders, 78*, 101643.

Walsh, L., Lydon, S., & Healy, O. (2014). Employment and vocational skills among individuals with autism spectrum disorder: Predictors, impact, and interventions. *Journal of Autism and Developmental Disabilities, 1*, 266–275.

Wehman, P., & Brooke, V. (2013). Securing meaningful work in the community: Vocational internships, placements, and careers. In P. Wehman (Ed.), *Life beyond the classroom: Transition strategies for young people with disabilities* (pp. 310–338). Paul H. Brookes Pub. Co.

Wehman, P. (2013). *Life beyond the classroom: Transition strategies for young people with disabilities.* Paul H. Brookes Pub. Co.

Wehman, P., Schall, C., McDonough, J., Molinelli, A., Riehle, E., Ham, W., & Thiss, W. R. (2013). Project SEARCH for youth with autism spectrum disorders: Increasing competitive employment on transition from high school. *Journal of Positive Behavior Interventions, 15*(3), 144–155.

Wehman, Sima, A. P., Ketchum, J., West, M. D., Chan, F., & Luecking, R. (2015). Predictors of successful transition from school to employment for youth with disabilities. *Journal of Occupational Rehabilitation, 25*(2), 323–334. https://doi.org/10.1007/s10926-014-9541-6.

Wehmeyer, M. L., & Shogren, K. A. (2013). Self-determination: Getting students involved in leadership. In P. Wehman (Ed.), *Life beyond the classroom: Transition strategies for young people with disabilities* (pp. 41–68). Paul H. Brookes Pub. Co.

Workforce Innovation and Opportunity Act, Pub. L. 113–128, 128 Stat. 1425 (2014).

22

# Empowering Families

Patricia Fingerhut

## GUIDING QUESTIONS

1. How do occupational therapy practitioners provide interventions to empower families?
2. What is meant by family-centered care, capacity building, and collaborative approaches?
3. How can occupational therapy practitioners use therapeutic use of self, coaching, and collaborative goal setting to empower children and families?

## KEY TERMS

Coaching
Collaboration
Collaborative approach
Family-centered care
Family capacity building
Family and professional collaboration
Self-efficacy
Strengths-based approach
Therapeutic use of self

## INTRODUCTION

Children are part of a family unit, and therefore, intervention for children and youth includes understanding and engaging the family. Working with families involves addressing outcomes for both the child and the family. Occupational therapy practitioners work closely with caregivers and families to empower them with knowledge and support to provide opportunities for their child's optimal development as well as the ability to thrive as a family. Effective outcomes for children and families employ interventions based on family-centered practice principles, which include collaborating with parents and caregivers throughout the occupational therapy process. This chapter focuses on interventions that use parent partnership and family-centered principles to empower families to enable children and youth to engage in their desired occupations.

Occupational therapy practitioners use a variety of family-centered approaches so that the caregiver develops the knowledge and skills to collaborate with team members to advocate for resources, create connections with their children, and understand their child's strengths and challenges. Empowering caregivers to interact, play, and support their child's skills and abilities adds to family life and enhances daily roles and routines. Each family differs in their values, expectations, style, and approach to parenting. Occupational therapy practitioners seek to understand the family and create strategies to reinforce family routines, values, and culture. They establish collaborative relationships with parents and caregivers to learn about the child and family's situation and lived experience, while also providing the family with information about the child's condition, options for intervention, help with accessing services, and advice about strategies to support daily activities (Baker et al., 2012; Smith et al., 2015). Occupational therapy practitioners provide these types of interventions along a continuum.

## CONTINUUM OF CAREGIVER-MEDIATED INTERVENTION APPROACHES

The caregiver-mediated approaches used by occupational therapy practitioners working with children and families can be described on a continuum from the practitioner acting as the expert and the caregiver as a recipient, to the practitioner engaging in a collaborative relationship with the parent or caregiver. See Fig. 22.1 for an illustration of this continuum. While there may be times for practitioners to provide information and give instructions using the "expert mode," this approach may distance families from the practitioner and does not promote parent engagement in the process. Rather, it assumes the practitioner is the expert who is "more skilled" than the parent and can "fix" the child in some way. This style assumes the occupational therapy practitioner has all the answers when they may only have some of the story and are not living with the child and experiencing the family.

The parents or caregivers have additional information and knowledge that must be considered for effective intervention planning. A collaborative family-centered approach provides a comprehensive perspective of the child's occupational performance. Occupational therapy practitioners seek to uncover the child and family's needs and to create solutions or strategies to foster occupational performance within the home and community environment. Therefore, they use a family-centered approach to engage the child and family in intervention designed to make a difference in the child and family's life.

Occupational therapy practitioners using a family-centered approach seek to understand the family and child. They collaborate with families on goals and discuss progress, family issues, and factors that support or interfere with the child's ability to do those things that are meaningful to the child and family. For example, practitioners using a family-centered approach may adjust the intervention plan

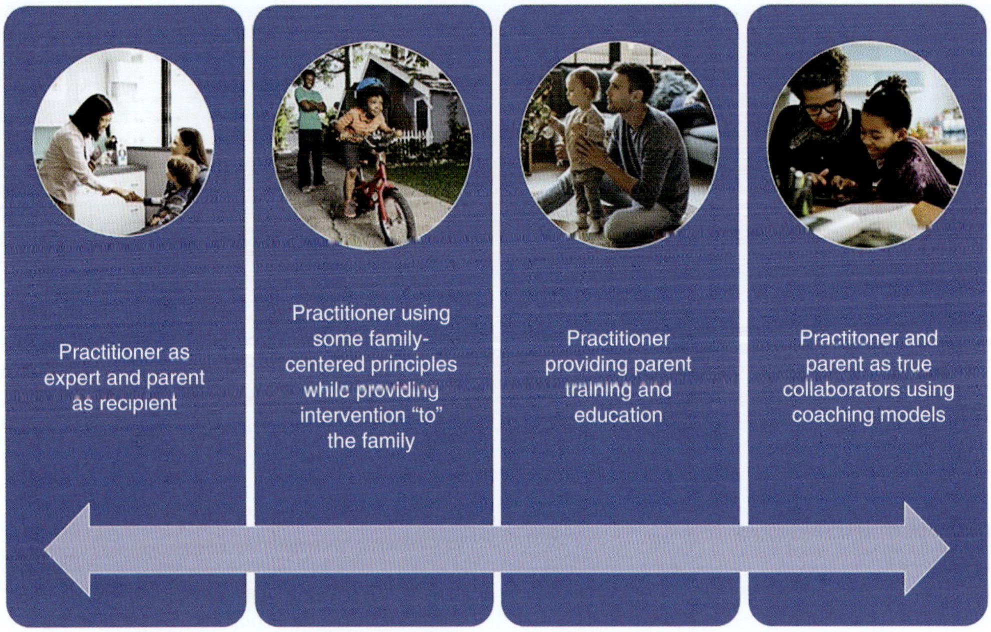


**Fig. 22.1** The continuum of occupational therapy approaches with children and families.

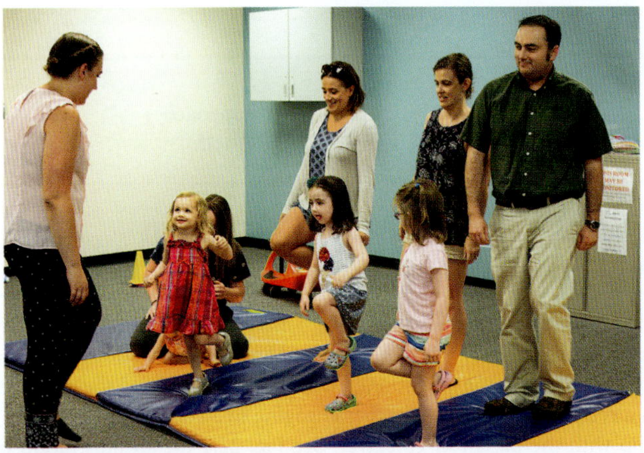

**Fig. 22.2** These parents engage in occupational therapy intervention by learning yoga poses with their toddlers.

when a caregiver reports they are concerned that the child is having trouble playing with his cousins at Sunday gatherings, so much that the family is contemplating not attending these valued events. A family may request that the practitioner prepare their child for a school project or provide strategies to adjust the child's bedtime routine. When using a family-centered approach, practitioners collaborate with families on strategies, allowing families to try out methods that may work and adjusting them to their home routines.

Occupational therapy practitioners balance family-centered care with capacity-building interventions, whereby they train parents and caregivers on strategies and techniques to support their children. For example, a practitioner may demonstrate feeding, positioning, exercise, and handling techniques to promote development (Fig. 22.2). They may educate caregivers on developmental milestones and play strategies. They also consult with families about motor, sensory, behavioral, and communication challenges.

Occupational therapy practitioners work with caregivers in all pediatric settings to facilitate outcomes for both the child and the family. This may involve working with the caregiver alone, in a caregiver and child dyad, or with the caregiver observing (Fig. 22.3A and B). Although interventions can be described on a continuum (from practitioner-led, to family-centered care, to parent training, to collaboration) most occupational therapy practitioners incorporate different elements at different times to meet the changing needs of the child, parents, and family throughout the intervention process. Caregiver-mediated approaches include family-centered practices, family capacity-building practices, and family and professional collaboration (Division of Early Childhood, 2014). See Case Example 22.1 comparing these three approaches.

## Family-Centered Care

**Family-centered care** is considered best practice in occupational therapy for children and youth (AOTA, 2020). The key features of family-centered care include building a collaborative relationship with families, creating goals together, and using knowledge of the family routine, values, expectations, beliefs, and culture when creating intervention plans (Barrios- Fernandez, 2022; Gafni-Lachter & Ben-Sasson, 2022; Popova et al., 2022). Family-centered care involves open communication, mutual trust and respect, the sharing of information with parents and families to allow shared decision-making, and the consideration and incorporation of family preferences and needs into intervention (Almasri et al., 2018; An & Palisano, 2014; King & Chiarello, 2014; Kuo et al., 2012).

Practitioners using family-centered care practices appreciate the family's impact on the child's well-being (King & Chiarello, 2014). They respect parents' knowledge of their child, acknowledging their resilience, and accepting their values while helping to build a network of social resources for families (Dunst & Dempsey, 2007). Practitioners following family-centered care philosophy treat families with dignity and respect and use **therapeutic use of self** to develop trusting relationships with families, which empower families and children to engage in their desired occupations. In relationship-building practices, occupational therapy practitioners actively listen, show compassion and respect, and believe in the family's capabilities (see Chapter 3 for more on the Intentional Relationship Model). Occupational therapy practitioners enable and promote the family's participation by individualizing their services, demonstrating flexibility in meeting family needs, and being responsive to family concerns (Fig. 22.4). Family-centered care models require collaboration between family members and health care providers, consideration of the family contexts, and provision of education and dedicated

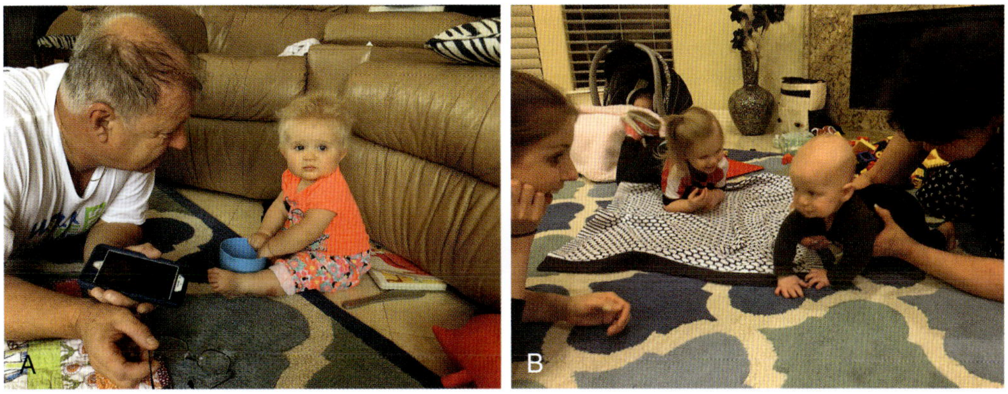


**Fig. 22.3** (A) The occupational therapy practitioner shows the child's grandparent how to play with the child while promoting sitting. (B) The practitioner shows the parent how to promote crawling and sitting during play.

## CASE EXAMPLE 22.1 CAREGIVER-MEDIATED CARE APPROACHES

DeAngelo is a 9-month-old boy with congenital issues at birth resulting in severe brain damage. His mother (Tanika) is a 16-year-old girl, who lives with her mother in a low-economic area. She attends the sessions at the outpatient occupational therapy clinic using public transportation by herself. The therapist uses elements from all three caregiver-mediated approaches to engage address DeAngelo's and Tanika's needs.

**Family-Centered Care:** The therapist takes the time to understand Tanika's goals for her son and understand their life situation. The therapist evaluates DeAngelo's current development along with his motor, processing, and sensory skills. The therapist explores the family routine, concerns, and available resources to identify supports and barriers.

DeAngelo has limited voluntary movement, does not startle, and is not responsive to movement, sounds, or touch. He will turn his head slightly when placed on his belly. He receives tube feedings for nutrition but will not suck from a bottle. DeAngelo is clean, dressed in new clothing, and Tanika holds him gently while she takes off his coat. She looks closely at her infant son. The therapist uses a strengths-based approach to support Tanika and praises her for taking such good care of her son. They discuss doctor's appointments and future milestones. Tanika does not work but receives public assistance and lives with her mother. She is solely responsible for taking care of DeAngelo.

The therapist is concerned that Tanika has minimal social and emotional support. As they continue in the therapy sessions, the therapist recommends Tanika discuss her situation with the social worker and look to her future, as it is important to take care of her needs too. Throughout the sessions, the therapist considers how to support Tanika. For example, she provides a bath seat, toys from a lending program, and resources on support groups with other mothers who have children with disabilities.

**Family Capacity Building:** Tanika wants to learn how to care for her son and facilitate his development. The therapist provides education on developmental milestones and trains Tanika on handling techniques to support DeAngelo's development. They review range of motion and stretching activities, and the therapist provides ideas for play. After receiving doctor's approval, they work on teaching DeAngelo to suck from a bottle. Throughout the process, the therapist provides adaptive equipment to position DeAngelo so he can observe and reach objects. The therapist demonstrates activities to promote responses. Tanika enjoys learning about child development and is patient and kind in her interactions with DeAngelo. Each week the therapist reinforces Tanika's efforts and complements her follow-through and care of DeAngelo. The therapist reminds Tanika that she is doing a great job caring for DeAngelo and acknowledges the progress (although limited) that he has made.

**Professional and Family Collaboration:** As the relationship develops, Tanika shares her concerns regarding DeAngelo's progress. The therapist takes the time to let Tanika express her concerns and talk through what this means. Together, they acknowledge that occupational therapy intervention is moving toward making accommodations (such as use of adaptive positioning devices and medical stroller) to make it easier for Tanika to provide care. The therapist empathizes with Tanika and agrees that this may be the best course of therapy. The therapist also reassures Tanika that they can continue to try to stimulate DeAngelo's development and reassess as needed.

Tanika would like to meet with the social worker and requests the therapist be present. Throughout the intervention process, the therapist allows Tanika to make decisions and set the therapy goals. The therapist provides information, support, and together, they decide the next steps for DeAngelo. This case (by Jane Clifford O'Brien) is based on a true story, but the names and some of the specifics have been changed.

policies and procedures (Kokorelias et al., 2019). For there to be successful collaboration, the caregivers must be engaged in the process.

Parents and caregivers who receive family-centered occupational therapy services report positive feelings of self-efficacy (a belief in one's abilities and skills) and satisfaction with programming, parenting behaviors, child behavior, and child functioning (Gafni-Lachter & Ben-Sasson, 2022; Popova et al., 2022). Parents who are treated with respect and dignity and involved in trusting relationships develop positive self-efficacy, which leads to feeling empowered. Feeling empowered and positive regarding one's ability to care for their children with disabilities allows parents to problem solve, feel open to asking questions and finding solutions, and improves quality of life for the child and family (Fig. 22.5).

Multiple studies using qualitative methods and surveys have investigated what parents want from service providers. Parents of children with Down syndrome, cerebral palsy, autism, and other developmental and neurological disabilities reported that they wanted the following from practitioners: (1) a true partnership; (2) a dependable resource for specific, objective information; (3) flexibility in service delivery and communication style; (4) sensitivity and responsiveness to their concerns; (5) positive, optimistic attitudes; and (6) effectiveness in generating outcomes (Edwards et al., 2018; Hayles et al., 2015; Marshall et al., 2015; McWilliam et al., 2009; Scime et al., 2017).

Although parents report that they want family-centered care (which results in better outcomes), recent national surveys suggest that not all parents receive services that are family centered, and significant regional, geographic, and socioeconomic disparities exist (Almasri et al., 2018; Azuine et al., 2015; Kuo et al., 2012). Cunningham and Rosenbaum (2014) used the *Measures of Processes of Care* to measure perceptions of parents and providers' self-efficacy (i.e., confidence) in implementing family-centered care. Feedback from parents and providers over the past 20 years suggests that some aspects of family-centered care are managed well, such as the provision of services in respectful partnerships with families, but other areas, such as providing information to parents and families, are not routinely family centered (Cunningham & Rosenbaum, 2014). Novak and Honan (2019) found that only 13% of pediatric occupational therapy interventions focused on the parent and the parent's daily interactions with the child. This suggests that professionals need to deliberately apply aspects of family-centered care in practice and evaluate their own services to determine if they are practicing family-centered care.

**Collaborative Assessment and Goal Setting.** Before the occupational therapy practitioner and caregiver can begin to address children's challenges, they must work together to identify the scope of the problem. In occupational therapy, the process often begins with the occupational profile. This caregiver interview experience sets the tone for the parent-practitioner relationship. Effective interviewing may provide as much information to the caregiver as the therapy practitioner gathers from the caregiver (Woods & Lindeman, 2008). Caregivers may need clarification on the purpose and scope of occupational therapy. Practitioners clearly describe the services that they can provide to the child. They engage in active listening, in-depth follow-up questions, continuing the conversation, proactive questioning about child development, questions that demonstrate that the parent has been heard, keeping the interview on track, attentive and open nonverbal behaviors, inclusion of social milieu of routines, seeking evaluative and interpretive opinions, and demonstrate empathy (McWilliam et al., 2009). When using a **strengths-based approach**, occupational therapy practitioners identify the child and family's strengths and challenges. Focusing on strengths empowers families to see positive traits in their children and family.

The practitioner and parents (and possibly the child) collaborate to create goals based on the child's challenges and current priorities. Practitioners creating collaborative goals often begin the process by asking parents global "big picture" questions, such as, "What would you like your child to do?" (Box 22.1 illustrates this process). They document the parent's response and continue to ask questions to better understand the parent's perspective. These probing questions clarify terms or behaviors, such as "What do you mean by 'stop misbehaving'? What does that look like? When does that occur?" The occupational therapy practitioner uses knowledge of occupational analysis to create short-term goals based on the long-term goal and to collaborate with the parent on this process. Questions such as, "What things does your

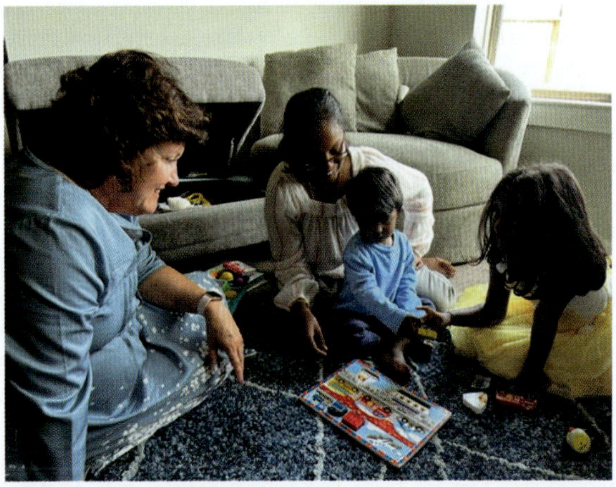

**Fig. 22.4** The practitioner shows flexibility and responsiveness by including the child's older sister in the occupational therapy session to meet the child and family's needs.

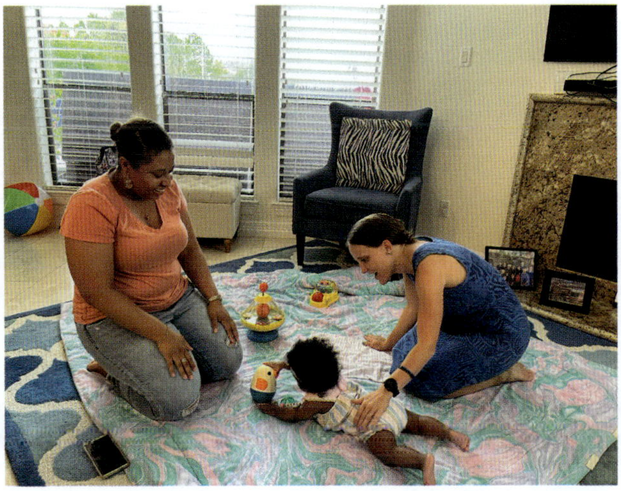

**Fig. 22.5** This young woman feels confident in her ability to play with her child. The practitioner shows her how to promote weight-bearing, hand skills, and play.

### BOX 22.1 Collaborative Goal Setting Example

**Occupational Profile:** Reason for referral, circumstances, situation

Kevin is a 3-year-old boy who "tantrums throughout the day." He lives with his parents and two older brothers (5 and 7 years). His mother expressed concern that "nothing makes him happy," and he disrupts outings and family meals, and the entire house is "tense."

**Assessment:** Child and family's strengths and challenges

Kevin is an active 3-year-old boy who played with toys and followed simple one-step directions from the therapist. His mother noted that Kevin can be playful and pleasant, but this is overshadowed by his tantrums, which have become more frequent. They live in the suburbs and have a large backyard, where Kevin often plays by himself. The therapist observed that Kevin expressed his needs with one word (e.g., Give, Me, No). He moved in and out of positions with ease. The therapist noted sensory aversions to some tactile materials, and Kevin did not come near others.

**Goal:** What is your main concern? What would you like your child to do? What are your concerns?

Mother stated she was concerned that Kevin had frequent tantrums that were disrupting the family. She was concerned that Kevin would not make any friends, would not get along with his brothers, and that something was "wrong" with him.

**Behaviors**: How does that look like for your child? What would you like to see your child do in 1 month? How would you measure success? Does this behavior change in different places?

Upon closer questioning, the therapist learned that Kevin screams, throws toys, and refuses to follow directions when he has a "tantrum." The tantrums occur in many settings, and the family has had to leave events (such as movie, community events, and family dinners) because of his behavior. At home, Kevin mostly plays by himself (as his brothers do not want to "make him mad").

**Goals:** Within 1 month, for 4 out of 7 days, Kevin will play an activity of his choice at home for 30 minutes with one of his brothers, keeping a positive nature

This goal was created with Kevin's mother and starts at home where Kevin is currently having the most success. The therapist will evaluate his sensory needs and further determine what may be interfering with Kevin's ability to express himself, while the family plays with Kevin and begins to establish positive behaviors.

child need to do before they can do the goal?" or the practitioner can ask them to describe how they would complete that occupation and write down the steps (as short-term goals). Practitioners create multiple goals within a variety of domains to provide some flexibility in the intervention plan. They may decide to prioritize with the parents and child.

To provide family-centered intervention, it is essential to gather information from families on their priorities, needs, and specific routines. This is done through a variety of interviews and observational techniques. For example, the *Routines-Based Interview* (McWilliam et al., 2009), collects information on family members' routines, satisfaction with routines, and priorities for changing routines. *The Life Participation for Parents* (LPP) (Fingerhut, 2005, 2013; Fingerhut et al., 2019) is a parent self-report assessment that explores how parents participate in chosen occupations while raising a child with disabilities. Box 22.2 summarizes sample questions from the assessment. Gathering information using this instrument can be valuable for developing important family outcomes and measuring success of interventions that are of interest to the caregivers and that address their concerns (Fingerhut et al., 2019).

**Caregiver Engagement.** For successful parent engagement in family-centered care, parents need to have trust, confidence in practitioners, and hope in the process. They also need to feel supported, empowered, validated, and reassured (D'Arrigo et al., 2020). Parent engagement is influenced by a parent's readiness for therapy, the service's time demands and flexibility, and other priorities and concerns in the parent's life. Practitioners who exude confidence, communicate clearly, and show responsiveness to parent and child's needs gain trust and confidence from parents and families (Popova et al., 2022) (Fig. 22.6). Parents who are more engaged in the therapy process benefit from increased knowledge about development, participation in home programming, psychological well-being, and feeling more competent as a parent and report increased self-efficacy and sense of control (Allen et al., 2021; Cunningham & Rosenbaum, 2014). Popova et al., (2022) trained families and therapists on relationship-building skills (using concepts from the Intentional Relationship Model; Taylor, 2020) during family-centered practice. They found that practitioners and parent interactions were aligned with family-centered care and that families wanted more information sharing (specific and general information). They also noted that practitioners used empathizing, encouraging, and instructing modes most frequently with families. Popova et al., (2022) suggest that there is an opportunity for practitioners to use collaborating, problem-solving, and advocating modes in practice.

**BOX 22.2 Life Participation for Parents**

The LPP (2005) includes 22 statements rated on a five-point Likert scale (strongly agree to strongly disagree) to indicate parents' view of their daily activities associated with having a child with a disability. Sample statement include:

1. Having a child with special needs affects my opportunities to engage in personal activities (e.g., hobbies, sports, leisure activities).
2. I feel I do a good job when I do the things a teacher/therapist might do for my child.
3. My child's need for emotional support is wearing me out (e.g., not able to entertain themselves, upset easily, cannot manage change in routine).
4. I am good at providing for my child's social activities.
5. Financial issues related to my child's special needs are a source of stress for our family.

Occupational therapy practitioners may find the LPP questionnaire useful in identifying areas of family concern that may otherwise go undetected (Fingerhut, 2005, 2013). They may use the findings to discuss resources and strategies to support the family. Practitioners may provide adaptations or modifications (or assistive technology) to improve the family's routines.

## Family Capacity Building

**Family capacity-building** practices include participatory opportunities and experiences afforded to families to strengthen existing parenting knowledge and skills and to promote the development of new parenting abilities that enhance parenting self-efficacy beliefs and practices. Family capacity building can involve both practitioner-led training and collaborative problem-solving with parents. Parent training to provide child intervention is generally professionally led, often with a preestablished curriculum, where the parents are provided information about their child's condition and intervention strategies (Miller-Kuhaneck & Watling, 2018) (Fig. 22.7A and B).

Two examples of preestablished curriculum where parents were trained to provide the intervention are as follows: (1) Woo and Leon (2013) trained parents to engage children in a sensorimotor enriched environment, and (2) Silva et al. (2016) trained parents in *Qigong Sensory Training* to reduce tactile abnormalities in children with autism spectrum disorder (ASD). Both studies showed achievement in targeted child-related skills. In both these studies, the parents provided the therapy for their children. Occupational therapy practitioners directed the treatment. Box 22.3 highlights two other parent training programs to benefit children and families.

Occupational therapy practitioners can use a variety of training approaches to empower parents and families and develop their skills for engaging their child. Ward et al. (2020) completed a systematic review of parental coaching approaches used for parents of children 0–5 years with disabilities (excluding the diagnosis of ASD). The authors categorized the approaches to coaching into three categories. (1) expert as coach, (2) parent observation of expert with another practitioner guiding the identification of the strategies, and (3) group model for training with individual coaching to apply the strategies to their specific child. All the studies reviewed utilized coaching techniques of illustration and action or practice and listening, observing, suggesting options, and providing information.

Successful outcomes in family-centered therapy require engagement of the caregivers who are providing the intervention (Carr et al., 2016; D'Arrigo et al., 2020; Gmmash et al., 2021) (Fig. 22.8A–C). Parents need to learn many skills, which can be challenging, and not all parents are receptive or able to develop the skills. However, children

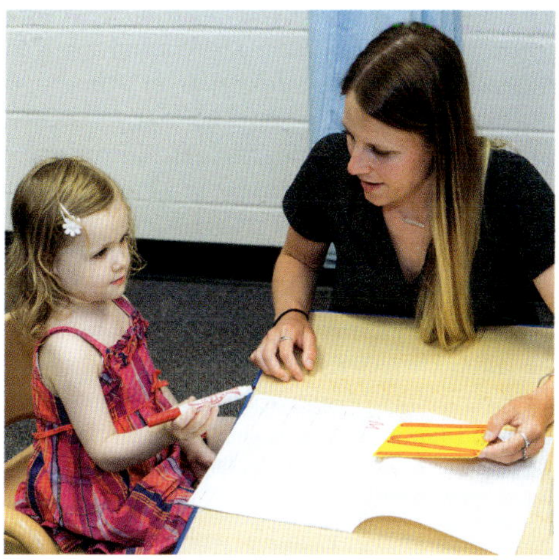

Fig. 22.6 The practitioner shows confidence, attention to the child, and responsiveness to the child's cues while providing occupational therapy intervention to this young girl.

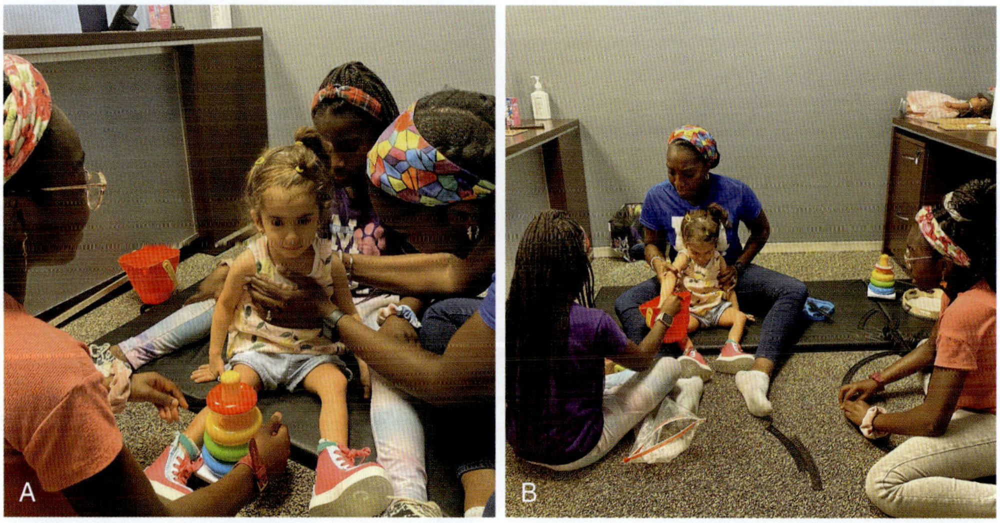


**Fig. 22.7** (A and B) The therapist trains the family on strategies to engage the child in daily activities.

> **BOX 22.3 Family Capacity-building Programs**
>
> **Emotion-Focused Parent Training** teaches parents to attend to their emotional experiences by (a) acknowledging their presence, (b) labeling the emotion, (c) validating the experience, and (d) meeting the emotional need (Knatz et al., 2015). This training can be conducted with parents individually or in groups; however, children are not present in the training sessions.
>
> **Cognitive-Functional (Cog-Fun) intervention** is an intervention used by occupational therapy practitioners certified in the approach. It is designed for children with ADHD and executive functioning difficulties. The approach involves both child and parent in nonthreatening playful activities designed to develop executive strategies, promote positive engagement, learn metacognitive language strategies, and provide necessary modifications to transfer skills to the home setting. Parents participating with their child in Cog-Fun intervention reported positive self-efficacy in comparison to parents who did not participate in the intervention (Hahn-Markowitz et al., 2018).

whose parents are more engaged in the intervention have better outcomes (Cunningham & Rosenbaum, 2014; Praphatthanakunwong et al., 2018). Therefore, occupational therapy practitioners seek to engage parents and families in intervention by addressing their goals, developing a trusting relationship, meeting families where they are at, respecting their circumstances, valuing parent and family input, being responsive to family, providing information in a timely manner, and establishing a therapeutic relationship. They engage parents and family members at their level, considering multiple factors that may influence their engagement. See Case Example 22.2 for an example of family capacity building.

Occupational therapy practitioners consider the family's current situation when creating capacity-building interventions, requiring parents or caregivers to learn how to implement interventions. They consider the family characteristics including marital status, socioeconomic status, availability of support systems, degree of difficulty of interventions, and family makeup when determining the best intervention approach for parents and caregivers. When training caregivers, the practitioner first trains the caregiver who is present most often for the targeted occupation. For example, with permission from parents, the practitioner trains the daycare worker who will be feeding the child two out of three meals and a snack, as well as family members (including siblings or grandparents, if appropriate).

Occupational therapy practitioners use training to reinforce concepts learned in the occupational therapy session. Parents enjoy playing with their children, which involves spontaneous interactions free from rules and controlled by the child. Children with disabilities benefit from unstructured play with parents. Therefore, training programs that can be integrated into daily routines and support the child's daily activities, such as engaging in play activities to promote hand use, are preferred. Allowing parents and caregivers to reinforce skills empowers them to feel competent and successful, promoting their willingness to engage in the intervention process. For example, as one practitioner was playing with a child and facilitating rotational patterns and weight-bearing in standing, the toddler almost took a step. To empower the parents, the practitioner moved away and asked the mother to encourage standing and walking at home. The practitioner asked the parent to demonstrate the "home program" before they left (as they did each session). As the mother demonstrated the activity, the toddler took his first step! In this example, the practitioner empowered the mother by stepping aside and letting them have this moment. The practitioner celebrated this success with the parent who was thrilled. Family-centered practice involves enabling parents and families to be successful and celebrating those successes. The therapeutic relationship is about the client and family (Taylor, 2020).

When engaging families in capacity-building practices, practitioners check in frequently to make sure that they are not requiring too much from the family. Home interventions are designed to use the child's newly learned or emerging skills in the home for occupational performance. Parents should not be expected to be the "therapist" but rather reinforce skills. For example, if an infant has trouble bringing his spoon to mouth in therapy, the practitioner may decide to have the family practice play in sand with spoons and provide the child with finger foods (so he can pick them up himself) at mealtimes rather than requesting the family struggle with an intervention. Some families may request more elaborate information or home programs. The practitioner individualizes programs to meet the child and family's needs.

## Family and Professional Collaboration

**Family and professional collaboration** builds relationships between families and professionals who work together to achieve mutually agreed upon outcomes and goals that promote family competencies and support the development of the child. Aspects of a **collaborative approach** (collaboration, structured problem-solving, and emotional support) were incorporated into the development of the *Parental*

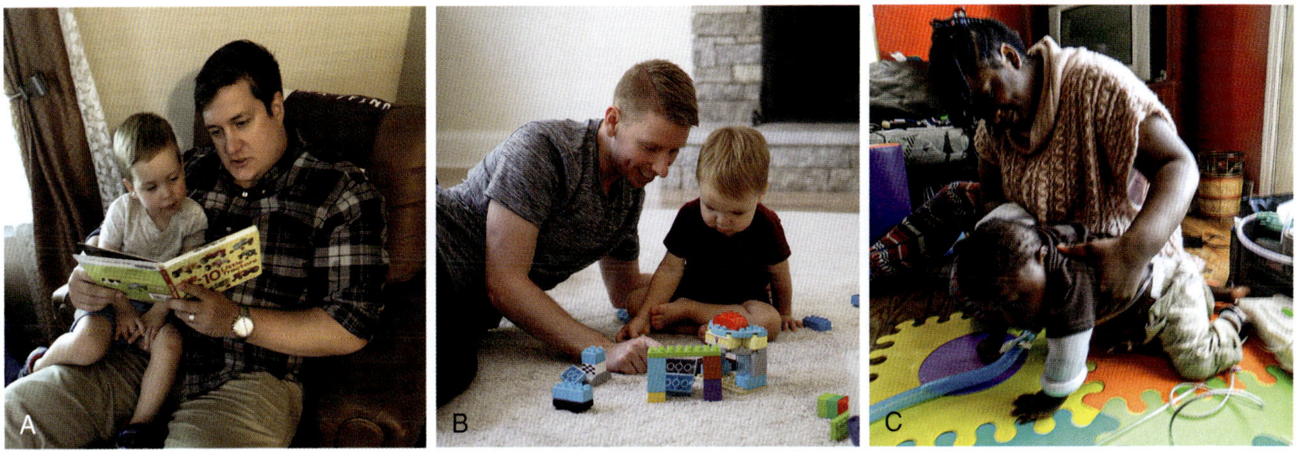


**Fig. 22.8** Children whose parents are engaged in intervention have better outcomes. (A) This father reads to his toddler. (B) This father plays with Legos with his young child. (C) This mother shows the practitioner how far the child has progressed in play.

### CASE EXAMPLE 22.2 FAMILY CAPACITY BUILDING

Cal is a 30-month-old boy referred to early intervention for developmental delays and behavioral challenges. He lives with his mother (Kerry), his 1-year-old brother, and the mother's new boyfriend in a second-floor inner city apartment. A home visit revealed the apartment to be unsafe for the children, as the windows were open and accessible to children, and the mother was caring for a friend's untrained adult pit bull (who was aggressive).

The occupational therapist met with the family and child. Cal did not follow one-step directions but ran around the room, picking up toys, dropping and throwing toys, and uttering nonsensical words. His mother did not attempt to change his behavior and remarked that this was typical, and she noted "he has always acted like this." Her infant remained in the stroller for the session.

The occupational therapist treated Cal individually to discover what was interfering with this ability to participate in daily activities. His mother watched the sessions from a one-way mirror where the social worker answered her questions and pointed out behavioral strategies that the therapist used. At the end of the session, the therapist reinforced the use of the strategies and asked her to try to use them at home. Kerry followed through with the suggestions and returned with questions and comments about what worked for her at home. Meanwhile the social worker informed her she must get rid of the dog and lock the windows shut. Kerry followed through with those suggestions. Over time, she implemented every suggestion and engaged in the home programs from speech therapy, occupational therapy, social work, and education. Cal showed great improvement in his behavior and was able to join the weekly group sessions. He followed simple one- to two-step directions and began communicating more clearly. His mother established a schedule for her children with help from the occupational therapist. She wanted to reduce television viewing. The therapist recommended replacing television viewing with coloring or fine-motor activities to prepare Cal for school. As they decreased television, Cal's language improved, although he often repeated a nonsensical phrase in a rhythmic way. Later, the team learned that he was mimicking "Beetlejuice," as that was his favorite show. This explained many of his behaviors. Over time, he stopped this behavior and entered regular 4-year-old kindergarten.

Kerry listened to other parents in the support groups, went to Al-Anon meetings to deal with her boyfriend's drinking, and eventually felt empowered enough to ask him to leave. Kerry was eager to learn but needed role models and support. The early intervention team represented a variety of professionals around her age, who treated her respectfully and honestly. Kerry built up her capacity to work with others, address her family situation, and make positive changes in her life. This case illustrates how building honest and trusting relationships with families can empower families. This case (by Jane Clifford O'Brien) is based on a true story, but the names and some of the specifics have been changed.

*Occupational Executive Training* (POET) model designed to address performance needs of children with executive functioning difficulty and their families. Frisch and colleagues conducted a study using the POET intervention whereby both parents conducted weekly individual sessions in quiet rooms at child development centers and private occupational therapy clinics. The parents described the approach as organized, consistent, sharing, accessible, and providing emotional support. The study had a high attendance and adherence rate for carryover of the activities in the home (Frisch et al., 2020). Mollo and colleagues taught mindfulness training strategies to parents of adolescents with executive functioning deficits. Their findings indicated improved outcomes in more consistent parenting skills, increased mindfulness, decreased parenting stress, increased self-competency and confidence, and positive shifts in attitudes toward the adolescent (Mollo et al., 2018).

**Collaboration** involves shifting the power to the client and allowing the client (or parent) to set the goals (even if the therapist disagrees) (Taylor, 2020). Therapists using the collaborative mode seek ongoing feedback from parents and children about the therapy process and about the therapist's performance. This method of practice empowers parents and caregivers to make decisions about their child that fit within their family structure and address their child's needs (Fig. 22.9). Collaboration requires the practitioner to inform the parent or family about options and discuss reasoning while allowing the parent to make the decisions, thereby supporting autonomy and choice, which is empowering (Taylor, 2020). Furthermore, parents are encouraged and empowered as the occupational therapy practitioner shows trust and confidence in their decisions, which further supports their confidence in making decisions over time. Occupational therapy practitioners using collaboration mode encourage parents and caregivers to use their own judgment. They must be okay with decisions that they do not agree with and continue to support the parent. This approach works well for parents who need control and want to drive the goals of therapy (Taylor, 2020). Early intervention guidelines recommend that occupational therapy practitioners use collaboration to empower parents to manage, advocate, and oversee their child's routines, occupational choices, health, and well-being. Occupational therapy practitioners may decide that a family or parent is not ready to make decisions about all aspects of the intervention process. In this case, the practitioner may decide to involve parents in collaborating by making decisions during the sessions and increasing the amount of collaboration over time. As parents and caregivers experience their decisions supporting their child positively, they feel encouraged to

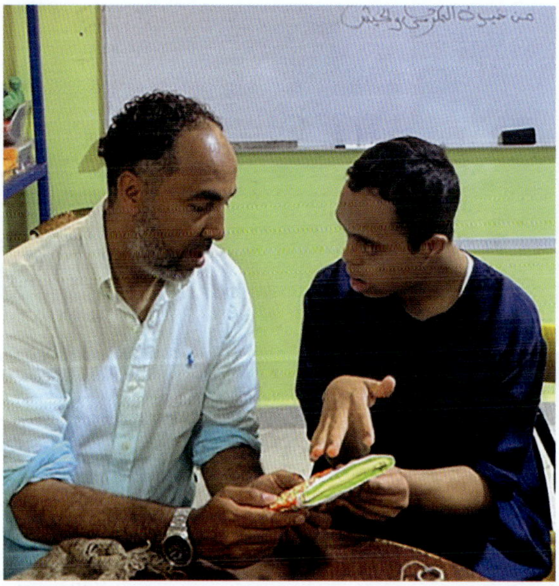

**Fig. 22.9** The therapist shifts power to the client to promote decision-making and empowerment.

engage more in the process. See Case Example 22.3 illustrating professional and family collaboration.

Occupational therapy practitioners create opportunities for parents and family to develop skills and capacity through collaborative discussion, exploring and trialing options, and reflection. Although the practitioners' knowledge and experiences are part of the collaboration, the goal is not to teach the parent or provide knowledge from an expert perspective but to identify family concerns and work collaboratively with the families to identify and trial potential strategies for intervention. This collaborative approach often uses coaching methods to encourage problem-solving, which leads to increased competence and sense of achievement, resulting in improved quality of life and feelings of control and empowerment.

## COACHING

Coaching is used in family-centered care, family capacity building, and during family and professional collaboration. **Coaching** is a collaborative process using observation, action, reflection, and feedback. Occupational therapy practitioners use coaching to promote family-centered practice (Allen et al., 2021; Kessler & Graham, 2015; Kim et al., 2023; Miller-Kuhaneck & Watling, 2018; Potvin et al., 2021). Parent coaching is an adult learning approach designed to build parents' capacity to support their child's development through improving existing skills, developing new skills, and enhancing problem-solving capabilities for future application (Ward et al., 2020). This type of intervention occurs within the family context, promotes caregiver-directed goals and solutions, and focuses on building parents' capacity to problem solve, reflect on their actions, determine effectiveness, and provide intervention within daily routines (Dunn et al., 2018; Dunn et al., 2012; Graham, 2010). Coaching is an effective approach to use when providing occupational therapy services for children and their families via telehealth (Caplan-Colon, 2021; Little et al., 2018; Pijarnvanit & Sriphetcharawut, 2023; Wallisch et al., 2019) (see Box 22.4).

Gmmash and colleagues interviewed parents of children receiving early intervention by providers who used coaching practices of joint planning, observation, practice, reflection, and feedback. Parents reported that modeling of the techniques was the most beneficial strategy for intervention and that they most often implemented home activities that were part of the family's routine and the child enjoyed (Gmmash et al., 2021) (Fig. 22.10). Parents reported improved self-efficacy after the coaching sessions.

### CASE EXAMPLE 22.3 PROFESSIONAL AND FAMILY COLLABORATION

Terry was a mother of three young boys; the youngest, 3-year-old Gavin, had an unknown neurological condition interfering with his ability to sit unsupported, feed himself, and play. While Gavin's medical diagnosis was cerebral palsy, he presented differently, and his condition was getting worse over time. Terry and her husband were managing the care of their children, but the uncertainty of Gavin's condition and the care demands were adding to the stress of their marriage. As the holiday season approached, Terry came to occupational therapy one session looking overwhelmed and tired. She expressed her concern for her child and frustration that his condition seemed worse when a medical professional informed her that cerebral palsy was not a progressive disorder. She noted that Gavin was not sleeping through the night and that she had not slept well in weeks.

The occupational therapist listened to Terry and empathized. The therapist noted the same concerns about Gavin so made a referral to the neurologist (who worked at the same hospital). The occupational therapist expressed concerns that the child was losing weight and not eating well and provided documentation in the referral of this decline.

The therapist also expressed concern for Terry's sleep routine. Since the occupational therapy students at local university were looking for holiday service projects, the therapist and Terry brainstormed the idea of the students providing "free" babysitting services for children with disabilities. The student group liked this idea of providing a service to the community, and Terry was the first recipient. Terry was very appreciative of her night out with her husband, and the occupational therapy students enjoyed giving back to the community.

The neurologist saw Gavin the following week and hospitalized him. The neurologist noted that the referral and documentation from occupational and physical therapy provided a clear perspective that further medical testing was warranted. Although the new diagnosis of a progressive neurological disorder was devastating, Terry and her family felt relieved that they now had a diagnosis and that the medical professionals listened to them.

This case illustrates the layers of collaboration between professionals and family members. The case is based on a true story (by Jane Clifford O'Brien), but the names are not real, and some of the specifics have been altered.

### BOX 22.4 Parent Coaching and Telehealth

Parent coaching practices can be delivered in person or through telehealth. Parent coaching through telehealth results in gains in child performance, improved parental self-efficacy, and parental satisfaction. Parents reported that telehealth was useful, convenient, and effective (Caplan-Colon, 2021; Little et al., 2018; Pijarnvanit & Sriphetcharawut, 2023; Wallisch et al., 2019).

Types of collaborative coaching used by occupational therapy practitioners include *occupational performance coaching, occupation-based coaching, health coaching, solution-focused coaching*, and *coaching in context* (Kistler et al., 2021). These coaching methods are based on collaborative and mutual discovery approaches between parents and practitioners. These interventions work well with principles of family-centered and occupation-based care that are central to pediatric occupational therapy practice.

### Occupational Performance Coaching

***Occupational Performance Coaching*** **(OPC)** is a specific intervention strategy described as "a process whereby parents are guided in solving problems related to achieving self-identified goals" (Graham et al.,

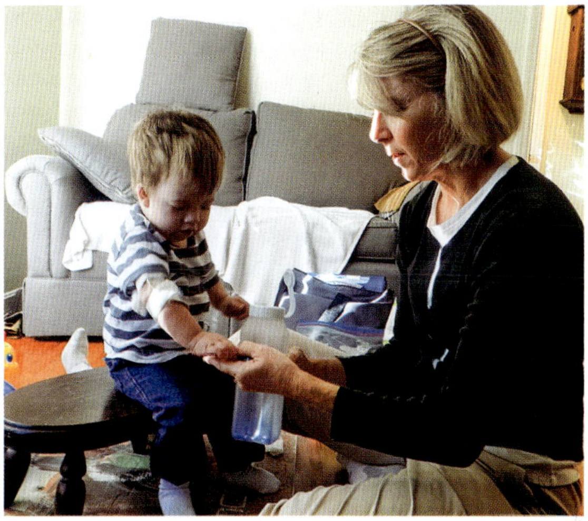

**Fig. 22.10** The therapist models how to promote dressing when coaching the caregiver on ways to promote the child's participation.

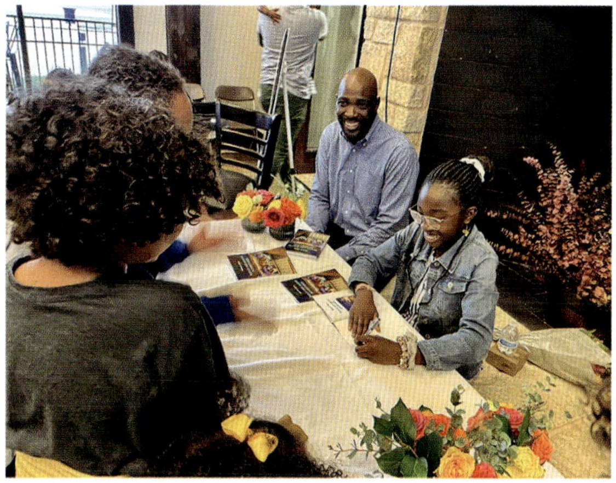

**Fig. 22.11** The practitioner coaches the student, allowing the student to make decisions and follow their plan. The practitioner is there for support and assistance as needed.

2009, p. 16). OPC intervention draws on the enablement framework of disability. This approach focuses on three domains: (a) emotional support, (b) information exchange, and (c) a structured process (Graham et al., 2010). The following six steps are used to coach parents in developing occupational performance for their children:

1) set goals
2) explore options
3) plan action
4) carry out plan
5) check performance
6) generalize

The OPC intervention emphasizes a collaborative partnership with the parent, enablement through parental self-discovery, and parent-directed intervention. OPC encourages parents to develop their own strategies based on their goals and circumstances rather than implementing practitioners' recommendations (Dunn et al., 2012; Graham et al., 2014, 2016; Kessler & Graham, 2015; Little et al., 2018).

Dunn et al. (2018) describe the guiding principles of OPC as (1) situate coaching in client's everyday life, (2) seek understanding by working collaboratively with client, (3) foster client's deep thinking about own life, and (4) explore resources with client. The practitioner using OPC (1) supports the client to pick goals because this makes goals meaningful and motivates clients, (2) focuses on problem-solving and identifying solutions, (3) situates the work in authentic contexts to foster generalization, and (4) uses reflective questioning and guided discovery to support the client to find solutions for their own challenges (Dunn et al., 2018).

Many of the aspects of this approach are shared with other family-centered care strategies such as promoting a collaborative relationship, allowing for client experimentation, reflecting on the usefulness of behaviors, focusing on strengths, supporting responsiveness to the impact of behavior and plans, promoting the client's ability to make plans, and promoting the client's ability to evaluate effectiveness (Fig. 22.11). The characteristics that "must not occur" in OPC include the use of traditional or protocol strategies, focus on isolated skills, and practitioners making goals, plans, activities, or otherwise telling the child or family what to do. Demonstration occurs after prior discussion with the client, and activities should always be a part of the child's authentic context or routines. Dunn and colleagues examined the effectiveness of this approach with parents of children with autism using telehealth delivery. They reported fidelity of intervention design, training, delivery, and receipt of OPC for families of children with autism using telehealth delivery (Dunn et al., 2018).

Angelin et al. (2021) demonstrated the effectiveness of OPC in a deeply traditional culture of India using a group approach. Following the Graham et al. (2009) protocol, children with ASD, attention deficit hyperactivity disorder (ADHD), intellectual disability, and sensory issues and their mothers received 10 group sessions of OPC in addition to standard therapy. The children and mothers who received the OPC showed significantly more improvement in children's performance, mother's performance, and mother's satisfaction than children and mothers receiving standard therapy alone. Mothers in the OPC group reported improved feelings of self-competence and performance in their parenting role. However, they recounted numerous environmental barriers that prevented improvement in sense of efficacy.

Mothers who participated in OPC reported they found benefits of the individual coaching approach (Foster et al., 2013; Graham et al., 2014, 2016). The mothers identified the benefits of learning to reflect and be mindful, which allowed them to feel more effective in addressing their child's behaviors (Foster et al., 2013). The mothers learned a variety of personal strategies, such as intentionally adjusting their own emotional state or attitude to modify the situation, ignoring negative or noncoping behaviors, modifying the child's task by increasing scaffolding or expectations, adding structure to routines, and utilizing a variety of learning strategies such as modeling, demonstration, explanation, and visualization; these strategies were also effective (Foster et al., 2013). They also reported the benefits of learning specific child-focused strategies, such as collaborating with the child by consulting them on their needs and ideas and negotiating task approaches. Similarly, offering children choices often promoted child success.

Graham et al. (2018) interviewed occupational and physical therapy practitioners regarding their perceptions of using OPC in practice. Occupational therapy practitioners reported that the approach enhanced their skills in therapeutic listening, meaning-focused goal setting, and encouraging caregiver participation in therapy. Occupational therapy practitioners described challenges in adopting the OPC approach, specifically in sharing power and not being as quick to offer an "expert" opinion, instead relying on the parent to describe and evaluate solutions they have tried or are considering (Graham et al., 2018). This was empowering for the parents, but practitioners felt ethical dilemmas when they strongly disagreed with the parents' ideas. Practitioners also needed to re-evaluate their time use. The OPC approach required more time in goal setting and rapport building with a greater focus on identifying caregivers' priorities resulting in less "hands-on" time with the child.

### Occupation-Based Coaching

*Occupation-based coaching* supports caregivers to create strategies that enhance their child's participation in daily activities (Kim et al., 2023; Little et al., 2018). Occupation-based coaching has been shown to improve caregiver knowledge and competence and to improve client participation, performance, and competence (Allen et al., 2021; Foster et al., 2013; Kessler & Graham, 2015; Potvin et al., 2021). Occupation-based coaching focuses on the family's strengths and supports children in participating in family roles (Foster et al., 2013; Miller-Kuhaneck & Watling, 2018). Practitioners using this method provide support to build on the family strengths and resources (Foster et al., 2013). They guide caregivers to master skills in natural environments to facilitate the child's participation (Simpson, 2015). Occupation-based coaching is incorporated into family routines throughout the week (Little et al., 2018; Wallisch et al., 2019).

### Health Coaching

*Health coaching* (Ogourtsova et al., 2019; Sprecher et al., 2022; Thom et al., 2014) uses multiple methods to inform children and families on matters of health. A program can be provided as an adjunct to primary care, via a clinician called a health coach. It also can be presented as a structured educational program delivered via telehealth or other online means. Generally, health coaching is a goal-oriented, client-centered partnership focused on health that works through a process of client empowerment. Health coaching may be delivered to parents with or without their child present, or it may be delivered in a group format (Ogourtsova et al., 2019). The expected outcomes of health coaching can be parent or child focused. One finding reported that health coaching by someone other than the primary care provider improved the parents' trust in the primary care provider (Thom et al., 2014). Another finding revealed that families who received healthcare coaching had fewer visits to the emergency room (Sprecher et al., 2022).

### Solution-Focused Coaching

*Solution-focused coaching* grew out of a variety of therapeutic approaches in psychology. The basic tenets of solution-focused coaching include:

1) Problems or challenges are not thought of as pathology but as an outcome of a limited behavioral repertoire.
2) Focus on creating solutions rather than trying to understand the root cause of the problem.
3) The child or parent is considered the expert on their life, needs, and desires.
4) Each coaching session is an opportunity for the coach to learn more about the child and the parent.
5) The coach helps the child and parent recognize and utilize resources.
6) Change can happen rapidly.
7) The child and the parent will work on goals (that they deem meaningful) outside of the sessions.
8) The approach promotes orienting the child and parent toward the future (goals).
9) The coach influences and encourages the child and parent to think in positive ways (i.e., looking for solutions rather than focusing on reasons).
10) The process is interactive and engages the child and parent (Grant, 2006, 2012, 2022).

Specifically designed for pediatric rehabilitation, solution-focused coaching in pediatric rehabilitation (Baldwin et al., 2013) integrates coaching and brief solution-focused therapy. The approach is strengths based and relational. Solution-focused coaching has a goal-oriented focus that includes positive reframing and strategic questioning so that clients are empowered to envision a future that they desire and then create and develop strategies and solutions to achieve that envisioned future (Baldwin et al., 2013). The specific steps to this approach include setting the stage, forming the relationship, envisioning the future, goal discovery, strategy creation, plan confirmation, and action/reflection cycles. Participants using this approach describe it as collaborative and report that it enhanced their abilities, improved their mindsets, encouraged their community participation, and promoted their engagement (King et al., 2019). Participants also developed skills, gained knowledge, grew in confidence, and reported increased self-efficacy and self-determination (King et al., 2019).

### Coaching in Context

Coaching in Context (Potvin et al., 2021) is an interprofessional coaching method that relies on skillful conversation that is client centered, powerful, and rooted in positive psychology. The coach must be fully present, engage in active listening, and provide reflective questioning. The coach and coachee (i.e., child and parent) together create action plans and solutions to problems that interfere with desired activities. This method uses motivational interviewing and is also solution focused. To date in occupational therapy, it has primarily been used with families of children who have had a spinal cord injury (Cadematori et al., 2021; Kim et al., 2023).

## FEATURES OF EFFECTIVE INTERVENTIONS WITH FAMILIES

There are a variety of effective interventions that focus on families, and they are similar in some key features. Effective interventions for children and youth include partnerships, typical routine daily activities, enabling or empowering caregivers, and a focus on family and child strengths. These approaches are effective for improving parent outcomes related to knowledge and self-efficacy, as well as child outcomes of overall function, feeding, cognition, and social skills (Novak & Honan, 2019). **Strengths-based approaches** empower parents by emphasizing the strengths of the child and using those capacities to develop strategies for promoting improved performance (Steiner, 2011). Occupational therapy practitioners teach children, parents, and family members to identify the strengths of the child and family and to problem solve using these strengths as part of the intervention, rather than focusing on the child's "problems" and deficits.

They emphasize the child's strengths in interactions with the child and others. They provide feedback on the child's effort and strengths for the session. For example, if a child had some difficulty maintaining attention to one task, a therapist could say to a parent, "he seems to be having difficulty attending today." In a strengths-based approach, however, the therapist might say something like "he seems to have a lot of different interests and that's a good sign. I am noticing how he seems equally interested in a few different toys." Then the therapist might follow this with a statement such as "a good way to try to get his attention when he is playing like this is to…". Using a strengths-based approach by considering how directions and instructions are phrased can influence the child's and family's perspective and sense of self.

### Contextually Based Intervention

Family-centered practice recommends practitioners provide intervention within the child's natural environment (e.g., home, daycare, school). Practitioners therefore engage children in activities delivered in the typical daily environments of the child and following typical routines (Fig. 22.12A and B). The environment provides cues and opportunities for meaningful repetition. Occupational therapy practitioners identify interventions that can be carried out within the typical daily routine using activities that are engaging to the child and with people who are engaging as well. For example interventions may be more effective if siblings are involved (Fig. 22.13A and B). Parents are more

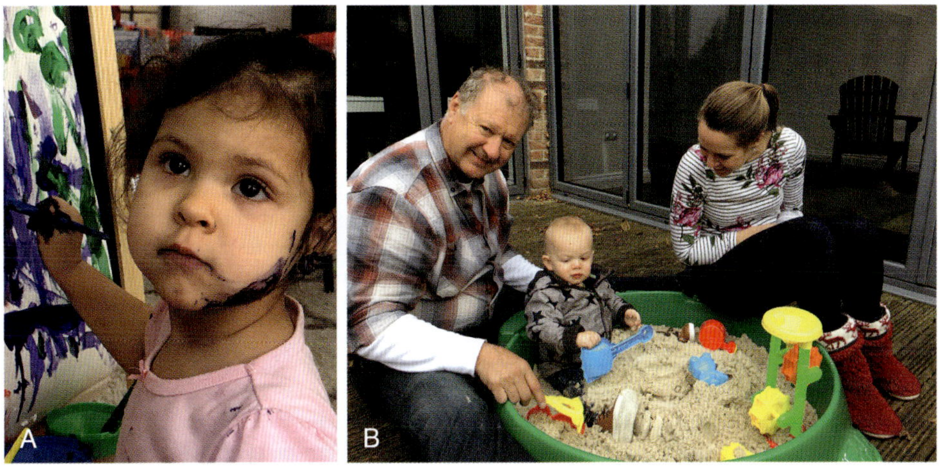

Fig. 22.12 (A) This child shows her creativity and gets a little messy at day care, a natural environment for this child. Creative play activities are part of the natural routine in the classroom. (B) The family encourages the child to play in the sandbox in their back yard, a typical play environment for this family.

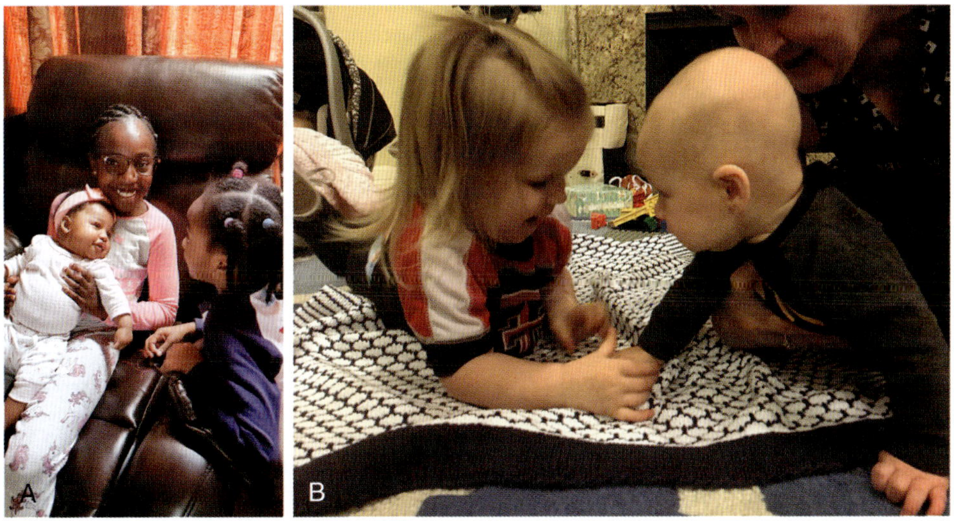

Fig. 22.13 (A and B) The occupational therapy practitioner providing intervention in the home may want to include siblings in the session to promote family involvement.

likely to engage their child in activities that are part of their routines and occur in their natural environment. Engaging children in activities within their environment and as part of their family routine results in significant improvements in participation for children with ASD and lower distress and defensive responding, and parents reported higher self-efficacy (Dunn et al., 2012; Law et al., 2011).

The *context therapy* approach (Darrah et al., 2011) is both routine and context based. The goals and intervention are functional and address changes in task or environment, rather than remediation of the child. Families (caregivers) are involved in setting goals and in identifying relevant tasks, constraints, and facilitators related to the task and environment. Occupational therapy intervention includes teaching families how to support and promote children's engagement in desired activities in their natural environments (Azari et al., 2019; Law et al., 2011).

## EVIDENCE FOR SPECIFIC CAREGIVER-MEDIATED APPROACHES

Caregiver-mediated approaches (such as family-centered care, family capacity building, and family and professional collaboration) result in positive parental outcomes including improving parental competence, quality of life, self-efficacy, and empowerment while reducing stress (Division for Early Childhood, 2014; Foster et al., 2013; Novak, 2014). For children, these approaches lead to improved performance in activities of daily living and social participation, as well as behavior, motor, academic, and social-emotional skills (Ingersoll et al., 2017; Mercer, 2017; Oono et al., 2013; Tanner et al., 2020).

Parent-mediated approaches used to develop skills for children with ASD primarily have a basis in behavioral theories or in social pragmatic theories. The social pragmatic approaches tend to use a parent-mediated model and focus on helping children develop social communication in appropriate social contexts instead of targeting the behavior (Mercer, 2017). Systematic reviews of parent-mediated intervention for children with ASD found positive outcomes for child goals of improved communication, behavior, play, adaptive functioning, and autism symptoms and parental goals of decreased stress and increased self-efficacy (Althoff et al., 2019; Ingersoll et al., 2017; Oono et al., 2013). Parent-mediated interventions improved motor skills for children with cerebral palsy and improved parent satisfaction with therapy (Tanner et al., 2020).

## SUMMARY

Occupational therapy practice with children and adolescents involves providing outcomes for the entire family. Using family-centered principles and a variety of effective parent and family-mediated intervention approaches can empower parents and families to provide the necessary support for the child while living life to the fullest.

1. Occupational therapy practitioners use a variety of approaches (i.e., family centered practices, family capacity-building practices, and family and professional collaboration) so that the caregiver develops the knowledge and skills to collaborate with team members to advocate for resources, create connections with their children, and understand their child's strengths and challenges. Empowering caregivers to interact, play, and support their child's skills and abilities adds to family life and enhances daily roles and routines. Occupational therapy practitioners seek to understand the family and to create strategies to reinforce family routines, values, and culture. They establish collaborative relationships with parents and caregivers to learn about the child and family's situation and lived experience, while also providing the family with information about the child's condition, options for intervention, help with accessing services, and advice about strategies to support daily activities (Baker et al., 2012; Smith et al., 2015).
2. The key features of **family-centered care** include building a collaborative relationship with families, creating goals together, and using knowledge of the family routine, values, expectations, beliefs, and culture when creating intervention plans (Barrios- Fernandez, 2022; Gafni-Lachter & Ben-Sasson, 2022; Popova et al., 2022). **Family capacity-building** practices include participatory opportunities and experiences afforded to families to strengthen existing parenting knowledge and skills and to promote the development of new parenting abilities that enhance parenting self-efficacy beliefs and practices. **Collaborative approaches** build relationships between families and professionals who work together to achieve mutually agreed upon outcomes and goals that promote family competencies and support the development of the child.
3. Practitioners following family centered care philosophy treat families with dignity and respect and use **therapeutic use of self** to develop trusting relationships with families, which empower families and children to engage in their desired occupations. In relationship-building practices, occupational therapy practitioners actively listen, show compassion and respect, and believe in the family's capabilities. **Coaching** is used in family-centered care, family capacity building, and during family and professional collaboration. Coaching is a collaborative process using observation, action, reflection, and feedback. Occupational therapy practitioners use coaching to promote family-centered practice (Allen et al., 2021; Kessler & Graham, 2015; Kim et al., 2023; Potvin et al., 2021). **Collaborating on goal setting** promotes the family's participation by assuring the goals are meaningful to the family and child. Listening to the family's concerns empowers families to engage and problem solve.

## REFERENCES

Allen, S., Knott, F., Branson, A., & Lane, S. (2021). Coaching parents of children with sensory integration difficulties: A scoping review. *Occupational Therapy International*, 1–10.

Almasri, N., An, M., & Palisano, R. (2018). Parents' perception of receiving family-centered care for their children with physical disabilities: A meta-analysis. *Physical and Occupational Therapy in Pediatrics, 38*(4), 427–443.

Althoff, C., Dammann, C., Hope, S., & Ausderau, K. (2019). Parent-mediated interventions for children with autism spectrum disorder: A systematic review. *American Journal of Occupational Therapy, 73*(3), 1–7.

American Occupational Therapy Association. (2020). Occupational therapy practice framework: Domain and process (4th ed.). *American Journal of Occupational Therapy, 74*(Suppl. 2), 7412410010.

An, M., & Palisano, R. (2014). Family-professional collaboration in pediatric rehabilitation: A practice model. *Disability & Rehabilitation, 36*(5), 434–440.

Angelin, S., Sugi, S., & Rajendran, K. (2021). Occupational performance coaching for mothers of children with disabilities in India. *Canadian Journal of Occupational Therapy, 88*(1), 38–47.

Azari, P., Hosseini, S. A., Rassafiani, M., Samadi, S. A., Hoseinzadeh, S., & Dunn, W. (2019). Contextual intervention adapted for autism spectrum disorder: An RCT of a parenting program with parents of children diagnosed with autism spectrum disorder (ASD). *Iran Journal of Child Neurology, 13*(4), 19–35.

Azuine, R., Singh, G., Ghandour, R., & Kogan, M. (2015). Geographic, racial/ethnic, and sociodemographic disparities in parent-reported receipt of family-centered care among US Children. *International Journal of Family Medicine, 2015*,168521.

Baker, T., Haines, S., Yost, J., DiClaudio, S., Braun, C., & Holt, S. (2012). The role of family-centered therapy when used with physical or occupational therapy in children with congenital or acquired disorders. *Physical Therapy Reviews, 17*(1), 29–36.

Baldwin, P., King, G., Evans, J., McDougall, S., Tucker, M. A., & Servais, M. (2013). Solution-focused coaching in pediatric rehabilitation: An integrated model for practice. *Physical & Occupational Therapy in Pediatrics, 33*(4), 467–483.

Barrios-Fernandez, S. (2022). Overcoming the barriers towards a family-based occupational therapy: A call to action. *British Journal of Occupational Therapy, 85*(12), 921–922.

Cadematori, C., Alpajora, B., Sivori, T., Betz, S., Gerhardt, N., Dunn, W., & Mulcahey, M. J. (2021). Preliminary examination of coaching in context with clients with spinal cord injury. *Spinal Cord Series and Cases, 7*(1), 27.

Caplan-Colon, L. (2021). Coaching parents on feeding techniques via telepractice. *The ASHA LeaderLive*. https://leader.pubs.asha.org/do/10.1044/leader.IPP.26012021.42/full/.

Carr, T., Shih, W., Lawton, K., Lord, C., King, B., & Kasari, C. (2016). The relationship between treatment attendance, adherence, and outcome in a caregiver-mediated intervention for low-resourced families of young children with autism spectrum disorder. *Autism, 20*(6), 643–652.

Cunningham, B., & Rosenbaum, P. (2014). Measures of processes of care: A review of 20 years of research. *Developmental Medicine and Child Neurology, 56*(5), 445–452.

D'Arrigo, R., Copley, J., Poulsen, A., & Ziviani, J. (2020). Parent engagement and disengagement in paediatric settings: An occupational therapy perspective. *Disability and Rehabilitation, 42*(20), 2882–2893.

Darrah, J., Law, M., Polk, N., Wilson, B., Russell, D., Walter, S., Rosenbaum, P., & Galupp, B. (2011). Context therapy: A new intervention approach for children with cerebral palsy. *Developmental Medicine & Child Neurology, 53*, 615–620.

Division for Early Childhood. (2014). Recommended practices in early intervention/early childhood special education 2014. http://www.dec-sped.org/recommendedpractices.

Dunn, W., Cox, J., Foster, L., Mische-Lawson, L., & Tanquary, J. (2012). Impact of a contextual intervention on child participation and parent competence among children with autism spectrum disorders: A pretest–posttest repeated-measures design. *American Journal of Occupational Therapy, 66*, 520–528.

Dunn, W., Little, L., Pope, E., & Wallisch, A. (2018). Establishing fidelity of occupational performance coaching. *OTJR: Occupation, Participation and Health, 38*(2), 96–104.

Dunst, C. J., & Dempsey, I. (2007). Family-professional partnerships and parenting competence, confidence, and enjoyment. *International Journal of Disability, Development and Education, 54*(3), 305–318.

Edwards, A., Brebner, C., McCormack, P., & MacDougall, C. (2018). From 'parent' to 'expert': How parents of children with autism spectrum disorder make decisions about which interventions to access. *Journal of Autism and Developmental Disorders, 48*(6), 2122–2138.

Fingerhut, P. E., DaLomba, E. J., & Li, C. Y. (2019). Responsiveness of Life Participation for Parents (LPP®): A tool for family-centered rehabilitation. *Physical & Occupational Therapy in Pediatrics, 39*(5), 543–552.

Fingerhut, P. E. (2005). Life Participation for Parents (LPP). https://veipd.org/earlyintervention/wp-content/uploads/2012/12/Life-Participation-for-Parents-and-description.pdf.

Fingerhut, P. E. (2013). Life Participation for Parents: A tool for family-centered occupational therapy. *American Journal of Occupational Therapy, 67*, 37–44. .

Foster, L., Dunn, W., & Mische Lawson, L. (2013). Coaching mothers of children with autism: A qualitative study for occupational therapy practice. *Physical & Occupational Therapy in Pediatrics, 33*(2), 253–263.

Frisch, C., Rosenblum, S., & Tirosh, E. (2020). Parental occupational executive training: Feasibility and parental perceptions. *OTJR: Occupation, Participation and Health, 40*(3), 203–210.

Gafni-Lachter, L., & Ben-Sasson, A. (2022). Promoting family-centered care: A provider training effectiveness study. *American Journal of Occupational Therapy, 76*(3), 7603205120.

Gmmash, A., Effgen, S., Skubik-Peplaski, C., & Lane, J. (2021). Parental adherence to home activities in early intervention for young children with delayed motor development. *Physical Therapy, 101*, 1–11.

Graham, F., Boland, P., Ziviani, J., & Rodger, S. (2018). Occupational therapists' and physiotherapists' perceptions of implementing Occupational Performance Coaching. *Disability and Rehabilitation, 40*(12), 1386–1392.

Graham, F., Rodger, S., & Ziviani, J. (2009). Coaching parents to enable children's participation: An approach for working with parents and their children. *Australian Occupational Therapy Journal, 56*, 16–23.

Graham, F., Rodger, S., & Ziviani, J. (2010). Enabling occupational performance of children through coaching parents: Three case reports. *Physical & Occupational Therapy in Pediatrics, 30*(1), 4–15.

Graham, F., Rodger, S., Ziviani, J., & Jones, V. (2016). Strategies identified as effective by mothers during occupational performance coaching. *Physical & Occupational Therapy in Pediatrics, 36*(3), 247–259.

Graham, F., Rodger, S., & Ziviani, J. (2014). Mothers' experiences of engaging in Occupational Performance Coaching. *British Journal of Occupational Therapy, 77*(4), 189–197.

Grant, A. M. (2012). Making positive change: A randomized study comparing solution-focused vs. problem-focused coaching questions. *Journal of Systemic Therapies, 31*(2), 21–35.

Grant, A. M. (2006). Solution-focused coaching. Excellence in coaching. *The Industry Guide*, 73–90.

Grant, A. M. (2022). Steps to solutions: A process for putting solution–focused coaching principles into practice. *Coaching Practiced*, 299–310.

Hahn-Markowitz, J., Berger, I., Manor, I., & Maeir, A. (2018). Cognitive-Functional (Cog-Fun) dyadic intervention for children with ADHD and their parents: Impact on parenting self-efficacy. *Physical & Occupational Therapy in Pediatrics, 38*(4), 444–456.

Hayles, E., Harvey, D., Plummer, D., & Jones, A. (2015). Parents' experiences of health care for their children with cerebral palsy. *Quality Health Research, 25*(8), 1139–1154.

Ingersoll, B., Wainer, A., Berger, N., & Walton, K. (2017). Efficacy of low intensity, therapist-implemented Project ImPACT for increasing social communication skills in young children with ASD. *Developmental Neurorehabilitation, 20*(8), 502–510.

Kessler, D., & Graham, F. (2015). The use of coaching in occupational therapy: An integrative review. *Australian Occupational Therapy Journal, 62*, 160–176.

Kim, R. Y., Johnson, M., & Mulcahey, M. J. (2023). Coaching in context: Parent perspectives. *Coaching: An International Journal of Theory, Research and Practice, 16*(1), 16–30.

King, G., & Chiarello, L. (2014). Family-centered care for children with cerebral palsy: Conceptual and practical considerations to advance care and practice. *Journal of Child Neurology, 29*(8), 1046–1054.

King, G., Schwellnus, H., Servais, M., & Baldwin, P. (2019). Solution-focused coaching in pediatric rehabilitation: Investigating transformative experiences and outcomes for families. *Physical & Occupational Therapy in Pediatrics, 39*(1), 16–32.

Kistler, B., Lynam, D., Mistek, M., Okerson, M., Pettigrew, T., Sweet, G., Ferraro, M., & Potvin, M. (2021). State of knowledge on the use of coaching in occupational therapy: A scoping review. *Student Papers & Posters*. Paper 79 https://jdc.jefferson.edu/student_papers/7930.12175.

Knatz, S., Braden, A., & Boutelle, K. (2015). Parent coaching model for adolescents with emotional eating. *Eating Disorders, 23*, 377–386.

Kokorelias, K. M., Gignac, M. A., Naglie, G., & Cameron, J. I. (2019). Towards a universal model of family centered care: A scoping review. *BMC Health Services Research, 19*, 1–11.

Kuo, D., Houtrow, A., Arango, P., Kuhlthau, K., Simmons, J., & Neff, J. (2012). Family-centered care: Current applications and future directions in pediatric health care. *Maternal and Child Health Journal, 16*(2), 297–305.

Law, M. C., Darrah, J., Pollock, N., Wilson, B., Russell, D. J., Rosenbaurm, P., & Galuppi, B. (2011). Focus on function: A cluster, randomized controlled trial comparing child- versus context-focused intervention for young children with cerebral palsy. *Developmental Medicine and Child Neurology, 53*, 621–629.

Little, L. M., Pope, E., Wallisch, A., & Dunn, W. (2018). Occupation-based coaching by means of telehealth for families of young children with autism spectrum disorder. *American Journal of Occupational Therapy, 72*, 7202205020p1–7202205020p7.

Marshall, J., Tanner, J., Kozyr, Y., & Kirby, R. (2015). Services and supports for young children with down syndrome: Parent and provider perspectives. *Child: Care, Health and Development, 41*(3), 365–373.

McWilliam, R., Casey, A., & Sims, J. (2009). The Routines-Based Interview: A method for gathering information and assessing needs. *Infants & Young Children, 22*(3), 224–233.

Mercer, J. (2017). Examining DIR/Floortime™ as a treatment for children with autism spectrum disorders. *Research on Social Work Practice, 27*(5), 625–635.

Miller-Kuhaneck, H., & Watling, R. (2018). Parental or teacher education and coaching to support function and participation of children and youth with sensory processing and sensory integration challenges: A systematic review. *American Journal of Occupational Therapy, 72*, 7201190030p1–7201190030p11.

Mollo, K., Merizalde, B., & Lape, J. (2018). Increasing competency for parents of adolescents with executive functioning deficits: Enhancing occupational performance with mindfulness. *Open Journal of Occupational Therapy, 6*(3).

Novak, I., & Honan, I. (2019). Effectiveness of paediatric occupational therapy for children with disabilities: A systematic review. *Australian Occupational Therapy Journal, 66*, 258–273.

Novak, I. (2014). New evidence in coaching Interventions. *Physical & Occupational Therapy in Pediatrics, 34*(2), 132–137.

Ogourtsova, T., O'Donnell, M., De Souza Silva, W., & Majnemer, A. (2019). Health coaching for parents of children with developmental disabilities: A systematic review. *Developmental Medicine and Child Neurology, 61*(11), 1259–1265.

Oono, I. P., Honey, E. J., & McConachie, H. (2013). Parent-mediated early intervention for young children with autism spectrum disorder (ASD). *Evidence-Based Child Health, 8*(6), 2380–2479.

Pijarnvanit, P., & Sriphetcharawut, S. (2023). The effects of telehealth parent coaching on occupational performance and executive function of children with attention-deficit/hyperactivity disorders, and parent self-efficacy: A preliminary study. *Occupational Therapy in Health Care, 38*(3), 783–799. https://doi.org/10.1080/07380577.2023.2169976.

Popova, E. S., O'Brien, J. C., & Taylor, R. R. (2022). Communicating with intention: Therapist and parent perspectives on family-centered care in early intervention. *American Journal of Occupational Therapy, 75*(5), 7605205130.

Potvin, M. C., Mulcahey, M. J., & Gerhardt, N. (2021). Coaching in context. *Department of occupational therapy faculty papers*. Paper 79 https://jdc.jefferson.edu/otfp/79.

Praphatthanakunwong, N., Kiatrungrit, K., Hongsanguansri, S., & Nopmaneejumruslers, K. (2018). Factors associated with parent engagement in DIR/Floortime for treatment of children with autism spectrum disorder. *General Psychiatry, 31*(2), e000009.

Scime, N., Bartlett, D., Brunton, L., & Palisano, R. (2017). Parents' experiences and perceptions when classifying their children with cerebral palsy: Recommendations for service providers. *Physical & Occupational Therapy in Pediatrics, 37*(3), 252–267.

Silva, L., Schalock, M., Gabrielsen, K., & Hd, G. (2016). One- and two-year outcomes of treating preschool children with autism with Qigong Massage Protocol: An observational follow-along study. *Alternative & Integrative Medicine, 5*(2), 1–10.

Simpson, D. (2015). Coaching as a family-centered, occupational therapy intervention for autism: A literature review. *Journal of Occupational Therapy, Schools, & Early Intervention, 8*, 102–125.

Smith, J., Cheater, F., & Bekker, H. (2015). Parents' experiences of living with a child with a long-term condition: A rapid structured review of the literature. *Health Expectations, 18*(4), 452–474.

Sprecher, E., Toomey, S., Epee-Bounya, A., Hernandez, B., Le, T., & Conroy, K. (2022). Randomized controlled trial of health coaching for parents of children with medical complexity. *Academic Pediatrics, 22*(8), 1482–1488.

Steiner, A. M. (2011). A strength-based approach to parent education for children with autism. *Journal of Positive Behavior Interventions, 13*(3), 178–190. .

Tanner, K., Schmidt, E., Martin, K., & Bassi, M. (2020). Interventions within the scope of occupational therapy practice to improve motor performance for children ages 0–5 years: A systematic review. *American Journal of Occupational Therapy, 74*, 7402180060p1–7402180060p40.

Taylor, R. R. (2020). *The intentional relationship: Occupational therapy and use of self* (2nd ed.). F.A. Davis.

Thom, D. H., Hessler, D., Willard-Grace, R., Bodenheimer, T., Najmabadi, A., Araujo, C., & Chen, E. H. (2014). Does health coaching change patients' trust in their primary care provider? *Patient Education and Counseling, 96*(1), 135–138.

Wallisch, A., Little, L., Pope, E., & Dunn, W. (2019). Parent perspectives of an occupational therapy telehealth intervention. *International Journal of Telerehabilitation, 11*(1), 15.

Ward, R., Reynolds, J., Pieterse, B., Elliott, C., Boyd, R., & Miller, L. (2020). Utilization of coaching practices in early interventions in children at risk of developmental disability/delay: A systematic review. *Disability & Rehabilitation, 42*(20), 2846–2867.

Woo, C., & Leon, M. (2013). Environmental enrichment as an effective treatment for autism: A randomized controlled trial. *Behavioral Neuroscience, 127*(4), 487–497. .

Woods, J. J., & Lindeman, D. P. (2008). Gathering and giving information with families. *Infants & Young Children, 21*(4), 272–284.

23

# Using Telehealth in Pediatric Occupational Therapy

Jana Cason

## GUIDING QUESTIONS

1. How is telehealth used in pediatric occupational therapy (OT) practice?
2. How is the OT process adapted when services are delivered through telehealth?
3. What telehealth resources exist for pediatric OT practitioners?

## KEY TERMS

Asynchronous telehealth
Blended/hybrid model
E-helper
Hub and spoke model
Synchronous telehealth
Telehealth

## INTRODUCTION

Telehealth describes the use of information and communication technologies to deliver services when occupational therapy (OT) practitioners and clients are in different physical locations at the time of service (American Occupational Therapy Association [AOTA], 2018). The COVID-19 pandemic brought telehealth to the forefront of OT practice, after limited use the previous 2 decades (AOTA, 2005; Abbott-Gaffney et al., 2022). Regulatory changes in response to the public health emergency (e.g., policies and payment) overcame long-standing telehealth barriers. Looking to the future, telehealth will continue to be an integral way OT services are provided. Both evaluation (see Chapter 9) and intervention can be completed via telehealth. Benefits of this model include improved access to services, flexibility of services (at the times family routines naturally occur; shorter and more frequent visits), and collaboration with caregivers and other professionals. In pediatrics, evidence supports the use of telehealth in early intervention (EI), school-based practice, outpatient clinics, and other community-based settings to improve developmental outcomes and caregiver engagement.

## TELEHEALTH IN EARLY INTERVENTION

As described in Chapter 15, in the United States, EI services are governed by Part C of the Individuals with Disabilities Education Act (IDEA) of 2004, P.L. 108–446. This law was amended in 2015 through the Every Student Succeeds Act, P.L. 114–195 (U.S. Department of Education [a], n.d.). Through IDEA Part C, OT practitioners provide services to children birth through 2 years of age who have an identified disability or who are at risk for developmental delay. OT practitioners providing EI services must adhere to the Health Insurance Portability and Accountability Act of 1996 (HIPAA) with requirements to protect health information. In a telehealth service delivery model, this includes using a HIPAA-compliant videoconferencing platform and having policies and procedures in place to protect health information on devices and in electronic communications (see Box 23.1).

Evidence for telehealth in EI services provided by OT practitioners dates back over 2 decades (Wakeford, 2002), with subsequent articles supporting the use of telehealth to overcome practitioner shortages and other access barriers and to improve child outcomes (Cason, 2009, Cason et al., 2012, Heimerl & Rasch, 2009; Kronberg et al., 2021; Little et al., 2018). According to Cason (2011), telehealth facilitates “assessment, communication, collaboration, coaching, role-release, and mobilization of resources and family supports” (Cason, 2011, p. 22). Further, telehealth-delivered occupation-based coaching increases caregiver efficacy, caregiver identified goals for young children, child learning opportunities in natural environments and routines, child participation, and positive child-caregiver interactions (Kronberg et al., 2021; Little et al., 2018). Using telehealth in EI promotes best practices, including the use of a caregiver coaching model. See Box 23.2 for a list of benefits associated with telehealth EI services.

### Telehealth Facilitates Coaching and Collaboration

Telehealth facilitates the use of a coaching model within a family-centered framework. Collaboration through caregiver coaching is a central tenet of EI services (Seruya et al., 2022). In the caregiver coaching model, practitioners guide caregivers in a process of joint planning, observation, action, reflection, and feedback (Rush & Shelden, 2020). This approach empowers caregivers to implement therapeutic strategies within their child’s daily routines, resulting in positive child outcomes and increased opportunities for the child to practice new skills.

EI services provided through telehealth promote a coaching model and family participation, support child and family outcomes, and result in high levels of family satisfaction (Kronberg et al., 2021; Little et al., 2018; Wallisch et al., 2019). For example, an OT practitioner may use telehealth to coach a caregiver on strategies to assist a child in gaining independence in self-feeding (see Fig. 23.1). Using an electronic tablet with videoconferencing software, the practitioner can observe the child’s position, caregiver-child interactions, observe the child engaged in the occupation, provide instruction on therapeutic techniques (e.g., active assistance, backward chaining, postural supports), and observe implementation of the therapeutic techniques. The practitioner can

### BOX 23.1 Example of HIPAA-compliant Videoconferencing Platforms and Policies and Procedures

**Videoconferencing Platforms**

- Most HIPAA-compliant videoconferencing platforms are subscription based. A few examples of HIPAA-compliant videoconferencing platforms include Doxy.me, Simple Practice, WebEx for healthcare, and Zoom for healthcare.
- To be HIPAA compliant, videoconferencing platforms must provide a Business Associate Agreement (BAA) indicating they will maintain compliance with security and privacy requirements of HIPAA related to protected health information. Additional features include end-to-end encryption, password-protected access, and other security features.

**Policies and Procedures**

- Connect for telehealth session from private setting (e.g., office with closed door).
- Communicate with caregiver through secure email/messaging services.
- Enable device security features (e.g., user authentication/password, antivirus/malware detection software with updates, firewall, automatic log-off, remote lock).
- Use password-protected Wi-Fi connection and do not use public Wi-Fi access.
- Avoid accessing telehealth and protected health information on shared devices.

### BOX 23.2 Benefits of Telehealth in Early Intervention Services

**Telehealth in EI Services:**

- Improves access to services otherwise unavailable (e.g., provider shortages)
- Allows flexibility of services (e.g., at the times family routines naturally occur; shorter and more frequent visits)
- Promotes a coaching model and family-centered services
- Enhances knowledge and skills of local providers through consultation and collaboration with remote practitioners who have specialized knowledge and expertise
- Facilitates more efficient use of interpreters with potential cost savings due to decreased travel
- Enables participation by family members who would otherwise not be able to participate in therapy sessions or IFSP meetings
- Supports training and role-release to other providers through telehealth consultations and co-treatments
- Permits family and IFSP team members to view, practice, and implement intervention strategies, if therapy sessions are recorded and securely archived in an educational record

provide feedback, discuss the caregiver's experience and concerns, and problem-solve strategies for skill progression.

Telehealth also fosters collaboration with specialists, remote practitioners, and other members of the child's Individualized Family Service Plan (IFSP) team through interdisciplinary evaluation, care coordination, and team-to-team consultation. Collaboration with remote practitioners and specialists, not otherwise available within the community, builds capacity among local practitioners (see Case Example 23.1).

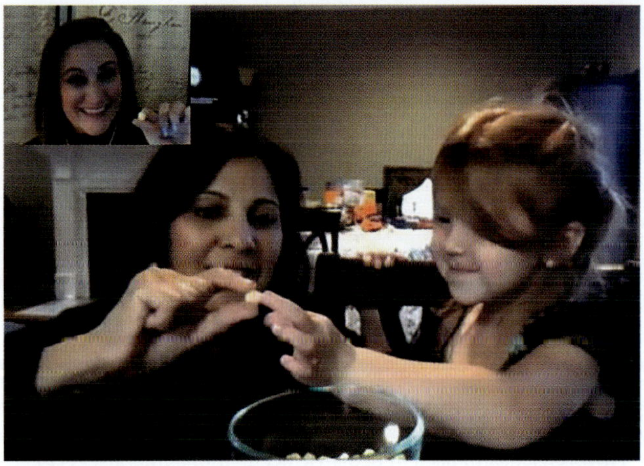

**Fig. 23.1** An occupational therapist uses telehealth technologies to coach a parent on therapeutic techniques to implement in the child's natural environment.

## Telehealth Models in Early Intervention

Telehealth EI services may use a *synchronous, asynchronous*, or **blended/hybrid model**. **Synchronous telehealth** occurs in real time through videoconferencing or phone-based (audio only) services. Synchronous telehealth facilitates live caregiver interactions, joint problem-solving, progression of home program activities, and remote participation in IFSP team meetings. **Asynchronous telehealth** augments in-person or synchronous telehealth services and may include use of publishers' online portals for administration of assessments (Pearson, 2022; WPS, 2022), email, text messaging, or the use of recorded video to promote skill development.

Selection of telehealth service delivery models should be based on clinical and ethical reasoning with consideration for the family's preferences, the complexity of the child's needs, and the nature of the interventions to be provided (AOTA, 2018). In some cases, telehealth may be used exclusively, whereas in other cases, an in-person model or **blended/hybrid model** (i.e., some services provided in person and other services provided through telehealth) may be indicated. OT practitioners should consult the policies of their organization and payer sources regarding the use of synchronous and asynchronous telehealth and adhere to all relevant policies, as well as state and federal laws.

## Telehealth Technologies in Early Intervention

Telehealth technologies in EI include a combination of hardware and software. Hardware refers to devices (e.g., computer, electronic tablet, smartphone, headset, microphone), whereas software refers to programs and applications ("apps") downloaded on devices. Families may access telehealth technologies for EI services in several ways.

- *Available technology*: Employing technology (e.g., computer, smartphone, electronic tablet) that families already use in their daily life results in increased comfort and familiarity with the technology.
- *Loaning technology to families*: Some EI programs loan equipment to families (e.g., electronic tablets) for use during telehealth sessions.
- *Technology brought in during co-treatments*: Nonoccupational therapy professionals on a child's IFSP team may bring technology to use during therapy sessions to facilitate consultation and co-treatment with a remote OT practitioner.
- *Technology at community sites*: When barriers prevent access to technology in the home, (e.g., high-speed internet is unavailable), it is possible to leverage existing technology within a child's community (e.g., community health center, private room in library). However,

## CASE EXAMPLE 23.1 EARLY INTERVENTION: AMELIA

### Background

Amelia is a 24-month-old child referred to an EI program by her pediatrician because of concerns with gross and fine motor development, feeding, and suspected sensory processing differences. Amelia enjoys music and age-appropriate books. Some strengths include the ability to follow one- to two-step directions, drink from a cup without a lid with minimal spillage, and sleep 10–12 hours each night. Problem areas for Amelia, as reported by her mother, include uncooperative behaviors, "extreme meltdowns," whining and fussing, feeding problems associated with aversion to food textures, and poor balance. Although she sat independently at 6 months of age, she did not reach for and grasp an object until 8 months of age. She rolled from back to stomach at 9 months of age and began crawling at 11 months.

### Assessment

A transdisciplinary, arena assessment model was used to determine Amelia's eligibility for services, present levels of development, and to facilitate intervention planning. In this model professionals from different disciplines assessed Amelia simultaneously, using skilled observations and standardized assessments. The evaluation team consisted of a physical therapist and developmental interventionist. Participation by an occupational therapist was indicated; however, Amelia lives in a rural community with no access to an OT practitioner trained in EI. The nearest hospital or outpatient rehabilitation clinic with a therapist onsite was a 50-minute drive from the family's home.

### Telehealth

The EI program in Amelia's area recently began using telehealth as a service delivery model to improve access to services for children living in rural and underserved areas. Amelia's mother gave consent for the use of videoconferencing to augment Amelia's EI services delivered in person. The physical therapist brought an electronic tablet with secure videoconferencing software to the family's home to enable the occupational therapist to participate virtually in the arena assessment.

During the assessment, Amelia was pleasant. She preferred not to be touched or held. The physical therapist took the lead in the arena assessment with the educational specialist (sometimes referred to as a developmental interventionist) assuming an observatory role. Amelia interacted with the examiner with caution after a brief period of ignoring her. Her mother remained in the room and participated in the assessment. The occupational therapist interviewed Amelia's mother via videoconferencing to obtain a sensorimotor history. Her mother reported that Amelia had difficulty with being touched and pulled away when touched. Sometimes she stiffened and arched her back when held. Amelia's mother reported that she was irritable when held and resisted having her hair or face washed. Amelia was bothered by noises, such as those from the vacuum cleaner and hair dryer. Although her aversion to sound had improved, she remained apprehensive of toys with noises. Amelia became anxious in situations with auditory and visual stimulation, such as a shopping mall. Amelia enjoyed swinging and other activities with movement.

During the arena assessment, which consisted of a criterion-referenced, five-area assessment by the EI team, the occupational therapist observed Amelia via videoconferencing technology. The occupational therapist noted that when handled, Amelia exhibited a mildly defensive reaction to touch. The occupational therapist asked the lead examiner (the physical therapist) to place a piece of tape on Amelia's hand. Amelia cried when the piece of tape was placed on the back of her hand. She seemed unable to plan the movements needed to remove the tape. Although she seemed to be visually oriented, visual tracking was delayed and inconsistent. Amelia enjoyed vestibular input as she was held and moved up and down or in circular motions by her mother under the direction of the lead examiner. She also enjoyed upside-down positions. Through videoconferencing, her mother completed the Sensory Profile 2 with the occupational therapist, and Amelia's sensory responses placed her in the Sensory Sensitivity and Sensation Avoiding quadrants.

### Summary and Interpretation

The arena assessment confirmed the pediatrician's concerns associated with Amelia's gross and fine motor development, feeding, and sensory processing and established eligibility for EI services. Based on the occupational therapist's observations and Amelia's scores on the Sensory Profile 2 and the motor and adaptive subtests of the criterion-referenced assessment, the occupational therapist concluded that Amelia experienced significant difficulties in receiving and modulating sensory information. This was evident particularly in her irritability and intolerance to touch and auditory stimulation. Inadequate adaptive motor function and feeding difficulties stemming from aversion to textures seemed to be related to her hypersensitivity. Amelia's tactile sensitivity probably contributed to her fine motor delays. Amelia's short-term goals were as follows: using sensory strategies to help her prepare for activities, Amelia would demonstrate (1) consuming an increased number of foods and variety of textures; (2) improved tolerance of touch, as demonstrated by improved affect when she is held or touched; and (3) improved play skills so that she could engage in a social play interaction for 10 minutes. See Table 23.1 for the priority areas, goals, and associated interventions.

### Intervention

The team recommended weekly OT for Amelia, which became part of her IFSP. A modified computer capable of videoconferencing and an internet access card not accessible for other uses was loaned to the family to facilitate remote OT services, which would otherwise be unavailable to Amelia and her family because of provider shortages in her area. The occupational therapist provided sensory-based strategies and recommendations to be implemented by Amelia's parents during daily routines. Co-visits through technology occurred with the physical therapist or educational specialist who was with the family in the home. The occupational therapist, working within a transdisciplinary practice model, collaborated with Amelia's parents and providers to support implementation of strategies and recommendations in Amelia's natural environments.

The occupational therapist recommended play-based activities that incorporated vestibular, proprioceptive, and tactile input (as accepted). Intervention included coaching Amelia's parents and other providers to incorporate sensory strategies, such as crawling activities, sand and water play, and activities that encouraged the use of both hands at the midline to facilitate cooperative, bilateral hand use. The occupational therapist provided Amelia's mother with reading material and a video to help her understand how sensory processing affects behavior.

Amelia responded well to the intervention approach and began to show indications of more efficient sensory processing and the ability to modulate sensory input. Within a few weeks, Amelia began to mold to her mother when she held her and was less irritable and more relaxed in situations with auditory stimulation. After 3 months of therapy, Amelia's mother reported increased cuddling and noticeable improvement in eating. She attempted a greater variety of foods and displayed fewer aversions; feeding time was shorter; and it was no longer necessary to use the television as a diversion to get her to eat. Amelia began to interact more with her older sister and began to explore her environment. Play skills and hand use also appeared to increase as evidenced by more complex independent play, including imaginative play with dolls and constructive play with puzzles and building blocks. Amelia also demonstrated improved social interaction with same-aged peers during community outings and at home with her older sister.

### Implications

The use of a telehealth service delivery model allowed Amelia's family to access OT services otherwise not available because of provider shortages in her area. Videoconferencing facilitated consultation, collaboration, and coaching among Amelia's EI providers and family and promoted improved outcomes by ensuring that the distinct perspective and contributions of OT services were available to Amelia's IFSP team.

**TABLE 23.1 Sample Goals and Interventions for Amelia and Her Family**

| Caregivers' Priorities | Goal | Interventions |
|---|---|---|
| Consume an increased number of foods and variety of textures | Amelia will eat four new foods and tolerate a variety of textures during mealtimes. | • Encourage play with food ("finger painting" with food, poking holes in JELL-O or pudding with pretzel sticks)<br>• Begin with preferred textures and slightly modify (e.g., add granola to yogurt)<br>• Introduce alternate brands for variation of consistency (e.g., yogurts, diced fruit)<br>• Consistently offer opportunities to try new foods<br>• Encourage Amelia to help with food prep, especially with "messy" foods |
| Improve tolerance of touch (not cry or get upset when held or touched) | Amelia will demonstrate improved tolerance of touch, as evident by remaining calm when held or touched. | • OT will provide "sensory diet" (individualized sensory input throughout the day)<br>• "Heavy work" activities (carrying heavy backpack, books, activities requiring pushing/pulling) to provide calming input<br>• Desensitization activities (play in textures like rice, sand, or beans)<br>• Avoid "light touch"; provide deep pressure/firm touch<br>• Playful use of vibration (end of vibrating toothbrush, massager) on body and face (as tolerated) |
| Improve play skills | Amelia will initiate and maintain play with peers including turn taking and sharing toys with minimal prompting. | • Sand and water play (provide opportunities for socialization and increased sensory exploration to promote tolerance of textures)<br>• Developmentally appropriate games that involve turn taking and social interaction<br>• Modeling and use of verbal and physical prompts |

with the expansion of internet access and affordable mobile technologies, it is less common to leverage technology within the community to provide EI services through telehealth (Cason, 2009).

In addition to access, there are other technology-related considerations for EI telehealth-delivered services. Built-in desktop and laptop computer cameras work well for conversation but do not capture angles needed for tabletop or motor-based activities. To capture alternate angles, mobile devices (smartphone or electronic tablet) may be needed. Multiple devices can be used during videoconferencing to capture different angles. For example, an OT practitioner may alternate between a built-in camera on a desktop computer for seated, conversation-based interactions and a mobile camera for demonstrating movement-based activities to a child and caregiver. If the OT practitioner or caregiver is joining through videoconferencing with two devices, it is important to connect the audio to only one device. This is because if audio is connected to both devices and they are in close physical proximity, audio feedback will occur. Placement of the devices for optimal viewing and safety (e.g., adequate space for movement without obstructions within the environment) is also an important consideration.

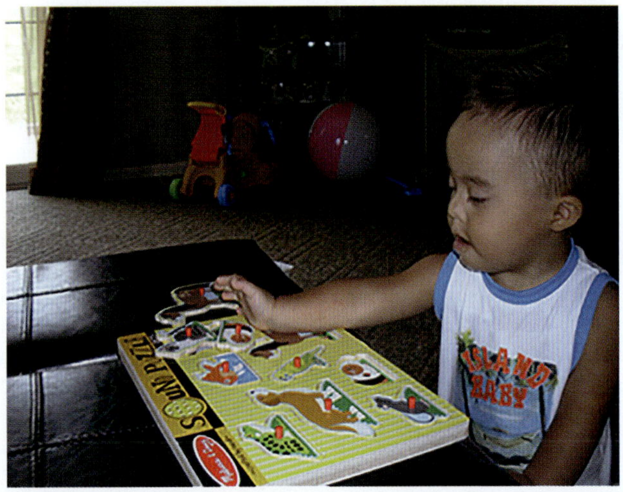

**Fig. 23.2** By planning telehealth OT interventions using materials and toys at home, the child can practice with family members to improve targeted skills.

## Telehealth Occupational Therapy Intervention in Early Intervention

Telehealth OT intervention in EI mirrors in-person intervention using a caregiver coaching model. For more information on the caregiver coaching model, see Chapter 22. Telehealth EI OT interventions should use materials the child and family have available within their home (Fig. 23.2). By using materials and toys at home, the child can practice with family members to improve targeted skills. During the evaluation, a materials checklist can be used to identify materials families have available and to guide intervention planning. See Fig. 23.3 for a materials checklist example for EI.

Materials commonly used in OT telehealth EI therapy sessions include small manipulatives such as pieces of cereal, beans, and rice; empty egg cartons, paper towel and toilet paper tubes; disposable cups; straws; empty food and drink containers of assorted sizes; bubble wrap/packaging materials; socks used for sorting by size/color or rolled into balls; and toys available in the home (e.g., bubbles, play dough, blocks, books, puzzles, nesting cups, shape sorters, dolls, etc.). It is beneficial for practitioners to have similar items on hand as the child and caregiver during the therapy session to be able to model and provide demonstrations of specific therapeutic strategies. Dolls and inflated balloons are especially helpful for OT practitioners to use to visually demonstrate child positioning and the amount of pressure to be applied during manual interventions. See Box 23.3 for examples of OT telehealth EI intervention ideas.

When working on activities of daily living (ADL) such as toileting, dressing, and/or bathing, do not have the child undressed on camera. Instead, use simulated activities, caregiver coaching, and target foundational skills (e.g., fine motor, range of motion, functional balance) needed for success with ADL (AOTA, 2018). See Fig. 23.4. For example, Little et al. (2020) used self-directed online educational modules and individualized caregiver coaching through telehealth to increase toileting skills in children with autism.

## Summary of Telehealth Occupational Therapy in Early Intervention

Telehealth in EI facilitates family-centered services using a caregiver coaching model. Evidence supports the use of telehealth for the delivery of OT services in EI. Benefits include improved access to services, increased opportunities for collaboration among IFSP team members,

**EI Occupational therapy materials checklist**

I will plan our occupational therapy sessions using items you already have in your home. Please click on the box to mark the items you have available, then save the file, and send it back to me. I will use this information to plan our therapy sessions.

- ❑ Balls (any size)
- ❑ Blocks for stacking and copying designs
- ❑ Books
- ❑ Bubbles
- ❑ Bubble wrap/air pillow packing material
- ❑ Cotton balls
- ❑ Crayons
- ❑ Clothespins
- ❑ Coat hanger for clothespin activity
- ❑ Empty plastic drink/food containers with lids
- ❑ Empty toilet paper, paper towel, or wrapping paper tubes
- ❑ Flashlights (hand puppets and visual games)
- ❑ Laundry basket
- ❑ Magna doodle or Magic board
- ❑ Measuring cups or nesting cups
- ❑ Muffin tin
- ❑ Plastic or paper cups
- ❑ Plastic or paper plates
- ❑ Playdough
- ❑ Playing cards
- ❑ Popsicle sticks
- ❑ Pots and pans
- ❑ Puzzles (large piece)
- ❑ Rice and/or beans
- ❑ Rubber bands
- ❑ Shape sorter
- ❑ Straws
- ❑ Tongs
- ❑ Turkey baster

**Favorite toys**

**List:**

**Favorite music/songs**

**List:**

**Available technology**

- ❑ Desktop computer with built in camera
- ❑ Laptop computer with built in camera
- ❑ Electronic tablet (e.g., iPad or iPad mini)
- ❑ Smartphone
- ❑ External computer camera
- ❑ Internet service

Adapted with permission from TelehealthShare LLC.

**Fig. 23.3** Example of a materials checklist to guide intervention planning.

increased caregiver efficacy and child-caregiver interactions, and positive child outcomes. For more information about the role of OT practitioners in EI, see Chapter 15.

## TELEHEALTH IN SCHOOL-BASED PRACTICE

As described in Chapter 15, school-based OT services in the United States are governed by Part B of the IDEA of 2004. As highlighted in the previous section, this law was amended in 2015 through the Every Student Succeeds Act (ESSA), P.L. 114–95 (U.S. Department of Education [b], n.d.). Through IDEA Part B, OT practitioners provide services in educational settings to children ages 3–21 years who have been identified with a disability. Other federal laws relevant to school-based practice include Section 504 of the Rehabilitation Act of 1973 (U.S. Department of Education [c], n.d.). This law requires schools to provide "free and appropriate education" to students regardless of disability (U.S. Department of Education [b], n.d.). HIPAA and the Family Educational Rights and Privacy Act require policies and procedures to protect privacy, security, and confidentiality of protected information defined within the laws.

OT practitioners may use telehealth in traditional brick-and-mortar schools or in online school settings (e.g., private or charter online schools, online public schools). Telehealth supports direct interventions with children; group therapy; consultation and follow up with teachers, parents, and administrators; and participation in Individualized Education Program (IEP) meetings. Evidence demonstrates that use of telehealth improves handwriting and school performance (Criss, 2013); symptoms of developmental dyslexia (Pecini et al., 2019); and educational outcomes for school-age children with autism (Little et al., 2018).

### Telehealth Models and Technologies for School-Based Practice

Telehealth OT services in school-based practice primarily use a direct intervention model, rather than the caregiver coaching model used in EI services. Depending on the developmental age of the child, a

**BOX 23.3 Telehealth OT Intervention Ideas for the Early Intervention Setting**

**Adaptive Skill: Self-Feeding**

Use telehealth to coach caregivers on appropriate foods to practice self-feeding (e.g., finger feeding, use of spoon/fork). For example, observe the caregiver giving the child dry pieces of cereal to practice finger feeding. If the child is grasping with the full hand, instruct the caregiver to place a few pieces of cereal in a small container or empty egg carton to facilitate use of pincer grasp. When teaching self-feeding with a spoon, brainstorm with the caregiver which thick foods (e.g., pudding, yogurt) the child may enjoy eating, as the thicker foods stick to the spoon and improve success. Similarly, when targeting self-feeding with a fork, encourage the caregiver to have the child use a metal-tined child sized fork, if available, and easy-to-poke foods such as small soft cheese cubes or bites of meat cut to a safe size. Observe the child and caregiver through videoconferencing, provide coaching and modeling, feedback, and strategies to grade the activity.

**Fine Motor Skill: Release Objects Into Containers**

Explore with the caregiver available containers in the home (e.g., empty oatmeal canister, plastic orange juice container). Instruct the caregiver on optimal positioning of the child during the activity. Provide verbal cuing and modeling to teach the child how to remove the lid and initially grade the activity down by having the caregiver place the lid loosely on the container. Demonstrate for the caregiver how to assist the child to place objects into the container, with the caregiver using physical and verbal prompts as needed. Grade the activity through strategic placement of the container (e.g., require midline crossing, overhead reach), size of objects placed in the container, and size of the container (smaller/larger or with wide or narrow opening). Through telehealth, OT practitioners can coach caregivers on activities and therapeutic strategies to promote fine motor skills using a variety of household objects and toys.

**Motor Planning and Functional Mobility**

When targeting motor planning and functional mobility, obstacle courses can be constructed using sofa cushions, pillows, chairs, blankets, and other objects (e.g., books, canned food) to create a path for the child to crawl over, under, and around. Using telehealth, the OT practitioner can help the caregiver construct the obstacle course, anticipate and address any safety concerns (e.g., corners of furniture, hard surfaces, fall risks), observe the child and caregiver while the child completes the obstacle course, and provide feedback and additional therapeutic strategies to incorporate into the activity.

**Constructive and Imaginary Play Using Household Objects**

Constructive play involves using materials to build and create, while imaginary play incorporates make-believe, imagination, and unstructured role-play. An OT practitioner using telehealth may collaborate with the caregiver to identify objects in the home that can be used for constructive and imaginary play; coach the caregiver in structuring the environment and play activity; and provide modeling, verbal cuing, and feedback. Household items that can be incorporated into constructive and imaginary play may include, but are not limited to, plastic cups for building, leaves or utensils for sorting and creating designs, homemade edible playdough, sock puppets, and play with large cardboard boxes decorated into a car, cafe, or other imaginary setting.

caregiver (e.g., aide, teacher, parent) may assist the child as an **e-helper**. In this role, the caregiver provides technical support, setup of therapy materials, facilitates transitions between therapeutic activities, and provides verbal cueing and physical assistance as needed.

Like EI services, telehealth school-based OT services may be *synchronous, asynchronous, or blended/hybrid*. *Synchronous telehealth* most commonly uses videoconferencing with the OT practitioner and child. OT intervention through videoconferencing may use a variety of software features including screen share, annotation (drawing/stamp tool), applications ("apps"), online videos and therapeutic games, and the videoconferencing platform's chat feature to share weblinks and files.

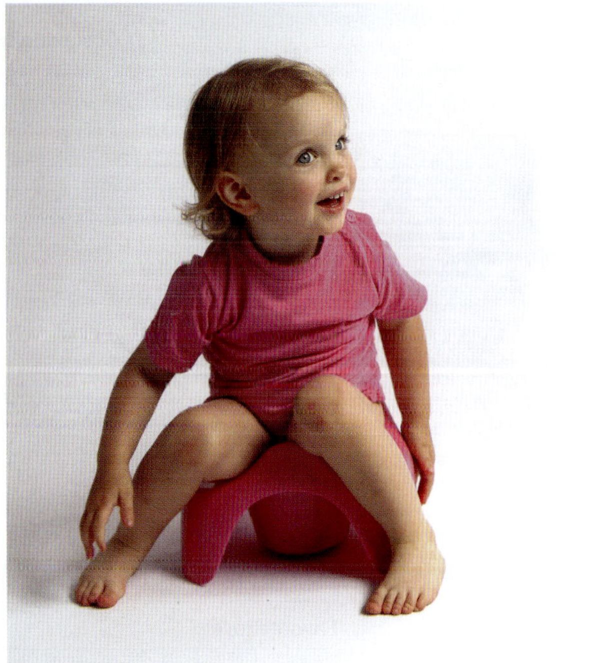

**Fig. 23.4** When working on ADL such as toileting, bathing, and dressing through telehealth, do not have the child undressed on camera. Instead, use simulated activities, caregiver coaching, and target foundational skills needed to complete the ADL.

*Asynchronous telehealth* may include administration of questionnaire-based assessments; recorded data from apps or online programs; video demonstrations; and communications by email, text, or secure messaging. For example, a student aide can record a student's response to an individualized sensory diet recommended by the OT practitioner. Through the school's secure online portal, the aide sends the recording to the OT practitioner for review and asks for additional strategies to optimize the student's attention to task during seated class work.

Telehealth hardware may include a computer, electronic tablet, smartphone, headset, microphone, and document camera for viewing worksheets, books, or other objects placed in the camera's view. "Homemade" document cameras can be made using an external computer camera or mobile device with instructions available online through a general search of the topic. An external computer camera or mobile device (e.g., electronic tablet, smartphone) can also provide alternate viewing angles during telehealth OT evaluations and interventions. A wireless headset with built-in microphone enables movement-based activity while enhancing audio quality and privacy.

## Telehealth School-Based Occupational Therapy Intervention

OT practitioners providing telehealth school-based services most often provide direct services to children and consultation with teachers, administrators, and caregivers. It is beneficial for the child and practitioner to have the same materials available during the OT session. The practitioner will often provide a demonstration for the child using the materials. Some pediatric outpatient clinics and school settings provide therapeutic materials (e.g., an "OT Toolkit") to children who receive occupational therapy services through telehealth. Items may include small manipulatives (e.g., dice, fidgets), bubble wrap, child-sized scissors, tongs, putty, and other therapy materials. OT interventions for school-age children may address social participation, ADLs, motor planning/bilateral coordination, strength, fine motor skills, handwriting, keyboarding, use of assistive technology, visual perception/visual-motor skills, sensory processing, emotional regulation, executive function, and other areas within the purview of OT. See Box 23.4 for an example of telehealth OT intervention ideas for the school-age population. Case Example 23.2 illustrates the use of telehealth with a school-aged child.

### Resources for Telehealth School-Based Occupational Therapy Practice

There are many online communities where OT practitioners share telehealth intervention ideas and telehealth tips and strategies. These can be found on popular social media platforms (e.g., Facebook, Instagram, Pinterest) and YouTube channels. Additionally, there are numerous telehealth resources produced by AOTA for school-based OT practitioners. Members of the American Occupational Therapy Association benefit from AOTA's virtual school-based service delivery decision guides (AOTA, 2021b). These include resources related to legal, ethical, and procedural telehealth considerations; strategies to embed IEP goals into daily routines; delivery of virtual group OT services; considerations for telehealth evaluations, progress monitoring, and documentation in the school setting; and strategies for collaborating with school team members through telehealth (AOTA, 2021b). See Box 23.5 for additional resources for telehealth pediatric OT practice.

## TELEHEALTH IN HOSPITAL AND PEDIATRIC COMMUNITY-BASED SETTINGS

Telehealth programs in hospital and pediatric outpatient settings use many of the same assessments, technologies, and interventions already presented for EI and school-based practice. Benefits of telehealth in hospital and pediatric outpatient settings include improved access to services, provision of services in natural environments and contexts, flexibility in frequency and duration of services, and decreased travel for families.

### Hospital and Community Feeding Clinics

A pioneering study by Clawson et al. (2008) explored the feasibility of using telehealth to provide initial screening and specialized services for children with complex pediatric feeding disorders. The children, families, and local health care professionals participated in videoconferencing with a team of interdisciplinary specialists at a hospital-based feeding clinic (Clawson et al., 2008). The study found that telehealth reduced the burden to families (e.g., eliminating travel to the hospital-based feeding clinic), and there was high family satisfaction with services. Of the children who received community-based services through telehealth, outcomes were improved acceptance of food variety and age-appropriate foods, increased oral-motor strength and swallowing ability, decreased supplemental and/or tube feedings, and reduced caregiver burden (Clawson et al., 2008).

A later study by Luscombe et al. (2021) explored clinician's experiences using telehealth to treat complex pediatric feeding disorders. The feeding clinic used a **hub and spoke model** where services were provided from a specialized feeding clinic (the hub) to clients at community-based sites (spokes). There were several benefits associated with telehealth. These included improved professional skill and confidence of community-based practitioners, interdisciplinary collaboration, increased access to specialized services and convenience for families, improved attendance, opportunity for family involvement due to the elimination of travel, and enhanced continuity of care (Luscombe et al., 2021).

### Pediatric Outpatient and Community Settings

In pediatric outpatient and community settings, telehealth enhances skills for daily living, including skills needed for employment in young adults with disabilities. Conner et al. (2021) examined the efficacy, feasibility, and acceptability of a hybrid group soft-skills training program to support employment for young adults with high-functioning autism compared to in-person training. Results indicated similar efficacy between the two delivery models with increased satisfaction, perceived confidence, and improvement in soft skills in the hybrid group (Conner et al., 2021).

## TELEHEALTH PRACTICE CONSIDERATIONS FOR THE OCCUPATIONAL THERAPY PROCESS

Though the OT process (AOTA, 2020) is the same when services are provided through telehealth, there are some important practice considerations. These practice considerations for OT services delivered through telehealth in the United States relate to HIPAA compliance,

### BOX 23.4 Telehealth OT Intervention Ideas for the School-age Population

**Fine Motor Skills**

Incorporate materials children have available and their interests in fine motor activities. For example, a child may enjoy feeding a "tennis ball" monster with coins to target finger dexterity and translation from palm-to-finger and finger-to-palm. Make a treasure hunt by having the child or caregiver bury treasure (coins/small manipulatives) into playdough or theraputty. Many children enjoy guessing how many drops of water will fill a coin using an eye dropper or medicine dropper and then testing their guess, an activity that targets fine motor skills, attention to task, and counting. Practice pinch patterns and sorting (by color or shape) with small pieces of cereal. Target fine motor skills by folding, tearing, crumpling, pinching, and incorporating fine motor games using paper, including junk mail or scrap paper.

**Visual-Motor and Handwriting**

Children may complete online worksheets and therapeutic activities targeting visual-motor and handwriting skills using screen share and annotation (i.e., a drawing tool commonly available in videoconferencing platforms). Clinics and schools may also purchase workbooks for children to use during telehealth OT sessions. Individual worksheets can be mailed or emailed to caregivers to print, as permitted by the copyright holder. Handwriting curriculums can be adapted for telehealth using screen share and digital assets or observing children using the materials in their natural environments.

**Multisensory Keyboarding Interventions**

Develop finger strength, isolation, coordination, and other skills needed for keyboarding through therapeutic activities and keyboarding practice. OT interventions may include use of bubble wrap (popping bubbles with individual fingers), games for finger isolation, and keyboarding practice with online keyboard programs. A mobile camera (e.g., via a smartphone, electronic tablet, or external camera) should be used to view the child's hands and finger placement for tabletop and keyboarding activities.

**Emotional Regulation**

Programs for emotional regulation (e.g., The Zones of Regulation, The Alert Program® can be incorporated through screen share and digital assets available from publishers or with physical materials (e.g., books, charts) provided to the child. Video social stories may be incorporated through screen sharing. Help children make their own social story books by copying or personalizing social story scripts and adding digital or hand-drawn pictures. Coping strategies can be taught and practiced in synchronous OT telehealth sessions or asynchronously through recorded videos and training modules.

*See the TelehealthShare YouTube channel for excerpts of telehealth OT sessions with the school-age population, intervention ideas using common household items, and telehealth tech tips (https://www.youtube.com/c/TelehealthShare/videos).

## CASE EXAMPLE 23.2 SCHOOL-BASED PRACTICE: SAM

### Background

Sam is a kindergarten student. He was referred for an OT evaluation due to concerns in the areas of fine motor skills, sensory processing, and self-regulation. His chronological age is 5 years, 8 months.

### Telehealth Assessment

Sam completed an OT evaluation through telehealth (i.e., videoconferencing with caregiver present) to determine if services were warranted to support his participation in an online school environment. Sam was cooperative, participated throughout the evaluation, demonstrated intermittent eye contact, and followed one-step directions with moderate verbal and visual cues. Observation of Sam's participation and behaviors during the evaluation indicated that his performance was likely an accurate reflection of his actual abilities.

Areas assessed included fine motor, visual-motor, visual perceptual, handwriting, keyboarding, and mouse skills; sensory processing; and executive functioning. Assessment information was obtained through caregiver interview/input; skilled clinical observations; Beery-Buktenica Developmental Test of Visual Motor Integration, 6th Edition (BEERY VMI); Functional Fine Motor Assessment (FFMA); and Sensory Processing Measure (SPM). The findings are reported below.

Table 23.2 shows Sam's score's on the BEERY VMI. Sam scored in the below average range for the overall visual-motor assessment, in the average range on the visual perception subtest, and in the low range on the motor subtest. These results indicate Sam may have difficulty with manipulating a writing instrument, handwriting performance, copying/drawing shapes, and creating art projects.

The Functional Fine Motor Assessment (FFMA) is a telehealth assessment of functional fine motor skills that can be used in the educational environment (Criss, 2020). It includes structured observation of in-hand manipulation, finger isolation, grasp, handwriting, keyboarding, and mouse skills. Student performance is compared to developmental age and grade expectations based on existing research and literature. Sam demonstrated age-appropriate in-hand manipulation and finger isolation skills. During the evaluation, Sam used a right-handed palmar supinate when using a writing tool. With this grasp, the pencil is held in a fist with thumb toward ceiling. He was observed using whole arm movements during writing and drawing/coloring activities.

Sam demonstrated below age-appropriate skill for pressure on paper, memory recall for letter formation, alignment to line, spacing between letters, spacing between words, letter size, writing speed, typing using home row hand placement, typing speed, and dragging using a mouse/trackpad.

Results of the Sensory Processing Measure (SPM) were as follows: typical performance (typical) for social participation, vision, hearing, touch, planning and ideas, and total sensory systems. Despite a "typical" score in the areas of visual, auditory, planning and ideation, and overall sensory systems, concerns were noted by parent and further observed by clinician during the OT evaluation indicating some concerns in those sensory areas. Mild to moderate problems ("some problems"; 1 standard deviation below the mean) were identified for body awareness and balance and motion.

### Summary and Interpretation

Sam demonstrates various strengths and areas for growth as evidenced by assessment data. Strengths include average to above average visual perceptual skills. Challenges, and therefore areas for growth, are in the areas of ADL performance, visual-motor skills, fine motor skills, executive functioning, sensory processing (body awareness, balance, and motion), and emotional/self-regulation.

While the IEP team will collectively, given all the evaluation data, make the determination regarding whether OT services are warranted, based upon data and observations from the assessment, they determined that Sam may benefit from OT services.

The occupational therapist recommended the following specifically designed instruction and/or modifications: modeling/cueing with opportunities for repeated practice, multisensory instructional strategies, instruction in self-regulation/self-monitoring strategies, visual/verbal prompts and cues, and developmentally sequenced multisensory review of keyboarding/handwriting skills. Table 23.3 includes Sam's goals, objectives, and sample intervention activities.

### Intervention

The team recommended OT services for Sam, which became part of his IEP. Because Sam attends school in an online school environment (from his home), a desktop computer and electronic tablet were used to participate in telehealth OT sessions. The occupational therapist recommended educationally based activities that targeted ADLs, visual-motor, fine motor, and executive functioning. Strategies for sensory processing (e.g., sensory diet and activities to improve body awareness and self-regulation) were incorporated into the telehealth sessions and provided as part of a home program. The occupational therapist, working within an interdisciplinary practice model, collaborated with Sam's parents, teacher, and other IEP team members. Sam responded well to OT interventions through telehealth as evidenced by progress toward educational goals outlined in his IEP.

### Implications

The use of telehealth facilitated consultation, collaboration, and direct intervention for Sam and allowed him access to OT services to support his participation in the online education setting.

### TABLE 23.2 Sam's Scores on the BEERY VMI

| Test | Raw Score | Standard Score | Interpretation |
|---|---|---|---|
| Beery VMI (overall) | 11 | 80 | Below average (80–84) |
| Subtest: Visual perception | 15 | 92 | Average (85–115) |
| Subtest: Motor coordination | 11 | 76 | Low (70–79) |

licensure, informed consent, and payment. Whether services are provided in person or through telehealth, the practitioner must have processes in place to assure HIPAA compliance. Specific to telehealth, this includes using a HIPAA-compliant videoconferencing platform where the vendor provides a Business Associate Agreement (BAA). This agreement indicates the vendor will adhere to HIPAA requirements to protect health information. Additionally, OT practitioners should hold the appropriate license(s) when engaging in interstate practice. The OT Compact facilitates interstate practice by granting licensed occupational therapy practitioners' privilege to practice within member states; however, not all states participate in the OT Compact (OTCompact.org, 2022). Additionally, clients must provide informed consent to receive services through telehealth. Requirements for the consent process vary by state.

The COVID-19 pandemic resulted in rapid expansion of payment for services provided through telehealth (AOTA, 2021a). Prior to initiating services through telehealth, payer coverage for telehealth OT services should be confirmed. Payers may require use of a specific

TABLE 23.3 **Sample Goals, Objectives, and Interventions for Sam**

| Long Term Goal | Objectives | Telehealth OT Interventions |
|---|---|---|
| Sam will write all uppercase letters independently from memory with 199% legibility as measured by therapist/teacher data sheets, within 1 year. | Sam will participate in 15 minutes non-preferred daily activity with less than 2 verbal cues by his teacher/parent to redirect to task, demonstrating improved emotional regulation and attention, within 6 months. | • Instruction, modeling, and practice of sensory and executive functioning supports to aid in increased self-regulation, body awareness, and motor planning/ideation to enable Sam to attend and engage in school tasks.<br>• Implementation of sensory diet/home program to enhance coping and emotional regulation. |
| | Sam will complete an age-appropriate art project independently, including cutting within 1/8 inch of the lines, within 6 months. | • Gross motor interventions (with caregiver participation for safety) to improve body awareness and motor planning/ideation which are important for fine motor, cutting, handwriting skills.<br>• Fine motor interventions using small manipulatives (e.g., coins, beads, theraputty/playdough) to improve fine motor skills<br>• Instruction and guided practice with scissors (grading activity for shapes and line width) to promote coordination and visual motor integration.<br>• Instruction and guided practice with ADLs using small fasteners/closures (e.g., zippers, snaps, buttons) to reinforce and add practice of fine motor, visual motor skills. |
| | Using a visual aid, Sam will write all uppercase letters using appropriate sizing in 50% of the letters, within 6 months. | • Handwriting instruction and guided practice using structured handwriting programs to practice and reinforce handwriting skills.<br>• Writing practice on slanted/vertical surface to enhance proprioceptive feedback and encourage wrist extension for handwriting.<br>• 'Air writing' to improve recall for letter formation.<br>• Motor interventions to enhance the ability to grade pressure on paper. |
| | Sam will identify 13/26 letters on a keyboard independently with 80% accuracy in 3/3 trials, within 6 months. | • Keyboarding instruction and guided practice using structured keyboarding programs to provide compensatory approach to handwriting.<br>• Motor-based interventions addressing fine motor skills, finger strength and isolation, and motor planning/ideation to improve handwriting and/or keyboarding so Sam may communicate in written format for academics. |

BOX 23.5 **Resources for Telehealth**

AOTA telehealth resources are available at www.aota.org/telehealth

- Telehealth Decision Guide
- Telehealth Ethics Advisory Opinion
- Telehealth Position Paper
- Virtual School-Based Services via Telehealth
  - Introduction
  - Legal, ethical, and procedural concerns
  - Embedding IEP goals in daily routines
  - Evaluation considerations for delivering virtual OT services via telehealth in the schools
  - Progress monitoring and documentation during virtual school-based OT service delivery via telehealth
  - Collaborating with school team members during virtual OT service delivery via telehealth

Pediatric OT telehealth books from AOTA press

- Telehealth and Occupational Therapy in Early Intervention
- Telehealth and Occupational Therapy in Schools

National Center for Hearing Assessment and Management (https://infant-hearing.org/ti101/index.html): free, self-paced, narrated online telehealth EI training courses for families, providers, and administrators.

Teleshare videos are available at https://www.youtube.com/c/Telehealth-Share/videos.

modifier or place of service code to designate a telehealth service delivery model.

## Planning for Occupational Therapy Intervention Through Telehealth

The intervention plan may include providing OT services exclusively through telehealth or through a hybrid/blended service delivery model. An important component of intervention planning for telehealth is determining what materials the child will have available for OT interventions. A scavenger hunt or materials checklist can be used to assist with intervention planning. Prior to each session, the practitioner should communicate with caregivers about any materials they need to provide. It is important to have an alternate plan in case the child does not have the materials available at the start of the session. An online activity or movement-based activity that does not require materials is helpful as an alternate plan.

When incorporating movement-based activities, the child's safety must be a priority. There should be unobstructed space in the child's environment for the planned activities. Sofa pillows or cushions may be used to create a soft barrier between the child and furniture. The OT practitioner should be confident in the caregiver's ability to both provide hands-on support as needed and to maintain the child's safety during movement-based therapeutic activities.

The use of a PowerPoint or Google slide deck to plan and guide the therapy session is a useful strategy. See Fig. 23.5 for a sample slide deck of a telehealth OT session with a school-aged child. The slide

A PowerPoint/Google slide deck is a great tool to guide telehealth OT sessions. It shifts some of the session planning to the client or caregiver. Below are screenshots of a therapy session template for telehealth. It can be easily adapted for other populations and interventions. The template includes the following headings:

**Slide 1: Catching up** – Use this slide to connect with the child and learn how things have been going since the last session (exploring the child's week/day, any new concerns, how the home program/therapy strategies were implemented, etc.)

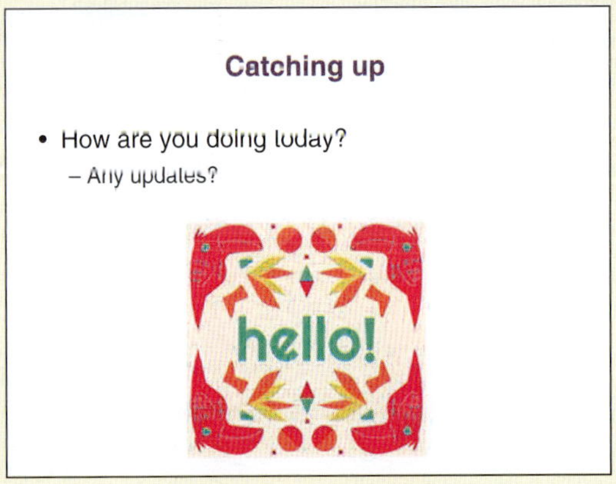
Catching up
• How are you doing today?
– Any updates?
hello!

**Slide 2: Warm up activity (gross motor)** – On this slide, provide visuals depicting activities (text/pictures) and have the child select two; encourage the child to select one 'tricky one' or one 'new one'. If you are wanting to target specific skills, have the child select one activity, and you select the other. When you update and save the PowerPoint for the next session, change the font color on specific activities you want to target in the next session.

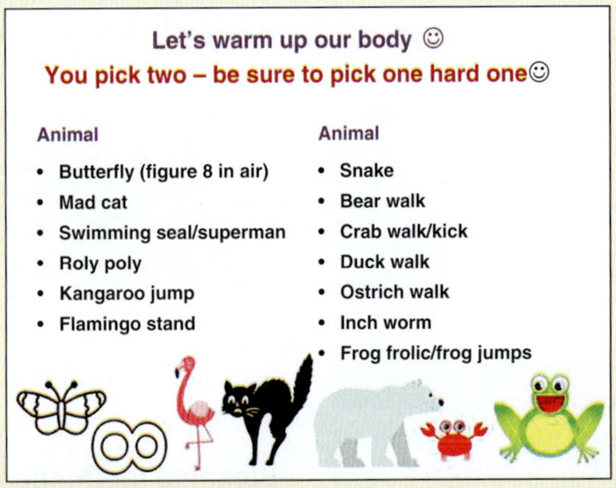
Let's warm up our body ☺
You pick two – be sure to pick one hard one☺
Animal
• Butterfly (figure 8 in air)
• Mad cat
• Swimming seal/superman
• Roly poly
• Kangaroo jump
• Flamingo stand
Animal
• Snake
• Bear walk
• Crab walk/kick
• Duck walk
• Ostrich walk
• Inch worm
• Frog frolic/frog jumps

**Slide 3: Warm up activity (fine motor)** – Customize this slide with activities that align with materials the child has available. To engage the child and caregiver in session planning and to assure the child is prepared with materials at the start of the session, ask the child to select two activities for the next session and have those materials ready. Pediatric clients are excited to show which activities they selected and almost always have their materials ready.

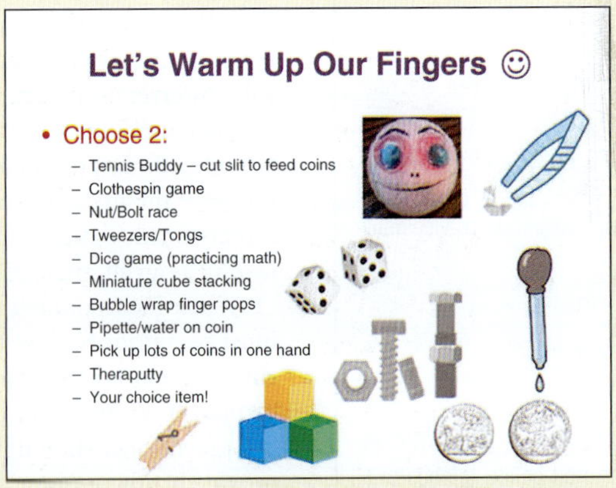
Let's Warm Up Our Fingers ☺
• Choose 2:
– Tennis Buddy – cut slit to feed coins
– Clothespin game
– Nut/Bolt race
– Tweezers/Tongs
– Dice game (practicing math)
– Miniature cube stacking
– Bubble wrap finger pops
– Pipette/water on coin
– Pick up lots of coins in one hand
– Theraputty
– Your choice item!

**Fig. 23.5** Example slide deck for telehealth OT session with school-aged child material. (Adapted with permission. Original blog post by Jana Cason (2022) for TelehealthShare's blog, *Tips and tricks to reduce planning time for telehealth sessions.*)

**Slide 4: Handwriting** – If the pediatric client has handwriting goals, customize this slide with an image of the handwriting curriculum workbook. At the end of the session, update the page number with the starting point for the next session.

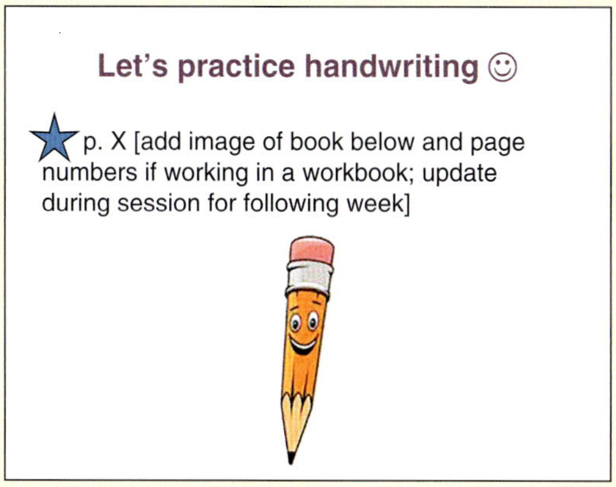


**Slide 5: Visual perception** – Online activities from Eye Can Learn (eyecanlearn.com) target a variety of visual-perceptual skills (e.g., tracking, visual discrimination, visual spatial relations, figure ground, visual closure, visual form constancy). Use screen sharing and annotation tools to enable the child to complete visual perceptual activities related to therapy goals during the OT telehealth session. When you update and save the PowerPoint, change the font color on the specific visual perceptual skills you want to target for the next session.

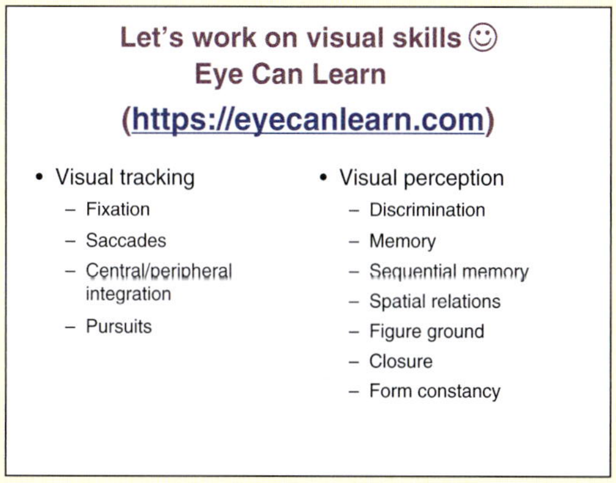


**Slide 6: Target new skills** – Add images of activities for motor skills (e.g., catching/kicking ball, jumping jacks, etc.) aligned with the child's goals. Give choices and encourage the child to select between two activities or select the order of activities.

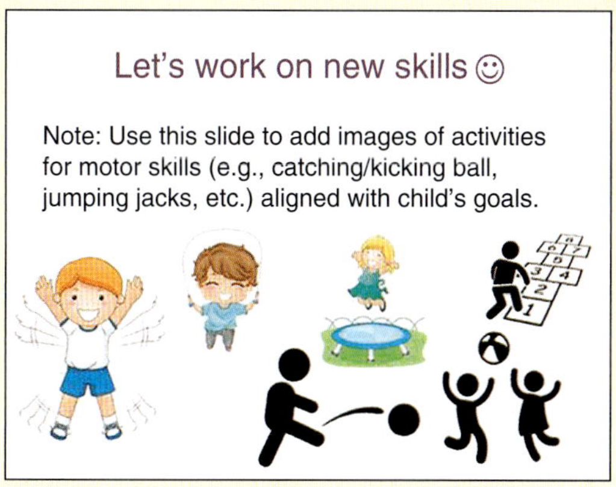


**Fig. 23.5, Cont'd**

**Slide 7: More therapy fun** – Customize this slide with online games/activities that align with targeted skill areas (e.g., visual-motor, life skills, sensory processing, handwriting, executive functioning, emotional regulation, keyboarding).

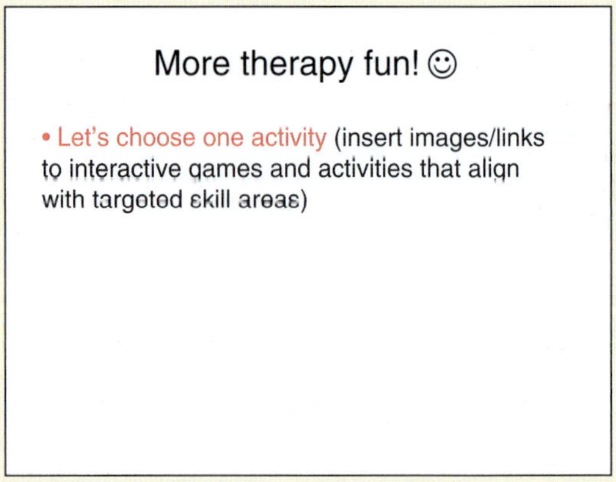
More therapy fun! ☺
• Let's choose one activity (insert images/links to interactive games and activities that align with targeted skill areas)

**Slide 8: Free choice activity** – Save the last 5-10 minutes of the therapy session for the child to select a 'free choice' activity, usually a preferred online therapeutic game or activity. For each child, customize a 'free choice menu' that the child can use to select a free choice activity. In this way, you know that any activity selected will be therapeutic and align with the child's goals. The free choice activity serves as a motivator during the session (e.g., "Let's stay on task so we have time for the free choice activity").

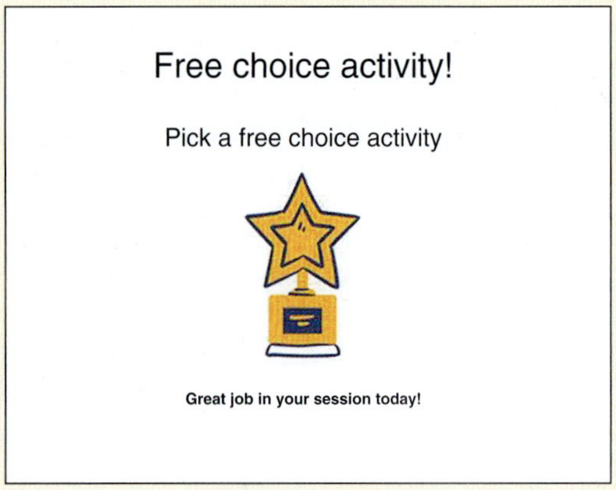
Free choice activity!
Pick a free choice activity
Great job in your session today!

**Fig. 23.5, Cont'd**

deck should be customized for the child based on the child's goals and therapy materials available. The slide deck does not need to be visible throughout the session; rather, it can be pulled up on a shared screen to facilitate flow and transition between activities. The OT practitioner can update the slides during the session. Opening the customized file at the next session, with previously highlighted activities and updated page numbers, serves as a prompt and facilitates the flow of the therapy session. To decrease session planning time, encourage the child to select activities from a choice of activities on the slides. Children enjoy the opportunity to make choices and are often eager to share their selection at the beginning of the session. This strategy shifts a portion of the planning and material preparation to the child and caregiver.

## Intervention Implementation

Prior to initiating the telehealth OT session, the practitioner should open any files, videos, or other material to screen share during the session. Close any computer programs not to be used during the session. When the child joins the session, make "eye contact" by looking directly into the camera. After initial greetings, assure that the technology is working properly (the child can see and hear the practitioner and vice versa). Discuss implementation of any previous recommendations (e.g., therapeutic strategies, home program) and any new concerns. Engage in planned activities. If the practitioner will be demonstrating tabletop, movement-based, or keyboarding activities, an alternate camera view is needed. In this case, there will need to be a shift between the built-in camera and an external camera (laptop, electronic tablet, or smartphone) positioned to capture the desired view.

The practitioner may need to ask the child or caregiver to reposition the camera/device in order to observe the child engaged in therapeutic activities. For example, a practitioner planned fine motor and handwriting activities for an OT session with a child. The child joined the session through videoconferencing on a desktop computer. The child initially talked to the OT practitioner through the desktop's built-in camera. However, in order to see the child engaged in the fine motor and handwriting activities, the child also logged into the OT session using a Chromebook computer. The practitioner directed the child to slide the Chromebook forward and partially close the Chromebook. This allowed the Chromebook's built-in camera to capture the child's hands and the table surface. The OT practitioner was able to see the child's face and talk to the child through the desktop computer camera and see the child's hands and tabletop surface through the Chromebook camera. The OT practitioner provided verbal cues and directions while observing the child engaged in the tabletop activities. In another scenario, a child joined an OT telehealth session using an electronic tablet. To capture movement-based activity, the child's caregiver positioned the device on a shelf providing a full view of the room and the child's movements. The practitioner coached the child's caregiver, who then implemented the therapeutic activities and provided physical assistance and verbal prompts, as directed. Toward the end of the telehealth session, the OT practitioner reviewed the activities and skills targeted, discussed home program activities, and planned for the next session.

### Assessment of Outcomes

Assessment of outcomes involves monitoring the child's progress toward desired outcomes and completing a re-evaluation at a designated time period (e.g., 6 months after initiation of services in an outpatient setting). The re-evaluation may use the same assessments used during the initial evaluation. The re-evaluation may lead to continuation of OT services, discharge from services, or a referral to other services (AOTA, 2020). For a structured approach to assessing telehealth outcomes at the individual, group, and population level, readers are directed to the PACE Framework (Little et al., 2021a; 2021b). This framework provides OT outcomes, operational definitions, and outcome measures aligned with telehealth. Research should continue to assess outcomes of telehealth OT services to inform practice and healthcare policy.

### Acknowledgment

The author would like to acknowledge Christine T. Myers, PhD, OTR/L, FAOTA, FNAP for contributions to Case Example 23.1 and Cassie R. Swihart Thein, OTD, OTR/L, CTP, who provided an evaluation report used to inform Case Example 23.2.

## SUMMARY

Telehealth has been effectively used to deliver pediatric OT services in EI, school-based practice, pediatric hospital and outpatient clinics, and other community-based settings. Benefits of a telehealth service delivery model include delivery of family-centered services in natural contexts, improved access to OT services and specialists, interdisciplinary collaboration, increased caregiver efficacy, and positive child outcomes. The COVID-19 pandemic resulted in widespread adoption of telehealth in OT. Looking to the future, telehealth will continue to be an integral service delivery model for OT practice.

1. Telehealth is used in pediatric OT practice to provide synchronous, asynchronous, and blended/hybrid services in EI, schools, hospitals, outpatient clinics, and other community-based settings.
2. The OT process includes consultation and screening, development of the occupational profile, analysis of occupational performance, synthesis of evaluation process, intervention implementation, and assessment of outcomes. Adaptions to the OT process when services are delivered through telehealth may include the following:
   a. completing the caregiver interview using videoconferencing or phone;
   b. using publishers' online evaluation platform and digital assessment materials;
   c. mailing materials (response forms or standardized materials) prior to the evaluation and/or incorporating digital assets through screen sharing during the evaluation;
   d. selecting and positioning technologies for optimal engagement; and
   e. communicating with caregivers prior to therapy sessions about any needed materials (e.g., fine motor manipulatives, pencil/crayon, and paper).
3. Many telehealth resources exist for pediatric OT practitioners. These include AOTA telehealth resources (www.aota.org/telehealth); continuing education courses, training modules, and books; social media resources (e.g., Facebook, Instagram, Pinterest); and telehealth-related YouTube channels (e.g., TelehealthShare).

## REFERENCES

Abbott-Gaffney, C. R., Gafni-Lachter, L., Cason, J., Sheaffer, K., Harasink, R., Donehower, K., & Jacobs, K. (2022). Toward successful future use of telehealth in occupational therapy practice: What the COVID-19 rapid shift revealed. *Work, 71*(2), 385–394. https://doi.org/10.3233/WOR-210789.

American Occupational Therapy Association. (2020). Occupational therapy practice framework: Domain and process—Fourth Edition. *American Journal of Occupational Therapy, 74*(Suppl. 2), 7412410010.

American Occupational Therapy Association. (2021a). COVID-19 state updates: Summary of telehealth, insurance, and licensure developments; and comprehensive state-by-state chart. https://www.aota.org/advocacy/advocacy-news/state/state-news/covid-19-summary-telehealth-insurance-licensure.

American Occupational Therapy Association. (2021b). COVID-19 virtual school-based services. https://www.aota.org/practice/clinical-topics/covid-19/covid-19-virtual-school-based-services.

American Occupational Therapy Association. (2018). Telehealth in occupational therapy [Position paper]. *American Journal of Occupational Therapy, 72*(Suppl. 2), 7212410059. https://doi.org/10.5014/ajot.2018.72S219.

American Occupational Therapy Association. (2005). Telerehabilitation position paper. *American Journal of Occupational Therapy, 59*(6), 656–660. https://doi.org/10.5014/ajot.59.6.656.

Cason, J. (2009). A pilot telerehabilitation program: Delivering early intervention services to rural families. *International Journal of Telerehabilitation, 1*(1), 29–38. https://doi.org/10.5195/ijt.2009.6007.

Cason, J., Behl, D., & Ringwalt, S. (2012). Overview of states' use of telehealth for the delivery of early intervention (IDEA Part C) services. *International Journal of Telerehabilitation, 4*(2), 39–46. https://doi.org/10.5195/ijt.2012.6105.

Cason, J. (2011). Telerehabilitation: An adjunct service delivery model for early intervention services. *International Journal of Telerehabilitation, 3*(1), 19–30. https://doi.org/10.5195/ijt.2011.6071.

Cason, J. (2022). *Tips and tricks to reduce planning time for telehealth sessions.* https://telehealthshare.myshopify.com/blogs/telehealth/tips-and-tricks-to-reduce-planning-time-for-telehealth-sessions.

Clawson, B., Selden, M., Lacks, M., Deaton, A. V., Hall, B., & Bach, R. (2008). Complex pediatric feeding disorders: Using teleconferencing technology to improve access to a treatment program. *Pediatric Nursing, 34*(3), 213–216.

Conner, A., Dizdarevic, S., Gonzalez, I., Knece, Z., & Koedam, H. (2021). Hybrid versus face-to-face delivery of group soft-skills training for young adults with high-functioning autism. *American Journal of Occupational Therapy, 75*(Suppl. 2), 7512515345. https://doi.org/10.5014/ajot.2021.75S2-RP345.

Criss, M. J. (2020). *Telehealth fine motor assessment-functional skills.* https://www.yourtherapysource.com/product/telehealth-fine-motor-assessment-functional-skills/.

Criss, M. J. (2013). School-based telerehabilitation in occupational therapy: Using telerehabilitation technologies to promote improvements in student performance. *International Journal of Telerehabilitation, 5*(1), 39–46. https://doi.org/10.5195/ijt.2013.6115.

Heimerl, S., & Rasch, N. (2009). Delivering developmental occupational therapy consultation services through telehealth. *Developmental Disabilities Special Interest Section Quarterly, 32*(3), 1–4.

Kronberg, J., Tierney, E., Wallisch, A., & Little, L. M. (2021). Early intervention service delivery via telehealth during COVID-19: A research-practice partnership. *International Journal of Telerehabilitation, 13*(1), 1–8. https://doi.org/10.5195/ijt.2021.6363.

Little, L. M., Cason, J., Pickett, K. A., & Proffitt, R. (2021a). Keeping PACE with the new normal: A framework for telehealth practice, research, and policy. *OT Practice, 26*(8), 10–15.

Little, L. M., Pickett, K. A., Proffitt, R., & Cason, J. (2021b). Keeping PACE with 21st century healthcare: A framework for telehealth research, practice, and program evaluation in occupational therapy. *International Journal of Telerehabilitation, 13*(1), 1–20. https://doi.org/10.5195/ijt.2021.6379.

Little, L. M., Pope, E., Wallisch, A., & Dunn, W. (2018). Occupation-based coaching by means of telehealth for families of young children with autism spectrum disorder. *American Journal of Occupational Therapy, 72*(2), 7202205020. https://doi.org/10.5014/ajot.2018.024786.

Little, L., Wallisch, A., Dunn, W., & Tomchek, S. (2020). A telehealth intervention to increase toilet training in autism. *American Journal of Occupational Therapy, 74*(Suppl. 1), 7411520511. https://doi.org/10.5014/ajot.2020.74S1-RP401E.

Luscombe, G. M., Hawthorn, J., Wu, A., Green, B., & Munro, A. (2021). Empowering clinicians in smaller sites': A qualitative study of clinician's experiences with a rural virtual Paediatric feeding clinic. *Australian Journal of Rural Health, 29*, 742–752. https://doi.org/10.1111/ajr.12781.

OTCompact.org. (2022). *About.* https://otcompact.org/about/#:~:text=The%20Occupational%20Therapy%20Licensure%20Compact,interstate%20practice%20of%20occupational%20therapy.

Pearson. (2022). *Staying connected through telepractice.* https://www.pearsonassessments.com/professional-assessments/digital-solutions/telepractice/about.html.

Pecini, C., Spoglianti, S., Bonetti, S., Di Lieto, M. C., Guaran, F., Martinelli, A., Gasperini, F., Cristofani, P., Casalini, C., Mazzotti, S., Salvadorini, R., Bargagna, S., Palladino, P., Cismondo, D., Verga, A., Zorzi, C., Brizzolara, D., Vio, C., & Chilosi, A. M. (2019). Training RAN or reading? A telerehabilitation study on developmental dyslexia. *Dyslexia, 25*(3), 318–331. https://doi.org/10.1002/dys.1619.

Rush, D. D., & Shelden, M. L. (2020). *The early childhood coaching handbook.* Baltimore, MD: Paul H. Brookes Publishing.

Seruya, F. M., Feit, E., Tirado, A., Ottomanelli, D., & Celio, M. (2022). Caregiver coaching in early intervention: A scoping review. *American Journal of Occupational Therapy, 76*(4), 7604205070. https://doi.org/10.5014/ajot.2022.049143.

U.S. Department of Education (a) (n.d.). *Every Student Succeeds Act (ESSA).* https://www.ed.gov/essa?src=rn.

U.S. Department of Education (b) (n.d.). *Individuals with Disabilities Education Act, Sec. 303.321(a).* https://sites.ed.gov/idea/about-idea/.

U.S. Department of Education (c) (n.d.). *The Rehabilitation Act of 1973.* https://www2.ed.gov/policy/speced/reg/narrative.html.

Wakeford, L. (2002). Telehealth technology for children with special needs. *OT Practice, 7*(21), 12–16.

Wallisch, A., Little, L., Pope, E., & Dunn, W. (2019). Parent perspectives of an occupational therapy telehealth intervention. *International Journal of Telerehabilitation, 11*(1), 15–22. https://doi.org/10.5195/ijt.2019.6274.

Western Psychological Services [WPS]. (2022). *Assessment telepractice overview.* https://pages.wpspublish.com/telepractice-101.

24

# Social-Emotional Learning

*Colleen Cameron Whiting, Renee Allen, and Mim Oshsensbein*

## GUIDING QUESTIONS

1. How do occupational therapy practitioners promote self-awareness, self-management, social awareness, relationships skills, and responsible decision-making competencies in children and youth?
2. How do occupational therapy practitioners implement a public health, trauma-responsive, relational approach to promote social-emotional learning?
3. What strategies based on the Collaborative for Academic, Social, and Emotional Learning interventions can occupational therapy practitioners use to promote critical skills needed for life satisfaction?

## KEY TERMS

Interoception
Relationship skills
Responsible decision-making
Self-awareness
Self-management
Self-regulation
Serve and Return
Social awareness
Social-emotional learning (SEL)
Social interaction skills

## OCCUPATIONAL THERAPY'S ROLE IN SOCIAL-EMOTIONAL LEARNING

Social and emotional development impacts a child's successful performance and participation in all occupations. Adequate social and emotional functioning supports overall wellness starting in childhood and continuing throughout the lifespan (Jones et al., 2019). Thus, wherever occupational therapy practitioners practice, they are called to use a public health, trauma-responsive, relational (rather than behavioral) approach to promote social and emotional development. Occupational therapy practitioners are well positioned to holistically support the child's well-being through occupational engagement in collaboration with other disciplines (AOTA, 2020).

The Collaborative for Academic, Social, and Emotional Learning (CASEL) has become the leading framework for exploring evidence-based social and emotional learning strategies to promote the critical skills needed for life effectiveness (CASEL, 2020). This framework has been used to develop learning standards and competencies regarding social and emotional development for preschool through high school-aged children around the world. As defined by CASEL, **social-emotional learning (SEL)** involves five core dynamically related competencies: self-awareness, self-management, social awareness, relationship skills, and responsible decision-making. Occupational therapy practitioners are ideally equipped to support these competencies with their knowledge of mental health, contextual, psychosocial, and performance factors that influence occupational performance and participation and their ability to evaluate the person-occupation-environment transaction.

This chapter explores how the client-centered occupational therapy practitioner can support each of the CASEL SEL competencies necessary to improve participation and performance in valued roles and meaningful activities for the child and adolescent. A variety of risk factors, as listed in Box 24.1, impact the child's social-emotional development. The key concepts and core assumptions of social-emotional intervention that span across the ages and competencies are highlighted in Box 24.2. Organized using a developmental perspective, the chapter acknowledges how these competencies shift in presentation and complexity depending on the child's age and abilities. Evidence-informed interventions are detailed throughout the chapter, providing specific examples for each competency for adapting the environments, tasks, and routines, coaching, utilizing universal support, designing and implementing programs, leading groups, and providing direct service (Kannenberg et al., 2017).

## OCCUPATIONAL THERAPY INTERVENTION FOR EACH COMPETENCY ACROSS CHILDHOOD AND ADOLESCENCE

Occupational therapy practitioners emphasize SEL to promote a child's engagement in their desired meaningful activities, such as play,

**BOX 24.1 Established Risk Factors for Social-Emotional Development Delay**

- Preterm birth
- Developmental, motor, and intellectual disorders
- Neurodivergence, including conditions, such as autism spectrum disorder, ADHD, intellectual and developmental disabilities, sensory processing disorder, and giftedness
- Adverse childhood experiences
- Children at risk for trauma due to substance abuse in the family, economic stress, homelessness, identification as LGBTQIA+ as youth, or social isolation

Adapted from: Kingsley, K., Sagester, G., & Weaver, L. L. (2020). Interventions supporting mental health and positive behavior in children ages birth–5 yr: A systematic review. *American Journal of Occupational Therapy, 74,* 7402180050. National Children's Traumatic Stress Network. (2021). Populations at risk. https://www.nctsn.org/what-is-child-trauma/populations-at-risk

academics, activities of daily living, instrumental activities of daily living, sleep and rest, health management, leisure, and social participation (AOTA, 2020). They address motor (e.g., how a person moves or interacts with objects), process (e.g., how a person organizes objects, time, and space, applies knowledge, or adapts), and **social interaction skills** (e.g., how person uses verbal and nonverbal skills to communicate, including initiating, terminating, producing, physically supporting, and adapting to social situations) (AOTA, 2020). They facilitate a child's ability to engage in a variety of activities by supporting the child's abilities to make decisions, be aware of their actions, manage emotions, and communicate with others. They use their knowledge of the multiple factors that influence occupational performance to address the five dynamically related competencies outlined in CASEL. The following is a description of the competencies with examples of how occupational therapy practitioners intervene.

## Self-Awareness

**Self-awareness** refers to the ability to accurately recognize one's emotions and thoughts and their influences on behavior. This includes accurately evaluating one's strengths and limitations and possessing a well-grounded sense of confidence and optimism (CASEL, 2020).

**Self-Awareness in Infants and Toddlers.** Self-awareness emerges during the first 3 years of development. Internal and external perceptual experiences from physical interactions with their sensory, motor, and relational environments help young children move from a prereflective sense of self, present at birth, to a reflective sense of self that can incorporate an emerging self-identity (Stern, 1985). A self-other distinction also begins to develop through interpersonal interactions, in which the infant plays a primary interactive role through both initiating and responding to a social partner (Fogel & Garvey, 2007; Montirosso & McGlone, 2020). Older toddlers can begin to use internal state talk to describe the perceptions and feelings of themselves and others, setting the stage for the theory of mind capacity in preschool (Feldman, 2007).

Initial self-awareness opportunities are best facilitated through everyday physical and relational exploration embedded in natural environments (Dunst et al., 2001). The occupational therapy practitioner can assess both the child's exploration skills and the affordances of the space to create opportunities for self-self or self-object understanding (Pierce et al., 2009). For an infant, this may mean assessing a safe place for the infant to lay unrestrained to explore its body or objects that are within or just out of reach (see Fig. 24.1). For a toddler with more mobility, the occupational therapy practitioner and parent can collaborate on opportunities in the home space for mastery and success to be embedded safely (Pierce et al., 2009).

**BOX 24.2 Key Concepts to Implement Social-Emotional Learning Interventions Throughout the Lifespan**

The following key concepts are recommended when providing intervention to address SEL challenges in children and youth.

1. Prioritize therapeutic use of self and establish connections with children and youth as essential to occupational therapy process and outcomes.
2. Support the child's emotional state and regulation throughout the session. Anticipate and observe responses to the intervention that may require modifications to keep the child engaged and feeling challenged, but supported and comfortable.
3. Individualize the timing and content (top-down/bottom-up) of intervention activities to the specific child.
4. Apply culturally informed, neurodiversity-affirming practices, avoiding ableist programming and language, and remaining open to cultural differences and nonnormative social styles.
   - Social interaction may look different for a non-Western family, for someone that is nonspeaking and using augmentative assistive communication with physical and sensory challenges, for an autistic child that uses echolalia to communicate and finds eye contact uncomfortable, or for someone with a mental illness that experiences social situations as anxiety producing.
   - Seek feedback from children and families during the course of therapy, so you can adjust your style if needed.
5. Integrate teaching and practice of new skills within the context of meaningful occupation in natural environments.
6. Encourage caregivers to develop their own regulation supports and tools.
   - Caregivers can only be effective in coregulation with their child if they themselves are regulated.
7. Communicate and engage with a multidisciplinary team of professional providers each with their own skill set and perspectives.
   - Ask questions and seek support from team members.
   - Discuss challenges and seek feedback.
   - Listen to others' perspectives. Provide your findings and perspectives.
8. Maintain a growth mindset, presume competence, and reflect upon sessions.
9. Engage children in strength-based programming to support self-determination.
10. Use a strength-based perspective when discussing concepts with children, caregivers, and other team members.
    - Team members and caregivers may view children differently after hearing about their strengths.
    - Children benefit from hearing about their strengths.
11. Use a dynamic systems approach and bioecological model of development to understand and address SEL.
    - A child's ability to gain social-emotional skills is impacted by a complex combination of continuously changing multidirectional influences.
    - A child's unique executive functioning, temperament, relationships, environmental circumstances, and cultural and community affordances all impact social-emotional competency development.
    - Address factors influencing SEL in therapy sessions by engaging the child in meaningful, fun, and appropriate occupation-based activities.
12. Engage family and caregivers in supporting children and youth by reinforcing skills, concepts, and processes from occupational therapy sessions in daily routines.

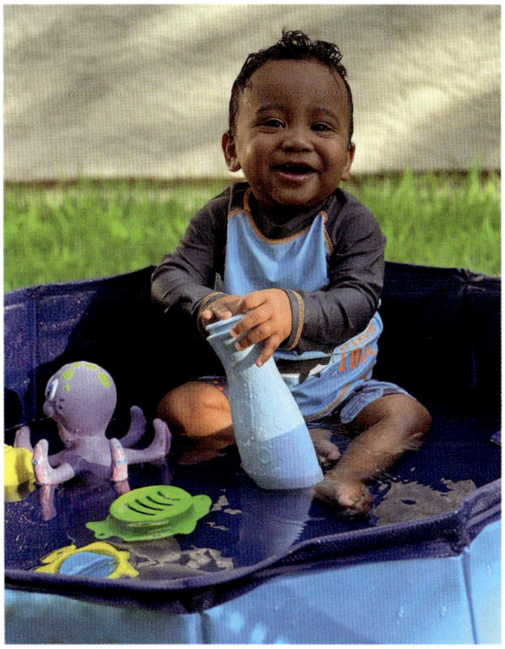

**Fig. 24.1** Baby is able to safely explore objects just within his reach.

Because the development of infants and toddlers is intrinsically tied to their caregiving context, interventions discussed at this age primarily involve collaboration between the occupational therapy practitioner and the caregiver. To promote self-awareness, the practitioner can use a combination of education, modeling, and coaching techniques empowering caregivers to embed opportunities for self-awareness and mastery into a child's play and routine. Box 24.3 highlights suggestions for coaching throughout childhood for all the competencies. Another important area for coaching combines neurobiology and language development research to promote self-awareness and emerging emotional awareness. The occupational therapy practitioner can coach caregivers on how to help the young child to connect their internal and external feeling states within the context of their natural routines. Interoceptive awareness, both discriminative and affective, has been linked to self-perception later in life (Montirosso & McGlone, 2020; Mulcahy et al., 2019). In addition, the frequency of using language to describe desires and feeling states during infancy and toddlerhood has been correlated with emotional awareness at 6 years old irrespective of language ability (Dunn et al., 1991).

Quality parent-child interaction is linked to social competence (Feldman et al., 2013). DeGangi (2017) describes how practitioners can use the Child-Centered Activity model to facilitate a child's sense of self during a parent-child engagement. In this evidence-based program, parents are coached to dedicate 15–20 minutes a day to allowing the infant or toddler to initiate all the interactions during the play. The parent is guided to dedicate noninterrupted time, follow the child's lead, and explore the child's interests without judgment. This nondirective play, which focuses on a child's internal locus of control versus external directions, was shown to be more effective than structured therapy or the control at improving inattention and irritability (DeGangi & Greenspan, 1997).

**Self-Awareness in Preschool- and School-Age Children.** In preschool, many children come to identify a basic range of emotions that they feel themselves and recognize in others (Rosanbalm & Murray, 2017b). As children age, they start to differentiate between more complex emotions, recognize the intensity of their emotions, and understand that they can use their thinking to regulate their emotions. Social behavior within occupational engagement is often driven by their emotions, and having an emotionally competent caregiver/teacher that is attuned and ready to provide support is critical to developing the child's capacity for emotional awareness (Denham & Bassett, 2019; Poulou et al., 2022) For a child, having a caring adult willing to teach about emotions and discuss emotions openly, can be transformational (Brackett, 2019). Teachers and other adults, including occupational therapy practitioners, may be trained in and then provide specific programming such as the RULER program which fosters emotional self-awareness and emotional literacy (see https://www.rulerapproach.org/) (Brackett et al., 2019; Hoffmann et al., 2020).

When considering the environment, the literature suggests that access to green spaces or natural areas has a positive association with stress reduction and mental well-being for school-age children, leaving children more available for self-reflection (see Fig. 24.2) (Chawla et al., 2014; McCormick, 2017). The occupational therapy practitioner can advocate for an inclusive playground with green spaces and increased recess times to align with recommendations regarding time spent in nature as well as in outdoor play areas (Christiana et al., 2016). They can also promote equitable opportunities for extracurricular and leisure activities related to the child's interests and strengths, leaning on the relationship between occupational engagement and satisfaction to identity affirmation and positive mental health.

To facilitate self-awareness within classrooms and homes, the occupational therapy practitioner can provide staff and caregiver training on **interoception** and the value of emotional literacy (recognizing emotions and using words to express more complex feelings). Interoception refers to an awareness of internal body states, which include both physical and emotional (Neff, 2023). For example, people sense when they are hungry, tired, happy, sad, calm, or anxious. Children and youth may sense when they are starting to feel ill. Poor interoception can lead to difficulty maintaining homeostasis (e.g., attending to body functions) and perceiving self and others, poor self-regulation and emotional regulation, and relationships affecting health and wellness (Neff, 2023). Therefore, occupational therapy practitioners engage children and youth in activities to understand and listen to body cues. They encourage children to recognize and communicate their emotions and feelings.

Lessons about interoception can be utilized throughout the day, using curricula such as The Interoception Curriculum (see Fig. 24.3) (Mahler, 2018; Mahler et al., 2022). To increase their interoceptive awareness, children need to learn to connect their feelings in their body to an emotion and to the urge to act. See Case Example 24.1 for an example of an occupational therapy practitioner working with kindergarten-age children to support their awareness of interoception. An example is helping the child to identify what brings them joy (see Fig. 24.4) and what body signals tell them. Practitioners can also help others understand that neurodivergent children who have alexithymia (trouble identifying and describing their emotions) may need options outside traditional emotion labels to identify how they are feeling.

There are a variety of visual supports that the occupational therapy practitioner can promote. Check-in spots located in various environments can provide pictures of faces with different emotions for the child to select instead of using words to describe how they are feeling. An "emotion thermometer" can be used for the child to identify the emotion's intensity (see Fig. 24.5). Many practitioners pair this strategy with "the size of the problem" visual, with which the child is guided to compare the intensity of their emotional response to the demands of the situation. It is imperative that the adult support does not attribute shame if a child identifies that their emotional response was not aligned with the size of the problem or encourage the child to "mask" how they are feeling. Instead, the practitioner can direct focus with the child on a growth mindset, brainstorming supports to help the child persist through difficult tasks.

## BOX 24.3 Strategies to Use Occupational Performance Coaching to Facilitate Social-Emotional Learning

Occupational therapy practitioners use a variety of occupational performance coaching strategies within occupational therapy interventions to promote SEL. They begin by understanding the child or youth's level of ability and adjust activities to promote learning by doing. Occupational Performance Coaching requires practitioners to engage in therapeutic use of self to motivate, encourage, support, and guide children and youth in developing social-emotional skills. Following is a list of strategies that can be adjusted for a variety of activities.

**Self-Awareness**

- Create opportunities for sensory, motor, and relational exploration.
- Support mastery and problem-solving in the natural environment.
- Incorporate feeling vocabulary/body talk into conversation (e.g., "Is your belly hungry?").
- Permit, without dismissal or judgment, the child's age-appropriate expression of feelings.
- Help the child label and understand their emotions through reflection.
- "Watch, wait, and wonder" with the child.
- Provide encouragement for the child's effort instead of praising the outcome.
- Connect physical and interoceptive sensations to feelings.
- Establish check-ins (notice heartbeat, body sensations, breathing rate, and felt body temperature).
- Label their own emotional state and how they know.
- Bring attention to youth's personal strengths and point out the strengths of others.

**Self-Management**

- Attune to the child's unique body signals.
- Anticipate and use contingent responses to the child's signals.
- Play exciting games (peek-a-boo and chase) while also providing re-regulating opportunities.
- Coregulate a child whose self-regulation skills are not developed or available.
- Acquire and use self-calming strategies when interacting with the child.
- Teach the child to notice body signals during regulatory changes and emotional experiences.
- Identify what activities/experiences help the child feel good and "empty their cup."
- Spend time connecting and letting them share about a special interest area.
- Collaborate with the child to determine the need to upregulate or downregulate.
- Validate the youth's emotional experience without minimization or dismissal.
- Model cognitive-based problem-solving (when youth is in a regulated state).

**Social Awareness**

- Talk out loud to infants about their routine as they go through it.
- Read books and sing songs that are culturally affirming.
- Have toddlers "help" with home routines such as cooking, cleaning, and laundry.
- Model empathy and the norms of expressing gratitude, repairing, and intimacy.
- Provide age appropriate support to understand new social experiences.
- Support pretend play games that incorporate familiar social and emotional scenarios.
- Ask questions such as "How would I feel if that happened to me?"
- Cue the child to notice others' nonverbal signs of how they are feeling
- Ask what is the "group plan" to bring voice to an unspoken expectation in social situations.
- Suggest examples of some prosocial behaviors in which the child could engage.

**Relationship Skills**

- Match the parent's affective and nurturing gestures to the individual differences of the child.
- Provide predictable interactive exchanges with the infant and toddler.
- Be a safe and secure "home base" for the child to explore uncertain places and people.
- Help the child to successfully form new family, peer, and community relationships.
- Create opportunities for shared joy and pleasure that invite social engagement.
- Group desks and offer toys and games to encourage cooperation and interaction.
- Provide partner reading and games or assign buddies for recess time.
- Apply and model conflict resolution techniques.

**Responsible Decision-Making**

- Use consistent, nonthreatening cues to encourage or discourage a young child's actions.
- Clearly communicate expectations by teaching the rules of the child's natural environments.
- Use play and stories to teach social problem-solving.
- Utilize naturalistic positive social reinforcement (e.g., "Great job using walking feet.").
- Offer guided choices.
- Provide opportunities to experience natural consequences.
- Coach the child to consider various strategies when navigating group goals or desires.
- Scaffold executive skills to support adolescent decision-making.
- Ask youth to provide their opinions on family plans, and acknowledge their contributions.

**Self-Awareness in Adolescents.** Gains in complex reasoning skills, increased importance of social affiliations outside the family unit, and an urge to experiment and test boundaries allows adolescents to explore self-identity in novel and profound ways compared to previous stages. Adolescence is considered an intensive period for occupation-related and self-identity development wherein individuals experience occupational changes that assist with the transition into adulthood (Clarkson et al., 2021; Tal-Saban & Maeir, 2021). These changes prompt exploring and questioning self-identity: *Who am I? Where do I fit in? Where do I want to be, to go?* This often occurs in the context of identifying and pursuing academic goals, vocational interests, social opportunities, and peer interactions. The practitioner is in a unique position to facilitate self-identity formation in adolescence by promoting self-awareness through occupational development.

Robust interoceptive and emotional awareness in adolescence is necessary for self-awareness development. Hence, the occupational therapy practitioner can make supporting these two areas a priority in the culture and context of the school environment. Occupational therapy practitioners' implementation of programs like Emotion Coaching helps adolescents understand the different emotions experienced, why they occur, and strategies to manage their responses (Rose et al., 2015). Practitioners train teachers in the use of five steps designed to build empathy in relationships with students, thereby modeling prosocial emotional intelligence: (1) being aware of the child's emotions; (2) recognizing emotion as an opportunity for intimacy and teaching; (3) listening empathetically and validating a child's feelings; (4) helping the child verbally label emotions; and (5) setting limits while helping the child problem solve. Students exposed to Emotion Coaching-trained

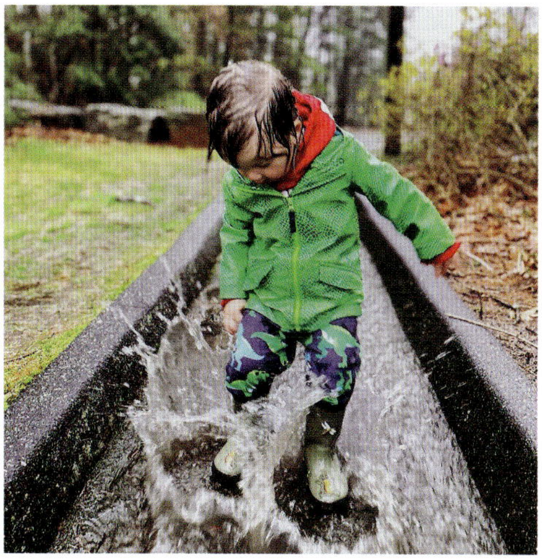

**Fig. 24.2** Child feeling empowered in outdoor play.

teachers were found to have increased academic and social successes, improved classroom behaviors, and more developed emotional regulation and resilience (Rose et al., 2015).

The occupational therapy practitioner can find a variety of opportunities to promote the development of positive, empowered self-awareness within adolescent school and community milieus. School-based groups designed by the clinician and implemented at the universal level (by practitioner-trained teachers or the clinician themselves) can facilitate the positive development of self-awareness through recognizing character strengths and emotion identification. One such evidence-based group curriculum, Strengths Gym (Proctor et al., 2011), provides exercises that encourage adolescent students to build their personal strengths, learn new strengths, and recognize strengths in others. The occupational therapy practitioner can further expand on adolescent-identified strengths by promoting engagement in school-based or extracurricular opportunities. For example, if the adolescent identifies a strength in singing, the clinician could support them in connecting with an activity such as the drama club's musical.

## Self-Management and Self-Regulation

**Self-management** refers to the ability to regulate one's emotions, thoughts, and behaviors effectively in different situations. This includes

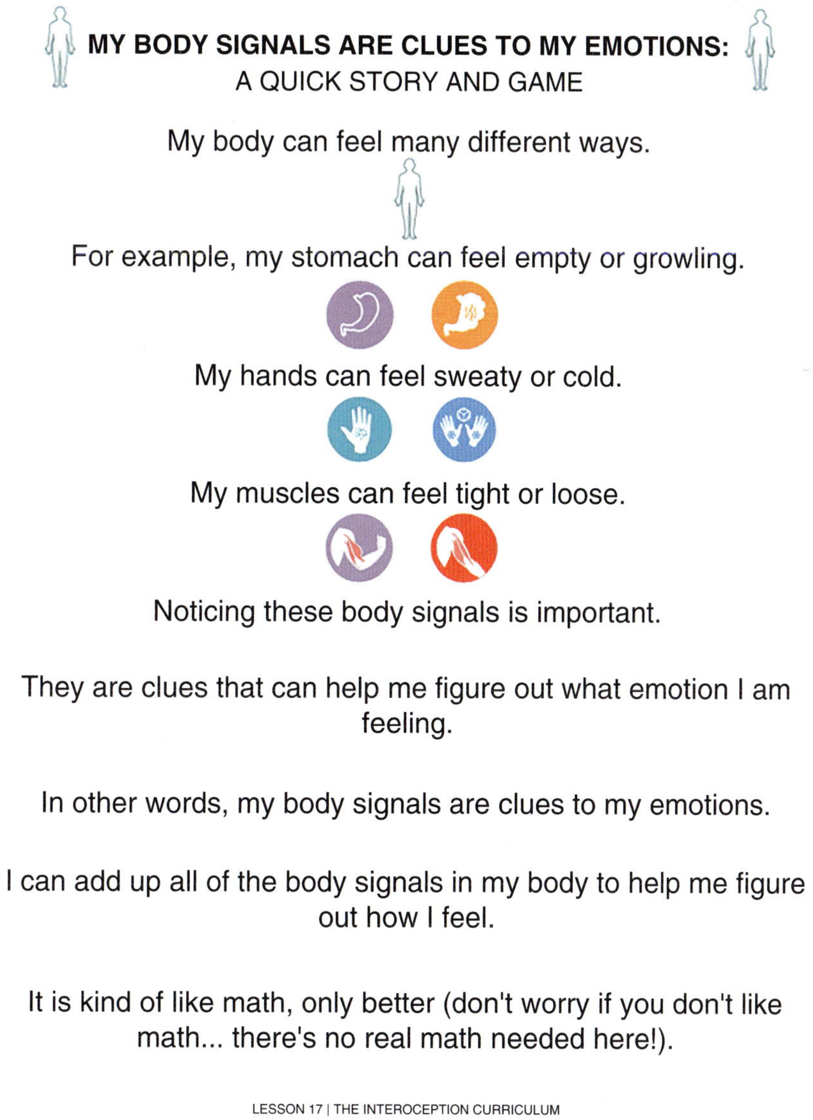


**Fig. 24.3** Example of Mahler's interoception curriculum.

## CASE EXAMPLE 24.1 SOCIAL-EMOTIONAL PROGRAMMING IN SCHOOL

The occupational therapy practitioner identified that the current kindergarten cohort was presenting with challenges in their social-emotional development. She asked the school psychologist and speech and language pathologist if they would like to develop a whole grade initiative with her. They drafted a plan for six 30-minute sessions and received approval from the administration.

The Kindergarten Social-Emotional-Regulation Initiative began, rotating to a new kindergarten class every 6 weeks. The goal of the intervention was to enhance the students' social and emotional learning, provide a common vocabulary throughout the class and the school, and give teachers ideas for incidental or quick activities within their classrooms. Each discipline provided 10-minute lessons, and students rotated through the stations. The speech and language pathologist used adaptations of the Social Thinking methodology (Winner & Crooke, 2009; see https://www.socialthinking.com/), and the school psychologist focused on elements from the MindUp curriculum (see https://mindup.org/). The occupational therapy practitioner engaged children in hands-on, active learning experiences that supported their development of interoceptive awareness and self-regulation. The occupational therapy practitioner helped them to identify their "triggers" (what left them feeling frustrated, annoyed, sad, or unable to concentrate) as well as their "glimmers" (what helped them feel ready to learn, play, and happy) (Dana, 2018; Porges, 2011). They selected their own tools for their "toolbox" of regulation from a variety of sensory, relational, movement, thinking, and engagement in occupation options. The students tried out different sensory experiences, noting how they affected their arousal level, their emotion, and their ability to participate in school. They also explored relational supports such as taking a walk with a friend or reading a book together. The students noted how doing a body scan and thinking about positive affirmations may help. Physical activity and engaging in a meaningful activity were both recognized as affecting their arousal level and ability to self-manage.

Students and teachers who participated in the 6-week programs provided feedback. The teachers and students reported finding the program invaluable and fun! Plans were made to repeat the program every year.

managing stress, controlling impulses, motivating oneself, and setting and working toward achieving personal and academic goals (CASEL, 2020). **Self-Regulation** refers to the conscious and unconscious ability to manage states, emotions, behaviors, and attention in an adaptive way, promoting successful and meaningful occupations and relationships.

**Self-Management and Self-Regulation in Infants and Toddlers.** Self-management has its foundations set in infancy, starting with the basic need to establish physiologic regulation. Infants are born with some self-regulatory capacities such as gaze aversion, crying, and sucking. However, infants remain highly dependent on the presence of a nurturing caregiver (i.e., co-regulator) to achieve regulation (Lupien et al., 2009; Rosanbalm & Murray, 2017a; Tronick & Beeghly, 2011). Coregulation is the "interactive process of regulatory support that can occur within the context of a caring relationship" (Rosanbalm & Murray, 2017a, p. 1). This coregulation through parental attunement and touch, which is responsive to the child's needs and desires, has a significant impact on the development of the social brain (Feldman, 2007; Jackson et al., 2022). The experience of regulation through coregulation and caregiver-infant synchrony gradually fosters the development of self-regulation.

Environments can serve as barriers and supports for a young child's regulation. The occupational therapy practitioner should assess a child's response to the physical, sensory, and relational demands of the child's natural environments. The regulatory systems of premature

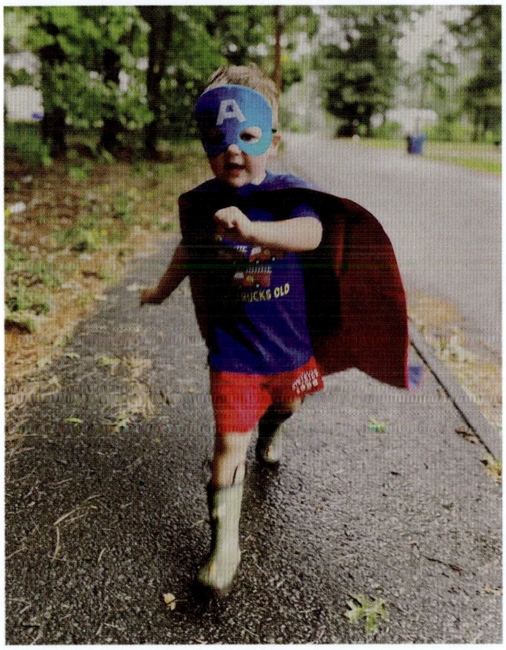


**Fig. 24.4** Child enjoying his experience dressing up as a superhero. Practitioners can assist children in learning about what brings them joy.

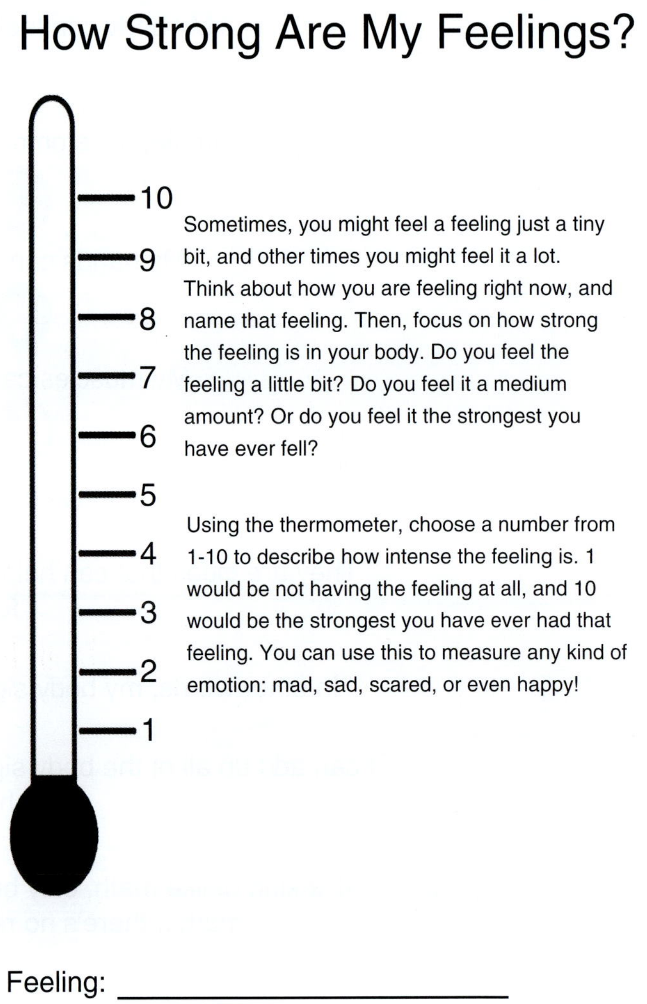


**Fig. 24.5** Example of an emotion thermometer.

infants, whose sensory systems may not be fully developed, are particularly affected by their environments (Jackson et al., 2022). The occupational therapist who works in the NICU can recommend environmental changes such as closing the shades and limiting intrusive and unpredictable noises. The early intervention practitioner can also assess home and community environments to determine which environmental characteristics support a child's regulation and then adapt the environment accordingly.

Parent coaching to support coregulation and parent-child synchrony is another potential focus of home-based occupational therapy intervention (Feldman, 2007; Kingsley et al., 2020). The occupational therapy practitioner can help the parent observe how proximity, gaze, vocalization, touch, affect, and behavior impact the child's ability to stay regulated and engaged with the caregiver (Calkins, 2011; Feldman, 2007). For both infants and toddlers, identifying which strategies are the most re-regulating for a child is a unique opportunity for the home-based practitioner. Practitioners frequently ask parents questions to inform specific strategies and routines that work for the child and family. Some questions may be the following:

- Does the child calm to oral strategies such as nutritive or nonnutritive sucking, chewing, or blowing?
- Does the child calm to quieter speech, rhythmic music, or white noise?
- Does the child respond to proprioceptive input such as deep pressure massage, big hugs, joint compressions, swaddling, weighted toys or lap pads, or moving "heavy items" around the house?
- Does the baby or toddler calm to linear rocking or swinging or vibration? How much time does the child need to settle?

Helping a child and family identify patterns of sensory support for calming, reorganization, and sleep can support a child's development of self-management skills. As the young child gains more self-management competencies, the practitioner can support the parent in grading the amount of coregulation needed during different challenges.

Occupational therapy practitioners trained in touch-based therapies can coach parents to use these physical modalities to improve regulation (Kingsley et al., 2020). Kangaroo Care is an intervention used with premature infants in the NICU. It encourages caregivers to use skin-to-skin contact, gentle movement, familiar voice, and smell stimulation while holding the infant up against their chest (Case-Smith, 2013). The occupational therapy practitioner can assist with positioning the baby and coaching the parent to regulate themselves while in this supportive position. The practitioner trained in infant massage, such as Baby's First Massage, can coach the parents on techniques that can help the infant's body to regulate (Kingsley et al., 2020). Other body-based interventions such as qigong massage have been shown to improve young autistic children's capacity for self-regulation (Silva et al., 2011).

**Self-Management and Self-Regulation in Preschool-Age and School-Age Children.** The rapid growth of the brain in preschool through elementary school years affords a new capacity for self-management and self-regulation (Rosanbalm & Murray, 2017a). Each child has individual differences that affect their capacity as well as their need for co-regulation, as coregulation continues to play an important role in helping the child feel safe and connected (Parris et al., 2014). Future participation and performance in occupations as well as the development of relationships rely on children being able to understand, regulate, and appropriately express their emotions (Blankson et al., 2017; Eisenberg et al., 2003).

Caregivers are charged with creating positive, safe, physical, social, emotional, and sensory environments. Children can have very strong emotional and physical reactions to their environment. The occupational therapy practitioner works with the teacher/caregiver and child to design more sensory-supportive environments (Whiting et al., 2021). Environmental elements that support regulation from the child's perspective include warm neutral colors, controlled noise, dimmable lights, and/or alternative seating options (e.g., comfy chair, hammock). Every Moment Counts (see Chapter 15) offers an environmental assessment that can be a helpful guide for this process (Bazyk, 2022). Practitioners may need to advocate that children have multiple spaces in different environments (e.g., home, school, community) that provide a space for them to be comfortable. Children may benefit from a calming corner that includes various sensory experiences such as a rocking chair, bean bag, music, scented lotions, fidget toys, oral motor options, and pinwheels (Whiting, 2018). Adding access to sensory rooms with items such as these has reduced seclusion and restraint in inpatient psychiatric settings (Sutton et al., 2013). A co-regulating adult should be available to go to the space with the child to provide compassionate support while maintaining awareness of their own state of arousal and emotion and its influence on the child.

When creating a culture at the classroom level for all students, research in the trauma field speaks to the importance of predictability for regulation, while research suggests adults proactively provide support for autistic children instead of waiting for dysregulation (Whiting, 2018). Examples of using this approach include taking the time to connect during arrival routines, infusion of positive affirmations, and a visual of the day's activities. Another example is using a visual support such as the "Get ready, Do, Done Model" when preparing to complete a task. The practitioner using this model may ask the student to answer questions such as: What will it look like when this is done? What steps do I need to take to complete this? and What materials, time, and actions do I need for the doing part of task planning (Ward & Jacobsen, 2014). The student moves on to executing the task only after they answer each question. The occupational therapy practitioner also considers what sensory input would be helpful to build into a predictable routine or performance pattern throughout the day for a particular child who is struggling to stay regulated. Recommendations are individualized and include the child's input.

Occupational therapy practitioners are intentional about the choice of tasks for each child. Drawing from the Neurosequential Model of Therapeutics, proactively planning daily use of repetitive, rhythmical body-based interactive activities done together as a group facilitates a functional regulated state and sense of cohesion (Perry, 2009). When entering a new environment, transitioning, taking a break, or having a difficult time staying engaged, the occupational therapy practitioner can offer suggestions of activities for the group such as chants, stomping of feet, drumming, yoga, and ball toss games to support self-management (Cahill et al., 2020).

At the group and universal levels, beginning to use systematic cognitive-behavioral approaches as well as embedding associated activities affords opportunities to expand the child's discrimination, awareness, and vocabulary regarding regulation (Blackwell et al., 2014). The "How Does Your Engine Run–The Alert Program" guides children to identify and change how alert they feel using an engine analogy to describe if their engine is running "high," "low," or just right" (Williams & Shellenberger, 1996). The Zones of Regulation program builds on this to draw the connection between one's triggers, arousal level, and one's emotions (see Fig. 24.6) (Kuypers, 2011). Care must be taken to discuss both the "engine" and "zones" in nonjudgmental terms. There are no "bad" zones, and the goal is not to stay at one level of arousal. The practitioner helps children and youth understand whether their arousal level matches the situation and learn strategies to modify their arousal when necessary.

Sensory tools, mindfulness, meditation, and body scans, as well as proactive strategies such as using healthy sleep, nutrition, and physical activity routines, support a regulated state for performance and

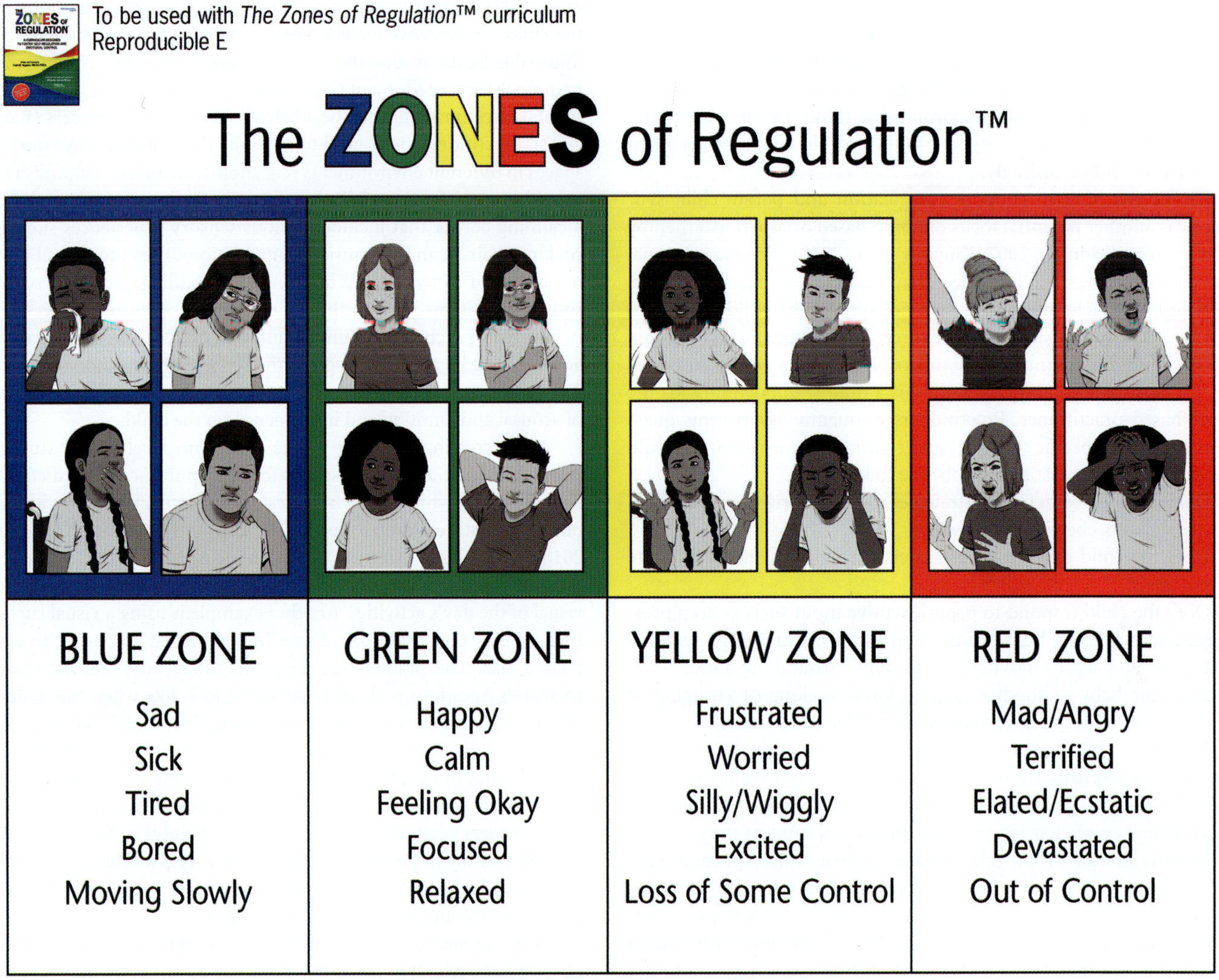



From *The Zones of Regulation*™ by Leah M. Kuypers • Available at www.socialthinking.com

**Fig. 24.6** Description of the different zones from Zones of Regulation.

participation. Older children can learn to manage the connection between their own body signals and their signs of regulation and dysregulation. The evidence-based MindUP curriculum discusses how the brain works and explains that when the nervous system has been triggered to protect, it flips the thinking part of the brain offline and lets the emotional part of the brain take over (Hawn Foundation, 2011; Schonert-Reichl et al., 2015). MindUP is one of many SEL programs that include lessons that the occupational therapy practitioner can deliver and then model how to use strategies such as deep breathing (in which the child is encouraged to focus on lengthening the breath out), relaxation techniques, imagery, or positive self-talk (Rosanbalm & Murray, 2017a). Another example of a potential universal support is the 12-week mindfulness-based Kindness Curriculum for promoting the development of self-regulation, which uses literature, music, and movement to present the concepts (Flook et al., 2015).

The occupational therapy practitioner acts as a behavioral detective to uncover and reveal the underlying challenges to the child's regulation and can help families and teachers identify a child's signs of regulation and dysregulation (a quiet body is not always a regulated system). Using a visual "cup" analogy, practitioners can teach that some children, due to prior trauma or challenges with mental health, have a smaller cup, one that overflows more quickly when they are triggered by a certain event or an accumulation of stress. When a child's cup is full, and they become dysregulated, the Neurosequential Model of Therapeutics guides the adult to first address the child's ability to self-regulate (e.g., provide strategies for the child to practice) using a bottom-up approach and later move to top-down strategies that allow the child to reason and self-regulate (Perry, 2009) (see Case Example 24.2).

Trauma can disrupt a child's sensory integration and processing development and, in turn, their ability to maintain an appropriate arousal level, self-regulate, and adapt to challenges in their environment (Diamant et al., 2020; Whiting, 2018). A child who has experienced trauma can demonstrate over-responsivity and under-responsivity to sensory stimuli (sensory modulation), impaired interoception or reading of internal body signals, and challenges in posture and praxis (or motor planning) due to difficulties with sensory perception (sensory discrimination) (Howard et al., 2020; Schulz & Vögele, 2015; Van der Kolk, 2003). Sensory integration intervention drawn from Ayres Sensory Integration® (Ayres, 1979) and the STAR Frame of Reference (Miller et al., 2018), and aligned with trauma-responsive principles, can be utilized by a trained occupational therapy practitioner to facilitate sensory processing to support self-management (see Fig. 24.7) (see Chapter 27).

## CASE EXAMPLE 24.2 APPLYING THE NEUROSEQUENTIAL MODEL

Mateo was in the fifth grade, a kind and empathetic young man with a significant history of trauma. Mateo often found himself in situations where he was triggered in the school setting and would shut down and ask to go to the nurse or just hide in the bathroom. The occupational therapy practitioner was asked to provide some guidance to help Mateo remain in the classroom and complete his work. First, the practitioner met with Mateo, and he shared that he loved music and liked the feeling of being in a contained space when he was upset. The practitioner worked with the teacher to make these options readily available to Mateo.

Using a proactive approach, the practitioner and teacher also identified movement opportunities during the day that Mateo reported he enjoyed and helped him to feel engaged in the class community. The occupational therapy practitioner then coached the teacher on how to use trauma-sensitive care with Mateo when he was dysregulated with Perry's (2009) regulate, relate, and reason model (i.e., Neurosequential model) as outlined below.

*Step 1 – Regulate:* The practitioner suggested that the teacher focus on being present for Mateo and not try to change how he was feeling but rather validate his feelings, offer a supportive physical environment with sensory tools, and suggest some mindful breathing if needed.

*Step 2 – Relate:* The occupational therapy practitioner guided the teacher to attune to Mateo, empathize, and reestablish a sense of safety for him by nurturing him through verbal and nonverbal communication.

*Step 3 – Reason:* The practitioner coached the teacher to engage in reflection with Mateo to better understand the reason behind the behavior, collaborate to create a solution, and develop a plan for next time.

After a month, the occupational therapy practitioner met with Mateo to hear his lived experience. He commented, "I still struggle not to get overwhelmed, but my teacher is helping school feel safer for me now." The practitioner continued to support Mateo by reaching out to the school team, including the mental health professionals, to consult on how to further cultivate this feeling, recognizing this needed to be an ongoing conversation. Mateo's availability to be engaged and successful in the school setting continued to fluctuate, but the team had a plan.

**Self-Management and Self-Regulation in Adolescents.** Adolescents have a growing need for effective self-management as youth move closer to adult-level expectations, roles, and responsibilities (including first-time jobs and volunteer pursuits). Self-management at this stage of life requires the adolescent to further develop self-regulation and emotional regulation in the face of physiologic dysregulators, like increased hormone production. Youth are expected to effectively engage their still developing executive functioning skills (such as planning, organization, and goal setting) in occupations driven by intrinsic motivations and growing external demands and expectations set by family, school, and community. Successful performance and the ability to meet these expectations are complicated by emerging inhibitory and logic systems and heightened sensitivity to rewards (Griffin, 2017).

The use of coregulation remains vital at this stage due to these maturational limitations on the developing brain circuitry and connectivity. The occupational therapy practitioner can coach coregulation techniques that promote adolescent emotional regulation and utilize group-based curricula to harness this stage's interest and desire for peer interaction (Murray et al., 2015). Along with Zones of Regulation (Kuypers, 2011), the Sensory Connection (Moore, 2005) addresses self-regulation development in older adolescents and adults. It incorporates sensory modalities, individual strengths, and interests to support the development of effective emotional

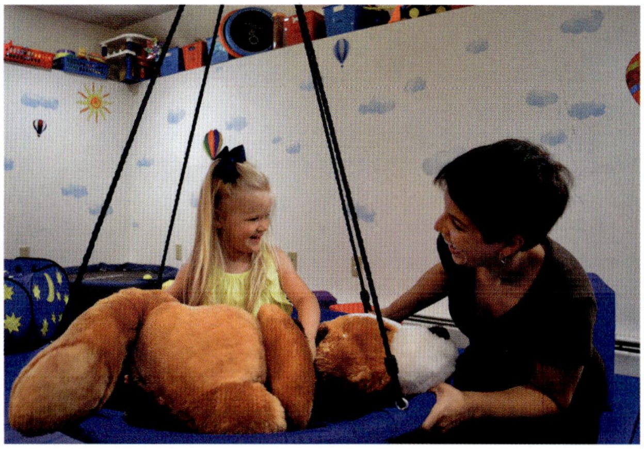

**Fig. 24.7** Using movement and therapeutic use of self, the occupational therapy practitioner is helping the child to regulate.

regulation, coping strategies, and healthy leisure and success-oriented activities.

Adolescent self-management requires higher-level executive functioning skills built on strong foundations of emotional regulation and inhibitory control. Executive functioning skills such as organization, planning, time management, goal setting, and problem-solving are implicit in the idea of self-management. At the individual service level, the practitioner can use occupationally based interventions to support and enhance the development and effective application of executive functioning. Based on the original Cog-Fun intervention, the Teen Cog-Fun for adolescents incorporates neurocognitive and psychiatric rehabilitation principles within an occupational therapy framework (Levanon-Erez et al., 2019). This intervention tool helps the teen to identify their own challenges, self-monitor during task performance, and learn self-management strategies. Use of the Cog-Fun or Teen Cog-Fun has been shown to promote occupational performance, executive functioning, and strategy behavior (Levanon-Erez et al., 2019). Other strategies to support executive functioning include using explicit instructions, task analysis, scaffolding instruction, breaking tasks into smaller, manageable pieces to be addressed on a timeline, and grading the complexity of the task.

## Social Awareness

Social awareness is the ability to take the perspective of and empathize with others from diverse backgrounds and cultures; to understand social and ethical norms for behavior; and to recognize family, school, and community resources and supports (CASEL, 2020).

**Social Awareness in Infants and Toddlers.** Infants begin social learning at birth. Infants' early development of sensory perceptions supports detecting and generating affective signaling in line with the cultural norms of their caregivers (Feldman, 2007, 2020). Through their interactions, experiences, and observations, infants learn the predictable patterns of social relationships and environments. The developing ability to interpret and use sensory-affective cueing (such as eye gaze, facial expression, pitch volume, and body language) and interoceptive perception to understand and facilitate adaptive communication sets the stage for affective prosody (e.g., conveying and understanding emotion nonverbally) and empathy (Mulcahy et al., 2019). As representational play develops, toddlers internalize these affective social norms of communicating and living through their play routines, such as pretending to care for a baby doll or "cook" a meal for a family member.

**BOX 24.4 Aspects of Emotional Expression and Coregulation That Differ Across Cultures**

- Animation
- Directness of eye contact
- Directness of questions
- Formality (customs, dress, or relationships)
- Meaning of words
- Physical proximity
- Touching
- Use of gestures
- Volume of speech

Adapted from: Day, M & Parlakian, R. (2004). *How culture shapes social-emotional development: Implications for practice in infant-family programs.* Washington, DC: Zero to Three Center for Program Excellence.

Interventions to support a young child's sense of social awareness require the practitioner to be cognizant of the social norms in the environment and cultural systems surrounding the child (see Box 24.4) (Feldman, 2007). Childrearing practices and goals vary considerably between Western independence-oriented cultures and Eastern and Native American community-oriented cultures (Feldman, 2007; Tsethlikai et al., 2018). Collaboration with the parent on culturally acceptable ways for the child and the caregiver to engage in co-occupation within the home environment and routines supports natural opportunities for the child to gain social awareness. The practitioner addresses mismatches between cultural norms and expectations between environments and relationships the young child encounters.

Joint attention is also foundational to emerging social awareness. Case-Smith's (2013) systematic review of interventions to promote social-emotional learning found that the most effective way to promote joint attention is to follow the child's lead, allowing them to select the activity and set the pace, by using positive affect and by prompting and socially reinforcing the child's joint attention.

**Social Awareness in Preschool- and School-Age Children.** Children in preschool are just beginning to understand social rules, initiate prosocial behavior, and show early signs of empathy that help support their occupational engagement (Rosanbalm & Murray, 2017b). Meanwhile, older children start to be able to adapt to more complex social situations and have a more robust ability for perspective-taking. The occupational therapy practitioner can model using an inquisitive mindset to learn more about their peers' social and cultural identities as well as how to have compassionate interactions with others.

Using the premise of positive psychology, the practitioner can coach teachers and caregivers on ways to foster connection and kindness among peers and prosocial behaviors to improve well-being (Datu et al., 2022). One approach is to tie these concepts to literacy, such as in the text "How Full is Your Bucket?" (Rath & Reckmeyer, 2009). After reading the book, the practitioner could coach the family or class to "fill each other's buckets" by engaging in prosocial behavior. The practitioner could also work with administrators to adopt a school-wide prosocial classroom model for which classroom management practices are student centered, and teachers learn to effectively respond to children's emotional needs, connect with them, and guide their behavior by using their own social and emotional competence (Jennings & Greenberg, 2009).

A variety of strategies can be used within occupational therapy sessions to enhance a child's social awareness. The Social Thinking curriculum increases awareness of unwritten social rules. Responses to social interactions are described as "expected," or "unexpected," and the "group plan" as compared to the "individual plan," and things you say and think are discussed as being in a "bubble" to help the child visualize their own and others' perspectives (Winner, 2005). This can help those who struggle with theory of mind to conceptualize what others are thinking. Additionally, emotion identification picture cards can be used to help the child learn to identify what people can look like while experiencing different emotions.

**Social Awareness in Adolescents.** Youth often have heightened emotions with social hypersensitivity, fueled by emerging understanding and attempts at applying social nuance to various contexts and situations, sometimes resulting in success, sometimes in "a learning experience." Engagement in risk taking behavior and difficulty taking others' perspectives may result. Facilitating social awareness guides them toward increased successful application of behaviors and social interactions that serve them in the engagement of meaningful occupations. For example, recognizing a teacher's expectations of respectful classroom behavior leads to a youth's increased use of cooperative and prosocial behaviors in the classroom setting, resulting in an improved academic experience.

At the universal level, the clinician can facilitate both environmental modifications and the development of groups to support social awareness development. Environmentally, clinicians can ensure the use of materials and visuals representative of various abilities and diversity. Practitioner-designed groups, utilizing character strength interventions, promote an increased understanding of others' perspectives and development of prosocial behaviors (perspective-taking, empathy, cooperation, sense of gratitude). These tools emphasize and promote individual differences and are thus more relevant to the adolescent's personal interactions and occupations (Lavy, 2020). Expanding on existing character strengths gives them the confidence to explore/develop other strength areas and recognize the strengths in others (Park & Peterson, 2008). Curricula like the evidence-based Youth Gratitude Project (Greater Good Science Center, n.d.) can be used to promote greater social awareness through the identification of character strengths in self and recognition of strengths in others.

The use of occupational mapping promotes self-awareness in direct-service models. Here, practitioner and adolescent collaborate to identify and explore social norms in the adolescent's natural contexts and environments. For example, the clinician and adolescent client could explore the expectations of self and others in the context of a high school basketball game or then look at what is expected by self and others during a date. Mapping of relevant social experiences allows for safe and explicit probing and examination of implicit social-cultural beliefs and socially enforced rules that the adolescent may otherwise have difficulty identifying or making sense of. This increased awareness can then be applied to the development of more explicit relationship skills.

## Relationship and Social Interaction Skills

**Relationship skills** include the ability to establish and maintain healthy and rewarding relationships with diverse individuals and groups. This includes communicating clearly, listening actively, cooperating, resisting inappropriate social pressure, negotiating conflict constructively, and seeking and offering help when needed (CASEL, 2020). **Social interaction skills** refer to effectively using both verbal and nonverbal skills to communicate, including initiating and terminating, producing, physically supporting, shaping content of, maintaining flow of, verbally supporting, and adapting social interaction (AOTA, 2020).

**Relationship and Social Interaction Skills in Infants and Toddlers.** In the first 3 years of life, infants and toddlers learn through lived experience how to form close and secure relationships. By 2–3 months, caregivers and infants participate in serve-and-return interactions that begin to have predictable patterns and rhythms (Feldman, 2007). "**Serve and return** interactions shape brain architecture. When an infant or young child babbles, gestures, or cries, and an adult responds appropriately with eye contact, words, or a hug, neural connections are built and strengthened in the child's brain that support the development of communication and social skills. Much like a lively game of tennis, volleyball, or Ping-Pong, this back-and-forth is both fun and capacity-building. When caregivers are sensitive and responsive to a young child's signals and needs, they provide an environment rich in serve and return experiences" (Center on the Developing Child, 2024).Through these interactions, the physical and relational needs of the infant are met forming the foundation for secure attachment (Case-Smith, 2013). Attachment relationships established in the first 6 months of life impact social relationships throughout childhood and adulthood (Kerr et al., 2019). Relationship skills continue to develop through early childhood, as social networks begin to incorporate siblings, extended family, daycare providers, and community members.

In promoting early social interaction skills, the occupational therapy practitioner is tasked with optimizing the environment for relational interactions. With infants, the occupational therapy practitioner can evaluate the environment and choose places with the least amount of competing stimulation and the most amount of postural support for face-to-face interactions. Car seats, high chairs, changing tables, rocking chairs, and blankets are all places that can offer supportive positioning for interaction. As toddlers gain mobility and can initiate interactions, environmental opportunities for engaging and relating increase. The practitioner can assess community environments where children and youth engage in new opportunities to practice relationship skills such as parks, playgrounds, libraries, and gyms. See Case Example 24.3 for an example of supporting a toddler with social interactions at the park.

Increased parent sensitivity can improve the quality of the attachment relationship (De Falco et al., 2014; Landry et al., 2006). Occupational therapy practitioners can use modeling, coaching, and feedback with parents to support responsiveness, sensitivity, and flexibility in relationship-focused interventions (Case-Smith, 2013; Kingsley et al., 2020). Equipped with the knowledge of sensory and motor development, the occupational therapy practitioner is in a unique position on the team to help a family identify subtle social cues and to facilitate the use of assistive technology to allow the child with limited mobility opportunities for social interaction.

The ability to initiate, respond, and maintain cycles of serve-and-return social exchanges is important to a relationship and social-emotional development yet is compromised in neurodivergent children (Ho & Lin, 2020). The Developmental Individual Relationship (DIR/Floortime Model) has resulted in improvement in parent-child interactions with autistic children (Ho & Lin, 2020; Reis et al., 2018; Solomon et al., 2014). This play-based, parent and teacher coaching intervention joins the child in their interest, accommodates their developmental and communication readiness, and works to expand the child's capacity to sustain relatedness with increasing complexity (Wieder & Greenspan, 2003). The DIR model lends itself toward interventions offered by early intervention practitioners in the home with primary caregivers who can be trained to use this methodology frequently throughout the day (Barenberg et al., 2022).

Early intervention and community centers frequently offer group-based infant-parent programs focused on parenting skills, caretaking, and attachment. Occupational therapy practitioners can support or run "Mommy and Me" playgroups for children with and without disabilities that offer opportunities for improving parent-child, parent-parent, and child-peer relationships.

### CASE EXAMPLE 24.3 SOCIAL INTERACTION SKILLS: SELF-REGULATION

Through early intervention home visits, the occupational therapy practitioner worked with Joey, a 25-month-old boy who aggressed against peers at the park, especially when on the slide. Joey was slow to get off the bottom of the slide because he did not like the feeling of the dirt on his skin. Often other children did not wait for him and would crash into him, both touching him and knocking him into the dirt.

The practitioner addressed the child's tactile over-responsivity by engaging the child in a variety of sensory activities. The practitioner also addressed the home environment so that it would be less stimulating to the child. For example, they suggested the parents provide Joey with a quiet corner, with pillows and blankets for him to play, and opportunities for Joey to make choices and communicate his needs. The practitioner also addressed challenges with self-regulation by providing opportunities for the child to engage in strategies during play (for example, they practiced counting to three after asking for a toy, taking deep breaths, and blowing bubbles to practice waiting). They practiced telling each other how they felt. The practitioner worked with the child for 6 months using this bottom-up approach to provide the child with strategies to self-regulate.

Once Joey showed that he could use words and some strategies to remain emotionally regulated, they went to the park to see if Joey could play with others (a top-down approach). They started the park visit with his mother pushing him in the swing from in front. Joey calmed with the linear swinging. Next, the practitioner, mother, and Joey went over to the playground structure with the slide. The practitioner noticed his mother's clenched jaw and nervous hesitation as well as Joey's extra requests for his mom's help near the structure when they saw other children playing there. Taking deep breaths near mom and giving her words of validation and support, the practitioner encouraged her to proceed. The practitioner reminded her of how successful he had been playing in the dirt recently and how well he did the previous week on the slide by himself. They knew the last piece he had to manage was the social piece. The occupational therapy practitioner followed him to the top of the slide and coached him to say "go ahead" to two other children so he could have extra time and to watch them go and get off. Joey successfully managed the slide and hopped off the quickest he had ever dismounted. He wanted to repeat it, so they allowed him to go alone. He successfully allowed one child to go ahead and then slid down independently. On the third time another child followed him down and Joey crashed into the dirt. His mother and the practitioner were prepared for this possibility. Instead of picking him up and whisking him away, his mother calmly and empathetically said "uh oh, you've got this" and modeled how he could brush off the dirt from his hands. The other boy said "sorry," and after getting a big hug from his mother, Joey returned to the slide for another few rounds smiling and taking turns with the other children.

**Relationship and Social Interaction Skills in Preschool- and School-Age Children.** When children enter preschool, peer relationships become their newest connection. Together they engage in parallel occupations, play, and make friends. These friendships have been cited as a protective factor against future bullying (Bayer et al., 2018). However, for those children with vulnerable mental health, their relationship with their teacher can determine future success in school and the prevalence of internalizing problems (Sabol & Pianta, 2012; Zatto & Hoglund, 2019). Teacher-student relationships also impact the children's ability to stay regulated in the school setting (Cadima et al., 2016).

First to consider is how to modify environments and tasks. In the school, home, and community settings, the occupational therapy practitioner can coach caregivers and teachers to champion social opportunities and foster inclusion to facilitate building relationships and social interaction skills for children (Case-Smith, 2013). The school-based practitioner can serve as a consultant to embed relationship-building activities into authentic contexts, such as the lunchroom and recess. For example, offering chalk activities at recess provides a social opportunity to children who love art while supporting sensory regulation. Family nights can be organized in the community to engage families in a meaningful activity together, such as designing a nightly yoga routine or completing a craft. Furthermore, occupational therapy practitioners can create or facilitate afterschool programs to provide opportunities for structured leisure time with others.

The occupational therapy practitioner can help develop routines that support relationship building and a positive climate in the school and home. For example, at the end of the school day or after dinner, the teacher/caregiver can take the child aside to note a proud moment the child had that day as well as a proud moment that the adult had of the child. Occupational therapy practitioners also educate adults about the importance of setting aside dedicated time to connect with the child in their various settings and incorporating safe touch for parents with socially anxious children (Brummelman et al., 2019; Wieder & Greenspan, 2003). At home, families can be encouraged to participate in co-occupation by gardening together, playing outside in the snow, reading together as part of the nighttime routine, or engaging in leisure time completing puzzles (see Fig. 24.8A and B). Additionally, family meals provide quality family time as opportunities for social skill development (DeGrace et al., 2016).

The school-based occupational therapy practitioner can serve on the district committee that chooses curricula and available programs for implementation. Whole school curricula such as the Responsive Classroom value relationships in the child's school experience as much as academics (Rimm-Kaufman & Chiu, 2007). One facet of the Responsive Classroom incorporates daily practices such as community-building morning meetings to promote positive relationships. Theraplay has similar morning meeting activities with their Sunshine Circles, which have been shown to support social-emotional development with improved cooperation, friendships, and solving social problems (Booth & Jernberg, 2010; Tucker et al., 2017).

Groups to facilitate social interaction skills are best run with a multidisciplinary team. Caregivers should be incorporated whenever possible, and the team promotes generalization of skills to other settings. Children who participate in group programs, particularly those that were activity based with opportunities for co-occupation, as opposed to individual programs, were more successful in improving their social skills (Tanner et al., 2015). Examples of specific activities include swimming, gardening, and improvisational theater (Güeita-Rodríguez et al., 2021; Mass, 2019). Peer-mediated interventions, in which the peer serves as the therapeutic agent, can also be effective in helping autistic students and those with attention deficit hyperactivity disorder (ADHD) enhance their social skills and connections with others (Chang & Locke, 2016; Fox et al., 2020; Tanner et al., 2015). Incorporating sensory-based strategies into group programs has been shown to improve peer interactions and responding behaviors (Templeton et al., 2019). With programs like "Learn to Play," incorporating child-led play provides opportunities for developing social flexibility such as following the plan of a peer or gaining insight into their perspective (Rosanbalm & Murray, 2017a; Stagnitti et al., 2012).

Using principles from Bandura's social cognitive theory, children can implicitly learn social skills by observing others. The occupational therapy practitioner can provide "just right challenges" for social situations in the group that fade as the child increases their sense of competency, aligning with self-determination theory. The practitioner can do this by promoting joint attention, having the participants choose the goal of the group, allowing the child to choose from activities that are meaningful and intrinsically motivating to them, determining the pace of the activity, and building relationships with their peers (Case-Smith, 2013). Themes to guide the activities may be chosen to connect with participants' special interest areas.

The occupational therapy practitioner additionally considers specific skill-building approaches. Video modeling, which has its roots in social learning theory, supports social interactions of children with ADHD, intellectual impairment, and autism who have a strength in imitation (Hetzroni & Banin, 2017; Qi et al., 2018; Wilkes-Gillan et al., 2021). The practitioner utilizing video modeling first works with the child to identify what social situation they are having trouble navigating. Then, by videotaping a peer or themselves engaging in the identified social interaction, the child can review the video (as often as needed or desired) and focus their attention on the intricacies of a specific interaction. Another approach involves scripting short phrases for use in certain social situations, such as greetings or making a request, which can help children in conversations (Hume et al., 2021). Social stories (short narratives about what may occur and how to experience success) offer solutions to anticipated challenges in social situations. Developing and reading social stories has a positive impact on social skills (Gray, 2000; Karkhaneh et al., 2010). Bringing in outside resources, such as animal-assisted intervention has been noted to improve autistic children's social interactions (O'Haire, 2017). In addition, several computer-based interventions, such as virtual reality, can provide engaging opportunities for autistic children to practice interactions in a safe, controlled manner (Pandey & Vaughn, 2021; Tanner et al., 2015).

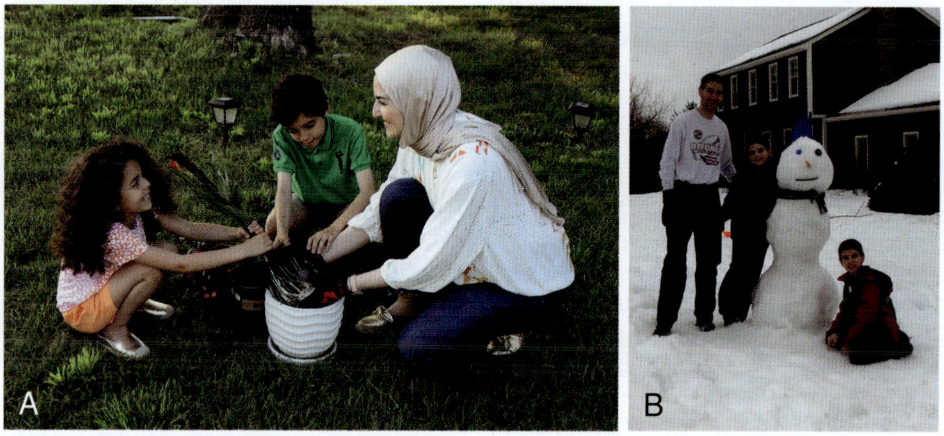

**Fig. 24.8** (A) Family gardening together. (B) Family making a snowman together.

**Relationship and Social Interaction Skills in Adolescents.** Positive parent and teacher-student relationships promote feelings of safety and security and are vital in the development of relationship and social interaction skills for adolescents (Murray et al., 2015). Peer influence can be important given the adolescent's proclivity toward peer interaction and the weight given to peer perspectives. Peers can expand positive development through encouragement, modeling, guidance, and advocacy or negatively impact development by reinforcing risk-taking, poor decision-making, and emotional and behavioral dysregulation.

As a universal initiative, occupational therapy practitioners can introduce relationship-building tools for educators to use in the classroom. These tools can be a powerful addition to the classroom routine. Micro-Moments or the 2 × 10 (developed by Raymond Wlodkowski) have been shown to improve overall class performance and behavior, improve a student's ability to socially engage in school and, in turn, increase academic performance, self-efficacy, and self-esteem (Coauette et al., 2021). This strategy involves the teacher taking two uninterrupted minutes each day for 10 consecutive days to provide positive, focused attention to a student or group of students. During this time, the teacher shares their own interests, asks questions, and tells stories, without discussing school, academics, or behavior.

Group-based programs geared toward adolescents tend to cluster around play-based or cognitive interventions. For the occupational therapy practitioner working with adolescents, it is helpful to conceptualize play as a state of mind, one that provides a sense of joy and flow. The occupational therapy practitioner can integrate a wide range of youth-identified areas of interests and strengths around which to base intervention. Meaningful youth-led play (often in the form of role-playing) can lead to improved social skills and social competence (Gutman et al., 2012). Development of play skills opens opportunities for social interactions with peers such as those facilitated through the "Imagine Create Belong" programs that use open-ended materials to facilitate ideas for play to create shared meaning (Goldingay et al., 2020).

Alternatively, Goldingay et al. (2020) found improved communication and conflict resolution by having participants demonstrate a skill and then use it in role plays, group activities, and structured tasks. Another role-play-based, teacher-facilitated social skills intervention, known as the Program for the Education and Enrichment of Relational Skills, looks to improve social functioning for autistic adolescents by focusing on making and keeping friends as well as managing conflict (Laugeson et al., 2014). A study of its use revealed improvements in the areas of social responsiveness, social communication, social motivation, social awareness, and social cognition. For neurodivergent adolescents, cognitive interventions improved social and emotional engagement while play-based interventions impacted more of a range of social interaction skills (Goldingay et al., 2020). Both types of intervention showed gains in executive function skills needed for social awareness, which supports the development and integration of relationship skills.

The developmental gains made in cognitive reasoning during adolescence, as well as the focus on the development and importance of interpersonal relationships, require the clinician to understand and apply therapeutic use of self to maximize the benefit of occupational therapy intervention. The Intentional Relationship Model (IRM; Taylor, 2020) promotes the clinician's understanding of the role of the interpersonal events occurring within a session and informs the practitioner's intentional acts and interpersonal reasoning to support children and their families (see Chapter 3). By providing guidance for interpersonal reasoning, IRM supports practitioners in determining appropriate interactive styles and modes to be used with adolescent clients, which is as impactful as the therapeutic activity itself.

## Responsible Decision-Making

Responsible decision-making is the ability to make constructive and respectful choices about personal behavior and social interactions based on ethical standards, safety concerns, social norms, realistic evaluation of consequences of various actions, and the well-being of self and others (CASEL, 2020).

**Responsible Decision-Making in Infants and Toddlers.** Responsible decision-making begins in early childhood. Typically, infants and toddlers have lived experiences of testing boundaries and experience the consequences through play and exploration. These embodied experiences of situations, actions, and consequences are stored and used for future decision-making (Barbey & Grafman, 2011). In young children, caregivers are a primary source of teaching and enforcing normative behavior. Infants as young as 10–12 months will socially reference a primary caregiver to encourage or prohibit behavior in uncertain circumstances (Sorce et al., 1985). When toddlers become mobile, they are socialized to know what appropriate behavior during familiar occupational routines is, such as eating and playing, and can learn to adapt to the social expectations of new surroundings by the age of 3 years (Kopp, 1982).

Environmental interventions for responsible decision-making with infants and toddlers require analyzing the home environment for safe exploration opportunities. Environments that allow child-safe opportunities for trial and error, while also setting firm boundaries like baby gates, around what is truly not safe, are important for infants and toddlers to have an embodied experience of learned decision-making (Adolph & Hoch, 2019).

Young children with impaired self-awareness and social awareness may not perceive the affordances of an environment or the social signaling of a caregiver and therefore may not respond accordingly to social norms. A child whose self-regulatory capacity is not developed may not be able to adhere to the social expectations of an environment or situation. The occupational therapy practitioner can work directly with caregivers to better understand the young child's capacity for responsible decision-making in different environments and occupations based on the child's unique profile. The practitioner can also help caregivers to match their social cueing to the unique needs of the child. For example, if a child is over-responsive to sound, the occupational therapy practitioner might guide a parent to lower their voice pitch or use nonverbal visual signaling to deter or promote a child's behavior, so as not to startle them.

**Responsible Decision-Making in Preschool- and School-Age Children.** Preschool-age children need significant assistance to solve the majority of their interpersonal disagreements as they are just starting to learn to problem solve simple situations (Rosanbalm & Murray, 2017b). As they move on in their school years, children become more adept at making responsible decisions and become flexible in their thinking. Children at this age benefit from having clear boundaries in addition to structured, predictable environments to guide their decision-making (Rosanbalm & Murray, 2017a). Opportunities to learn and achieve are key to developing a child's sense of agency (Ruscoe et al., 2018).

Regarding universal support, the occupational therapy practitioner can join the school district's committee that selects the SEL curriculum and advocate for a choice that relies on relationship-based approaches. One example is Conscious Discipline, which is focused on safety, connection, and problem-solving, seeing connectedness as governing behavior, as opposed to compliance and consequences for dysregulated behavior (Bailey, 2004). In all settings, the occupational therapy practitioner can encourage positive risk-taking in play and sensory and motor exploration, which offers opportunities to make decisions in a safe, supported environment.

Occupational therapy needs to continue to be client centered and to support agency for this age range. At a basic level, this includes honoring body autonomy. Furthermore, the practitioner can elevate the child's voice, share power with the child by offering them opportunities to contribute to decision-making and choices, and advocate for themselves (Gurdal & Sorbring, 2018). The occupational therapy practitioner is also charged with ensuring that nonspeaking children have meaningful communication support and that all forms of communication are honored. When setting goals, it is imperative to include the child's input. In fact, child-determined goals have been shown to not only increase intrinsic motivation but also have a positive impact on the attainment of goals (O'Connor et al., 2021). Practitioners can survey students to find out self-motivating goals as supported by self-determination theory.

Approaches that use a cognitive-behavioral methodology can uphold the decision-making process. For example, behavior contingency mapping, in the form of a graphic organizer, is drawn out to help the child consider the consequences of two different possible plans of action. Similarly, the Situation, Options, Consequences, Choices, Strategies, and Simulation, developed by Jan Roosa (1995), coaches the child to consider potential problems in social situations, which options are available to solve the problem, think through the consequences, and decide on a course of action. Drawing on perspective-taking, social behavior mapping explores the social impact of expected and unexpected behavior in response to a problem (Winner et al., 2007). Another approach is to team with caregivers to coach them on how to model strategies and provide practice and support to encourage growth, such as offering a "redo" for disrespectful behavior to repair (Parris et al., 2014).

**Responsible Decision-Making in Adolescents.** Changes in brain structure and function during adolescence propel us toward adulthood and the levels of functional independence and interdependence associated with that stage of life. The cognitive development of formal operations allows adolescents to consider their choices, weigh actions against consequences, reflect on how their choices and actions affect their lives, and consider the viewpoints of other people (Merlger & Patton, 2007). The adolescent paradox of continued development and simultaneous higher-level application is supported by multiple components. Neurological changes, relational influences, and opportunities for engagement and participation in the wider community out of the home and away from the direct influence and support of caregivers and teachers push adolescents to rely on themselves (see Fig. 24.9). Adolescents may make decisions based on emotions alone or potential rewards as opposed to actively reducing impulsivity and thinking through consequences (Ciranka & Van den Bos, 2019; van Hoorn et al., 2019). Ubiquitous to adolescence is the profound influence of peers and a need for acceptance (Ciranka & Van den Bos, 2019). This can have both positive and negative outcomes. Over time, the adolescent becomes more adept at resisting peer influence, relying more on personal value systems and awareness of the impact of their actions on others (Van Hoorn et al., 2019).

Parental control over decision-making can vary according to culture. The occupational therapy practitioner can engage parent coaching models that acknowledge and respect culture-based variations while supporting parents in scaffolding support for responsible decision-making (Hair et al., 2002). Here, coaching focuses on supporting parents in creating effective scaffolding for youth, resulting in the eventual ability of the adolescent to decide on their own.

The support of adolescent decision-making is paramount in areas of salience to the adolescent stage: dating, reproductive health, and social media use. Occupational therapy practitioners are well positioned to contribute to collaborative teams addressing adolescent sexual identity, health, and safety. They may explore issues with teens related to sexuality and dating, identifying appropriate privacy boundaries, and create safe and supportive environments for teens in which to express their sexual identity (Krantz et al., 2016). Increased use of social media and its implications adds more complex layers to adolescent decision-making. Programs such as the "Comfortable in our Body" delivered to teens in a community-based workshop celebrate the diversity of appearances and give tips for healthier social media behaviors (Mumber et al., 2022).

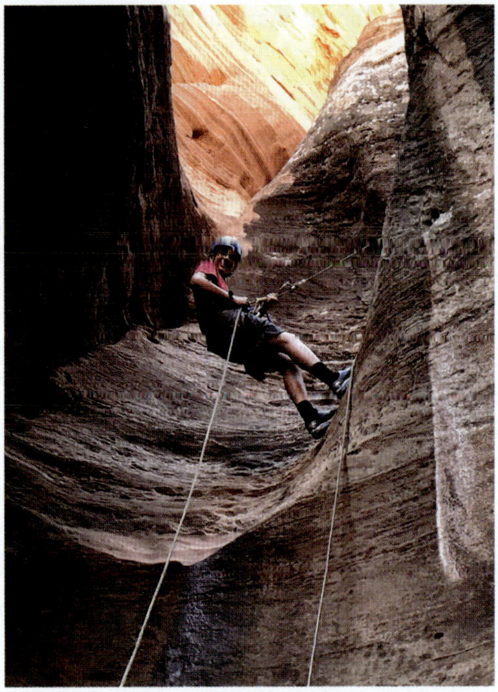

**Fig. 24.9** An adolescent making independent decisions.

Decision-making relies on the development of multiple pieces that are integrated and used to inform choices in service of desired short-range and long-range outcomes. The Cognitive Orientation to Daily Occupation Performance (CO-OP) approach (see Chapter 26) is effective in promoting the dynamic performance of many of these component pieces: self-analysis of skill development, metacognition, self-efficacy, and meaningful daily life outcomes (Kraversky, 2020). This top-down approach focuses on supporting the client's ability to identify, develop, and use cognitive strategies to perform daily activities. In keeping with the developmental trajectory of adolescence, the CO-OP acknowledges the essential role of parents, caregivers, and teachers in their perspectives of the adolescent's strengths and needs, expected collaboration with the clinician, and learning to identify actions that assist with generalization and transfer of cognitive strategies and skills (Kraversky, 2020).

Adolescent autonomous motivation and agency can be facilitated through the inclusion of youth in collaborative goal setting. Implementing evidence-based tools, such as Goal Attainment Scaling (Kiresuk et al., 1994), provides the practitioner with a structured and measurable way to engage in positive goal development with the adolescent client. Working directly with adolescents at risk of emotional or behavior disorders on self-determination skills can support youth to transition to adulthood, utilizing discussion and activities around getting to know oneself, valuing oneself, setting long- and short-term goals by making a collage, role-play using assertiveness skills, and engaging in a self-determined activity (Hojati Abed et al., 2021).

## SUMMARY

Understanding SEL through a developmental lens highlights the need for occupational therapy's holistic approach to prevention and positive mental health promotion throughout childhood and adolescence. Social-emotional competencies and social interaction skills are required for the child to participate in a multitude of settings. SEL requires collaboration and communication among various professionals and family members with multiple perspectives. The occupational therapy practitioner prioritizes the child's perspective and lived experiences when designing SEL goals and interventions that support their unique profile. In all settings, the practitioner is called to facilitate social-emotional development to improve the child's occupational participation and performance. If this is not the culture of the practice setting, the practitioner needs to advocate for their vital role in this area. Through SEL support, occupational therapy practitioners empower children with agency, resiliency, and enhanced quality of life.

1. Social emotional learning (SEL) impacts a child and adolescent's successful participation and performance across settings. CASEL has become the leading framework for exploring evidence-based SEL strategies to promote the critical skills needed for life effectiveness (CASEL, 2020). It identifies the five core competencies of self-awareness, self-management, social awareness, relationships skills, and responsible decision-making. Occupational therapy practitioners are ideally equipped to support these competencies with their knowledge of mental health, contextual, psychosocial, and performance factors that influence occupational performance and participation and their ability to evaluate the person-occupation-environment transaction.
2. Occupational therapy practitioners use a public health, trauma-responsive, relational (rather than behavioral) approach to promote social and emotional development. They holistically support the child and adolescent's well-being through occupational engagement in collaboration with other disciplines (AOTA, 2020). They may remove barriers (e.g., physical, emotional, social, safety) and proactively implement universal support for social-emotional development before looking at individualized interventions for challenges. Evidence-informed interventions for each competency include adapting the environments, tasks, and routines, coaching, utilizing universal support, designing and implementing programs, leading groups, and providing direct service.
3. Occupational therapy practitioners create individualized intervention plans to support growth in social and emotional learning by understanding the child and adolescent's strengths, challenges, and goals. They integrate teaching and practicing of new skills within the context of meaningful, fun, and appropriate occupation-based activities in natural environments. Practitioners use a strengths-based, developmental approach to collaborate with the child, family, teacher, and caregivers, and meet the child where they are, prioritizing therapeutic use of self and engagement in connection.

## REFERENCES


Adolph, K. E., & Hoch, J. E. (2019). Motor development: Embodied, embedded, enculturated, and enabling. *Annual Review of Psychology*, *70*, 141–164.

American Occupational Therapy Association. (2020). Occupational therapy practice framework: Domain and process (4th ed.). *American Journal of Occupational Therapy*, *74*(2, Suppl. l), 7412410010p1–7412410010p87.

Ayres, A. J. (1979). *Sensory integration and the child*. Western Psychological Services.

Bailey, R. A. (2004). *Conscious discipline*. Loving Guidance.

Barbey, A. K., & Grafman, J. (2011). An integrative cognitive neuroscience theory of social reasoning and moral judgment. *Wiley Interdisciplinary Reviews. Cognitive Science*, *2*(1), 55–67.

Barenberg, B., Casler, M., & Hasslebrook, B. (2022). What is the effectiveness of a DIR/Floortime occupational therapy intervention program for improving parent-child social interaction in children with autism spectrum disorder? Creighton University. *Critically Appraised Topic*. http://hdl.handle.net/10504/136320.

Bayer, Mundy, L., Stokes, I., Hearps, S., Allen, N., & Patton, G. (2018). Bullying, mental health and friendship in Australian primary school children. *Child and Adolescent Mental Health*, *23*(4), 334–340.

Bazyk, S. (2022). *Every moment counts*. https://everymomentcounts.org/comfortable-cafeteria/.

Blackwell, A. L., Yeager, D. C., Mische-Lawson, L., Bird, R. J., & Cook, D. M. (2014). Teaching children self-regulation skills within the early childhood education environment: A feasibility study. *Journal of Occupational Therapy, Schools, & Early Intervention*, *7*(3–4), 204–224.

Blankson, A. N., Weaver, J. M., Leerkes, E. M., O'Brien, M., Calkins, S. D., & Marcovitch, S. (2017). Cognitive and emotional processes as predictors of a successful transition into school. *Early Education & Development*, *28*(1), 1–20.

Booth, P., & Jernberg, A. (2010). *Theraplay®: Helping parents and children build better relationships through attachment-based play* (3rd ed.). Jossey-Bass.

Brackett, M. (2019). *Permission to feel: Unlocking the power of emotions to help our kids, ourselves, and our society thrive*. Celadon Books.

Brackett, M. A., Bailey, C. S., Hoffman, J. D., & Simmons, D. N. (2019). RULER: A theory-driven, systemic approach to social, emotional, and academic learning. *Educational Psychologist*, *54*(3), 144–161.

Brummelman, E., Terburg, D., Smit, M., Bögels, S. M., & Bos, P. A. (2019). Parental touch reduces social vigilance in children. *Developmental Cognitive Neuroscience*, *35*, 87–93.

Cadima, J., Verschueren, K., Leal, T., & Guedes, C. (2016). Classroom interactions, dyadic teacher-child relationships, and self-regulation in socially disadvantaged young children. *Journal of Abnormal Child Psychology*, *44*(1), 7–17.

Cahill, S. M., Egan, B. E., & Seber, J. (2020). Activity- and occupation-based interventions to support mental health, positive behavior, and social participation for children and youth: A systematic review. *American Journal of Occupational Therapy*, *74*, 7402180020.

Calkins, S. D. (2011). Caregiving as coregulation: Psychobiological processes and child functioning. In A. Booth, S. M. McHale, & N. S. Landale (Eds.), *Biosocial foundations of family processes. National symposium on family issues* (pp. 49–59). Springer Science.

Case-Smith, J. (2013). Systematic review of interventions to promote social-emotional development in young children with or at risk for disability. *American Journal of Occupational Therapy Association*, *67*(4), 395–404.

Chang, Y. C., & Locke, J. (2016). A systematic review of peer-mediated interventions for children with autism spectrum disorder. *Research in Autism Spectrum Disorders*, *27*, 1–10.

Chawla, L., Keena, K., Pevec, I., & Stanley, E. (2014). Green schoolyards as havens from stress and resources for resilience in childhood and adolescence. *Health & Place*, *28*, 1–13.

Christiana, R. W., Battista, R. A., James, J. J., & Bergman, S. M. (2016). Pediatrician prescriptions for outdoor physical activity among children: A pilot study. *Preventive Medicine Reports*, *5*, 100–105.

Ciranka, S., & Van den Bos, W. (2019). Social influence in adolescent decision-making: A formal framework. *Frontiers in Psychology*, *10*, Article 1915.

Clarkson, C., Boshoff, K., & Kernot, J. (2021). Occupational therapy interventions for adolescents: A scoping review. *The Allied Health Scholar*, *2*(1), 51–102.

Coauette, S., Ekre, K., & Stagg, B. (2021). Impact of social skills groups on school aged children with emotional disturbance. *Critically Appraised Topics*, *26*. https://commons.und.edu/cat-papers/26.

Collaborative for Academic, Social, and Emotional Learning (CASEL). (2020). *What is the CASEL framework?*. https://casel.org/fundamentals-of-sel/what-is-the-casel-framework/.

Dana, D. (2018). *The polyvagal theory in therapy: Engaging the rhythm of regulation*. W W Norton & Co.

Datu, J., Mateo, N. J., & Natale, S. (2022). The mental health benefits of kindness-oriented schools: School kindness is associated with increased belongingness and well-being in Filipino high school students. *Child Psychiatry and Human Development, 54*, 1075–1081.

Day, M., & Parlakian, R. (2004). *How culture shapes social-emotional development: Applications for practice in infant-family programs*. Zero to Three Center for Program Excellence.

De Falco, S., Emer, A., Martini, L., Rigo, P., Pruner, S., & Venuti, P. (2014). Predictors of mother–child interaction quality and child attachment security in at-risk families. *Frontiers in Psychology, 5*, Article 898.

DeGangi, G. A. (2017). Addressing attachment and problems of intimacy: How to build healthy emotional connections. In *Pediatric disorders of regulation in affect and behavior*(2nd ed.) (pp. 427–477). Academic Press.

DeGangi, G. A., & Greenspan, S. I. (1997). The effectiveness of short-term interventions in treatment of inattention and irritability in toddlers. *Journal of Developmental and Learning Disorders, 1*(2), 277–298.

DeGrace, B. W., Foust, R. E., Sisson, S. B., & Lora, K. R. (2016). Benefits of family meals for children with special therapeutic and behavioral needs. *American Journal of Occupational Therapy, 70*(3), 7003350010p1–7003350010p6.

Denham, S. A., & Bassett, H. H. (2019). Early childhood teachers' socialization of children's emotional competence. *Journal of Research in Innovative Teaching & Learning, 12*(2), 133–150.

Diamant, R., Ruiz, H., & Holmes, K. (2020). Relationships between sensory processing behaviors, executive function, and temperament characteristics for effortful control in school-age children. *American Journal of Occupational Therapy, 74*(S1). 74115052371 .

Dunn, J., Brown, J., & Beardsall, L. (1991). Family talk about feeling states and children's later understanding of others' emotions. *Developmental Psychology, 27*(3), 448–455.

Dunst, C. J., Bruder, M. B., Trivette, C. M., Hamby, D., Raab, M., & McLean, M. (2001). Characteristics and consequences of everyday natural learning opportunities. *Topics in Early Childhood Special Education, 21*(2), 68–92.

Eisenberg, N., Valiente, C., Morris, A. S., Fabes, R. A., Cumberland, A., Reiser, M., Gershoff, E. T., Shepard, S. A., & Losoya, S. (2003). Longitudinal relations among parental emotional expressivity, children's regulation, and quality of socioemotional functioning. *Developmental Psychology, 39*(1), 3–19.

Feldman, R. (2007). Parent-infant synchrony and the construction of shared timing; physiological precursors, developmental outcomes, and risk conditions. *The Journal of Child Psychology and Psychiatry and Allied Disciplines, 48*(3–4), 329–354.

Feldman, R. (2020). What is resilience: An affiliative neuroscience approach. *World Psychiatry, 19*, 132–150.

Feldman, R., Bamberger, E., & Kanat-Maymon, Y. (2013). Parent specific reciprocity from infancy to adolescence shapes children's social competence and dialogical skills. *Attachment & Human Development, 15*(4), 407–423.

Flook, L., Goldberg, S. B., Pinger, L., & Davidson, R. J. (2015). Promoting prosocial behavior and self-regulatory skills in preschool children through a mindfulness-based Kindness Curriculum. *Developmental Psychology, 51*(1), 44–51.

Fogel, A., & Garvey, A. (2007). Alive communication. *Infant Behavior and Development, 30*, 251–257.

Fox, A., Dishman, S., Valicek, M., Ratcliff, K., & Hilton, C. (2020). Effectiveness of social skills interventions incorporating peer interactions for children with attention deficit hyperactivity disorder: A systematic review. *American Journal of Occupational Therapy, 74*(2), 7402180070p1–7402180070p19.

Goldingay, S., Stagnitti, K., Robertson, N., Pepin, G., Sheppard, L., & Dean, B. (2020). Implicit play or explicit cognitive behaviour therapy: The impact of intervention approaches to facilitate social skills development in adolescents. *Australian Occupational Therapy Journal, 67*, 360–372.

Gray, C. (2000). *Writing social stories with Carol Gray*. Non Basic Stock Line.

Greater Good Science Center. (n.d.). *Thanks! A strengths-based gratitude curriculum for tweens and teens*. https://ggsc.berkeley.edu/images/uploads/GGSC_Gratitude_Curriculum_MS_HS.pdf

Griffin, A. (2017). Adolescent neurological development and implications for health and well-being. *Healthcare, 5*(4), 62.

Güeita-Rodríguez, J., Ogonowska-Slodownik, A., Morgulec-Adamowicz, N., Martín-Prades, M. L., Cuenca-Zaldívar, J. N., & Palacios-Ceña, D. (2021). Effects of aquatic therapy for children with Autism Spectrum Disorder on social competence and quality of life: A mixed methods study. *International Journal of Environmental Research and Public Health, 18*(6), 3126.

Gurdal, S., & Sorbring, E. (2018). Children's agency in parent-child, teacher-pupil and peer relationship contexts. *International Journal of Qualitative Studies on Health and Well-Being, 13*(Suppl. 1), 1565239.

Gutman, S. A., Raphael-Greenfield, E. I., & Rao, A. K. (2012). Effect of a motor-based role-play intervention on the social behaviors of adolescents with high-functioning autism: Multiple-baseline single-subject design. *American Journal of Occupational Therapy, 66*(5), 529–537.

Hair, E. C., Jager, J., & Garrett, S. B. (2002). Helping teens develop healthy social skills and relationships: What the research shows about navigating adolescence. *Child Trends Research Brief.*

Harvard University's, Center on the Developing Child. (2024). Serve and return. https://developingchild.harvard.edu/science/key-concepts/serve-and-return/. [Accessed 23 September 2024].

Hawn Foundation. (2011). *The MindUP curriculum: Brain-focused strategies for learning and living*. Scholastic.

Hetzroni, & Banin, I. (2017). The effect of educational software, video modeling and group discussion on social–skill acquisition among students with mild intellectual disabilities. *Journal of Applied Research in Intellectual Disabilities, 30*(4), 757–773.

Ho, M., & Lin, L. (2020). Efficacy of parent-training programs for preschool children with autism spectrum disorder: A randomized controlled trial. *Research in Autism Spectrum Disorders, 71*, 101495.

Hoffmann, J. D, Brackett, M. A., Bailey, C. S., & Wilner, C. J. (2020). Teaching emotion regulation in schools: Translating research into practice with the RULER approach to social and emotional learning. *Emotion, 20*(1), 105–109. https://doi.org/10.1037/emo0000649.

Hojati Abed, E., Shafaroodi, N., Akbarfahimi, M., Zareiyan, A., & Parand, A. (2021). Effect of occupational therapy on self-determination skills of adolescents at risk of emotional and behavioral disorders: A randomized controlled trial. *Medical Journal of the Islamic Republic of Iran, 35*, 57.

Howard, A. R. H., Lynch, A. K., Call, C. D., & Cross, D. R. (2020). Sensory processing in children with a history of maltreatment: An occupational therapy perspective. *Vulnerable Children and Youth Studies, 15*(1), 60–67.

Hume, K., Steinbrenner, J. R., Odom, S. L., Morin, K. L., Nowell, S. W., Tomaszewski, B., Szendrey, S., McIntyre, N. S., Yücesoy-Özkan, S., & Savage, M. N. (2021). Evidence-based practices for children, youth, and young adults with autism: Third generation review. *Journal of Autism and Developmental Disorders, 51*(11), 4013–4032.

Jackson, E. E., McGlone, F. P., & Haggarty, C. J. (2022). The social brain has a nerve: Insights from attachment and autistic phenotypes. *Current Opinion in Behavioral Sciences, 45.*

Jennings, P. A., & Greenberg, M. T. (2009). The prosocial classroom: Teacher social and emotional competence in relation to student and classroom outcomes. *Review of Educational Research, 79*(1), 491–525.

Jones, S. M., McGarrah, M. W., & Kahn, J. (2019). Social and emotional learning: A principled science of human development in context. *Educational Psychologist, 54*(3), 129–143.

Kannenberg, Fette, C., & Burson, K. (2017). Mental health promotion, prevention, and intervention in occupational therapy practice. *American Journal of Occupational Therapy, 71*(Suppl. 2), 7112410035p1–7112410035p19.

Karkhaneh, M., Clark, B., Ospina, M. B., Seida, J. C., Smith, V., & Hartling, L. (2010). Social stories ™ to improve social skills in children with autism spectrum disorder: A systematic review. *Autism: The International Journal of Research and Practice, 14*(6), 641–662.

Kerr, K. L., Ratliff, E. L., Cosgrove, K. T., Bodurka, J., Morris, A. S., & Kyle Simmons, W. (2019). Parental influences on neural mechanisms underlying emotion regulation. *Trends in Neuroscience and Education, 16*, 100118.

Kingsley, K., Sagester, G., & Weaver, L. L. (2020). Interventions supporting mental health and positive behavior in children ages birth–5 yr: A systematic review. *American Journal of Occupational Therapy, 74*, 7402180050.

Kiresuk, T. J., Smith, A., & Cardillo, J. E. (1994). *Goal attainment scaling: Applications, theory, and measurement*. Lawrence Erlbaum Associates.

Kopp, C. B. (1982). Antecedents of self-regulation: A developmental perspective. *Developmental Psychology, 18*(2), 199–214.

Krantz, G., Tolan, V., Pontarelli, K., & Cahill, S. M. (2016). What do adolescents with developmental disabilities learn about sexuality and sating? A potential role for occupational therapy. *The Open Journal of Occupational Therapy, 4*(2).

Kraversky, D. G. (2020). Cognitive orientation to daily occupational performance (CO-OP) approach: Evidence-based, occupation-centered intervention for children. *American Occupational Therapy Association*. Article code CEA0720 .

Kuypers, L. (2011). *The zones of regulation*. Think Social Publishing.

Landry, S. H., Smith, K. E., & Swank, P. R. (2006). Responsive parenting: Establishing early foundations for social, communication, and independent problem-solving skills. *Developmental Psychology, 42*(4), 627–642.

Laugeson, E. A., Ellingsen, R., Sanderson, J., Tucci, L., & Bates, S. (2014). The ABC's of teaching social skills to adolescents with autism spectrum disorder in the classroom: The UCLA PEERS® Program. *Journal of Autism and Developmental Disorders, 44*(9), 2244–2256.

Lavy, S. (2020). A review of character strengths interventions in twenty-first century school: Their importance and how they can be fostered. *Applied Research in Quality of Life, 15*(2), 573–596.

Levanon-Erez, N., Kampf-Sherf, O., & Maeir, A. (2019). Occupational therapy metacognitive intervention for adolescents with ADHD: Teen cognitive-functional (Cog-Fun) feasibility study. *British Journal of Occupational Therapy, 82*(10), 618–629.

Lupien, S. J., McEwen, B. S., Gunnar, M. R., & Heim, C. (2009). Effects of stress throughout the lifespan on the brain, behaviour and cognition. *Nature Reviews Neuroscience, 10*(6), 434–445.

Maas, C. (2019). Improvisational theatre and occupational therapy for children with autism spectrum disorder. *International Journal of Disability, Development and Education, 68*(1), 10–25.

Mahler, K. (2018). *The interoception curriculum: A step-by-step guide to developing mindful self-regulation*. AAPC Publishing.

Mahler, K., Hample, K., Jones, C., Sensenig, J., Thomasco, P., & Hilton, C. (2022). Impact of an interoception-based program on emotion regulation in autistic children. *Occupational Therapy International*.

McCormick, R. (2017). Does access to green space impact the mental well-being of children: A systematic review. *Journal of Pediatric Nursing, 37*, 3–7.

Merlger, A., & Patton, W. (2007). Adolescents talking about personal responsibility. *The Journal of Student Wellbeing, 1*(1).

Miller, L. J., Schoen, S. A., & Spielmann, V. A. (2018). A frame of reference for sensory processing difficulties: Sensory therapies and research (STAR). In P. Kramer, J. Hinojosa, & T. Howe (Eds.), *Frames of reference for pediatric occupational therapy* (4th ed.) (pp. 159–202). Lippincott Williams & Wilkins.

Montirosso, R., & McGlone, F. (2020). The body comes first. Embodied reparation and the co-creation of infant bodily self. *Neuroscience & Biobehavioral Reviews* (13), 77–87.

Moore, K. M. (2005). *The sensory connection program*. Therapro.

Mulcahy, J. S., Davies, M., Quadt, L., Critchley, H. D., & Garfinkel, S. N. (2019). Interoceptive awareness mitigates deficits in emotional prosody recognition in Autism. *Biological Psychology, 146*, 107711.

Mumber, H. E., Rashid, S., Carey, G., Navarro, A., Oh, E., Nasir, M., & Lee, M. S. (2022). Impact of a comfortable in our skin interactive workshop on social media awareness and self-confidence in adolescents. *Pediatric Dermatology, 39*(4), 553–556.

Murray, D. W., Rosanbalm, K., Christopoulos, C., & Hamoudi, A. (2015). *Self-regularion and toxic stress report 1: Foundations for understanding self-regulation from an applied developmental perspective. OPRE Report #2015-21*. Washington, DC: Office of Planning, Research and Evaluation, Administration for Children and Families, U.S. Department of Health and Human Services. https://www.acf.hhs.gov/sites/default/files/documents/report_1_foundations_paper_final_012715_submitted_508_0.pdf.

Neff, M. A. (2023). *What is interoception and how to improve yours*. https://neurodivergentinsights.com/blog/what-is-interoception.

O'Connor, D., Lynch, H., & Boyle, B. (2021). A qualitative study of child participation in decision-making: Exploring rights-based approaches in pediatric occupational therapy. *PLoS One, 16*(12), e0260975.

O'Haire, M. (2017). Research on animal-assisted intervention and autism spectrum disorder, 2012-2015. *Applied Developmental Science, 21*(3), 200–216.

Occupational Performance Coaching (OPC). University of Otago. https://www.otago.ac.nz/wellington/research/groups/rehabilitation-teaching-and-research-unit-rtru/occupational-performance-coaching-opc. (Accessed 02 November 2024).

Pandey, V., & Vaughn, L. (2021). The potential of virtual reality in social skills training for autism: Bridging the gap between research and adoption of virtual reality in occupational therapy practice. *The Open Journal of Occupational Therapy, 9*(3), 1–12.

Park, N., & Peterson, C. (2008). Positive psychology and character strengths: Application to strengths-based school counseling. *Professional School Counseling, 12*(2).

Parris, S. R., Milton, H. S., Harlow, J. G., Cross, D. R., & Purvis, K. B. (2014). The importance of addressing complex trauma in schools: Implementing trust-based relational intervention in elementary school. *Contemporary School Psychology, 19*(3), 157–164.

Perry, B. D. (2009). Examining child maltreatment through a neurodevelopmental lens: Clinical applications of the neurosequential model of therapeutics. *Journal of Loss & Trauma, 14*(4), 240–255.

Pierce, D., Munier, V., & Myers, C. T. (2009). Informing early intervention through an occupational science description of infant-toddler interactions with home space. *American Journal of Occupational Therapy, 63*, 273–287. https://doi.org/10.5014/ajot.63.3.273.

Porges, S. W. (2011). *The polyvagal theory: Neurophysiological foundations of emotions, attachment, communication, and self-regulation*. W W Norton & Co.

Poulou, M. S., Garner, P. W., & Bassett, H. H. (2022). Teachers' emotional expressiveness and classroom management practices: Associations with young students' social–emotional and behavioral competence. *Psychology in the School, 59*, 557–573.

Proctor, C., Tsukayama, E., Wood, A. M., Maltby, J., Eades, J. F., & Linley, P. A. (2011). Strengths gym: The impact of a character strengths-based intervention on the life satisfaction and well-being of adolescents. *The Journal of Positive Psychology, 6*(5), 377–388.

Qi, C. H., Barton, E. E., Collier, M., Lin, Y., & Montoya, C. (2018). A systematic review of single case research studies on using video modeling interventions to improve social communication skills for individuals with autism spectrum disorder. *Focus on Autism and Other Developmental Disabilities, 33*(4), 249–257.

Rath, T., & Reckmeyer, M. (2009). *How full is your bucket? For kids*. Simon and Schuster.

Reis, H., Pereira, A., & Almeida, L. (2018). Intervention effects on communication skills and sensory regulation on children with ASD. *Journal of Occupational Therapy, Schools, & Early Intervention, 11*(3), 346–359.

Rimm-Kaufman, S., & Chiu, Y.-J. I. (2007). Promoting social and academic competence in the classroom: An intervention study examining the contribution of the Responsive Classroom approach. *Psychology in the Schools, 44*(4), 397–413.

Roosa, J. B. (1995). *Men on the move: Competence and cooperation conflict resolution and beyond*. Author.

Rosanbalm, K. D., & Murray, D. W. (2017a). *Caregiver coregulation across development: A practice brief. OPRE Brief #2017-80*. Washington, DC: Office of Planning, Research, and Evaluation, Administration for Children and Families, US, Department of Health and Human Services.

Rosanbalm, K. D., & Murray, D. W. (2017b). *Promoting self-regulation in early childhood: A practice brief. OPRE Brief #2017-79*. Washington, DC: Office of Planning, Research, and Evaluation, Administration for Children and Families, US, Department of Health and Human Services.

Rose, J., Gilbert, L., & McGuire-Snieckus, R. (2015). Emotion coaching - a strategy for promoting behavioural self-regulation in children/young people in schools: A pilot study. *European Journal of Social & Behavioural Sciences, XIII*, 1766–1790.

Ruscoe, A., Barblett, L., & Parrath-Pugh, C. (2018). Sharing power with children: Repositioning children as agentic learners. *Australian Journal of Early Childhood, 13*(3), 63–71.

Sabol, T. J., & Pianta, R. C. (2012). Recent trends in research on teacher–child relationships. *Attachment & Human Development, 14*(3), 213–231.

Schonert-Reichl, K. A., Oberle, E., Lawlor, M. S., Abbott, D., Thomson, K., Oberlander, T. F., & Diamond, A. (2015). Enhancing cognitive and social-emotional development through a simple-to-administer mindfulness-based school program for elementary school children: A randomized controlled trial. *Developmental Psychology, 51*(1), 52–66.

Schulz, A., & Vögele, C. (2015). Interoception and stress. *Frontiers in Psychology, 6*, 993.

Silva, L. M., Schalock, M., & Gabrielsen, K. (2011). Early intervention for autism with a parent-delivered Qigong massage program: A randomized controlled trial. *American Journal of Occupational Therapy, 65*, 550–559.

Solomon, R., Van Egeren, L. A., Mahoney, G., Quon Huber, M. S., & Zimmerman, P. (2014). PLAY Project home consultation intervention program for young children with autism spectrum disorders: A randomized controlled trial. *Journal of Developmental and Behavioral Pediatrics, 35*(8), 475–485.

Sorce, J. F., Emde, R. N., Campos, J. J., & Klinnert, M. D. (1985). Maternal emotional signaling: Its effect on the visual cliff behavior of 1-year-olds. *Developmental Psychology, 21*(1), 195–200.

Stagnitti, K., O'Connor, C., & Sheppard, L. (2012). Impact of the Learn to Play program on play, social competence and language for children aged 5-8 years who attend a specialist school. *Australian Occupational Therapy Journal, 59*(4), 302–311.

Stern, D. (1985). *The interpersonal world of the Infant.* Basic Book.

Sutton, D., Wilson, M., Van Kessel, K., & Vanderpyl, J. (2013). Optimizing arousal to manage aggression: A pilot study of sensory modulation. *International Journal of Mental Health Nursing, 22*, 500–511.

Tal-Saban, M., & Maeir, A. (2021). Adolescents' self-perceptions of occupational strengths and difficulties. *American Journal of Occupational Therapy, 75*(2).

Tanner, K., Hand, B. N., O'Toole, G., & Lane, A. E. (2015). Effectiveness of interventions to improve social participation, play, leisure, and restricted and repetitive behaviors in people with autism spectrum disorder: A systematic review. *American Journal of Occupational Therapy, 69*(5), 6905180010p1–6905180010p12.

Taylor, R. R. (2020). *The intentional relationship: Occupational therapy and use of self* (2nd ed.). FA Davis.

Templeton, O., Charney, L., Bennett, H., Betz, M., Byrne, K., & Duffy, J. (2019). The effect of sensory-based strategies and social-skill training on social skills among preschool children with autism spectrum disorder. *American Journal of Occupational Therapy, 73*(4_Suppl. 1), 7311515359p1.

Tronick, E., & Beeghly, M. (2011). Infants' meaning making and the development of mental health problems. *American Psychologist, 66*(2), 107–119.

Tsethlikai, M., Murray, D. W., Meyer, A. L., & Sparrow, J. (2018). *Reflections on the relevance of "self-regulation" for Native communities* (OPRE Brief No. 2018-64) United States, Administration for Children and Families, Office of Planning, Research and Evaluation. https://www.acf.hhs.gov/sites/default/files/opre/native_self_regulation_brief_accessible_508.pdf.

Tucker, C., Schieffer, K., Wills, T. J., Hull, C., & Murphy, Q. (2017). Enhancing social-emotional skills in at-risk preschool students through Theraplay based groups: The Sunshine Circle Model. *International Journal of Play Therapy, 26*(4), 185. https://psycnet.apa.org/doi/10.1037/pla0000054

Van der Kolk, B. A. (2003). The neurobiology of childhood trauma and abuse. *Child and Adolescent Psychiatric Clinics of North America, 12*, 293–317, ix .

van Hoorn, J., Shablack, H., Lindquist, K. A., & Telzer, E. H. (2019). Incorporating the social context into neurocognitive models of adolescent decision-making: A neuroimaging meta-analysis. *Neuroscience & Biobehavioral Reviews, 101*, 129–142.

Ward, S., & Jacobsen, K. (2014). A clinical model for developing executive function skills. *Perspectives on Language Learning and Education, 21*(2), 72–84.

Whiting, C. C. (2018). Trauma and the role of the school-based occupational therapist. *Journal of Occupational Therapy, Schools, & Early Intervention, 11*(3), 291–301.

Whiting, C. C., Ochsenbein, M., Schoen, S., & Spielmann, V. (2021). A Multi-tiered and multi-dimensional approach to intervention in schools: Recommendations for children with sensory integration and processing challenges. *Journal of Occupational Therapy, Schools, & Early Intervention, 15*(3), 314–327.

Wieder, S., & Greenspan, S. I. (2003). Climbing the symbolic ladder in the DIR model through Floor Time/Interactive play. *Autism, 7*(4), 425–435.

Wilkes Gillan, Cordier, R., Chen, Y., Swanton, R., Mahoney, N., Trimboli, C., Yule, E., & Tam, E. (2021). A systematic review of video–modeling interventions for children and adolescents with attention–deficit hyperactivity disorder. *Australian Occupational Therapy Journal, 68*(5), 454–471.

Williams, M. S., & Shellenberger, S. (1996). *How does your engine run?: A leader's guide to the alert program for self-regulation.* TherapyWorks, Inc.

Winner, M. (2005). *Think social.* Think Social Publishing.

Winner, M. G., Bosmeijer, J., & Horras, J. (2007). *Social behavior mapping.* Gray Center.

Winner, M. G., & Crooke, P. J. (2009). Social thinking: A developmental treatment approach for students with social learning/social pragmatic challenges. *Perspectives on Language Learning and Education, 16*(2), 62–69.

Zatto, B. R., & Hoglund, W. L. (2019). Children's internalizing problems and teacher–child relationship quality across preschool. *Early Childhood Research Quarterly, 49*, 28–39.

25

# Approaches for Managing Challenging Behavior

*Renee Watling*

## GUIDING QUESTIONS

1. What are challenging behaviors that occupational therapy practitioners may address?
2. How do occupational therapy practitioners address challenging behaviors to support children and youth's engagement in meaningful activities?
3. What are the principles of behavioral therapy approaches?

## KEY TERMS

Antecedents
Antecedent intervention
Behavior
Behavior theory
Behavior service plan (BSP)
Behavioral analysis
Challenging behavior
Consequences
Consequence-based intervention
Functional communication training
Pivotal response training
Positive behavioral intervention and supports (PBIS)
Reinforcement
Setting events

## INTRODUCTION

Application of behavioral approaches for pediatric clients who receive occupational therapy has grown as the frequency of challenging behaviors encountered among children and youth has increased and as advocates for behavioral methods have been more vocal. In fact, many scientific and professional agencies recommend widespread use of behavioral approaches for challenging behaviors, and many state agencies have adopted them as best practices. However, self-advocates question the value of these approaches, describing personal experiences of trauma and conflict between personal values and methodological philosophies that underpin behaviorism (McGill & Robinson, 2021; Milton, 2018; Sandoval-Norton & Shkedy, 2019; and see Editor's Note 25.1). Because behavioral approaches are commonly used by other team members in addressing children's challenging behaviors, occupational therapy practitioners must understand behavior theory, including behavioral perspectives about factors that influence human behavior, as well as the aims of recommended interventions and their expected outcomes. By understanding approaches used by other professionals, occupational therapy providers can more effectively collaborate and can more clearly communicate about the value of occupational approaches to promote client goal achievement. This chapter presents behavioral approaches to challenging behaviors and describes how they might be provided for children and adolescents. Case examples illustrate selected strategies that occupational therapy practitioners may use to address behavioral challenges with children and adolescents.

## UNDERSTANDING BEHAVIOR

The term behavior refers to what a person does, including overt, observable actions, such as moving, talking, or playing a game, as well as covert, unobservable actions, such as thinking about something, experiencing emotion, or being confused. The domain of occupational therapy includes both overt and covert behaviors with concern for any behavior that interferes with occupational engagement. Children's engagement in daily life experiences creates the building blocks for learning, growth, development, and productive occupation. When engagement in daily life may be disrupted by challenging behavior, occupational therapy practitioners identify and intervene with those variables, aiming to influence the individual's behavior and engagement patterns. Fig. 25.1A–E shows a range of child behaviors that can interfere with engagement in daily life activities.

Within society, the appropriateness of a behavior is usually interpreted according to a social standard or expectation and is judged to be positive when it is in accordance with social expectations, or to be negative, problematic, or challenging when it does not conform to social norms or causes others in the vicinity to feel threatened or experience harm. For example, in a public school building, it is inappropriate and unacceptable for a student to leave the classroom and go to the playground when the teacher passes out a work assignment; however, the same behavior would be appropriate and desirable in response to the recess bell. Even behaviors such as playing with cars by lining them up along a seam in the carpet or carrying a Band-Aid everywhere and refusing to set it down, though not disruptive to the context or harmful to others, can be identified as challenging because they interfere with the child's occupational engagement and do not comply with social norms.

The literature is replete with definitions of challenging behavior. Most of these definitions stem from the work of Smith and Fox (2003) and encompass the ideas that challenging behaviors are not socially acceptable; can cause physical harm, disruption, or destruction; or can affect education or living environments (O'Regan et al., 2022, pp. 1–20; Rahn et al., 2017). All children display inappropriate or challenging

## EDITOR'S NOTE 25.1 AMERICAN MEDICAL ASSOCIATION'S RESOLUTION REGARDING APPLIED BEHAVIORAL ANALYSIS

Since 2023, a process has been unfolding that has led to changes in the American Medical Association's (AMA) recommendations regarding applied behavioral analysis. First, the AMA House of Delegates put forth a resolution proposed by the medical student section of the AMA, calling for the AMA to support further development of new interventions, the availability of a full range of services, and coverage for evidence-based interventions while removing the specific inclusion of applied behavioral analysis (ABA) intervention. The rationale for the resolution, called resolution 706, questioned the evidence for ABA, supported an individual's rights to engage in behavior that is nonharmful and that may serve the individual as a coping mechanism, contemplated the ethics of seeking to make someone behave more "normally" and of changing someone's behavior without their consent, considered the preferences and well-being of autistic individuals who have described the trauma they endured because of ABA, similarly considered the evidence for a relationship between ABA and PTSD and suicide in autistic individuals, and cited concerns with the profitability of ABA services and its growth as a large money-making industry. The Council of Autism Service Providers suggested that those responsible for the resolution had an anti-ABA agenda and that they used flawed research to support it. The resolution was sent to committee and was amended and revised. In June of 2024, the AMA voted on a revised resolution that passed. This revised "706" does not specifically remove support for ABA but instead expands support to all evidence based approaches. The final resolution that passed also acknowledged the evidence for developmental relationship-based interventions.

Occupational therapy practitioners are urged to examine the evidence for themselves, consider the profession's code of ethics and humanistic philosophy, and selectively engage in the use of behavioral interventions in a judicious manner, only when the client understands and has agreed to the approaches, and when use of the approaches is directly informed by client-generated data.

See https://www.ama-assn.org/system/files/a23-706.pdf for the resolution document and see the explanation and rebuttal from the Council of Autism Service Providers https://www.casproviders.org/news/correcting-the-record-the-ama-did-not-remove-support-for-aba. The full resolution proposal is outlined in the AMA House of Delegates Handbook (pp. 1187–1189) available at https://www.ama-assn.org/system/files/a23-combined-handbook.pdf and the final version is available at https://www.ama-assn.org/system/files/a23-refcomm-g-annotated.pdf.

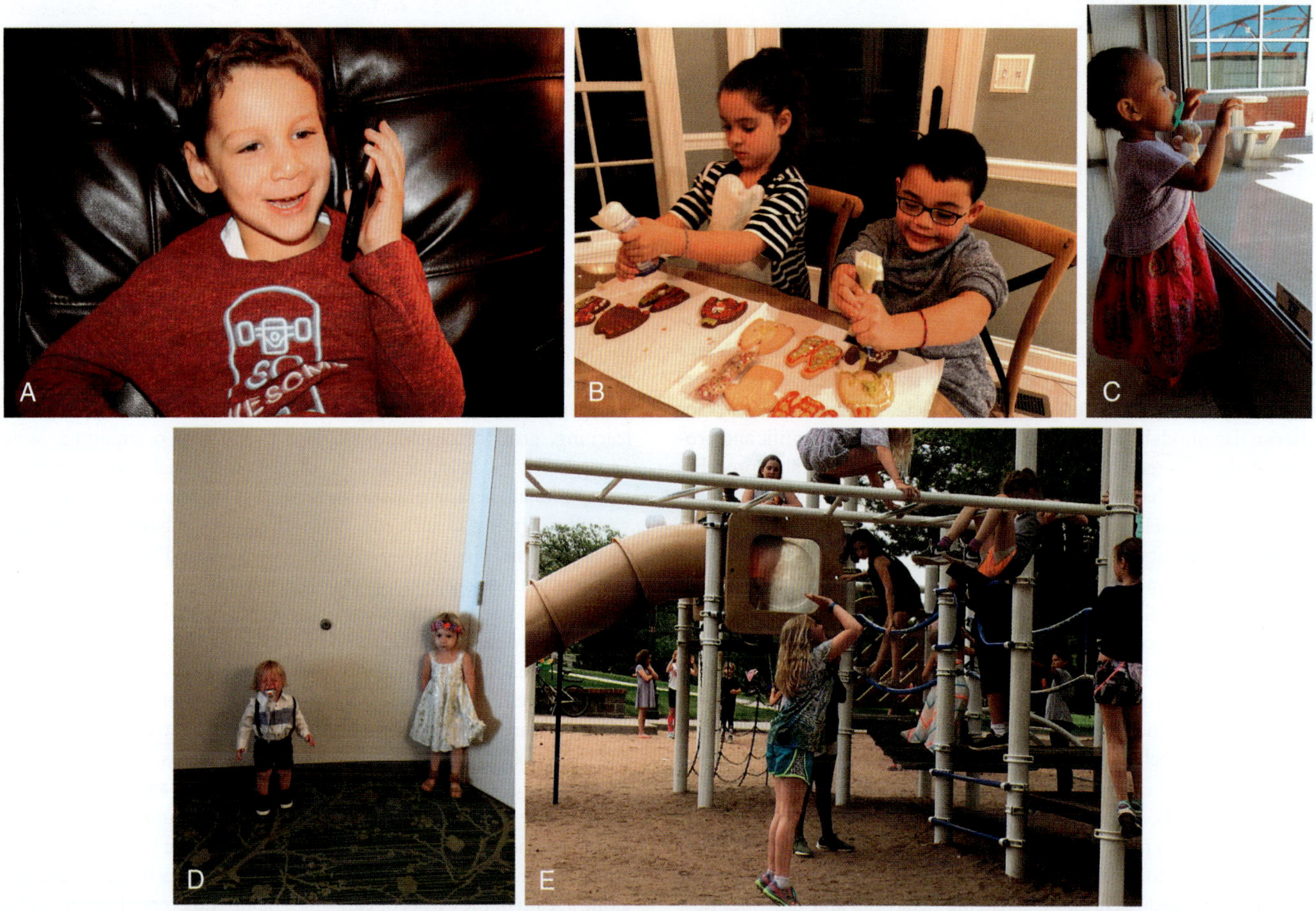


**Fig. 25.1** (A–E) Children engage in all forms of behavior: positive functional behaviors, inappropriate behaviors, nonfunctional behaviors, and challenging behaviors.

behaviors at times as they grow through the various ages and stages of childhood, and such behaviors frequently are not cause for concern. However, attention must be given when such behaviors are of an intensity, frequency, or duration that they interfere with the child's ability to engage and participate in daily life activities, when they are disruptive to the engagement and participation of others, or when the behaviors place the child or others at risk for injury (O'Regan et al., 2022, pp. 1–20). See Case Example 25.1 for an example of challenging behaviors.

For many years, researchers and practitioners focused on changing or removing challenging behaviors of people who function differently than the social norm or whose behaviors make them appear to be a threat to others. Such behavior change may be appropriate when safety or harm to self or others is a concern. However, nonproductivity-oriented behaviors such as repetitive movements, humming, and finger tapping are expressions of the individual's nervous system state and may serve regulatory functions (Dawson et al., 2022; Kapp et al., 2019).

> **CASE EXAMPLE 25.1 SAMUEL AND TREVON**
>
> Samuel is a 2.5-year-old boy who lives with his mother, father, and 6-year-old brother. Samuel enjoys staying at home to play with his toys or watch movies. He plays by himself for unlimited periods of time. He spends many hours a day driving his cars and trucks back and forth while side lying and watching the wheels turn. If his brother plays with the cars, Samuel screams uncontrollably until the car is returned to him. Another of Samuel's favorite activities is playing with balls. He pulls the basket of balls to the top of the stairs where he bounces them off the wall and down the stairs into the family room over and over. If someone else retrieves one of the balls or tries to engage Samuel in a ball game, an ear-piercing scream is heard before Samuel deteriorates into a kicking, screaming tantrum.
>
> Samuel's brother Trevon is 6 years old. He attends kindergarten 5 days each week, where he follows the classroom routine, engages with teacher-directed activities, and plays side by side with his peers. At home, Trevon plays by himself for up to 30 min at a time. He prefers activities such as coloring and playing with dinosaur figurines. His favorite color is blue, and his coloring pictures consist of all shades of the hue. His favorite dinosaur is a Tyrannosaurus rex, and Trevon can recite a number of known facts about this creature. When a visitor comes to the family home, Trevon inundates the person with incessant talk about the T-rex. His eye contact is spontaneous but fleeting. He is easily distracted, looking away from a task to investigate all noise or movement around him. When approached by others, Trevon gives a quick, "Hi," and then directs his gaze to the person's shoulder and begins reciting facts about the T-rex.
>
> Samuel eats approximately 10 different foods. His diet is restricted by his own preferences for certain tastes and textures and by intolerance for gluten. His mother is careful to prepare foods that are gluten-free and that she knows Samuel will eat. He can use a spoon and fork moderately well but prefers to use his fingers. He refuses all fruits, vegetables, and dairy products. His mother has expressed concern about Samuel's nutrition. His behavioral rigidity considerably impacts the family's daily life. He does well on weekdays during the school year while his brother is at school. On school days, Samuel accompanies his mother on errands to one familiar place at a time if she brings favorite toys and a snack. If his mother tries to combine two errands into one trip, Samuel tantrums and refuses to exit the car. Samuel's behavior is much more erratic on weekends and holidays, when the schedule is inconsistent, and more people are in the home.
>
> Both Samuel and Trevon are diagnosed with developmental disabilities.

From a client-centered perspective, therapists do not try to change such behaviors merely for the comfort of others. Rather, intervention approaches should align with the individual's strengths, aim to develop skills that support successful engagement in desired and meaningful occupations, and target achievement of client-identified goals. For these reasons, this chapter aims to give both entering and experienced occupational therapy practitioners the knowledge needed to apply clinical reasoning and critical analysis to situations in which client behavior disrupts occupational performance to guide decision-making about the need for intervention as well as selection of intervention methods.

As referrals for intervention to address challenging and problem behaviors have increased, it has become increasingly expected that occupational therapy practitioners are knowledgeable about and skilled in addressing such behaviors among their clients. Knowledge of challenging behavior and the strategies to facilitate behavior change has emerged from the fields of education and psychology. Occupational therapy practitioners can benefit by learning from these professions and selectively applying that knowledge to supplement their evaluation of client behaviors, inform their clinical decision-making, and enhance their ability to collaborate with clients and other team members.

Over the past 3 decades, behavioral intervention methods have gained considerable popularity as their effectiveness is found in programs for children with autism spectrum disorder and other conditions (e.g., Carr, 2016; Lovass, 1987; Martinez et al., 2016). This robust body of research provides a wealth of knowledge that occupational therapy practitioners can use to understand behavioral perspectives regarding why challenging behaviors occur, strategies for prevention, and approaches for intervening when challenging behaviors occur.

As evidence-based practitioners, it is crucial to recognize that many behavioral approaches do not align with occupational therapy's client-centered philosophy and emphasis on engagement in meaningful occupation. Thus, incorporating behavioral approaches into occupational therapy services should only occur with thorough understanding of the approach, a clear aim for using the approach, agreement of the client that the approach is acceptable to them, and a specific plan for evaluating outcomes.

## Challenging Behavior

Evidence shows that 90% of early childhood and licensed childcare teachers report having at least one child with challenging behavior in their classroom, but that on average, there are four children with challenging behaviors in each school classroom (Granja et al., 2018). The nature of behaviors changes with age, with older children displaying more serious challenging behavior than younger children. Among school age children with disabilities, challenging behavior occurs in 48%–60% of those with intellectual developmental disorders and in up to 90% of autistic children (Simo-Pinatella et al., 2018). In a 4-year longitudinal study, Nicholls et al., 2023 examined the stability of challenging behaviors and the relationship between challenging behaviors and functional characteristics among more than 200 children 4–19 years of age with intellectual disability. Results showed that behaviors including aggression/destruction, self-injury, and general challenging behavior were stable across the 4-year period, but that the prevalence of stereotyped behaviors increased significantly. Additionally, Nicholls et al., 2023 reported consistent relationships between adaptive skills and specific challenging behaviors with higher rates of self-injury, aggression, and stereotypy being associated with lower rates of adaptive skills.

As indicated from the findings reported above (Nicholls et al., 2023), challenging and problem behavior can take many forms. Passive behaviors such as noncompliance, withdrawal, avoidance, inattention, or lack of response are not overtly disruptive but still interfere with occupational performance and participation (Lipschultz & Wilder, 2017). Active behaviors such as direct refusal to engage, opposition, aggression toward people or property, or self-injurious behavior not only interfere with occupational performance and participation but can also be disruptive or harmful to self or others (Hong & Matson, 2020; Newcomb & Hagopian, 2018). See Fig. 25.2 for examples of aggressive behavior. Both passive and active forms of challenging behavior can be difficult to manage and require attention and intervention by caregivers and service providers. See Table 25.1 for frequency data for selected challenging behaviors among children with and without diagnoses.

## Contributions from Behavior Theory

Decades of research examining animal and human responses to external stimuli (e.g., Pavlov, 1927; Skinner, 1953; Watson, 1913) have contributed to the development of **behavior theory** and particularly to the understanding of operant conditioning. These concepts describe human behavior as shaped through an individual's interaction with the environment as they respond to external cues and learn from the effect of their actions (McLeod, 2017). These stimulus-response relationships, in which the individual experiences a stimulus that evinces

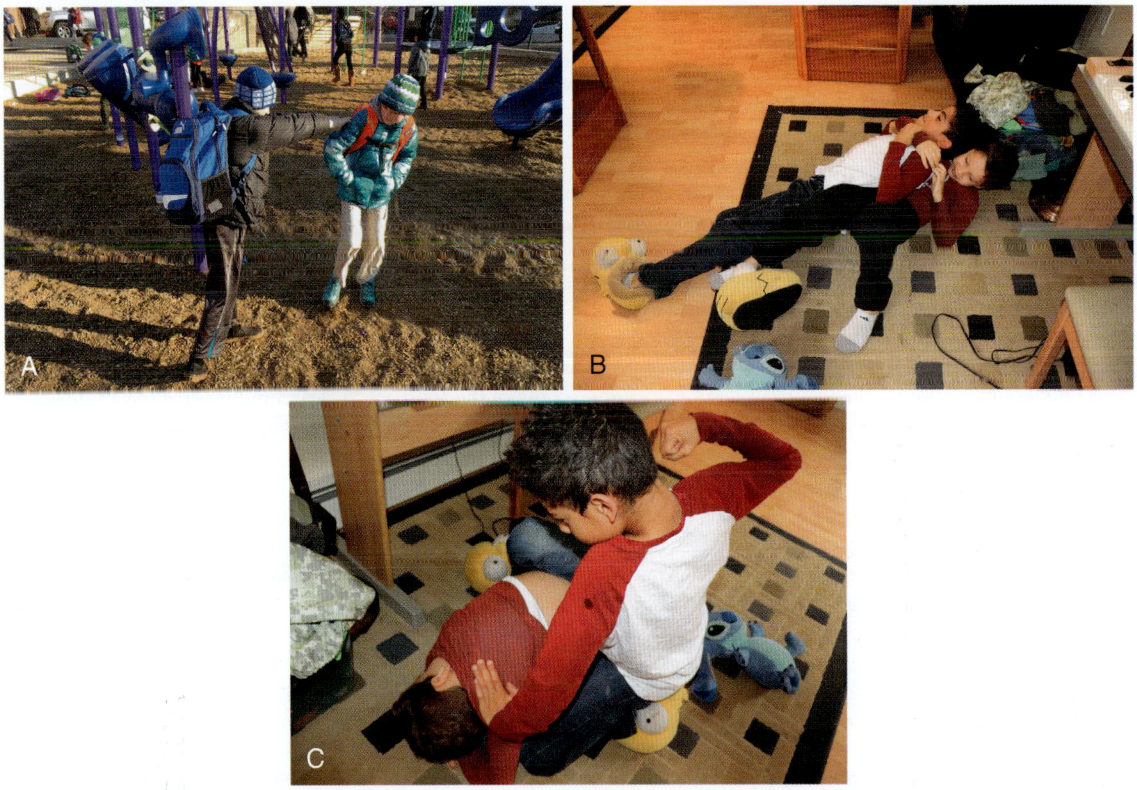

**Fig. 25.2** (A–C) Challenging behavior can include aggression that places the child or others at risk.

**TABLE 25.1 Selected Types and Frequencies of Problem Behaviors Among Children With and Without Diagnoses**

| Population | Behavior Type | Frequency Behavior Is Reported (%) |
|---|---|---|
| Early childhood (0–5 years) | Impulsivity that disrupts classroom | 51 |
| | Refusal to cooperate or follow directions | 47 |
| | Aggression (hitting, biting, throwing) | 38 |
| | Withdrawal or sadness limiting engagement | 26 |
| Special education (5–19 years) | Disruptive | 51 |
| | Aggression toward others | 43 |
| | Stereotypy | 33 |
| | Self-injury | 28 |
| | Withdrawn | 26 |

a behavioral response, provide the basis for learned behaviors. The individual learns which behaviors lead to pleasurable or positive outcomes and which lead to negative or unpleasant outcomes. Those behaviors that lead to outcomes which the individual finds pleasurable are strengthened and likely to occur again, while behaviors that lead to unpleasant results are weakened and are less likely to occur again. Classical behaviorism describes this relationship between observed behaviors and the environmental variables that elicit and maintain them as the A-B-C relationship. See Table 25.2 for behavioral terminology and definitions. Case Example 25.1 illustrates these concepts.

**TABLE 25.2 Behavioral Terminology and Definitions**

| Behavior Component | Description |
|---|---|
| Setting events | Physical, social, or physiologic conditions or events that predispose the individual to evincing a behavior and that increase the likelihood that an antecedent will trigger the behavior |
| Antecedents | Stimuli that immediately precede and lead to a behavior |
| Consequences | Stimuli that follow and strengthen a behavior |
| Topography | Description of the behavior that details what is seen when the behavior occurs |
| Frequency | The rate at which a behavior occurs |
| Intensity | The degree of force or effort with which a behavior occurs |
| Duration | The amount of time for which a behavior occurs |
| Reinforcement | Responses that make a target behavior more likely to occur in the future |

The *A-B-C relationship* describes the variables that make up the behavior learning process. *A* represents the antecedents to the behavior. **Antecedents** are those stimuli that occur prior to a behavior and that elicit or trigger the behavior occurrence (Iovannone et al., 2017). Identifying the antecedents to a behavior helps explain what causes the behavior. Antecedents can occur immediately prior to the behavior and serve as a trigger for the behavior, or they can be separated from the behavior by time and space. Just as human behavior is highly individualized, so are the antecedents that trigger the behaviors. Common antecedents are contextual, including a particular person, room, visual stimulus, or sound. Other common antecedents are cognitive, motor, communicative, or social performance demands.

*B* represents the behavior itself. It includes three primary characteristics: the topography, or *form*, of the behavior, including what is seen when the behavior is observed; the frequency of the behavior's occurrence; and the duration for which the behavior occurs. Each of these characteristics should be included when developing objective and thorough descriptions of behaviors.

*C* represents the consequences of the behavior. **Consequences** are those events that occur following a behavior and that result in strengthening or maintaining the behavior. Most often, the consequences are events that occur immediately following the behavior, such as giving a child the toy he requested when he uses the word "please." Consequences affect the likelihood that the behavior will occur in the future. Common consequences include eye contact, attention, verbal interaction, physical engagement, removal from a situation or a performance demand, receiving a desired object, or access to a desired event.

**Setting events** are those events that may not immediately cause the behavior to occur but that set the stage for the behavior to emerge if other triggers also occur (Iovannone et al., 2017; Robertson & Coy, 2019). Setting events act like priming a pump, where once they occur, the challenging behavior is much more likely to occur. In other words, setting events are part of a chain of events that eventually lead to the behavior happening. Examples of setting events are as follows.

- Oversleeping
- Illness
- Spilling milk at breakfast
- Disruption in the expected schedule
- Experiencing conflict earlier in the day
- Feeling anxious about an upcoming event

Understanding the setting events that predispose the individual to stress or heightened arousal helps the occupational therapy practitioner recognize situations in which the challenging behaviors are more likely to occur and affords the opportunity to proactively implement strategies to counteract the setting event and reduce the likelihood that the behavior will occur.

Occupational therapy practitioners bring an appreciation for the role of sensory processing and sensory integration to their conceptualization of factors that influence behavior. Because of the neurophysiological mechanisms involved in processing and integrating sensation, sensory stimuli have a direct effect on arousal, which in turn affects behavior (Watling et al., 2018). In behavioral terminology, this relationship functions as a setting event. For children who have challenges in processing and integrating sensory stimuli, experiencing sensation can lead to hyperresponsivity and heightened arousal, both of which set the stage for challenging behavior. For more information on sensory processing and sensory integration, see Chapters 27 and 28. See Box 25.1 for internal and external factors that can function as setting events.

### BOX 25.1 Internal and External Factors that May Function as Setting Events

| Internal Factors | External Factors |
|---|---|
| Emotional state: anxious, unhappy, dissatisfied | Ambient sensory input such as flickering light |
| Fatigue | Change in schedule |
| Hunger | Task demands greater than skill level |
| Illness | Unfamiliar person |
| Frustration | Unfamiliar place |
| Pain | Ineffective communication |
| Poor emotional regulation | Ineffective interpersonal interactions |
| Poor self-regulation | Absence of meaning in tasks |
| Poor sensory processing | |
| Poor interoception | |

## Behavior Always Has a Purpose

In most everyday situations, people view inappropriate or challenging behavior as inconvenient and irritating to those in the surrounding environment. Have you ever sat in a restaurant at a table next to a screaming toddler or in the movie theater behind a person using a cell phone? These behaviors do not present real threats, but people view them as problematic.

To best understand and address changing a behavior, one must first determine the underlying purpose of the behavior (Hong & Matson, 2020); for example, is the child confused by too many choices, overwhelmed by environmental stimuli, experiencing pain, or lacking the necessary language skills to convey a message? Deciphering the purpose of a given episode of challenging behavior can be difficult. Most challenging behaviors are reactive, and the person performing the behavior usually does not have insight into the motivation for or purpose of the behavior. Professionals well-versed in behavioral theory can uncover the purpose by analyzing the antecedent and consequent variables surrounding the behavior and determining which are connected to the behavior in a manner that strengthens or sustains it (Newcomb & Hagopian, 2018) using a process called **Behavioral analysis**.

Decades of behavioral research have identified four primary purposes, or *functions*, of challenging behavior: attention, alone/nonsocial, escape, and tangible (Newcomb & Hagopian, 2018). See Table 25.3 for examples of how the behaviors serve the child's purpose. The attention function is in effect when the behavior results in the individual receiving attention from or achieving reciprocal interaction with others, such as when a child receives teacher attention in response to acting out during class. Behavior has an alone/nonsocial function when it results in the absence of any form of attention from others, including prompts for performance. An example of the alone/nonsocial function is a child who does not want the teacher to call on them, so they withdraw in class. In this example, the event (speaking in class) is removed as the child withdraws. The child receives a reward for the nonsocial behavior or for "escaping." This escape function results in removal of an undesired object, event, or demand in response to the child's behavior, such as removing an assignment sheet from the student's desk when he displays self-injurious behavior. Finally, a behavior has a tangible function when the behavior results in the child obtaining a desired object or event, such continuing to use an iPad because of whining.

Some behaviorists recognize an additional function of behavior, often referred to as automatic reinforcement, which occurs via the sensory input received through self-stimulatory or stereotypic behaviors (Hong & Matson, 2020) such as body rocking, finger flicking, bouncing on toes, or covering ears. Behaviors may have a single function or multiple functions; this should be determined through the Functional Behavior Assessment (FBA).

## Functional Behavior Assessment

A *Functional Behavior Assessment (FBA)* is a systematic process designed to identify the variables in the A-B-C relationship so that they can be analyzed to determine which ones are maintaining the behavior. Once the professional identifies the variables maintaining the behavior, they can address them in intervention (Hong & Matson, 2020). The FBA process involves five steps.

**TABLE 25.3 Functions of Behaviors and Examples**

| Function of Behavior | Examples of How Each Function Might Be Fulfilled |
|---|---|
| Attention | Verbal praise, smiles, eye contact, positive comments, joking, joining into what child is doing |
| Alone/nonsocial | Absence of attention examples given above, allowed to seclude in study carrel, tent, or other hideaway; absence of questions, prompts to engage, or instructions to work |
| Escape | Removal of a task or performance demand, removal of a person, or removal of the student from the environment |
| Tangible | Acquire a snack, token, preferred activity, sticker, or prize |
| Sensory | Experience a visual, auditory, tactile, or vestibular input |

Functions are best identified through analysis of the individual's behavior and systematic testing of the hypothesized function to determine its effect on the target behavior.

1. team building and goal setting
2. functional assessment of the behavior
3. hypothesis formulation
4. development of the comprehensive support plan
5. implementation and outcome monitoring of the plan, including refining the plan as needed

During the first step of the FBA, a team of individuals gathers to address the challenging behavior. Ideally, the team includes the child's parents or caregivers as recognized experts on the child and as partners in the intervention process, along with other professionals who work with the child on a consistent basis. Occupational therapy practitioners should be part of the FBA process when they have personal knowledge of the child or adolescent and direct experience with the target behavior. The team collaborates to identify desired outcomes for the child as a foundation for addressing the behavior.

Step two involves the comprehensive functional assessment of the challenging behavior. Efforts focus on clearly and completely describing the behavior, the context(s) in which it occurs, the antecedents and consequences that maintain the behavior, and the functions of the behavior. The goal of this step is to understand the purpose of the behavior and conditions under which the behavior is most and least likely to occur. Data are systematically collected by interviewing people who have direct knowledge of the child and experience with the behavior, observing the child where and when the behavior is most likely to occur, reviewing records in which the behavior has been documented, and gathering information about contextual variables such as health or changes in other environments or activity schedules. Fig. 25.3 shows an adult observing a child behaving in his natural environment to better understand his behaviors as part of intervention planning.

Third, the team formulates a hypothesis about the behavior, including explicitly stating the antecedents, consequences, and function of the behavior. The hypothesis statement emerges from the information gathered in step two.

In the fourth step, the team develops a comprehensive **behavior service plan (BSP)** that outlines the intervention(s) plan. The BSP plan itself has four elements.

1. the functional assessment of behavior including hypothesized functions of the behavior

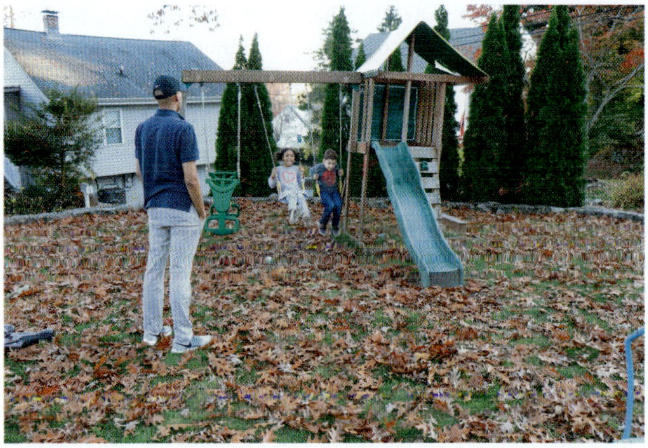

**Fig. 25.3** The function of a challenging behavior is best determined through data collection consisting of direct observation and interviewing people familiar with the behavior. This adult is directly observing the interaction of these siblings in their natural environment.

2. the specific individualized intervention strategies that will be used to address the behaviors
3. strategies that will be applied throughout the day
4. evidence that the plan is consistent with the values and resources of the child receiving support and the persons providing support (Iovannone et al., 2017)

Fifth, the team implements the plan, collects outcomes data, and evaluates the effectiveness of the plan. If the child is not progressing toward the outcomes identified in step one, the team modifies the plan and collects outcome data again. Case Example 25.2 provides an illustration of an FBA.

## INTERVENTIONS BASED ON BEHAVIOR THEORY

Interventions using behavioral methods can have two primary aims: building desired behaviors or reducing challenging behaviors. While occupational therapy practitioners and other professionals seek to address both aims, the approach they use to intervention is guided by their profession's underlying philosophies and values. According to behavioral approaches, **antecedent interventions** are more effective at building desired behaviors. These approaches occur before the onset of a challenging behavior and aim to reduce the need for the challenging behavior (Steinbrenner et al., 2020). For example, if the child uses self-injurious behavior to receive adult attention, proactively giving adult attention for desired and nonchallenging behaviors such as entering the classroom or joining in a conversation can meet the same function without the child self-injuring. **Consequence-based interventions** are another option. However, since these methods occur after the child demonstrates a behavior, consequence methods could inadvertently lead to strengthening a challenging behavior, thus it is best to use consequence-based interventions in response to desired behaviors.

### Antecedent Interventions

Antecedent interventions have distinct advantages over other approaches for both reducing challenging behaviors and promoting desired behaviors (Wood et al., 2018). By removing or modifying environmental events that maintain challenging behavior, challenging behavior may be subverted before it occurs, allowing the individual to spend more time in functional occupational behavior (Steinbrenner et al., 2020). In addition, antecedent approaches may have a quick effect (Wood et al., 2018) and can enhance the overall environment, establishing a context that is positive, orderly, and motivating for all

## CASE EXAMPLE 25.2 SIDDARTH

7-year-old Siddarth was at risk of being suspended from his second-grade classroom because of uncontrollable aggressive outbursts that included yelling at the teacher, refusing to complete schoolwork, overturning desks, and throwing school supplies. The behaviors had been building throughout the fall and culminated with punching the teacher in early November. An FBA was immediately initiated. The teacher, behavior specialist, principal, parents, and occupational therapist met to identify the behaviors of concern and desired outcome for intervention. The plan for data collection included observation of Siddarth in the classroom, on the playground, and in the cafeteria by the behavior specialist.

The occupational therapist observed Siddarth's handwriting abilities in October at the request of the classroom teacher. At that time, she noted that Siddarth used a mature tripod grasp, formed letters correctly, and exhibited good upper extremity positioning and postural support for handwriting tasks. Siddarth performed handwriting activities without difficulty when copying from a sample or when writing personal information such as his name but showed signs of anxiety when he was asked to write creatively. The occupational therapist documented that he "seemed unable to generate ideas or topics to write about, and he became flushed, fidgeted with his pencil, and stated that the assignment was 'stupid.'"

During the FBA the behavior specialist noted that signs of anxiety often preceded Siddarth's behavioral outbursts and that the outbursts were worse later in the day during the creative writing lessons. Siddarth also showed signs of anxiety during collaborative work activities. When group work was assigned, Siddarth fidgeted with materials in his desk and did not join his group until specifically instructed by the teacher. He did not join in the group discussions or participate in work activities; rather, he remained at the fringe of the group. If his participation was requested by a peer or instructed by the teacher, Siddarth fidgeted and looked around anxiously, often giving excuses for not working. If pushed to participate, he verbally refused with increased vocal intensity and volume and sometimes shoved a desk or chair.

The FBA team reconvened after the observation period. The behavior specialist reported his findings and the occupational therapist contributed her observations noting that Siddarth seemed to have difficulty with flexible thinking, especially when also under performance pressure. The team hypothesized that the aggressive behaviors were a result of poor ability to cope with anxiety and that writing and social situations were anxiety producing for Siddarth. The FBA team then worked together to develop a plan to better match writing and social demands to Siddarth's abilities, provide support during writing assignments, and provide intervention to develop social skills that would support his ability to participate in group learning activities.

In addition to modifications the teacher made to assignments, the occupational therapist recommended modifying the classroom environment to decrease anxiety-producing situations and add coping supports. She also designed a program aimed to help Siddarth develop improved self-regulation of behavior, body scheme, fine motor coordination, and social skills. Some classroom-wide strategies were implemented, including seated isometric exercises for the entire class at key times during the school day, regularly scheduled dimmed lighting and whispered voice times, and a "cozy corner" for independent use by students. The occupational therapist also worked with Siddarth, his teacher, and the school counselor to identify two peers with whom Siddarth could work to build his social skills. She provided training sessions with the students, teacher, and counselor including instruction on teamwork, complimenting, turn-taking, and collaboration. Data collection forms were used to track Siddarth's behavior. A change in the frequency and intensity of Siddarth's behavior was seen almost immediately, and within 3 weeks of implementing the program, Siddarth's inappropriate behavior diminished to occasional verbal outbursts with no physical aggression.

(Steinbrenner et al., 2020; Wood et al., 2018). As shown in Fig. 25.4, peers may deliver antecedents to desired behaviors.

The team may implement antecedent approaches for an individual or more broadly, such as within a classroom or an entire school. It is important that the team develop individualized antecedent approaches in response to the FBA and aim to identify and reduce or remove the triggers for the challenging behaviors so that they become less frequent. Generalized antecedent approaches involve implementation of contextual conditions known to promote positive behaviors by reducing common stressors and introducing positive and supportive environments. See Table 25.4 for examples of contextual and individual antecedent approaches. Functional communication training and pivotal response training are examples of two antecedent interventions used in practice, as explained in Case Example 25.2.

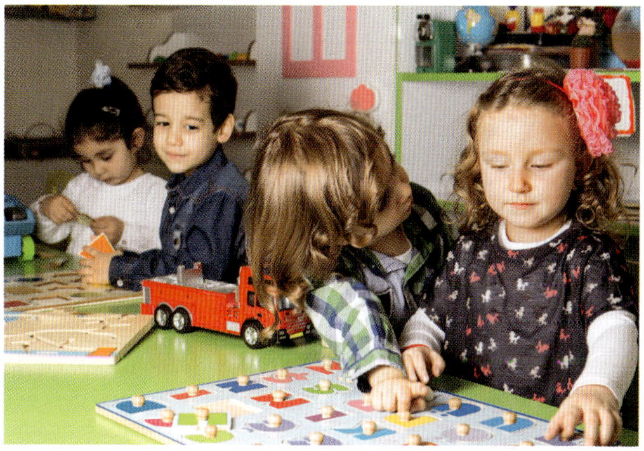

Fig. 25.4 Antecedent interventions can include peers and can be as simple as gesturing to provide a cue before the child makes an error.

**Functional Communication Training.** Functional communication training (FCT) involves teaching specific, functional strategies for communication that result in the individual acquiring the same result as is typically acquired using a challenging or undesired behavior (Gerow et al., 2018; Ghaemmaghami & Hanley, 2020). For example, if a student typically escapes from doing math worksheets by verbally protesting and flopping on the floor, the therapist may instruct the student to express disinterest in completing the math worksheet through a different communication method. In instances such as this, it is important to develop a response strategy that honors the student's communicative abilities and achieves the instructional target of helping the student learn the math lesson (Gerow et al., 2018). The child is taught a method of communication that is consistent with their strengths and a method that is accessible to the individual regardless of the context. This may include picture cards, sentence strips, gestures, or voice output devices. FCT diminishes the impact of ineffective communication and enables the child to influence the context in a positive way, reducing challenging behaviors while also building a sense of self-efficacy and empowerment.

**Pivotal Response Training.** The concept of pivotal behaviors is like that of functional communication in that it recognizes that certain behaviors are fundamental for success in daily life. Pivotal response training aims to teach these behaviors, motivation, responding to multiple cues, self-management, and self-initiations, through systematic application of applied behavioral methods (Steinbrenner et al., 2020). Pivotal behaviors positively influence a child's ability to access learning or engage in social participation. For example, a child benefits from learning how and when to request help or ask for

**TABLE 25.4 Common Contextual and Individual Antecedent Approaches to Reduce Problem Behavior**

| Contextual Antecedents | Individual Antecedents |
|---|---|
| Clear rules and expectations that apply to all | Match tasks to the individual's developmental and cognitive level to ensure capability and to maximize possibility of success |
| Predictable schedules to ease anxiety about activity sequences | Allow modes of task completion that tap into the child's strengths |
| Support transitions with predictability and advanced information | Provide individualized support for transitions that is matched to the child's unique characteristics |
| Consistent environmental arrangement and features | Provision of individualized environmental modifications to remove antecedents for child's specific challenging behavior |
| Frequent and consistent praise for appropriate group or class-wide behavior | Deliver frequent behavior- and task specific praise to alleviate the child's stress related to performance expectations |
| Incorporate interests and preferred activities of the group | Customize learning tasks or therapeutic activities to include the child's preferred interests |
| Arrange instruction so that brief, easy tasks are interspersed with challenging tasks | Allow child's interests to drive task selection |
| Offer multiple opportunities to respond to cues and performance demands | Offer multiple opportunities for choice |
| Incorporate regular opportunities for physical exercise and movement | Provide regular opportunities for preferred forms of physical exercise and scaffold as needed |
| Provide scheduled and frequent adult attention to the group | Provide child-focused attention consistently throughout the day that is not contingent on task performance |
| Minimize waiting times and unstructured time in the daily schedule | Provide materials for purposeful engagement during waiting |
| Arrange seating to support attention to teacher | Position child in a location and orientation that supports their individual sensory needs and learning style |
| Minimize sensory features known to be distracting or irritating | Remove all sensory features of the environment known to be setting events for the child and provide a sensory-free zone the child can retreat to when feeling overstimulated |

clarification regarding expectations across multiple contexts and situations. Children who learn these behaviors do not need to use challenging behaviors to get their desired outcomes. Children are taught pivotal behaviors in low-pressure situations to support acquisition of the skill prior to their facing a demand to use the skill in a higher-stakes context. Pivotal response training is considered a naturalistic intervention because it is implemented during regular daily activities and within natural environments (Steinbrenner et al., 2020).

**Specific Environmental Modifications.** Select antecedent strategies use modification of some aspect of the environment as the main component of the intervention. All such methods aim to prevent challenging behavior by altering the environment to remove the conditions that elicit the challenging behavior. *Environmental modifications* can be especially helpful in supporting transitions between activities, a time during which challenging behavior is common. Visual schedules, timers, and representational objects, described later, can be useful strategies to support successful transitions. A wide range of other environmental modifications can also support success in meeting daily performance expectations. Environmental modifications should be based on the child's strengths and preferences and in accordance with their FBA. Case Example 25.4 illustrates how environmental modifications can support a child's behavioral goals.

**Visual Schedules.** *Visual schedules* are a commonly used and effective method for supporting successful transitions and reducing challenging behaviors (Lory, Rispoli, et al., 2020; Zimmerman et al., 2017). These are particularly useful in situations where the schedule remains similar from day to day or week to week, or to represent changes in the schedule for a child who has difficulty tolerating change. Either picture icons or word cards can be arranged on a schedule board to represent the sequence of activities or events that is going to occur. Children can follow the visual representation of the sequence. Depending on a given child's abilities, they can learn to use the visual schedule independently, or they can use the schedule to decide what to do next. Visual schedules may represent activity sequences with no time allotted. They may include the time only, day of week, time of day, and the activity that will be occurring. Visual schedules can be removable cards that allow the practitioner to easily modify the child's schedule. They can be displayed on poster boards mounted to the wall or in a binder or notebook for easy transport. The practitioners create a visual schedule that is individualized to the child and their capabilities and needs. Evidence suggests that children who use visual schedules have less challenging behavior (Zimmerman et al., 2017).

**Signals.** *Signals* provide an objective indicator that something is about to occur. Because a signal operates independently of an adult once it is set, children do not view them as imposed by the adult, which removes pressure and alleviates performance anxiety that can contribute to challenging behavior (Watling, 2005). Use of signals can be explicitly (e.g., show it to the child and inform them of what will happen, for example, "The timer will make a beeping sound. When you hear the beeping sound, it will be time to clean up the blocks and come to the table for snack.") or implicitly taught (e.g., implement the signal and expose the child to its use through repetition). Case Example 25.3 (Sonara) provides an example of using a timer as a signal.

Once a child has learned to complete activities using a signal, the practitioner can apply this to a variety of contexts and situations. Signals might include static means, such as posting a colored index card or placing a wristband on the child, or dynamic tools such as

## CASE EXAMPLE 25.3 SONARA

Sonara is a 4-year-old girl with autism. She enjoys playing with alphabet blocks and her toy piano. Sonara has extreme difficulty concluding her play to transition to a different activity. When a transition is imposed on her, Sonara demonstrates one of two predictable responses: a complete lack of response as if she did not hear the instruction or extreme refusal to transition expressed by screaming and stamping feet. At times, the behavior can escalate into a full-blown tantrum including hitting, kicking, dropping to the floor, and throwing toys.

Sonara is enrolled in a preschool classroom for children with developmental disabilities. Transition between activities occurs multiple times each day as the children engage in different play centers, circle time, snack time, and outdoor play. Sonara's difficulties with transitions often disrupt the class.

The occupational therapist works with Sonara on a weekly basis and introduces a timer to help her learn how to conclude an activity. Within 3 days, Sonara consistently responds when the timer signals. She alerts to the sound, discontinues her activity, and turns the timer off. Sometimes she returns to her activity and reengages, but when cued by the teacher or occupational therapist, she is able to transition to the next activity. By the end of 9 school days, Sonara reliably alerts to the sound of the timer, discontinues her activity, and consults a visual schedule to determine what she is to do next. She then activates the timer for a preset duration of time and transitions to the activity indicated on her schedule.

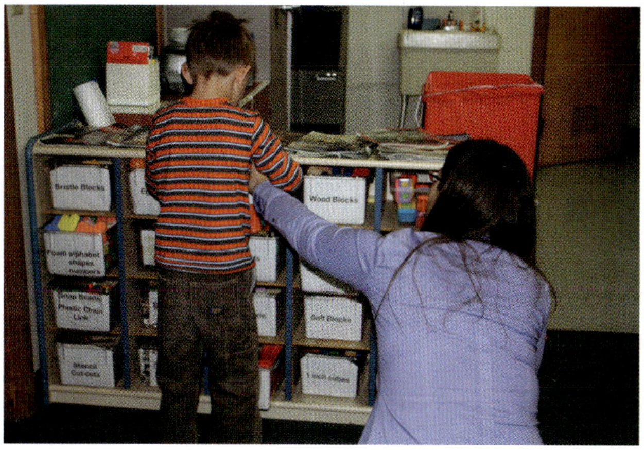

**Fig. 25.5** Tier one interventions, such as organizing materials into easily accessible and clearly labeled boxes, benefit all students.

Time Timer, a standard alarm clock, timer on a digital device, or an hourglass (Campos et al., 2022). Children can learn to utilize signals themselves as a way to self-monitor their use of time and compliance with time limits and to support attending events that occur at a specific time such as going to the bus stop, getting ready for bed, or leaving for a social event.

**Representational Objects.** *Representational objects* offer another strategy for supporting transitions (Thelen & Klifman, 2011; Watling, 2005). In this method, the practitioner gathers concrete objects that clearly represent the various activities or events that make up the child's day. When the child needs to transition to another activity, the practitioner or adult shows them the relevant representational object and simple verbal instructions. For example, the occupational therapy practitioner may hand the child a crayon and say, "Time for art." The child may take the object and carry it with them to the location where the designated activity will occur. The use of representational objects is flexible and may be combined with transition routines, visual schedules, and timers in the manner that best supports the child's success.

**Positive Behavioral Intervention and Supports.** Positive behavioral intervention and supports (PBIS; initially known as positive behavior support, PBS) is an approach to managing the behavior of individuals and groups that involves incorporating principles of applied behavior analysis via antecedent approaches (Kincaid et al., 2016). As a movement away from consequence-based approaches, PBS emerged in the 1980s to address problem behaviors that interfered with function and detracted from quality of life. The primary strategies involve environmental modifications to remove or reduce behavior triggers. PBIS has been identified in the 2004 reaffirmation of the amendments to the Individuals with Disabilities Education Act (IDEA) as an evidence-based preventive program for children whose behaviors impede their own learning or the learning of others (20 USC §1414[d][3][B][i]). PBIS has since developed into a framework with standards of practice.

The PBIS framework includes three tiers of support. Tier one includes school-wide strategies for all students, such as social and emotional learning or bully prevention programs. Tier one interventions are designed to prevent new cases of challenging behavior from occurring. Strategies may include creating an organized environment to support learning, arranging the physical environment to promote engagement and positive behavior, and providing instruction in communication and social skills to support social interaction and participation. Fig. 25.5 shows a tier one intervention strategy that promotes positive behaviors within the classroom.

Tier two involves strategies aimed at reducing current occurrences of challenging behavior. These interventions are targeted at students who are identified as at risk for more serious behaviors and can involve more focused strategies such as group social skills interventions, classroom management systems such as working together to earn group privileges or rewards, or check-in/check-out systems in which the students check in with an adult and receive daily goals upon arriving at school and then check out, which includes reviewing goals at the end of the day.

Tier three interventions are provided to individual students to reduce more intense or problematic behaviors and improve quality of life. Strategies at this level include the FBA process with resulting intervention plan and outcomes measurement, wraparound planning, strategies to address individual antecedents, and teaching replacement behaviors to reduce the effectiveness of established challenging behavior. Helpful resources for PBIS, including intervention ideas, can be found at https://www.pbisworld.com and https://www.pbis.org.

## Consequence Interventions

Consequence interventions aim to impact behavior by addressing those situations or stimuli that occur after, or as the result of, a child's behavior. Consequence approaches include three primary methods: punishment, extinction, and reinforcement. *Punishment* involves the child experiencing an aversive consequence after exhibiting a challenging behavior (Lipschultz & Wilder, 2017). The aversive consequence can be the occurrence of an unpleasant or negative stimulus or the removal of a pleasant or preferred stimulus. *Extinction* occurs when the variables reinforcing a behavior are no longer present, causing the behavior to gradually fade away (Lipschultz & Wilder, 2017). Erturk et al. (2018) found that consequence-based interventions were highly effective in reducing self-injurious behaviors among children with developmental disabilities.

**Reinforcement.** Reinforcement is a consequence-based behavioral technology that can strengthen desired behaviors and weaken undesired behaviors. Reinforcement can take different forms depending on the target behavior and desired result. Positive and negative reinforcement both aim to strengthen behavior but do so through different mechanisms. *Positive reinforcement* involves adding something pleasant or desirable to increase the likelihood of a behavior occurring, such as giving the child a preferred object when they use good manners to request it (Lipschultz & Wilder, 2017). *Negative reinforcement* involves taking away something unpleasant to increase the desired behavior, such as allowing the child to leave the dinner table after eating two bites of food.

Because every behavior has a response, every behavior is reinforced in some way. *Differential reinforcement* involves intentionally using reinforcement to strengthen a desired behavior while simultaneously removing reinforcement from undesired or challenging behaviors (Steinbrenner et al., 2020). Differential reinforcement provides a rewarding consequence for behaviors that take the place of the child's challenging behavior. Reinforcement is differentially applied to three types of behaviors: those that are incompatible with the target behavior, called *differential reinforcement of incompatible*; those that are alternative and could replace the target behavior, called *differential reinforcement of alternative*, or other behaviors that are not related to the target behavior but are positive in nature, called *differential reinforcement of other*. For example, if a child raises his hand and verbally requests a break rather than being disruptive or aggressive, then he receives praise, and he may take a break. Teaching and differentially reinforcing desired behaviors strengthens them (Reeves et al., 2017), and simultaneous removal of reinforcement from challenging behaviors weakens them, leading to the child having a repertoire of desired and functional behaviors. Adults can be positive reinforcers by taking time to listen and respond as shown in Fig. 25.6.

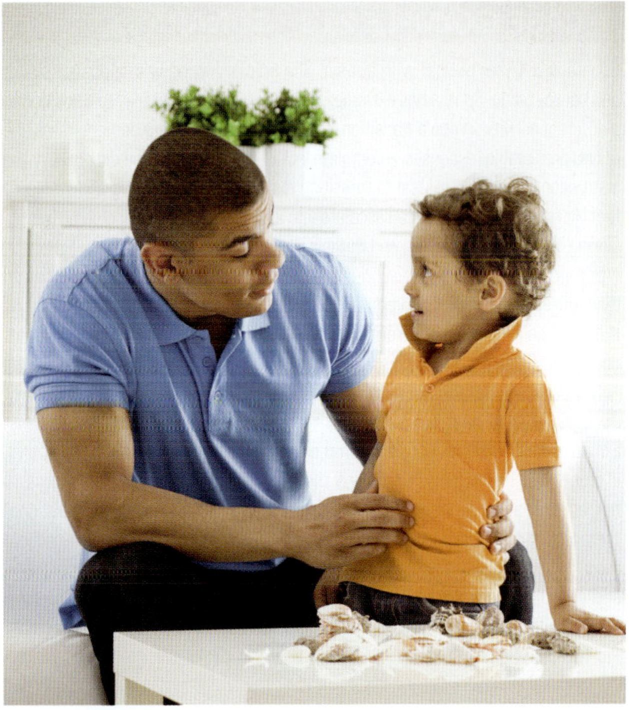

**Fig. 25.6** Adult attention is a powerful reinforcer that can be used strategically to strengthen desired behaviors. (Copyright iStock Photo.)

*Noncontingent reinforcement* is an antecedent-based approach that is useful when the aim is to decrease a challenging behavior (Steinbrenner et al., 2020). The practitioner delivers reinforcement to the child at fixed intervals rather than making reinforcement contingent on a specific behavior. The reinforcement used should match the function of the targeted challenging behavior. By providing reinforcement in this manner, the student receives the desired result on a frequent basis without needing to display the challenging behavior. For example, if a student frequently says inappropriate comments during teacher instruction and teacher attention is the consequence that is reinforcing the behavior, the teacher can provide attention at a high frequency prior to and during the beginning of instruction so that the student does not need to speak out during the lesson.

The power of reinforcement to effect behavior change has more than 50 years of empirical support (e.g., Koegel et al., 1995; Wolf et al., 1964; Zannolli & Daggett, 1998), which identifies crucial aspects of implementation such as timing, method, frequency, and form of reinforcement. However, occupational therapy practitioners typically are not trained in these techniques (Watling & Schwartz, 2004). Because positive reinforcement strengthens a behavior, practitioners must be cognizant of inadvertently reinforcing undesired behaviors by allowing a child to escape from or avoid a demand because of the undesired behavior. Strategic and effective use of reinforcement can increase desired behaviors and reduce challenging behaviors, thereby supporting client engagement in therapeutic activities.

**Contingency Methods.** *Contingency methods* are a group of consequence interventions that proactively implement a specific response-consequence relationship (also called *if-then*; e.g., if the child does X, then Y will occur) that is designed to elicit a desired behavior (Poling & Li, 2019). Children may resist engaging in tasks that they do not enjoy. Resistance can take various forms including, but not limited to, withdrawal, refusal, avoidance, and aggression, which limit occupational engagement and reduce opportunities for learning. Contingency methods such as offering rewards or using a token economy can help elicit participation in nonpreferred activities. Contingency methods are based on the principle of allowing access to a desired event only after performance of, or compliance with, a directive, instruction, or rule. For example, during intervention a child who enjoys blowing bubbles may have to complete therapist-directed task such as pencil and paper work before playing with bubbles. Contingency approaches are used in everyday life for children such as when a child puts on his coat before going outside to play. Children and youth may be more motivated to complete mandatory tasks and be more compliant if they can earn a desired item or activity. As soon as the child completes the mandatory activity, they should receive the reward. It is also important to judge how long the child engages in the mandatory task. For example, parents may allow teens to watch a television show if they help with chores. However, the teen may lose interest in the reward (television show) if the chores are too difficult or time consuming.

These contingency management approaches are used strategically by occupational therapy practitioners to manage challenging behaviors. For example, using contingencies can be complicated when a child tries to negotiate the demands or displays undesired behaviors to avoid the contingency. It is important that the practitioner avoids engaging the child in power struggles during these times. Instead, the practitioner matter-of-factly adheres to the contingency in place and ensures that the child does not gain access to the desired event or activity unless they have completed the required task.

**Token Economies.** Token economies involve systems in which the child earns tokens for desired behaviors and then uses the tokens as currency to purchase desired activities, items, or opportunities (Ackerman et al., 2020). Practitioners define and teach these systems to the child. They specify the behaviors for which children can earn tokens and determine the number of tokens each behavior is worth. For example, a child might earn one token for engaging in seat work for 3 min without needing redirection or earn two tokens for spontaneously sharing art supplies with another child. In addition, they explain the privileges or items that the child can purchase with the tokens and the cost of each at the outset of establishing the token economy. For example, they may indicate that children may exchange tokens for privileges such as 2 min of play with a preferred toy, a piece of candy, or the opportunity to play a game on the computer. They explain to the children that they must earn tokens to engage in certain privileges.

Therapists adjust the complexity of token economies depending on the child's developmental and cognitive age. A simple system may involve merely earning tokens and purchasing rewards, while more complex systems may incorporate the child relinquishing tokens for episodes of undesired behaviors (see Case Example 25.4). In this type of system, the child earns one color of token for desired behaviors and another color for undesired behaviors. The tokens for desired behavior have purchasing value, and those for undesired behavior decrease purchasing value. For example, a child might earn one green token for every 2 min that he remains seated during independent work time and one red token each time he moves out of his chair. At the end of a 10-minute work period, the child has four green tokens and two red tokens. Each red token cancels out one green token, leaving the child with two tokens for that period.

## BEHAVIOR METHODS AND OCCUPATIONAL THERAPY'S HOLISTIC APPROACH

Use of behavioral methods within occupational therapy can be at odds with the profession's holistic perspective of the client (Freidman et al., 2022; Scheibel & Watling, 2016; Welch & Polatajko, 2016; see Freidman et al., 2022 for an overview of philosophical differences and suggestions for effective collaboration with behavioral professionals). In addition to external factors and observable behaviors, occupational therapy practitioners consider internal factors such as physiologic arousal, sensory processing patterns, temperament, volition, and emotional state (Watling, 2017). Practitioners considering incorporating behavioral methods into their occupational therapy sessions must use their clinical reasoning skills to consider the effect of all internal and external factors on the child's occupational functioning.

In addition, occupational therapy practitioners emphasize occupational engagement to achieve client goals. Children with challenging behaviors may have limited engagement due to their behaviors, which in turn restricts learning and skill development. Thus, occupational therapy practitioners should specifically address building client skills that promote occupational engagement and individualizing expectations for performance. This approach is consistent with the concept of pivotal behaviors in that new skills provide the child

### CASE EXAMPLE 25.4 ARIF

Arif is a 10-year-old boy enrolled in the third grade. The classroom teacher states that Arif often has difficulty with attention to tasks, following directions, and completing assigned work. Arif constantly fidgets with clothing and does not sit still in a chair. They are frequently sent to the principal's office for disrespecting the teacher's authority and having an uncooperative attitude. Arif often has a scowl on their face and does not greet others or participate in social interactions. Verbal comments are negative and demeaning toward others, often leading to arguments between students in the classroom. When given a compliment or praise, Arif deflects these comments by stating a rule that was broken or promise not kept. A recent psychological evaluation resulted in a diagnosis of oppositional defiant disorder. The classroom teacher requested an occupational therapy evaluation to address Arif's difficulty in performing the handwriting required to complete schoolwork and a behavior specialist consultation to help with strategies for behavior management.

The occupational therapy evaluation identified poor development of intrinsic hand musculature as well as difficulties in processing visual, auditory, and tactile sensation such that behavior and fine motor performance were affected. The occupational therapist recommended antecedent fine motor skills training and environmental modifications to Arif's classroom to address sensitivity to bright lights, ambient noise, and unexpected touch.

The behavior specialist completed observations of Arif in the classroom, library, gym, and playground. She reported that Arif's behaviors seemed to be maintained by teacher attention and recommended a behavioral intervention plan consisting of noncontingent reinforcement, differential reinforcement, and a class-wide contingency plan in which the entire class earns extra recess each week if there are no student arguments. The behavior specialist provided the teacher with appropriate materials and data collection sheets for the behavior plan.

The teacher agreed with the behavior specialist recommendations and began implementing the behavior plan immediately. She was reluctant to make changes to the classroom because she did not want to provide any special treatment to Arif, fearing that it would make his behaviors worse. The occupational therapist explained the connections between sensory processing and behavior to the teacher and behavior specialist, including the way in which poor sensory processing can be a setting event for challenging behavior. Upon hearing this explanation, the behavior specialist understood the occupational therapist's rationale for environmental modifications and agreed to add them to the behavior plan.

The placement of Arif's desk was moved from the center of the classroom to the side near the teacher's desk to reduce the possibility of unexpected touch and give them a better view of others in the room, so they would know if someone was approaching. Arif could wear sunglasses in class during work time to reduce the glare from the overhead lighting and headphones to block ambient noise. The occupational therapist collaborated with the classroom teacher to develop an activity plan that incorporated regular opportunities for movement and physical activity for the whole class as well as individual activities to meet Arif's need for increased proprioceptive input. In addition, she conducted an in-service for the school staff instructing them on the relationship between poor sensory processing and ineffective behavioral regulation, the importance of addressing sensory needs as a first step in helping children more effectively regulate behavioral responses to others, and the need to intentionally teach performance skills the child is lacking to reduce anxiety.

In addition to addressing Arif's sensory needs, the occupational therapist recommended establishing a behavior contract outlining expectations for appropriate interactions with the teacher, school staff, and other children. The contract would allow Arif to be involved in identifying rewards and consequences for inappropriate behaviors. The behavior specialist agreed with the recommendation, and the team collaborated to develop a contract that was acceptable to all parties.

A primary feature of Arif's behavior contract was a token economy tied to the specific positive behaviors that Arif was expected to display. Arif earned a green token for each desired behavior and a red token for undesired behavior. The contract also specified graduated consequences for not abiding with the contract. Green tokens were earned for specific occurrences of appropriate interactions with others and for maintaining appropriate on-task classroom behavior for a specified duration of time. Red tokens were given to Arif for occurrences of inappropriate social interactions with peers or adults, off-task behavior, swearing, and noncompliance with the teacher's instructions. Tokens were counted and exchanged at the end of each school day for a choice from the school prize box, 5 min of free choice from a specified set of activities, and opportunities for special activities such as ice cream with the principal.

**BOX 25.2 Individual Strategies to Mitigate Effects of Setting Events**

| Teach New Skills/ Pivotal Behaviors | Individualize Expectations | Address Physical Needs |
|---|---|---|
| Build friendship skills | Tailor expectations to developmental level and capacity | Ensure consistent and sufficient sleep |
| Teach self-care and responsibility | Use clear, understandable directions | Provide good nutrition |
| Teach functional communication of wants, needs, dislikes | Specify what the child should do | Consider possibility of illness or pain |
| Scaffold problem-solving skills | Redirect child to desired behavior or task | Modify context or task to address sensory needs |
| Teach social skills: waiting, sharing, turn-taking, cooperation | Incorporate child's interests and strengths | Ensure adequate exercise |
| Teach emotional skills: emotional understanding and expression, empathy, self-calming, self-management, and problem-solving | Know and respond to child's emotional expressions | |
| Teach strategies for self-managing free time | Ensure child has access to and utilizes individualized visual supports | |

with flexible abilities that children can apply in multiple contexts (Box 25.2). Further, when children build new skills and encounter realistic performance expectations, they develop a sense of self-efficacy that supports positive behaviors.

Incorporation of the child's strengths and preferred interests into occupational therapy intervention activities is consistent with the profession's value on personal meaning. Inclusion of personally meaningful activities promotes desired behavior and helps prevent problem behavior because using activities consistent with strengths and preferences can increase the child's interest and motivation to engage in the activities. This in turn leads to greater efficiency in learning and using new behaviors, as well as reducing escape and noncompliance behaviors (Patten Koenig, 2019). Providing clients with access to preferred activities also enables the child to act as his own change agent and self-extinguish challenging behaviors such as aggression (Lory, Mason, et al., 2020; Piven & Derakhshanrad, 2017). Fig. 25.7 shows children engaged in a preferred activity with the teacher.

With their knowledge of human development and psychosocial functions, occupational therapy practitioners recognize that all children display a range of behaviors, including functional, socially appropriate behaviors and challenging behaviors that interfere with function. Thus, when practitioners intervene to address challenging behavior, the target outcome often is to reduce the behaviors to a manageable level, so the child is able to experience an improved quality of life and enjoy functional and productive occupational engagement, rather than to completely eliminate the behavior. However, if the behavior presents a threat to the safety of the child or others, intervention aims

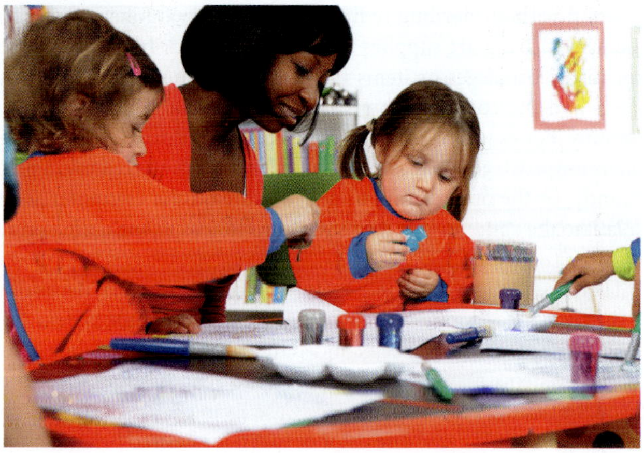

**Fig. 25.7** Incorporating a child's preferred interests into therapeutic activities increases motivation, reduces anxiety, and can minimize challenging behavior. (Copyright iStock Photo.)

to reduce the behavior to the lowest rate possible. Case Example 25.4 illustrates the use of behavioral approaches in occupational therapy.

Occupational therapy's emphasis on *therapeutic use of self* provides another tool that practitioners use when addressing challenging behaviors. See Chapter 3 regarding the intentional relationship. Through the therapeutic relationship, the practitioner can convey noncontingent validation of the child, indicating their acceptance and valuing of the child as a person regardless of behavioral profile. Communicating belief in the child's ability to succeed can improve self-esteem and a sense of self-worth (Patten Koenig, 2019). The occupational therapy practitioner conveys a respect for the child's choices throughout the course of intervention. The occupational therapy practitioner follows the child's lead while striving to challenge the child so that they reach their goals. This art of therapy requires occupational therapy practitioners to use clinical reasoning and therapeutic use of self. Creating flexible intervention plans to address the child's needs and tap into the child's interests and motivations allows practitioners to avoid power struggles and issues regarding compliance.

The practitioner uses the therapist-client interactions strategically to support the child in whatever challenge they are experiencing and to communicate belief in the child's ability to achieve their desires. Effective therapeutic use of self leads to a partnership between the practitioner and the client that is empowering and encouraging (Taylor, 2020). The power of these experiences can help prevent misbehaviors that are associated with feelings of despair and low self-esteem.

## Collaboration with Other Professionals to Manage Behavior

Due to the pervasive nature of behavior challenges, all professionals on a child's intervention team will encounter and need to address any challenging behaviors that are present. A cohesive and consistent approach to behavior intervention implemented by all team members offers the best support for the child. Intentional and proactive collaboration is the best strategy for achieving this aim (Watling & Jones, 2018).

*Collaboration* among team members, while recognized as crucial, requires effort. Knowledge about and preparation for collaboration can differ among professionals, as can the personal perspectives of the individual practitioners. A range of strategies have been identified to support effective collaboration among intervention team members. These include the following.

- Building rapport by respecting peer knowledge and contributions
- Demonstrating respect when disagreements occur

- Seeking common ground by learning about the other professional
- Educating others about your value by knowing and articulating your scope of practice
- Fostering unity by conducting services with fidelity and working to build trust with other professionals
- Gaining trust by understanding and articulating the evidence for your interventions
- Identifying roles of each professional in a manner that defines and values the contributions of each team member
- Taking a proactive approach to problem-solve any conflicts that occur (Watling & Jones, 2018)

Intentional pursuit of effective collaboration can be particularly important in cases where there is overlap in scope of practice. This is often the case between occupational therapy and applied behavior analysis in providing services for children with challenging behavior. Behavior analysts use behavior analytic approaches to improve behaviors that are socially significant (APBA, 2017; Watling & Jones, 2018) and addresses any behavior the person needs to perform, including those for adaptive behavior, self-care, work, social engagement, education participation, and overall well-being (APBA, 2017). These socially significant behaviors directly overlap with the domain of occupational therapy, which addresses person-, context-, and occupation-based factors to enhance or enable child participation in the broad range of environments, activities, and situations that the child encounters throughout the day (AOTA, 2020). Further, the techniques used by behavior analysts include both individual and system-wide interventions, which often contrast with the client-centered, occupation-based methods, frames of reference, therapeutic use of self, and clinical reasoning used by the occupational therapy practitioner to address the interconnected health, wellness, performance, participation, and quality of life of their clients (AOTA, 2020).

Without intention, this combination of overlap in practice domains and contrasting approaches to intervention can lead to dissension among team members in planning and delivering services. Thus, practitioners must work together to pursue and promote collaboration to ensure best practice and maximal benefit for the child. (Also see Table 25.1 for additional resources occupational therapy practitioners can use for understanding and implementing behavioral approaches.)

## SUMMARY

Contributions from behavior theory help identify and understand the factors that trigger and maintain a child's challenging behaviors. Occupational therapy practitioners should consider these concepts along with their professional knowledge and skills in task analysis, human behavior, and occupational engagement and participation to effectively analyze problem behavior, develop intervention plans, and implement therapeutic strategies to address challenging behaviors while maintaining a client-centered, occupationally based approach to services. Occupational therapy practitioners can adopt strategies to successfully collaborate with caregivers and other service providers to provide coordinated and comprehensive interventions. Occupational therapy practitioners bring a holistic occupational perspective to understanding a client's behaviors, making them key contributors to designing and implementing positive behavioral support programs in home, school, and community environments.

1. A behavior is often considered challenging when it does not conform to social norms or causes others in the vicinity to feel threatened or experience harm.
2. Occupational therapy practitioners may address behaviors such as noncompliance, withdrawal, avoidance, inattention, or lack of response, refusal to engage, opposition, aggression toward people or property, or self-injurious behavior. They use positive reinforcement when designing client-centered occupation-based intervention. They provide children with choices to promote self-determination. They may teach children new skills or pivotal behaviors, individualize expectations, address physical needs, and match activities with the child. Occupational therapy practitioners support children's strengths to promote choice, problem-solving, and engagement in meaningful activities. They use therapeutic use of self to identify behaviors and adapting or modifying the context to support the child's participation.
3. Occupational therapy practitioners use behavioral theory judiciously, in collaboration with the rest of the team, and in accordance with occupational therapy philosophy. They identify the child's strengths and challenges and work with team members to create achievable goals. They use positive reinforcements, motivating activities, and an awareness of the child's responses to create positive experiences and opportunities for the child to develop self-awareness and self-efficacy. Occupational therapy practitioners engage children in meaningful activities of which they are successful, which is reinforcing and helps children develop a sense of competency.

## REFERENCES


Ackerman, K. B., Samudre, M., & Allday, R. A. (2020). Practical components for getting the most from a token economy. *Teaching Exceptional Children, 52*(4), 242–249.

American Occupational Therapy Association. (2020). Occupational therapy practice framework: Domain and process. *American Journal of Occupational Therapy, 74*(Suppl. 2), 7412410010. https://doi.org/10.5014/ajot.2020.74S2001.

Association of Professional Behavior Analysts. (2017). *Identifying applied behavior analysis interventions.* https://www.APBAHome.net.

Campos, C., Bloom, S. E., Kollin, L., & Weyman, J. R. (2022). Comparing the effects of static and dynamic signals during multiple schedules. *Behavioral Interventions,* 1–15.

Carr, M. (2016). Self-management of challenging behaviours associated with autism spectrum disorder: A meta-analysis. *Australian Psychologist, 51,* 316–333. https://doi.org/10.1111/ap.12227.

Dawson, G., Franz, L., & Brandsen, S. (2022). At a Crossroads—reconsidering the goals of autism early behavioral intervention from a neurodiversity perspective. *Journal of the American Medical Association Pediatrics, 176*(9), 839–840.

Erturk, B., Machalieck, W., & Drew, C. (2018). Self-injurious behavior in children with developmental disabilities: A systematic review of behavioral intervention literature. *Behavior Modification, 42*(4), 498–542. https://doi.org/10.1177/0145445517741474.

Friedman, Z. L., Akselrud, R., Goldman, M., Horowitz, R., Moradi, S., & Seror, E. (2022). Charting a path to collaboration: Experiences of occupational therapy and applied behavior analysis professionals. In *Journal of Occupational Therapy, Schools, & Early Intervention.*

Gerow, S., Davis, T., Radhakrishnan, S., Gregori, E., & Rivera, G. (2018). Functional communication training: The strength of evidence across disabilities. *Exceptional Children, 85*(1), 86–103.

Ghaemmaghami, M., & Hanley, G. P. (2020). Functional communication training: From efficacy to effectiveness. *Journal of Applied Behavioral Analysis, 54*(1), 122–143.

Granja, M. R., Smith, S., Nguyen, U., & Grifa, B. (2018). *Learning about young children's challenging behavior and impacts on programs and families: A state-wide survey of Virginia's early care and education teachers.* In National Center for Children in Poverty, Mailman School of Public Health, Columbia University.

Hong, E., & Matson, J. L. (2020). An evaluation of the functions of challenging behavior in toddlers with and without Autism Spectrum Disorder. *Journal of Developmental and Physical Disabilities, 33*, 85–97.

Iovannone, R., Anderson, C., & Scott, T. (2017). Understanding setting events: What they are and how to identify them. *Beyond Behavior, 26*(3), 105–112.

Kapp, S. K., Steward, R., Crane, L., Elliott, D., Elphick, C., Pellicano, E., & Russell, G. (2019). People should be allowed to do what they like': Autistic adults' views and experiences of stimming. *Autism, 23*(7), 1782–1792.

Kincaid, D., Dunlap, G., Kern, L., Lane, K. L., Bambara, L. M., Brown, F., Fox, L., & Knoster, T. P. (2016). Positive behavior support: A proposal for updating and refining the definition. *Journal of Positive Behavior Interventions, 18*, 69–73. https://doi.org/10.1177/1098300715604826.

Koegel, R. L., Koegel, L. K., Frea, W. D., & Smith, A. E. (1995). Emerging interventions of children with autism: Longitudinal and lifestyle implications. In R. L. Koegel, & L. K. Koegel (Eds.), *Teaching children with autism: Strategies for initiating positive interactions and improving learning opportunities* (pp. 1–16). Brookes.

Lipschultz, J. L., & Wilder, D. A. (2017). Behavioral assessment and treatment of noncompliance: A review of the literature. *Education & Treatment of Children, 40*, 263–298.

Lory, C., Mason, R. A., Davis, J. L., Wang, D., Kim, S. Y., Gregori, E., & David, M. (2020). A meta-analysis of challenging behavior Interventions for students with developmental disabilities in inclusive school settings. *Journal of Autism and Developmental Disorders, 50*(4), 1221–1237.

Lory, C., Rispoli, M., Gregori, E., Kim, S. Y., & David, M. (2020). Reducing escape-maintained challenging behavior in children with autism spectrum disorder through visual activity schedule and instructional choice. *Education & Treatment of Children, 43*(2), 201–217.

Lovaas, O. I. (1987). Behavioral treatment and normal educational and intellectual functioning in young autistic children. *Journal of Consulting and Clinical Psychology, 55*(1), 3–9.

Martinez, J. R., Werch, B. L., & Conroy, M. A. (2016). School-based interventions targeting challenging behaviors exhibited by young children with autism spectrum disorder: A systematic literature review. *Education and Training in Autism and Developmental Disabilities, 51*, 265–280.

McGill, O., & Robinson, A. (2021). "Recalling hidden harms": Autistic experiences of childhood applied behavioural analysis (ABA). *Advances in Autism, 7*(4), 269–282.

McLeod, S. A. (2017). *Behaviorist approach.* https://www.simplypsychology.org/behaviorism.htm.

Milton, D. (2018). *A critique of the use of applied behavioural analysis (ABA): On behalf of the neurodiversity manifesto steering group.* https://kar.kent.ac.uk/id/eprint/69268.

Newcomb, E. T., & Hagopian, L. P. (2018). Treatment of severe problem behaviour in children with autism spectrum disorder and intellectual disabilities. *International Review of Psychiatry, 30*(1), 96–109.

Nicholls, G., Bailey, T., Grindle, C. F., & Hastings, R. (2023). Challenging behaviour and its risk factors in children and young people in a special school setting: A four wave longitudinal study. *Journal of Applied Research in Intellectual Disabilities*, 366–373. https://doi.org/10.1111/jar.13066.

O'Regan, O., Doyle, Y., Murray, M., McCarthy, V. J., & Saab, M. M. (2022). Reducing challenging behaviours among children and adolescents with intellectual disabilities in community settings: A systematic review of interventions. *International Journal of Developmental Disabilities.*

Patten Koenig, K. (2019). A strength-based frame of reference for autistic individuals. In P. Kramer, J. Hinojosa, & T. Howe (Eds.), *Frames of reference for pediatric occupational therapy* (4th ed.) (pp. 496–523). Wolters Kluwer.

Pavlov, I. P. (1927). *Conditioned reflexes.* Oxford University Press.

Piven, E. F., & Derakhshanrad, S. A. (2017). A case study demonstrating reduction of aggressive client behaviors using the neuro-occupation model: Addressing professional burnout through nonlinear thinking. *Occupational Therapy in Mental Health, 33*, 179–194. https://doi.org/10.1080/0164212X.2017.1278734.

Poling, A., & Li, A. (2019). Commit heresy: Stop using "contingency. *Behavior Analysis in Practice, 13*(1), 226–231.

Rahn, N. L., Grygas Coogle, C., Hanna, A., & Lewellen, T. (2017). Evidence-based practices to reduce challenging behaviors of young children with autism. *Young Exceptional Children, 20*(4), 166–178.

Reeves, L. M., Umbreit, J., Ferro, J. B., & Liaupsin, C. J. (2017). The role of the replacement behavior in function-based intervention. *Education and Training in Autism and Developmental Disabilities, 52*(3), 305–316.

Robertson, R. E., & Coy, J. N. (2019). Your student is hungry, tired, angry-now what? Addressing distal setting events in the classroom. *Teaching Exceptional Children, 51*(5), 361–371.

Sandoval-Norton, A. H., & Shkedy, G. (2019). How much compliance is too much compliance: Is long-term ABA therapy abuse? *Cogent Psychology, 6*(1),1641258.

Scheibel, G., & Watling, R. (2016). Collaborating with behavior analysts on the autism service delivery team. *OT Practice, 21*(7), 15–19.

Simo-Pinatella, D., Mumbardo-Adam, C., Lowe, K., Jones, E., Cortina, A., Alomar-Kurz, E., & Rodriguez, C. O. (2018). Exploring youth's problem behavior prevalence in educational settings: Piloting the process. *Advances in Neurodevelopmental Disorders, 2*, 142–150. https://doi.org/10.1007/s41252-017-0042-4.

Skinner, B. F. (1953). *Science and human behavior.* MacMillan.

Smith, B., & Fox, L. (2003). *Systems of service delivery: Synthesis of evidence relevant to young children at risk of or who have challenging behavior.* Center for Evidence-Based Practice: Young Children with Challenging Behavior, University of South Florida.

Steinbrenner, J. R., Hume, K., Odom, S. L., Morin, K. L., Nowell, S. W., Tomaszewski, B., Szendrey, S., McIntyre, N. S., Yücesoy-Özkan, S., & Savage, M. N. (2020). *Evidence-based practices for children, youth, and young adults with autism.* The University of North Carolina at Chapel Hill, Frank Porter Graham Child Development Institute, National Clearinghouse on Autism Evidence and Practice Review Team.

Taylor, R. R. (2020). *The intentional relationship: Occupational therapy and use of self* (2nd ed.). F.A. Davis.

Thelen, P., & Klifman, T. (2011). Using daily transition strategies to support all children. *Young Children, 66*, 92–98.

Watling, R. (2017). Combining occupational therapy and behavioral approaches to intervention for challenging behaviors in pediatric therapy. In *Medbridge: Web-based continuing education.*

Watling, R. (August 22, 2005). Interventions for common behavior problems in children with disabilities. *OT Practice, 10*, 12–15.

Watling, R., & Jones, C. (2018). Managing challenging behaviors in pediatric clients: Occupational therapy – behavior analyst collaboration. *Medbridge: Web-based continuing education.*

Watling, R., Kuhaneck, H., Parham, L. D., & Schaaf, R. C. (2018). *Occupational therapy practice guidelines for children and youth with challenges in sensory integration and sensory processing.* AOTA Press. https://doi.org/10.7139/2017.978-1-56900-483-8..

Watling, R., & Schwartz, I. S. (2004). The issue is: Understanding and implementing positive reinforcement as an intervention strategy for children with disabilities. *American Journal of Occupational Therapy, 58*, 113–116.

Watson, J. B. (1913). Psychology as the behaviorist views it. *Psychological Review, 20*, 158–177. https://doi.org/10.1037/h0074428.

Welch, C. D., & Polatajko, H. J. (2016). The issue is—applied behavior analysis, autism, and occupational therapy: A search for understanding. *American Journal of Occupational Therapy, 70*,7004360020.

Wolf, M. M., Risley, T. R., & Mees, H. (1964). Application of operant conditioning procedures to the behavior problems of an autistic child. *Behavior Research and Therapy, 1*, 305–312.

Wood, C. L., Kisinger, K. W., Brosh, C. R., Fisher, L. B., & Muharib, R. (2018). Stopping behavior before it starts: Antecedent interventions for challenging behavior. *Teaching Exceptional Children, 50*(6), 356–363.

Zannolli, K., & Daggett. (1998). The effects of reinforcement rate on the spontaneous social initiations of socially withdrawn preschoolers. *Journal of Applied Behavior Analysis, 31*, 117–125.

Zimmerman, K. N., Ledford, J. R., & Barton, E. E. (2017). Using visual activity schedules for young children with challenging behavior. *Journal of Early Intervention, 39*(4), 339–358.

# 26

# Cognitive-Based Interventions

*Jolien van den Houten, Angela Mandich, Jessie Wilson, and Kaitlyn Carmichael*

## GUIDING QUESTIONS

1. What concepts, principles, and key features define a cognitive-based intervention?
2. What do the terms cognition and metacognition mean?
3. What are the seven key features of the Cognitive Orientation to daily Occupational Performance (CO-OP) approach?
4. How are cognitive strategies applied in occupational therapy practice?
5. Why use cognitive-based approaches?

## KEY TERMS

**Cognitive Orientation to daily Occupational Performance (CO-OP)**
**Cognitive strategies**
**Concept mapping**
**Discovery learning**
**Dynamic performance analysis (DPA)**
**Global strategies**
**Guided discovery learning**
**Instrumental Enrichment program**
**Metacognition**
**Neuroplasticity**
**Performance-based approaches**
**Personalized strategies**
**Scaffolding**
**Self-coaching**
**Self-determination**

## COGNITIVE-BASED INTERVENTIONS

Cognitive-based interventions have their historical beginnings in disciplines of education and psychology and have been used with pediatric populations for several decades. Pediatric occupational therapy practitioners recognize the effectiveness of cognitive-based approaches in supporting children in meeting a variety of occupational performance goals. In pediatric occupational therapy, cognitive-based interventions focus on the development of strategies to support children in engaging in their desired occupations, such as activities of daily living, instrumental activities of daily living, play, academics, work, leisure, and social participation.

Two main cognitive-based approaches are used: cognitive-based approaches that attempt to change faulty or delayed cognitive processes, such as cognitive behavior therapy, and cognitive-based approaches that focus on enabling occupational performance, such as the Cognitive Orientation to daily Occupational Performance (CO-OP) approach. These **performance-based approaches** have also been called "top-down" approaches in the occupational therapy literature. Their focus is to assist the child in identifying, developing, and utilizing cognitive strategies to perform activities of daily living (Dawson et al., 2017; Missiuna et al., 1997; Polatajko & Mandich, 2004). Performance-based approaches are seen as complex interventions, meaning that they consist of several interacting key features supporting mechanisms of change in performing (Skidmore et al., 2017). Table 26.1 defines general terminology that is used in cognitive and related literature and provides an overview of key concepts (Missiuna et al., 1997). Table 26.2 provides an overview of the theories underpinning cognitive interventions.

A number of different cognitive-based interventions have been described in the broader literature; however, they all share similar tenants (Bouffard & Wall, 1990). Bouffard and Wall (1990) proposed a five-step problem-solving framework to guide motor skill acquisition that includes the following:

- problem identification'
- problem representation
- plan construction
- plan execution
- evaluation of progress

Henderson and Sugden (1992) also proposed an approach to motor skill acquisition, called the cognitive motor approach. This approach centered on a three-step information-processing framework. The first step is *movement planning* and requires the child to understand the task and its demands and to decide if the task is achievable. This requires the child to gain information through sensory and perceptual processes, including vision and kinesthesia, and then to translate this information into a plan. The next step is *movement execution*, which involves the child enacting their motor plan and is dependent on the interaction of the person, task, and environment (O'Brien, 2015). During the final step, *movement evaluation*, the child monitors their progress in achieving their desired motor performance. The cognitive motor approach is effective in improving the functional skills of children with developmental coordination disorder (DCD; Wright & Sugden, 1998).

Expanding on the principles highlighted in the cognitive-based approaches listed above, the CO-OP was developed (Dawson et al., 2017; Polatajko & Mandich, 2004). This approach uses a learning-based perspective on skill acquisition and occupational performance and is the focus of this chapter.

**TABLE 26.1 Definitions for Terminology Used in Cognitive-Based Interventions**

| Term | Definition | Application to Occupational Therapy |
|---|---|---|
| Cognitive-based approaches | Cognition is a person's ability to acquire and use information to adapt to environmental demands (Lidz, 1987). | Cognitive-based approaches address performance challenges by working collaboratively with children to enable them to identify and recognize cognitive processes and use strategies when completing meaningful daily activities (Mandich et al., 2004). |
| Declarative Knowledge | Declarative knowledge is knowledge about things; it is the knowledge that is often explicitly known and can be consciously brought to the attention of the learner (Bloom et al., 1956; Seger, 1994). | Declarative knowledge includes rules and facts about a skill and is often used during the initial stages of learning (Seger, 1994). Children begin by identifying the steps of a task or rules of social engagement. With practice (rehearsal and verbalization), declarative knowledge converts to procedural. |
| Procedural Knowledge | Procedural knowledge is the implicit knowledge about how to complete a task (Seger, 1994). | Procedural knowledge is acquired through the repetition of an activity and observed through enhanced task performance (Seger, 1994). Children complete the steps or sequence of an activity fluidly as they understand "how" the activity is performed through practice. |
| Metacognition | Metacognition refers to knowledge concerning one's own cognitive processes, performance, and outcomes (Flavell, 1979). Metacognition is made up of metacognitive knowledge and self-regulation (Flavell, 1979). | Through metacognition, children generalize and transfer cognitive skills to meet changing contextual demands. (Missiuna et al., 1997). Metacognitive strategies are employed when a task becomes too difficult relative to the child's skill level, and they have to select appropriate cognitive strategies, monitor, and evaluate their performance (Missiuna et al., 1997). Cognitive-based occupational therapy intervention directly addresses and enhances the child's metacognition skills. |
| Metacognitive Knowledge | Metacognitive knowledge consists of one's awareness of the cognitive processes that are employed to learn and perform a new task (Flavell, 1979; Missiuna et al., 1997). | This is the individual's ability to reflect on how they are learning (e.g., mnemonics, rehearsal, imagery, practice) to retain new information (Toglia et al., 2012). |
| Self-Regulation | Self-regulation is the individual's influence over their own thought processes and affective constructs like emotional states, motivation, and patterns of behavior (Bandura, 1982; Hunt & Reed, 2017). It is the process of selecting, monitoring, and evaluating the effectiveness of cognitive strategies (Polatajko & Mandich, 2004). | To demonstrate self-regulation, an individual who encounters a challenge pauses, selects a different strategy, applies it, and evaluates the performance outcome (Missiuna et al., 1997). The ability to self-regulate allows for skill transfer and generalization to occur. |
| Cognitive strategies | Strategies are cognitive processes (consciously employed and controllable by the learner; Pressley & Harris, 2006) that allow the person to achieve a task. Cognitive strategies are a "mental plan of action that helps a person to learn, problem solve, and perform" (Toglia et al., 2012). | Cognitive strategies support skill acquisition or reacquisition. They help individuals regulate and manage challenges in learning and performance, playing a key role in achieving a higher level of task performance (Toglia et al., 2012). Occupational therapy practitioners engage children in a variety of cognitive strategies to support their daily activities. |
| Neuroplasticity | Neuroplasticity refers to the "ability of the nervous system to respond to intrinsic or extrinsic stimuli by reorganizing its structure, function, and connections." (Cramer et al., 2011, p. 1592). | Occupational therapy interventions that are meaningful, occupation based, and repeated often in the natural context promote neuroplasticity. By guiding the child to identify the performance issue, set a feasible goal, and plan for reaching that goal, the occupational therapy practitioner encourages the child's own problem-solving and investment in achieving that goal. In (re-)learning activities, children are challenged to use their cognitive abilities in a variety of challenging practices. This process stimulates active learning, resulting in reorganization of the brain (i.e., neuroplasticity), resulting in generalization and transfer (Dawson, 2017). |

## COGNITIVE ORIENTATION TO DAILY OCCUPATIONAL PERFORMANCE

The CO-OP is described as "a client-centered, performance-based, problem-solving approach that enables skill acquisition through a process of strategy use and guided discovery" (Polatajko & Mandich, 2004). Research (see Table 26.3 for a review of evidence) suggests that the CO-OP approach is effective for improving occupational performance in children.

CO-OP places emphasis on the interaction between individual and environmental factors to promote children's successful participation in daily activities. Developed within an evidence-based framework, CO-OP draws on behavioral and cognitive psychology, health, human movement science, and occupational therapy to achieve its objectives (Dawson et al., 2017; Polatajko & Mandich, 2004). Case Example 26.1 provides an overview of the use of the CO-OP approach to support a child's handwriting performance in school.

### Primary Objectives of CO-OP

The overall goal of the CO-OP approach is to enable children to engage in occupational performance for optimal participation in all required day-to-day situations (Dawson et al., 2017). To that end, CO-OP focuses on cognition as a performance support (Polatajko & Mandich, 2004). Evidence suggests that the CO-OP approach is effective in meeting its four objectives: (1) skill acquisition; (2) cognitive strategy use; (3) generalization; and (4) transfer of learning (Houldin et al., 2017; Novak & Honan, 2019).

**TABLE 26.2 Theoretical Foundations of Cognitive-Based Approaches**

| Theorist and Key Contributions | Description of Concepts |
|---|---|
| L.S. Vygotsky (1896–1932)<br>• Development of problem-solving (talking out loud to thinking internally before acting)<br>• Learning as part of social interaction<br>• Active participation of the child<br>• Zone of proximal development<br>• Scaffolding | Vygotsky, a Russian psychologist, believed that cognitive development occurred through the gradual internalization of concepts and relationships. He noted that younger children used overt speech (talking out loud) when they were problem-solving through a difficult task. In contrast, older children seemed to think about a solution internally before acting (Missiuna et al., 2001). When comparing the problem-solving dialogs (internal and overt) of the older and younger children, he concluded they were similar and deduced that, as development occurs, children gradually internalize their thought processes (Vygotsky, 1987).<br>Vygotsky also viewed learning as being embedded in social and cultural contexts. He underscored the necessity of cooperative dialogs between adults and children in the learning process and saw these communicative opportunities as a way of developing children's internal dialogs (Bouffard & Wall, 1990). According to Vygotsky, an important component of the learning process involves the participation of the child, and the child's active engagement in the learning and developmental process enables success. Vygotsky viewed the learning process as a "circular reaction" where action and motivation influence one another and contribute to the child's learning and development (Vygotsky, 1987).<br>The **zone of proximal development** is the range of skills that the child can achieve through social interaction with a more competent individual. A child's developmental skills fall into a "zone, or range, of skills which differ contingent upon the social interactions accompanying the activity, rather than a specific skill level" (Humphry & Womack, 2013). Therefore, each stage of a child's development is characterized by different modes of social interaction. In therapeutic practice, this concept of intentional and graded adult feedback to promote a child's skill is referred to as **scaffolding**. |
| Alexander Luria (1902–1977)<br>• Problem-solving process<br>• Development is complex and dynamic<br>• Many factors (e.g., environmental, social, and culture) influence child development<br>• Social interactions are important for development | Luria believed that a child's development could not be simply explained through a natural inborn process, but that development is a complex and dynamic relationship between many factors, including the child's social and cultural environment(s) as also referred to as "nurture." Luria delineated how individuals explore problems and learn new concepts, identifying five stages in an individual's problem-solving process:<br>1. discovery of the problem<br>2. investigation of the problem<br>3. selection of an alternative strategy<br>4. attempt to solve the problem<br>5. comparison of results of the solution (Luria, 1959, 1961)<br>According to Luria, children use overt verbalization of process steps when learning a new skill, which eventually fades into covert speech as the child rehearses the process steps of the new activity. Luria hypothesized that the speech system is formed in the process of the child's social interactions with an adult and is a powerful means of change and systemic organization of human mental processes (Luria, 1959, 1961). |
| Meichenbaum<br>• Self-instructional strategies as problem-solving<br>• GOAL-PLAN-DO-CHECK process as a problem-solving pathway<br>• Scaffolding to promote generalization of cognitive strategies | Meichenbaum further emphasized the importance of speech and adult guidance in driving the development of cognitive strategies (Meichenbaum, 1977; Meichenbaum & Goodman, 1971). Hypothesizing that internal speech can regulate one's behavior, he proposed that a child could follow self-instructional steps to assist in behavior regulation (Meichenbaum & Goodman, 1971). This problem-solving pathway included the child identifying a goal, developing a plan, enacting the plan, and then evaluating its success (Meichenbaum & Goodman, 1971). These steps are modeled by a more competent adult and then verbalized out loud by the child. Through adult guidance and functional practice and rehearsal, the steps of GOAL-PLAN-DO-CHECK are internalized and recalled covertly by the child when performing a task (Meichenbaum & Goodman, 1971). Meichenbaum also utilized scaffolding to help with the generalization of the newly formed cognitive strategies. |
| Bandura<br>• Metacognition<br>• Empowerment fosters goal commitment and intrinsic motivation<br>• Engagement of child in learning process<br>• Social interactions promote learning<br>• Discovery learning | Bandura (1982) believed that a child's experiences performing an activity contribute extensively to their self-perceptions. Through the development of **metacognitive** abilities, the thinking about one's own thinking, children learn to evaluate their performance of an activity and reflect on their areas of strength and weakness. When setting new goals based on their identified areas of difficulty, children begin to feel empowered. Empowerment fosters increased goal commitment, enhanced performance, and the intrinsic motivation to set new meaningful goals (Bandura, 1982).<br>Like Vygotsky and Bruner, Bandura believed that the individual child was the main motivator for cognitive development, that children were hard-wired to learn, and that these intrinsic capabilities emerged through interactions with others (Goodley & Runswick-Cole, 2010). Therefore, engagement of the child in the learning process and interaction with social partners are key to a child's successful learning (Goodley & Runswick-Cole, 2010). Learning occurs through the result of experience, and information is interpreted through the lens of the individual's values and beliefs.<br>Contributions from the fields of cognitive, educational, psychology, and neuroscience have brought to light the foundational elements of discovery learning and the understanding that children display optimal learning when they are allowed to reflect on their participation in their chosen occupations (Tudge & Winterhoff, 1993). |

**TABLE 26.3 Examining Selected Evidence of the CO-OP Model**

| Authors/Date | Study Purpose | Sample | Interventions/Measures | Findings |
|---|---|---|---|---|
| Butchereit et al. (2022) | 1. To identify and categorize strategies used by children with HMD to support skill acquisition during CO-OP<br>2. To review the possible underlying mechanisms that might contribute to the cognitive strategies, to facilitate further studies for developing focused rehabilitation approaches | Review total of 40 randomly selected hours of video footage of CO-OP sessions delivered to six participants (age 6–19 years) over 10 intervention sessions | An observational recording sheet was applied to identify systematically the participants' or therapist's verbalizations of cognitive strategies during the therapy | Strategies used by HMD participants included distraction, externally focused attention, internally focused attention, emotion self-regulation, motor imagery, and mental self-guidance; we postulate different underlying working mechanisms for these strategies, which have implications for the therapeutic management of children and young people with HMD including dystonia |
| Cameron et al. (2017) | To determine if CO-OP is a feasible approach to be used with children with cerebral palsy (CP) and to determine the effects of CO-OP when compared to usual occupational therapy practice with this population | 18 children, ages 7–12 with CP (9 in each treatment group); pilot randomized control study | 10 weekly intervention sessions in their home; COPM, PQRS | All children in the CO-OP group were able to learn the strategies and achieve their goals, demonstrating the feasibility of the approach with this population<br>Both approaches equally promoted skill acquisition and maintenance at follow-up (effect size suggests that CO-OP may show some advantage for skill transfer and maintenance) |
| Gharebaghy et al. (2015) | To examine the influence of a 12-week intervention using CO-OP with six children with ADHD | Six children, ages 7–12 years with ADHD; single case experimental design | 12-week intervention using CO-OP, COPM, Goal Attainment Scale, and BOTMP | Improvements in both goals and motor performance following intervention, providing support for the use of CO-OP with this population |
| Izadi-Najafabadi et al (2022) | To determine if CO-OP is effective in improving performance and transfer of motor learning in children with DCD (with/without ADHD) and whether outcomes were maintained post intervention | 37 children with DCD and 41 children with co-occurring ADHD<br>Ages: 8–12 years | Randomized treatment or waitlist<br>Treatment: 1 h of intervention once weekly for 10 weeks<br>COPM, PQRS, and BOTMP | Significant improvement in motor performance and movement quality; 3 months after treatment, children maintained their gains, but only children with developmental coordination disorder showed transfer of learning to overall motor skills |
| Peny-Dahlstrand et al. (2023) | To investigate effectiveness of CO-OP in children with CP and SB with executive dysfunctions and explore generalization and transfer | 38 children, ages 7–16 | 10 sessions with CO-OP or treatment as usual.<br>COPM- COSA interviews, PQRS, BRIEF, and D-KEFS | Significantly higher outcomes for trained and untrained goals with the CO-OP approach; CO-OP shows transfer to new activities and situations<br>Sessions by video link can be added to the intervention |
| Thornton et al. (2016) | To determine of a 10-week, group-based, CO-OP intervention improved outcome measures across the impairment, activity and participation levels across the International Classification of Functioning, Disability and Health (ICF) framework | 20 male children, ages 8–10 years | 10 weekly CO-OP sessions (10 participants); control group of 10 regular activity sessions; quasi-experimental, pre-/posttest measure related to impairments (MABC-2 motor overflow assessment), activity (handwriting speed test), and participation (COPM and Goal Attainment Scale) | The strategies implemented in the CO-OP treatment group, targeted toward individualized goal attainment, show that CO-OP, when run in a group environment, can lead to improvements across all areas of the ICF |

***Summary:*** Overall, the findings from these studies provide evidence for the use of the CO-OP approach in improving the performance of children ages 5–15 with *ADHD*, Attention-deficit hyperactivity disorder; *ASD*, autism spectrum disorder; *CP*, cerebral palsy; *DCD*, developmental coordination disorderl; *HMD*, hyperkinetic movement disorders; *SB*, spina bifida, and other fine and gross motor delays, in both individual and group settings. Studies are ongoing to examine the use of CO-OP with other pediatric populations and various age ranges. The evidence to date suggests that CO-OP is effective in helping children with a variety of performance problems learn to use cognitive strategies to learn to perform the skills they choose and to generalize and transfer these skills to other performance areas.

*ABI*, Acquired brain injury; *ADHD*, attention-deficit hyperactivity disorder; *AMPS*, assessment of motor processing skills; *AS*, Asperger syndrome; *BOTMP*, Bruininks-Oseretsky test of motor proficiency; *CO-OP*, cognitive orientation to daily occupational performance; *COPM*, Canadian occupational performance measure; *CP*, cerebral palsy; *DCD*, developmental coordination disorder; *HMD*, hyperkinetic movement disorders; *ICF*, international classification of functioning, disability and health (ICF) framework; *MABC*, movement assessment battery for children; *PDD*, pervasive developmental disorder; *PQRS*, performance quality rating scale; *SB*, spina bifida; *VABS*, Vineland adaptive behavior scales; *VMI*, visual motor integration.

### CASE EXAMPLE 26.1 HANDWRITING PERFORMANCE

Matty is a 9-year-old boy who was referred for an occupational therapy assessment within the school setting to address difficulties with his printing skills. Matty displays challenges with placement and spacing between words, which significantly affects the overall legibility of his written work and his overall academic performance. He received 10 occupational therapy sessions by his school-based occupational therapist. During this time, the practitioner worked with him on his printing skills, using the CO-OP approach and the "GOAL-PLAN-DO-CHECK" framework. Within this framework, Matty identified his own concerns with his printing skills and generated his own solutions to resolve the problematic aspects of his handwriting. With verbal guidance from the practitioner, he identified that sometimes all his letters do not sit on the line and at other times all his words run together.

To work on Matty's goal to improve his handwriting, the practitioner analyzed his performance (see Goal and Breakdown Points). Then the practitioner guided Matty in identifying personalized strategies tailored for him along with a plan for how to implement the strategies (see Strategy Use). They created activities, including teaching his sisters how to print, making a scrapbook, using paper with a highlighted baseline to act as a visual cue for letter placement, using a finger space between words, and securing a "printing checklist" onto his desk to remind him of letter placement and spacing. Using these activities and strategies, Matty improved these specific areas of his printing within the classroom environment.

**GOAL AND BREAKDOWN POINTS**

| GOAL | Breakdown Points |
|---|---|
| Improve the quality of his handwriting | • Poor letter formation<br>• Words are too close together<br>• Difficulty making sure his letters sit on the line correctly (baseline orientation) |

**STRATEGY USE**

| Personalized Strategy | Plan | Activities to Reinforce the Strategy |
|---|---|---|
| Task specification/ modification | • Finish the letter<br>• Make the letter larger | • Having a writing checklist secured to his desk to prompt him of the important strategies that he had developed |
| Supplementing task knowledge | • "There should always be a finger space between your words" | • Teach younger sister how to print by role-playing that he's the teacher<br>• Making scrapbook of summer vacation |
| Attention to doing | • "Where do you need your letters to sit" | • Teaching student, teacher, and parent to highlight baseline of paper to help with attention to doing |

In a typical CO-OP program, the child selects three occupations or activities to learn over 10 intervention sessions. The occupations are chosen by the child, in collaboration with their care givers, and may include activities such as handwriting, cycling, tying shoelaces, or cutting. Through customized intervention, cognitive strategies are used to solve performance issues and enable skill development within the occupations. The second objective of CO-OP is to coach the child how to use these strategies to achieve their goals. Over the course of the intervention, children learn a problem-solving strategy that enables them to discover and identify strategies that will support their performance. The third objective of CO-OP is to facilitate generalization of the occupation to other settings, including home and school. Once the child has obtained the skills required to perform the identified occupation, the focus of therapy shifts to facilitating generalization of the learning beyond the therapy situation. The final objective of CO-OP is the transfer of the learning to other occupations. Since only three occupations are addressed during a CO-OP intervention, it is important that children learn to adapt their skills and strategies to other new occupations that they confront in contexts of daily life (Houldin et al., 2017; Polatajko & Mandich, 2004).

## Who Benefits From CO-OP?

The CO-OP approach was initially developed for use with children with Developmental Coordination Disorder (DCD; Miller et al., 2001) and has been shown to be an effective intervention for use with this population (Bernie & Rodger, 2004; Gill et al., 2022; Izadi-Najafabadi et al., 2022; Ward & Rodger, 2004). More recently, CO-OP has been used with children with spina bifida (SB), high-functioning autism spectrum disorder (ASD), traumatic brain injuries, attention deficit hyperactivity disorder (ADHD), cerebral palsy (CP), hyperkinetic movement disorder (HMD), and fine and gross motor skill delays (Cameron et al., 2017; Cameron, Schwellnus, & Polatajko, 2017; Gharebaghy et al., 2015; Hahn-Markowitz et al., 2011; Missiuna et al., 2010; Novak et al., 2020; Peny-Dahlstrand et al., 2020, 2023; Rodger, 2017; Rodger et al., 2007; Ziviani et al., 2015). Research supports the use of CO-OP for these populations and demonstrates positive occupational performance outcomes when used with a pediatric population. Recent literature also highlights the effectiveness of implementing the CO-OP approach in a group format with children and adolescents with DCD and ASD (Krajenbrink et al., 2022; Martini et al., 2014; Thornton et al., 2016).

For the CO-OP approach to be successful, the child must be able to understand the cognitive framework and be able to apply cognitive strategies (Polatajko et al., 2001). Although a certain level of cognitive functioning is required for the CO-OP approach to be successful, cognitive interventions can often be modified based on the client and the specific population. For example, although CO-OP is a verbally mediated metacognitive framework; for children who may experience challenges with articulating their problem-solving process (language impairments), or for those who approach problems in a different way (visual learners), the CO-OP can be utilized effectively to enable them to overtly demonstrate the selection, application, and evaluation of their cognitive strategies. However, CO-OP must include parent support and inclusion within the therapeutic process.

Evidence is emerging exploring the use of concept mapping as a way to visually represent the problem-solving processes undertaken throughout the implementation of the CO-OP approach. Concept maps are graphic tools that act as a visual tool to organize and represent knowledge (Ricon, 2010; Wilson et al., 2014). Using concept maps as a way for individuals to communicate their problem-solving without relying heavily on their expressive language skills allows more opportunities for children/adolescents of various abilities to successfully engage in the CO-OP intervention (Wilson et al., 2014). Fig. 26.1 illustrates how concept mapping may be used with the CO-OP model in practice. See Case Example 26.2 of using concept mapping in occupational therapy practice.

## Goals for CO-OP Intervention

CO-OP has been used to address a variety of child-chosen occupations across self-care, productivity, and leisure domains. A key feature of the CO-OP approach is its focus on client-chosen goals determined through administration of the Canadian Occupational Performance

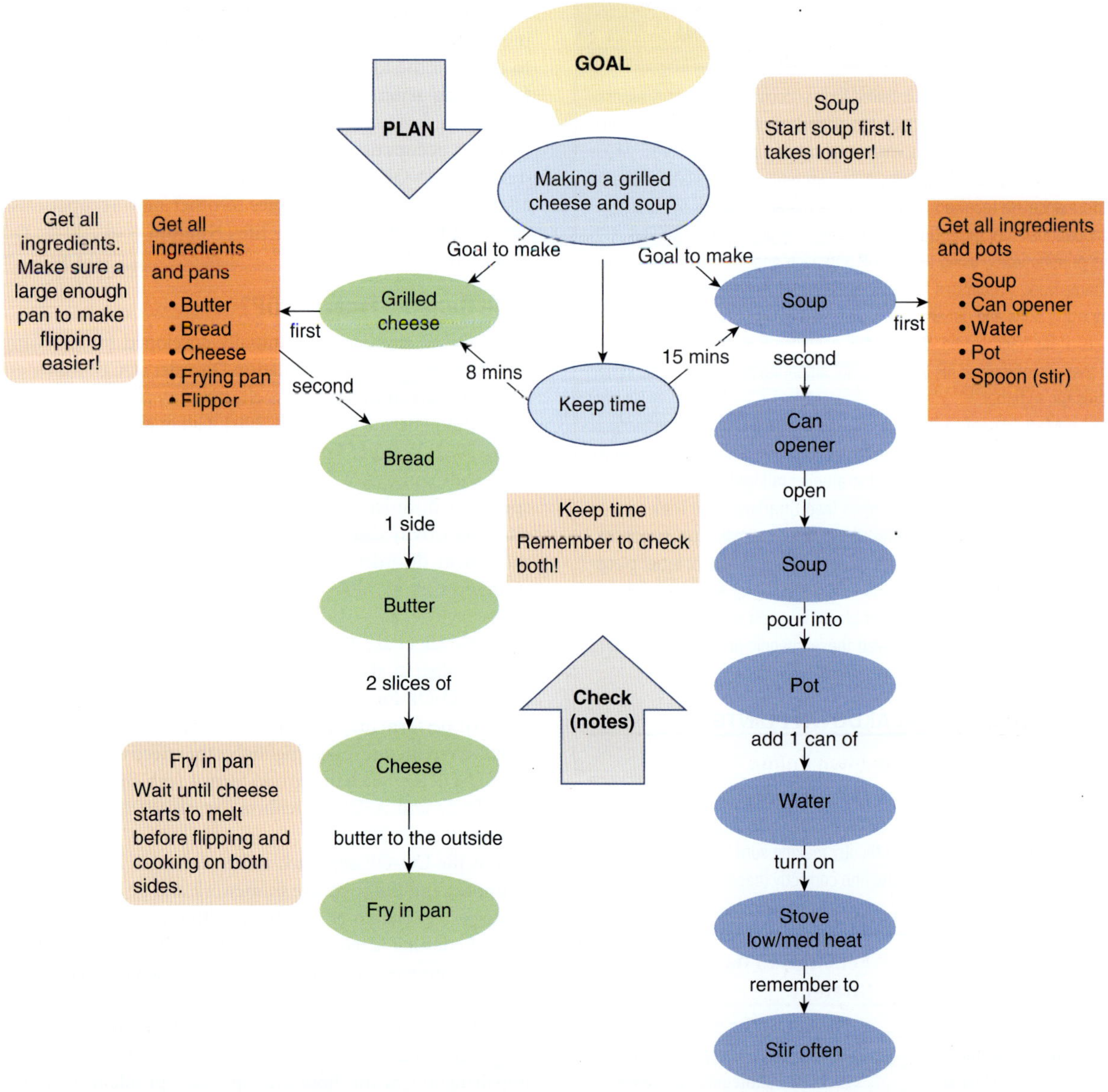


**Fig. 26.1** The occupational therapist begins by creating a concept map with Peter of meal preparation.

> ### CASE EXAMPLE 26.2 CONCEPT MAPPING AS A METHOD TO ENGAGE IN PROBLEM-SOLVING
>
> Peter is a 16-year-old who has ASD and attends mainstream schooling. Peter experiences difficulties with planning and preparing dinner on the days his father works late, which Peter reports to be frustrating. He told the occupational therapy practitioner that he would like to be able to plan and prepare meals so that he does not always have to eat takeaway when he goes to university next year. Peter had difficulty articulating his challenges for completing this activity or identifying the "points of breakdown" but focused on the details of temperatures and his struggles with preparing multiple dishes at the same time (e.g., soup and a grilled cheese). Together, the therapist and Peter created a concept map of meal preparation (Fig. 26.1).

Measure (COPM), the Pediatric Activity Card Sort (PACS), or other occupationally focused goal-setting tools. A variety of evaluation tools can be used by the occupational therapy practitioners to ensure meaningful goal selection, monitor skill acquisition, and demonstrate improvements in occupational performance. Box 26.1 describes the assessments often used with the CO-OP. Originally, the CO-OP approach focused on targeting motor performance goals that are deemed important by the child in achieving competency in their daily occupations within the home, school, and community contexts. These goals could fall into the category of self-care occupations like brushing teeth and tying shoelaces, preparing meals, or socializing with friends (Cameron et al., 2017; Cameron, Schwellnus, & Polatajko, 2017; Peny-Dahlstrand et al., 2023). Other children may choose to work on goals related to school productivity. These could include handwriting, dressing for outside recesses (snow pants and jackets), and participating in physical education classes (Cameron et al., 2017; Cameron, Schwellnus, & Polatajko, 2017; Thornton et al., 2016; Ward & Rodger, 2004).

The CO-OP has been used as a successful intervention approach when helping children achieve competency in a variety of sports and/or activities like soccer, bike riding, and handball (Thornton et al., 2016; Ward & Rodger, 2004). Beyond motor-based goals, the CO-OP approach also can address organizational and social skill goals like

## BOX 26.1 Assessments Used in CO-OP Approach

**Daily Activity Log**

The daily activity log is a tool used to record the activities a child identifies as important over the course of a day The child client is asked to complete the daily activity log, with the assistance of parents or caregivers if necessary, thinking about a typical day. The completed daily activity log provides the occupational therapy practitioner with information on the client's typical day and is used to initiate the process of goal setting.

**Pediatric Activity Card Sort**

The Pediatric Activity Card Sort (PACS; (Mandich et al., 2004) is a picture-based assessment used to determine the child's level of occupational engagement. The visual nature of the assessment is useful when setting client-centered goals with young clients, aligning with the key feature of the CO-OP approach.

**Canadian Occupational Performance Measure**

The Canadian Occupational Performance Measure (COPM; (Law et al., 1998) is a semistructured interview to better understand client's performance goals, their perceived performance, and satisfaction in their performance. Clients identify three goals and their satisfaction with their performance. The occupational therapy practitioner uses the information obtained from the daily activity log and the Activity Card Sort (ACS)/PACS to initiate the COPM interview and to help guide the questions asked to ensure that meaningful goals are identified. COPM can be administered with children (Verkerk et al., 2023).

**Performance Quality Rating Scale**

Performance Quality Rating Scale (PQRS; Henry & Polatajko, 2003; Martini & Polatajko, 1998; Miller et al., 2001) is an observation-based rating scale used to measure performance and change in performance. This assessment allows for the objective rating of the quality of the child's occupational performance before and after intervention.

**Other Assessments to Measure Performance Changes**

Movement Assessment Battery for Children (Movement ABC-2), Bruininks-Oseretsky Test of Motor Proficiency (BOTMP), Behavior Rating Inventory of Executive Function (BRIEF), Social Skills Rating Scales (SSRS), Vineland Adaptive Behavioral Scales (VABS), and handwriting assessments. The Child Occupational Self-Assessment (COSA) can also be used for goal-setting purposes as it interviews children to determine what activities they value (i.e., important to them) and their perceived competence (i.e., how well they feel they complete the activity; Peny-Dahlstrand et al, 2023; Rodger et al., 2007,2008; Thornton et al., 2016). See Appendix A for more information on pediatric assessments.

making decisions, managing daily routines, getting ready for school, learning internet banking, managing interpersonal conflict at school, and completing homework (Hunt & Reed, 2017; Peny-Dahlstrand et al., 2020; Rodger et al., 2007, 2008).

## Key Features of the CO-OP Approach

Essential to the effectiveness of CO-OP is that the child and occupational therapy practitioner are fully engaged in the approach as it has been specified in the intervention protocol (Polatajko & Mandich, 2004). CO-OP is comprised of seven key elements, referred to as key features. The concepts are illustrated in Fig. 26.2.

The first key feature is goal identification. The client goals are established in collaboration with child and family and focus on occupations the child wants, needs, or is expected to perform. The child is actively engaged in the goal-setting process to ensure motivation. In the CO-OP approach, the child's perspective is integral to the therapy process. As such, the child is actively engaged in choosing the goals (Hunt & Reed, 2017; Polatajko & Mandich, 2004).

The second key feature of CO-OP is **dynamic performance analysis (DPA)** (Dawson et al., 2017; Polatajko et al., 2000). DPA acknowledges that performance is the result of the interaction between the person, environment, and the occupation. At the start of the intervention the practitioner analyzes the child performing the task and documents the performance problems or performance breakdowns. In doing so, the practitioner focuses on the fit between client abilities, skills, and actions and the task and environmental demands and supports. During the intervention sessions the child takes the lead in doing their own performance analysis. The focus of CO-OP is on performance, and correcting performance problems or breakdown, not on underlying component skills. Once the practitioner has identified the initial performance breakdown points, they use cognitive strategies to bridge the gap between ability and skill proficiency. See student online learning site for materials and video resources that review DPA.

The third feature of CO-OP is cognitive strategies that are used to support skill acquisition, generalization, and transfer. Cognitive strategies are cognitive operations beyond those that are inherent to the task itself. In the CO-OP approach, the child uses cognitive strategies to problem solve a performance issue and monitor the outcome. In other words, the strategies promote **metacognition**, which refers to thinking about one's thinking (Flavell, 1979). Two types of strategies are used in the CO-OP approach: global and personalized specific. **Global strategies** are intended to be used over long periods of time in a variety of different contexts. The global or executive strategy GOAL-PLAN-DO-CHECK (GPDC) used in CO-OP was developed by Camp et al. (1976) and used by Meichenbaum (1977):

GOAL: What do I want to do?
PLAN: How am I going to do it?
DO: Do it!
CHECK: How well did my plan work? Do I need to revise my plan?

In CO-OP, the child is taught to use the mnemonic GPDC to support the solving of occupational performance problems. During the first therapy session, the child is introduced to the GPDC strategy and is directly taught how to use it. To ensure that the child understands the global strategy, the child is asked to teach the occupational therapy practitioner an activity using this new framework. See Fig. 26.3 for an illustration of the concept map using GPDC strategy. Often a puppet, a bracelet, or a visual representation is used to teach a global strategy. The global strategy frames each intervention session. Initially, the practitioner takes the lead in using the GPDC strategy. As the child learns the strategy, the child gradually begins to initiate strategy use. Through the process of overtly talking oneself through an occupation, the steps become internalized and eventually covert; therefore, speech guides behavior (Dawson et al., 2017; Miller et al., 2001; Polatajko & Mandich, 2004).

The second type of strategies used in CO-OP is domain specific. Domain-specific strategies (DSS) also called **personalized strategies** are specific to a task or part of a task. See Table 26.4 for a comprehensive list of personalized cognitive strategies that can be used within the CO-OP approach. All are nested in verbal guidance. The goal is to lead the child from early reliance on the practitioner's verbal guidance to the independent use of cognitive problem-solving strategies through self-talk. Therefore, as the intervention progresses, the practitioner encourages the child to talk himself through a sequence. Verbalization ensures that the cognitive mechanisms that distinguish it from other approaches are used, that the strategies are brought to the attention of the child, that the child understands the role of the strategies, and that the child can use the strategies independently, in the absence of the occupational therapy practitioner. Once the child and practitioner have identified the strategies, the occupational therapy practitioner reinforces their use during

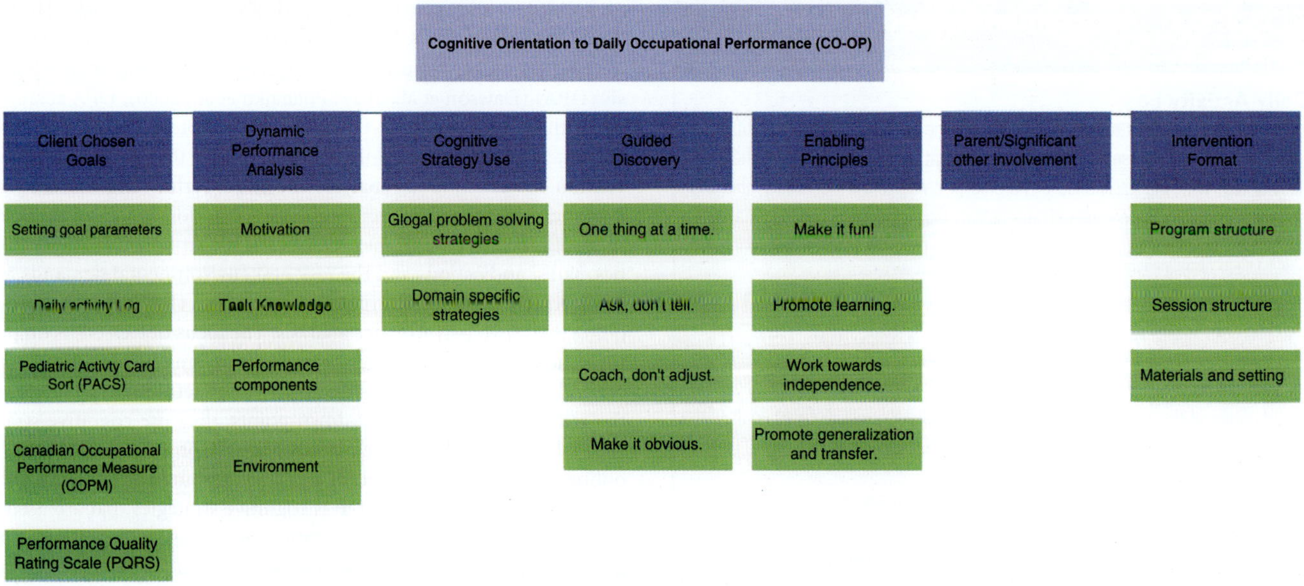


**Fig. 26.2** CO-OP is comprised of seven key elements, referred to as key features.

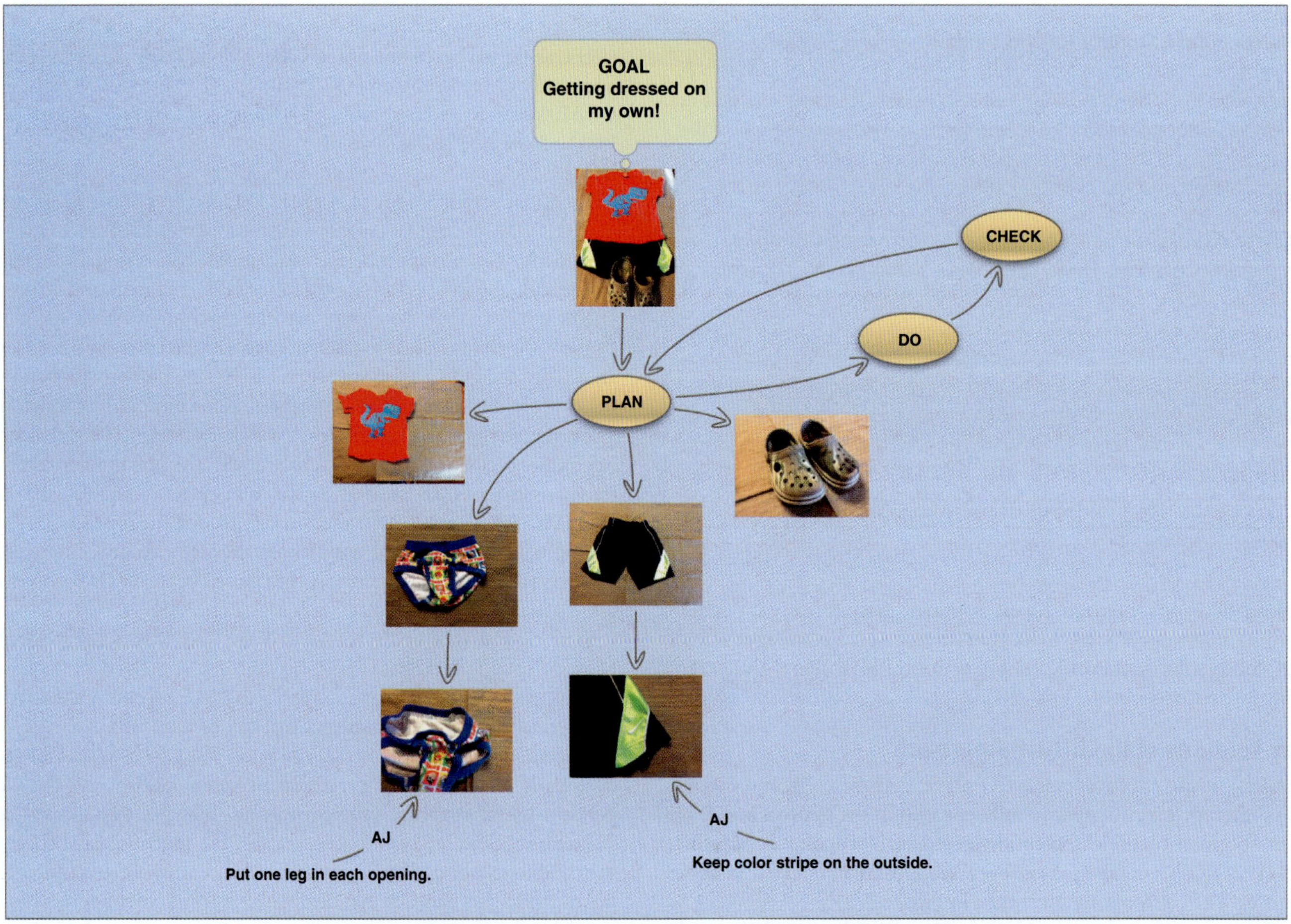


**Fig. 26.3** An illustration of the concept map for GOAL-PLAN-DO-CHECK.

## TABLE 26.4 Defining and Describing Personalized Cognitive Strategies

| Personalized Strategy | Description | Clinical Examples |
|---|---|---|
| **(1) External Sensory and Environmental Strategies** | | |
| Sensory cues or prompts from the environment that the individual provides to him/herself/themselves to help guide skill acquisition | Tactile, visual, auditory, and/or kinesthetic cues | Pictures, vibrations (from buzzer or other external device), alarms, or any other modality that attracts the learner's attention and guides them through the steps of a task or prompts their memory or previously learned motor patterns (Toglia et al., 2012) |
| **(2) Mental or Self-Verbalization Strategies** | | |
| Self-coaching | Encouragement, positive self-talk, strength-based thinking to help increase persistence and/or to control and regulate the learner's emotions | "I can do this!"<br>"Stay calm and focused ...."<br>"Only a few more times, and I will have it!" |
| Self-guidance | Providing instruction to him/herself to assist in completing a new/difficult task, cueing oneself and reminders to prepare for or complete an activity | Talking oneself through the steps of an activity, talking aloud through the problem-solving process, self-talk |
| Self-questioning | Identifying and asking him/herself or visualizing key questions relating to the activity or task performance | Picturing in your "mind's eye" key transition points of an activity, identifying and asking him/herself specific areas of difficulty experienced in each task |
| Distraction | Drawing the attention away from focusing on the performance | By thinking of something else or doing a dual task like counting from 100 backward, verbalization of history (former presidents), geographic facts (cities in Europe), or listening to music |
| Emotion regulation | Verbal or visual cues to reduce anxiety or tension | Prior to or during the performance cues on positive thinking, happy occasions, breathing |
| Imagery | Mental images that are created to represent physical objects, actions, experiences, or events | Creation of images, symbols, or representations that have direct meaning to the client; can also include imaging textures, sounds, smells, and kinesthetic feelings of movement |
| Association | Relating previous knowledge to relevant information about task | Associations can arise from previous experiences, recognition of physical similarities, and knowledge of categories |
| Rote script | A rote pattern of words or phrases that are meaningful to the client and can help to guide a sequence of actions or improve the recall of information | Some motor pattern rote scripts might include "dribble, dribble, shoot" (basketball) or "slide down, climb up, slide down" (making an "x" in printing) |
| Elaboration | Increase and add new information and relate it back to previous knowledge | Can include the expansion and addition of images, symbols, actions, images, words, or sentences; it also includes verbal and mental processes |
| Mnemonic techniques | Associating pictures, words, phrases, or images to cue an action or enhance memory recall | "Bunny ears" when tying shoes<br>"Helper hand" when printing and completing bilateral cutting activities |
| Rehearsal | Repeating information visually or mentally to aid in retention of important information related to the given task/occupation | Repeating key words/actions out loud, creating internalized visual images of the task procedure, and visually carrying out the task in a repeated manner |
| Reconstruction | Involves mental and verbal processes and involves the learner thinking back to a previous task, experience, or context to guide their performance in a new situation | The learner reconstructs experiences, activities, or contexts through imaging, replaying, and/or verbalizing |
| Anticipation | Preparing for a new activity through imagining or verbalizing possible outcomes, areas of difficulty, or scenarios the learner might encounter | Before a client goes to school, they anticipate loud noises, crowds, visual distractions, and possible "safe spots" to collect their thoughts when feeling overwhelmed |
| Knowledge | Identifying, acknowledging, and reflecting on what the individual knows about a given task | Observing the individual completing the task, conducting assessment/interview to discover how much the learner knows and understands regarding task sequence and demands |
| Translation | Converting written instructions and directions into different mediums to meet the individual's unique learning needs | Creating visual images/schedules explaining written information, chunking directions together into smaller steps |
| **(3) Task Modification and Specification Strategies** | | |
| Finger pointing | Similar to attention to doing but limited to pointing with one's finger directly at relevant task stimuli to enhancing timing within a task or refocus the learner's attention | As the individual is reading (either book, task directions, etc.), have the learner point at each word as they read to slow down the pace at which they are acquiring new information and to ensure they do not skip ahead |

*Continued*

**TABLE 26.4 Defining and Describing Personalized Cognitive Strategies—cont'd**

| *Personalized Strategy* | *Description* | *Clinical Examples* |
|---|---|---|
| Task simplification | Simplifying or breaking apart the parts of a task into more manageable pieces | When printing, the learner writes their name, date, and title at the top of the page and then the teacher scribes the rest of the assignment |
| Lists | Creating and/or using a list of steps to help guide task performance and/or cue actions | The list can be comprised of audio, visual, or written steps; for example, written list/script that is left by the phone that walks the learner through the socially appropriate steps to carry out when answering the phone |
| Task specification | Discussion regarding the specifics of a task, its components, or relevant features prior to engaging in the activity | These specifications should highlight those areas that require special attention, planning, or consideration; for example, placing an "x" where the child hangs his book bag or places his lunch bag |
| Attention to doing | Identifying the specific and relevant cues or features that need to be attended to when completing the task | An example might include "Where do you need to start your letters?" (printing) |
| Pacing strategies | Activities that assist with the timing of tasks | Some examples might include humming a song, taking breaks, counting out loud or to oneself, or tapping one's foot |
| Stimuli reduction | Removing or decreasing the amount and number of stimuli present at a given time | Covering or removing a part of task stimuli; e.g., when reading a page of information, placing a blank sheet over of the rest of the lines of text (hiding it), so that the reader can focus on one line at a time |
| Organization | Restructuring and reorganizing task materials or steps so that they are grouped together in a more logical or meaningful way | Commonly referred to as categorization or association; reorganizing a list of chores so that all the ones that need to be completed in the morning are together, and all the ones that need to be completed in the evening are together |

Adapted and referenced from Butchereit, K., Manzini, M., Polatajko, H. J., Lin, J.-P., McClelland, V. M., & Gimeno, H. (2022). Harnessing cognitive strategy use for functional problems and proposed underlying mechanisms in childhood-onset dystonia. *European Journal of Paediatric Neurology, 41*, 1–7. https://doi.org/10.1016/j.ejpn.2022.08.007; Polatajko, H. J., & Mandich, A. D. (2004). *Enabling occupation in children: The cognitive orientation to daily occupational performance (CO-OP) approach.* CAOT; Toglia, J. P. (2011). The dynamic interactional model of cognition in cognitive rehabilitation. In N. Katz (Ed.), *Cognition, occupation and participation across the life span: Neuroscience, neurorehabilitation and models of intervention in occupational therapy* (3rd ed., pp. 161–201); and AOTA Press; and Toglia, J. P., Rodger, S. A., & Polatajko, H. J. (2012). Anatomy of cognitive strategies: A therapist's primer for enabling occupational performance. *Canadian Journal of Occupational Therapy, 79*, 225–236.

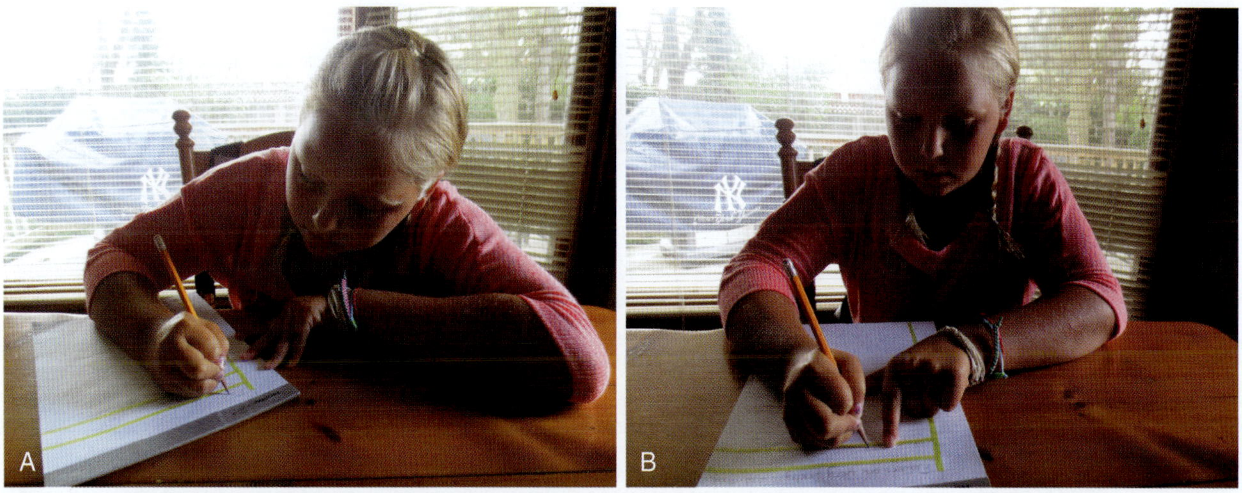

**Fig. 26.4** (A and B) The occupational therapist highlights the margin and finger space as a strategy that the child can complete on her own.

the intervention sessions. For example, the occupational therapy practitioner highlights the margin and finger space as a strategy that the child can complete on her own (Fig. 26.4A and B).

The next key feature of CO-OP is guided discovery. In the **guided discovery** process the learner is helped to identify a problem to solve; he is not given the solution but is provided with hints, coaching, feedback, or modeling to identify a solution. In CO-OP, the process of guided discovery is closely linked with the process of strategy use. It is used in conjunction with dynamic performance analysis (DPA), a process primarily to identify when the child becomes "stuck" and to elucidate the plan within the Goal Plan Do Check (GPDC) problem-solving process. Guiding the child to discover the plans and the personalized strategies increases the likelihood that he will attribute the success of the plans to himself, supporting self-efficacy (Dawson et al., 2017; Polatajko & Mandich, 2004). If the child becomes stuck when performing the occupation, the practitioner questions the child to discover a plan, enact the plan, and then evaluate the plan to see if it worked. As such, guided discovery supports both skill acquisition and strategy use.

Guided discovery has four main elements: (1) "One thing at a time"; (2) "Ask, don't tell!"; (3) "Coach, don't adjust!"; and (4) "Make it obvious!" (Dawson et al., 2017; Polatajko & Mandich, 2004).

**One thing at a time.** When a child is having difficulty performing an occupation, often several performance problems exist. Since CO-OP is embedded in a learning paradigm and skills are learned, not developed, it is important to keep the intervention and the client focused on only "one thing at a time."

**Ask, don't tell.** When a child discovers the solution to a performance problem, the child is likely to remember that solution and use it more often than when he or she is told the solution. Through Socratic questioning the child is taught to critically think, analyze, and evaluate solutions. Asking questions helps the child focus on the relevant aspects of the performance, and strategy identification is facilitated.

**Coach, don't adjust.** One of the most important components of the CO-OP approach involves adjusting the task or the environment to support occupational performance and skill acquisition. Many occupational therapy practitioners intuitively adjust a variety of factors including body positions, chair position, or equipment to ensure success. Often this leads to success within therapy sessions and in the presence of the occupational therapy practitioner, but the child may not be aware of these enabling strategies and may find it difficult to achieve success in the absence of the practitioner. Within the CO-OP intervention, the practitioner brings these adjustments to the child's attention by guiding the child to discover the personal, task, or environmental adjustments that will improve occupational performance.

**Make it obvious.** Often, children do not readily learn from observation and may have difficulty identifying the important components of a task. Therefore, when working with a child using the CO-OP approach, the part of the occupation the child needs to attend to is "made obvious" by the occupational therapy practitioner. The practitioner emphasizes the strategy that the child discovers by talking about it with the child. The practitioner makes the relationship between strategy use and outcome obvious to the child.

The fifth key feature of CO-OP consists of the four enabling principles that are used throughout the intervention. These four enabling principles include: (1) make it fun; (2) promote learning; (3) work toward independence; and (4) promote generalization and transfer. These enabling principles are important in engaging the child in therapy.

Parent or caregiver involvement is essential throughout the CO-OP therapeutic process. The primary role of parents or caregivers is to support the child in learning the occupations and the strategies and to facilitate the generalization and transfer of these to the home, school, and other environments.

The CO-OP program involves 10 intervention sessions. In the first phase of the CO-OP process, the child identifies three goals to address during intervention, and then the practitioner establishes the child's performance baseline on these chosen goals. Subsequently, the occupational therapy practitioner teaches the child the GPDC strategy, and then it is applied to the child's three goals. The GPDC strategy is then used to identify the personalized strategies. Once therapy is complete, the occupational therapy practitioner reevaluates the child's performance. Case Example 26.3 describes use of the CO-OP approach to address self-care. Fig. 26.5A–G illustrate the progression involved in brushing one's teeth.

Case Example 26.4 illustrates the use of the CO-OP approach to address leisure and play. This example includes a description of the role of the environment on addressing occupational performance and includes home programs and parental support to reinforce learning.

## COGNITIVE STRATEGIES USED WITHIN OCCUPATIONAL THERAPY

There are a variety of specific cognitive strategies that can be used within occupational therapy practice.

### Scaffolding

Scaffolding emphasizes communication between adults and children in the effort to develop children's internal dialogs. This, in turn, helps guide their own actions in the acquisition of new skills (Berk & Schanker, 2006). In cognitive-based approaches, the progression of moving skill acquisition from an overt to covert process demonstrates the increasing independence of the child in their understanding of activity demands, in using problem-solving strategies, and in coping with failures (Meichenbaum, 1977). Through scaffolding the practitioner modifies an occupation to create the just-right fit between the child's ability level and the activity demands. A clinical example of strategies moving from an overt to covert process is when a child is learning how to hit a baseball. Initially the child may articulate aloud the steps required to successfully swing a bat to hit a baseball during practice. "Keep my eye on the ball," "swing through the ball," and "take my time" are examples of self-coaching, a personalized strategy that over time fades to an internalized (covert) strategy or becomes tacit knowledge. Therefore, the child no longer needs to overtly articulate the steps and/or process of hitting a baseball but instead uses internal dialog, imagery, or other (cognitive) strategies covertly to maximize task performance.

### Discovery Learning

Discovery learning is a related educational-based cognitive approach that proposes that children construct their own knowledge by drawing on their past experiences and through interacting directly with the activity and the environment(s; Bruner, 1961). Discovery learning is similar to task exploration; however, through the addition of instructional scaffolding by the practitioner, it can more accurately be described as guided discovery (Pressley et al., 2003). In guided discovery learning, the occupational therapy practitioner assumes the role as a facilitator or the "more competent other" needed for learning. Rather than providing direct instruction, the practitioner allows the client to generate his or her own answers through tailoring the activity and the environment to the individual (Pressley et al., 2003). Occupational therapy practitioners pose questions to the child as they complete an activity, offering them the opportunity to approach an activity by generating and prioritizing their own strategies, while at the same time, the practitioner reduces the amount of support/guidance they are providing. In doing so, they can illuminate important components and concepts related to the activity. As a child engages in guided discovery learning, they take control over their performance, and the occupational therapy practitioner reduces the amount of support/guidance provided (Pressley & Harris, 2006). As they increase competence and experience success, guided discovery learning shifts the individual's reinforcement for learning from an external to a more internal locus, and "The child is now in a position to experience success and failures not as a reward or punishment, but as information" (Bruner, 1961). Guided discovery learning offers opportunities for the

## CASE EXAMPLE 26.3 SELF-CARE

Sarah is a 10-year-old girl who was referred for an occupational therapy assessment of her fine motor skills. Sarah demonstrates difficulties completing a variety of self-care activities such as tying her shoes, buttoning buttons, and zipping zippers. An assessment of Sarah's fine motor skills revealed challenges with in-hand manipulation skills and bilateral motor coordination skills impacting her ability to be independent in a variety of areas.

Sarah received services from an occupational therapy practitioner for 10 sessions. The practitioner used the CO-OP approach to support skill acquisition. Together, Sarah and the practitioner created dressing goals and identified key points of challenge (or breakdown points). The chart below describes the goal and breakdown points. During the first session, the practitioner introduced the GOAL-PLAN-DO-CHECK (GPDC) framework and applied it to familiar activities that Sarah was successful at completing. This helped Sarah learn the GPDC strategy.

The therapist completed a dynamic performance analysis to better understand Sarah's motivation, task knowledge, and current occupational performance. The analysis informed them of the areas of dressing that were challenging for Sarah, which are also referred to as breakdown points. They (parents, child, and therapist) identified a variety of personalized strategies (e.g., attention to doing, motor mnemonic, feeling the movement, verbal instruction and self-guidance, and body position) to assist in skill acquisition (tying shoes, buttoning, zipping) for dressing that were included (see Strategy Use). They created specific ways to address the strategies and created activities to reinforce strategy use. Each session, the occupational therapy practitioner engaged Sarah in challenging (but novel and fun) activities where she used the GPDC along with the personalized-specific strategies. The practitioner guided Sarah through questioning and promoting problem-solving and the use of the strategies. After each session, Sarah reflected on her performance and identified the next steps. Sarah's parents were involved in following up with home routines to support Sarah's progress. Sarah mastered the three selected skills within the 10 therapy sessions.

**GOAL AND BREAKDOWN POINTS**

| GOAL | Breakdown Points |
|---|---|
| Tying her shoes | • Forming the loops<br>• Manipulating the laces in her hands (holding the one still and looping the other around or holding two loops at the same time)<br>• Tying the final knot |
| Buttoning buttons | • Grasping the button while holding the fabric steady with her other hand<br>• Aligning the button with the correct hole<br>• Pulling the button through the hole |
| Doing up and undoing her zippers | • Holding the zipper stable with one hand and manipulating the other side of the zipper with her other hand<br>• Pushing the end of the zipper all the way into the pull tab (having it grab so that the zipper does not split) |

**STRATEGY USE**

| Personalized Strategy | Plan | Activities to Reinforce the Strategy |
|---|---|---|
| Attention to doing | • Making an X<br>• Glue my loop to the shoe | • Tying soccer cleats and figure skates |
| Motor mnemonic | • Make a bunny ear | • Tying her doll's shoes and indoor gym shoes at school |
| Feeling the movement | • "Feel the edge of the button and grip that as you pull it through the hole"<br>• "Feel the end of the zipper fit snugly into the pull tab before pulling up" | • Buttoning her doll clothing and helping her younger brother with dressing in the morning<br>• Putting sleeping bag back together when camping |
| Verbal rote script | • "Hole one ... button one, hole two ... button two, hole three ... button three" | • Buttoning doll clothing and helping her younger brother with dressing in the morning |
| Body position | • "Pinch the pull tab between your index finger and thumb" | • Buttoning (pinching the button to manipulate more effectively) |

child to ask questions and generate ideas that can be further tested or researched (Bruner, 1961). Through the shifting of the child's motivation for learning from an external to internal locus of control, guided discovery aids in enhancing the learner's level of self-efficacy (Ryan & Deci, 2000).

Neuroscience also supports the benefits from discovery learning. Processing information by the child, derived from its engagement in learning, promotes the reorganization of neural networks. These networks form the neurological foundation for children to participate optimally, allowing the child to perform in new situations and participate optimally (Dawson et al., 2017). More knowledge on how learning takes place is provided by theory on **neuroplasticity** explaining the ability of the brain to adapt to new demands by reorganizing brain structure, function, and connections (Gill et al., 2022). The cognitive-based CO-OP intervention has a positive effect on structure and function of the brain of children with DCD, specifically related to the cerebellum and associated networks (Gill et al., 2022).

### Instrumental Enrichment

The **Instrumental Enrichment program** is based on the notion that an individual's cognitive performance can be modified through intentional mediated interventions (Ben-Hur & Feuerstein, 2011; Kozulin et al., 2010). When an adult selects and organizes environmental stimuli so that it is congruent with the child's level of learning, the child's learning is optimized (Ben-Hur & Feuerstein, 2011; Kozulin et al., 2010). Children learn when adults are mediators, assisting the child to derive generalized meaning from life experiences (Feuerstein et al., 1980). Feuerstein et al. (1980) and Haywood (1987) developed mediation techniques for adults to use to help children make sense of their life experiences. These techniques include process questioning, bridging, comparison/describing, modeling, challenging, and elaborated feedback (Feuerstein et al., 1980; Missiuna et al., 2001). These mediation techniques provide a method through which the child learns to bridge newly acquired cognitive strategies into daily living situations. Occupational therapy practitioners can use mediated learning to promote a child's ability to generalize new learning to his or her daily routine.

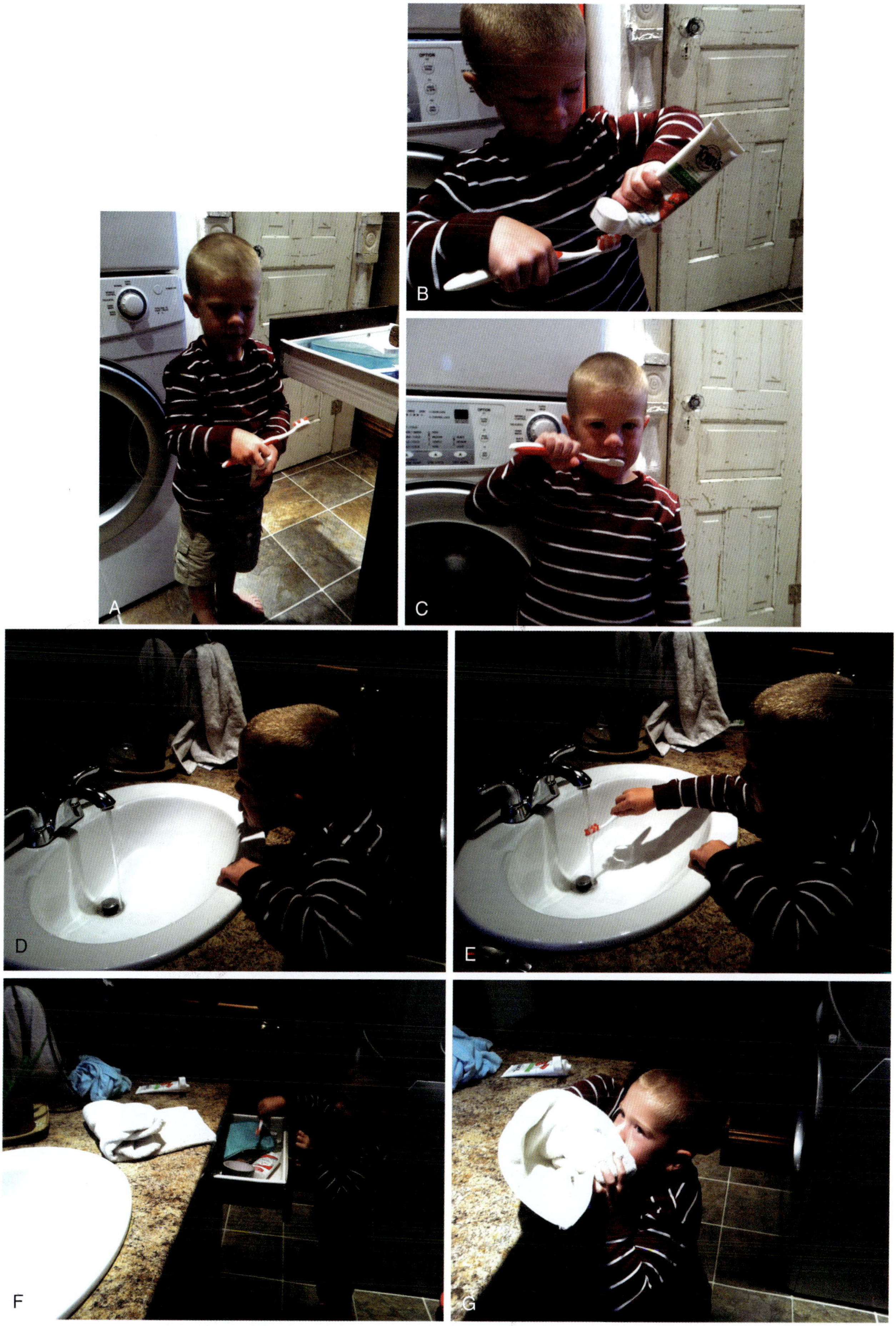

**Fig. 26.5** (A–G) Illustrated is a self-care progression of brushing one's teeth.

## CASE EXAMPLE 26.4 LEISURE AND PLAY

The Cognitive Orientation to Daily Occupational Performance (CO-OP) can be used to promote leisure and play skills such as riding a scooter (Fig. 26.6A) or bicycle (Fig. 26.6B).

Sam is a 7-year-old boy who has a diagnosis of Developmental Coordination Disorder (DCD). He was referred for private occupational therapy services, with one goal in mind: learning to ride his new bike. After completing the Canadian Occupational Performance Measure (COPM), the occupational therapy practitioner realized that Sam was highly motivated to acquire the skills to complete the activity successfully. The therapist used the Cognitive CO-OP approach as the framework for Sam's 12 therapy sessions.

They focused on task components of bike riding as the "just right challenge for him." The occupational therapy practitioner completed a dynamic performance analysis (DPA) to determine points that were challenging (i.e., breakdown points) for Sam (see Goal and Breakdown Points). Next, they identified personalized cognitive strategies (e.g., body position, feeling the movement, attention to doing, mnemonic, task modification) to help Sam navigate through the motor learning process (see Strategy Use). They provided a plan for how the strategies would be implemented (such as "keep my feet moving") and activities to reinforce the strategies. During the intervention sessions, the practitioner used his bicycle with training wheels and engaged Sam in a variety of activities to reinforce the strategies. The occupational therapy practitioner provided encouragement, adjusted activities as needed, and provided coaching. The practitioner allowed Sam to problem solve throughout. At the end of each session, Sam reflected on his performance and identified the next steps.

Sam collaborated in the therapeutic process to improve his skill acquisition, retention, and transfer of learning. Sam completed "homework" to practice the skill of bike riding at home using the cognitive strategies that he learned during the intervention sessions. The home program also encouraged involvement of Sam's family in the learning process to reinforce skill retention, generalization, and transfer. After succeeding at each "step" of bike riding (determined through task analysis), Sam rode his bike in a controlled environment (i.e., padded surface, with a helmet on, no obstacles). Once Sam was competent in this space, he practiced his newly developed skills in an open environment (on his street at home) to learn how to manage environmental obstacles (i.e., street signs, curbs, traffic, etc.) using his cognitive strategies.

### GOAL AND BREAKDOWN POINTS

| GOAL | Breakdown Points |
|---|---|
| Riding his bike | • Taking off from a stopped position (balancing bike and starting to pedal)<br>• Turning the bike while pedaling at the same time<br>• Remember to pedal backward to stop his bike |

### STRATEGY USE

| Personalized Strategy | Plan | Activities to Reinforce the Strategy |
|---|---|---|
| Body position | • Keep my feet moving<br>• Sit up with hands straight holding handles | • Running or playing volleyball or badminton |
| Feeling the movement | • "Feel your body lean to the side as you turn the corner"<br>• "Feel the forward power (motion) as you start pedaling" | • Enhancing body awareness and positioning to improve task performance in sports |
| Attention to doing | • "Look ahead to where you are going to turn … where are you going?" | • Roller blading and skateboarding |
| Verbal motor mnemonic | • "Step back" | • Stopping the bike, stopping when using roller blades |
| Task specification/ modification | • Use training wheels until confident with balance and control of the bike | • Understanding that when learning new skills that support from equipment or a person is useful for gaining confidence in task performance |

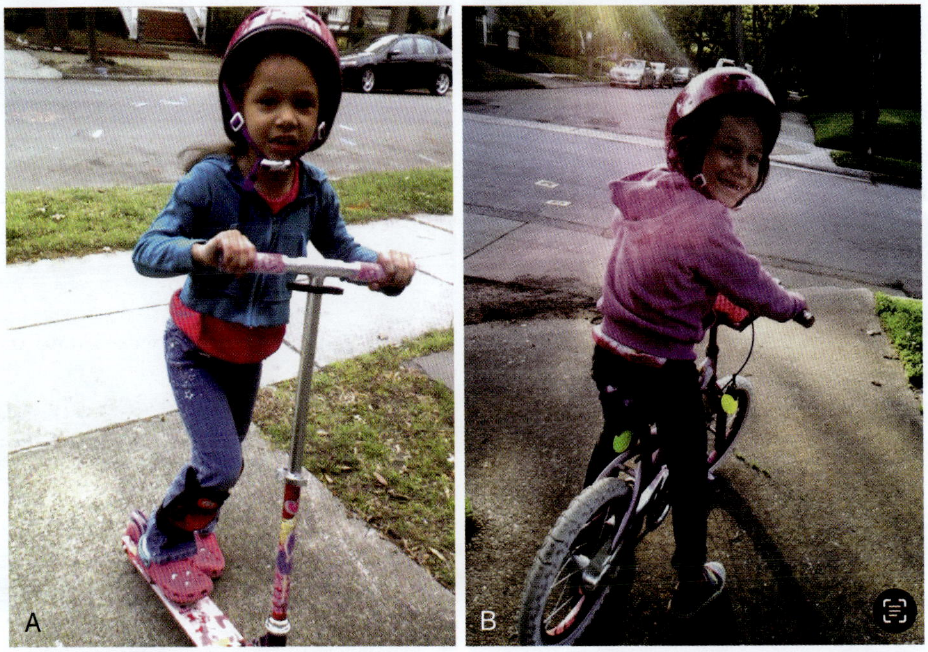

**Fig. 26.6** The CO-OP approach can be used to help children achieve leisure pursuits such as riding a scooter (A) or bicycle (B).

## RATIONALE FOR USING COGNITIVE-BASED APPROACHES

Cognitive-based approaches not only are effective for improving a variety of skills, but they also may be beneficial for a host of other reasons as well. Cognitive approaches may improve motivation and generalization of skills across environments, and they can be used across the lifespan.

### Motivation

People engage in occupation based on choice and personal motivation. The occupations in which a child chooses to engage play a role in defining who they are and directly influence personal identity and the development of one's self (Christiansen, 2004). Motivation plays a large role in this and is thought to influence learning, persistence, and the willingness to participate in therapy sessions (Dweck, 1986). Activity and curiosity (intrinsic motivation) is supported by adults facilitating the child's autonomy and competence (Ryan & Deci, 2000). Intervention goals therefore need to reflect occupations that the child identifies as being important and that they desire to improve (Miller et al., 2001). These elements resonate with the values and beliefs in client-centered practice and reflect the views of Meichenbaum (1977) who highlighted the importance of the child being an active collaborator in the therapeutic process (Miller et al., 2001).

Children who experience illness and/or a disability are often restricted in the occupations in which they can participate. Environmental, physical, and institutional barriers inhibit full engagement in many occupations. Participating in daily occupations brings meaning to lives, offers a sense of accomplishment, is a determinant of health, and establishes a rhythm in lives (Polgar & Landry, 2004). When an individual is unable to participate in a chosen occupation, lower self-esteem or self-efficacy, a decreased sense of independence, and an overall loss of motivation may result (Bandura, 1982; Gage & Polatajko, 1996). Cognitive-based interventions and adult-guided discovery learning focus on child-generated ideas, maintain the child's internal locus of control, and promote the child's self-efficacy. They offer individuals choice and control, which allow children to derive a sense of self-determination and empowerment (Polgar & Landry, 2004). **Self-determination** is a concept from psychology theory on "motivation" that refers to the ability of making choices and managing life issue and leads to freedom to make choices and a positive sense of well-being (Ryan & Deci, 2000).

### Generalization and Transfer

**Generalization** is defined as the ability of an individual to apply what they have learned in therapeutic rehabilitation to different real-life environments and activities (Sufrin, 1984; Toglia, 1991). Occupational therapy interventions focus on developing abilities that generalize to many situations to support independence and self-determination (McEwen & Houldin, 2017). Both internal and external factors affect the generalization of skills. External (to the learner) factors include the environmental context, the nature of the task, and the learning criteria of the activity. The internal factors that directly affect generalization are the learner's metacognition, their processing strategies, and their characteristics (Jenkins, 1979; McEwen & Houldin, 2017; Toglia, 1991). A multicontextual or complex approach promotes skill generalization (Skidmore et al., 2017; Toglia, 1991). Scaffolding through adult feedback can help a child generalize and transfer newly developed skills to different environments and tasks (Missiuna et al., 2001). Therapeutic intervention approaches focus on the generalization and transfer of skills through the following means:

- Maintaining client motivation ensures that the child applies the strategies to different tasks. Children are collaborators in the therapeutic process. Occupational therapy practitioners promote motivation and aid in the transfer of skills to the child's natural environments and daily activities (Meichenbaum, 1977; Polatajko et al., 2001).
- Contextually relevant practice exposes children to many different transfer experiences, which allows the child to understand the commonalities among situations and tasks (McEwen & Houldin, 2017; Toglia, 1991). Finding these commonalities among tasks and environments promotes generalization.
- Direct exposure to the task allows the child to engage directly in the task or occupation that they desire to improve (Bernie & Rodger, 2004; Perry, 1998).

The occupational therapy practitioner uses DPA to solve performance problems and identify possible solutions. The practitioner builds on the child's involvement by analyzing the effects of person, activity, and environmental constraints and possibilities on performance (Dawson et al., 2017). Through DPA the child gains a deeper understanding of the task and environmental demands and explores solutions to performance problems. The process of analyzing performance eventually becomes internalized by the child through scaffolding, which allows the child to "check" their occupational performance on an ongoing basis (Skidmore et al., 2017). The child can then take the newly developed skills and transfer them to other tasks and environments.

### Lifelong Development

The occupations that individuals participate in over time can be defined as their occupational trajectories (Martini et al., 2014). Individuals' occupational trajectories are fluid in nature and can change due to different life transitions. Some examples of life transitions include moving to a different grade in school, leaving home for postsecondary education, or getting a job. As children grow, develop, and mature, they experience different activities that might become barriers to their occupational success (Martini et al., 2014). Using a cognitive-based approach to guide therapeutic intervention recognizes the importance of self-determination and supports children independently applying cognitive strategies to different environments and activities (Polatajko & Mandich, 2004; Ryan & Deci, 2000; Toglia, 2011). As children encounter transition points in their lives and as their occupations change, so can the cognitive strategies that they employ.

## SUMMARY

Occupational therapy practitioners use cognitive-based interventions to address motor, cognitive, and social skills that interfere with the child's ability to participate in desired occupations. Cognitive-based interventions that focus on occupational performance, such as the CO-OP approach, provide children with strategies and problem-solving techniques that they can use in a variety of situations. Cognitive-based approaches teach children strategies through doing, which promotes the acquisition of new skills, leading to generalization and transfer of these skills.

1. Cognitive-based approaches focus on the development of strategies (including problem-solving and reflection) to accomplish a chosen task. Cognitive-based interventions rely on child processing, problem-solving, and using strategies to overcome performance challenges. These approaches help children create and understand the requirements (motor, sensory, cognitive, and organizational) and expectations for success. Cognitive-based interventions focus on working on the goals identified by the child

and their family, therefore enhancing motivation, skill retention, generalization, and transfer. The child understands the activity and its demands and engages in strategies to complete the activity. They reflect upon their performance and adjust accordingly. Performance may be related to motor, sensory, social-emotional, or cognitive skills.

2. *Cognition* refers to the process of acquiring knowledge and understanding through thought, experience, and the senses (https://en.wikipedia.org/wiki/Cognition). It refers to understanding, discovering, creating, synthesizing, problem-solving, and perceiving. *Metacognition* refers to thinking about one's thinking (Flavell, 1979).
3. The seven key features of CO-OP include the following:
   - Goal identification: The occupational therapy practitioner works with child and family to establish meaningful goals. The child's perspective is key, and the child is actively involved in choosing goals.
   - Dynamic performance analysis: The practitioner analyzes the child's abilities, skills, and actions and the task and environmental demands and supports.
   - Cognitive strategy use: Children are taught global and personalized strategies. Global strategy includes GPDC. Personalized strategies or domain-specific ones are used to problem solve performance issues and monitor outcomes.
   - Guided discovery: The practitioner uses guided discovery to encourage the child to identify a problem to solve and to develop solutions by providing hints, coaching, feedback, or modeling.
   - Enabling principles: Enabling principles used during the intervention process include (1) make it fun, (2) promote learning, (3) work toward independence, and (4) promote generalization and transfer.
   - Parent or caregiver involvement: The primary role of parents or caregivers is to support the child in learning occupations and the strategies and to facilitate the generalization and transfer of these to the home, school, and other environments.
   - Intervention format: The CO-OP program involves 10 intervention sessions that include identifying goals, learning strategies, implementing strategies, and measuring outcomes.
4. Cognitive strategies are the implicit mental processes that guide learning. When an activity is challenging, the child must use metacognitive strategies to select appropriate cognitive strategies, monitor, and evaluate their application. Once a strategy becomes automatic and can be efficiently used, the child does not have to think about it or monitor the strategies consciously.
5. Cognitive-based approaches focus on the development of strategies to support children in engaging in their desired occupations, such as activities of daily living, instrumental activities of daily living, play, academics, work, leisure, and social participation. Cognitive approaches are designed to teach children organization, decision-making, and problem-solving skills that enable them to discover and identify strategies that they can use to support their performance across environments over time.

## REFERENCES


Bandura, A. (1982). Self-efficacy mechanism in human agency. *American Psychologist, 37*, 122–147.

Ben-Hur, M., & Feuerstein, R. (2011). Feuerstein's new program for the facilitation of cognitive development in young children. *Journal of Cognitive Education and Psychology, 10*(3), 224–237.

Berk, L. L., & Schanker, S. G. (2006). *Child development* (2nd ed.). Pearson Education Inc.

Bernie, C., & Rodger, S. (2004). Cognitive strategy use in school-aged children with developmental coordination disorder. *Physical and Occupational Therapy in Pediatrics, 24*(4), 23–45.

Bloom, B. S., Engelhart, M. D., Furst, E. J., Hill, W. H., & Krathwohl, D. R. (1956). *Taxonomy of educational objectives. Handbook I: Cognitive domain.* David McKay.

Bouffard, M., & Wall, A. E. (1990). A problem-solving approach to movement skill acquisition: Implications for special populations. In G. Reid (Ed.), *Problems in movement control.* Elsevier Science.

Bruner, J. S. (1961). The act of discovery. *Harvard Educational Review, 31*, 21–32.

Butchereit, K., Manzini, M., Polatajko, H. J., Lin, J.-P., McClelland, V. M., & Gimeno, H. (2022). Harnessing cognitive strategy use for functional problems and proposed underlying mechanisms in childhood-onset dystonia. *European Journal of Paediatric Neurology, 41*, 1–7. https//doi.org/10.1016/j.ejpn.2022.08.007.

Cameron, D., Craig, T., Edwards, B., Missiuna, C., Schwellnus, H., & Polatajko, H. J. (2017). Cognitive orientation to daily occupational performance (CO-OP): A new approach for children with cerebral palsy. *Physical and Occupational Therapy in Pediatrics, 37*(2), 183–198. https://doi.org/10.1080/01942638.2016.1185500.

Cameron, D., Schwellnus, H., & Polatajko, H. (2017). Using the CO-OP approach: Cerebral palsy. In D. R. Dawson, S. E. McEwen, & H. J. Polatajko (Eds.), *Cognitive orientation to daily performance in occupational therapy.* AOTA Press.

Camp, B., Blom, G., Herbert, F., & VanDoorwick, W. (1976). *Think aloud: A program for developing self-control in young aggressive boys.* Unpublished manuscript. University of Colorado School of Medicine.

Christiansen, C. (2004). Occupation and identity: Becoming who we are through what we do. In C. H. Christiansen, & E. A. Townsend (Eds.), *Introduction to occupation the art and science of living* (pp. 121–139). Prentice Hall.

Cramer, S. C., Sur, M., Dobkin, B. H., O'Brien, C., Sanger, T. D., Trojanowski, J. Q., Rumsey, M. J., Hicks, R., Cameron, J., Chen, D., Chen, W. G., Cohen, L. G., deCharms, C., Duffy, C. J., Eden, G. F., Fetz, E. E., Filart, R., Freund, M., Grant, S. J., & Vinogradov, S. (2011). Harnessing neuroplasticity for clinical applications. *Brain, 134*, 1591–1609.

Dawson, D. R., McEwen, S. E., & Polatajko, H. J. (Eds.). (2017). *Cognitive orientation to daily performance in occupational therapy.* AOTA Press.

Dweck, C. S. (1986). Motivational processes affecting learning. *American Psychologist, 41*(10), 1040.

Feuerstein, R., Hoffman, M., & Miller, R. (1980). *Instrumental enrichment: An intervention program for cognitive modifiability.* University Park Press.

Flavell, J. (1979). Metacognition and cognitive monitoring: A new area of cognitive developmental inquiry. *American Psychologist, 34*, 906–911.

Gage, M., & Polatajko, H. (1996). Enhancing occupational performance through an understanding of perceived self-efficacy. In R. P. Fleming-Cottrell (Ed.), *Perspectives on purposeful activity: Foundation and future of occupational therapy* (pp. 367–371). American Occupational Therapy Association.

Gharebaghy, S., Rassafiani, M., & Cameron, D. (2015). Effect of cognitive intervention on children with ADHD. *Physical and Occupational Therapy in Pediatrics, 35*(1), 13–23.

Gill, K. K., Lang, D., & Zwicker, J. G. (2022). Cerebellar differences after rehabilitation in children with developmental coordination disorder. *Brain Science, 12*, 856.

Goodley, D., & Runswick-Cole, K. (2010). Emancipating play: Disabled children, development and deconstruction. *Disability and Society, 25*(4), 499–512.

Hahn-Markowitz, J., Manor, I., & Maeir, A. (2011). Effectiveness of cognitive–functional (Cog–Fun) intervention with children with attention deficit hyperactivity disorder: A pilot study. *American Journal of Occupational Therapy*, *65*, 384–392.

Haywood, H. C. (1987). A meditational teaching style. *The Thinking Teacher*, *4*(1), 1–6.

Henderson, S. E., & Sugden, D. (1992). *The movement assessment battery for children*. The Psychological Corporation Ltd.

Henry, L., & Polatajko, H. J. (2003). *Exploring the inter-rater reliability of the performance quality rating scale* (Canada).

Houldin, A., Mcewen, S., Howell, M., & Polatajko, H. (2017). The cognitive orientation to daily occupational performance approach and transfer: A scoping review. *OTJR: Occupation, Participation and Health*, *38* 153944921773605.

Humphry, R., & Womack, J. (2013). Transformations of occupations: A life course perspective. In B. A. Boyt Schell, G. Gillen, M. E. Scaffa, & E. S. Cohn (Eds.), *Willard and Spackman's occupational therapy* (12th ed.) (pp. 60–72). Lippincott, Williams and Wilkins.

Hunt, A. W., & Reed, N. (2017). Goal setting in the CO-OP approach context. In D. R. Dawson, S. E. McEwen, & H. J. Polatajko (Eds.), *Cognitive orientation to daily performance in occupational therapy* (pp. 43–60). AOTA Press.

Izadi-Najafabadi, I., Gunton, C., Dureno, Z., & Zwicker, J. (2022). Effectiveness of cognitive orientation to daily occupational performance intervention in improving motor skills of children with developmental coordination disorder: A randomized waitlist-control trial. *Clinical Rehabilitation*, *36*(6), 1–13.

Jenkins, R. L. (1979). The influence of children in family decision-making: Parents' perceptions. *Advances in Consumer Research*, *6*(1), 413–418.

Kozulin, A., Lebeer, J., Madella-Noja, A., Gonzalez, F., Jeffrey, I., Rosenthal, N., & Koslowsky, M. (2010). Cognitive modifiability of children with developmental disabilities: A multicenter study using Feuerstein's Instrumental Enrichment—Basic program. *Research in Developmental Disabilities*, *31*, 551–559.

Krajenbrink, H., Lust, L., Heeswijk van, J., Aarts, P., & Steenbergen, B. (2022). Benefits of an intensive individual CO-OP intervention in a group setting for children with DCD. *Occupational Therapy International*, *2022*, 1–12.

Law, M., Baptiste, S., Carswell, A., McColl, M. A., Polatajko, H., & Pollock, N. (1998). *Canadian occupational performance measure* (3rd ed.). CAOT Publications ACE.

Lidz, C. (1987). *Dynamic assessment: An interactional approach to evaluating learning potential*. Guildford Press.

Luria, A. (1959). The directive function of speech in development. *Word*, *18*, 341–352.

Luria, A. (1961). *The role of speech in the regulations of normal and abnormal behaviors*. Liveright.

Mandich, A., Polatajko, H., Miller, L., & Baum, C. M. (2004). *The pediatric activity card sort (PACS)*. Canadian Occupational Therapy Association.

Martini, R., Mandich, A., & Green, D. (2014). Implementing a modified cognitive orientation to daily occupational performance approach for use in a group format. *British Journal of Occupational Therapy*, *77*(4), 214–219.

Martini, R., & Polatajko, H. J. (1998). Verbal self-guidance as a treatment approach for children with developmental coordination disorder: A systematic replication study. *Occupational Therapy Journal of Research*, *18*(4), 157–181.

McEwen, S. E., & Houldin, A. (2017). Generalization and transfer in the CO-OP approach. In D. R. Dawson, S. E. McEwen, & H. J. Polatajko (Eds.), *Cognitive orientation to daily performance in occupational therapy* (pp. 32–42). AOTA Press.

Meichenbaum, D. (1977). *Cognitive-behavioral modification: An integrative approach*. Plenum Press.

Meichenbaum, D., & Goodman, J. (1971). Training impulsive children to talk to themselves: A means of developing self-control. *Journal of Abnormal Psychology*, *77*, 115–126.

Miller, L. T., Polatajko, H. J., Missiuna, C., Mandich, A. D., & Macnab, J. J. (2001). A pilot trial of a cognitive treatment for children with developmental coordination disorder. *Human Movement Science*, *20*, 183–210.

Missiuna, C., DeMatteo, C., Hanna, S., Mandich, A., Law, M., Mahoney, W., & Scott, L. (2010). Exploring the use of cognitive intervention for children with acquired brain injury. *Physical and Occupational Therapy in Pediatrics*, *30*(3), 205–219.

Missiuna, C., Malloy-Miller, T., & Mandich, A. (1997). Cognitive, or "top-down", approaches to intervention. *Keeping Current*, *97*(1).

Missiuna, C., Mandich, A. D., Polatajko, H. J., & Malloy-Miller, T. (2001). Cognitive orientation to daily occupational performance (CO-OP): Part I—theoretical foundations. *Physical and Occupational Therapy in Pediatrics*, *20*(2/3), 69–81.

Novak, I., & Honan, I. (2019). Effectiveness of paediatric occupational therapy for children with disabilities: A systematic review. *Australian Occupational Therapy Journal*, *66*(3), 258–273 Epub April 10, 2019.

Novak, I., Morgan, C., Fahey, M., Finch-Edmondson, M., Galea, C., Hines, A., Langdon, K., Namara, M. M., Paton, M. C., Popat, H., Shore, B., Khamis, A., Stanton, E., Finemore, O. P., Tricks, A., Te Velde, A., Dark, L., Morton, N., & Badawi, N. (2020). State of the evidence traffic lights 2019: Systematic review of interventions for preventing and treating children with cerebral palsy. *Current Neurology and Neuroscience Reports*, *20*(2), 3.

O'Brien, J. (2015). Application of motor control/motor learning to practice. In J. Case-Smith, & J. Clifford O'Brien (Eds.), *Occupational therapy for children and adolescents* (6th ed.) (pp. 193–219). Elsevier.

Peny-Dahlstrand, M., Bergqvist, L., Hofgren, C., Himmelmann, K., & Öhrvall, A. M. (2020). Potential benefits of the cognitive orientation to daily occupational performance approach in young adults with spina bifida or cerebral palsy: A feasibility study. *Disability & Rehabilitation*, *42*(2), 228–239.

Peny-Dahlstrand, M., Hofgren, C., Lindquist, B., Bergqvist, L., Himmelmann, K., Opheim, A., Sjöwall, D., Brock, K., & Öhrvall, A. M. (2023). The cognitive orientation to daily occupational performance (CO-OP) approach is superior to ordinary treatment for achievement of goals and transfer effects in children with cerebral palsy and spina bifida – a randomized controlled trial. *Disability and Rehabilitation*, *45*(3), 822–831.

Perry, S. B. (1998). Clinical implications of a dynamic systems theory. *Neurology Report*, *24*, 4–10.

Polatajko, H. J., Mandich, A. D., Missiuna, C., Miller, L. T., Macnab, J. J., Malloy-Miller, T., & Kinsella, E. A. (2001). Cognitive approach to daily occupational performance (CO-OP): Part III- protocol in brief. *Physical and Occupational Therapy in Pediatrics*, *20*(2/3), 107–123.

Polatajko, H. J., & Mandich, A. D. (2004). *Enabling occupation in children: The cognitive orientation to daily occupational performance (CO-OP) approach*. CAOT.

Polatajko, H. J., Mandich, A. D., Missiuna, C., Miller, L. T., Macnab, J. J., Malloy-Miller, T., & Kinsella, E. A. (2000). Cognitive approach to daily occupational performance (CO-OP): Part III- protocol in brief. *Physical and Occupational Therapy in Pediatrics*, *20*(2/3), 107–123.

Polgar, J. M., & Landry, J. E. (2004). Occupations as a means for individual and group participation in life. In C. H. Christiansen, & E. A. Townsend (Eds.), *Introduction to occupation the art and science of living* (pp. 197–220). Prentice Hall.

Pressley, M., Roehrig, A. D., Raphael, L., Dolezal, S., Bohn, C., Mohan, L., Wharton-McDonald, R., Bogner, K., & Hogan, K. (2003). Teaching processes in elementary and secondary education. In W. M. Reynolds, & G. E. Miller (Eds.), *Handbook of psychology volume 7: Educational psychology*. John Wiley and Sons Inc.

Pressley, M., & Harris, K.R. (2006). Cognitive strategies introduction: From basic research to classroom instruction. In Anderman E., Winne P.H., Alexander P.A., & Corno L. (Eds.), *Handbook of educational psychology* (2nd ed., pp. 265-286). Lawrence Erlbaum.

Ricon, T. (2010). Using concept maps in cognitive treatment for children with developmental coordination disorder. *Health*, *2*(7), 685–691.

Rodger, S. (2017). Chapter 6: Autism spectrum disorder. In D. R. Dawson, S. E. McEwen, & H. J. Polatajko (Eds.), *Cognitive orientation to daily performance in occupational therapy*. AOTA Press.

Rodger, S., Ireland, S., & Vun, M. (2008). Can cognitive orientation to daily occupational performance (CO-OP) help children with Asperger's syndrome to master social and organisational goals? *British Journal of Occupational Therapy*, *71*(1), 23–32.

Rodger, S., Springfield, E., & Polatajko, H. (2007). Cognitive orientation for daily occupational performance approach for children with Asperger's syndrome: A case report. *Physical and Occupational Therapy in Pediatrics*, *27*(4), 7–22.

Ryan, R. M., & Deci, E. L. (2000). Self-determination theory and the facilitation of intrinsic motivation, social development, and well-being. *American Psychologist*, *55*(1), 68–78.

Seger, C. A. (1994). Implicit learning. *Psychological Bulletin*, *115*(2), 163.

Skidmore, E. R., McEwen, S. E., Green, D., Houten van den, J., Dawson, D. R., & Polatajko, H. J. (2017). Essential elements and key features of the CO-OP Approach. In D. R. Dawson, S. E. McEwen, & H. J. Polatajko (Eds.), *Cognitive orientation to daily performance in occupational therapy*. AOTA Press.

Sufrin, E. M. (1984). The physical rehabilitation of the brain injured elderly. In B. A. Edelstein, & E. T. Couture (Eds.), *Behavioral assessment and rehabilitation of the traumatically brain-damaged* (pp. 191–221). Plenum.

Thornton, A., Licari, M., Reid, S., Armstrong, J., Fallows, R., & Elliot, C. (2016). Cognitive orientation to (daily) occupational performance intervention leads to improvements in impairments, activity and participation in children with developmental coordination disorder. *Disability and Rehabilitation*, *38*(10), 979–986.

Toglia, J. P. (1991). Generalization of treatment: A multicontext approach to cognitive perceptual impairment in adults with brain injury. *American Journal of Occupational Therapy*, *45*(6), 505–516.

Toglia, J. P., Rodger, S. A., & Polatajko, H. J. (2012). Anatomy of cognitive strategies: A therapist's primer for enabling occupational performance. *Canadian Journal of Occupational Therapy*, *79*, 225–236.

Toglia, J. P. (2011). The dynamic interactional model of cognition in cognitive rehabilitation. In N. Katz (Ed.), *Cognition, occupation and participation across the life span: Neuroscience, neurorehabilitation and models of intervention in occupational therapy* (3rd ed.) (pp. 161–201). AOTA Press.

Tudge, J. R. H., & Winterhoff, P. A. (1993). Vygotsky, Piaget, and Bandura: Perspectives on the relations between the social world and cognitive development. *Human Development*, *36*, 61–81.

Verkerk, G., van der Molen-Meulmeester, L., van Hartingsveldt, M., & Alsem, M. (2023). Instructions for administering the Canadian occupational performance measure with children themselves. *Physical and Occupational Therapy in Pediatrics*, *43*(1), 58–73.

Vygotsky, L. S. (1987). Thinking and speech. In R. W. Reiber, & A. S. Carton (Eds.), *The collected works of L.S. Vygotsky* (pp. 29–38). Plenum Press.

Ward, A., & Rodger, S. (2004). The application of cognitive orientation to daily occupational performance (CO-OP) with children 5–7 years with developmental coordination disorder. *British Journal of Occupational Therapy*, *67*(6), 256–264.

Wilson, J., Mandich, A., Magalhaes, L., Polgar, J., & Holmes, J. (2014). *Concept mapping and the Cognitive Orientation to daily Occupational Performance (CO-OP) approach as an intervention framework for adolescents with autism spectrum disorder (ASD)* (Doctoral dissertation). Retrieved from: Electronic Thesis and Dissertation Repository. 2379. http://ir.lib.uwo.ca/etd/2379.

Wright, H. C., & Sugden, D. A. (1998). A school-based intervention programme for children with developmental coordination disorder. *European Journal of Physical Education*, *3*, 35–50.

Ziviani, J., Polatajko, H., & Rodger, S. (2015). Embedding goal setting in practice the CO-OP approach. In A. A. Poulsen, J. Ziviani, & M. Cuskelly (Eds.), *Goal setting and motivation in therapy engaging children and parents* (pp. 80–88). Jessica Kingsley Publishers.

27

# Ayres Sensory Integration Intervention

*Diane Parham and Zoe Mailloux*

## GUIDING QUESTIONS

1. What are the key elements of occupational therapy using ASI intervention with fidelity?
2. What are the expected outcomes of this intervention?
3. What kinds of evidence are available on the effectiveness of ASI intervention, how strong is the evidence, and where can this evidence be found?

## KEY TERMS

**Active participation**
**Adaptive response**
**Ayres Sensory Integration (ASI)**
**Fidelity**
**Inner drive**
**Just right challenge**
**Neuroplasticity**

## AYRES SENSORY INTEGRATION INTERVENTION

The term **Ayres Sensory Integration (ASI)** intervention refers to the individualized occupational therapy practice approach that A. Jean Ayres, OTR, PhD developed specifically to remediate sensory integrative problems of children (Roley et al., 2007). Early in her career as an occupational therapist, Dr. Ayres became interested in conducting research to better understand and help children who were identified as having learning disabilities and, later in her career, children diagnosed by physicians as having autism spectrum disorders. Building on the knowledge that she gained from several decades of practice, test development, and research, she developed the theory that some children experience difficulties with learning or behavior due to disordered processing of sensory information in the brain. To help remediate the difficulties that these children experience, Dr. Ayres developed an intervention approach that is now known as ASI intervention. Box 27.1 outlines the tenets of this approach that are part of the intervention process and described in the following section.

In ASI intervention, the occupational therapy practitioner presents activity challenges that are individually tailored to improve sensory integration capacities of the child. These challenges are embedded within the context of play. In occupational therapy sessions that utilize sensory integration procedures, the practitioner tailors the therapy environment for the individual child by setting up equipment in a manner that will be appealing to the child and will elicit the child's engagement in play. At the same time, the occupational therapy practitioner embeds challenges within activities, so that they are just beyond what the child can easily do. The child experiences the therapy session as a time to play, while the practitioner continuously adjusts activities to make them easier or more challenging, depending on the child's responses.

The findings of a thorough sensory integration evaluation are critical in planning sensory integration intervention. Evaluation findings identify the child's sensory difficulties as well as their strengths (see Chapter 9 for more information about evaluating a child regarding their sensory difficulties). This information, along with the reasons for why the child was referred to occupational therapy, guides the types of activity challenges that the practitioner will prioritize during therapy sessions.

For the child, a sensory integration therapy session will be experienced as a time to play, while for the practitioner, the session requires engaging the child in play activities that present "**just right challenges**," – activities that are not so easy that the child does not have to exert much attention to the tasks, but also not so difficult that the child is unable to engage in the activity with some degree of success (Gaylard, 1966; Kuhaneck & Spitzer, 2024; Lindquist et al., 1982; Mack et al., 1982; Michelman, 1974). Ultimately, this intervention is designed to help a child gain confidence and competencies that directly carry over to everyday occupations at home, in play, at school, or in the community.

ASI intervention is applied on an individual basis because the occupational therapy practitioner must adjust therapeutic activities moment by moment in relation to the individual child's interest in the activity or response to a specific challenge or sensory experience (Clark et al., 1989; Kimball, 1999; Koomar & Bundy, 2002). This requires the occupational therapy practitioner to continually focus attention on the child while being mindful of opportunities in the environment for eliciting adaptive responses (see Box 27.2; Fig. 27.1). Of particular importance is the delicate interplay between the potential therapeutic value of an activity and the child's motivation to engage in it. Therefore, the occupational therapy practitioner's session plan is fluid, changing according to the child's behaviors. The occupational therapy practitioner establishes a relationship with the child that fosters the child's inner drive to actively explore the environment and to master challenges posed by the environment. Because of the high degree of personal attention continuously given to the child during the therapy

### BOX 27.1 Basic Tenets of Ayres Sensory Integration Intervention

1. Sensory input can be used systematically to elicit an adaptive response.
2. Registration of meaningful sensory input is necessary before an adaptive response can be made.
3. An adaptive response contributes to the development of sensory integration.
4. Better organization of adaptive responses enhances the child's general behavioral organization.
5. More mature and complex patterns of behavior emerge from consolidation of simpler behaviors.
6. The more inner-directed a child's activities are, the greater is the potential for the activities to improve neural organization.

### BOX 27.2 An Adaptive Response

Ayres provides an example of learning to ride a bicycle to illustrate an adaptive response (Ayres, 1979) (see Fig. 27.1). The child must integrate sensations, particularly from the vestibular and proprioceptive systems, to learn how to balance on the bicycle. The vestibular, proprioceptive, and visual senses must accurately and quickly detect when the child begins to fall and then must be rapidly integrated with each other to produce motor reactions that counteract the direction of the fall. Eventually, often after many trials of falling, the child integrates sensory information efficiently enough to make the appropriate weight shifts over the bicycle to maintain balance. This adaptive response, and those that follow, enable the child to balance effectively to ride the bike. The child's nervous system has changed in how it integrates multisensory information to produce refined, dynamic balancing, so the child is now more adept at bicycle riding.

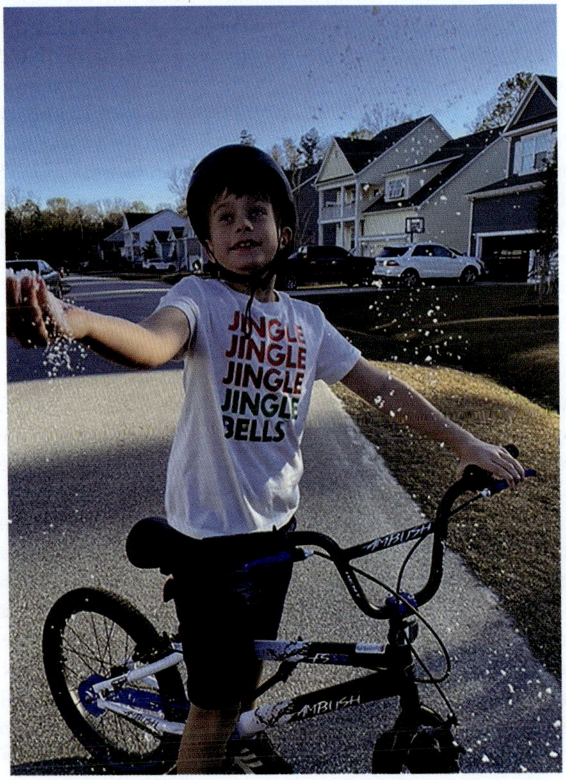


**Fig. 27.1** Riding a bike requires children to integrate visual, vestibular, and proprioceptive sensations to master the coordination, timing, sequencing, safety awareness, and speed. (Photo courtesy Patricia Schaefer.)

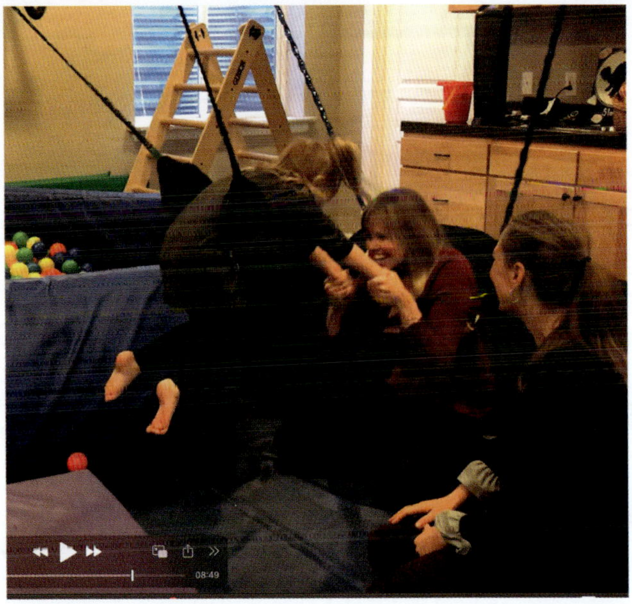


**Fig. 27.2** This young girl is challenged to engage in a play session that requires her to respond to vestibular, tactile, and proprioceptive input. She is actively engaged and leading the activity, as the occupational therapist monitors her responses and adjusts the environment to challenge her as needed.

session, a fine gradient of complexity can be built into therapeutic activities while simultaneously ensuring that the child's interests are prioritized, and the child experiences success with a growing sense of "I can do it!" (Fig. 27.2).

The occupational therapy practitioner's job is to create an environment that evokes increasingly complex **adaptive responses** from the child. In this intervention, it is critical that the child must be actively engaged in each activity. The practitioner generally does not "do something to the child." Instead, the practitioner sets up equipment and activities in the therapy room that will entice the child to actively engage with them in ways that will be therapeutically beneficial. To accomplish this, the occupational therapy practitioner respects the child's needs and interests while structuring opportunities to help the child successfully meet a challenge. An example is a child who needs to develop more efficient righting and equilibrium reactions and chooses to sit and swing on a platform swing (a square wooden platform, usually padded with carpeting, that is suspended from the ceiling by ropes). The occupational therapy practitioner may allow the child to swing awhile to become accustomed to the vestibular sensations. Once the child seems comfortable, the occupational therapy practitioner steps in to jiggle the swing to stimulate the desired equilibrium responses. However, if the child responds to this challenge with signs of anxiety, fear, or instability (appearing a bit "floppy" and unstable, which might pose danger of falling off), the occupational therapy practitioner needs to intervene quickly to reduce anxiety, enhance safety, and help the child to enjoy the sensations of swinging or rotating motions. The occupational therapy practitioner might set an inner tube horizontally on the swing platform. This allows the child to lean back against the inner tube for greater stability (ensuring safety), while sitting upon the platform swing. In this example, the inner tube supports the child's stability while sitting and swinging on the platform. The lower part of the child's body is more secure, increasing feelings of security and enhancing safety, while simultaneously the child's upper body is free to make the required righting reactions to maintain an upright seated position while swinging in different directions. Therapeutic activities

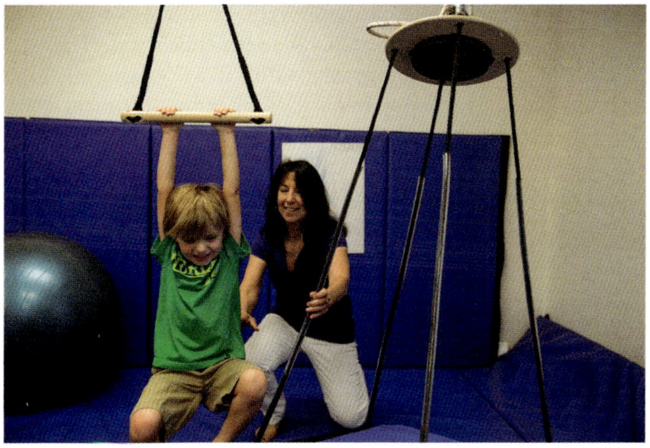

**Fig. 27.3** Ayres Sensory Integration (ASI) intervention requires that the therapist attend closely to the child on a moment-by-moment basis to ensure that therapeutic activities are individually tailored to changing needs and interests of the child.

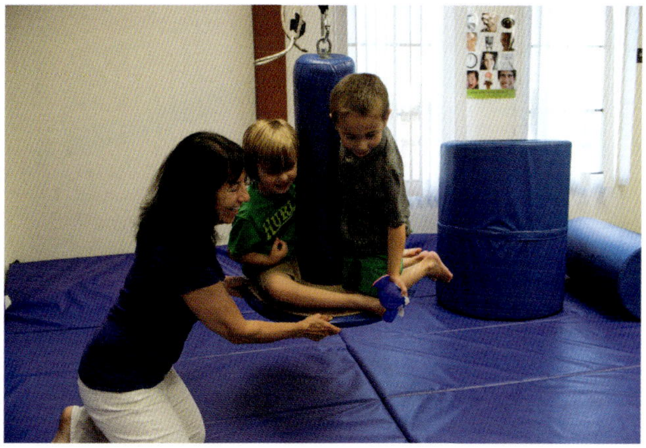

**Fig. 27.4** Rather than passively imposing vestibular input on the child, classic sensory integration treatment emphasizes active participation and self-direction of the child.

thus emerge from the interaction between the occupational therapy practitioner and the child. Such individualized treatment can be fully realized only with one-to-one interaction between the occupational therapy practitioner and the child. Please see Fig. 27.3 for an illustration of this one-to-one interaction.

Occupational therapy using ASI intervention capitalizes on the **inner drive** of the child during intervention (Ayres, 1973, 1979; Clark et al., 1989; Koomar & Bundy, 2002). Self-direction on the part of the child is encouraged because therapeutic gains are maximized if the child is fully invested as an active participant. This is not the same as permitting the child to engage in free play with no adult guidance. The optimal therapy situation is one in which a balance is struck between the structure provided by the occupational therapy practitioner and freedom of choice on the part of the child (Ayres, 1973, 1979). Drawing on the child's interests and imagination is often key to encouraging greater effort on a difficult task or staying with a challenging activity for a longer time. However, because children with sensory integrative problems do not always demonstrate inner drive toward growth-inducing activities, it may be necessary to modify activities and find ways to entice such children toward interaction. When facilitating engagement in children with autism or other children whose inner drive is limited, the occupational therapy practitioner may need to frequently initiate activities and guide the child on how to perform them. Occasionally, an occupational therapy practitioner may use a more "directed" approach in the context of a particular activity, to show a child that the challenging activity is possible not only to achieve but also to enjoy. In situations in which the occupational therapy practitioner intervenes by directing the child, the occupational therapy practitioner always looks for opportunities in which the child can increase his or her active engagement and control of the activity, including supporting the child's initiation of a new activity.

**Active participation** is also emphasized because the brain responds differently and learns more effectively when an individual is actively involved in a task, rather than merely receiving passive stimulation. Therefore, in ASI intervention, the occupational therapy practitioner actively engages the child to the greatest degree possible. For example, sensory integration theory posits that a child experiences a greater degree of integration from pumping a swing or pulling on a rope to make it go, than from being swung passively.

Maximal active involvement generally takes place when therapeutic activities are at just the right level of complexity, at which the child not only feels comfortable and nonthreatened but also experiences some challenge that requires effort. The course of therapy usually begins with activities for which the child feels comfortable and competent, and then it moves toward increasing challenges and presenting novel ways to engage in an activity. For example, for children with gravitational insecurity, therapy usually begins with activities close to the ground and with physical support from the practitioner (such as holding the child at the hips as the child moves) in order to help the child feel secure. Gradually, over weeks of therapy, activities that require stepping or climbing upon elevated surfaces are introduced as the practitioner subtly reduces and eventually withdraws continuous physical support. Introducing the "just right" level of challenge, while respecting the child's need to feel secure and allowing the child to have degree of control, is a key to maximizing the child's active involvement in therapy (see Fig. 27.4).

At times, sensory experiences may be initiated and provided by the occupational therapy practitioner to help prepare a child for more complex or challenging activities that they may later perform. For example, a child with autism may show improved awareness and interest in movement activities after receiving passive vestibular sensation on a swing that the occupational therapy practitioner has moved in a linear or rotary fashion (Slavik et al., 1984). The increased awareness of the joys and affordances of movement will also likely mean that the child has greater awareness of the environment. In this way, therapist-initiated sensory experiences can be a steppingstone toward the child's active involvement in an activity. Another example is the use of carefully introduced tactile activities as a means for reducing tactile defensiveness and improving the child's comfort in situations and activities that involve frequent tactile contact with objects and people (Ayres, 1973). Overall, therapist-directed or induced sensory experiences are a limited component of a sensory integrative treatment program and are used only as a step toward facilitating more active participation. See Case Example 27.1 for an example of ASI intervention in practice.

## Ayres Sensory Integration Setting

The setting in which ASI takes place, including the availability of specialized therapeutic equipment, is another important aspect of this type of intervention (May-Benson et al., 2014; Slavik & Chew, 1990; Walker, 1991). A therapy room that is designed for ASI contains large activity areas with an array of specialized equipment (May-Benson et al., 2014). The availability of suspended equipment is a hallmark of this treatment approach (Clark et al., 1989; Koomar & Bundy, 2002). Suspended equipment provides rich opportunities for engaging and challenging the vestibular system. In addition, equipment and

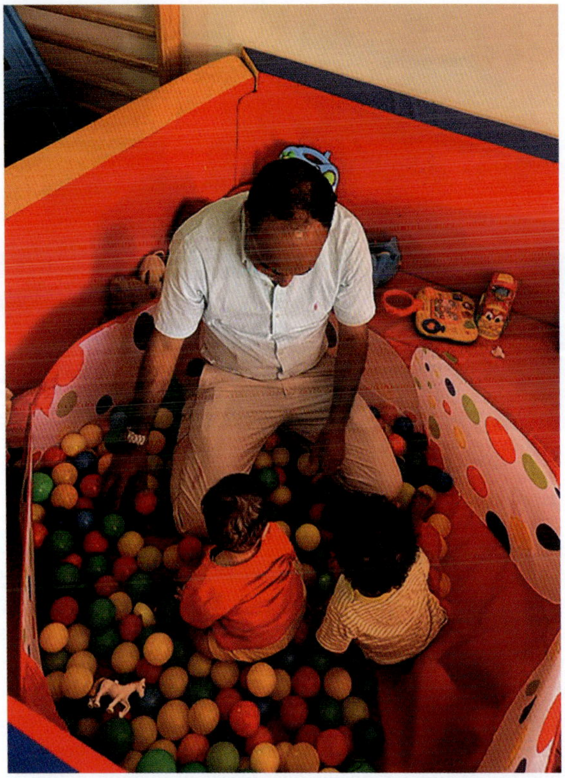

**Fig. 27.5** The setting in which ASI intervention takes place provides a variety of sensory experiences.

materials are available that provide a variety of somatosensory activities, including tactile, vibratory, and proprioceptive input. Mats and large pillows are used for safety. Overall, this special environment provides the child with a safe and interesting place in which to explore his or her capabilities. At the same time the equipment and setting provide the occupational therapy practitioner with a tool kit and workshop for creating sensory experiences that are enticing to the child and for gently guiding the child toward activities that challenge perception, dynamic postural control, and motor planning. The environments created for ASI incorporate essential features of enriched environments including multiple sensory experiences, novelty in the environment, and active engagement in challenging cognitive, sensory, and motor tasks (Fig. 27.5).

## A Word of Caution Regarding the Use of Vestibular and Tactile Stimulation

Vestibular and tactile stimulation are powerful inputs that can have profound effects on the physiologic state. For example, activation of the vestibular system, usually in the form of linear movement, is commonly introduced early during treatment for many children because it is believed to have an organizing effect on other sensory systems (Ayres, 1973, 1979) (Fig. 27.6). However, it can have a disturbing and disorganizing effect on the child if used without careful monitoring of the child's response. Vestibular system activation may produce strong autonomic responses, manifested as blanching and nausea. It directly influences arousal level and, if not regulated carefully, may produce hyperactive, distractible states or lethargic, drowsy states. These responses may occur immediately or sometime later depending on the child's processing.

Because ASI intervention emphasizes active participation on the part of the child, vestibular stimulation is rarely passively imposed on the child. Whenever vestibular stimulation is used, the occupational therapy practitioner constantly monitors the child's responses and frequently adjusts the activity in response to the child's state. For example, if a child is actively rotating while sitting in a tire swing and begins to exhibit mild signs of autonomic activation, the occupational therapy practitioner might intervene by acting to reduce the intensity of the swinging, guide the child to shift to slow linear swinging, or increase proprioceptive input by offering the child a trapeze to pull. This latter strategy (increasing proprioceptive input) is derived from animal research showing that proprioceptive input has an inhibitory effect on vestibular activation (Fredrickson et al., 1966). Knowledge of the effects of vestibular stimulation and its interactions with other sensory systems is critical in this treatment approach.

Similarly, tactile stimulation during ASI is informed by knowledge about this sensory system and how it interacts with arousal processes as well as other sensory systems. Passive tactile stimulation is not often used. Imposing tactile stimulation on a child who is tactile defensive may lead to a state of greater sensitization, in which the child becomes increasingly more defensive instead of habituating. Instead of using passive tactile stimulation, tactile stimuli are usually incorporated into the materials and surfaces that the child contacts while engaging in activities under their active control, for example, through manipulation of objects with varying shapes and textures or through contact with surfaces that have diverse textures.

## Summary of Essential Features of ASI Intervention

To summarize the essential features of ASI intervention, therapeutic activities are neither predetermined nor are they simply free play. The flow of the treatment session involves collaboration between the occupational therapy practitioner and child in which the practitioner encourages and supports the child in a way that moves the child toward therapeutic goals. This all takes place within a special environment that is safe yet challenging. To determine if a child can benefit from ASI intervention, a comprehensive occupational therapy assessment, including an in-depth evaluation of sensory integration, must be conducted (see Chapter 9 for more information about comprehensive evaluation and specific assessments for sensory functions). Assessment findings are used to determine whether ASI is appropriate and desirable for the individual child. If so, assessment findings guide treatment planning (Schaaf et al., 2012). Because challenges in sensory integration are often identified early in life and can affect occupational performance over many phases of development, ASI intervention may be appropriate for extended or intermittent periods across childhood.

Because of the highly specialized and complex nature of the ASI approach, application of this approach requires training beyond entry level practice in occupational therapy (Watling el al., 2011). A mentorship process is the best preparation for learning how to clinically apply sensory integration principles (Koomar & Bundy, 2002). Self-study of professional and scholarly resources relevant to this area of practice is also important in developing professional competencies. In addition, ongoing personal study and discussion with peers are highly recommended after acquiring advanced training, to hone clinical expertise and explore emerging evidence in the field.

Although ASI intervention often occurs within specialized therapy centers, many of the concepts can be applied in other settings as well. School-based occupational therapy practitioners have found ways to incorporate the central principles of ASI into the educational setting, including bringing specialized equipment into classrooms, therapy rooms, and playgrounds in ways that help organize and prepare a child for learning (Whiting et al., 2023). Successful therapy programs frequently involve helping families understand and use the sensory integration concepts that support and facilitate their children's success by developing activities at home and identifying resources within the

## CASE EXAMPLE 27.1 KAREN

### History

Karen was born after a full-term pregnancy complicated by gestational diabetes. Labor, which was induced at 40 weeks, was prolonged, and it was believed that Karen broke her right collarbone during delivery. Karen achieved her early motor and language milestones within the average age ranges. However, she was described as an irritable baby who had difficulty breastfeeding, startled easily, and could be calmed only by swinging. Karen attended a parent cooperative child development program as a toddler, and at 4 years of age, she was eligible for a special education preschool program through her school district. She has not been given any specific medical or educational diagnosis.

### Reason for Referral

Karen's mother expressed concern about Karen's fine and gross motor skills to a neurologist, who referred Karen for an occupational therapy assessment when she was 4 years of age. When asked why she was seeking an evaluation for Karen, her mother wrote, "Up until recently I had been very patiently waiting for normal development to occur (for example, handedness, fine motor). The school psychologist feels that this still may occur, but I am convinced that something isn't right. Karen's increasing frustration and decreasing belief in herself prompted me to seek evaluations. While a part of me wishes to have a 'normal child,' the other part will be relieved to find that the child I have had so many doubts about since infancy does indeed have some behaviors and actions that are unusual."

### Evaluation Procedure

The SIPT was administered in one testing session. Karen was also observed in a clinical therapy setting and at home. In addition, Karen's mother was interviewed, and she completed a developmental and sensory history on which she provided detailed accounts of Karen's early and current sensorimotor, language, cognitive, social, and self-care development.

### Evaluation Results

On the SIPT, Karen scored below average for age expectations on seven of 17 tests. This profile was generated through computer scoring by the test publisher. The unit of measure represented by the scores is a statistical measure called a *standard deviation*, which represents how different the child's score is from that of an average child of the same age. The closer a child's score is to zero on the horizontal axis, the closer to average is the child's performance on that test. Karen's scores are plotted as solid squares that are connected by a dark line on the computer-generated profile. Scores falling below −1.0 on the horizontal axis are possibly indicative of dysfunction.

One of Karen's scores was low on a motor-free visual perception test (space visualization), and it was noted that she had difficulty fitting a geometric form into a puzzle board during this test. Her mother reported that Karen knew colors at 18 months of age but had trouble learning shapes. However, she was reported to have a strong visual memory for roads, signs, and faces. These findings suggested difficulty with spatial orientation of objects but relative strengths in visual memory.

Karen had several low scores and showed signs of difficulty performing on several of the tests of somatosensory and vestibular processing. A low score on finger identification suggested inefficient tactile feedback involving the hands. This was corroborated by observations of poor manipulative skills during activities such as buttoning and using utensils. She was also observed to have signs of tactile defensiveness, also corroborated by her mother's report. Her low score on Kinesthesia, as well as her difficulty in exerting the appropriate amount of pressure on a pencil and in positioning her body for dressing, suggested problems with proprioceptive feedback.

Karen's lowest score on the SIPT was on the Postrotary Nystagmus test (−2.2 standard deviations). This low score, as well as below-average scores on Standing and Walking Balance, observations of poor functional balance in dressing and playground activities, a tendency not to cross her body midline, poor bilateral coordination in activities such as cutting, and reports that she never appeared to get dizzy, pointed to the probability of vestibular processing problems.

Karen showed above-average performance on a praxis test on which she could rely on verbal directions. However, tests of motor planning that were more somatosensory dependent (Oral Praxis and Postural Praxis) were substantially more difficult for her. Karen was unable to ride a tricycle, pump a swing, or skip. She had extreme difficulty planning her movements to dress herself or even letting someone else dress her. She also had a great deal of difficulty using utensils during eating and often choked on food and drinks. Writing skills were particularly difficult for Karen, and her lack of hand preference, immature grasp, and hesitancy to cross her midline hampered her attempts at drawing or writing.

Karen was reported to be a social child who was liked by adults and younger peers. However, her mother worried that she did not seem able to "pick up on the hints and unwritten rules of her peers" and was "definitely starting to march to her own beat." She noticed increasing signs of frustration that she thought were beginning to impinge on Karen's willingness to participate with peers.

Overall, the evaluation results suggested problems in sensory processing of some aspects of visual, tactile, proprioceptive, and vestibular sensory information. These difficulties were seen as related to somatodyspraxia, poor balance and bilateral integration, difficulties with specific gross and fine motor skills, and emerging concerns around socialization. Karen's strengths included age-appropriate cognitive and language skills, good ability to motor plan actions using verbal directions, and an exceptionally supportive and involved family.

### Recommendation

Based on the evaluation results and a meeting of Karen's Individualized Education Program team, who met shortly after the assessment, it was recommended that Karen receive individual occupational therapy using a sensory integration approach to enhance foundational sensory and motor processes. Because of her significant sensory integrative problems and need for a specialized approach, the therapy was recommended to initially occur in a setting equipped for Ayres Sensory Integration (ASI) intervention.

### Occupational Therapy Program

In the first 6 months of individual occupational therapy, an ASI approach was used that included individualized, carefully selected therapeutic activities aimed at enhancing visual, tactile, proprioceptive, and vestibular sensory processing. As part of her intervention program, Karen's occupational therapy practitioner provided her with graded challenges to praxis, bilateral coordination, and balance.

After 6 months of therapy, Karen has decreasing tactile defensiveness, a reduced tendency to choke on food, acquisition of the ability to ride a tricycle, and an improved ability to plan new or unusual motor actions. Although these are significant gains for Karen, she continues to exhibit substantial difficulties with many aspects of sensory processing, general motor planning ability, and many age-appropriate fine and gross motor skills. If she continues to respond to occupational therapy using an ASI approach, it is expected that by the beginning of the next school year (in about 6 months), she will have improved in basic sensory and motor functions to the extent that some specific skill training will become more appropriate. It is likely that at that time some therapy will occur at school with the introduction of a consultation program for her teacher. Her parents have already begun a home program, which appears to support the gains she is making through direct services. Karen's young age and initial positive response to therapy make her an optimal candidate for application of the sensory integration approach, and her long-term outlook is excellent.

community that reinforce the experiences emphasized during therapy (Schaaf & Mailloux, 2015).

## Expected Outcomes of ASI Intervention

Occupational therapy aims to improve a child's health and quality of life through engagement in meaningful and important occupations or activities. To accomplish this with a young child who has sensory integrative problems, the occupational therapy practitioner usually first aims to improve sensory integrative functions through direct ASI intervention. Based on the premise of neuroplasticity in the young and developing brain, sensory integration theory holds that many of the child's sensory integration functions improve with individually tailored therapeutic activities that provide opportunities for exploration and challenge. In addition to addressing the underlying sensory integration problems, occupational therapy practitioners also often help the child develop specific skills and strategies to minimize the effects of the problems the child is experiencing and to help the child cope with the current day-to-day demands. Finally, consulting with parents and teachers to allow for carryover of direct intervention and to plan modifications of activities, routines, and environments is an important component of any intervention program involving children. Often direct intervention, specific skill training, and consultation are thoughtfully combined in an intervention plan that is designed to meet the needs of the child and family. Fig. 27.7A and B show children engaging in successful adaptive responses through play.

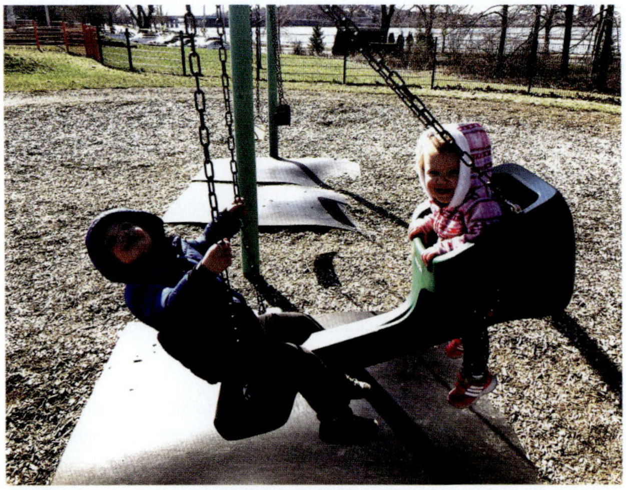

Fig. 27.6 These young children enjoy the organizing sensation of linear vestibular movement provided by the swing.

The child's goals and objectives target specific occupations, such as eating, play, rest, work, and self-care, in which positive changes are expected. For example, a toddler who tends to be overstimulated much of the time because of severe sensory reactivity difficulties may consequently have difficulty falling and staying asleep. Sleep deprivation can aggravate hyperreactivity and behavior problems for the child and can also disrupt occupational performance of other family members. A goal may be for the child to acquire more predictable sleep patterns with adequate amounts of sleep. A related objective might be that the child will accept unpredictable sensations such as household sounds, change in room temperature, or the texture of sheets and blankets to successfully nap without interruption for at least 1 hour for 3 days per week. The intervention could involve direct remediation to reduce the sensory defensiveness, as well as parent coaching on strategies such as calming activities, a predictable activity schedule including a specific rest time ritual, and creation of an arousal-reducing environment after lunch (e.g., lights dimmed and noise reduced and screened with rhythmic sounds or "white noise"). Expected outcomes are summarized in Table 27.1.

## Evidence of Effectiveness of ASI Intervention

A recent systematic review of ASI intervention found strong evidence of its effectiveness in improving participation of children with sensory integration difficulties, specifically those with a diagnosis of autism spectrum disorder (Schaaf et al., 2018). One important characteristic

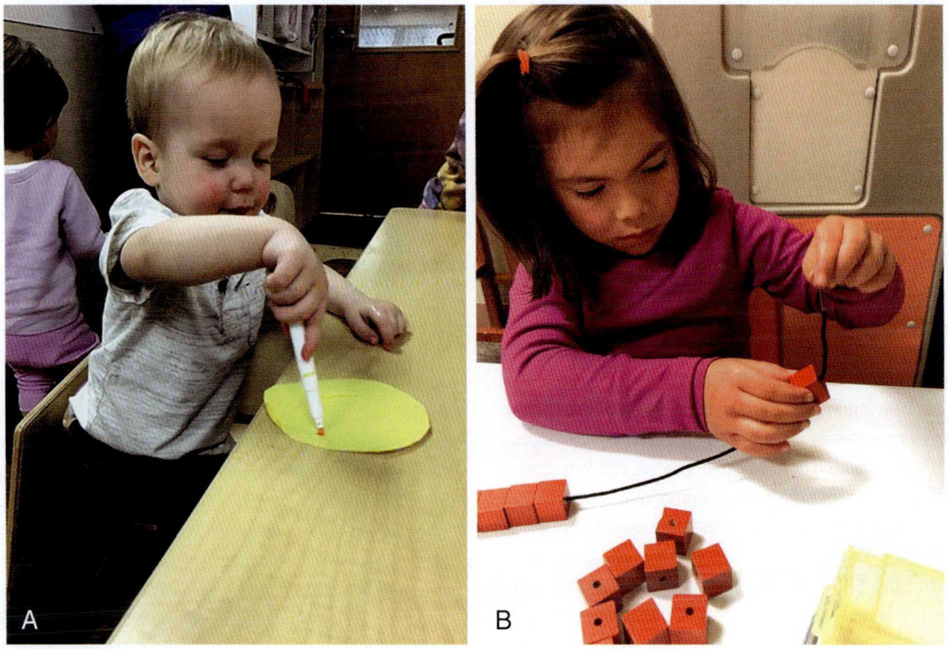

Fig. 27.7 (A) This preschooler experiements with holding a pen to make marks on paper. This activity requires the integration of tactile, proprioceptive, and visual sensations, in addition to postural stability. (B) This young girl can concentrate on stringing beads, which requires tactile, vestibular, and proprioceptive processing. ((A) Photo courtesy Kathryn Loukas.)

**TABLE 27.1 Expected Outcomes of Occupational Therapy Using a Sensory Integration Approach**

| Expected Outcome | Explanation | Example |
|---|---|---|
| Increase in the frequency or duration of adaptive responses | Increasing the duration and frequency of adaptive responses is an important outcome of sensory integration because functional behavior and skills are developed by mastering simple adaptive responses. The Ayres Sensory Integration (ASI) intervention approach intensively focuses on the child's acquisition of higher-level adaptive responses. | A child who has difficulty staying with an activity for more than a few seconds tends to shift from one activity to another, thus never having the chance to fully process the sensation and develop purposeful actions in response to it. A desirable outcome for that child might be to remain involved in a simple activity, such as swinging, for longer periods of time. |
| Development of increasingly more complex adaptive responses | More complex adaptive responses may require timing and sequencing, as well as integration of various sensory functions.<br>The result is an improvement in the child's ability to make judgments about the environment, what can be done with objects, and which specific actions need to be taken to accomplish a goal. | An example is a child releasing grasp while swinging on a trapeze, and then at just the right moment, jumping off to land on a pillow. This is more complex than simply holding on, or letting go of the trapeze at random times. |
| Improvement in gross and fine motor skills | The child who makes consistent and more complex adaptive responses shows evidence of improved sensory integration. Moreover, this child meets new challenges with greater self-confidence. A net result of these gains frequently is greater mastery in the motor domain. | An example is the child with a vestibular processing problem who exhibits greater competency and interest in playground activities and sports after individual ASI intervention, even though these activities were not practiced during therapy. Motor skills may be among the earliest complex skills to show measurable change in response to an ASI approach, probably because extensive motor activity is inherent in this intervention approach (Andelin et al., 2021; Ottenbacher, 1982). |
| Improvement in cognitive, language, and academic performance | Although cognitive, language, and academic skills are not usually the specific objectives of ASI, improvement in these domains has been detected in some effectiveness studies involving the provision of ASI intervention (Ayres, 1972; 1978; Ayres & Mailloux, 1981; Magrun et al., 1981; Ray et al., 1989). Application of ASI therapeutic procedures is thought to generate broad-based changes in these areas secondary to enhancement of sensory reactivity, perception, postural control, or praxis (Ayres, 1979; Cabbay & King, 1989). | Improvement in sensory reactivity may lead to a better ability to attend to language and academic tasks; thus improvements in these areas may follow.<br>A child who has a vestibular processing disorder may improve in postural control and equilibrium, freeing the child to concentrate more efficiently on academic learning, without the distraction of frequent loss of sitting balance or loss of place while copying from the blackboard. |
| Increase in self-confidence and self-esteem | The outcome of therapy that encourages successful, self-directed experiences is a child who perceives the self as a competent actor in the world. Ayres asserted that enhanced ability to make adaptive responses promotes self-actualization by allowing the child to experience the joy of accomplishing a task that previously could not be done (Ayres, 1979).<br>Mastery of such activities is expected to result in feelings of personal control that, in turn, lead to increased willingness to take risks and try new things (Ayres, 1979; Cohn et al., 2000). | A child with gravitational insecurity may experience not only fear responses to climbing and movement activities but also feelings of failure and frustration when limited in participating in the play of peers. In such a case, improvement in these areas would lead to an increase in self-confidence and comfort in one's physical body, accompanied by a general boost in feelings of self-efficacy and worth. |
| Enhanced occupational engagement and social participation | As the child develops general sensory integrative capabilities and improved strategies for planning action, gains are seen in relation to the ability to master self-care tasks, cope with daily routines, and organize behavior more generally (Ayres, 1979). | Intervention may help the child who is overly sensitive to touch or movement respond to sensations in a more adaptive manner. As a result, the child approaches and engages in the challenges of everyday occupations, such as getting ready for school in the morning, sharing a table with others in the school cafeteria, behaving appropriately in the classroom, and playing with friends on the playground with greater security and confidence (Kuhaneck et al., 2023). |

*Continued*

**TABLE 27.1 Expected Outcomes of Occupational Therapy Using a Sensory Integration Approach—cont'd**

| Expected Outcome | Explanation | Example |
|---|---|---|
| Enhanced family life | When children with sensory integrative problems experience positive changes during intervention, their lives and the lives of other family members may be enhanced. One possible by-product of intervention based on ASI principles is that parents gain a better understanding of their children's behavior and begin to generate their own strategies for organizing family routines in a way that supports the entire family system. An important outcome of sensory integrative intervention, then, may include changes in parents' understanding of the child, leading to new coping strategies and alleviation of parental stress (Cohn & Cermak, 1998). In her studies of parental perspectives, Cohn has found that an important outcome of the sensory integrative approach is that parents tend to "reframe" their view and expectations of their children in a positive manner (Cohn, 2001). | For example, behavior that is interpreted as bizarre, such as insisting on wearing tight rubber bands on the arms, may be reframed as a meaningful strategy that the child uses to obtain deep pressure input for self-calming (Anderson, 1993). Instead of viewing the behavior as a frustrating sign of pathology that should be eliminated, reframing may lead the parents to explore other ways that they could provide the child with the deep pressure experiences that he or she seeks. |

of this review, as opposed to some earlier reviews, was the use of very specific inclusion and exclusion criteria to ensure that ASI intervention was provided appropriately in each of the studies analyzed. When reading studies of ASI intervention effectiveness, practitioners need to be aware of methodologic limitations that are common in research on interventions for children with developmental, learning, and behavioral challenges (May-Benson & Koomar, 2010; Miller, 2003; Mulligan, 2003). For example, a common limitation in some effectiveness studies of ASI is that children may have been provided this intervention without confirming whether they actually have any problems with sensory integration, based on a thorough assessment using several methods, such as standardized tests, structured clinical observations, and norm-referenced parent and/or teacher questionnaires. Another common limitation is that the intervention provided in a study may have been called sensory integration but was not actually provided in a manner that matches the defining characteristics of ASI (Parham et al., 2007). This type of limitation is called a fidelity problem. In intervention research, the term **fidelity** refers to the extent to which the intervention provided in a study is faithful to the key elements of the intervention approach.

A reliable and valid fidelity instrument, the Fidelity Measure for ASI Intervention, was developed to provide researchers with a rigorous method for ensuring that ASI intervention would be applied appropriately (May-Benson et al., 2014; Parham et al., 2011). The Fidelity Measure addresses two main aspects of ASI intervention: (1) structural elements and (2) process elements. Structural elements include features such as availability of a variety of sensory integration therapeutic equipment in the therapy room; procedures for maintaining safe use of therapeutic equipment; adequate space in the therapy room to ensure safety; and systematic documentation of essential information such as reasons for referral, assessment findings, recommendations based on referral and assessment information, and documentation briefly describing activities provided within therapy sessions and how these relate to specific goals. Process elements include activities the therapist is responsible for doing throughout ASI therapy sessions (Parham et al., 2011). In action, these elements occur simultaneously and interactively. See Box 27.3 for a description of the process elements.

Because rigorous research has verified the effectiveness of ASI intervention for children with autism, the National Clearinghouse on Autism Evidence and Practice at the University of North Carolina at Chapel Hill identified ASI intervention as an "evidence-based practice" for children with autism spectrum disorders (Steinbrenner et al., 2020). It is important to note that the systematic review of ASI effectiveness cited earlier (Schaaf et al., 2018) included only the studies that met the criteria for fidelity described in the Fidelity Measure for ASI Intervention, in order to verify that the Intervention provided in the study was truly ASI intervention (Schaaf et al., 2014; Schoen et al., 2019).

An important issue in intervention trials is the maintenance of long-term gains after completion of a period of ASI intervention. An encouraging finding reported by Wilson and Kaplan (1994) suggests that children with learning difficulties who receive sensory integration intervention may obtain long-term benefits that are not obtained by children who receive other interventions. Although this study was published long before development of the Fidelity Measure for ASI Intervention, a systematic review of fidelity in sensory integration research found that the intervention in this study included most of the key fidelity elements of ASI identified by Parham et al. (2007). Although no significant differences in outcomes were found between the two intervention groups in the original study (i.e., both the ASI and tutoring groups made significant gains) (Wilson et al., 1992), at follow-up, 2 years later, only the children who had received ASI maintained the gains that they had made after intervention. Maintenance of intervention gains is a critical issue that is relevant to the cost-effectiveness of intervention. Additional studies are needed to measure long-term outcomes of ASI.

Although randomized clinical trials are the gold standard of effectiveness studies, other research designs examining intervention outcomes also make valuable contributions to understanding the effects of sensory integration intervention. In research using single-subject designs, a child serves as their own control and is monitored repeatedly before intervention (the baseline phase) and during intervention. An advantage to this approach is that behavioral outcomes can be highly individualized and tracked over time to provide an understanding of each child's response to intervention. For example, Linderman and Stewart (1999) measured three behavioral outcomes of ASI for two preschool children with pervasive developmental disorders. Each outcome was observed in the child's home and was tailored to address functional issues for each child (e.g., response to holding and hugging for one child and functional communication during mealtime for the other). Results indicated significant improvements between baseline and intervention phases for five of the

**BOX 27.3 The Process Elements of Ayres Sensory Integration According to the Fidelity Measure (Parham et al., 2011)**

1. *Ensures physical safety:* The physical space arrangement and materials in the therapy room, as well as the occupational therapy practitioner's actions, ensure the child's physical safety.
2. *Presents sensory opportunities:* Using therapeutic equipment, materials, and activities, the occupational therapy practitioner provides the child with sensory-rich activities, particularly those that involve body-centered (tactile, proprioceptive, and vestibular) sensory experiences.
3. *Supports sensory modulation for attaining and maintaining a regulated state:* The occupational therapy practitioner modifies sensory conditions and activity challenges to help the child attain optimal arousal, alertness, and affect for engagement in activities.
4. *Challenges postural, ocular, oral, and/or bilateral motor control:* Using assessment data regarding areas of need, the occupational therapy practitioner introduces, supports, or modifies activities to provide challenges to these areas of motor control.
5. *Challenges praxis and organization of behavior:* Using assessment data regarding areas of need, the occupational therapy practitioner introduces, supports, or modifies activities to challenge the child's motor planning, ideation, and/or ability to plan and engage in organized activities.
6. *Collaborates in activity choice:* The occupational therapy practitioner strives to share control with the child in choosing, modifying, or changing activities; ultimately the goal is that activities are chosen collaboratively by the occupational therapy practitioner and child.
7. *Tailors activity to present just right challenge:* To ensure the child's optimal engagement, the practitioner tailors activities so that they are at the "just right" level of challenge, by suggesting or supporting an increase or decrease in task complexity, so that the activity is not too difficult or too easy for the child to do independently or with practitioner support.
8. *Ensures that activities are successful:* The occupational therapy practitioner strives to provide challenges in which the child will experience feelings of success.
9. *Supports child's intrinsic motivation to play:* The child's intrinsic motivation to play is prioritized in the ASI approach, so the occupational therapy practitioner creates a setting that supports play to fully engage the child in the intervention.
10. *Establishes a therapeutic alliance with the child:* In ASI, a strong positive relationship between the child and occupational therapy practitioner is essential; therefore, the occupational therapy practitioner establishes an interpersonal connection with the child, forming a therapeutic alliance that entails working together in a mutually enjoyable partnership.

six outcomes measured. These results are encouraging, but they should be considered tentative because of the small number of participants and the absence of a fidelity measure.

There have been other recent studies using single-subject research designs with subjects with autism or a sensory-based motor disorder (Andelin et al., 2021; Kuhaneck et al., 2023). These authors found gains in motor skills and changes in the frequency of varied forms of play following ASI intervention. A third study noted improved child playfulness and parental support of playfulness following ASI with parent training; however the changes were not maintained (Waldman-Levi & Kuhaneck, 2023).

Future studies can build on current research to explore questions regarding characteristics of children who are the best candidates for ASI intervention, the types of outcomes that can be expected, and the most effective dosages. It would be reasonable to expect different intervention outcomes for children with different types or severity of sensory integration difficulties or with concomitant developmental or medical diagnoses; however, these factors have not been systematically addressed since Ayres's pioneering research (Ayres, 1972, 1978; Ayres & Mailloux, 1981; Ayres & Tickle, 1980). Research addressing this issue could help practitioners predict who will best respond to individual ASI intervention and who may be better served by other intervention approaches. The effectiveness of systematically combining individual ASI intervention with other interventions, such as specific sensory techniques, sensory environmental modifications at home or in the classroom, cognitive interventions, and parent coaching or education, also needs further research. Finally, long-term maintenance of gains, particularly those related to social participation outcomes, is an important issue that should be addressed in future research.

## Measuring Outcomes of ASI Intervention

Because every child with a sensory integrative problem is unique, the expected outcomes of an ASI approach are individualized and diverse. Goals are often stated as objectives that target observed behaviors of the child. Fig. 27.8A and B shows children who met their goals. These objectives should contain a specific description of the desired behavior, including the context of the behavior and an objective way to measure the behavior, for example, by timing how long the child can sustain an activity or with what percentage of success she can perform it after a specified number of attempts. Some good examples of measurable outcomes that target child-specific behaviors are provided by single-subject studies (Andelin et al., 2021; Case-Smith & Bryan, 1999; Kuhaneck et al., 2023; Linderman & Stewart, 1999).

Additionally, outcomes are sometimes measured using standardized tests. In fact, some subtests of the Sensory Integration and Praxis Test (SIPT) (e.g., Design Copying, Standing and Walking Balance, and most of the praxis tests) are good measures of change because of their strong test-retest reliability, in addition to being relevant to concerns that are commonly voiced by parents and teachers. However, standardized tests often do not address key occupational issues. When used, care must be taken to select a test that is likely to be sensitive to the kinds of changes expected for the child. Sometimes changes in raw scores are more informative than changes in standardized scores because raw score change is a direct measure of the child's improvement in skill relative to performance at initial assessment. Comparing the child's performance to normative data may not detect actual changes in performance.

Goal attainment scaling (GAS) is an alternative to standardized tests that addresses the uniquely individualized nature of expected outcomes of ASI. Goal attainment scaling provides a means to prioritize goals that are specifically relevant to individuals and their families and to quantify the results using a standard metric that allows comparison of achievement across different types of goals. Evidence indicates that this approach is useful for capturing outcomes of ASI intervention programs (Mailloux et al., 2007).

## Other Interventions for Children With Sensory Integrative Challenges

In addition to ASI intervention, occupational therapy practitioners may introduce other interventions to help a child with sensory integration difficulties. For example, educating parents or teachers to understand the child's sensory characteristics, and how they influence the child's behavior, is an important component of any intervention program for children (see Fig. 27.9). This may lead parents and teachers to create new ideas for how to modify activities, routines, and environments in ways that are tailored to support the child's participation. Often ASI intervention, specific skill training, and parent/teacher education or coaching are all thoughtfully included in a treatment plan that is designed to meet the needs of the child and family.

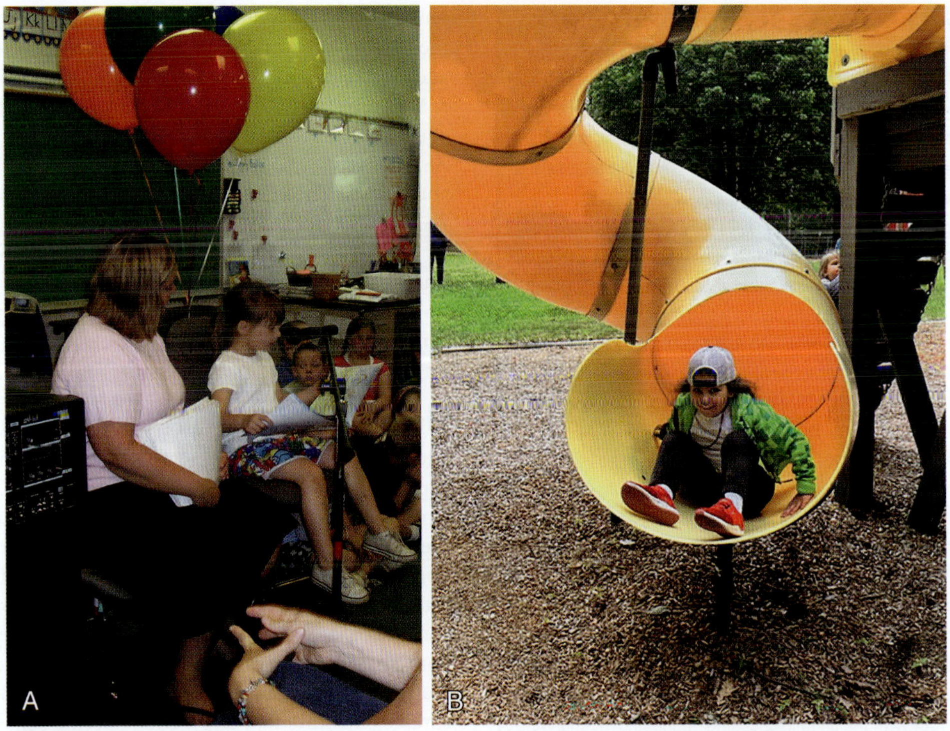


**Fig. 27.8** (A) This first grader can sit in front of the class, attend, read her story, and engage in the classroom experience with her peers. (B) This young child plays on the playground equipment (i.e., climbs up and slides down the slide) by herself. ((A) Photo courtesy Jane OBrien. (B) Photo courtesy Carol Lambdin-Pattavina.)

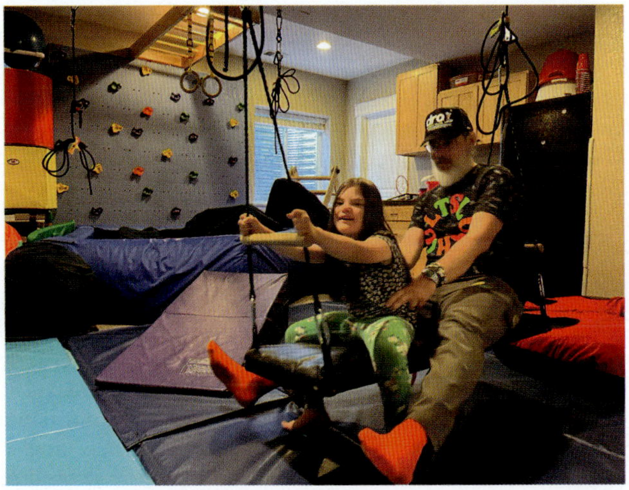

**Fig. 27.9** Occupational therapy practitioners educate parents about the child's sensory processing strengths and challenges, so they can understand their child and support them. In this session, the therapist involves the young girl's father in the session. (Photo courtesy Renee Allen.)

## SUMMARY

Ayres Sensory Integration intervention, created by Dr. A. Jean Ayres, is an approach used frequently by occupational therapists. Children who have difficulty processing sensory information (e.g., visual, tactile, auditory, vestibular, proprioceptive, and taste) experience challenges in movement, organization, timing, and planning. They may over- or under-respond to sensory stimuli that interferes with their ability to engage in daily tasks. For example, children may be reluctant to try new movements, or they may respond negatively to noises, touch, movement, or sounds, affecting their ability to attend to directions or complete academic or home tasks. Children with sensory integration dysfunction exhibit a cluster of sensory challenges that interfere with their daily functioning. Occupational therapy practitioners using this approach receive additional training and follow fidelity measures for best practice.

1. The Fidelity Measure for ASI Intervention can be used to ensure that when ASI intervention is provided, the process of intervention

as well as the occupational therapy practitioner's qualifications and the therapeutic environment are appropriate. ASI intervention may be appropriate when assessment results indicate a known pattern of sensory integration difficulty for children with a wide range of learning and behavioral challenges. Occupational therapy practitioners using ASI provide the just right challenge by facilitating an adaptive response from the child through activities that challenge vestibular, tactile, and proprioception. The child is an active participant and has choice throughout the playful sessions.

2. Challenges in sensory integration affect occupational performance. Increasing sensory integration functions through ASI addresses the underlying sensory integration challenges to develop specific skills and strategies to enable the child to experience success, health, and quality of life through engagement in meaningful and important occupations and activities. ASI is designed to help children gain confidence and competencies that directly carry over to everyday occupations at home, at school, or in the community.
3. The best evidence of effectiveness of ASI intervention uses rigorous research design, including fidelity checks, and provides encouraging evidence of effectiveness, particularly when goal attainment scaling is used. Other interventions that are used in conjunction with or instead of ASI intervention include specific skill training, group skill training, specific sensory techniques, sensory environmental modifications, cognitive interventions, occupation-based interventions, and teacher or parent education and coaching. Outcomes vary for these diverse interventions, but a growing body of evidence provides valuable information to guide the practitioner's decision-making and recommendations.

## REFERENCES


Andelin, L., Reynolds, S., & Schoen, S. (2021). Effectiveness of occupational therapy using a sensory integration approach: A multiple-baseline design study. *American Journal of Occupational Therapy, 75*(6), 7506205030. https://doi.org/10.5014/ajot.2021.044917.

Anderson, E. L. (1993). *Parental perceptions of the influence of occupational therapy utilizing sensory integration techniques on the daily living skills of children with autism (Unpublished master's thesis)*. Los Angeles: University of Southern California.

Ayres, A. J. (1972). Improving academic scores through sensory integration. *Journal of Learning Disabilities, 5*, 338–343.

Ayres, A. J. (1978). Learning disabilities and the vestibular system. *Journal of Learning Disabilities, 11*(1), 30–41.

Ayres, A. J., & Mailloux, Z. (1981). Influence of sensory integration procedures on language development. *American Journal of Occupational Therapy, 35*(6), 383–390.

Ayres, A. J. (1973). *Sensory integration and learning disorders*. Western Psychological Services.

Ayres, A. J. (1979). *Sensory integration and the child*. Western Psychological Services.

Ayres, A. J., & Tickle, L. (1980). Hyperresponsivity to touch and vestibular stimuli as a predictor of positive response to sensory integration procedures in autistic children. *American Journal of Occupational Therapy, 34*, 375–381.

Cabbay, M., & King, L. J. (1989). Sensory integration and perception: The foundation for concept formation. *Occupational Therapy in Practice*, 18–27.

Case-Smith, J., & Bryan, T. (1999). The effects of occupational therapy with sensory integration emphasis on preschool-age children with autism. *American Journal of Occupational Therapy, 53*, 489–497.

Clark, F. A., Mailloux, Z., & Parham, D. (1989). Sensory integration and children with learning disorders. In P. N. Pratt, & A. S. Allen (Eds.), *Occupational therapy for children* (2nd ed.) (pp. 457–509). Mosby.

Cohn, E. S. (2001). Parent perspectives of occupational therapy using a sensory integration approach. *American Journal of Occupational Therapy, 55*, 285–294. https://doi.org/10.5014/ajot.55.3.285.

Cohn, E. S., & Cermak, S. A. (1998). Including the family perspective in sensory integration outcomes research. *American Journal of Occupational Therapy, 52*(7), 540–546. https://doi.org/10.5014/ajot.52.7.540.

Cohn, E. S., Miller, L. J., & Tickle-Degnen, L. (2000). Parental hopes for therapy outcomes; Children with sensory modulation disorders. *American Journal of Occupational Therapy, 54*, 36–43. https://doi.org/10.5014/ajot.54.1.36.

Fredrickson, J. M., Schwartz, D. W., & Kornhuber, H. H. (1966). Convergence and interaction of vestibular and deep somatic afferents upon neurons in the vestibular nuclei of the cat. *Acta Oto-Laryngologica, 61*, 168–188.

Gaylard, A. (1966). Treatment of children with perceptual problems: An introduction to the role of the occupational therapist. *Canadian Journal of Occupational Therapy, 32*(2), 53–61.

Kimball, J. G. (1999). Sensory integrative frame of reference. In P. Kramer, & J. Hinojosa (Eds.), *Frames of for pediatric occupational therapy* (pp. 169–204). Williams & Wilkins.

Koomar, J. A., & Bundy, A. C. (2002). Creating direct intervention from theory. In A. C. Bundy, S. J. Lane, & E. A. Murray (Eds.), *Sensory integration: Theory and practice* (2nd ed.) (pp. 261–308). F. A. Davis.

Kuhaneck, H., & Spitzer, S. L. (2024). The importnace of conceptual origins: The case of the just-right challenge. *American Journal of Occupational Therapy, 78*(4), 78–4185110. https://doi.org/10.5014/ajot.2024.050616.

Kuhaneck, H. M., Watling, R., & Glennon, T. J. (2023). Ayres Sensory Integration® for addressing play in autistic children: A multiple-baseline examination. *American Journal of Occupational Therapy, 77*(2). https://doi.org/10.5014/ajot.2023.050169. 7702205080.

Linderman, T. M., & Stewart, K. B. (1999). Sensory integrative-based occupational therapy and functional outcomes in young children with pervasive developmental disorders: A single-subject study. *American Journal of Occupational Therapy, 53*, 207 213.

Lindquist, J. E., Mack, W., & Parham, L. D. (1982). A synthesis of occupational behavior and sensory integration concepts in theory and practice, Part 2: Clinical applications. *American Journal of Occupational Therapy, 36*(7), 433–437.

Mack, W., Lindquist, J. E., & Parham, L. D. (1982). A synthesis of occupational behavior and sensory integration concepts in theory and practice, Part 1. Theoretical foundations. *American Journal of Occupational Therapy, 36*(6), 365–374.

Magrun, M., Ottenbacher, K., McCue, S., & Keefe, R. (1981). Effects of vestibular stimulation on spontaneous use of verbal language in developmentally delayed children. *American Journal of Occupational Therapy, 35*(2), 101–104. https://doi.org/10.5014/ajot.35.2.101.

Mailloux, Z., et al. (2007). The issue is—goal attainment scaling as a measure of meaningful outcomes for children with sensory integration disorders. *American Journal of Occupational Therapy, 61*(2), 254–259.

May-Benson, T. A., et al. (2014). Structural elements of the Ayres Sensory Integration fidelity measure. *American Journal of Occupational Therapy, 68*, 506–513.

May-Benson, T. A., & Koomar, J. A. (2010). Systematic review of the research evidence examining the effectiveness of interventions using a sensory integrative approach for children. *American Journal of Occupational Therapy, 64*, 403–414.

Michelman, S. S. (1974). Play and the deficit child. In M. Reilly (Ed.), *Play as exploratory learning* (pp. 157–207). Sage Publications.

Miller, L. J. (2003). Empirical evidence related to therapies for sensory processing impairments. *National Association of School Psychologist Communique, 31*(5), 34–37.

Mulligan, S. (2003). Examination of the evidence for occupational therapy using a sensory integration framework with children: Part two. *Sensory Integration Special Interest Section Quarterly, 26*(2), 1–5.

Ottenbacher, K. (1982). Sensory integration therapy: Affect or effect. *American Journal of Occupational Therapy, 36*(9), 571–578. https://doi.org/10.5014/ajot.36.9.571.

Parham, L. D., et al. (2011). Development of a fidelity measure for research on Ayres Sensory Integration. *American Journal of Occupational Therapy, 65*, 133–142.

Parham, L. D., et al. (2007). Fidelity in sensory integration intervention research. *American Journal of Occupational Therapy, 61*, 216–227.

Ray, T. C., King, L. K., & Grandin, T. (1989). The effectiveness of self-initiated vestibular stimulation in producing speech sounds in an autistic child. *Occupational Therapy Journal of Research, 8*, 186–190.

Roley, S. S., et al. (2007). Understanding Ayres Sensory Integration. *Occupational Therapy Practice, 12*(17), CE1–CE8.

Schaaf, R. C., Dumont, R. L., Arbesman, M., & May-Benson, T. A. (2018). *Efficacy of occupational therapy using Ayres Sensory Integration: A systematic.*

Schaaf, R. C., et al. (2014). An intervention for sensory difficulties in children with autism: A randomized trial. *Journal of Autism and Developmental Disorders, 44*(7), 1493–1506.

Schaaf, R. C., Hunt, J., & Benevides, T. (2012). Occupational therapy using sensory integration to improve participation of a child with autism: A case report. *American Journal of Occupational Therapy, 66*, 547–555.

Schaaf, R., & Mailloux, Z. (2015). *Promoting participation for children with autism: A clinician's guide for implementing Ayres Sensory Integration.* AOTA.

Schoen, S., et al. (2019). A systematic review of Ayres Sensory Integration intervention for children with autism. *Autism Research, 12*, 6–19.

Slavik, B. A., & Chew, T. (1990). The design of a sensory integration treatment facility: The Ayres Clinic as a model. In S. C. Merrill (Ed.), *Environment: Implications for occupational therapy practice* (pp. 85–101). American Occupational Therapy Association.

Slavik, B. A., et al. (1984). Vestibular stimulation and eye contact in autistic children. *Neuropediatrics, 15*, 333–336.

Steinbrenner, J. R., et al. (2020). *Evidence-based practices for children, youth, and young adults with Autism.* The University of North Carolina at Chapel Hill, Frank Porter Graham Child Development Institute, National Clearinghouse on Autism Evidence and Practice Review Team, 120.

Waldman-Levi, A., & Kuhaneck, H. (2023). Father–child playfulness: A secondary analysis of a multiple-baseline single-subject study of three children with autism spectrum disorder. *American Journal of Occupational Therapy, 77*(2).

Walker, K. F. (1991). Sensory integrative therapy in a limited space: An adaptation of the Ayres Clinic design. *Sensory Integration Special Interest Section Newsletter, 14*(3) 1, 2, 4.

Watling, R., et al. (2011). *Occupational therapy practice guidelines for children and adolescents with challenges in sensory processing and sensory integration.* AOTA Press.

Whiting, C. C., Schoen, S. A., & Niemeyer, L. (2023). A sensory integration intervention in the school setting to support performance and participation: A multiple-baseline study. *American Journal of Occupational Therapy, 77*, 7702205060.

Wilson, B. N., et al. (1992). The efficacy of sensory integration treatment compared to tutoring. *Physical and Occupational Therapy in Pediatrics, 12*, 1–36.

Wilson, B. N., & Kaplan, B. J. (1994). Follow-up assessment of children receiving sensory integration treatment. *Occupational Therapy Journal of Research, 14*, 244–266.

## FURTHER READING

Omairi, C., Mailloux, Z., Antoniuk, S. A., & Schaaf, R. (2022). Occupational therapy using Ayres Sensory Integration®: A randomized controlled trial in Brazil. *American Journal of Occupational Therapy, 76*(4).

28

# Specific Sensory Techniques, Environmental Modifications, and Related Interventions: A Multifaceted Approach to Intervention for Children and Youth With Challenges in Sensory Integration and Sensory Processing

*L. Diane Parham Trigg and Heather Miller Kuhaneck*

## GUIDING QUESTIONS

1. What are specific sensory techniques and related interventions?
2. What evidence is available to support their use?
3. How should occupational therapy practitioners consider their use as part of comprehensive intervention?

## KEY TERMS

Alert Program
Astronaut Program
Cognitive Orientation to Daily Occupational Performance (CO-OP)
Qigong massage
Reflex Integration
Sensory diet
Specific sensory techniques
Therapeutic listening
Wilbarger Protocol

## INTRODUCTION TO SPECIFIC SENSORY TECHNIQUES AND RELATED INTERVENTIONS

For children who have been identified as having challenges in sensory integration and processing (see Chapter 9), occupational therapy practitioners may introduce a variety of interventions in combination with, or as an adjunct to, Ayres Sensory Integration Intervention (ASI) (see Chapter 27) (Reynolds et al., 2017; Watling et al., 2018). Often these intervention activities would be provided at home by a parent or primary caregiver who has been trained by a qualified occupational therapist. Some of these activities may be provided at school, under the supervision of an occupational therapist, or by a teacher or teacher assistant who has been trained by an occupational therapist with post-professional training in sensory integration. In situations where ASI is not accessible, the occupational therapist may consider coaching parents via email or phone in how to embed sensory-rich activities and just right challenges during daily routines, in addition to educating parents and teachers about the lived experiences of the child who has sensory challenges. The decisions about which interventions to use to address these challenges are guided by research evidence supporting (or not supporting) the intervention, the therapist's professional reasoning, the child's needs, the caregiver's needs, the practice setting, and accessibility to an occupational therapy-sensory integration practice setting. A multifaceted approach to children with challenges in sensory integration and sensory processing includes treating the client in all of the client's contexts including home and school, and it also includes the caregivers and other members of the client's support system (Reynolds et al., 2017). A comprehensive multifaceted intervention approach includes not only the traditional therapist-led, child-focused interventions (sensory, behavioral, cognitive, and biomechanical), but it also includes any required environmental supports, adaptations to tasks and activities that are warranted, and the provision of education that allows caregivers or teachers to take over the implementation of certain interventions in consultation with the practitioner (see Fig. 28.1) (Reynolds et al., 2017). Although a variety of terms exists, the AOTA *Practice Guidelines for Children and Youth with Challenges in Sensory Integration and Sensory Processing* (Watling et al., 2018) categorize these additional interventions as specific sensory techniques, sensory environmental modifications, education and coaching, cognitive interventions, and occupation-based interventions. This chapter will describe each type and present current evidence that supports or does not support their use.

### Specific Sensory Techniques

In the AOTA *Practice Guidelines for Children and Youth with Challenges in Sensory Integration and Sensory Processing*, the term **specific sensory techniques** refers to interventions that involve application of specific types of sensory stimuli that are controlled and delivered in a predetermined manner, usually according to a prescribed schedule, protocol, or sequence (Watling et al., 2018). A **specific sensory technique** does not provide other elements required of ASI intervention, such as challenging the child's praxis and organization of behavior, collaborating with the child in activity choice, tailoring an activity to present a just right challenge, or supporting the child's intrinsic motivation to play (Parham et al., 2011). Typically, their expected outcomes (Table 28.1) relate to behavior, attention, and arousal. Most sensory techniques

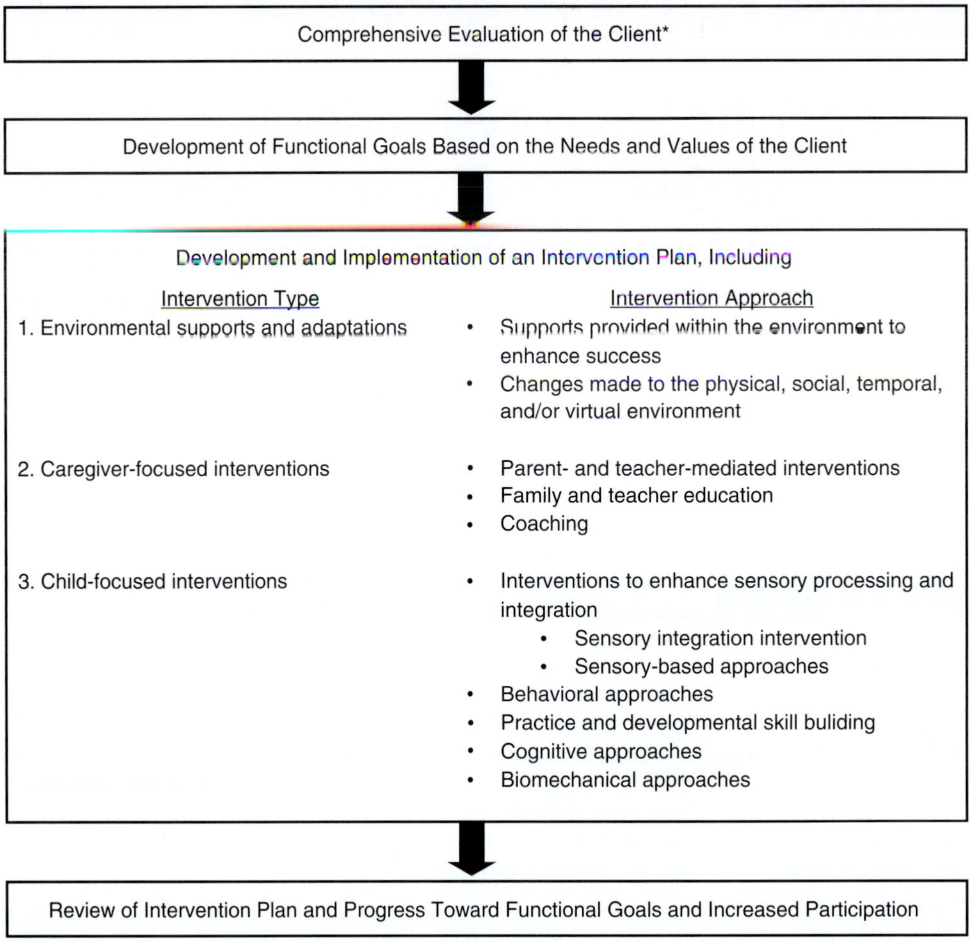


**Fig. 28.1** A multifaceted approach to children with challenges with sensory processing and integration. (Adapted from Reynolds, S., Glennon, T. J., Ausderau, K., Bendixen, R. M., Heather Kuhaneck, Pfeiffer, B., Watling, R., Wilkinson, K., & Bodison, S. C. (2017). Using a multifaceted approach to working with children who have differences in sensory processing and integration. *American Journal of Occupational Therapy 71*(2), p1–p10.)

**TABLE 28.1 Descriptions and Expected Outcomes for a Selection of Specific Sensory Techniques**

| Technique | Description | Expected Outcome |
|---|---|---|
| Astronaut Program | Application of rotary vestibular stimulation combined with sound stimulation, along with prescribed activities that provide strong proprioceptive input by challenging postural control and bilateral coordination | Improved sensory modulation and self-regulation, improvements in attention, and behavior |
| Hug Machine | Self-administered deep touch pressure input across the sides for the body, while controlling the intensity and duration of the touch pressure input | Calming of arousal level, improvements in attention, and behavior |
| Therapeutic listening | Combines sound-based intervention with sensory integrative activities; the sound intervention uses patterns of sounds in music to impact the nervous system | Increased attention, balance, body awareness and social engagement; improved organization and regulation of behavior |
| Weighted vests | Provides both tactile and proprioceptive input as the child actively moves about while wearing the vest | Calming of arousal level and improvements in attention and behavior |
| Wilbarger Protocol | Brushing arms and legs with a surgical scrub brush using stroking motions in a particular direction and sequence, followed by manual compression of specific joints, every 2 h | Improved sensory modulation and self-regulation and improved attention and behavior |

focus on a specific sensory system or a combination of two sensory systems. Generally, sensory techniques involve the passive application of sensory stimuli, although in some cases the child may self-administer the sensory input. They are occasionally used within an ASI approach to alter arousal level (Bodison & Parham, 2018). For example, during an ASI therapy session, the therapist might guide an overstimulated, disorganized child to lie on a very large square pillow (large enough for the child to lay upon it, so that the therapist can fold the pillow over the child in order to apply steady deep pressure over the child's body. This strategy is used to help the child calm down and become centered and ready for organized therapeutic play. Usually, the therapist presents this as a pretend play activity, e.g., "Let's make you into a sandwich!"

Specific sensory techniques generally are applied by the occupational therapist or by the teacher, aide, or the parent under the guidance of an occupational therapist. They should be therapist led or therapist supported (Bodison & Parham, 2018), depending on the level of therapist involvement during provision of the intervention. Often these techniques begin as therapist led, but become therapist supported as a caregiver, teacher, or child takes over the implementation after being trained by the occupational therapist.

Specific sensory techniques are sometimes used throughout the day to create a sensory diet. A **sensory diet** is an intervention program that involves provision of individualized sensory experiences and activities throughout the day to support optimal functioning of the child with sensory integration challenges. The term "sensory diet" was coined by Wilbarger (1984) to describe a program of scheduled activities that would be individualized to address a child's sensory needs to help the child regulate behavior. Using a nutritional diet as a metaphor, a sensory diet is created based on knowledge about the complex relationship between sensation and function (Wilbarger, 1995). Within this lens, it is proposed that all people require the appropriate amount and type of sensory input for their optimal arousal level to perform at their best (Wilbarger & Wilbarger, 1991). Although the term "sensory diet" is sometimes misinterpreted as simply a rigid brushing protocol, ideally the therapeutic sensory diet aims to provide an optimal combination of sensory-based activities throughout the day, tailored to the appropriate intensities and frequencies for the specific child. Studies on sensory diets have primarily been single-subject research or pre-post, although they have documented some improvements in students with autism and reduced fussiness in infants (Jorge et al., 2013; Pingale et al., 2019, 2022).

**Somatosensory Techniques.** Somatosensory techniques involve the controlled application of tactile, proprioceptive, or combined tactile and proprioceptive input. Examples include massage, brushing the skin, use of a device or special garment to apply compression to the body, having the child wear a weighted vest, and reflex integration training. However, most of these interventions are not supported by high-quality, peer-reviewed published research, primarily because high-quality research has not yet been conducted to determine their efficacy. Well-designed clinical trials are needed to determine which of these interventions may be effective, for whom they are effective, costs in terms of time and money, and expected outcomes.

***Massage.*** Infant and child massage protocols, specifically the massage programs pioneered by Tiffany Field (2016; 1995), are an exception, because these interventions have been supported by high-quality research for many years. More recent well-designed randomized clinical trials have provided strong evidence that a specific type of massage, Qigong massage, is effective for preschoolers with autism spectrum disorders (Silva et al., 2009, 2011, 2015). Both the Field and the Silva massage protocols require formal training. It is important to bear in mind that the occupational therapists delivering the massage intervention in the Silva studies had completed 50–80 h of training before research implementation. During the intervention period of the studies, they provided instruction and ongoing monitoring to parents, who provided the massage on a daily basis.

Currently, the specific sensory techniques with the strongest research support are somatosensory interventions involving massage protocols. Two randomized controlled trials (RCTs) examined effects of a simple massage protocol developed by Tiffany Field that could be administered by any trained health professional (Escalona et al., 2001; Field et al., 1997). Both studies indicated that this intervention produced improvements in tactile reactivity and reductions in problem behaviors among children with autism, perhaps related to improved sleep of participants receiving the massage. RCTs of **Qigong massage** (derived from traditional Chinese medicine) have also found positive for children with autism when provided by occupational therapists trained in this particular intervention. This intervention was designed to improve sensory processing, physiologic self-regulation, and sleep of children with autism. Significant improvements in behavior of children with autism were indicated after individualized delivery of a 5-month Qigong massage regimen by trained occupational therapists or by parents who were trained and coached by occupational therapists (Silva et al., 2009; Silva et al., 2011). A systematic review (Bodison & Parham, 2018) concluded that Qigong massage embedded in daily routines at home, with supervision from an occupational therapists, has strong evidence of effectiveness for preschoolers with autism spectrum disorder (ASD), due to the availability of three well-designed RCTs reporting positive outcomes for this intervention (Silva et al., 2009, 2011, 2015).

***Wilbarger Protocol.*** In the **Wilbarger Protocol** (also called the *deep pressure proprioceptive technique*), an adult provides touch pressure stimuli by brushing arms and legs with a surgical scrub brush using stroking motions in a particular direction and sequence, followed by manual compression of specific joints, every 2 h (Wilbarger et al., 2020) (Fig. 28.2). Expected outcomes for the Wilbarger Protocol include improved sensory modulation and self-regulation and general improvements in attention, learning, and behavior. However, not all children experience the Wilbarger Protocol as comfortable. If a child rejects this protocol (i.e., moves away from the brush, pushes away the brush or the person holding the brush, cries, tantrums, or hits the provider) after several attempts over the course of a week, it should be discontinued rather than imposed on a distressed child.

Research on the effectiveness of the **Wilbarger Protocol** is limited to case reports, studies that are weak in rigor, and unpublished Master's theses or doctoral dissertations (Wilbarger et al., 2020). Although many of these studies report positive outcomes, because the research designs are not rigorous and sample sizes are small, the Wilbarger Protocol

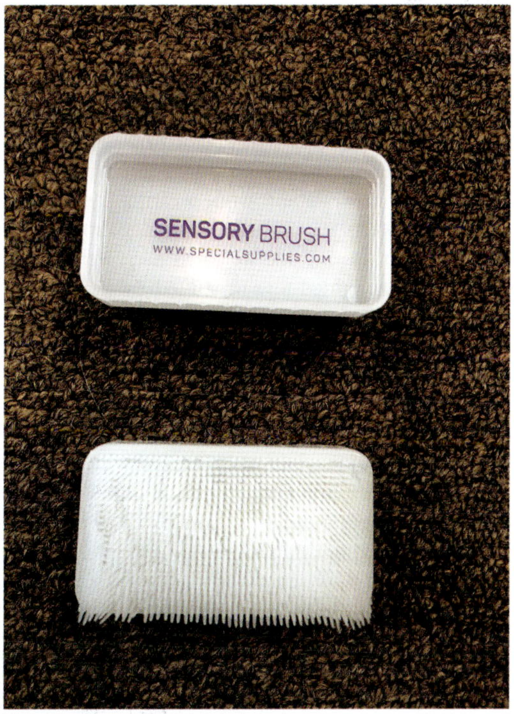


**Fig. 28.2** The Wilbarger Protocol requires the use of a particular surgical scrub brush.

is not recommended as an evidence-based intervention. Similarly, research on the effectiveness of the Astronaut Program is quite limited, so it is not recommended at the present time. However, one small case study examined the effects of this program on balance, posture, and in-seat movement (Katzenellenbogen et al., 2021). The authors documented different patterns of changes for children who initially were able to tolerate rotary movement versus those who were overreactive initially. Research on effectiveness of swinging for supporting child arousal level and attention is currently very limited and inconclusive (Bodison & Parham, 2018), so it is not recommended at this time as a stand-alone intervention.

***The Hug Machine.*** Some somatosensory techniques involve self-administration of deep touch pressure across the body using special devices. Deep pressure techniques are thought to have a short-term calming effect, which may serve to help decrease anxiety or arousal level in the immediate situation (Edelson et al., 1999). Temple Grandin's squeeze or Hug Machine was designed so that a child or adult can self-administer deep touch pressure input across the sides for the body, while controlling the intensity and duration of the touch pressure input (Edelson et al., 1999) (see https://www.grandin.com/inc/squeeze-11.html for a schematic of the machine designed by Grandin). Recently the Hug Machine has been adapted to a device that can be used while on public transportation, to make using transportation more comfortable and less anxiety-provoking for those on the autism spectrum (Afif et al., 2022; Afif et al., 2021; Maula et al., 2021).

A small RCT that evaluated use of the Grandin Hug Machine for 6 weeks by children with ASD found that participants who used this machine showed evidence of reduction in self-perceived anxiety and decreased arousal/reactivity, as measured by electrodermal responses (Edelson et al., 1999). The adapted seated inflatable version of the Hug Machine appears to reduce difficult behaviors, heart rate, and galvanic skin response (a measure of sympathetic stress response) when worn by children on the spectrum (Afif et al., 2021, 2022; Maula et al., 2021). An experimental study of a similar device that provided self-administered deep pressure around the circumference of the body showed that it had a calming effect with decreased subjective anxiety and increase in perceived relaxation (Krauss, 1987).

***Weighted Items.*** Another technique for providing somatosensory input is to have the child wear or use weighted items. The most used item of this type is the weighted vest. A weighted vest may be worn according to a prescribed schedule or while engaged in specific activities. This provides both deep pressure and proprioceptive input as the child actively moves about while wearing the vest. Typically, the vest weighs between 5%–15% of the child's body weight (Fig. 28.3). Other applications include weighted hats, weighted lap pads, weighted neck rolls, weighted toys or stuffed animals, and weighted blankets (Bolic Baric et al., 2021; Gringras et al., 2014; Larsson et al., 2021, 2022).

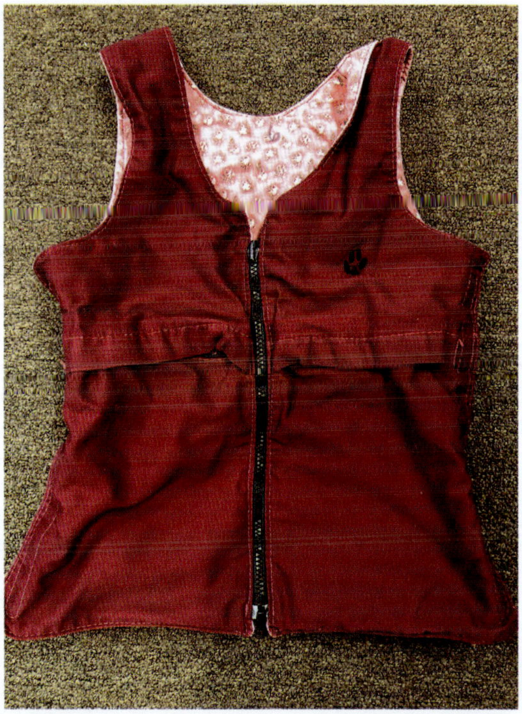

**Fig. 28.3** Weighted vests are meant to provide additional touch pressure input to the area under the vest, and additional proprioceptive input because of the added weight increases joint compression as the child moves about.

The use of weighted vests to improve attention to task and in-seat classroom behaviors may be the most often studied sensory technique. No high-quality research is currently available that evaluates effectiveness of weighted vests in the contexts of everyday life at home and in school. Limited evidence is available in favor of the use of weighted vests to support classroom participation of children with ADHD (Buckle et al., 2011). Although a large (N = 110) well-designed RCT reported significantly positive effects of weighted vests on attention of children with ADHD, these results might not generalize to everyday life settings such as home and school, because the outcome measure in this study was performance on controlled laboratory tasks rather than functional performance in the children's classrooms, homes, or neighborhoods (Lin et al., 2014). However, when considered together, these two studies suggest that perhaps the deep touch pressure of the vest supports the ability of children with attention difficulties to attend to cognitive tasks, thereby helping them to engage in classroom activities at school. Future research is needed to determine whether these results can be generalized to other schools, home, and neighborhood settings. In these RCTs, the vest was weighted to 10% of the child's body weight before wearing. Another well-designed study found no effect for the weighted vest for children with ADHD (Macphee et al., 2019). The inconsistent findings of these studies suggest that wearing a weighted vest may have differential effects across diagnostic groups, may vary by the percentage of weight of the vest (some use 5%, some 10%, and some 15%), and may vary because they examine different outcomes. However, most of the studies of effects of weighted vests were for children with ASD. Many used single-subject research designs, and most did not report any improvements in behavior, which were the expected outcomes (Hodgetts et al., 2011a, 2011b; Cox et al., 2009; Fertel-Daly et al., 2001; Harry et al., 2019; Kane et al., 2004; Leew et al., 2010; Reichow et al., 2010).

Similarly, the evidence for weighted blankets does not strongly support their use (Gringras et al., 2014; Larsson et al., 2022; Lönn et al., 2023). However, parent reports and adult retrospective reports suggest that some families and individuals may find them helpful (Bolic Baric et al., 2021; Larsson et al., 2021). As for other weighted items, currently there is little or no evidence to support their use and limited evidence for their lack of effectiveness (Zimmerman et al., 2019).

Based on the current research, wearing a weighted vest generally is not recommended at the present time, as research has consistently found that this intervention does not seem to benefit children with autism, Because they are inexpensive and do not present any known adverse effects, therapists may consider a trial period of weighted vest use for children with ADHD, on a case-by-case basis, with careful monitoring of effects for each child to determine whether the child seems to benefit from this sensory technique. Occupational therapists should consider on a case-by-case basis whether a trial period of wearing a weighted vest may be helpful for the child who is receiving their services. If no positive changes in behavior are evident after 2 or 3 weeks of wearing the weighted vest at school, at home, and/or in community settings such as restaurants, shops, or playgrounds, then wearing the vest should be discontinued.

***Reflex Integration Training.*** The Masgutova Neurosensorimotor Reflex Integration (MNRI) method is comprised of several integration programs, each designed to reinforce and optimize the integration of primary motor reflex patterns. It is proposed to restore normal interpretive function to each functional sensory system. Improvement in interpretive function, in turn, can work to improve emotional and behavioral regulation and enhance the maturation and integration process for primary motor reflex patterns. Studies have documented atypical reflexes in children with neurodevelopmental disorders and related these reflexes to motor skills and issues such as dyspraxia, vestibular disorders, and postural disorders, but the minimal research to date documenting improvements in reflexes after this intervention have been pre-post designs without control groups (Masgutova et al., 2016a; Masgutova et al., 2015, 2015; Pecuch et al., 2020; 2021).

**Vestibular Techniques.** Vestibular techniques stimulate the vestibular receptors of the inner ear (i.e., the semicircular canals and the otolith organs). Specifically, vestibular interventions involve the provision of rotary movement of the body through space (as in spinning around while seated on a rotating chair), angular movement (such as moving in an arc on a swing attached by two ropes), linear movement of the body through space (e.g., jumping up and down on a trampoline or sliding straight down a playground slide), or a combination of these types of movement. As for other sensory techniques, vestibular techniques used alone are not the same as ASI intervention because they lack many of the essential ASI fidelity elements, such as challenging praxis and motor planning, collaborating on activity choice, individualizing the activity to present a just right challenge, and supporting the child's intrinsic motivation to play (Parham et al., 2011).

The Astronaut Program involves the application of rotary vestibular stimulation combined with sound stimulation, along with prescribed activities that provide strong proprioceptive input by challenging postural control and bilateral coordination (Wilbarger et al., 2020). At the time of this writing, the authors are not aware of any peer-reviewed research studies evaluating the effects of this program that have been published in high-quality research journals. Expected outcomes for the Astronaut Program are similar to those of the Wilbarger brushing technique: improved sensory modulation and self-regulation and general improvements in attention, learning, and behavior. However, therapists should be mindful that this intervention is not supported by research, and that intense vestibular stimulation may not be appropriate for many children, particularly those who are generally hypersensitive and easily overwhelmed by intense vestibular stimulation, such as spinning while seated on a swing or on a suspended inner tube.

Occupational therapists sometimes use *swinging* back and forth (not the same as spinning, which is rotating) to help regulate a child's alertness or attention. Swinging is a sensory technique that involves primarily linear vestibular input (if slow and low to the ground), but it may also be angular if swinging fast and high in an arc of movement. It is thought to differentially affect a child's arousal level depending on velocity and predictability. Slow, consistent linear movement (such as gently rocking a baby in a cradle) tends to be calming due to its inhibitory effect on arousal, whereas fast swinging is thought to increase arousal level and attention, especially when the swinging involves unpredictable changes in velocity or direction of movement through space. Another application of vestibular input is the provision of dynamic seating that provides increased vestibular and somatosensory stimuli to support attention in the classroom. This input is usually provided by having the child sit on a therapy ball or an inflatable disk-like cushion in place of a conventional chair.

**Auditory Techniques.** Auditory techniques are usually called auditory programs, listening programs, sound-based interventions, or sound therapy. These typically involve complex applications of music delivered through headphones or other listening systems. Usually, the selected auditory stimuli are selected based on the child's presenting pattern of sensory difficulties or from an audiogram. These interventions usually involve multiple sessions over a time frame in which a specific sequence of filtered music is presented over time. Generally, the child is not guided or prompted to make any responses to the stimulation beyond simply listening. Originally developed by physicians as an individual therapy, occupational therapists and other professionals have developed versions that can be used alone, during ASI intervention sessions, or while participating in other interventions. Sound-based interventions target a variety of outcomes, including sensory reactivity, self-regulation, attention, improved language, and adaptive functioning.

High-quality, rigorous research studies examining the effectiveness of sound-based interventions have not been published in peer-reviewed research journals at the time of this writing. This does not mean that the intervention is not effective; it simply means that we do not have adequate evidence to strongly recommend this intervention as effective, at the present time. Although parents may report qualitative improvements from auditory interventions (Chiu & Li, 2017; Slevin et al., 2020), published research studies have used a variety of auditory intervention programs and research designs involving children, including randomized clinical trials (RCTs), but most of these studies have produced no significant benefits (Bazyk et al., 2010; Gee et al., 2014; Hall & Case-Smith, 2007; Mudford & Cullen, 2005; Sinha et al., 2011; Slevin et al., 2020). A large systematic review of effectiveness studies on auditory integration training programs concluded that these interventions probably are not effective (Sinha et al., 2011), and a more recent review noted that there was limited evidence to support their use (Villasenor et al., 2018).

However, results of a relatively recent RCT involving young children indicated that children who received the Therapeutic Listening Program benefitted from this intervention with regard to sensory processing (Slevin et al., 2020). In a single-subject design study of the Integrated Listening Systems intervention, positive changes in arousal level were documented in five of the seven subjects who participated (Schoen et al., 2015).

## Sensory Environmental Modifications and Supports

Children and youth with sensory integration challenges will usually benefit from recommendations for sensory environmental modifications in conjunction with direct intervention. These recommendations are designed to help cope with and manage sensory input arising from stimuli such as sound, lighting, physical contact with other people, odors, and visual distractions in environments such as classrooms, playgrounds, cafeterias, auditoriums, or museums. This is particularly important for children with sensory hyperreactivity, as they tend to be strongly affected by sensory environmental characteristics that others may not notice. Environmental modifications may enhance or add sensory stimuli to the environment, or conversely, they may reduce or remove it, for example, using noise attenuating headphones, sunglasses, study carrels, light covers, and classroom soundproofing (Reynolds et al., 2017). School and classroom environments, in particular, tend to be exceptionally noisy (Kuhaneck & Kelleher, 2015; Minelli et al., 2022). This can create stress, impacting arousal, attention, and performance, especially for those on the autism spectrum (Gentil-Gutiérrez et al., 2021; Keith et al., 2018; Mallory & Keehn, 2021). Environmental modifications potentially can make an important contribution to the child's functioning by reducing distress and anxiety, thereby supporting attention, behavior, and, ultimately, the ability to participate successfully in academic and social activities.

The effectiveness of sensory environmental modifications has just begun to be studied in the last 10 years or so. Results so far are encouraging, although very limited, and the environmental modifications used in these studies are intended primarily for children on the autism spectrum (Cermak et al., 2015; Dargue et al., 2021; Krieger et al., 2018; Martin, 2016; Pfeiffer et al., 2019; Ruiz-Rodrigo et al., 2023). One well-designed RCT examined the effects of modifying the auditory and visual aspects of a dental office while providing deep touch pressure via a weighted blanket to children with ASD and typical children (the control group) as they received routine dental cleanings (Cermak et al., 2015). Outcomes included significant improvements in child-reported measures of pain intensity and sensory discomfort, as well as improved participation in dental cleaning. Reduction of stress and anxiety, as measured by changes in electrodermal responses, showed a moderate to large effect size after intervention, for the children with ASD. These findings suggest that the environmental adaptations reduced physiologic stress of participants, improving their ability to tolerate and appropriately participate in routine dental cleaning.

Modifications in school environments have been successful, as well. Kinnealey et al. (2012) conducted a small study of four adolescent males with sensory hyperreactivity, three of whom had autism, to examine whether modifications to classroom sound and lighting would improve their attention and perceptions of classroom experiences (Kinnealey et al., 2012). The intervention consisted of replacing fluorescent lights with halogen lighting and installing sound-absorbing walls, which decreased the decibel levels within the room. Results indicated that all students demonstrated increased attention to academic tasks while in the modified classroom. In daily journals, the students expressed comfort and pleasure with the altered environment. Another well-designed single-subject study documented physiologic changes in children on the spectrum when they wore noise attenuating headphones in their natural environments such as at school (Pfeiffer et al., 2019). More studies such as this are needed to identify the kinds of sensory environmental modifications that are most successful and cost effective in improving participation of children with sensory integration challenges across diverse environmental settings.

Positive short-term effects of sitting on a "therapy ball chair" (also called stability ball) in the classroom have been documented in a few single-case experimental design studies of children with autism spectrum or attention-deficit disorders, with immediate benefits related to in-seat behavior, attention to task, and productivity in academic tasks for some but not all children (Bagatell et al., 2010; Fedewa & Erwin, 2011; Schilling & Schwartz, 2004). However, a recent study documented that students in a third-grade classroom were on task less frequently when sitting on the ball chairs (Hulac et al., 2022). Another study comparing a regular chair, a therapy ball, and an "active chair" found that the therapy ball led to the "least proper" seat behavior (Stanic et al., 2022). However, in this last study, which was well designed and used physiologic outcome measures in addition to cognitive and behavioral ones, the "active chair" was found to improve performance for those with ADHD. The authors describe this active chair as one that "does not restrict leg movement and at the same time stabilizes the torso, thus enabling writing and solving tasks despite increased activity" (Stanic et al., 2022, pp. 3).

It may be that therapy balls are most effective when used selectively with consideration for the sensory integration characteristics of the individual child. In one study of children with autism, the best responder to a ball chair was a child who demonstrated strong vestibular-proprioceptive sensory seeking (Bagatell et al., 2010). Perhaps this strategy was effective for this child because therapy balls generate more sensory input via vestibular and proprioceptive sensory input than conventional classroom chairs, leading to increased alertness and attention as compared with conventional classroom chairs. Conversely, use of a therapy ball was not helpful for a child in this study who had poor postural stability. It may be that, for this child, sitting on a ball chair created stress and distraction due to the extra challenge that this intervention imposes on postural control. These findings underscore the importance of conducting a thorough evaluation of sensory integration before selecting sensory techniques for a particular child and then carefully monitoring outcomes to ensure that the child's responses are moving toward desired goals. Research on use of therapy cushions (inflatable disks placed in the child's chair to sit on) has not produced consistent positive benefits, but they may offer a more practical alternative to therapy balls in some classrooms (Schilling & Schwartz, 2004; Umeda & Deitz, 2011).

The first rigorous examination of the effects of ball chairs and weighted vests for children with ADHD in the classroom, in comparison to medications and other control conditions, has documented no behavioral changes in following rules or in accuracy of completion of worksheets (math, reading, or language) with the sensory interventions (MacPhee et al., 2019). This research was a within-subjects study completed over a 6-week period with 64 participants using a 2 × 3 research design, where 2 = medication (methylphenidate or placebo) and 3 = OT intervention (stability ball or weighted vest). The study was conducted in a summer classroom, and treatment fidelity was assessed. These initial findings indicated that ball chairs and weighted vests probably are not effective for many children with ADHD. Still, it may be worthwhile to provide an initial trial period for selected children with ADHD, as it is possible that some children may benefit from weighted vests, which are relatively inexpensive and do not produce negative side effects.

## Education and Coaching

Educating, coaching, or consulting with parents or teachers has been an important aspect of occupational therapy practice for children with sensory integration difficulties since the inception of this practice area. These interventions usually focus on guiding the parent or teacher to modify environments, adjust daily routines, reframe challenging child behaviors, or embed sensory interventions or experiences within the home or classroom to support the development or behavior of children with sensory integration challenges.

Sensory integrative problems are complex and are often misinterpreted as solely behavioral, psychological, or emotional. Helping family members, teachers, and other professionals understand the sensory integrative nature of the problem can be a powerful means toward helping the child. When the child's behavior is explained in sensory terms using everyday language, a new understanding of the child often ensues. Cermak (2001) aptly referred to this process as *demystification*, and others have used the term *reframing* (Niehues et al., 1991). Caregivers commonly express relief at finally understanding puzzling and frustrating behaviors, and they may experience release from feeling that they have caused these problems through a maladaptive parenting style. This insight opens the door to discovering simple strategies that can be used throughout the day that help the child feel more comfortable and participate more fully in everyday occupations. Teachers also may appreciate having an alternative way to view child behaviors, especially when this new perspective is coupled with classroom strategies that promote responses from the child that are more productive. Children also stand to benefit greatly from understanding their own sensory characteristics. Because individual differences in sensory integration may be lifelong tendencies, it is critical that the child with sensory processing differences learn to construct their daily routines and organize the sensory aspects of their work and play activities and environments to live as comfortably and successfully as possible (Dunn, 2001).

Through educating, coaching, and collaborating with those who are in ongoing contact with the child, the therapist can provide critical information and recommend implementation of specific strategies to influence the child's life positively across a variety of settings. Indirect intervention in the form of consultation is an important way that education and coaching is provided and should be included in a comprehensive occupational therapy program for the child with sensory integration challenges. Whenever individual ASI intervention is provided, consultation with parents and/or teachers should also be provided.

In many situations, the first step in the consultation process should be to help caregivers and teachers better understand sensory integration in general, as well as how sensory integration concepts apply to specific children. This can be achieved through individual meetings with parents or teachers, parent/teacher conferences, group experiential sessions, lecture and discussion groups, professional in-services, and ongoing education programs. Helping adults in a child's life to understand their own sensory integrative processes is often an effective way to make new sensory integration concepts meaningful. Williams and Shellenberger (1994) use this tactic in their Alert Program. Before implementing the program with children, the adults who will administer the program participate in a training program designed to develop self-awareness and insight into their own sensory characteristics and preferences.

Perhaps the most important component of any consultation program is providing guidance for identifying, preventing, and coping with the specific challenges in everyday life that stem from a child's sensory integrative problems. Sometimes specific activities can be suggested that help a child prepare for a challenging task. For example, a child who has tactile defensiveness may more readily engage in activities such as finger painting or sand play if firm touch pressure is applied to the skin before the activity. Modifying the activity might involve providing tools to use with the paint or sand to give the child a ready "break" from the unpleasant sensation. A home program that includes gradual introduction of tactile sensation in a safe place, such as the bathtub, can also help reduce negative reactions. The therapist can also promote success in activities by suggesting individualized ways to help a child through difficult tasks. For example, some children with dyspraxia are likely to be more successful in completing a novel task when they receive verbal directions, whereas others respond optimally to visual demonstrations, and still others need physical assistance with the motions. Determining which method or combination of methods is most likely to help the individual child can assist adults in facilitating success.

Consultation involves collaboration with parents or teachers to embed individualized sensory experiences at strategic time points throughout the day to support the child's alertness or calming at appropriate times. For example, a child might engage in physical activity before school to boost arousal level, chewing gum while in class to support sustained attention, and a deep pressure massage to promote calming on returning home. Development of an appropriate regime requires ongoing education and coaching of the adults who implement this intervention. The same therapist qualifications needed to provide individual ASI intervention are desirable in providing consultation. The occupational therapist should be well versed in sensory integration concepts to explain them in simple yet accurate and meaningful terms. Furthermore, the therapist needs to fully understand the child's sensory integrative difficulties and use this understanding to predict what the child's likely responses will be to various activities and situations. Therefore, the occupational therapist needs to conduct a comprehensive assessment of the child before making any suggestions to identify the sensory interventions that are likely to be most helpful, and to consider any precautions that might apply. Also, it is imperative that the occupational therapist have excellent communication skills and respect for the various people and environments that are involved.

Expected outcomes of consultation, coaching, and education for parents or teachers depend on the individual child's presenting problems, the family or school team's goals, and the focus of the consultation. For instance, helping a teacher understand how best to seat a child in class (e.g., on a therapy ball chair versus a firm wooden chair or in the front corner of the room near the teacher's desk versus the back of the room) may make it easier for the child to attend to instruction in the classroom. Desired outcomes might be measured as increased time on tasks, increased time in seat, decreased number of disruptive behaviors in class, or improved performance in academic tasks.

Often during consultation for individual children, occupational therapists become aware of sensory features within home, school, or community environments that can be modified in ways that benefit all of the children who live, work, and play there. In such situations, occupational therapists should consider using their knowledge of sensory integration to advocate for environmental changes that will benefit all children. For example, playgrounds or backyards may be modified to stimulate development of praxis and playfulness for all the children by providing equipment and materials that can present sensorimotor challenges at varying levels of complexity and can be played with in many ways (Bundy et al., 2008). Adjustments to school environments may be especially important because children spend large amounts of time in this environment. These may include alterations in lighting, sound, or types and amount of sensory stimulation present in different areas. Additionally, daily routines with key sensory components may benefit all children in a classroom. For example, research indicates that children generally have better attention to demanding academic tasks when they engage in physical activity breaks throughout the day, which boosts ability to sustain attention to cognitively challenging tasks (Barros et al., 2009; Jarrett, 2003). Initial morning routines involving sensorimotor activity may assist in preparing children for the cognitive work ahead in the school day, and regularly scheduled recess periods allow for physical activity to prepare children to return to the classroom refreshed and ready to work (Hopkins, 2010).

The research on outcomes resulting from consultation involving changes to daily environments or routines so far is consistently positive (Allen et al., 2021; Azari et al., 2019; Heyburn et al., 2022; Little et al., 2018; Wallisch et al., 2019). Studies report improved child behavior and participation, parental satisfaction with the interventions, parental empowerment, and greater feelings of self-efficacy. These interventions have been successfully implemented by telehealth as well. Consultation and training in a group format may also reduce practitioners' workload as it takes less time than one-on-one intervention (Heyburn et al., 2022).

## Cognitive Interventions

Cognitive interventions focus on teaching specific strategies or procedures to the child to support successful performance or participation. These interventions differ from ASI intervention because they do not include fidelity process elements that are essential in ASI, for example, collaborating with the child in activity choice, challenging the child's postural control or bilateral coordination, or supporting the child's intrinsic motivation to play.

An example of a cognitive intervention is the **Alert Program** for Self-Regulation, which was developed by occupational therapists Williams and Shellenberger (Williams & Shellenberger, 1994). This program applies sensory integration concepts to teach children how to self-manage their arousal levels for better participation. Provided individually or within a group, classroom, or online format, the Alert Program helps children learn to recognize how they feel when their levels of alertness and arousal change throughout the day. Using this awareness, participants then learn to monitor their arousal levels in a variety of settings and to identify the sensory experiences that they can use to change their level of alertness to function more optimally. This approach particularly seems to be useful in school settings and as an adjunct to individual ASI. In a survey of types of services provided by occupational therapists to children with emotional disturbances in public schools, Barnes et al. (2003) found that nearly 47% of respondents reported using the Alert Program individually or in groups. More recently, the Alert Program has been expanded to include a version for adolescents and adults.

Positive outcomes for children with emotional disturbance and those with fetal alcohol syndrome disorder (FASD) have been reported following programming with the Alert Program delivered within a classroom setting (Barnes et al., 2008; Wagner et al., 2017, 2019) or delivered by a primary caregiver (Wells et al., 2012). A review of the evidence for this program included six studies and suggested the program improved self-regulation in the schools (Gill et al., 2018). It is likely that this intervention is effective for other children with self-regulatory difficulties, not only for those with FASD, but research is needed to verify this.

A cognitive intervention called **Cognitive Orientation to Daily Occupational Performance (CO-OP)** (see Chapter 26) is supported by research as an effective intervention for improving motor performance of children with developmental coordination disorder, but none of the studies to date have examined whether the participants had sensory integration challenges (Pfeiffer, Frolek Clark, & Arbesman, 2018). Research on the effectiveness of CO-OP for children with sensory integration-based dyspraxia would be helpful in ascertaining whether this specific population is likely to benefit from this intervention.

## Occupation-Based Interventions With Strong Sensory Input

Occupation-based interventions use engagement in ordinary daily activities or leisure activities that provide strong sensory input as therapeutic agents. Examples of occupation-based interventions that provide strong sensory input include household chores, such as carrying heavy laundry or vacuuming, meal preparation such as kneading or rolling dough, gardening, or yard work with digging/shoveling or hauling with a wheelbarrow or tarp, and leisure such as swimming, music or dance, art such as ceramics, bowling, horseback riding, or yoga.

A systematic review that focused on leisure activities found that two occupation-based interventions, horseback riding and yoga, are supported by research as beneficial for some children and youth with documented sensory integration difficulties or sensory processing differences (Pfeiffer et al., 2018). Horseback riding has led to improvements in social and sensory functioning of children with ASD (Bass et al., 2009; Ward et al., 2013) and in improved motor skills as well (Zhao et al., 2022). Parents of children with disabilities report yoga to beneficial (Lovrić et al., 2020), and evidence suggests yoga may improve pulse rate and reduce distress, suggesting that it perhaps leads to a reduction in anxiety (Rè et al., 2014). Yoga also produced significant reductions in maladaptive behaviors in students on the autism spectrum (Koenig et al., 2012). Minimal research has been completed on swimming as leisure or a family activity (as opposed to aquatic therapy); however, one very small (n = 3 subjects with autism) pre-post study without a control group documented improved behavior following swimming lessons (Musiyenko et al., 2020).

Occupation-based interventions for children and youth with sensory integration challenges are encouraging but limited in scope at the present time. Moreover, these interventions are quite diverse, so outcomes can be expected to vary across the specific interventions. Currently, research on horseback riding presents moderate evidence of sensory and social participation benefits for children with ASD who have sensory challenges, but its effectiveness for children with other kinds of sensory integration conditions, such as postural and bilateral coordination difficulties or dyspraxia, apparently has not yet been examined. Evidence of effectiveness of yoga is positive but tentative due to the limited research design. Many other occupation-based interventions may be effective for children and youth with sensory integration challenges, but research that evaluates their efficacy is not yet available. This is an area of occupational therapy research that is greatly needed to inform best practices for serving children with sensory integration challenges.

## Emerging Interventions

In addition to the interventions discussed in this chapter, new applications of sensory integration theory are emerging, for example, collaborations among occupational therapists, psychologists, and other professionals such as art therapists to merge sensory integration knowledge and techniques into psychotherapeutic interventions for children and youth who have experienced trauma (Koomar, 2009). Other emerging applications of sensory integration knowledge aim to promote the well-being of communities as well as individual children, for example, through playground design and school-wide routines that support the emotional, physical, intellectual, and social development of all children. For these as well as established interventions for children with sensory integration difficulties, research will continue to be important in discerning the extent to which an intervention is helpful, how it is helpful, and for whom it is helpful.

# SUMMARY

A comprehensive intervention approach for children with challenges with sensory integration and processing includes not only the traditional therapist-led, child-focused interventions but also may include specific sensory techniques, sensory environmental modifications, education and coaching, cognitive interventions, and occupation-based interventions. Occupational therapy practitioners must evaluate the evidence for each of these approaches and consider the individual needs of each child and situation before determining the "mix" of interventions that are appropriate and that support the occupational therapy focus on occupation.

- Specific sensory techniques and related interventions include approaches such as the use of weighted items, the Wilbarger Protocol, sensory diets, massage, auditory interventions such as the Therapeutic Listening Program, the Hug Machine, the Astronaut Program, sensory environmental modifications, parent and teacher coaching and consultation, and sensory heavy leisure occupations such as horseback riding and yoga.
- In many cases, evidence to support their use is minimal or nonexistent, and practitioners must be cautious with their use. In other

cases, evidence is strong. Practitioners must evaluate each approach and strategy for each situation and collect individual client data regarding effectiveness, if selected interventions are implemented knowing there is little research evidence.

- Occupational therapy practitioners may consider their use as part of a comprehensive intervention plan but must consider their relationship to occupation and resist using many of these interventions as stand-alone strategies. Practitioners must also openly discuss their use with clients and their families, honestly describing the current level of evidence for their use, and gain client and family consent to engage in strategies on a trial basis while collecting individual data for the specific child.

## REFERENCES


Afif, I. Y., Manik, A. R., Munthe, K., Maula, M. I., Ammarullah, M. I., Jamari, J., & Winarni, T. I. (2022). Physiological effect of deep pressure in reducing anxiety of children with ASD during traveling: A public transportation setting. *Bioengineering, 9*(4), 157.

Afif, I. Y., Maula, M. I., Aliyafi, M. B., Aji, A. L., Winarni, T. I., & Jamari, J. (2021). Design of hug machine portable seat for autistic children in public transport application. In *IOP conference series: Materials science and engineering* (p. 1096). IOP Publishing.

Allen, S., Knott, F. J., Branson, A., & Lane, S. J. (2021). Coaching parents of children with sensory integration difficulties: A scoping review. In *Occupational Therapy International.*

Azari, Z. P., Hosseini, S. A., Rassafiani, M., Samadi, S. A., Hoseinzadeh, S., & Winnie, D. U. N. N. (2019). Contextual intervention adapted for autism spectrum disorder: An RCT of a parenting program with parents of children diagnosed with autism spectrum disorder (ASD). *Iranian Journal of Child Neurology, 13*(4), 19.

Bagatell, N., et al. (2010). Effectiveness of therapy ball chairs on classroom participation in children with autism spectrum disorders. *American Journal of Occupational Therapy, 64*, 895–903.

Barnes, K. J., Beck, A. J., Vogel, K. A., Grice, K. O., & Murphy, D. (2003). Perceptions regarding school-based occupational therapy for children with emotional disturbances. *American Journal of Occupational Therapy, 57*, 337–341.

Barnes, K. J., Vogel, K. A., Beck, A. J., Schoenfeld, H. B., & Owen, S. V. (2008). Self-regulation strategies of children with emotional disturbance. *Physical & Occupational Therapy in Pediatrics, 28*(4), 369–387.

Barros, R. M., Silver, E. J., & Stein, R. F. K. (2009). School recess and group classroom behavior. *Pediatrics, 123*, 431–436.

Bass, M. M., Duchowny, C. A., & Llabre, M. M. (2009). The effect of therapeutic horseback riding on social functioning in children with autism. *Journal of Autism and Developmental Disorders, 39*, 1261–1267.

Bazyk, S., Cimino, J., Hayes, K., Goodman, G., & Farrell, P. (2010). The use of therapeutic listening with preschoolers with developmental disabilities: A look at the outcomes. *Journal of Occupational Therapy, Schools, & Early Intervention, 3*(2), 124–138.

Bodison, S. C., & Parham, L. D. (2018). Specific sensory techniques and sensory environmental modifications for children and youth with sensory integration difficulties: A systematic review. *American Journal of Occupational Therapy, 72*(1), p1–p11. https://doi.org/10.5014/ajot.2018.029413.

Bolic Baric, V., Skuthälla, S., Pettersson, M., Gustafsson, P. A., & Kjellberg, A. (2021). The effectiveness of weighted blankets on sleep and everyday activities - a retrospective follow-up study of children and adults with attention deficit hyperactivity disorder and/or autism spectrum disorder. *Scandinavian Journal of Occupational Therapy, 29*, 1–11.

Buckle, F., Franzsen, D., & Bester, J. (2011). The effect of the wearing of weighted vests on the sensory behaviour of learners diagnosed with attention deficit hyperactivity disorder within a school context. *South African Journal of Occupational Therapy, 41*(3), 37–41.

Bundy, A. C., et al. (2008). Playful interaction: Occupational therapy for all children on the school playground. *American Journal of Occupational Therapy, 62*, 522–527.

Cermak, S. A., Stein Duker, L. I., Williams, M. E., Dawson, M. E., Lane, C. J., & Polido, J. C. (2015). Sensory adapted dental environments to enhance oral care for children with autism spectrum disorders: A randomized controlled pilot study. *Journal of Autism and Developmental Disorders, 45*, 2876–2888.

Cermak, S. A. (2001). The effects of deprivation on processing, play and praxis. In S. S. Roley, E. I. Blanche, & R. C. Schaaf (Eds.), *Understanding the nature of sensory integration with diverse populations* (pp. 385–408). San Antonio, TX: Therapy Skill Builders.

Chiu, E. C., & Li, C. P. (2017). A sound-based intervention for children with sensory processing disorders in Taiwan. *Neuropsychiatry, 7*(5), 759–765.

Cox, A. L., et al. (2009). The effects of weighted vest on appropriate in-seat behaviors of elementary-age students with autism and severe to profound intellectual disabilities. *Focus on Autism and Other Developmental Disabilities, 24*, 17–26.

Dargue, N., Adams, D., & Simpson, K. (2021). Can characteristics of the physical environment impact engagement in learning activities in children with autism? A systematic review. *Review Journal of Autism and Developmental Disorders*, 1–17.

Dunn, W. W. (2001). The sensations of everyday life: Empirical, theoretical, and pragmatic considerations. *American Journal of Occupational Therapy, 55*, 608–620.

Edelson, S. M., Edelson, M. G., & Kerr, D. (1999). Physiological and behavioral changes of deep pressure: A pilot study investigating the efficacy of temple grandin's hug machine. *American Journal of Occupational Therapy, 53*(2), 145–152.

Escalona, A., et al. (2001). Brief report: Improvements in the behavior of children with autism following massage therapy. *Journal of Autism and Developmental Disorders, 31*, 5.

Fedewa, A. L., & Erwin, H. E. (2011). Stability balls and students with attention and hyperactivity concerns: Implications for on-task and in-seat behavior. *American Journal of Occupational Therapy, 65*, 393–399.

Fertel-Daly, D., Bedell, G., & Hinojosa, J. (2001). Effects of a weighted vest on attention to task and self-stimulatory behaviors in preschoolers with pervasive developmental disorders. *American Journal of Occupational Therapy, 55*, 620–640.

Field, T., et al. (1997). Autistic children's attentiveness and responsivity improve after touch therapy. *Journal of Autism and Developmental Disorders, 27*, 333–338.

Field, T. (1995). Massage therapy for infants and children. *Journal of Developmental and Behavioral Pediatrics, 16*(2), 105–111.

Field, T. (2016). Massage therapy research review. *Complementary Therapies in Clinical Practice, 24*, 19–31.

Gee, B. M., Thompson, K., & St John, H. (2014). Efficacy of a sound–based intervention with a child with an autism spectrum disorder and auditory sensory over–responsivity. *Occupational Therapy International, 21*(1), 12–20.

Gentil-Gutiérrez, A., Cuesta-Gómez, J. L., Rodríguez-Fernández, P., & González-Bernal, J. J. (2021). Implication of the sensory environment in children with autism spectrum disorder: Perspectives from school. *International Journal of Environmental Research and Public Health, 18*(14), 7670.

Gill, K., Thompson-Hodgetts, S., & Rasmussen, C. (2018). A critical review of research on the Alert Program®. *Journal of Occupational Therapy, Schools, & Early Intervention, 11*(2), 212–228.

Gringras, P., Green, D., Wright, B., Rush, C., Sparrowhawk, M., Pratt, K., Allgar, V., Hooke, N., Moore, D., Zaiwalla, Z., & Wiggs, L. (2014). Weighted blankets and sleep in autistic children--a randomized controlled trial. *Pediatrics, 134*(2), 298–306.

Hall, L., & Case-Smith, J. (2007). The effect of sound-based intervention on children with sensory processing disorders and visual-motor delays. *American Journal of Occupational Therapy, 61*, 209–215.

Harry, J. R., Eggleston, J. D., Lidstone, D. E., & Dufek, J. S. (2019). Weighted vest use to improve movement control during walking in children with autism. *Translational Journal of the American College of Sports Medicine, 4*(10), 64–73.

Heyburn, K., Shaw, D., Carbert, K., & Thompson-Hodgetts, S. (2022). “Sensory in-Service”: An exploratory evaluation of a group-based, caregiver intervention for children with sensory processing difficulties. *Physical & Occupational Therapy in Pediatrics*, 1–15.

Hodgetts, S., Magill-Evans, J., & Misiaszek, J. E. (2011a). Effects of weighted vests on classroom behavior for children with autism and cognitive impairments. *Research in Autism Spectrum Disorders, 5*, 495–505.

Hodgetts, S., Magill-Evans, J., & Misiaszek, J. E. (2011b). Weighted vests, stereotyped behaviors and arousal in children with autism. *Journal of Autism and Developmental Disorders, 41*, 805–814.

Hopkins, G. (2010). The 4th R: Making the case for recess. Retrieved from http://ofprincipalconcern-educationworld.blogspot.com/2010/03/fourth-r-making-case-for-recess.html.

Hulac, D. M., Mickelson, L. R., Briesch, A. M., Marocca, H., Hartjes, C., Anderson, K., & Ederveen, K. (2022). Stability balls and student on-task behavior. *Journal of Behavioral Education, 31*, 543–560. https://doi.org/10.1007/s10864-020-09412-3.

Jarrett, O. S. (2003). Recess in elementary school: What does the research say? *ERIC Digest*. Retrieved from www.ericdigests.org/2003-2/recess.html.

Jorge, J., de Witt, P. A., & Franzsen, D. (2013). The effect of a two-week sensory diet on fussy infants with regulatory sensory processing disorder. *South African Journal of Occupational Therapy, 43*(3), 28–34.

Kane, A., Luiselli, J. K., Dearborn, S., & Young, N. (2004). Wearing a weighted vest as intervention for children with autism/pervasive developmental disorder: Behavioral assessment of stereotype and attention to task. *Scientific Review of Mental Health Practice, 3*(2), 19–24.

Katzenellenbogen, G., Franzsen, D., & van der Linde, J. (2021). Postural control in children receiving intervention using the Astronaut Training Protocol. *South African Journal of Occupational Therapy, 51*(2), 65–73.

Keith, J. M., Jamieson, J. P., & Bennetto, L. (2018). The influence of noise on autonomic arousal and cognitive performance in adolescents with autism spectrum disorder. *Journal of Autism and Developmental Disorders, 49*, 113–126.

Kinnealey, M., et al. (2012). Effect of classroom modification on attention and engagement of students with autism or dyspraxia. *American Journal of Occupational Therapy, 66*, 511–519.

Koenig, K. P., Buckley-Reen, A., & Garg, S. (2012). Efficacy of the get ready to learn yoga program among children with autism spectrum disorders: A pretest–posttest control group design. *American Journal of Occupational Therapy, 66*(5), 538–546.

Koomar, J. (2009). Trauma- and attachment-informed sensory integration assessment and intervention. *Special Interest Section Quarterly: Sensory Integration, 32*(4), 1–4.

Krauss, K. E. (1987). The effects of deep pressure touch on anxiety. *American Journal of Occupational Therapy, 41*, 366–373.

Krieger, B., Piškur, B., Schulze, C., Jakobs, U., Beurskens, A., & Moser, A. (2018). Supporting and hindering environments for participation of adolescents diagnosed with autism spectrum disorder: A scoping review. *PLoS One, 13*(8),e0202071.

Kuhaneck, H. M., & Kelleher, J. (2015). Development of the classroom sensory environment assessment (CSEA). *American Journal of Occupational Therapy, 69*(6), p1–p9.

Lönn, M., Aili, K., Svedberg, P., Nygren, J., Jarbin, H., & Larsson, I. (2023). Experiences of using weighted blankets among children with ADHD and sleeping difficulties. *Occupational Therapy International*,1945290.

Larsson, I., Aili, K., Nygren, J. M., Jarbin, H., & Svedberg, P. (2021). Parents' experiences of weighted blankets' impact on children with attention-deficit/hyperactivity disorder (ADHD) and sleep problems-A qualitative study. *International Journal of Environmental Research Public Health, 18*(24),12959.

Larsson, I., Aili, K., Nygren, J. M., Johansson, P., Jarbin, H., & Svedberg, P. (2022). Sleep: Intervention with weighted blankets for children with attention deficit hyperactivity disorder (ADHD) and sleep problems: Study protocol for a randomised control trial. *BMJ Open, 12*(1),e047509.

Leew, S. V., Stein, N. G., & Gibbard, W. B. (2010). Weighted vests' effect on social attention for toddlers with autism spectrum disorders. *Canadian Journal of Occupational Therapy, 77*, 113–124.

Lin, H. Y., Lee, P., Chang, W. D., & Hong, F. Y. (2014). Effects of weighted vests on attention, impulse control, and on-task behavior in children with attention deficit hyperactivity disorder. *American Journal of Occupational Therapy, 68*(2), 149–158.

Little, L. M., Pope, E., Wallisch, A., & Dunn, W. (2018). Occupation-based coaching by means of telehealth for families of young children with autism spectrum disorder. *American Journal of Occupational Therapy, 72*,7202205020.

Lovrić, R., Farčić, N., Mikšić, Š., & Gvozdanović Debeljak, A. (2020). Parental perception of changes in basic life needs of children with disabilities after six months of therapeutic horseback riding: A qualitative study. *International Journal of Environmental Research and Public Health, 17*(4), 1213.

Macphee, F. L., Merrill, B. M., Altszuler, A. R., Ramos, M. C., Gnagy, E. M., Greiner, A. R., Coxe, S., Raiker, J. S., Coles, E., Burger, L., & Pelham, W. E. (2019). The effect of weighted vests and stability balls with and without psychostimulant medication on classroom outcomes for children with ADHD. *School Psychology Review, 48*(3), 276–289. https://doi.org/10.17105/SPR-2017-0151.V48-3.

Mallory, C., & Keehn, B. (2021). Implications of sensory processing and attentional differences associated with autism in academic settings: An integrative review. *Frontiers in Psychiatry, 12*:695825.

Martin, C. S. (2016). Exploring the impact of the design of the physical classroom environment on young children with autism spectrum disorder (ASD). *Journal of Research in Special Educational Needs, 16*(4), 280–298.

Masgutova, S., Akhmatova, N., Sadowska, L., Shackleford, P., & Akhmatov, E. (2016). Progress with neurosensorimotor reflex integration for children with Autism Spectrum Disorder. *Journal of Neurology and Psychology, 4*(2), 14.

Masgutova, S. K., Akhmatova, N. K., Sadowska, L., Shackleford, P., & Akhmatov, E. A. (2016). Neurosensorimotor reflex integration for autism: A new therapy modality paradigm. *Journal of Pediatric Neurological Disorders, 2*(1), 1–12.

Masgutova, S., Sadowska, L., Kowalewska, J., Masgutov, D., Akhmatova, N., & Filipowski, H. (2015). Use of a neurosensorimotor reflex integration program to improve reflex patterns of children with down syndrome. *Journal of Neurology and Neurosciences, 6*(4), 59.

Maula, M. I., Aji, A. L., Aliyafi, M. B., Afif, I. Y., Ammarullah, M. I., Winarni, T. I., & Jamari, J. (2021). The subjective comfort test of autism hug machine portable seat. *Journal of Intellectual Disability, Diagnosis, and Treatment, 9*, 182–188.

Minelli, G., Puglisi, G. E., & Astolfi, A. (2022). Acoustical parameters for learning in classroom: A review. *Building and Environment, 208*, 108582.

Mudford, O. C., & Cullen, C. (2005). *Auditory integration training: A critical review*. Controversial Therapies for Developmental Disabilities, 373–384.

Musiyenko, O. V., Chopyk, R. V., & Kizlo, N. B. (2020). Influence of swimming on sensory functioning, quality of life and behavior of children with autism. *Health, Sport, Rehabilitation, 6*(3), 60–69.

Niehues, A. N., Bundy, A. C., Mattingly, C. F., & Lawlor, M. C. (1991). Making a difference: Occupational therapy in the public schools. *Occupational Therapy Journal of Research, 11*(4), 195–212.

Parham, L. D., Roley, S. S., May-Benson, T. A., Koomar, J., Brett-Green, B., Burke, J. P., … Schaaf, R. C. (2011). Development of a fidelity measure for research on the effectiveness of the Ayres Sensory Integration® intervention. *American Journal of Occupational Therapy, 65*(2), 133–142.

Pecuch, A., Gieysztor, E., Telenga, M., Wolańska, E., Kowal, M., & Paprocka-Borowicz, M. (2020). Primitive reflex activity in relation to the sensory profile in healthy preschool children. *International Journal of Environmental Research and Public Health, 17*(21), 8210.

Pecuch, A., Gieysztor, E., Wolańska, E., Telenga, M., & Paprocka-Borowicz, M. (2021). Primitive reflex activity in relation to motor skills in healthy preschool children. *Brain Sciences, 11*(8), 967.

Pfeiffer, B., Clark, G. F., & Arbesman, M. (2018). Effectiveness of cognitive and occupation-based interventions for children with challenges in sensory processing and integration: A systematic review. *American Journal of Occupational Therapy, 72*(1), p1–p9.

Pfeiffer, B., Stein Duker, L., Murphy, A., & Shui, C. (2019). Effectiveness of noise-attenuating headphones on physiological responses for children with autism spectrum disorders. *Frontiers in Integrative Neuroscience, 65*.

Pingale, V., Fletcher, T., & Candler, C. (2019). The effects of sensory diets on children's classroom behaviors. *Journal of Occupational Therapy, Schools, & Early Intervention, 12*(2), 225–238.

Pingale, V., Fletcher, T. S., Candler, C., Pickens, N., & Dunlap, K. (2022). Effects of sensory diets: A single subject study. *Journal of Occupational Therapy, Schools, & Early Intervention, 15*(2), 165–180.

Re, P., McConnell, J. W., Reidinger, G., Schweit, R., & Hendron, A. (2014). Effects of yoga on patients in an adolescent mental health hospital and the relationship between those effects and the patients' sensory–processing patterns. *Journal of Child and Adolescent Psychiatric Nursing, 27*(4), 175–182.

Reichow, B., et al. (2010). Effects of weighted vests on the engagement of children with developmental delays and autism. *Focus on Autism and Other Developmental Disabilities, 25*, 3–11.

Reynolds, S., Glennon, T. J., Ausderau, K., Bendixen, R. M., Kuhaneck, H. M., Pfeiffer, B., Watling, R., Wilkinson, K., & Bodison, S. C. (2017). Using a multifaceted approach to working with children who have differences in sensory processing and integration. *American Journal of Occupational Therapy, 71*(2), p1–p10. https://doi.org/10.5014/ajot.2017.019281.

Ruiz-Rodrigo, A., Morales, E., Louis-Delsoin, C., & Rousseau, J. (2023). Parents' perceptions of the impact of the home environment on youth living with an Autism Spectrum Disorder. *Journal of Accessibility and Design for All, 13*(1), 43–68.

Schilling, D. L., & Schwartz, I. S. (2004). Alternative seating for young children with autism spectrum disorder: Effects on classroom behavior. *Journal of Autism and Developmental Disorders, 34*, 423–432.

Schoen, S. A., Miller, L. J., & Sullivan, J. (2015). A pilot study of integrated listening systems for children with sensory processing problems. *Journal of Occupational Therapy, Schools, & Early Intervention, 8*(3), 256–276.

Silva, L. M., Schalock, M., Ayres, R., Bunse, C., & Budden, S. (2009). Qigong massage treatment for sensory and self-regulation problems in young children with autism: A randomized controlled trial. *American Journal of Occupational Therapy, 63*(4), 423–432.

Silva, L. M., Schalock, M., & Gabrielsen, K. (2011). Early intervention for autism with a parent-delivered qigong massage program: A randomized controlled trial. *American Journal of Occupational Therapy, 65*(5), 550–559.

Silva, L. M., Schalock, M., Gabrielsen, K. R., Budden, S. S., Buenrostro, M., & Horton, G. (2015). Early intervention with a parent-delivered massage protocol directed at tactile abnormalities decreases severity of autism and improves child-to-parent interactions: A replication study. *Autism Research and Treatment, 2015.*

Sinha, Y., Silove, N., Hayen, A., & Williams, K. (2011). Auditory integration training and other sound therapies for autism spectrum disorders (ASD). *Cochrane Database of Systematic Reviews, 2011*(12).

Slevin, M., O'Connor, K., Segurado, R., & Murphy, J. F. A. (2020). Therapeutic listening for preterm children with sensory dysregulation, attention and cognitive problems. *Irish Medical Journal, 113*(1), 4.

Stanić, V., Žnidarič, T., Repovš, G., & Geršak, G. (2022). Dynamic seat assessment for enabled restlessness of children with learning difficulties. *Sensors, 22*(9), 3170.

Umeda, C., & Deitz, J. (2011). Effects of therapy cushions on classroom behaviors of children with autism spectrum disorder. *American Journal of Occupational Therapy, 65*, 152–159.

Villasenor, R. F., Smith, S. L., & Jewell, V. D. (2018). A systematic review of sound-based intervention programs to improve participation in education for children with sensory processing and integration challenges. *Journal of Occupational Therapy, Schools, & Early Intervention, 11*(2), 172–191.

Wagner, B., Fitzpatrick, J., Symons, M., Jirikowic, T., Cross, D., & Latimer, J. (2017). The development of a culturally appropriate school based intervention for Australian aboriginal children living in remote communities: A formative evaluation of the Alert Program® intervention. *Australian Occupational Therapy Journal, 64*(3), 243–252.

Wagner, B., Olson, H. C., Symons, M., Mazzucchelli, T. G., Jirikowic, T., Latimer, J., … Fitzpatrick, J. (2019). Improving self-regulation and executive functioning skills in primary school children in a remote Australian aboriginal community: A pilot study of the Alert program. *Australian Journal of Education, 63*(1), 98–115.

Wallisch, A., Little, L., Pope, E., & Dunn, W. (2019). Parent perspectives of an occupational therapy telehealth intervention. *International Journal of Telerehabilitation, 11*(1), 15.

Ward, S. C., Whalon, K., Rusnak, K., Wendell, K., & Paschall, N. (2013). The association between therapeutic horseback riding and the social communication and sensory reactions of children with autism. *Journal of Autism and Developmental Disorders, 43*, 2190–2198.

Watling, R., Miller-Kuhaneck, H., Parham, L. D., & Schaaf, R. C. (2018). *Occupational therapy practice guidelines for children and youth with challenges in sensory integration and sensory processing.* AOTA Press. https://doi.org/10.7139/2017.978-1-56900-483-8..

Wells, A. M., et al. (2012). Neurocognitive habilitation therapy for children with fetal alcohol spectrum disorders: An adaptation of the Alert Program. *American Journal of Occupational Therapy, 66*, 24–34.

Wilbarger, J., Wilbarger, P., Williams, M., Shellenberger, S., McEwen, M., Gjesing, G., Osten, B., Kawar, M., Frick, S., Oetter, P., & Richter, E. (2020). Complementary programs for intervention. In A. C. Bundy, & S. Lane (Eds.), *Sensory integration theory and practice* (3rd ed.) (pp. 423–478). FA Davis.

Wilbarger, P. (1984). Planning an adequate "sensory diet" - application of sensory processing theory during the first year of life. *Zero to Three, 5*(1), 7–12.

Wilbarger, P. (1995). The sensory diet: Activity programs based on sensory processing theory. *Sensory Integration Special Interest Section Newsletter, 18*(2), 1–4.

Wilbarger, P., & Wilbarger, L. (1991). *Sensory defensiveness in children aged 2-12. Avanti Educational Programs.*

Williams, M. S., & Shellenberger, S. (1994). *"How does your engine run?" A leader's guide to the Alert Program for Self-regulation.* TherapyWorks.

Zhao, M., You, Y., Li, J., Healy, S., Taylor, A., Zhang, Z., … Zou, L. (2022). *The effects of therapeutic horseback riding program on motor skills in children with autism spectrum disorder.*

Zimmerman, K. N., Ledford, J. R., & Severini, K. E. (2019). Brief report: The effects of a weighted blanket on engagement for a student with ASD. *Focus on Autism and Other Developmental Disabilities, 34*(1), 15–19.

29

# Application of Motor Control and Motor Learning

*Katherine Dimitropoulou, Jane Clifford O'Brien, and Patty Coker-Bolt*

## GUIDING QUESTIONS

1. What are the key concepts and primary principles of motor control and motor learning theories?
2. How do principles of motor control inform occupational therapy evidence-based interventions for children with motor skill deficits?
3. Which child, occupation, and contextual factors influence motor skill acquisition and occupational performance?
4. What concepts of motor control and motor learning contribute to interventions such as CIMT and bimanual therapy?

## KEY TERMS

Agency
Constraint-induced movement training
Extrinsic feedback
Intrinsic feedback
Flexibility
Intensive bimanual therapy
Mental practice
Motor control
Motor learning
Motor skills
Prospectivity
Transfer of learning

## INTRODUCTION

Children use movement to learn about their bodies, explore their worlds, and develop motor, cognitive, sensory, emotional, and social skills (Adolph & Franchak, 2017; Comalli et al., 2016; Hoch et al., 2019). They use their bodies and movements intentionally for feeding, dressing, bathing, play, and academics (Fig. 29.1A and B). They spend abundant time and effort practicing their movements and skills while playing, interacting with peers, and as they access their environments (Adolph & Hoch, 2019; Goodway et al., 2019).

Children's movements and motor skills are variable, embedded in their plans and decisions about their activities and interactions within the context of daily occupations (Fig. 29.2A–D). Children's movements within daily occupations are goal directed (Frese & Sabini, 2021). Goal-directed movements are complex and influenced by many factors, such as sensory (e.g., visual information, tactile information), motor (e.g., range of motion, muscle strength), cognitive (e.g., attention, problem-solving), emotional (e.g., motivation), and environmental (e.g., objects used, tasks, peer interactions) contexts (Fiehler et al., 2019).

Children who have difficulties with their motor systems may take longer and often do not master movements they need for daily occupations; they may give up on expanding their motor skills to accomplish their goals; and they may not have the same opportunities to explore their surroundings (Hua et al., 2022; Nobre et al., 2023). Because movements and motor skills are central to participation, occupational therapy practitioners provide interventions to improve children's motor skills. These interventions often focus on mismatches between the child's abilities, the task, and the environment through evidence-based principles of motor control and learning (Fig. 29.3).

**Motor skills** are goal-directed actions in which children voluntarily engage in an activity that is meaningful to them. Children's daily lives consist of a plethora of goal-directed tasks that require skillful motor engagement. Reaching for a cup of water, building a Lego truck, or climbing a jungle gym ladder are some examples of everyday activities that engage a multitude of systems toward a desired goal. Skillful interaction with daily tasks to accomplish desired goals develops and is refined over time as children's bodies grow and their interactions with the world become more complex (Adolph & Hoch, 2019).

Two specific processes assist in the growing abilities and mastery of skillful behaviors: motor control and motor learning. The term **motor control** refers to how the body organizes and directs movement through dynamic interactions of multiple systems to accomplish a goal (Schmidt et al., 2018). The process of motor control addresses how the central nervous system organizes movement and how we can evaluate and characterize the nature, quality, and timing of movement (Shadmehr et al., 2010). **Motor learning** refers to the process, conditions, and rate in which a person learns motor skills. Person factors, task characteristics, and contexts influence the learning process (Krakauer et al., 2019). Motor learning research provides evidence of how learning occurs (e.g., person-task interaction conditions, task-environment conditions, level of practice needed) and whether newly learned motor responses are generalized and used in a variety of functional tasks (Jelsma et al., 2015; Jongbloed-Pereboom et al., 2015; Krebs et al., 2012). Children's motor skill learning is dynamic and adaptive as they develop, grow, and change interests and environments (Babik et al., 2022). Motor learning research examines the mechanisms of learning and learning processes in the context of occupations and development and focuses on the techniques and strategies that influence brain development for learning and adaptation (Risen et al., 2015).

Occupational therapy practitioners and researchers interested in motor control and motor learning examine the mechanisms, systems, strategies, and development of movement, motor performance, and functional abilities in daily tasks as well as causes of motor dysfunction (de Camargo Barros, Tani, & Correa, 2017). Motor control and

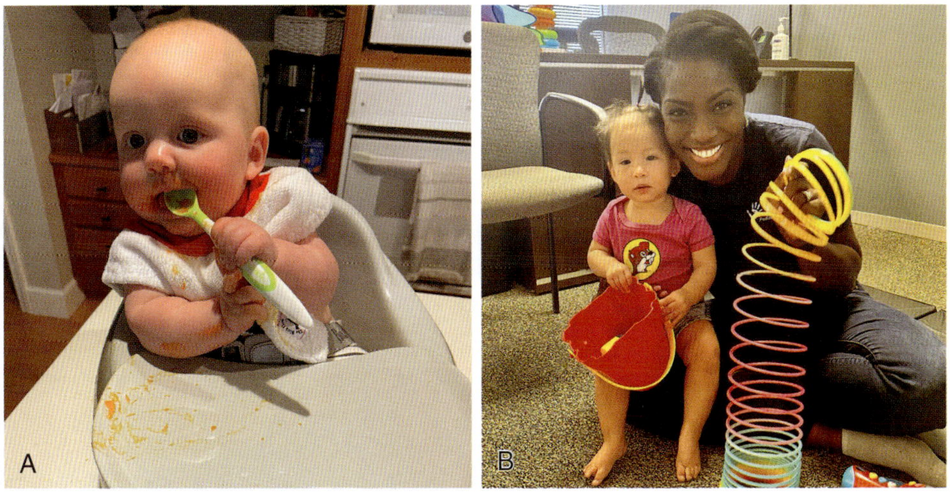

**Fig. 29.1** (A) Children use their hands for feeding. (B) Children hold objects during play. ((A) Photo courtesy Lauren Shain). (B) Photo courtesy Michelle Atanu.)

learning are integral to occupational engagement. Box 29.1 highlights the diversity of motor control and learning challenges found in children and adolescents and the functional consequences as they engage in daily occupations. Occupational therapy practitioners engage children in goal-directed tasks and daily occupations (Bo & Lee, 2013; Goncalves et al., 2018; Kearney & Judge, 2017; Kolovelonis et al., 2012). Thus, for occupational therapy practitioners, motor control and learning also pertain to the strategies and the nature of the tasks and environments that promote motor performance and skills (Chan et al., 2015; Gredin & Williams, 2016; Jongbloed-Pereboom et al., 2015; Maxwell et al., 2017). Understanding motor control and learning processes is essential to designing and applying interventions for children with disabilities to learn and retain motor skills as well as to use these skills in their occupations.

This chapter begins by describing the motor control process to provide readers with a systematic way to view children's movements. Then, the authors describe motor control and learning strategies that can be used to design activities and interventions in occupational therapy practice. This chapter has four sections: (1) principles of motor control and their application in pediatric clinical populations; (2) principles of motor learning and their application in pediatric clinical populations; (3) intervention strategies based on motor control/learning principles; and (4) specific existing pediatric evidence-based intervention protocols based on principles of motor control and learning.

## PRINCIPLES OF MOTOR CONTROL AND THEIR APPLICATION IN PEDIATRIC CLINICAL POPULATIONS

Occupational therapy practitioners acknowledge the dynamic nature of movement and consider influences of the child, occupation (including tasks), and environment, as illustrated in Fig. 29.3, to better support this fit. They evaluate children's strengths and areas that need improvement and support (see Chapter 9). They use clinical reasoning to decide how to support children's strengths while addressing factors hindering children's motor performance. They use task analysis to examine task demands for effective interactions. They identify environmental factors that can support or hinder children's performance.

Contemporary motor control approaches that are congruent with the occupational therapy perspective are based on dynamic systems and ecologic theories (see online resources for more information) and support children's active engagement in activity and the use of goal-directed tasks. Guiding principles of contemporary motor control approaches provide a useful context of examining motor behavior in the context of functional activities (see Box 29.2).

### Goal-Directed Movements

Infants, toddlers, children, and adolescents are internally motivated to move as they explore their bodies, objects, carry out important tasks, and interact with others and their environments. They reach and grasp objects, bang things together, crawl, walk, run (even if they stumble), dress, scribble, draw, write, build structures, engage in sports, etc., mastering movements and increasing their repertoire of motor behaviors to accomplish important goals. There are four important characteristics in motor performance that in typically developing children are present beginning in the first 3–4 months of life: agency, prospectivity, flexibility, and adaptability (Adolph & Hoch, 2019; Adolph & Robinson, 2015; Reddy et al., 2013; Von Hofsten, 2004). Persistent lack of agency, prospectivity, flexibility, and adaptability over the course of development leads to motor dysfunction.

**Agency.** The development of motor skills is driven by agency (Adolph & Kretch, 2015). Children practice, problem solve, develop strength, accuracy, timing, and coordination to control their movements with a purpose. *Agency* refers to the discovery in early childhood of the ability to control aspects of an event or an activity through one's own actions. Early on in life, classic studies demonstrate that infants discover that they can control and transform spontaneous waving and kicking movements to organized reaching and kicking goal-directed actions (Kelso, 2016; Kelso & Fuchs, 2016). Infants as early as 4 months can demonstrate an early grasp pattern as they randomly move their arms/hands, swiping toward a rattle. Getting the rattle (goal) and the discovery that their arms/hands can be moved in concerted ways and used to accomplish that goal (*agency*) lead to the first skillful reach and grasp patterns (D'Souza et al., 2017; Haggard, 2017). Early studies in children with motor deficits support that children with cerebral palsy (CP) used more supination when hitting a drum with their hand than when simply exercising (Van der Weel et al., 1991). Not only did children perform the task more efficiently, but they also engaged in the task for longer periods of time and activated more areas of the brain during the activity. Additional behavioral studies confirm that agency enhances

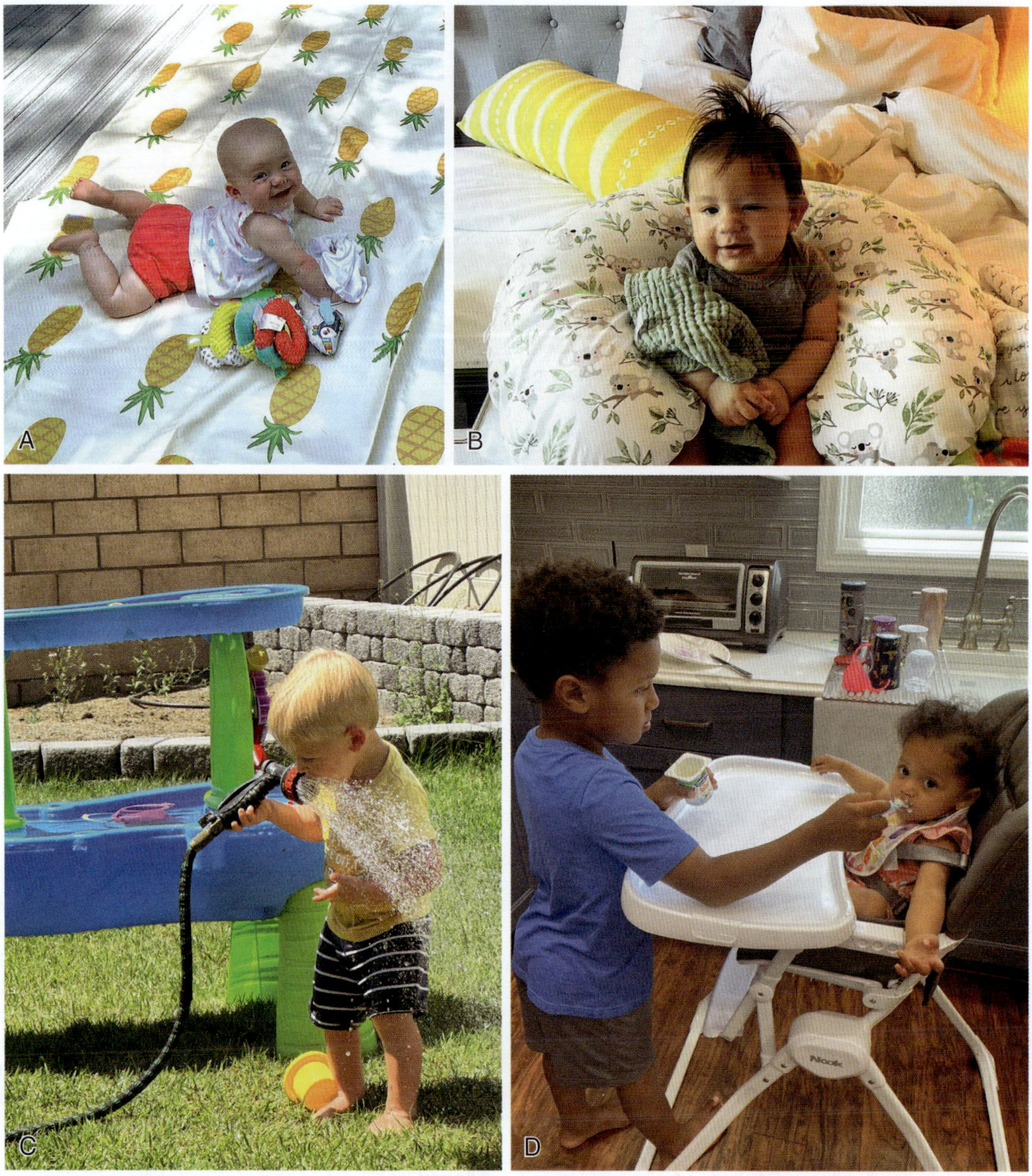


**Fig. 29.2** Children move in many positions (such as prone, sitting, kneeling, or standing) when playing. (A) This young infant enjoys playing on her tummy (prone position). (B) This infant needs some support to sit upright and play. (C) This toddler enjoys standing and moving during play. (D) This child stands to feed his little sister. ((A) Photo courtesy Lauren Shain. (B) Photo courtesy Krysta Rives. (C) Photo courtesy Sydney Bast Weldner. (D) Photo courtesy of Angela Olijumi.)

motor performance in the same population (Miller et al., 2016). Van de Winckel and colleagues found significantly more brain activation for both children with CP and typically developing children when they were engaged in active movement (grasp and release of an object) compared with passive movements (robot moved finger up and down) and tactile stimulation (stroking back of hand with sponge cotton cloth). The findings suggest engaging children in active tasks results in more brain activation for both typical children and clinical populations (Gaberova et al., 2019; Lee et al., 2013; Van de Winckel et al., 2013). When designing interventions, occupational therapy practitioners select activities that are within the children's interests, engage children in setting goals and make choices, provide children with clear results for their motor actions (salient outcomes), and provide opportunities for children to reflect and evaluate their motor actions and make decisions for future performance.

**Prospectivity.** Prospectivity is another important characteristic of skilled motor performance. It refers to planning motor actions in anticipation of task demands and consequences of behavior (Adolph, 2020; Adolph & Kretch, 2015). As infants learn more about their bodies and how objects move, they position their bodies, arms, and hands effectively and timely to successfully reach and grasp a moving rattle. Prospectivity is a developing skill and enables children to engage in increasingly complex motor tasks that require more than one step and/or that require timed coordination and accuracy, such as ball games, putting on a shirt, drawing letters, or playing basketball (Bäckström

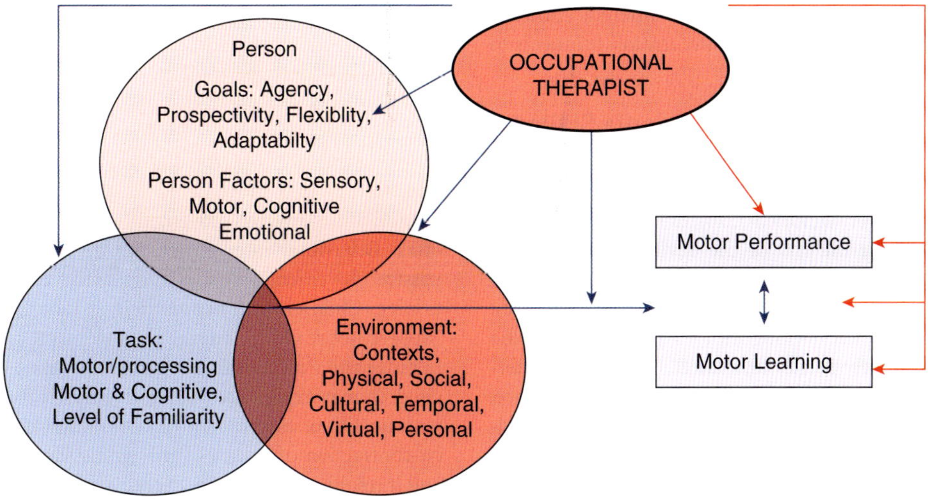


**Fig. 29.3** Motor control factors and the role of occupational therapy practitioner in the process.

## BOX 29.1 Examples of Motor Control Deficits

- Georgia is a 2-year-old girl who has difficulty playing on the playground. She is diagnosed with CP, right hemiplegia. She walks but her movements are slow. She leans to the left and drags her right toe on the ground. She walks with a wide base of support. She does not use her right hand when playing with her toys and has difficulty manipulating objects. The other children ran quickly past her. Georgia falls frequently. She looks frustrated at times, but she is eager and curious to engage in play with peers. She follows them around.
- Teagan is a 4-year-old boy with Down syndrome who loves to play T-ball. Teagan has low muscle tone throughout his body. His posture is asymmetric (he elevates his shoulders and leans to the left) when he runs. He runs with a wide-based gait and holds his arms close to his body for balance. He must take breaks when running around the bases. He holds objects using a palmar grasp and exhibits delay in the visual-perceptual skills that interferes with his fine motor performance. Teagan engages in parallel play with other children at the daycare center. When he does interact with his peers, he engages at a much younger level of play and/or frequently interferes in their play.
- Devin is a 10-year-old boy, diagnosed with Developmental Coordination Disorder (DCD), who has difficulty with fine motor tasks, such as tying his shoes, buttoning, and writing. He takes longer than his peers to get ready for recess. Devin has difficulty with balance and coordination skills and falls frequently. He cannot skip, hop, or ride a bicycle. Eye-hand coordination is poor as shown in his inability to catch a ball or play games such as baseball or Frisbee.

## BOX 29.2 Guiding Principles of Motor Control

- **Goal-directed movements** have common characteristics important for success:
  - *Agency*: the ability to control and monitor movements to serve a specific action and goal
  - *Prospectivity*: the ability to plan movements in anticipation of their outcomes
  - *Flexibility*: the ability to stop and alter strategies that do not work
  - *Adaptability*: the ability to transfer strategies from familiar to novel situations
- **Interactions among multiple systems underlie skilled motor behavior** (i.e., person, occupation, contexts) and are responsible for the control of motor actions at any given moment
  - *Person:* These are factors related to body structures and functions specific to each child (i.e., sensory, musculoskeletal, perceptual, cognitive/processing, and emotional skills).
  - *Tasks (with Occupation)*: Tasks are meaningful, impact the motor actions and children's ability to engage in occupations. Included are task nature, motor and cognitive demands, objects used and their properties, and level of familiarity for the child. Tasks can be modified and adapted to facilitate motor control and goal achievement.
  - *Contexts* include personal factors (e.g., age, sex/gender, socio-economic factors, cultural expectations) and environments (e.g., home, school, community). Contexts affect the expression of motor skills and the control and monitoring of motor actions for successful performance.

et al., 2021; Donath et al., 2015). Repeated errors that relate to the accuracy and timely execution of movements are indicators of lack of prospectivity. Prospectivity errors are also evident in tasks that require more than one step (multistep).

**Flexibility.** Flexibility refers to the ability to recognize errors in motor performance and shift strategies toward a better outcome (Adolph & Hoch, 2019). After some failed attempts toward the task goal, children will modify their movements (i.e., reach further, move slower, turn their wrists, flex their fingers) or adjust their posture (i.e., sit on floor, instead of standing) to successfully stop and grasp a rolling tennis ball. Daily tasks are inherently variable even if they are carried out in the same contexts. Thus, the use of the same strategies even if movements are not successful reveals lack of flexibility and relates to significant functional problems in everyday tasks. Children with autism spectrum disorder (ASD) often present lack of flexibility. They appear "stuck," using the same motor behavior in a task even if they are not successful with their goal (Mostert-Kerckhoffs et al., 2015).

**Adaptability.** *Adaptability* refers to the generation of new strategies to novel tasks and environments (transfer). Children with sensory, motor, and/or processing deficits (e.g., developmental coordination disorder [DCD]) often lack adaptability. They frequently carry out a task successfully within a specific context, but their repertoire of movements and their ability to adapt to different environmental demands does support the same performance in different contexts. Occupational therapy practitioners develop intervention protocols to support the development of these skills.

## Interactions Among Multiple Systems Underlie Skilled Motor Behavior

Children's movements are the results of interactions among many systems (i.e., person, task, and environment). Instead of focusing work on either personal factors or the task or the environment, occupational therapy practitioners consider all these components and their interactions when evaluating functional performance to design an intervention. For example, when working with a 5-year-old child who attends kindergarten, to improve letter formation, occupational therapy practitioners may work on improving the child's sitting balance, core strength, strength of arm/grasp patterns (person factors) or modify the task and start with a few letters that are easier to form and use an adaptive pencil grip (task adaptation); they may also recommend to add a slant board for writing on the student's desk in the classroom (environmental adaptation) to ergonomically support student's stamina and performance. This multilevel intervention can facilitate improvement of arm/hand muscle strength and movement coordination during handwriting and can result in faster and more legible writing samples, further motivating the child to practice these skills. The complexity of motor skills can be further illustrated by examining the system requirements for the complex motor tasks of biking or cutting with scissors (see online resources for video case studies and a checklist to examine system requirements). The following sections provide an overview of systems and how they influence motor skills.

**Person Factors.** Occupational therapy practitioners examine personal factors using knowledge of anatomy, biomechanics, neuroscience, and kinesiology to identify areas that may be interfering with motor performance. They develop goals based on the child's strengths, needs, and preferences.

***Sensory Systems.*** Sensory systems are important for accessing information and feedback to inform motor actions and facilitate performance (Adolph & Hoch, 2019; Cuturi & Gori, 2019; Steinberg et al., 2016). Visual, proprioceptive, vestibular, tactile, and auditory systems separately and in concert inform motor actions. For example, the visual system provides a plethora of information in the immediate and far space about objects and people and their interactions (de Sá et al., 2018; Sinno et al., 2021). The vestibular system provides a sense of movement in space and allows for timed motor responses to task demands. Integration across systems informs complex motor actions. For example, visual, vestibular, and kinesthetic information constantly interact to maintain balance control as children navigate a jungle gym in a noisy playground.

***Musculoskeletal System.*** Observation of a child's physical appearance provides the occupational therapy practitioner with an overview of musculoskeletal structures required for movement. Physical appearance includes symmetry between the right and left sides of the body, muscular structures (including range of motion), and physical stature. There are specific characteristics essential for understanding the musculoskeletal system: muscle tone, range of motion, strength, and posture.

Muscle tone refers to tension or the contraction state of a muscle at rest. Muscles are in partial contraction when at rest, maintaining a level of readiness to engage the body in different movements (Ganguly et al., 2021; Goo et al., 2018). This dynamic state is accomplished by reflexive activity and top-down control in the central nervous system. Muscle tone maintains posture for each body limb and the entire body. Typical muscle tone dynamically supports voluntary control of limbs in goal-directed tasks, allows movement into and out of positions with ease, fluidity of movement, and variety in movement. Tone abnormalities such as high (hypertonicity) or low tone (hypotonia) create significant problems with controlled voluntary movement and impact skilled motor control. Children with ***hypertonicity*** exhibit excessive muscle tone. Muscles are contracted at rest and/or present excessive contraction during quick movements. As a result, there is a limited range of motion and power of movement when engaging in voluntary motor tasks. Behavioral interventions to decrease tone may include slow passive movement and stretching, active range of motion, and positioning. Children with ***hypotonicity*** exhibit low muscle tone, muscles "appear not ready" to engage in movement, and movements are wide in range and slow, limiting control and timing of motor actions. Some children may experience fluctuating muscle tone, which also interferes with quality of motor control. Voluntary movement, which requires co-contraction of muscles (protagonists/antagonists), is not efficient, and it results in unplanned, excessive movements (e.g., the arm cannot reach straight forward toward a target).

The ability of joints is to actively move through the biomechanical range. Muscle tone problems such as hypertonicity, hypotonicity, etc., can alter the range of motion of specific joints and impact the child's ability to functionally use these joints to move and interact with objects. For example, limited abduction and opposition of the thumb in the hand prevents a child from being able to hold and lift a cup to drink water.

**Strength** is defined as the voluntary recruitment of muscle fibers to support motor actions that have some levels of resistance (Torres-Costoso et al., 2020). Strength is needed to perform movements against gravity or to pick up/carry objects of varying weights. A degree of trunk strength is required to maintain posture. Strength building programs entail movements *during activities*, often with added resistance or weight.

***Posture*** is the ability to control and maintain a specific position of a body segment (alignment) or of the entire body in space (Ivanenko & Gurfinkel, 2018; Shumway-Cook et al., 2023). It can be achieved by co-contraction of groups of muscles to keep a limb or the entire body in a specific position. Postural control is required for functional movement and involves an interplay between sensorimotor and musculoskeletal systems (Kiefer et al., 2021; Westcott & Burtner, 2004). Children stabilize their head, trunk, and legs to support arm and hand movements in everyday activities (e.g., to hold a cup). This stability is essential for refined movements, and it is dynamic and adaptable to support complex task demands (Hill et al., 2019; Westcott & Burtner, 2004). For example, keeping the head and body steady is essential for reaching. However, when reaching for a pair of pants to put on while standing, head and trunk stability postures dynamically change to support leaning forward to hold the pants with both hands toward the legs while standing briefly on one leg to slide the other through the pants. Given the dynamic nature of postural control, it is essential to evaluate it in stationary (e.g., sitting, standing) and dynamic movement tasks (e.g., sitting and reaching for an object, walking, and holding a cup, etc.).

Postural control problems differ across neurodevelopmental disorders (e.g., CP, DCD, ASD), affecting balance and coordination (Miller et al., 2019; Patel et al., 2020; Zoccante et al., 2021). For example, children with hemiplegic CP experience better head and trunk stability while reaching with the unaffected arm/hand for a cup rather than when using the affected side (Dimitropoulou & Gordon, 2020; Seyyar et al., 2019). Children with ASD have problems coordinating head and trunk stability to support skillful reaching for a cup, resulting in loss of balance or errors in reaching and grasping (Miller et al., 2019).

***Perceptual Systems.*** *Perception* refers to the ability to make sense of sensory stimuli and possibilities for action and interaction with the environment (Adolph & Young, 2021). During motor development, it is an iterative process of learning movements and movement combinations that can better accomplish task goals in variable environments. In the brain, perception entails information from the senses to be integrated to inform actions (Kandel et al., 2021). For example, visual, proprioceptive, and kinesthetic systems interact with motor systems to inform reaching for a cup. Children perceive the distance (vision), the cup size (vision), their body position (proprioception), and arm/hand movement (kinesthesia), and they can regulate hand/arm speed toward the cup and how the hand and fingers should be aligned (forming a grip) before they even reach the cup.

Perceptual problems can be evident for interpreting specific information from a sensory system and/or from integrating information across systems. For example, children with visual-perceptual problems may have difficulty finding their socks in a busy drawer (visual figure-ground discrimination) or are unable to recognize their shirt if it is crumpled, folded, and thrown on the ground (visual form constancy). Their dressing skills will be hindered by their ability to find their clothes. On the other hand, children with visual-perceptual and proprioceptive problems (combining perceptual information from both senses) may have difficulty recognizing if a shirt can fit them or have problems putting on their shirt correctly (put the shirt on backward or use multiple attempts to put their arms through the sleeves).

***Cognition/Processing Systems.*** Infants and children are curious and enjoy movement to explore and interact with their own bodies, activities, and their environments. Understanding a child's ability to *attend* to specific components of their own movement, the task, and the environment as well as their ability *to shift* their attention toward important information that can inform their strategies is essential. The child's tendency to *initiate* and *explore* tasks and strategies is critical for their ability to utilize known movements and action in novel situations. Children need to *problem solve* to produce smooth, coordinated movements and to move around obstacles or to adjust to situations that occur in the environment (Fernandes et al., 2016; Veldman et al., 2019). Children's engagement in goal-directed tasks is informed by prior experiences that allow for motor actions to be *prospectively guided* while open to new information and feedback. This process allows children to break down a task into steps, integrate feedback, modify existing or create new strategies, and plan and execute motor actions (motor planning). For the prospective process to work, two essential cognitive control skills need to be engaged: inhibitory control and strategy switching. *Inhibitory control* refers to the child's ability to gauge the task/environment demands and stop an internally prompted behavior that does not match these demands. *Strategy switching* is the ability to alter strategies to match the task demands. Inhibitory control and strategy switching are developing skills in childhood, but evidence of these abilities begins within the first year of life, especially in the context of motor actions (Schmidt et al., 2017).

Lastly, daily tasks that occur in natural environments require organization (i.e., sequencing of actions, efficiency) and multitasking. Even in simple daily activities such as eating cereal from a bowl with their family at breakfast, children need to organize and sequence multiple motor actions that are timely with the least amount of effort while being able to listen and/or participate in a conversation.

***Emotional Systems.*** Emotion is a psychological state that may affect motor performance. Individuals use emotional strategies to enhance their performance (Meunks et al., 2018; Murphy, 1994; Page et al., 1999; Rathunde, 2001). For example, athletes use the "power of positive thinking" to visualize achievement and subsequently exhibit improved motor performance as a result (Murphy, 1994). *Motivation*, *choice*, and *self-efficacy* are supporting emotional factors for success in motor actions. Motivation refers to the engagement and increased interest in a task and the motor actions associated with the task engagement (Lewthwaite & Wulf, 2017). Choice is the ability to select the level of engagement and task goals. Self-efficacy refers to one's belief in their abilities (Bandura & Schunk, 1981). Children who feel they will be successful are more apt to attempt new actions leading to improved neural plasticity. They engage in habits and routines that allow them to develop new skills (Kielhofner, 2008; Kramer, 2007; Taylor et al., 2024). They may move more confidently and try out new activities freely.

Conversely, children may have difficulty performing at their best when they are experiencing negative emotions such as *anxiety* or *fear*. Children may perform less effectively if they are feeling pushed or judged; they may be afraid of failure, thus may not explore or test their skills (Mahoney & Meyers, 2021). Children may want to perform an activity or skill and feel frustrated when they cannot. Watching the child's expressions during motor performance can provide cues to practitioners about the child's emotions and perceived task difficulty.

When children are overly stressed or afraid, the sympathetic nervous system is activated (e.g., increased heart rate, face redness), and their whole body begins to engage in stress response (increased cortisol levels), making it difficult for them to problem solve or learn a new motor skill (Cool & Zappetti, 2019; Dimitropoulou & Baxter, 2018). Children learn movement best when they are challenged at a level in which success is achievable and they are emotionally ready to engage in problem-solving.

**Tasks.** Occupational therapy practitioners refer to tasks as activities that are meaningful *for the child* and goal directed, supporting the individual's daily occupations. See Fig. 29.4A and B as children engage in the meaningful task of writing and drawing. Tasks can vary in their structure and demands and can challenge each child's motor performance differently. For example, washing the face can be easy for a typically developing 5-year-old child and a significant challenge for another 5-year-old child with hemiplegic CP. Thus, there is no universally accepted taxonomy for characterizing task complexity.

Occupational therapy practitioners follow general guidelines when they need to adjust the task complexity and always consider the specific child's needs before making decisions. Table 29.1 describes task categories based on information from existing literature (McIsaac et al., 2015) that focus on the motor, as well as the combined cognitive and motor (dual task) demands of a task, and the degree of children's familiarity with the task. (see Table 29.1).

Tasks can vary on the motor and processing demands. In this perspective, tasks can have low to high demands: (a) tasks can be unimanual (e.g., hold a toy with one hand) or bimanual (e.g., open a snack bag to retrieve a piece of banana); (b) tasks can differ in postural control requirements and be stationary (e.g., hold a ball) or dynamic (e.g., run and kick a ball); (c) tasks may have different requirements for coordination (degrees of freedom, speed, smoothness, force, and accuracy/precision): low demands for coordination and precision – discrete (e.g., simple tap to open a phone app) or high-level coordination and precision (jumping rope); (d) tasks can be close-ended, i.e., involve objects, people, and context that are stationary (e.g., scribble on a piece of paper) or open-ended (e.g., following with a stylus a moving target on an iPad screen).

Tasks can also pose dual demands: motor and cognitive: (a) tasks can be one step (e.g., draw a line) or multistep (e.g., draw a house); (b) tasks can have simple rules (e.g., place ball in container) or complex rules (e.g., playing a game of mini-golf); (c) tasks can be structured

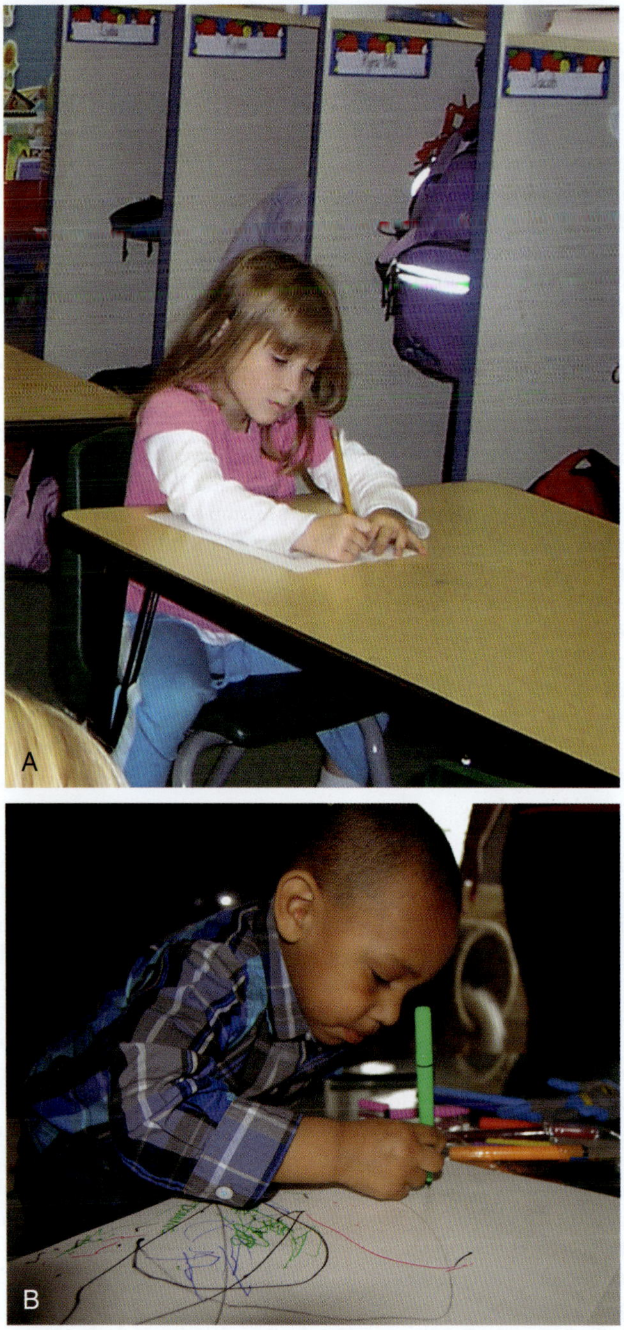

Fig. 29.4 (A and B) Children engage in the motor skill of writing to participate in academics. These activities are meaningful to them.

(e.g., follow step-by-step directions) or unstructured (e.g., create a game).; (d) single task (e.g., write a short text message on your phone) or multitasking (e.g., walking through a busy street while texting). See Table 29.1 for more examples.

Tasks may be along a spectrum of familiarity for children given their experiences. Familiar tasks are easier as children have developed strategies for how to carry them out. However, their growing bodies, curiosity, and variable environments expose them to tasks that can be somewhat or completely novel. Performance in these novel tasks is less skillful and requires present exploration of movements and strategies. Task novelty can pose a challenge for children with lack of exploratory skills. For example, children with ASD can become anxious, appear confused, make errors, or refuse altogether to engage in a novel daily activity.

For children, tasks need to be challenging enough to promote opportunities for performance but also new learning. This process is known as the "just right challenge." The goal of this process is to build on and expand skills that are already forming and learn new possible strategies. Occupational therapy practitioners can design the "just right challenge" task conditions for children by modifying components of task complexity and selecting tasks that may be novel or familiar. For example, when training a 3-year-old child to use utensils for the first time, you start with the form only (unimanual), while they are sitting (stationary posture), and have on the plate one to two pieces of solid food easy to get with the fork with no other distractions. As the child becomes familiar with the task and they are successful, you can introduce more challenges such as adding items that are smaller in size or starting a conversation. To gauge whether tasks pose the right level of challenge for a child, behavioral indicators can be helpful. When children are engaged, they can perform the task, they use exploratory strategies, and they actively seek information.

**Environmental Contexts.** Occupational therapy practitioners evaluate the physical, social, cultural, temporal, virtual, and personal contexts in which movement and occupational performance occur. For example, children may move successfully in a structured clinical setting but have difficulty navigating the uneven terrain outdoors. The light, terrain, setting, gravity, and novelty of the physical setting may influence a child's performance (Law et al., 2011). For example, children were more playful and moved more (as measured using ActiGraph units) at recess when novel objects (e.g., hay bales, tires) were introduced (Bundy et al., 2008). The social environment can place additional motor requirements on activities. For example, a child may perform "dance moves" in front of his family but show poor quality when in front of classmates at school. The social pressure of "performing" influences movement. Cultural expectations may influence motor actions. Children in different cultures can be exposed at different times in their development to demands of independence in carrying out daily activities. Temporal aspects include the developmental stage of the child. Younger children may be allowed to be "silly" in their motor performance, whereas adolescents may be expected to control movements more carefully for success. Virtual contexts include motor interactions with a computer screen. Playing video games can challenge children's motor performance in a different way than regular play. Visual and motor demands can be different and may need to be examined separately.

## PRINCIPLES OF MOTOR LEARNING

Motor learning explores the process of learning new motor skills while engaging in meaningful/goal-directed activities within supportive environments that allow children to problem solve. Motor learning is gradual. In the *initial stage*, children learn "what" to do, and they experiment with the shape of their movements and the impact of their movement (Gentile, 2000). This stage has a lot of trial and error. As the child becomes more and more familiar with the task in the specific context, they begin to develop strategies that support coordination (accuracy and timing), thereby gradually reducing the errors. The *later phase* of learning is characterized by "how" to do it, that is increasing coordination, flexibility in the strategies used, consistently improved performance, and efficiency in task execution (Gentile, 2000). The goal of this process is to learn a skill that can be used in different contexts (generalization or transfer learning).

In pediatrics, we examine the motor learning process and principles in the context of development. Motor learning principles refer to successful strategies that can be utilized to support the process of learning within a task/environment and transfer of learning across tasks and

TABLE 29.1 **Task Categories and Demands Grading and Adapting Activity**

| Task Categories | Lower Demand | Example | Higher Demand | Example |
|---|---|---|---|---|
| Motor/processing requirements | Unimanual | Carry a cup | Bimanual | Open a container to retrieve a toy |
| | Stationary | Stand on your two feet | Dynamic | Run as fast as you can |
| | Discrete | Tap the button to ring a bell | Continuous | Jumping rope |
| | Close-ended | Scribble on paper | Open-ended | Following with a stylus a moving target on an iPad screen |
| Motor and cognitive demands (dual task) | One step | Write your name | Multistep | Write a short paragraph |
| | Simple rules | Place one block on top of another | Complex rules | Play a game of Jenga |
| | Structured | Follow the guide to build a simple Lego set | Unstructured | Use free pieces of Lego to build a tree |
| | Single task | Use utensils to eat your food | Multitasking | Eat your food with utensils while talking to your family at the dinner table |
| Level of familiarity | Familiar | Walking | Novel | Roller blading |

environments (Krakauer et al., 2019). These strategies include type and amount of feedback and type and amount of practice. To quantify motor learning strategies for occupational therapy student work, O'Brien (2020) revised Williams' (2006) compilation of motor learning strategies based on current research. Table 29.2 provides a description of motor learning strategies that can be used in occupational therapy practice. The worksheet may be used in clinical practice to identify strategies utilized in treatment and their effectiveness to support children's learning of new motor skills.

## Meaning

Occupational therapy practitioners have historically viewed the meaningfulness of activities as essential to practice and acknowledge the benefits of purposeful activity in motivating clients to learn and perform (Fisher, 1998; Kielhofner, 2008; Taylor et al., 2024; Trombly, 1995). Meaning implies an emotional engagement to goal-directed action and is central to the motor learning process. Children's active participation in motor tasks is influenced by the extent to which they can identify their own interests, set goals, and believe that they can be effective and successful in those motor tasks (Fig. 29.5, A–C). Children are more motivated to challenge their motor skills if they find the activity important and fun and if they believe they can learn and be successful (Kielhofner, 2008; Kramer, 2007; Master et al., 2017; Taylor et al., 2024). In addition, children and youth participate for longer periods of time and perform more repetitions when activities are meaningful (Wright et al., 2005). Not only do they perform longer, but, in addition, the quality of movement improves when the activity has meaning to the child (Gordon et al., 2007). Several studies found that children with motor deficits wanted to participate in "regular" activities with friends (Cohn et al., 2000; O'Brien et al., 2009). These expressed interests suggest that occupational therapy practitioners promote meaningful physical activity for children who have motor impairments.

Hetu and Mercier (2012) examined the influence of purposeful activity by reviewing 35 articles. They suggest that clinicians use tasks with high object affordance to promote optimal motor performance. Consistent with the ecologic approach (see online resources), they defined object affordance tasks as those that included functional goals, consisted of the correct number of actual objects required, and these objects conveyed clear information for functional use. For example, the object is meaningful to the person (i.e., child's favorite toy), and the object suggests a specific motor action (e.g., flying a toy helicopter).

## Practice

Practice is a key element for learning and highly important in occupational therapy interventions. Structuring practice relative to the tasks (whole/part task), practice distribution, and intensity are all very important factors to take under consideration to promote learning. A considerable amount of research has been conducted on the use of practice to improve or develop motor skills (Chan et al., 2015; de Camargo Barros et al., 2017; Farhat et al., 2016; Hung et al., 2017).

**Practice Related to Task: Whole-Task Training.** Engaging in a whole activity facilitates multiple systems and interactions required for effective movement (Fig. 29.6). Overall, learning the whole motor task is more effective and motivating than learning only a part of the movement. Evidence suggests that typically developing children and children with neurodevelopmental problems perform whole tasks more efficiently and with better coordination than when they are asked to perform only a part or component of the movement (Emanuel et al., 2008). Chan et al. (2015) found that fifth graders learned better using whole practice. Van der Weel et al. (1991) found that children with CP used more supination when banging a drum than when simply exercising. Not only did children perform the task more efficiently, but they also engaged in the task for longer periods of time and activated more areas of the brain during the activity. In addition, functional magnetic resonance imaging studies indicate that more areas of the brain are activated when subjects engage in meaningful whole tasks versus parts of the tasks (Klingberg et al., 2002). Van de Winckel and colleagues found significantly more brain activation for both children with CP and typically developing children when they were engaged in active movement (grasp and release of an object) compared with passive movements (robot moved finger up and down) and tactile stimulation (stroking back of hand with sponge cotton cloth). The findings suggest engaging children in active tasks results in more brain activation for both typical children and children with CP (Lee et al., 2013; Van de Winckel et al., 2013).

Engaging in the whole activity requires children to process stimuli and respond to changes within and between systems (i.e., person, task, environment). The ability to respond in variable ways is a hallmark of goal-directed functional movement. Typically developing children, for example, use multiple strategies when moving, as opposed to children with DCD, who have been found to exhibit limited variability and adaptability in their movement (Mandich et al., 2001; Screws & Surburg, 1997; Taktek et al., 2008). Therefore, one goal of occupational

**TABLE 29.2 Occupational Therapy Motor Learning Strategies Worksheet (O'Brien, 2024)**

| Category | Strategy | Description of Observations |
|---|---|---|
| Meaning | • Skill has meaning or purpose to child.<br>• Child expresses interest in skills/chooses activities and skills.<br>• Child acknowledges abilities and self-efficacy (belief in skills).<br>• Child shows pleasure in activity.<br>• Child wants to demonstrate skill.<br>• Child indicates desire to complete skill or activity. | |
| Transfer of learning | • Skill experiences are presented in logical progression.<br>• Simple, foundational skills are practiced before more complex skills.<br>• Skill practice includes "real" life and simulated settings.<br>• Skills with similar components are more likely to show transfer effects.<br>• Practice in the natural context with actual objects is most effective.<br>• Child practices the "whole" movement within the natural context. | |
| Feedback<br>Modeling or demonstration | • Demonstration is best if it is given to the individual before practicing the skill and in the early stages of skill acquisition.<br>• Demonstration should be given throughout practice and as frequently as deemed helpful.<br>• The demonstration highlights one to three key features.<br>• Demonstration progresses from general movement to demonstration of subtle quality of movement.<br>• Allow child time to "figure it out." | |
| Feedback<br>Verbal instructions | • Verbal cues should be brief, to the point and involve one to three words.<br>• Verbal cues should be carefully timed to not interfere with performance.<br>• Verbal cues should emphasize key aspects of movement.<br>• Use words the child understands. | |
| Knowledge of results (KR) and knowledge of performance (KP) | • Use a variety of both KR and KP to facilitate learning.<br>• Balance between feedback that is error-based and that based on "appropriate" or "correct" characteristics of the performance.<br>• KP feedback can be descriptive or prescriptive.<br>• KP and KR should be given close in time to but after completion of the task, but not necessarily given 100% of the time.<br>• Learning is enhanced if KP/KR are given at least 50% of the time. | |
| Distribution and variability of skill practice | • Shorter, more frequent practice sessions are preferable to longer, less frequent practice.<br>• Frequent rest periods are preferable if a skill or task is complex.<br>• Practicing several tasks in the same session enhances skill acquisition.<br>• Practicing skills in several different environmental contexts promotes motor learning.<br>• Practitioners use clinical judgment (therapeutic reasoning) to recognize when practice is no longer producing changes and to introduce a new or different task. | |
| Whole versus part practice | • Practicing the whole skill is preferred.<br>• Whole practice may be preferable when the skill or task is simple; part practice may be preferable when the skill is more complex.<br>• If part practice is used, be sure parts practiced go together.<br>• To simplify a task, reduce the nature and/or complexity of the objects to be manipulated.<br>• Provide support to reduce attention or physical demands (i.e., provide trunk support during practice of different eye-hand coordination tasks).<br>• To simplify a task, provide auditory or rhythmic sounds or motions. This may help the learner feel or hear the appropriate "rhythm" of the movement<br>• Allow children to think about or feel movement while practicing; avoid extraneous tasks that distract them. | |
| Mental practice | • Mental practice (e.g., imagery, visualization) helps to facilitate acquisition of new skills as well as the relearning of old skills<br>• Mental practice helps the person to prepare to perform a task; it should be relatively short, not prolonged.<br>• Mental practice may include watching videos of the movement, discussing key parts, and visualizing.<br>• Walking the child through the movement slowly using keywords reinforces mental practice.<br>• Mental practice combined with physical practice works best. | |

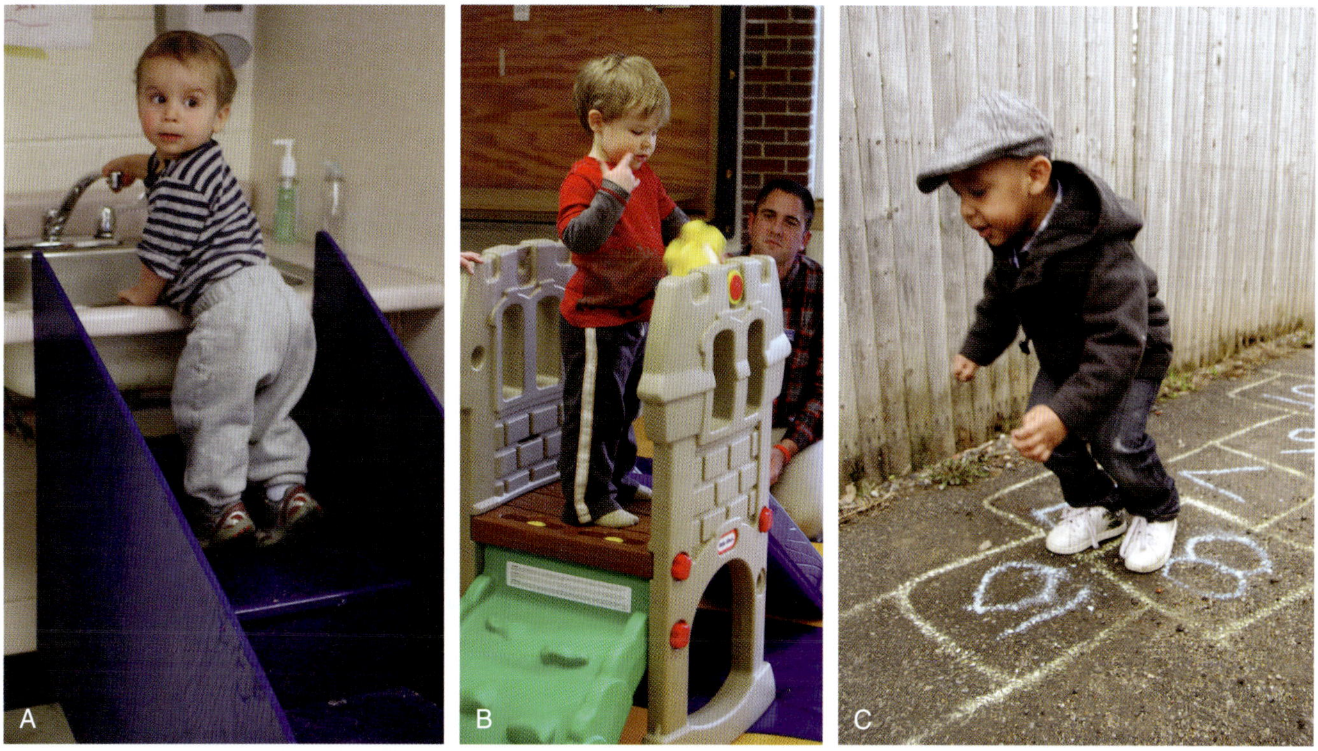

Fig. 29.5 Children are more likely to engage in a difficult task if they find it meaningful. (A) This young boy climbs and reaches over to wash his hands "all by himself." (B) This child climbs the castle with the encouragement of his father. (C) This young child is motivated to learn hopscotch, which requires motor planning, coordination, timing, and sequencing.

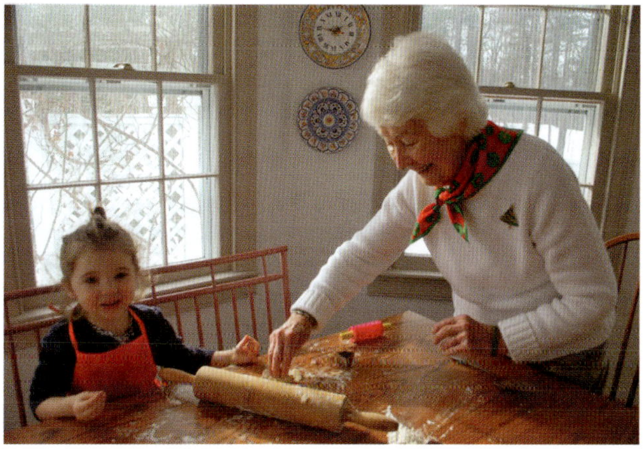

Fig. 29.6 Making cookies with grandma allows the child to engage in a variety of motor actions as part of the "whole task" of baking.

therapy intervention is to promote variability and flexibility in movements through whole training.

**Practice Related to Task: Part-Task Training.** Part-task training can be an effective way to enhance learning, especially in motor tasks that require multiple steps (sequential tasks) that can be difficult to plan and execute and at the initial stages of learning a complex movement. Parts of the task and movement that need to developed can be practiced separately (Hu & et al., 2005). Best practices suggest that parts of the tasks that are connected sequentially should be practiced together. In multistep tasks *part-task training* follows a shaping process. The child usually starts practicing only the final steps for a task that requires multiple steps. Part-task training progresses based on the child's success in the initial steps until the entire sequence is learned (Gordon et al., 2011). Part-task training creates conditions for learning a plan through a process of exploration (gathering information), agency (the child problem solves the task), and perceiving affordances (able to learn what possibilities for action are possible). In the study by Chan et al. (2015), first and third graders showed better learning with part practice (in contrast to the fifth graders, described above), suggesting occupational therapy practitioners consider the child's developmental level when choosing to engage a child in whole or part practice. The authors (Chan et al., 2015) hypothesized that this could be due to neural maturity, explicit learning, and coordination capabilities. In clinical populations, evidence-based interventions (such as intensive bimanual therapy, hand-arm bimanual intensive training [HABIT], and constraint-induced movement therapy [CIMT]) utilize a combination of whole-task and part-task training for designing activities to learn motor skills. Part-task training may be most effective for learning the foundational skills for movements but should be paired with whole learning and discovery learning to promote transfer of learning (Gredin & Williams, 2016).

## Practice Distribution and Intensity

***Blocked Versus Random Practice.*** *Blocked practice* distributions create conditions to engage the learners in sets of trials where movements and skills and important variations of these are practiced one at a time. There are practice trials (or amounts of time) for each skill or activity variation. *Random practice* is the exact opposite. All movements, task variations, etc., are practiced in a random order with the session.

***Massed Versus Distributed Practice.*** These refer to the intensity of practice. There are no well-established guidelines for determining intensity for skill learning in typically developing children or in clinical populations. In clinical practice, massed practice is usually a high-intensity few-breaks type of protocol. *Distributed practice* is defined as practice in which rest between trials is greater than the time of the trial and is most useful during the associative stage (Fig. 29.7A and B). However, the total time could remain the same between the two. High intensity (massed) promotes skill learning. This type of practice works best when the child is beginning to learn the movements, provided that fatigue does not become an issue. In children with hemiplegic CP, Gordon et al., 2011, supported that for lasting behavioral and neural pathway changes, children who participated in the HABIT had to complete at 90 hours of training for 5–7 weeks, with a minimum of 1.5 hours per session (massed practice).

**Mental Practice/Imagery.** Mental practice (also referred to as motor imagery or mental rehearsal) includes performing the skill in one's imagination, without any action involved. It consists of role playing, watching a video, or imagining. Mental practice is effective in teaching motor skills and retraining the timing and coordination of muscle group activity (Barhoun et al., 2019; Behrendt et al., 2021; Deecke, 1996; Doussoulin & Rehbein, 2011; Eaves et al., 2022; Marshall et al., 2020; Page et al., 1999; Steenbergen et al., 2020). It is most effective at the early and later stages of learning and may be task specific. It should be combined with action observation (Eaves et al., 2022) and further enhanced with physical practice (Frank et al., 2023). Much of the research on mental practice is conducted on athletes trying to maximize their performance (Murphy, 1994; Page et al., 1999). However, the techniques used may be beneficial to children with motor difficulties (Scott et al., 2021; Screws & Surburg, 1997; Steenbergen et al., 2013; Williams et al., 2013). Some positive results regarding motor performance were reported for children with attention-deficit disorder and DCD (Scott et al., 2021; Williams et al., 2013). Taktek and colleagues (2008) found performance (in throwing a ball) resulting from mental imagery combined with physical practice was equal during the retention phase but superior during the transfer of learning phase. The researchers examined visual and kinesthetic imagery in young children and found that they were both effective for children as young as 8 years old. Many theorists suggest imagery is effective because it requires cognitive processes and helps children to problem solve motor solutions (Eaves et al., 2022; Scott et al., 2021).

Children may experience stress when learning a new motor skill. Providing analogies allows children to visualize the skills and attend to other aspects of the task. Occupational therapy practitioners may easily incorporate analogies to teach children motor skills.

Recent evidence suggests that occupational therapy practitioners using mental practice consider the type of task, duration of mental practice, and time between practice and performance for retention (Eaves et al., 2022; Scott et al., 2021; Souto et al., 2020). Tasks in which the child has experience may be easier to imagine. However, the child may be able to imagine movements after observing them on a video or observing someone else perform them. Techniques of watching a video, pointing out components of the movement, or simply reviewing mentally how the movement will look in combination with physical practice may improve motor learning. Finally, practitioners should incorporate actual performance shortly after the mental practice for the best retention.

In clinical populations, motor imagery may be impaired. In a descriptive study, researchers compared EEG topographic maps in four typically developing children and four children with CP while they were engaged in motor execution and motor imagery tasks (Shin et al., 2012). The researchers asked the children to reach and grasp a small ball with their dominant hand, imagine hand movement needed to reach and grasp the ball, observe an animated reaching and grasping movement on the monitor, visualize the right-handed reaching and grasping movement, and create a "mental video" of the virtual hand movement. The authors found that different areas of the brain were activated during the imagery tasks for typical children and those with CP (Shin et al., 2012). Using mental practice as a strategy to introduce and practice motor skills in the contexts of tasks can be still beneficial and supportive of learning.

### Variability

Variability is inherent in activity (e.g., reaching for different objects, environmental stimuli) as well as within and between systems (e.g., interactions between visual and sensory systems). Movement occurs in a variety of contexts and requires that children adapt to environmental changes (using visual and auditory systems) or internal changes (perceived through vestibular and proprioceptive systems). For example, children may need to adjust movements in response to interpretations of visual input (e.g., the ball is coming quickly versus slowly); children may experience physiologic changes (e.g., low energy) affecting movement patterns. The environment may pose changes (e.g., weather, terrain, peers). Functional movement, the goal of motor control intervention, requires that children possess a variety of motor skills.

*Variable or random practice* is most effective for typically developing children and during the final stage of motor skill acquisition (Chua et al., 2019; Dhawale et al., 2017; Smits-Engelsman et al., 2020). Variable practice requires that learners repeat the same patterns but make small changes as necessary (Fig. 29.8). This type of practice increases the ability to adapt and generalize learning. In general, short, frequent practice is better than longer, less frequent practice because it decreases fatigue and increases reinforcement (Breslin et al., 2012). Persons with Down syndrome showed improvement in a simple reach (to a target) with variable practice (Jaric et al., 1993). An example of random practice includes intervention working on grasp and release while the child is engaged in a variety of play activities. This type of practice is most closely related to the actual occupation. The child must pick up and release toys during the play session. The child picks up a variety of objects: small blocks, large balls, light toys, and heavy scooter boards.

In certain children, variability of performance is too great, and the goal is to establish consistency in movements. Variability in movements can be measured by intra-individual variability. In a simple reaction time task to examine intra-individual variability, children with attention-deficit/hyperactivity disorder (ADHD) or dyslexia did not differ from each other but were more variable than typically developing children (Borella et al., 2011). Children with ADHD produced fewer writing sequences than did the children with dyslexia (controls were not significantly different from children with dyslexia). Excessive variability was found in the children with ADHD, and those with dyslexia had it interfere with consistency in handwriting performance.

Children with CP experience more variability in reaching patterns that interfere with their ability to complete bimanual activities effectively (Hung et al., 2017). Structured skill practice decreased the variability of their movement patterns and increased the quality of movement, whereas unstructured practice did not. Structured skill practice involves the practitioner scaffolding the movement (so the child is successful) and creating opportunities for the child to engage in the desired movement.

These findings support the need to encourage more accuracy in movements while allowing for variability for functional performance. Understanding the range of typical development and factors influencing movement is essential to designing effective intervention. Performing movements in multiple ways requires that children problem solve and self-correct. All children use problem-solving to develop

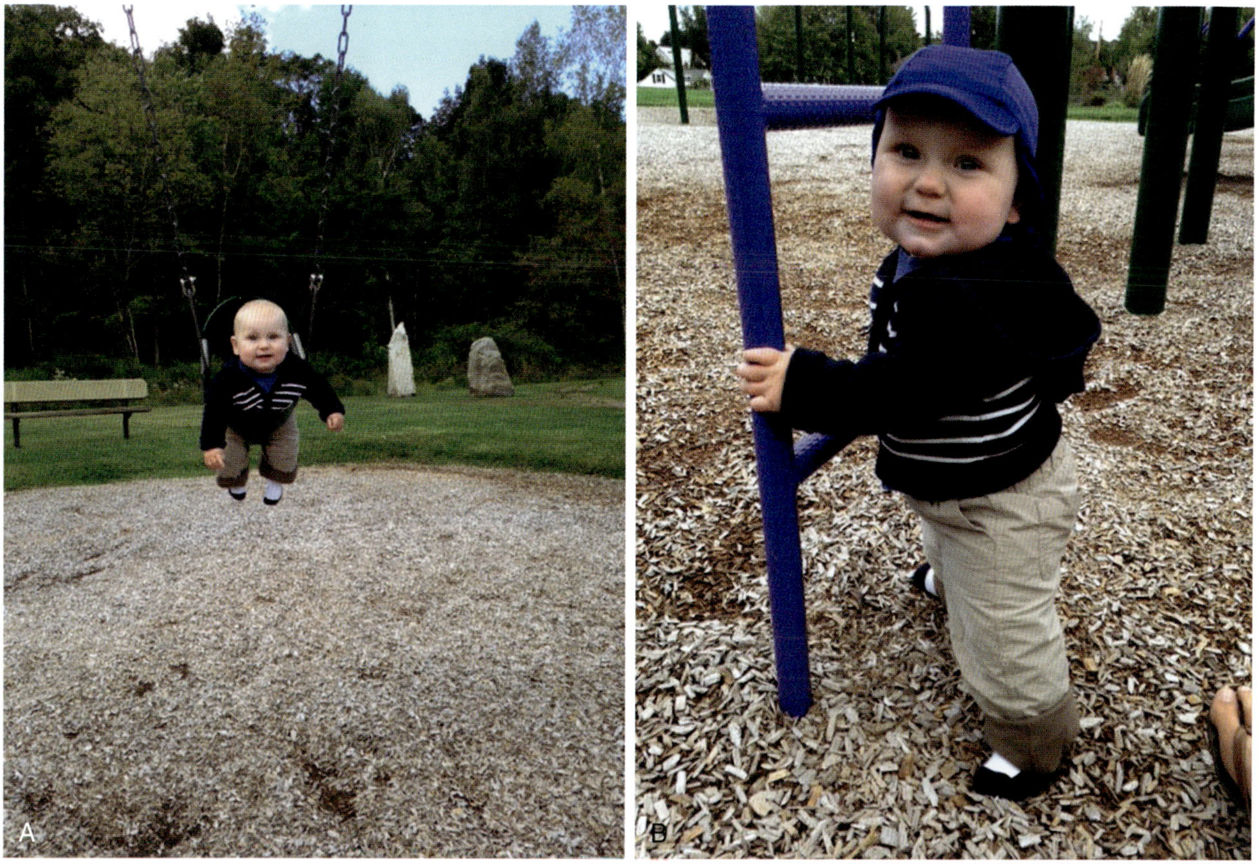

**Fig. 29.7** (A and B) This child takes breaks from learning to climb, with the engaging activity of swinging. This is an example of distributed practice.

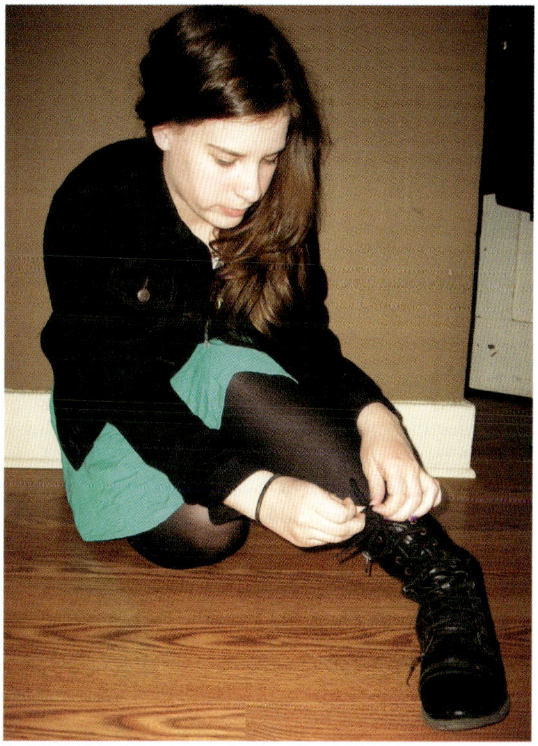

**Fig. 29.8** Variable practice. The child ties her shoes right before she goes outside to meet friends. She can tie different types of shoes (e.g., sneakers, boots), and although often she sits on the floor to complete the task, she can also tie her shoes in other positions.

and refine movement; therefore, problem-solving is an important part of motor control.

## Problem-Solving or Error-Based Learning

Improved retention of motor skills occurs when children problem solve and self-correct for motor errors (Bouffard & Wall, 1990; Missiuna & Mandich, 2002; Miyahara & Wafer, 2004; Polatajko et al., 2001). Children learn and retain motor skills better from intrinsically solving problems than they do from receiving external feedback during an action (such as hand-over-hand assistance). For example, to learn to build a sandcastle, the child problem solves his or her position in the sand and how to scoop and place the sand (Fig. 29.9A and B). The child is more likely to learn a new motor task in a meaningful, socially engaging activity. The child must position his or her body away from the structure and use adequate timing and force to make the castle of choice. Self-correcting enables children to rely on internal cues that indicate the effectiveness of movement and thereby help them adapt and modify movements in a variety of contexts.

Occupational therapy practitioners working to improve a child's motor performance provide many opportunities for the child to actively solve motor problems by doing, rather than repetitive practicing of a part of the movement. Setting up the environment to facilitate physical, social, and cognitive tasks encourages the child to discover how to move, explore options, and self-correct movement errors beneficial to motor learning. Children with disabilities must learn to adapt to new, different, or unexpected situations.

Children learn movement by making errors or mistakes and self-correcting (Banks et al., 2008; Sullivan et al., 2008). Therefore, occupational therapy practitioners sometimes allow the challenge to exceed

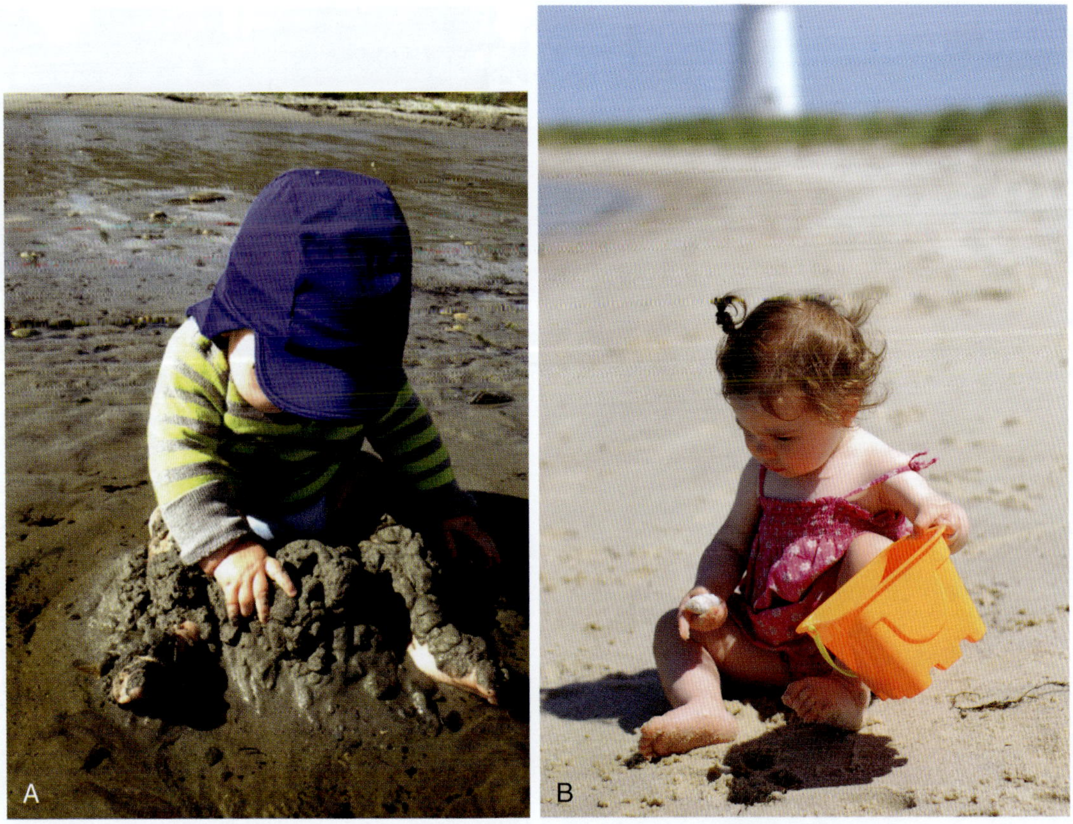

**Fig. 29.9** (A and B) Children building sandcastles must problem solve.

the capacity of the child, to give him or her the opportunity to make errors, correct them (if possible), and to learn from the experience. In the past, occupational therapy practitioners were hesitant to allow children to learn through making errors. However, making errors in controlled settings allows children to resolve problems and is important for facilitating motor skill learning. Encouraging children to explore, adjust movements, and evaluate their responses and reactions helps them learn and refine motor skills.

## Transfer of Learning

**Transfer of learning**, or generalization, refers to applying learning to new situations. The goal of occupational therapy intervention is that the child transfers learning performed in the clinic or intervention setting to a natural context. For example, after working on maneuvering a new wheelchair through an obstacle course at the clinic with ease, the occupational therapy practitioner hopes the child will be able to maneuver the wheelchair through the school hallway.

Children are best able to transfer motor skills when they have practiced the motor skill within the natural context or in the "real-world" situation. Therefore, the best way to help the child successfully maneuver his wheelchair through the school hallway is to practice in that setting. The occupational therapy practitioner may initially teach basic wheelchair skills to the child, then practice in the hallway after school hours (to decrease obstacles), and finally work up to maneuvering the wheelchair during class change. Research suggests that children transfer the task more quickly with this intervention strategy than with practicing in a clinic setting only (Sullivan et al., 2008). In addition, transfer of learning occurs more easily when the motor task is performed during a functional activity or actual occupation (Emanuel et al., 2008; Gordon et al., 2007; Painter et al., 1994). When selecting activities to practice, the occupational therapy practitioner recognizes that motor skills with similar components are more likely to transfer. For example, a child who has just successfully learned to throw a ball would more easily learn to throw a bean bag at a target.

## Feedback

Intrinsic feedback, which allows the child to self-correct, is most effective for sustaining motor performance and should be the goal of intervention sessions. Intrinsic feedback may be elicited through discovery, a situation in which the occupational therapy practitioner sets up the environment and the child is allowed to explore and discover, make errors, and consequently learn new ways of moving.

Children may require **extrinsic feedback** in the early stages of motor skill development. Extrinsic feedback consists of providing verbal cueing or physical guidance. *Demonstrative feedback* refers to modeling or imitating movements. Demonstrative feedback is best if it is provided before the child practices the movement, as well as throughout early stages of skill acquisition. The practitioner provides modeling without verbal commentary because simultaneous verbal cues can decrease the child's attention to the movement (Sullivan et al., 2008). Positive feedback results in better motor learning and perceived competence and serves to motivate children to continue to engage in the activity.

**Knowledge of Performance.** Feedback to improve movement is most helpful when it is specific and clear. *Knowledge of performance* helps children understand how they performed the desired movement that improves quality of movement (Bishop et al., 2018). Knowledge of performance is helpful in refining and adjusting motor skills and therefore is useful after the child has established basic skills. Practitioners may provide descriptive feedback to the child about performance of a specific task (i.e., writing), such as, "You held the pencil between thumb and fingers and pressed lightly" or practitioners may provide prescriptive feedback, such as, "Next time, press a little more." Descriptive feedback is more helpful for experienced performers, whereas beginners learn better with prescriptive feedback. During easy tasks, typical children benefited from knowledge of performance 33% of the time, whereas they benefited from knowledge of performance 100% of the time when the task was difficult (Sidaway et al., 2012). This study suggests that occupational therapy practitioners consider the complexity of the task with feedback frequency.

**Knowledge of Results.** Feedback related to the desired outcome helps children understand movement. Providing this knowledge is most effective when specific information on the movement's goal is stated. Thus saying, "Each button is lined up with its buttonhole" is preferred over, "Good job." *Knowledge of results* is motivating and encourages children to continue; it is most helpful when learning new motor tasks. Knowledge of results should not be provided after every trial (100% of the time), since the child becomes too reliant on it, and studies show children benefit from self-reflection (Schmidt et al., 2018). Children with CP were able to learn a new motor skill with 50% knowledge of results feedback; 100% knowledge of results feedback interfered with their learning (Hemayattalab & Rostami, 2010).

**Verbal Feedback.** Verbal praise and reinforcement are useful in motivating clients and changing behaviors but may be overused in clinical settings. Allowing children to make their own assessments of their performance is beneficial and will increase their sense of efficacy (Sullivan et al., 2008). Verbal feedback is best if provided immediately after completion of the task. Using one to three brief cue words that can be repeated easily by the performer is best. Knowledge of correct performance motivates a child to continue practicing, so such reinforcement may be used frequently. Positive feedback with specific cues improves performance, such as saying, "You pressed firmly with the pencil!"

## INTERVENTION STRATEGIES BASED ON MOTOR CONTROL/LEARNING PRINCIPLES

Occupational therapy practitioners consider motor skills in the context of goal-directed tasks. Tasks are embedded in children's occupations. Occupational therapy practitioners facilitate children's motor performance and learning by applying the principles discussed earlier in this chapter with their clinical reasoning skills and specific hands-on skills such as handling and facilitating to support every infant, child, and adolescent. Handling and facilitating using precise strategies are especially important to support motor performance and learning because the practitioners' assistance through handling and feedback through handling directly affect the process.

### Handling and Facilitating

Therapeutic handling is important to support children in the process of learning new motor strategies. Neurodevelopmental Treatment (NDT) is a hands-on approach that uses faciltation strategies to promote correct joint alignment and optimal movement trajectories for indviduals with neuromuscular problems. The NDT/Bobath approach is a holistic and interdisciplinary clinical practice model informed by current and evolving research that emphasizes individualized therapeutic handling based on an analysis of a child's movement during functional tasks. A practitioner using an NDT/Bobath approach assesses a child's activity and participation in specific tasks to help prioritize relevant strengths and impairments as a basis to establish achievable outcomes with the child and caregivers. The practitioner uses an in-depth understanding of typical and atypical development, and expertise in analysis of postural control, movement, activity, and participation throughout the lifespan, to formulate an intervention plan based on a child's strengths and areas of weakness or challenge. A practitioner uses therapeutic handling during evaluation and intervention to activate optimal sensorimotor processing, task performance, and skill acquisition while a child is engaged in a meaningful activity (Bierman et al., 2016). The key elements in NDT/Bobath treatment include facilitations (a practitioner using sensory inputs to improve motor performance), management of compensatory motor behavior, and a top-down assessment to determine what movement patterns may be needed to complete a specific functional task (Zanon et al., 2019).

Despite being one of the oldest and most frequently used interventions to treat children with CP, there is limited evidence that using an NDT/Bobath approach promotes functional improvement of children with neuromuscular disorders (Mayston, 2016). Based on the results of two recent randomized clinical trials, the effectiveness of NDT/Bobath approaches for children with CP is no different from usual and customary occupational and physical therapy for improving the motor function of children with CP (Zanon et al., 2019). The findings of a recent review indicate that the effectiveness of neurodevelopmental treatment for children with CP is unclear, and due to the lack of evidence, this intervention approach should be used with caution (Novak et al., 2020). A clinician should use a data-driven strategy to carefully observe a child's response to treatment and attainment of therapy goals. Practitioners may consider combining an NDT/Bobath approach with other types of treatments (i.e., goal-directed training, CIMT).

### Combining Motor Control and Learning Principles

To design their intervention protocols, occupational therapy practitioners combine their observations and clinical evaluation findings regarding the following:

- Child's agency, prospectivity, flexibility, adaptability, during motor performance with and across tasks and environments
- Child's person, task, environment factors, and their dynamic interaction
- The conditions needed to promote motor learning

Occupational therapy treatment directly engages children in tasks that include the following characteristics.

- Provide "just right challenge" and promote learning and development of skills
- Activities are within the children's interests
- Tasks utilize areas of strength to expand children's abilities
- Tasks are adapted (complexity level) (Tasks, in Principles of Motor Control and Their Application in Pediatric Clinical Populations) to provide opportunities for successful interactions, practice of skills, and feedback for performance to improve

Learning conditions are set up meeting the child's learning needs taking under consideration the following:

- Stage of learning (initial or later)
- Practice movement as part of the whole task with activities that are meaningful for the child
- Practice conditions (structure, distribution, intensity, and ability for mental imagery)
- Appropriate feedback (implicit or explicit)
- Problem-solving
- Variability level
- Transfer of learning to other activities/environments
- Environments are adapted and modified to facilitate access to tasks and support possibilities for successful performance and learning

The occupational therapy practitioner uses the occupation-centered practice model and motor learning principles to create intervention activities addressing the child's motor control for desired occupations. Motor learning principles suggest that children learn movement most effectively when (1) the movement is taught as a whole (versus part); (2) the movement is performed in variable situations; (3) the child is allowed to actively problem solve the actions required; and (4) the activity is meaningful to the child. It is important that the occupational therapy practitioner structure the intervention session, paying close attention to the goals of the intervention. See Box 29.3 for additional tips to design occupational therapy intervention addressing motor control using motor learning principles.

Children with CP who participated in a structured practice showed improved quality of performance compared with those who did not (Hung et al., 2017). Children (with and without disabilities) who received a fundamental motor skills program made significant progress in 6 weeks compared with a control group of children whose motor skills remained the same (Taunton et al., 2017). Other studies support the use of motor skills training programs using motor learning strategies for children with CP (Bleyenheuft et al., 2015, 2017; Law et al., 2011), and DCD (Farhat et al., 2016; Jelsma et al., 2015).

We provide an illustration of how to apply these principles to design specific activities in Table 29.3, and we provide two case studies with these principles and/or in combination with other frameworks (i.e., Model of Human Occupation [MOHO]). Case Example 29.1 provides a description using Kielhofner's MOHO (Kielhofner, 2008; Taylor et al., 2024) to plan occupational therapy intervention targeting motor control. Case Example 29.2 illustrates how occupational therapy practitioners may apply current motor control/motor learning principles and strategies to practice.

## SPECIFIC EXISTING PEDIATRIC EVIDENCE-BASED INTERVENTION PROTOCOLS BASED ON PRINCIPLES OF MOTOR CONTROL AND LEARNING

In addition to these principles, occupational therapy practitioners have available specific evidence-based pediatric protocols to develop expertise and utilize with specific pediatric populations.

### Occupation-Centered Practice Models

Occupation-centered practice models such as the MOHO (Kielhofner, 2008; Taylor et al., 2024), Person-Environment-Occupation-Performance (Christiansen et al., 2011), Occupational Adaptation (Grajo, 2017; Schkade & Schultz, 1992), and the Canadian Model of Occupational Performance and Engagement (Polatajko et al., 2007) guide one's thinking and help occupational therapy practitioners develop intervention that is fitting with the principles of dynamic systems and ecologic theory. Each of these models places the client and family at the center of decision-making while considering multiple systems and their impact on the child's abilities. See Chapter 9 for more information on the occupation-centered models of practice.

### Task-Specific Training

Task-specific training involves practicing the specific actions or activity (task) while considering the concepts of motor learning. Clients

**BOX 29.3 Tips for Designing Intervention Using Motor Control Concepts**

**Whole Learning Within the Child's Capacity and Interests**

- Play activities (e.g., crafts, dress-up, cooking, dance moves)
- Games
- Themed activities

**Variability**

- Develop occupations as goals (e.g., play with peers)
- Provide variety of activities or different ways to do tasks
- Same motor movement in different forms
- Vary the objects or placement
- Vary the requirements of the task
- Consider the social nature of the task
- Vary the environmental context (e.g., clinic versus playground)

**Problem-Solving**

- Set up activities with different degrees of difficulty
- Repeat movements, so child must figure it out
- Wait for child to figure it out

**Meaning**

- Select activities the child enjoys
- Offer choice
- Add novelty and creativity to sessions
- Offer activities in which the child is interested
- Engage child in activities that have significance in his/her life
- Engage child in creating his/her goals
- Allow time for self-reflection

**TABLE 29.3 Sample Intervention Activities**

| | Child | Task | Environment |
|---|---|---|---|
| Ride-on-car obstacle course | Require the child to challenge motor skills or perform for longer period of time.<br>Require the child to perform a less challenging motor task but a more challenging social task. | Change the type of "ride-on-car" so that it is easier or more difficult to operate. The car could be operated by pedaling, pushing, or walking or even motorized. These different cars change the task requirements. | Change the course so that it is a flat or hilly course or a grass-covered or tarred surface. |
| Follow the leader | Provide a one-on-one assistant to help the child complete the tasks. Provide pictures or cues to the child and vary the time required to follow. | Change the motor movements required when imitating the leader. The leader could walk slowly or hop on one foot. The leader could do bilateral activities or unimanual activities. | Perform game in a structured setting with few distractions. Vary the type of terrain or area that the children must "follow." |
| Safari trip | Provide hand-over-hand assistance or modify the tasks so the child can achieve the motor task. | Change the requirements for each stage of the trip. The child may have to reach, pull, throw, or push objects. | Perform the trip in a variety of settings (e.g., ball pit, trampoline, outside, inside). |

## CASE EXAMPLE 29.1 OCCUPATIONAL THERAPY INTERVENTION PLAN: MODEL OF HUMAN OCCUPATION AND MOTOR CONTROL

See accompanying video clip.

### Occupational Profile

Teagan is a 4-year-old boy who lives with his mothers and 7-year-old brother in a rural town. Both mothers are employed; one is a teacher, and the other is a business manager. Teagan has Down syndrome and had cardiac surgery at 7 months. He has not experienced any other health issues. He receives physical therapy and occupational therapy at preschool.

### Volition

Teagan loves to play T-ball and play outside with his brother. He follows his brother, imitates his play, and indicates what he would like to do. Teagan enjoys being outside at preschool and watches his peers but does not interact with them. They run quickly by him. His parents state that he is an active boy. They are concerned that he does not play with his peers.

### Habituation

Teagan attends a preschool for 4-year-old children. Teagan needs help getting dressed, and he is not toilet trained. He washes his face and hands. He feeds himself with a spoon (with spillage) and uses a sippy cup to drink. He participates in recreational T-ball. Teagan's parents report that he goes to bed at a reasonable hour (9:00 p.m.) during school days and awakes at 8:00 a.m. Teagan has chores to do each day, including picking up his plates after meals, putting his dirty clothes in the hamper, and walking the dog. He takes a 2-hour nap daily.

### Performance Capacity

Teagan's has low muscle tone throughout. His posture is asymmetric (he elevates his shoulders and leans) when he runs. He runs with a wide-based gait and holds his arms close to his body for balance. He falls frequently and shows difficulty moving around obstacles. He needs to take breaks when running around the bases in T-ball. His movements are slow, and he watches his peers play instead of engaging. Teagan climbs up the slide but does not slide down. Teagan engages in some parallel play with other children at day care. When he does interact with his peers, he plays at a much younger level and frequently interrupts and/or interferes in their play.

### Environment

The preschool is a playful environment with a large fenced-in playground with a large slide, swings, and grassy play area. The inside rooms are full of toys and child-friendly decorations, small tables, and child-sized chairs.

### Strengths

Teagan is a physically active 4-year-old boy who imitates his older brother's play. He enjoys rough play with his brother, playing T-ball, and water play.

### Areas for Improvement

Teagan does not play with his peers but rather watches them or interferes in their play (i.e., sits at the top of the slide). He spends outdoor playtime at preschool playing alone.

### Evaluation Results

Teagan's motor difficulties are interfering with his ability to engage in play with his peers. He has difficulty initiating movement, as observed by not moving down the slide. He falls frequently and has poor timing and sequencing of movements. Helping Teagan become more proficient in motor skills may improve his ability to keep up with peers on the playground.

### Intervention Plan

**Goals:** To improve initiation, timing, and sequencing of motor skills for play with peers.

1. At preschool, Teagan will initiate movement by climbing up and sliding down the slide five times consecutively (without stopping at the top for more than 10 seconds) within a 30-minute play session (initiation).
2. Teagan will complete a 4-step obstacle course (walk on balance board for 5 ft, reach and throw object in container × 3, crawl through tunnel for 5 ft, and run 10 ft) within 10 minutes without falling or requiring verbal cues (timing and sequencing).

### Analysis of Intervention

The occupational therapy practitioner used the MOHO and the principles of motor control and learning in this chapter (influenced by dynamic systems and ecologic theory) to understand Teagan's occupational needs. When developing client-centered goals, the occupational therapy practitioner considered Teagan's preference for playing outside and the parents' goal for Teagan to play with his peers. These goals helped Teagan establish positive habits and routines at preschool and provided him with confidence in his ability to play with peers (self-efficacy). The practitioner engaged Teagan in activity in his environment and trained the teacher and caregivers through modeling and instruction. The practitioner designed interventions to specifically improve his posture and to train visual/proprioceptive and vestibular systems to support his motor performance and prevent falls. Treatment also focused on the cognitive components influencing his motor performance: initiation, sequencing, and timing of motor actions for play. The occupational therapy practitioner also focused on activities that supported his emotional engagement (self-efficacy and motivation) but also provided the "just right challenge."

Therapy sessions included a variety of games (e.g., follow the leader, obstacle course parades in ride-on cars) where other children could participate. The occupational therapy practitioner determined that person factors (e.g., limited initiation, inadequate timing, and difficulty sequencing) interfered with Teagan's movement for play. Teagan's low muscle tone may result in poor postural control and subsequent difficulty with gross motor activities. Because Teagan engaged in rough play with his older brother at home, the practitioner hypothesized that the social environment at preschool was causing him to be "nervous" or "anxious" because the children ran quickly around him, seldom paying attention to him. The practitioner conducted a task analysis and concluded that activities involving complex motor tasks and multiple children (higher cognitive demands) were very difficult for him. The practitioner graded activities down to allow Teagan to practice new motor actions in a safe and fun setting. During these sessions, the practitioner adapted the course (environment), task (a car that was easier to move), or child requirements (allowing Teagan to perform a task differently) to help him be successful. Engaging Teagan in play activities that involved other children provided him with opportunities to socialize in nonthreatening and successful ways. For example, the practitioner gave him the opportunity to be the leader of the course, allowing him to practice prior to inviting other children. Teagan was proud that he could provide "tips" and directions for his peers. This helped develop his motivation for motor activities, further reinforcing practice and socialization.

receive feedback while they are practicing context-specific motor tasks (Fong et al., 2016). The focus of task-specific training is on function rather than impairment (Toovey et al., 2017). Task-specific training resonates with occupational therapy philosophy when creating intervention to expand the child's capacity in specific skills. According to Hubbard et al. (2009), occupational therapy practitioners using task-specific training follow these guidelines:

1. Training is relevant to the client and context.
2. Practice sequences are randomly ordered.
3. Training is repetitive within the context of the task.

## CASE EXAMPLE 29.2 OCCUPATIONAL THERAPY INTERVENTION PLAN: MOTOR LEARNING STRATEGIES

Paul is a 7-year-old boy referred to occupational therapy after his mother expressed concern that he has difficulty using his hands, completing schoolwork (e.g., coloring), and playing on the playground (e.g., climbing up the slide, getting on the swing). Paul has stomachaches in the mornings and does not want to go to school. He enjoys playing with trucks on the floor in the living room with his friend.

Paul is in the first grade. His teacher is concerned that Paul is not "picking up things" as quickly as his peers and noted he has trouble with handwriting and reading. She acknowledged that Paul verbally contributes to class.

### Occupational Performance

#### *Living Situation/Home Environment*

Paul lives with his parents and 2-year-old sister in a three-bedroom apartment. He has access to toys inside and outside. His home is child friendly. The backyard is fenced in and includes a swing set, slide, and sandbox. He does not ride a bike, swing, or go down the slide. He prefers to play indoors. If he must play outside, he likes to play with his trucks on the deck. His neighborhood has many children who frequently play together outside. He has one good friend, with whom he plays in the afternoons and sees at school. Paul participates in recreational soccer (although he says, "I'm not very good").

#### *Sensory*

Paul's poor balance and motor planning are interfering with his movement. Paul's body awareness is somewhat affected because he struggles to identify right-left, a skill expected at his age. His internal body awareness is not quite developed.

#### *Motor*

Paul's low muscle tone, poor postural control, and difficulty with timing and sequencing are interfering with his ability to move in a coordinated fashion (prospectivity issues). Paul shows some soft neurologic signs, such as associated reactions. He demonstrates poor standing balance with his eyes closed and poor dynamic balance. Paul ran with his feet apart (wide gait), and his arms did not swing consistently or in rhythm. He had difficulty changing positions as observed by stopping and reorienting himself as his friend ran around him. Paul showed poor sequencing and timing of movements—he could not jump with both feet together or catch a ball. He fell three times on the tires when he tried to balance on them during recess.

### Tasks (Motor Performance)

#### *Handwriting*

Paul held a pencil in a tight pronated grasp and made dark marks on the paper. He did not draw a straight line (3 inches) within the 0.25-inch markings—his line went over in more than five places. He printed his name slowly; spacing was inconsistent between letters; the letters were of uneven size; and he did not stay within the large, ruled lines. When writing, he sat with his feet on the floor, his back was rounded, and his face was close to the paper. He showed some associated reactions (e.g., facial movements) when writing. He could not perform alternating hand movements.

#### *Self-Care*

Paul independently donned his coat and hat. He had difficulty with buttoning it and required several minutes to accomplish it. He demonstrated beginning skills in tying his shoes, making multiple knots instead. He feeds himself but has difficulty with opening cartons and tearing packages. He washes his face and hands.

#### *Play*

Paul was the last child to go outside for recess. He played with his friend and watched others. His friend waited for him and frequently repeated, "Hurry up, Paul." Paul watched others on the swings and slides but did not try to interact with others. He played on the tires by himself.

### Environments

#### *School*

Paul attends a local elementary school; there are 15 students in his class. The teacher provides structure and is consistent. She expressed concern that Paul is falling behind his classmates (cognitive, person factor) and notes difficulty with handwriting and paying attention (cognitive, person factor) and getting things done in a timely manner. She commented that Paul is always the last one out the door, forgets things in the classroom (cognitive, person factor), and seems frustrated at time (emotions, person factor). However, she revealed that Paul is verbal, answers questions readily (cognitive, person factor), behaves well, and is polite.

### Assessment

Paul exhibits DCD, as his motor abilities are interfering with his daily activities of play, self-care, and academics. He is aware of his difficulties and experiencing frustration with an inability to keep up with his peers. He has changed his activity preferences (to indoor activities) and is beginning to resist going to school.

#### *Goals*

1. *Academic performance*: Paul will improve fine motor skills for academics.
   a. Paul will write his first name in a 2-inch by 3-inch rectangle on the upper-right-hand corner of his paper with 90% legibility.
   b. Given a verbal prompt, Paul will complete a short writing assignment (three lines) in 15 minutes with 80% legibility.
2. *Play*: Paul will improve motor skills to engage in play on playground with peers.
   a. Paul will show improved timing and sequencing by pumping a swing consecutively for 5 minutes on the school playground.
   b. Paul will demonstrate posture and balance for play as evidenced by remaining upright while climbing on at least 10 tires (on the playground tire hill) within a 30-minute play session.

### Analysis of Intervention Planning

The occupational therapy practitioner, Cora, a school-based practitioner, developed an intervention plan to help Paul play with his peers and perform in the classroom. These goals address the parents' concern that Paul is having "difficulty playing on the playground and doing anything with his hands." Cora hypothesized that helping Paul gain postural control, balance, timing, and sequencing through playground activities would provide a foundation for hand skills. Improving the quality, speed, and timing of his motor performance allows him to keep up with his peers. Engaging in successful activities contributes to his sense of competency and leads to a positive view of school. Because children spend so much of their day writing, Cora felt targeting handwriting would significantly affect his occupational performance in school.

Keeping in mind that children learn best when they are presented with the whole versus a part of the activity that is meaningful and carried out in natural contexts, Cora designed a variety of fun gross motor games for the playground. The intervention was designed to help Paul develop postural control, balance, timing, and sequencing while completing fun games with peers and helping him feel better about his abilities. Providing Paul with the opportunity to develop some basic skills will help him succeed on the playground. The practitioner graded and adapted activities to promote his success in this context.

Cora spent the first session recording baseline measurements directly related to the established goals. She recorded the time and legibility of Paul's performance of writing his name on his paper and writing three sentences after being given a verbal prompt ("Tell me about your favorite animal"). She also measured how many consecutive swings (back and forth) Paul could complete on the swing in 5 minutes and how many times he fell on the tires. Cora videotaped the baseline measurements, recorded the results, and documented her observations of the quality of his motor performance. This data provided her with solid measurements to determine the effectiveness of occupational therapy intervention.

## CASE EXAMPLE 29.2 OCCUPATIONAL THERAPY INTERVENTION PLAN: MOTOR LEARNING STRATEGIES—CONT'D

During the subsequent sessions, Cora designed fun activities to target postural control, balance, timing, and sequencing play by setting up a five-step obstacle course on the playground, which included Paul:

1. Climb over three tires (lined up on flat surface)
2. Run to the slide (10 ft)
3. Pick up an object sitting on the fourth rung of the slide
4. Swing back and forth two times on the swing
5. Run back to the starting line.

Cora used motor learning strategies by *demonstrating* the movement for each step before asking Paul to perform. Once she reviewed each step, she asked him to complete them in order. Paul made many mistakes but started to *problem solve* how to better perform toward the end of the course (evidence of initial stages of learning). On completion, he said, "Let me try it again and see if I can go faster." Cora provided some key points about the *part of the course* with which he had trouble (e.g., swinging). She cued him using one to three key words to "Pump back and forth." Providing one to three key words as *verbal feedback* after the child has performed is recommended for motor learning. Furthermore, allowing Paul to make and *learn from his own motor mistakes* allowed him to internalize the motor learning. This technique has been found to improve generalization. The practitioner periodically changed the format ("Just right challenge"), allowing Paul to make some revisions in the course, to ensure that the course was *meaningful*. For example, Paul added more tires to the course and requested that the toy be placed higher on the ladder.

Cora provided intervention in the *natural context*, which provides cues to the child and allows *for transfer of learning*. Cora waited to invite peers to join Paul so that he could develop competence in skills before the added social "pressure" and stimuli (grading task difficulty).

Cora in the classroom discussed with Paul about his writing and strategies that might help make it easier for him (allowing for agency). Paul suggested holding the paper down with his left thumb; he liked the idea of using a mechanical pencil with a new pencil grip. Using *mental practice strategies*, Cora asked Paul to visualize how he would complete his writing tasks in school. She suggested that he visualize his handwriting immediately before beginning the writing task.

In the therapy session, they played with a spirograph, using it to help Paul improve his handwriting grasp (blocked practice). The spirograph requires repetitive movement and is fun for children. It improves sequencing and allows the child to work on grip strength. This proved to be a nice activity to work on the mechanics of writing. Later in the intervention sessions, Cora and Paul worked on his "art portfolio" (meaning) creating art by drawing/coloring (variable practice).

Cora worked with Paul with a variety of activities to promote postural control, coordination, timing and sequencing (worked on person factors), and handwriting (activity-based training) that were meaningful and fun. Periodically, she stopped the spirograph activity and reviewed how to hold the pencil or reinforced correct posture (feedback; knowledge of performance/results). On the playground (activity-based training), she spent time explaining pumping and working on songs to improve timing and rhythm (feedback; knowledge of performance/results). Cora paid close attention to the nonverbal and verbal cues Paul gave her. If the activities were too challenging, she adapted them almost effortlessly. She used humor and paid attention to therapeutic use of self so that she could optimize the session. Cora was attentive to Paul, provided positive facial expressions, and encouraged gently.

She used a blocked practice schedule to teach the new skills, such as climbing to the top of the slide alternating one's feet and hands (bilaterally). As Paul became more competent, she used a distributed practice schedule and later a random or variable schedule. She focused on her goal to enable Paul to participate in play on the playground with peers and complete handwriting assignments with better quality and speed.

4. The goal is for the client to complete the whole task (occupation).
5. The client should be positively reinforced.

### Constraint-Induced Movement Therapy

**CIMT** is a therapeutic treatment approach used for children with unilateral motor weakness. CIMT requires restraint of the unaffected upper limb combined with 3 or more hours of a day of intensive task practice using the affected upper limb (Chen et al., 2014; Chiu & Ada, 2016; Ouyang et al., 2020) (see online resources for more evidence). Massed practice and shaping of more mature motor movement is provided for at least 2 consecutive weeks (14–21 days) by a professional with an understanding of rehabilitation techniques to improve motor function (Chen et al., 2014; Chiu & Ada, 2016). CIMT provides several components that are packaged together to maximize rehabilitation efforts and includes task-specific training. The essential elements of CIMT include (1) restraint of the stronger unaffected upper extremity (UE); (2) task-oriented mass practice of specific motor activities; and (3) shaping of more mature motor movement. The overall aim of CIMT is to reverse developmental disregard or learned nonuse of the affected extremity in children with unilateral motor weakness. Pediatric CIMT approaches also include a transfer package to bridge the child's unimanual skills to become part of real-word bimanual performance (Aarts et al., 2010; Deluca et al., 2012).

Accumulated evidence linking repetition and skill training to neuroplasticity has led to contemporary task-oriented training motor rehabilitation approaches (Gordon & Magill, 2012; Manning et al., 2016; Shumway-Cook et al., 2023). Task-oriented training approaches are based on the idea that motor rehabilitation for children with congenital or acquired unilateral motor weakness involves learning how to move; thus, the child is engaged as an active participant in a dynamic motor skill (re)learning process (Gordon & Magill, 2012). The child is presented with a clear functional goal (e.g., use hand to pull off socks, reach for a toy, or turn a doorknob), requiring the use of visual, perceptual, cognitive, and motor systems as he or she uses problem-solving to achieve the goal (Timmermans et al., 2010). The child repeatedly practices strategies for reaching, grasping, manipulating, and transporting real objects during meaningful activity sequences. Each practice trial provides information to the child (i.e., feedback), which forms the basis for strategizing the next attempt. For example, a child may attempt to reach toward and grasp a toy. If he is successful, he may use the same movement strategy again. If he is not successful, he may realize that a new movement strategy is needed. Over the course of practice sessions, task demands are optimally progressed according to the child's capability. This progression is critical to prevent failure of motor learning if tasks become overly simple or too difficult (Gordon & Magill, 2012). Task-oriented approaches also assume learning-dependent functional recovery and reversal of learned nonuse, which is measured in terms of the child's ability to perform functional tasks (Deluca et al., 2006).

CIMT includes specific task-oriented practice involving engagement in play or functional activities (Chen et al., 2014; Chiu & Ada, 2016; DeLuca et al., 2017; Ramey, Coker-Bolt, & DeLuca, 2013). The choice of activities and the movements they elicit are both important. Movement impairments of the involved upper limb are determined during the child's evaluation and prior to starting a CIMT program.

Movement impairments in the affected arm can include lack of shoulder flexion or abduction greater than 90 degrees, lack of supination of the forearm, poor wrist stability, inability to accurately reach objects, lack of functional grasp, or release. Unilateral treatment activities are then chosen to target deficits movements and engage the child in activities requiring more complex motor behaviors. Task demands are graded to ensure success, and the task is made more difficult once the child achieves successful performance in the majority trials. Directions specifying how the affected hand will be used during the activity (often providing choice to the child) are provided before the start of each task to prevent compensatory strategies (i.e., performing the activity using trunk compensation). CIMT is conducive to active problem-solving, given the increased degrees of freedom associated with the use of the affected arm and hand. Positive reinforcements and knowledge of results are used to motivate the child's engagement and performance (often with tangible rewards as well as praise), which reinforce target movements and behaviors.

### Intensive Bimanual Therapy

**Intensive bimanual therapy** retains the intensive structure and task practice at CIMT, but the focus is improving the ability to perform bimanual activities. This type of therapy uses carefully planned, repeated practice of two-handed, or bimanual, games, and activities to improve a child's ability to use their hands together in daily activities. It involves high-dosage, intensive, mass practice, similar to the dosage required for CIMT (>30 hours) and can be provided during individual or group therapy formats (Gordon, 2011). During bimanual therapy, object properties can be adapted to trigger goal-related perceptual and cognitive processes required for children to learn to recognize when two hands are required for task completion (Gordon, 2011; Gordon & Magill, 2012). The practitioner encourages the child to use both hands during bimanual tasks and discourages unimanual skills using only the stronger nonaffected upper limb. Therapy activities target bimanual movements such as those required to play with toys with two hands, transfer items between hands, remove or put on clothing, or carry or move toys. A recent study comparing CIMT and intensive bimanual training found that both approaches led to significant improvements in the quality of unimanual movement, bimanual capacity, and movement efficiency in children with hemiplegic CP (Klepper et al., 2017).

**Hand-Arm Bimanual Intensive Training.** A specific type of bimanual therapy is the HABIT protocol (Charles & Gordon, 2006) which includes a series of principles such as the increase of task difficulty based on individual child's performance, part-task practice of component movements necessary for a complex motor action, sequencing the motor movements to shape motor action, and working on whole-task learning toward the accomplishment of a functional goal. The main difference between the HABIT protocol and intensive bimanual therapy is the individualized nature of progressing through specific activities and the intensity of the protocol. Studies suggest that there should be at least 60 hours of intensive practice for neuroplasticity to occur. Friel et al. (2016) examined the effects of HABIT on manual skills and motor cortex plasticity in children with unilateral spastic CP. In this clinical trial, the authors compared structured skill training using the HABIT protocol (experimental group) versus unstructured hand use (controls). Each group received 90 hours of therapy that were spread over 3 weeks total time. The experimental group received HABIT (Charles & Gordon, 2006), and the control practice group engaged in bimanual activities but did not train in specific movements or functional goals. The groups were tested at three points in time (before, immediately after, and 6 months after training) using outcome measures of unimanual dexterity, bimanual ability, and functional goal performance. The authors also implemented single-pulse transcranial magnetic stimulation (TMS) to map the representation and excitability of the digit and wrist muscles of the affected hand at the same three time points. The data showed that both structured and unstructured training improved bimanual performance, as well as hand dexterity of the affected hand, and these improvements were evident at 6 months post practice. However, only the group that received structured training showed a significant increase in the size of the motor map of the affected hand and amplitude of the motor responses to TMS.

The findings further suggest that the changes in cortical plasticity for the experimental group were independent of the hemisphere of control (i.e., contralateral, or ipsilateral to the affected hand). This provides evidence that both hemispheres responded to the bimanual training. These data are in contrast with results from neuroplasticity studies of the CIMT that have shown that functional gains are less pronounced in children with ipsilateral than contralateral control of the affected hand (Kuhnke et al., 2008). Children who showed the strongest functional improvement also demonstrated the largest cortical motor map expansion, suggesting the existence of reorganization mechanisms that can be facilitated through rehabilitation (Mackey et al., 2014).

## SUMMARY

Motor control is essential to participation in feeding, dressing, bathing, toileting, academics, play, and instrumental activities of daily living. Occupational therapy practitioners address motor control issues of children who have a variety of movement deficits. Dynamic systems and ecologic theories suggest that multiple systems interact to influence movement. Extensive research in a variety of fields supports this contemporary approach and indicates that engaging children in whole, meaningful tasks in a supportive natural environment promotes brain plasticity. Occupational therapy practitioners use this knowledge to create intervention plans that promote motor control by engaging children in their desired occupations and using motor learning strategies to reinforce movement.

Motor learning strategies are based upon research and provide occupational therapy practitioners with techniques to use in practice. Motor learning strategies include information on type of practice, feedback, directions, how to promote transfer of learning, and how to facilitate mental rehearsal. Research on motor learning supports the importance of engaging children in meaningful activities and consideration of the environment. Contemporary motor control approaches (such as CIMT, intensive bimanual therapy such as HABIT, task-specific-training, and the cognitive orientation to daily occupational performance [CO-OP] model) are effective in improving movement in children. These approaches emphasize the intensity of intervention, referred to as dosage, specificity of goals, and use of motor learning strategies.

1. Children and youth exhibit better motor control when engaged in whole, meaningful tasks within the natural context using authentic objects. Occupational therapy practitioners use motor learning strategies to promote movement by engaging children in meaningful activities that include problem-solving, practice, mental

rehearsal, and considering the type of task, objects, feedback, and directions provided.

2. Contemporary motor control interventions support the idea that healthy motor performance is characterized by agency, prospectivity, flexibility, and adaptability. Movement is the result of interaction of person factors, task characteristics, and environmental systems. The principles include the following.
   - Goal-directed movements have common characteristics important for success: agency, prospectivity, flexibility, and adaptability.
   - Interactions among multiple systems underlie skilled motor behavior (i.e., person, occupation, contexts) and are responsible for the control of motor actions at any given moment.
3. The interaction between child, task, and contextual factors influences movement.
   - *Person:* These are factors related to body structures and functions specific to each child (i.e., sensory, musculoskeletal, perceptual, cognitive/processing, and emotional skills).
   - *Tasks (with Occupation)*: Tasks are meaningful, impact the motor actions and children's ability to engage in occupations. Included are the task nature, motor and cognitive demands, objects used and their properties, and level of familiarity for the child. Tasks can be modified and adapted to facilitate motor control and goal achievement.
   - *Contexts* include personal factors (e.g., age, sex/gender, socioeconomic factors, cultural expectations) and environments (e.g., home, school, community). Contexts affect the expression of motor skills and the control and monitoring of motor actions for successful performance.
4. Contemporary therapy approaches that show significant scientific rigor and use motor control and motor learning principles inform evidence-based interventions, such as CIMT and intensive bimanual therapy. The research evidence supports that providing the "just right challenge" within the natural environment and while engaged in meaningful whole activities supports motor performance and facilitates motor learning. Using an occupation-based model of practice interventions that allows the child to perform meaningful whole activities using real objects in the natural setting promotes motor performance and learning. Motor learning strategies (such as transfer of learning, feedback, practice, and mental rehearsal) are techniques to promote motor acquisition and motor control. Motor learning strategies help practitioners decide how and when to provide feedback and how to promote generalization of skills (transfer of learning). Practice information helps define which type of practice to provide at each stage of learning. Practitioners are encouraged to use evidence-based motor learning strategies to enhance a child's occupational performance.

## REFERENCES


Aarts, P. B., et al. (2010). Effectiveness of modified constraint-induced movement therapy in children with unilateral spastic cerebral palsy: A randomized controlled trial. *Neurorehabilitation and Neural Repair, 24*(6), 509–518.

Adolph, K. E. (2020). An ecological approach to learning in (not and) development. *Human Development, 63*(3–4), 180–201.

Adolph, K. E., & Franchak, J. M. (2017). The development of motor behavior. *Wiley Interdisciplinary Reviews: Cognitive Science, 8*(1–2), e1430.

Adolph, K. E., & Hoch, J. E. (2019). Motor development: Embodied, embedded, enculturated, and enabling. *Annual Review of Psychology, 70*, 141–164.

Adolph, K. E., & Kretch, K. S. (2015). Gibson's theory of perceptual learning. *International Encyclopedia of the Social and Behavioral Sciences, 10*, 127–134.

Adolph, K. E., & Robinson, S. R. (2015). Motor development. *Handbook of Child Psychology and Developmental Science*, 1–45.

Adolph, K. E., & Young, J. W. (2021). Learning to move in the real world. *Science, 373*(6555), 620–621.

Bäckström, A., Johansson, A. M., Rudolfsson, T., Rönnqvist, L., von Hofsten, C., Rosander, K., & Domellöf, E. (2021). Motor planning and movement execution during goal-directed sequential manual movements in 6-year-old children with autism spectrum disorder: A kinematic analysis. *Research in Developmental Disabilities, 115*, 104014.

Babik, I., Galloway, J. C., & Lobo, M. A. (2022). Early exploration of one's own body, exploration of objects, and motor, language, and cognitive development relate dynamically across the first two years of life. *Developmental Psychology, 58*(2), 222.

Bandura, A., & Schunk, D. H. (1981). Cultivating competence, self-efficacy, and intrinsic interest through proximal self-motivation. *Journal of Personality and Social Psychology, 41*(3), 586.

Banks, R., Rodger, S., & Polatajko, H. (2008). Mastering handwriting: How children with developmental coordination disorder succeed with CO-OP. *OTJR: Occupation, Participation and Health, 28*(3), 100–109.

Barhoun, P., Fuelscher, I., Kothe, E. J., He, J. L., Youssef, G. J., Enticott, P. G., & Hyde, C. (2019). Motor imagery in children with DCD: A systematic and meta-analytic review of hand-rotation task performance. *Neuroscience & Biobehavioral Reviews, 99*, 282–297.

Behrendt, F., Zumbrunnen, V., Brem, L., Suica, Z., Gäumann, S., Ziller, C., & Schuster-Amft, C. (2021). Effect of motor imagery training on motor learning in children and adolescents: A systematic review and meta-analysis. *International Journal of Environmental Research and Public Health, 18*(18), 9467.

Bierman, J. C., Franjoine, M. R., Hazzard, C. M., Howle, J. M., Stamer, M., Styer-Acevedo, J., & McElroy, J. (2016). *9 Neuro-Developmental Treatment Intervention—A Session View*, 150.

Bishop, J. C., Kelly, L. K., & Hull, M. (2018). Knowledge of performance feedback among boys with ADHD. *Research in Developmental Disabilities, 74*, 31–40.

Bleyenheuft, Y., Arnould, C., Brandao, M. B., Bleyenheuft, C., & Gordon, A. M. (2015). Hand and Arm Bimanual Intensive Therapy Including Lower Extremity (HABIT-ILE) in children with unilateral spastic cerebral palsy: A randomized trial. *Neurorehabilitation and Neural Repair, 29*(7), 645–657.

Bleyenheuft, Y., Ebner–Karestinos, D., Surana, B., Paradis, J., Sidiropoulos, A., Renders, A., & Gordon, A. M. (2017). Intensive upper and lower–extremity training for children with bilateral cerebral palsy: A quasi–randomized trial. *Developmental Medicine and Child Neurology, 59*(6), 625–633.

Bo, J., & Lee, C. M. (2013). Motor skill learning in children with developmental coordination disorder. *Research in Developmental Disabilities, 34*, 2047–2055.

Borella, E., et al. (2011). Increased intraindividual variability is a marker of ADHD but also of dyslexia: A study on handwriting. *Brain and Cognition, 77*, 33–39.

Bouffard, M., & Wall, A. E. (1990). A problem-solving approach to movement skill acquisition: Implications for special populations. In G. Reid (Ed.), *Problems in movement control* (pp. 107–131). Amsterdam: Elsevier Science.

Breslin, G., Hodges, N. J., Steenson, A., & Williams, A. M. (2012). Constant or variable practice: Recreating the especial skill effect. *Acta Psychologica, 140*(2), 154–157.

Bundy, A., et al. (2008). Playful interaction: Occupational therapy for all children on the school playground. *American Journal of Occupational Therapy, 62*(5), 522–528.

Chan, J. S. Y., Luo, Y., Yan, J. H., Cai, L., & Peng, K. (2015). Children's age modulates the effect of part and whole practice in motor learning. *Human Movement Science, 42*, 261–272.

Charles, J., & Gordon, A. M. (2006). Development of hand–arm bimanual intensive training (HABIT) for improving bimanual coordination in children with hemiplegic cerebral palsy. *Developmental Medicine and Child Neurology*, *48*(11), 931–936.

Chen, Y. P., Pope, S., Tyler, D., & Warren, G. L. (2014). Effectiveness of constraint-induced movement therapy on upper-extremity function in children with cerebral palsy: A systematic review and meta analysis of randomized controlled trials. *Clinical Rehabilitation*, *28*(10), 939–953.

Chiu, H. C., & Ada, L. (2016). Constraint-induced movement therapy improves upper limb activity and participation in hemiplegic cerebral palsy: A systematic review. *Journal of Physiotherapy*, *62*(3), 130–137.

Christiansen, C., Baum, C. M., & Bass, J. (2011). The person-environment-occupational performance model. In E. A. S. Duncan (Ed.), *Foundations for practice in occupational therapy* (5th ed.) (pp. 93–104). Elsevier.

Chua, L. K., Dimapilis, M. K., Iwatsuki, T., Abdollahipour, R., Lewthwaite, R., & Wulf, G. (2019). Practice variability promotes an external focus of attention and enhances motor skill learning. *Human Movement Science*, *64*, 307–319.

Cohn, E., Miller, L. J., & Tickle-Degnen, L. (2000). Parental hopes for therapy outcomes: Children with sensory modulation disorders. *American Journal of Occupational Therapy*, *54*, 36–43.

Comalli, D. M., Keen, R., Abraham, E. S., Foo, V. J., Lee, M. H., & Adolph, K. E. (2016). The development of tool use: Planning for end-state comfort. *Developmental Psychology*, *52*(11), 1878.

Cool, J., & Zappetti, D. (2019). The physiology of stress. *Medical student well-being: An essential guide*, 1–15.

Cuturi, L. F., & Gori, M. (2019). Biases in the visual and haptic subjective vertical reveal the role of proprioceptive/vestibular priors in child development. *Frontiers in Neurology*, *9*, 1151.

D'Souza, H., Cowie, D., Karmiloff–Smith, A., & Bremner, A. J. (2017). Specialization of the motor system in infancy: From broad tuning to selectively specialized purposeful actions. *Developmental Science*, *20*(4), e12409.

de Camargo Barros, J. A., Tani, G., & Corrêa, U. C. (2017). Effects of practice schedule and task specificity on the adaptive process of motor learning. *Human Movement Science*, *55*, 196–210.

de Sá, C. D. S. C., Boffino, C. C., Ramos, R. T., & Tanaka, C. (2018). Development of postural control and maturation of sensory systems in children of different ages a cross-sectional study. *Brazilian Journal of Physical Therapy*, *22*(1), 70–76.

Deecke, L. (1996). Planning, preparation, execution, and imagery of volitional action. *Cognitive Brain Research*, *3*, 59–64.

DeLuca, S. C., Case-Smith, J., Stevenson, R., & Ramey, S. L. (2012). Constraint-induced movement therapy (CIMT) for young children with cerebral palsy: Effects of therapeutic dosage. *Journal of Pediatric Rehabilitation Medicine*, *5*(2), 133–142.

Deluca, S. C., et al. (2006). Intensive pediatric constraint-induced therapy for children with cerebral palsy: Randomized, controlled, crossover trial. *Journal of Child Neurology*, *21*, 931–938.

DeLuca, S. C., Trucks, M. R., Wallace, D. A., & Ramey, S. L. (2017). Practice-based evidence from a clinical cohort that received pediatric constraint-induced movement therapy. *Journal of Pediatric Rehabilitation Medicine*, *10*, 37–46.

Dhawale, A. K., Smith, M. A., & Ölveczky, B. P. (2017). The role of variability in motor learning. *Annual Review of Neuroscience*, *40*, 479–498.

Dimitropoulou, K., & Gordon, A. (2020). Adaptation of motor action in children with hemiplegic cerebral palsy. *Journal of Clinical and Translational Science*, *4*, 92.

Dimitropoulou, K., & Baxter, M. (2018). Neural basis of adaptation: Motivation, intention, resilience, and goal-directed behaviors. In L. Grajo, & A. Biosselle (Eds.), *Adaptation through occupation: Multidimensional perspectives*. Slack.

Donath, L., Faude, O., Hagmann, S., Roth, R., & Zahner, L. (2015). Fundamental movement skills in preschoolers: A randomized controlled trial targeting object control proficiency. *Child: Care, Health and Development*, *41*(6), 1179–1187.

Doussoulin, S., & Rehbein, L. (2011). Motor imagery as a tool for motor skill training in children. *Motricidade*, *7*(3), 37–43.

Eaves, D. L., Hodges, N. J., Buckingham, G., Buccino, G., & Vogt, S. (2022). Enhancing motor imagery practice using synchronous action observation. *Psychological Research*, 1–17.

Emanuel, M., Jarus, T., & Bart, O. (2008). Effect of focus of attention and age on motor acquisition, retention, and transfer: A randomized trial. *Physical Therapy*, *88*, 251–260.

Farhat, F., Hsairi, I., Baati, H., Smits-Engelsman, B. C. M., Masmoudi, K., Mchirgui, R., ... Moalla, W. (2016). The effect of a motor skills training program in the improvement of practiced and non-practiced tasks performance in children with developmental coordination disorder (DCD). *Human Movement Science*, *46*, 10–22.

Fernandes, V. R., Ribeiro, M. L. S., Melo, T., de Tarso Maciel-Pinheiro, P., Guimarães, T. T., Araújo, N. B., & Deslandes, A. C. (2016). Motor coordination correlates with academic achievement and cognitive function in children. *Frontiers in Psychology*, *7*, 318.

Fiehler, K., Brenner, E., & Spering, M. (2019). Prediction in goal-directed action. *Journal of Vision*, *19*(9), 10.

Fisher, A. G. (1998). Uniting practice and theory in an occupational framework. *American Journal of Occupational Therapy*, *52*, 509–521.

Fong, S. S., Guo, X., Liu, K. P., Ki, W. Y., Louie, L. H., Chung, R. C., & Macfarlane, D. J. (2016). Task-specific balance training improves the sensory organisation of balance control in children with developmental coordination disorder: A randomised controlled trial. *Scientific Reports*, *6*(1), 20945.

Frank, C., Kluever, J., & Simonsmeier, B. A. (2023). Imagery training of motor actions in children and adolescents: A meta-analysis. *International Review of Sport and Exercise Psychology*, 1–22.

Frese, M., & Sabini, J. (Eds.). (2021). *Goal directed behavior: The concept of action in psychology*. Routledge.

Friel, K. M., et al. (2016). Skilled bimanual training drives motor cortex plasticity in children with unilateral cerebral palsy. *Neurorehabilitation and Neural Repair*, *30*(9), 834–844.

Gaberova, K., Pacheva, I., Timova, E., Petkova, A., Velkova, K., & Ivanov, I. (2019). An individualized approach to neuroplasticity after early unilateral brain damage. *Frontiers in Psychiatry*, *10*, 747.

Ganguly, J., Kulshreshtha, D., Almotiri, M., & Jog, M. (2021). Muscle tone physiology and abnormalities. *Toxins*, *13*(4), 282.

Gentile, A. M. (2000). Skill acquisition: Action, movement, and neuromotor processes. In J. H. Carr, & R. B. Shepherd (Eds.), *Movement science: Foundations for physical therapy in rehabilitation* (2nd ed.) (pp. 11–187). Aspen.

Goncalves, G. S., Cardozo, P. L., Valentini, N. C., & Chiviacowsky, S. (2018). Enhancing performance expectancies through positive comparative feedback facilitates the learning of basketball free throw in children. *Psychology of Sport and Exercise*, 174–177.

Goo, M., Tucker, K., & Johnston, L. M. (2018). Muscle tone assessments for children aged 0 to 12 years: A systematic review. *Developmental Medicine and Child Neurology*, *60*(7), 660–671.

Goodway, J. D., Ozmun, J. C., & Gallahue, D. L. (2019). *Understanding motor development: Infants, children, adolescents, adults*. Jones & Bartlett Learning.

Gordon, A., et al. (2007). Efficacy of hand-arm bimanual intensive therapy (HABIT) in children with hemiplegic cerebral palsy: A randomized control trial. *Developmental Medicine and Child Neurology*, *49*, 830–839.

Gordon, A., & Magill, R. (2012). Motor learning: Application of principles to pediatric rehabilitation. In S. K. Campbell, R. J. Palisane, & M. N. Orlin (Eds.), *Physical therapy for children* (4th ed.) (pp. 151–174). Elsevier.

Gordon, A. M., Hung, Y. C., Brandao, M., Ferre, C. L., Kuo, H. C., Friel, K., ... Charles, J. R. (2011). Bimanual training and constraint-induced movement therapy in children with hemiplegic cerebral palsy: A randomized trial. *Neurorehabilitation and Neural Repair*, *25*(8), 692–702.

Gordon, A. (2011). To constrain or not to constrain, and other stories of intensive upper extremity training for children with unilateral cerebral palsy. *Developmental Medicine and Child Neurology*, *53*(Suppl. 4), 56–61.

Grajo, L. (2017). Occupational adaptation. In P. Kramer, J. Hinojosa, & C. Royeen (Eds.), *Perspectives in human occupation* (pp. 287–311). FA Davis.

Gredin, V., & Williams, M. (2016). The relative effectiveness of various instructional approaches during the performance and learning of motor skills. *Journal of Motor Behavior, 48*, 86–96.

Haggard, P. (2017). Sense of agency in the human brain. *Nature Reviews Neuroscience, 18*(4), 196–207.

Hemayattalab, R., & Rostami, L. R. (2010). Effects of feedback on learning of motor skills in individuals with cerebral palsy. *Research in Developmental Disabilities, 31*, 212–217.

Hetu, S., & Mercier, C. (2012). Using purposeful tasks to improve motor performance: Does object affordance matter? *British Journal of Occupational Therapy, 75*(8), 367–376.

Hill, M. W., Wdowski, M. M., Pennell, A., Stodden, D. F., & Duncan, M. J. (2019). Dynamic postural control in children: Do the arms lend the legs a helping hand? *Frontiers in Physiology, 9*, 1932.

Hoch, J. E., O'Grady, S. M., & Adolph, K. E. (2019). It's the journey, not the destination: Locomotor exploration in infants. *Developmental Science, 22*(2), e12740.

Hu, Y., et al. (2005). A model of coupling between grip aperture and hand transport during human prehension. *Experimental Brain Research, 167*, 301–304.

Hua, J., Williams, G. J., Jin, H., Chen, J., Xu, M., Zhou, Y., & Du, W. (2022). Early motor milestones in infancy and later motor impairments: A population-based data linkage study. *Frontiers in Psychiatry, 13*, 31.

Hubbard, I. J., et al. (2009). Task-specific training: Evidence and translation to clinical practice. *Occupational Therapy International, 16*(3–4), 175–189.

Hung, Y.-C., Brandao, M. B., & Gordon, A. (2017). Structured skill practice during intensive bimanual training leads to better trunk and arm control than unstructured practice in children with unilateral spastic cerebral palsy. *Research in Developmental Disabilities, 60*, 65–76.

Ivanenko, Y., & Gurfinkel, V. S. (2018). Human postural control. *Frontiers in Neuroscience, 12*, 171.

Jaric, S., et al. (1993). Principles of learning single joint movements. II. Generalizing a learned behavior. *Experimental Brain Research, 94*, 514–521.

Jelsma, D., Ferguson, G. D., Smits-Engelsman, B. C., & Geuze, R. H. (2015). Short-term motor learning of dynamic balance control in children with probable Developmental Coordination Disorder. *Research in Developmental Disabilities, 38*, 213–222.

Jongbloed-Pereboom, M., Nijhuis-Van der Sanden, M. W. G., & Steenbergen, B. (2015). Implicit and explicit motor learning in children born very preterm and typically developing children: Effects of task, age, and working memory. *Physiotherapy, 101*, e693–e694.

Kandel, E. R., Koester, J. D., Mack, S. H., & Siegelbaum, S. A. (2021). *Principles of Neural Science*, 449–453.

Kearney, P. E., & Judge, P. (2017). Successful transfer of a motor learning strategy to a novel sport. *Journal of Perceptual and Motor Skills, 124*(5), 1009–1021.

Kelso, J. S., & Fuchs, A. (2016). The coordination dynamics of mobile conjugate reinforcement. *Biological Cybernetics, 110*, 41–53.

Kelso, J. S. (2016). On the self-organizing origins of agency. *Trends in Cognitive Sciences, 20*(7), 490–499.

Kiefer, A. W., Armitano-Lago, C. N., Cone, B. L., Bonnette, S., Rhea, C. K., Cummins-Sebree, S., & Riley, M. A. (2021). Postural control development from late childhood through young adulthood. *Gait & Posture, 86*, 169–173.

Kielhofner, G. (2008). *Model of human occupation: Theory and application* (4th ed.). F. A. Davis.

Klepper, S. E., Clayton, D., Gilb, M. C., & Khalil, N. (2017). Comparing unimanual and bimanual training in upper extremity function in children with unilateral cerebral palsy. *Pediatric Physical Therapy, 29*(4), 288–306.

Klingberg, T., Forssberg, H., & Westerberg, H. (2002). Increased brain activity in frontal and parietal cortex underlies the development of visuospatial working memory capacity during childhood. *Journal of Cognitive Neuroscience, 14*, 1–10.

Kolovelonis, A., Goudas, M., & Dermitzaki, I. (2012). The effects of self-talk and goal setting on self-regulation of learning a new motor skill in physical education. *International Journal of Sport and Exercise Psychology, 10*(3), 221–225.

Krakauer, J. W., Hadjiosif, A. M., Xu, J., Wong, A. L., & Haith, A. M. (2019). Motor learning. *Comprehensive Physiology, 9*(2), 613–663.

Kramer, J. M. (2007). Using a participatory action approach to identify habits and routines to support self-advocacy. *OTJR: Occupation, Participation and Health, 27*, 84S–85S.

Krebs, H. I., et al. (2012). Motor learning characterizes habilitation of children with hemiplegic cerebral palsy. *Neurorehabilitation and Neural Repair, 26*(7), 855–860.

Kuhnke, N., Juenger, H., Walther, M., Berweck, S., Mall, V., & Staudt, M. (2008). Do patients with congenital hemiparesis and ipsilateral corticospinal projections respond differently to constraint-induced movement therapy? *Developmental Medicine and Child Neurology, 50*(12), 898–903.

Law, M., et al. (2011). Focus on function: A cluster, randomized controlled trial comparing child- versus context-focused intervention for young children with cerebral palsy. *Developmental Medicine and Child Neurology, 53*(7), 621–629.

Lee, J. J., et al. (2013). Comparative neuroimaging in children with cerebral palsy using fMRI and a novel EEG-based brain mapping during a motor task—a preliminary investigation. *NeuroRehabilitation, 32*, 279–285.

Lewthwaite, R., & Wulf, G. (2017). Optimizing motivation and attention for motor performance and learning. *Current Opinion in Psychology, 16*, 38–42.

Mackey, A., Stinear, C., Stott, S., & Byblow, W. D. (2014). Upper limb function and cortical organization in youth with unilateral cerebral palsy. *Frontiers in Neurology, 5*, 117.

Mahoney, M. J., & Meyers, A. W. (2021). Anxiety and athletic performance: Traditional and cognitive-developmental perspectives. In *Anxiety in sports* (pp. 77–94). Taylor & Francis.

Mandich, A. D., et al. (2001). Treatment of children with developmental coordination disorder: What is the evidence? *Physical & Occupational Therapy in Pediatrics, 20*, 51–58.

Manning, K. Y., et al. (2016). Neuroplastic sensorimotor resting state network reorganization in children with hemiplegic cerebral palsy treated with constraint-induced movement therapy. *Journal of Child Neurology, 31*(2), 220–226.

Marshall, B., Wright, D. J., Holmes, P. S., Williams, J., & Wood, G. (2020). Combined action observation and motor imagery facilitates visuomotor adaptation in children with developmental coordination disorder. *Research in Developmental Disabilities, 98*, 103570.

Master, A., Cheryan, S., Mostcatelli, A., & Metlzoff, A. (2017). Programming experience promotes higher STEM motivation among first-grade girls. *Journal of Experimental Child Psychology, 160*, 92–106.

Maxwell, J. P., Capio, C. M., & Masters, R. S. (2017). Interaction between motor ability and skill learning in children: Application of implicit and explicit approaches. *European Journal of Sport Science, 17*(4), 407–416.

Mayston, M. (2016). Bobath and NeuroDevelopmental therapy: What is the future? *Developmental Medicine and Child Neurology, 58*(10), 994.

McIsaac, T. L., Lamberg, E. M., & Muratori, L. M. (2015). Building a framework for a dual task taxonomy. *BioMed Research International 2015*.

Meunks, K., Wigfield, A., & Eccles, J. S. (2018). I can do this! The development and calibration of children's expectations for success and competence beliefs. *Developmental Review, 48*, 24–39.

Miller, H. L., Caçola, P. M., Sherrod, G. M., Patterson, R. M., & Bugnariu, N. L. (2019). Children with Aautism Spectrum Disorder, Developmental Coordination Disorder, and typical development differ in characteristics of dynamic postural control: A preliminary study. *Gait & Posture, 67*, 9–11.

Miller, L., Ziviani, J., Ware, R. S., & Boyd, R. N. (2016). Does context matter? Mastery motivation and therapy engagement of children with cerebral palsy. *Physical & Occupational Therapy in Pediatrics, 36*(2), 155–170.

Missiuna, C., & Mandich, A. (2002). Integrating motor learning theories into practice. In S. Cermak, & D. Larkin (Eds.), *Developmental coordination disorder* (pp. 221–233). Delmar Thomson Learning.

Miyahara, M., & Wafer, A. (2004). Clinical intervention for children with developmental coordination disorder: A multiple case study. *Adapted Physical Activity Quarterly, 21*, 281–300.

Mostert-Kerckhoffs, M. A., Staal, W. G., Houben, R. H., & de Jonge, M. V. (2015). Stop and change: Inhibition and flexibility skills are related to repetitive behavior in children and young adults with autism spectrum disorders. *Journal of Autism and Dvelopmental Disorders, 45*, 3148–3158.

Murphy, S. M. (1994). Imagery interventions in sport. *Medicine & Science in Sports & Exercise, 26*, 486–494.

Nobre, G. C., Ramalho, M. H. D. S., Ribas, M. D. S., & Valentini, N. C. (2023). Motor, physical, and psychosocial parameters of children with and without developmental coordination disorder: A comparative and associative study. *International Journal of Environmental Research and Public Health, 20*(4), 2801.

Novak, I., Morgan, C., Fahey, M., Finch-Edmondson, M., Galea, C., Hines, A., … Badawi, N. (2020). State of the evidence traffic lights 2019: Systematic review of interventions for preventing and treating children with cerebral palsy. *Current Neurology and Neuroscience Reports, 20*, 1–21.

O'Brien, J., et al. (2009). Children with disabilities and their parents' views of occupational participation needs. *Occupational Therapy in Health Care, 25*, 1–17.

O'Brien, J. (2020). *Occupational therapy motor learning strategies worksheet*. Portland, ME: University of New England (unpublished worksheet).

Ouyang, R. G., Yang, C. N., Qu, Y. L., Koduri, M. P., & Chien, C. W. (2020). Effectiveness of hand-arm bimanual intensive training on upper extremity function in children with cerebral palsy: A systematic review. *European Journal of Paediatric Neurology, 25*, 17–28.

Page, S., Sime, W., & Nordell, K. (1999). The effects of imagery on female college swimmers' perceptions of anxiety. *The Sport Psychologist, 13*, 458–469.

Painter, M., Inman, K., & Vincent, W. (1994). Contextual interference effects: I. The acquisition and retention of motor tasks by individuals with mild mental handicaps. *Adapted Physical Activity Quarterly, 11*, 383–395.

Patel, D. R., Neelakantan, M., Pandher, K., & Merrick, J. (2020). Cerebral palsy in children: A clinical overview. *Translational Pediatrics, 9*(Suppl. 1), S125.

Polatajko, H. J., Townsend, E. A., & Craik, J. (2007). *Canadian model of occupational performance and engagement (CMOP-E)Enabling occupation II: Advancing an occupational therapy vision of health, well-being & justice through occupation, 23.*.

Polatajko, H., Mandich, A. D., Miller, L. T., et al. (2001). Cognitive orientation to daily occupational performance (CO-OP): Part II—the evidence. *Physical & Occupational Therapy in Pediatrics, 20*, 83–106.

Ramey, S. L., Coker-Bolt, P., & DeLuca, S. C. (Eds.). (2013). *Handbook of pediatric constraint-induced movement therapy (CIMT): A guide for occupational therapy and health care clinicians, researchers, and educators*. AOTA Press.

Rathunde, K. (2001). Toward a psychology of optimal human functioning: What positive psychology can learn from the "experiential turns" of James, Dewey, and Maslow. *Journal of Humanistic Psychology, 41*, 135–153.

Reddy, V., Markova, G., & Wallot, S. (2013). Anticipatory adjustments to being picked up in infancy. *PLoS One, 8*(6), e65289.

Risen, S. R., Barber, A. D., Mostofsky, S. H., & Suskauer, S. J. (2015). Altered functional connectivity in children with mild to moderate TBI relates to motor control. *Journal of Pediatric Rehabilitation Medicine, 8*(4), 309–319.

Schkade, J. K., & Schultz, S. (1992). Occupational adaptation: Toward a holistic approach for contemporary practice, part 1. *American Journal of Occupational Therapy, 46*(9), 829–837.

Schmidt, M., Egger, F., Benzing, V., Jäger, K., Conzelmann, A., Roebers, C. M., & Pesce, C. (2017). Disentangling the relationship between children's motor ability, executive function and academic achievement. *PLoS One, 12*(8):e0182845.

Schmidt, R. A., Lee, T. D., Winstein, C., Wulf, G., & Zelaznik, H. N. (2018). *Motor control and learning: A behavioral emphasis*. Human kinetics.

Scott, M. W., Wood, G., Holmes, P. S., Williams, J., Marshall, B., & Wright, D. J. (2021). Combined action observation and motor imagery: An intervention to combat the neural and behavioural deficits associated with developmental coordination disorder. *Neuroscience & Biobehavioral Reviews, 127*, 638–646.

Screws, D. P., & Surburg, P. R. (1997). Motor performance of children with mild mental disabilities after using mental imagery. *Adapted Physical Activity Quarterly, 14*, 119–130.

Seyyar, G., Aras, B., & Aras, O. (2019). Trunk control and functionality in children with spastic cerebral palsy. *Developmental Neurorehabilitation, 22*(2), 120–125.

Shadmehr, R., Smith, M. A., & Krakauer, J. W. (2010). Error correction, sensory prediction, and adaptation in motor control. *Annual Review of Neuroscience, 33*, 89–108.

Shin, Y. K., Lee, D. R., Hwang, H. J., You, S. J. H., & Im, C. H. (2012). A novel EEG-based brain mapping to determine cortical activation patterns in normal children and children with cerebral palsy during motor imagery tasks. *NeuroRehabilitation, 31*(4), 349–355.

Shumway-Cook, A., Woollacott, M. H., Rachwani, J., & Santamaria, V. (2023). Constraints on motor control: An overview of neurologic impairments. In *Motor control: Translating research into clinical practice* (6th ed.). Lippincott Williams & Wilkins.

Sidaway, B., Bates, J., Occhiogrosso, B., Schlagenhaufer, J., & Wilkes, D. (2012). Interaction of feedback frequency and task difficulty in children's motor skill learning. *Physical Therapy, 92*(7), 948–957.

Sinno, S., Dumas, G., Mallinson, A., Najem, F., Abouchacra, K. S., Nashner, L., & Perrin, P. (2021). Changes in the sensory weighting strategies in balance control throughout maturation in children. *Journal of the American Academy of Audiology, 32*(02), 122–136.

Smits-Engelsman, B., Bonney, E., & Ferguson, G. (2020). Motor skill learning in children with and without developmental coordination disorder. *Human Movement Science, 74*, 102687.

Souto, D. O., Cruz, T. K. F., Coutinho, K., Julio-Costa, A., Fontes, P. L. B., & Haase, V. G. (2020). Effect of motor imagery combined with physical practice on upper limb rehabilitation in children with hemiplegic cerebral palsy. *NeuroRehabilitation, 46*(1), 53–63.

Steenbergen, B., et al. (2013). Impaired motor planning and motor imagery in children with unilateral spastic cerebral palsy: Challenges for the future of pediatric rehabilitation. *Developmental Medicine and Child Neurology, 55*, 43–46.

Steenbergen, B., Krajenbrink, H., Lust, J., & Wilson, P. (2020). Motor imagery and action observation for predictive control in developmental coordination disorder. *Developmental Medicine and Child Neurology, 62*(12), 1352–1355.

Steinberg, N., Waddington, G., Adams, R., Karin, J., & Tirosh, O. (2016). The effect of textured ballet shoe insoles on ankle proprioception in dancers. *Physical Therapy in Sport, 17*, 38–44.

Sullivan, K., Kantuk, S., & Burtner, P. (2008). Motor learning in children: Feedback effects on skill acquisition. *Physical Therapy, 88*, 720–732.

Taktek, K., Zinsser, N., & St-John, B. (2008). Visual versus kinesthetic mental imagery: Efficacy for the retention and transfer of a closed motor skill in young children. *Canadian Journal of Experimental Psychology, 62*, 174–187.

Taunton, S., Brian, A., & True, L. (2017). Universally designed motor skill intervention for children with and without disabilities. *Journal Development and Physical Disabilities, 29*, 941–954.

Taylor, R. R., Bowyer, P., & Fisher, G. (2024). *Kielhofner's model of human occupation: Theory and application* (6th ed.). Wolters Kluwer.

Timmermans, A. A., Spooren, A. I., Kingma, H., & Seelen, H. A. (2010). Influence of task-oriented training content on skilled arm-hand performance in stroke: A systematic review. *Neurorehabilitation and Neural Repair, 24*(9), 858–870.

Toovey, R., Bernie, C., Harvey, A. R., McGinley, J. L., & Spittle, A. J. (2017). Task-specific gross motor skills training for ambulant school-aged children with cerebral palsy: A systematic review. *BMJ Paediatrics Open, 1*(1).

Torres-Costoso, A., López-Muñoz, P., Martínez-Vizcaíno, V., Álvarez-Bueno, C., & Cavero-Redondo, I. (2020). Association between muscular strength and bone health from children to young adults: A systematic review and meta-analysis. *Sports Medicine, 50*, 1163–1190.

Trombly, C. A. (1995). Occupation: Purposefulness and meaningfulness as therapeutic mechanisms. 1995 Eleanor Clarke Slagle Lecture. *American Journal of Occupational Therapy, 49*, 960–972.

Van de Winckel, A., et al. (2013). How does brain activation differ in children with unilateral cerebral palsy compared to typically developing children, during active and passive movements, and tactile stimulation? An fMRI study. *Research in Developmental Disabilities, 34*, 183–197.

Van der Weel, F. R., Van der Meer, A. L., & Lee, D. N. (1991). Effect of task on movement control in cerebral palsy: Implications for assessment and therapy. *Developmental Medicine and Child Neurology, 33*, 419–426.

Veldman, S. L., Santos, R., Jones, R. A., Sousa-Sá, E., & Okely, A. D. (2019). Associations between gross motor skills and cognitive development in toddlers. *Early Human Development, 132*, 39–44.

Von Hofsten, C. (2004). An action perspective on motor development. *Trends in Cognitive Sciences, 8*(6), 266–272.

Westcott, S. L., & Burtner, P. (2004). Postural control in children: Implications for pediatric practice. *Physical & Occupational Therapy in Pediatrics, 24*(1/2), 5–55.

Williams, H. (2006). Motor control. In J. Solomon, & J. O'Brien (Eds.), *Pediatric skills for occupational therapy assistants* (2nd ed.) (pp. 461–480). St. Louis, MO: Mosby.

Williams, J., et al. (2013). Motor imagery skills of children with attention deficit hyperactivity disorder and developmental coordination disorder. *Human Movement Science, 32*, 121–135.

Wright, M. G., Hunt, L. P., & Stanley, O. H. (2005). Object/wrist movements during manipulation in children with cerebral palsy. *Pediatric Rehabilitation, 8*(4), 263–271.

Zanon, M. A., Pacheco, R. L., Latorraca, C. D. O. C., Martimbianco, A. L. C., Pachito, D. V., & Riera, R. (2019). Neurodevelopmental treatment (Bobath) for children with cerebral palsy: A systematic review. *Journal of Child Neurology, 34*(11), 679–686.

Zoccante, L., Ciceri, M. L., Chamitava, L., Di Gennaro, G., Cazzoletti, L., Zanolin, M. E., & Colizzi, M. (2021). Postural control in childhood: Investigating the neurodevelopmental gradient hypothesis. *International Journal of Environmental Research and Public Health, 18*(4), 1693.

# 30

# Intervention for Fine Motor Skills

*Aimee Piller and Jane Clifford O'Brien*

## GUIDING QUESTIONS

1. What factors influence fine motor skill development in children and youth?
2. How do occupational therapy practitioners address fine motor challenges with children and youth?
3. How do occupational therapy practitioners use activity- or occupation-centered interventions to address fine motor challenges for children and youth?
4. What intervention approaches address fine motor skill development in children?

## KEY TERMS

**Bimanual hand use**
**Cylindrical grasp**
**Hook grasp**
**Inferior pincer grasp**
**Lateral grasp**
**Motor planning**
**Palmar grasp**
**Radial digital grasp**
**Raking grasp**
**Scissors grasp**
**Sensory processing**
**Stereognosis**
**Superior pincer grasp**
**Tactile perception**
**Three-jaw chuck**
**Visual-motor integration**

## INTRODUCTION

Infants use their hands to explore their environment, calm themselves, and communicate with others. For example, they suck their thumb to soothe, hold a bottle or breast, and grasp their caregiver's finger and rattles. Toddlers hold and manipulate objects and toys, grasp utensils, pull on their clothing, and begin to point and use their hands to wave and gesture. School-age children scribble, color, and write. They express themselves using their hands and make things such as sandcastles, block buildings, and collages. Children develop fine motor skills to zip, button, manipulate, and engage with objects. They use their hands to hold onto things and communicate via phones, tablets, and computers. They also use their hand skills to communicate in writing or through gesturing, to demonstrate emotions, and to make social connections. As they touch and feel things, they develop ideas, figure out how things work, and problem solve. They learn about textures, temperatures, and consistencies.

Occupational therapy practitioners are trained to analyze the motor, sensory, and cognitive factors that influence fine motor skills. They integrate knowledge of the sequence of fine motor development with a child's strengths and challenges and use knowledge of the task or occupation in relation to the environment, in combination with the cultural roles and expectations, to create intervention plans to support the child's occupational engagement. This chapter defines the motor, sensory, and cognitive factors that influence fine motor development (reach, grasp, in-hand manipulation, and bimanual hand use). The authors provide intervention approaches based on selected frames of references and strategies to address fine motor skills to promote handwriting and occupational performance.

## FINE MOTOR SKILLS

Fine motor skills allow children and youth to participate in daily occupations such as activities of daily living, instrumental activities of daily living, health management, rest and sleep, education, work, play, leisure, and social participation. Fine motor skills include movements such as reaching, grasping, releasing, manipulating, and engaging in bilateral hand skills. These require different levels of precision, timing, sequencing, and motor planning. Fine motor skills require the child to have proprioceptive awareness (i.e., sense of their muscles and joints, movement, and force), tactile discrimination (i.e., ability to feel and identify objects), and visual perceptual skills (i.e., seeing and identifying objects, colors, shapes, sizes). As children gain muscle control, sensory awareness, and cognition through practice, they become more precise in their fine motor movements, and the movements become more automatic. When children develop automaticity in movements, they are more able to quickly adapt to changes as needed, manipulate objects in flexible manner, and use the skill in a variety of situations. To illustrate the complexity involved in fine motor skills, Box 30.1 provides a task analysis of the components used to taking off one's shirt. Occupational therapy practitioners analyze fine motor skills by observing various upper extremity movements, including reach, release, grasp, in-hand manipulation, and bimanual hand use, that progress in precision as children practice and use them in daily activities (see Chapter 8 for the developmental progressions of fine motor skills and Chapter 9 for evaluation of fine motor skills).

Occupational therapy practitioners consider the "typical" developmental progression as a guideline and not a fixed progression as children progress at different rates. Understanding the factors that may interfere with the child's motor performance requires occupational

**BOX 30.1 Task Analysis of Pulling Off One's Shirt**

**Task:** Pulling one's shirt off
**Materials:** Shirt (pull over).
**Equipment:** May help to have the child sit in a chair
**Requirements:**

- Postural stability: Maintain upright posture (seated and standing)
- Bilateral upper extremity range of motion in shoulders, elbow, wrist, and fingers: to move through the full range to grasp shirt and pull over head
- Bilateral upper extremity shoulder and elbow flexion: shoulder flexion to move upper extremity so hands can grip shirt; elbow flexion and extension required
- Bilateral upper extremity wrist and hand movements: wrist flexion and extension to grasp and release shirt; hand movements of flexion, extension, thumb abduction, and adduction to grasp with thumb and fingers
- Bilateral upper extremity grasp:
    - Grip strength: palmar grip to grasp clothing, hold, and pull
- Cognitive: understand that they must pull shirt overhead (which may take some adjustment of hands); problem-solve when shirt becomes a little tight when neckline goes onto head when pulling it off
- Sequence: complete steps in order (first grasp shirt and then pull off)

**Contexts:** Taking off one's shirt is part of dressing. Children take clothes off before learning to put them on.

**Activity Demands**:

- Posture: sit or stand upright
- Sequence: first grasp, then pull
- Endurance: hands overhead causes exertion; time of this task is short (2–5 seconds) unless child struggles
- Motor: bilateral upper extremity range of motion, strength (to hold position, grasp, and pull up), and coordination (to pull over head and to readjust as needed)
- Sensory: child feels shirt being pulled up and feels when neckline has passed over their head to gauge how much longer to pull
- Cognitive: problem-solving throughout the task on where to position hands, how tightly to grasp, how to adjust as neckline moves onto head; understanding the sequence and what "off" means; communicating for help as needed

Adapted from Jane Clifford O'Brien & Solomon, J. W. (2022). Clinical application: Exercises and worksheets. In Jane Clifford O'Brien & J. Solomon (Eds.), *Occupational analysis and group process* (2nd ed., Worksheet 2.1, p. 207). Elsevier.

therapy practitioners to consider the child's progression, in addition to the child's motor, cognitive, sensory abilities, and their specific situation and experiences. In each of the following areas, growth can be supported by providing developmentally appropriate, playful, and motivating activities to encourage and support greater skill.

**Reaching and Release.** Reaching refers to extending one's arm to grasp objects out of reach, and it may also include bending one's trunk (AOTA, 2020). Reaching for an object requires sensory processing to anticipate and modify the position of the arm and hand based upon the characteristics of the object. A child must coordinate head movements to look at an object and coordinate the eyes and hands together to successfully reach for the object to grasp it (Shumway-Cook & Woollacott, 2017).

Infants reach for rattles, faces, bottles, or toys. At first the reach is inaccurate as they overreach or underreach. Over time, infants become more accurate with their reach using a direct reach. As children gain postural control, they may bend while reaching. They may reach with both arms (bilateral) or with one (unilateral). As children become more skilled at reaching, they may move while reaching (such as when playing a ball game).

Purposeful release follows reflexive release and initially lacks precision. As a child gains more control with posture and the upper extremities, release becomes more precise, allowing a child to place items in a hand or container and eventually to stack objects. Both reach and precise release rely on postural support to stabilize the body, allowing the child to isolate the upper extremity for movement (Shumway-Cook & Woollacott, 2017). Occupational therapy practitioners addressing reach and release may address postural stability through a variety of play activities to strengthen a child's trunk. They may strengthen the upper extremities for reach through repetitive play activities to improve strength and endurance. They may also provide adaptive seating to provide external support or alter positioning to reduce the strength required to reach against gravity.

**Grasping.** Grasping refers to the hand movement whereby a person picks up an object within their palm or between the fingers (AOTA, 2020). When grasping, the hand molds itself based on sensory feedback to match the shape of the object. Table 30.1 illustrates the variety of grasp patterns.

Palmar grasp (also referred to as gross grasp) is one of the earliest grasp patterns; the child uses most of the hand when picking up large objects. The palmar grasp reflex is present at birth (infant flexes fingers when an object is placed in the palm), which progresses to the voluntary palmar grasp. Infants use the palmar grasp to hold rattles, bottles, and toys. Toddlers may use the palmar grasp to initially hold markers, crayons, and spoons.

The hook grasp involves more of the distal portion of the fingers and less of the palm. Children use a hook grasp to carry items with handles, such as suitcases and bags. The cylindrical grasp is used to pick up objects such as cups, pegs, and toys as shown in Fig. 30.1. The **spherical grasp** uses the entire hand and is used to grasp spherical shaped objects, such as a ball. The spherical grasp differs from the palmar grasp (where child holds object in palm), as the child holds the object within their fingers resulting in a wide web space as the thumb abducts to surround the object.

As children develop hand strength, they begin to develop the ability to use their fingers to grasp items. Generally, development occurs proximally to distall—from the ulnar side of the hand to the radial side—and from whole movements to more precise movement. Infants often begin using a raking grasp that involves contacting objects in a raking finger motion with the ulnar side of the hand and moving it to the palm, as may be observed when picking up finger foods. Infants develop lateral grasp or scissors grasp, which is observed as they grasp small objects between their thumb and index finger on the radial side of the hand, which is used to stabilize an object with force (McPhee, 1987; Stival et al., 2019). Toddlers use a radial digital grasp to pick up slightly larger items. Since they do not yet have adequate wrist stability, they approach the object from the side. As wrist and upper extremity stability improves and hand muscles develop, they can approach the item from the top using a three-jaw chuck pattern. The child's web space when using a three-jaw chuck grasp becomes rounded, which is the precursor for grasps on writing utensils and feeding utensils. As wrist stability increases, children use an inferior pincer grasp to pick up small objects with the pads of their fingers, and later they use a superior or neat pincer grasp as the child picks up objects precisely with the tips of their index finger and thumb.

**TABLE 30.1 Common Grasp Patterns**

| Grasp Pattern | Use | Picture |
|---|---|---|
| Palmar | Grasp larger objects or objects that require strength; uses the entire hand | 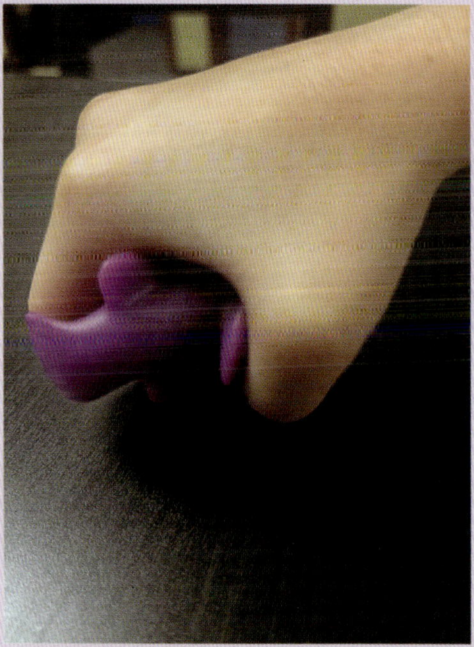 |
| Cylindrical | Grasp cylindrical objects of all sizes | 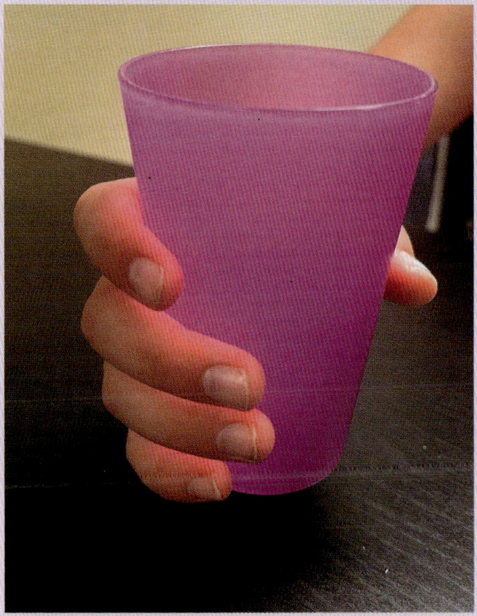 |
| Spherical | Grasp round objects; may consist of all fingers or only the first three fingers | 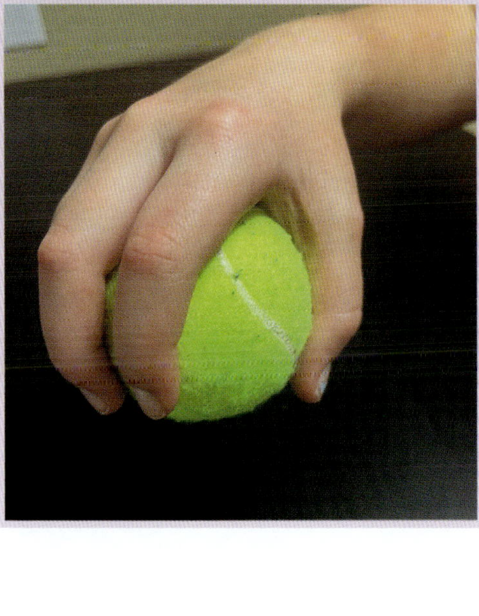 |

**TABLE 30.1 Common Grasp Patterns—cont'd**

| Grasp Pattern | Use | Picture |
|---|---|---|
| Lateral | Grasp with power on a small object | 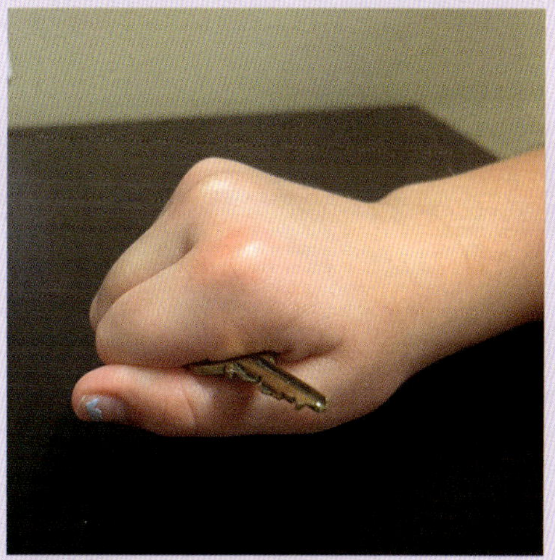 |
| Hook | Carry objects often using a handle | 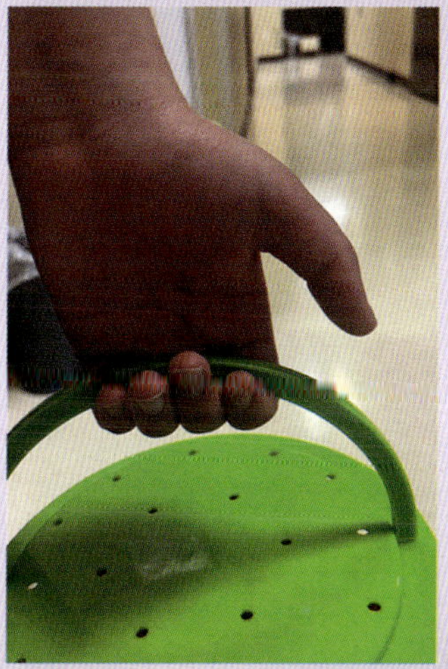 |
| Radial digital | Precursor to three-jaw chuck; approaches items from the side | 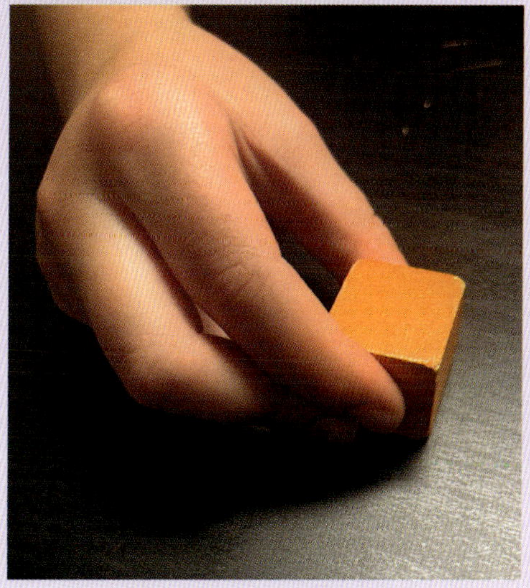 |

*Continued*

**TABLE 30.1 Common Grasp Patterns—cont'd**

| Grasp Pattern | Use | Picture |
|---|---|---|
| Three-jaw chuck | Grasp smaller objects that require precision such as blocks or a pencil | 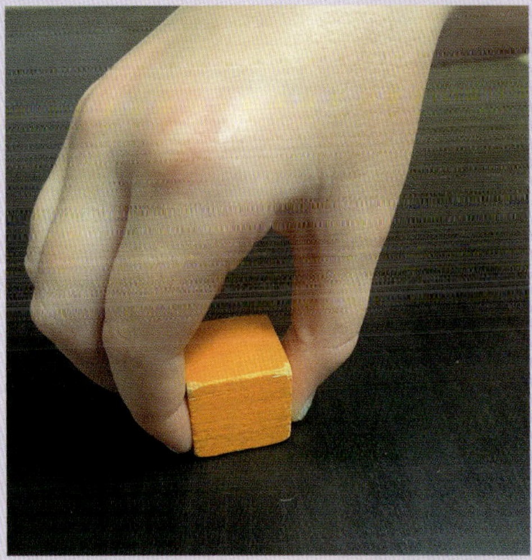 |
| Inferior pincer | Pick up small objects; uses pad of finger and thumb; develops prior to superior pincer | 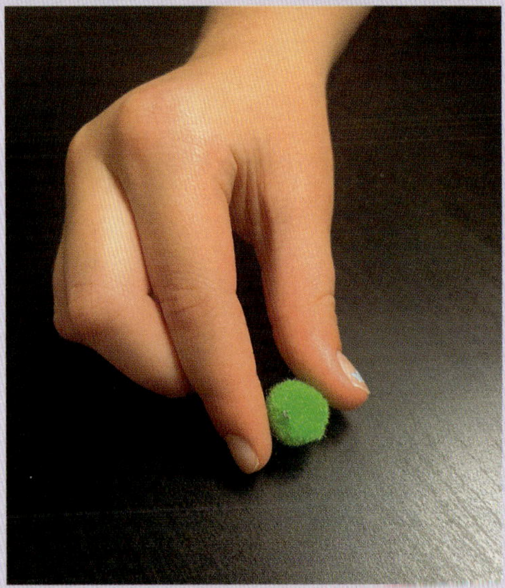 |
| Superior pincer | Pick up small objects with high levels of precision | 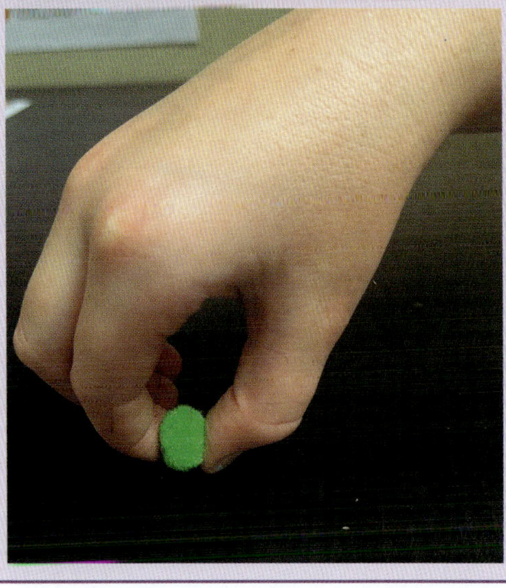 |

Adapted from McPhee, S. D. (1987). Functional hand evaluations: A review. *American Journal of Occupational Therapy*, *41*(3), 158–163. https://doi.org/10.5014/ajot.41.3.158; and Stival, F., Michieletto, S., Cognolato, M, Enrico, P., Muller, H., & Atzori, M. (2019). A quantitative taxonomy of human grasp. *Journal of NeuroEngineering and Rehabilitation*, *16*(1). https://doi.org/10.1186/s12984-019-0488-x.

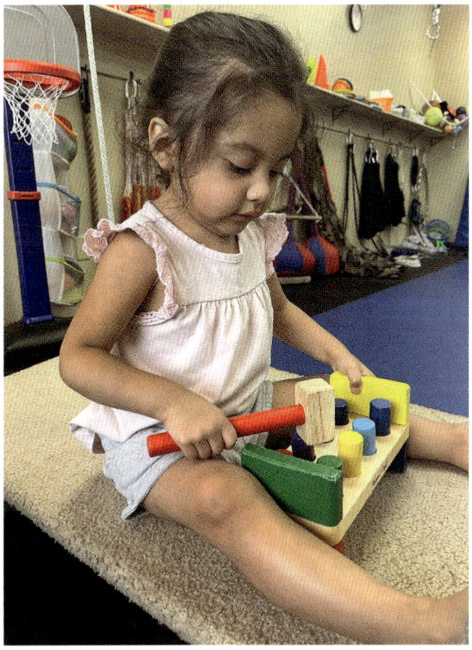

**Fig. 30.1** A child uses a cylindrical grasp to hold a tool during play.

**In-Hand Manipulation.** In-hand manipulation refers to the ability to manipulate and reposition small objects in one hand, using only the one hand. There are three main categories of in-hand manipulation skills: translation, shift, and rotation. ***Translation*** refers to the movement of objects from the palm to the finger or from the finger to the palm. For example, a child may move a piece of food placed in their palm to their fingertips to put in their mouth. Translation is also observed as a child moves a coin placed in their palm to their fingertips to place in a vending machine. ***Shift*** refers to the linear movement of an object, such as when repositioning one's hand on a pencil or pushing a cap off a marker while holding the marker with the same hand. ***Rotation*** involves flipping an item end over end or moving an object between the fingertips. For example, rotational movements are used when spinning a top, flipping a pencil, and holding a key ring to rotate one key for placement in the lock.

Additional skills that develop at approximately the same time as these three in-hand manipulation skills include separation of the sides of the hand and open web space. Although these are not specifically in-hand manipulation skills, as an object is not being manipulated or repositioned within the hand, they are also important for fine motor function, and they allow fine motor precision. **Separation of the sides of the hand** occurs when the radial side of the hand is engaged in precision fine motor skill while the ulnar side of the hand stabilizes in flexion. The radial side is generally the skilled side, and the ulnar side promotes stability or holding. The ulnar side of the hand stabilizes while the radial side performs grasp and manipulation. A child uses an **open web space** to make the rounded "OK" sign with the fingers. Being able to pinch small objects with force, without the thumb and index fingers joints collapsing under the strain, allows children to perform activities such as snapping their pants closed. Occupational therapy practitioners create activities so children may develop both sides of the hand and an open web space.

**Finger isolation**, the ability to use either one finger independently, such as for pointing with the index finger or pushing a button with the index or the thumb, is another important step in the fine motor progression. This skill develops earlier than the other in-hand manipulation skills but is often observed with them during play in the preschool years. Table 30.2 provides examples of activities to address each type of in-hand manipulation skill, and Table 30.3 provides examples of activities to address finger isolation, separation of the sides of the hands and development of open web space.

**TABLE 30.2 Activities to Address In-Hand Manipulation Skills**

| Manipulation Skill | Activities |
|---|---|
| Translation: palm to finger | • Moving small objects such as pegs, coins, chips individually from palm to fingers before placing in board or container<br>• Placing a magnetic chip on a wand by moving the chip from palm to finger<br>• Moving one coin from palm to fingertip to place it in coin bank<br>• Moving finger food from palm to fingertip to place in mouth<br>• Moving string to fingertips when lacing beads |
| Translation: finger to palm | • Crumpling paper<br>• Getting a coin or chip out of a container with fingertips and then moving it to hold in the hand<br>• Picking up a piece of food to hold in hand<br>• Taking a peg out of a peg board and holding it in the hand<br>• Picking up dice and moving to palm |
| Translation with stabilization | • Taking a peg out of a peg board and holding it in the hand and then getting another with the fingers while still holding the first<br>• Pulling magnetic chips from a wand by moving the chip from finger to palm, and then getting another while holding the first<br>• Playing jacks<br>• Putting coins into a piggy bank if holding some in the palm while doing so |
| Shift | • Turning pages of a book<br>• Repositioning a pencil by sliding fingers up or down the shaft<br>• Counting paper money<br>• Sorting cards<br>• Manipulating paper during cutting tasks<br>• Moving a sandwich or cookie during eating |
| Shift with stabilization | • Pushing the cap off a marker while holding the marker with the same hand<br>• Holding fabric while buttoning/snapping |
| Simple rotation | • Opening a water bottle<br>• Screwing and unscrewing nuts and bolts<br>• Removing and putting on a lid of a jar<br>• Rotating a puzzle piece before placing it in an insert puzzle<br>• Spinning a top |
| Complex rotation | • Flipping a pencil to write and erase<br>• Turning cubes to see each side<br>• Flipping a paper clip with fingers |
| Rotation with stabilization | • Holding key ring with keys to rotate one key for placement in the lock |

**TABLE 30.3 Activities to Address Additional Fine Motor Skills**

| Skills | Activities |
|---|---|
| Finger isolation | • Poking holes in pegboards<br>• Finger painting<br>• Fingerprint stamping<br>• Finger puppets<br>• I spy by pointing to objects<br>• Keypad games, toy cash register, calculator, keyboard<br>• Poking holes in playdough<br>• Finger spelling with American Sign Language |
| Separation of the sides of the hand | • Spinning a top<br>• Stringing beads with lace<br>• Cutting with scissors<br>• Writing or coloring with a tripod grasp |
| Open web space | • Pinching clothespins to hang toy clothing on a line<br>• Pinching knobs on toys<br>• Snapping clothing closed<br>• Pinching playdough or clay<br>• Closing Ziploc bags<br>• Picking up blocks or dominos using thumb and index finger<br>• Buttoning<br>• Making small balls of playdough<br>• Lacing cards |

Young children engage in activities using in-hand manipulation in play. For example, picking up and placing a small peg in a pegboard requires translation, and repositioning a puzzle piece often requires rotation. With practice, in-hand manipulation skills become automatic as youth complete daily living tasks such as buttoning, handling change, playing with small toys and objects, and using classroom tools. When there are difficulties with in-hand manipulation, children often must use two hands for a motor task rather than one, or they will use a surface, such as the table or their own trunk, to reposition an object in the hand. They may need to use assistive devices to complete daily tasks, such as buttoning, dressing, cutting, handwriting, or opening doors.

Precise and accurate in-hand manipulation requires motor planning and somatosensory processing (i.e., the ability to process tactile and proprioceptive sensory input). To reposition objects in the hand, the child must feel where in the hand the object is and how the fingers are moving the object. Sometimes children with poor in-hand manipulation skills have poor sensory processing. They may drop objects frequently or have difficulty using objects without relying on their visual skills to compensate.

Occupational therapy practitioners design intervention to support skill development through repetitive meaningful and playful practice, compensation (e.g., teaching child how to complete task more easily in a different way), or adaptation (e.g., providing assistive device so child does not have to use fine motor skills to complete task). Oftentimes, occupational therapy intervention uses skill training, compensation, and adaptations strategies together.

Occupational therapy practitioners create intervention activities to promote each of these areas by engaging children in fun and repetitive activities, such as crumpling paper for indoor "snowball fights," playing a game of jacks, or feeding a puppet monster pom-pom food (to address translation); counting play money or playing or sorting cards (to address shift); and winding up small toys, spinning tops, or removing and putting on jar lids (to address rotation). They create activities that the child finds meaningful.

Occupational therapy intervention is designed to allow the child to repeat skills in meaningful ways while engaging in a desired occupation. For example, a child engages in play that involves completing activities whereby they repeatedly use intrinsic muscles of the hand to manipulate objects leading to improved visual-motor integration, hand skill, processing, attention, cognition, and resulting in neuroplasticity. Case Example 30.1 provides an example of a client-centered occupation-based intervention session to address in-hand manipulation skills (translation, shift, and rotation).

**CASE EXAMPLE 30.1 CREATING AN OCCUPATION-BASED CLIENT-CENTERED INTERVENTION TO ADDRESS FINE MOTOR CHALLENGES**

Ezra is a 10-year-old boy with dyspraxia and learning disability. He has difficulties with in-hand manipulation skills that he needs to perform many school-related tasks. Ezra does not like to work on his handwriting and becomes easily frustrated. However, Ezra enjoys simple magic tricks. The occupational therapy practitioner created a session based on the child's interest in "magic." The practitioner demonstrated some fun "tricks" to the child that involve in-hand manipulation skills. The tricks involved movements such as moving a coin from fingertips to palm (translation), sorting cards (shift), and spinning a top (rotation).

The practitioner began with simple tricks and proceeded to more challenging ones during the session. After repeatedly practicing the card tricks, the child created a "demonstration" by ordering the tricks and presenting it to his brother and sister. The occupational therapy practitioner ended the session by asking the child to select a new "trick" to learn and present to his family over the week. Ezra was proud of his performance and stated that he will bring in his magic hat next week to show the practitioner.

**Bimanual Hand Use.** Bimanual hand use or **bilateral coordination** involves using both hands together. Infants bring hands to midline to grasp toys or bottles and to engage in imitation play such as clapping hands. Children grasp objects with two hands and bang them together, first symmetrically and then in an alternating pattern. Banging encourages differentiation of the upper extremities as the hands bang at different times or one hand may hold an object to bang while the other remains stationary. The baby is pleased with the success of banging and begins to bang items together at midline. Transferring objects (which develops by 9 months of age) from one hand to another is a building block for hand preference and bilateral tasks (CDC, 2022).

Midline crossing allows a child to reach across midline to grasp an object placed on the other side. This leads to specialization of one hand versus another. When a child has a hand preference, they reach across the midline of the body to grasp a tool for use with the preferred hand. The dominant hand performs the skilled movement, while the alternate hand provides stability or support. The child's preferred hand can be identified when observing them play with one-handed manipulatives, such as tops and windup toys, or use tools including crayons, toothbrush, and feeding utensils. By the age of 4–6 years of age, most children recognize their preferred hand (Sacrey et al., 2012). As children reach school age, they develop a preferred foot, eye, and ear to match the preferred hand in the development of laterality.

Rotational movement patterns in the first few years of life facilitate the development of midline crossing. For example, babies reach across the midline to prop in sitting and then rotate from sitting into quadruped, crossing the midline of the body. When a child does not cross midline, they pick up an object on the left with the left hand and an object on the right with the right hand, thus interfering with specialization of hand use.

## FACTORS INFLUENCING FINE MOTOR SKILLS

### Diagnosis or Condition

Children with a variety of pediatric conditions (e.g., cerebral palsy, Down syndrome, spina bifida, brachial palsy, congenital anomalies) may have atypical fine motor development. Similarly, children who have experienced physical or neurological trauma (e.g., burns, fractures, injuries, stroke, or brain injury) will likely also demonstrate altered fine motor performance. Occupational therapy practitioners do not treat conditions. However, they use knowledge of the child's condition as one of the factors that may influence their fine motor skills.

### Proximal Stability

Proximal stability at the trunk, shoulder, and elbow is necessary for developing hand skills for manipulation and grasping (Naider-Steinhart & Katz-Leurer, 2007; Wang et al., 2011). Adequate postural control allows for the body to maintain positions so that children can use their extremities. A stable trunk allows the extremity to move in isolation without losing stability of the rest of the body (Shumway-Cook & Woollacott, 2017). Children must have a stable shoulder girdle and adequate scapular stability and mobility to move the arm through space to retrieve, grasp, and manipulate objects (Colangelo & Shea, 2020).

A child with poor trunk control may use their upper extremities to support them in an upright position such as observed when infants prop themselves in sitting, interfering with the child's ability to use their hands for play, self-care, and object manipulation. Therefore, children who have poor trunk control may have difficulty with upper extremity movement as they try to maintain an upright position. Lack of trunk stability may result in limited upper extremity range of motion interfering with fine motor development.

Children can develop strength in the shoulder girdle through weight bearing on the upper extremities, such as when in quadruped position. Weight bearing with open hands also helps to develop intrinsic muscles that form the palmar arches and are necessary for in-hand manipulation skills. Providing children with opportunities to hold positions such as coloring and drawing in a prone position promotes shoulder stability for hand skills. Occupational therapy practitioners address postural strength in children through gross motor activities, or seating systems that provide needed support, so the child can use their extremities. For example, the practitioner may provide additional support to the child's high chair. A variety of adaptive seats exist to support children, so they can use their hands more effectively (such as a corner seat).

**Wrist Stability.** Developing stability at the wrist provides a foundation for writing and fine motor skills. Slight wrist extension is beneficial for writing and cutting and many precise fine motor tasks. Weakness in the wrist or an inability to hold the wrist stable can make manipulation of objects with the hands and fingers much more difficult. The elbow and wrist provide the stability required for the isolated movements of the interphalangeal joints of the fingers.

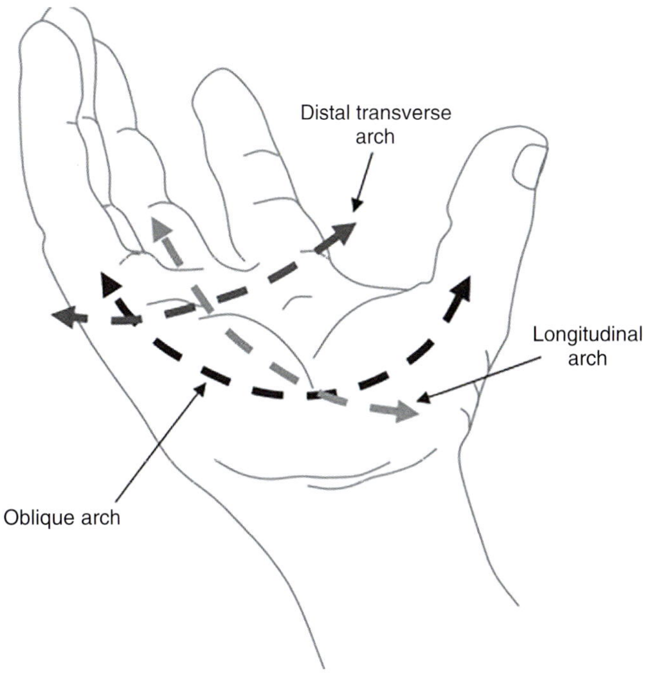


**Fig. 30.2** The three palmar arches of the hand support fine motor skills.

**TABLE 30.4 Motor Stability Activities for Children**

| Motor Function | Activity |
|---|---|
| Motor stability | • Mirrors and windows with shaving cream or dry erase markers<br>• Art easels<br>• Spraying mirrors and windows with spray bottle and wiping clean<br>• Taping paper to wall for drawing and coloring<br>• Painting on wall or large paper on a wall<br>• Vertical activities, such as slanted writing board, using three-ring binder to provide slanted surface |
| Wrist extension | • Painting/drawing on vertical surfaces<br>• Playing with Lite-Brite<br>• Shaving cream on a mirror or window<br>• Shaking rattles<br>• Batting a balloon with hand or racket<br>• Stringing beads<br>• Playing with Lego or Duplo |
| Palmar arches | • Hold many pegs, coins, or chips in the palm of the hand<br>• Manipulating dice<br>• Squeezing or moving stress balls in hand<br>• Holding and moving tennis ball in hand |

**Arches.** The intrinsic muscles of the hand form the arches that are used to grasp objects. Children who have underdeveloped or flat arches may display fine motor challenges. Typically, this is noted as an inability to bring the fingers together to grasp with all the fingertips and thumb. For example, to open a jar lid, you must get all the fingers and the thumb on the lid to turn it. To get into that position, the palm of the hand forms arches (Fig. 30.2). Table 30.4 provides examples of activities that can be used to address motor stability, wrist extension, and palmar arches.

**TABLE 30.5 Creative Theraputty Activities to Promote Hand Strength**

| Activity | Description |
|---|---|
| Treasure hunt | Hide small items such as pennies or pretend jewels in putty; pull the putty apart to find the items and place them in a container |
| Ice tray | Put putty into an ice tray with an item inside; pull the item out of the putty |
| Shapes and letter | Roll out putty into a snake; use it to shape into letters and shapes |
| Snake spikes | Roll out the putty into a snake; use fingers to pinch the putty to make "spikes" on the snakes back |
| Making cookies | Use hands to press the putty flat; use a rolling pin to make it flatter, press cookie cutters in the putty to make cookies |
| Cover the container | Put a lid on a plastic container; spread the putty over the container to cover it using fingers |
| Ziploc bag search | Place putty in Ziploc bag with small items; spread the putty in the bag to find the different items |
| Snowman | Pull the putty apart into approximately 1- to 2-inch sizes; roll them into a ball using the fingertips; stack them into snowmen or other shapes |
| Ice cream making | Roll the putty into a cylinder; hold with one hand and use the fingertips of the other hand to twist up into an ice cream cone |

## Strength and Endurance

A certain level of hand strength is required to hold and manipulate objects, such as opening a bottle, maintaining a sustained grip on an object, or squeezing a toy. When examining muscle strength for fine motor performance, the occupational therapy practitioner examines proximal (trunk, shoulder, and wrist) and distal (grasp and pinch) strength. If weakness is the issue, then improving a child's grip strength can allow them to hold toys more effectively, use a mature grasp on a crayon, or use a spoon to feed themselves. Improving pinch strength may encourage independence with snapping jeans closed.

Occupational therapy practitioners address hand strength in creative, repetitive, and meaningful activities that challenge the child to complete more repetitions with greater force to a point a fatigue (Rybski, 2012). Occupational therapy practitioners integrate strength training activities in play. For example, they may engage children in games to pick up more objects, squeeze items that get progressively more challenging, or engage in weight-bearing activities, such as crawling along an obstacle path that requires them to go further each time. Occupational therapy practitioners may focus on overall grip strength or focus on specific muscles, such as developing strength on the radial or ulnar side of the hand. By changing the position of the item, the therapist can address different muscles of the hand. Table 30.5 provides examples of creative hand strengthening activities using Theraputty.

Children develop fine motor endurance through repeated movements or extended holding of positions. Muscle endurance refers to the amount of time the child engages in the movement before fatiguing. In clinical practice, children who exhibit poor fine motor endurance may stop the activity, wring out their hands, or avoid engaging in the activity all together. Occupational therapy practitioners create fun, novel activities to engage children in interesting and challenging activities for a longer time. See Case Example 30.2, Cassidy, for an example of building endurance.

**CASE EXAMPLE 30.2 CASSIDY**

An occupational therapy student created a fine motor project to work on intrinsic muscle endurance for 9-year-old Cassidy who loved basketball. The session required Cassidy to build a "catapult" craft with elastic and Popsicle sticks and a small basketball that she could propel into the "hoop." Cassidy enjoyed the activity and invested in completing it within the session time. The occupational therapy student provided written directions and a sample of the end project, cued Cassidy as needed, and provided verbal encouragement. Cassidy engaged in 45 minutes of fine motor activity, reflected on her performance, and asked for additional activities like this to do at home. The student practitioner and Cassidy enjoyed the "competition" of propelling the ball into the hoop. This activity required repetitive in-hand manipulation skills with resistance to build strength and required attention, visual-motor integration, and endurance. See below for picture of the completed project. Here are the directions to build the catapult activity.

**Instructions** for the catapult activity:

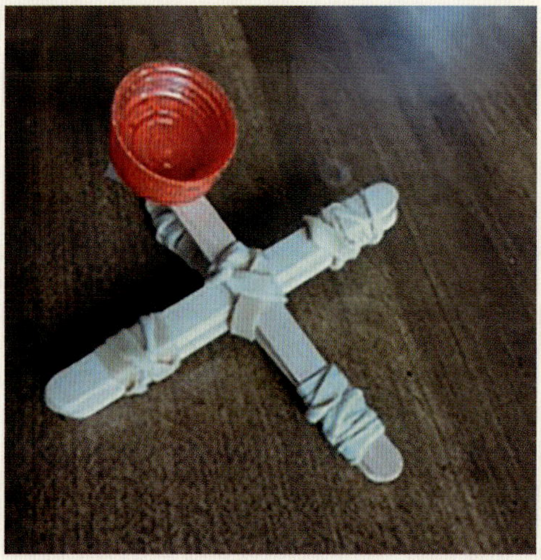

Simple craft stick catapult.

- Stack five craft sticks together and wrap a rubber band around each end.
- Stack two craft sticks and wrap a rubber band around only one end.
- Slide the five sticks in between the two sticks, as shown.
- Wrap a rubber band where the two sections meet to hold the catapult together.
- Attach a bottle cap to the top stick to hold the projectile.
- Place a projectile (mini-marshmallow, small ball of paper, etc.) in the cap, hold the stick down, and release!

*Source:* Retrieved from https://kids.discoveryplace.org/huntersville/stay-at-home-science/diy-catapult

## Visual-Motor Integration

**Visual-motor integration** refers to the ability to make sense of what you see to complete a motor response (e.g., copy, draw or write, stack blocks, string beads). Visual-motor integration is the integration of visual perception and motor skill, and it is an essential feature of many fine motor tasks and written communication. Visual perception requires the child develop spatial awareness (where things are in relation to other objects), figure ground (ability to identify objects in foreground from background), and visual closure (ability to identify what the object or picture is when you do not see the whole). Written communication (i.e., reproducing letters and numbers) requires children to integrate vision (e.g., acuity, awareness), visual memory, and visual perception with motor actions. Figs. 30.3 and 30.4 show children using simple visual-motor skills in play.

Visual-motor integration develops as children develop an awareness of themselves and the properties of objects as they engage in play activities, such as sorting shapes, identifying colors, and understanding

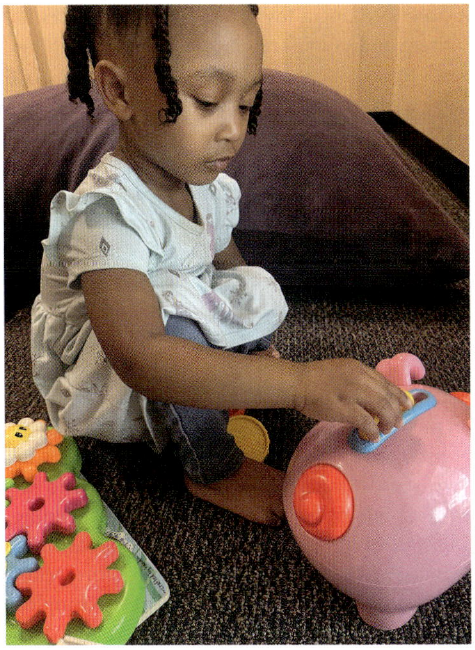

Fig. 30.3 A child uses visual perceptual skills (i.e., knowledge of figure ground, directionality) and in-hand manipulation skills as they move the "coin" to place it in the piggy bank.

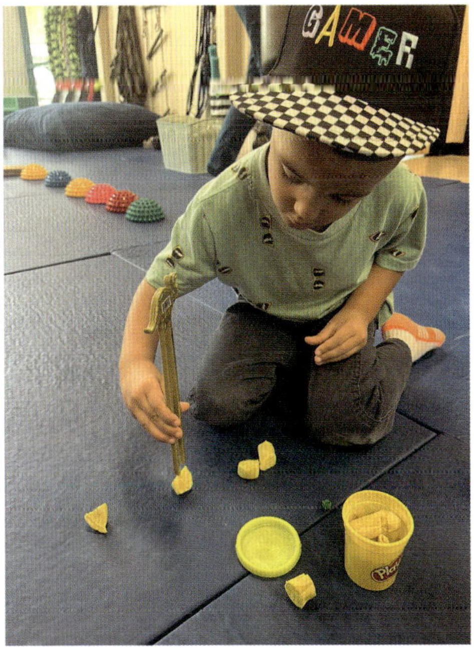


Fig. 30.4 Using tongs to pick up and place small objects is fun and requires visual-motor integration along with postural stability and hand strength. This activity may be adapted to address tripod grasp of a tool and separation of the sides of the hand.

how objects are used. For example, infants (around 1 year of age) begin to realize that objects that are out of sight still exist (i.e., object permanence). As children develop cognition, they realize that objects may be large or small, have different shapes, and have different purposes. They learn how to engage with objects, such as throwing a ball, shaking a rattle, or placing a block in the container. They learn directional concepts (on, above, over, in, under, and around) through gross motor play, which informs fine motor skills. Together, children integrate sensory (visual, touch, and kinesthesia), cognitive, and motor actions to engage

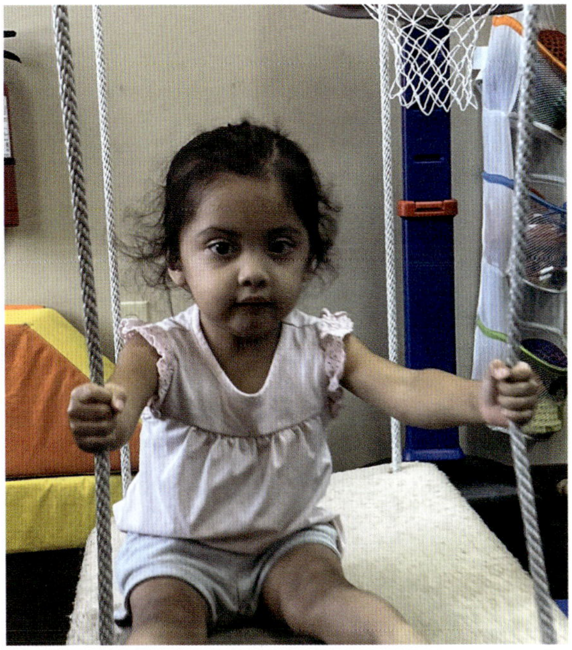

Fig. 30.5 A child responds to sensory changes when playing. For example, the child experiences changes in movement and body position while holding onto the swing (tactile and proprioception inputs) and adjusts to maintain upright posture (vestibular).

in fine motor movements with tools (such as pencils, keyboard, and clothing) to communicate, play, and engage in self-care.

## Sensory Integration

**Sensory integration** is necessary for accurate movement. Children make sense of sensory information from multiple senses at once and use it to act upon the environment effectively (Roley et al., 2020). For example, they visually see objects while processing vestibular and proprioceptive information to remain upright against gravity. They use sensation to accurately move their extremity to grasp an object and to engage the grasp with the correct amount of force. They make sense of what they see (visual perception) to form the movement. They contact the object and use tactile input to manipulate it. A child learns about the features of an object through stereognosis (i.e., the ability to recognize an item through touch), which develops when a child manipulates objects in the hand (Reed & Ziat, 2018). As children engage in activities, their sensory processing improves as the result of neuroplasticity. Fig. 30.5 shows a young child processing vestibular, proprioceptive, and tactile input as she swings and uses bilateral upper extremities to move herself.

Children use tactile and proprioceptive awareness when they manipulate small items and identify and learn about the features of objects. The hands have many tactile receptors necessary for refined fine motor movements. **Tactile perception** provides information about the shape, size, weight, and texture of an object, which is used to identify the object and provide information to motor centers of the brain as to what the hands should do to grasp, release, or manipulate the object. Children learn about objects through tactile exploration. **Stereognosis** (or haptic perception) is the ability to recognize an item through touch. It involves the use of somatosensory feedback and manipulation skills. Tactile play allows children to explore their environment and increase imagination and creativity (Howie, 2016). **Proprioceptive processing** is essential for grading the force of movements, including grasp and manipulation. When a child has difficulties in proprioceptive processing, they may grasp an object with increased force. They may also grasp

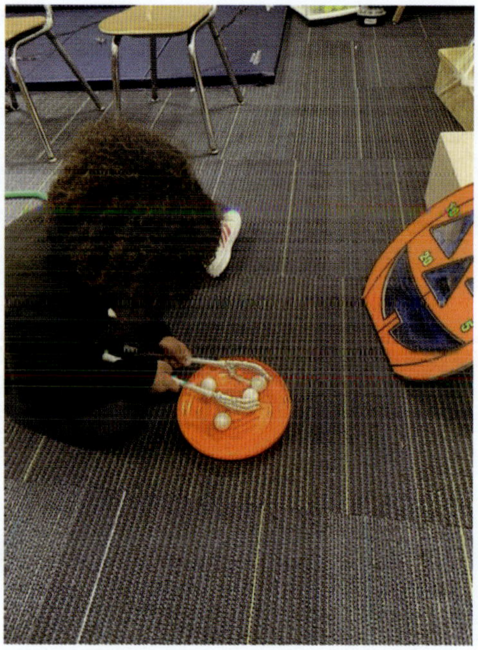

**Fig. 30.6** This child is motor planning as she attempts this novel activity for Halloween. She understands the idea is to lift the small ball with the skeleton hands. She must create a motor plan to do so and then implement it. Success with getting the balls into the pumpkin mouth depends on her ability to both formulate and implement a plan that can work. (*Source:* Photo courtesy of Angela N.)

the object so loosely that the items fall out of their hand. Providing resistance to the muscles and joints of the hand stimulates proprioception to allow the child to sense their position in space, leading to body awareness. Weighted objects may provide stimulation to the Golgi tendon organs to stimulate proprioception, allowing children to become more aware of their position in space for fine motor manipulations. Children rely on adequate tactile and proprioceptive processing to complete fine motor manipulation of objects (Seminara et al., 2019).

## Praxis

**Praxis** or motor planning refers to the ability to conceive of, plan, and execute a novel movement (Roley et al., 2020). Fine motor movements are complex and involve the manipulation and use of tools. For example, a child sees a spoon and creates a plan to use it to scoop their food. This involves understanding how one moves (kinesthesia) and acts upon the environment. Therefore, children have a sense of their bodies and how they act to accomplish movements. Motor planning also requires the child to understand objects and their uses.

Children with motor planning difficulties affecting fine motor skills may not intuitively or internally realize how their body works, the purpose of objects, and may have difficulty executing a motor plan (See Fig. 30.6). Occupational therapy practitioners working on motor planning for fine motor skills provide children with opportunities to practice the occupation within their natural environment. They provide verbal and demonstrative cues and engage the child in multiple repetitions. They may adjust the expectations or sequence of movements, so the child is successful. When promoting motor planning, practitioners allow children to problem solve and reflect upon their actions.

## Cognition

Fine motor skills progress as the child figures things out, such as how hitting a button turns on music, opening a box reveals a hidden surprise, or how inserting a toy into a container makes it "go away." Infants, children, and youth are curious about how things work and use their hands to make sense of things (Duncan et al., 2020). As skills progress, they require cognition to sequence steps, problem solve how to manipulate things, and carry out the actions. Along with motor skills, effective fine motor performance requires cognitive skills that include discrimination or naming an object, memory, processing, perception, and attention to details. Children associate the object or movement with past experiences, which allows them to reproduce the action. For example, a toddler may visually see a hat and cognitively process that by naming it and associating it with something that goes on one's head. The child reaches for the hat with the understanding that they will put it on their head and knowing where the top of their head is (directionality) as well as knowing that the open side of the hat must be placed on their head (so that hat fits). This requires body awareness and perhaps problem-solving if something goes wrong. Children combine cognitive, sensory, and motor skills when engaged in fine motor tasks related to handwriting, dressing, grooming, building toy structures, playing, and eating. Occupational therapy practitioners analyze the components of each task to identify areas for intervention with the understanding that children learn best when they complete the entire activity (such as putting the hat on) within their natural environment.

## Environment

Environmental factors include "aspects of the physical, social, and attitudinal surroundings" in which children live (AOTA, 2020, p. 76). Occupational therapy practitioners examine the physical setting to understand how it influences a child's fine motor performance. They consider the location and types of toys available and the child's physical needs. They determine the accessibility requirements, safety, and type of materials available to the child. For example, they consider if the space provided allows the child to access toys to manipulate. They examine the child's positioning to support fine motor development. For example, a child with poor upper extremity control may require an adapted seat to support their trunk, so they can use their hands for play. Children may require adapted toys to manipulate successfully.

Children enjoy engaging in social activities that can also promote fine motor skills, such as playing games opening and closing one's hands (such as peek-a-boo), and taking turns placing objects in one's palm with positive social responses by an adult may promote skills. Promoting positive social environments supports children's development. Occupational therapy practitioners use knowledge of social support (e.g., caregivers, parents, siblings, peers) to support children and youth. They also identify social barriers, such as accessibility issues, or limited knowledge of how to promote skill development or engage in play with a child. They may create home programs to promote engagement in fun games to support children.

Attitudinal factors may include other people's beliefs in the child's progress or potential. Political attitudes or policies may limit the resources available to children and their families. Occupational therapy practitioners promote positive attitudes and work with children, families, and society to understand each child's unique contributions. They pay attention to attitudes that may interfere with the child's achievements and advocate for children and families. For example, they may encourage others to see the child's strengths, engage in creative programming, advocate for services, and address attitudes that interfere with the child's goals. Occupational therapy practitioners view the entire landscape (child, occupation, and environment) when creating intervention plans to address fine motor performance. Providing occupation-based interventions promotes occupational performance.

## FINE MOTOR INTERVENTION: BODY FUNCTION VERSUS OCCUPATION BASED

Occupational therapy intervention is designed to empower children to develop their skills and abilities, so they can do those things they want and need to do. Fine motor activities are important for children, and children spend at least 37%–60% of the school day engaged in fine motor activities (Caramia et al., 2020). Occupational therapy practitioners address the motor, sensory, and cognitive factors influencing fine motor skills, the child's unique strengths and challenges, environmental supports and barriers, and desired occupations. They engage children in fine motor interventions that target (1) underlying capacities or foundational skills (such as strength, postural control, balance, and stability); (2) practice of small movements of the hand, fingers, wrists; and (3) activity-based interventions whereby children engage in handwriting, self-care (such as dressing, feeding, and hygiene), and play (Alaniz et al., 2015; Eddy et al., 2019; Grajo et al., 2020).

There is evidence that intervention focusing on developing underlying capacities (such as strength, coordination, grasp, and release) improves skills (Alaniz et al., 2015; Axford et al., 2018; Eddy et al., 2019; Mano et al., 2020). However, more research is required to examine how these capacities affect occupational performance (Alaniz et al., 2015; Eddy et al., 2019; Schneider et al., 2019). Alaniz et al. (2015) found that grip and pinch strength correlated with independence in functional activities for children with and without autism, although grip strength did not change handwriting legibility in children with autism. Prunty et al. (2020) did not find that grip strength and pen pressure contributed to the handwriting difficulties in children with developmental coordination disorder, suggesting underlying motor processes (such as cognitive motor planning) may be affecting performance. Several studies suggest interventions should not focus solely on grasp, release, or strength but on activity-based therapeutic interventions (Alhusaini et al., 2016; Grajo et al., 2020; Prunty et al., 2020).

Strong evidence supports therapeutic practice over sensorimotor activities to improve handwriting legibility (Grajo et al., 2020). Sensorimotor approaches include activities to address visual perception, kinesthesia, in-hand manipulation, visual-motor integration, and biomechanical features of handwriting (Grajo et al., 2020). Sensorimotor approaches engage children in activities to address underlying capacities (e.g., visual perception, kinesthesia) but do not directly target the child's occupational performance (i.e., handwriting, dressing, grooming). Therapeutic practice for handwriting includes paper and pencil activities with an emphasis on self evaluation techniques and the provision of performance feedback (Denton et al., 2006). Occupational therapy practitioners engage children in therapeutic practice whereby they tailor intervention to match the child's specific needs, engage the child in activities at their level, and challenge children sufficiently. Grajo et al. (2020) found strong evidence to support activity-based intervention in schools for handwriting intervention.

Practitioners plan interventions that are based on the unique strengths and challenges of children within their environments and culture. They create goals to address how the child uses fine motor skills in their daily occupations. They establish meaningful goals with children. Case Example 30.3, Ty, provides examples of occupation-based fine motor goals.

Research is needed to determine the appropriate dosage, intensity, and efficacy of interventions (Eddy et al., 2019). Dosage refers to the length of the intervention, such as longer sessions in a short amount of time versus short sessions over a longer period. Jackman et al. (2020) conducted a systematic review to determine the threshold dose of upper limb training for children with cerebral palsy and reported that children need to practice goals for more than 14–35 hours (face to face and home practice) to improve upper limb function. They found that interventions that do not set functional goals that involve actual practice of those goals needed more than 30–40 hours.

### CASE EXAMPLE 30.3 TY'S DRESSING GOALS

Ty is a 7-year-old boy with limited right upper extremity use resulting from a traumatic brain injury from a snowmobiling accident 3 months ago. This is interfering with his ability to use both hands together for activities of daily living (dressing, feeding, and grooming) and school (handwriting, sports, and carrying his backpack). The occupational therapist collaborated with Ty who would like to "dress himself for school." The therapist determined that his inability to use both hands together interfered with his success. The therapist created the following goals.

**Long-term goal:** Ty will dress himself for school within 20 minutes 5 days a week.

**Short-term goal:** Ty will use his right upper extremity as an assist in three out of five opportunities during therapy sessions.

During the therapy session, the therapist engaged Ty in bilateral manipulation activities through a variety of play activities and eventually worked on playing dress-up games to reach his long-term goal of timed dressing at home. The therapist also demonstrated some one-handed techniques to save time while dressing. Together, they played games of how fast they could put things into a bag holding with one hand and putting things in with the other hand. The therapist provided cues as needed, encouragement, and graded the activities to be challenging but not impossible for him to achieve.

Children can engage in motor training safely if they are supervised and do so with proper intensity (Stricker et al., 2020). Intensity refers to the degree of difficulty or number of repetitions of movement provided during the sessions. Research in sports performance literature suggests that high-intensity interventions (i.e., frequent repetitions in a short time) produce greater motor results in healthy populations (Atakan et al., 2021). Thus, occupational therapy practitioners seek to safely and carefully provide high-dosage and -intensity activity-based interventions to target fine motor performance in children and youth. Engaging children in activities that they repeat as part of their typical routine provides more practice, such as providing them with activities they use in school, home, or during play.

Since play is the primary role of children, engaging children in play situations that require them to develop their hand skills is an effective intervention approach. For example, children may be more apt to try novel activities that are playful. They may be motivated to put on a vest of their favorite character. Painting their own cardboard "playhouse" may be motivating and challenging while encouraging bilateral hand use and shoulder flexion/extension over time (thereby promoting strength, range of motion, and endurance). Occupational therapy practitioners engage children in fine motor skills during play, education, leisure, activities of daily living (such as self-care, hygiene, dressing, grooming), and social participation. Table 30.6 provides examples of how an occupational therapy practitioner may address fine motor challenges in children and youth when using principles from selected frames of reference.

There is evidence that occupational therapy fine motor programs improve hand skills in young children compared to general fine motor as addressed in regular preschool and play situations (Lust & Donica., 2011; Ohl et al., 2013). For children, participation in occupations improves with therapeutic practice in tasks that are intentionally focused on the child's goals (Cahill & Beisbier, 2020). Addressing fine motor skills with goal-directed, evidence-based interventions grounded in theory is an essential part of enhancing participation of children with fine motor

**TABLE 30.6 Frames of Reference for Occupational Therapy Intervention to Address Fine Motor Skills**

| Frame of References | Principles | Description | Sample Activities |
|---|---|---|---|
| Developmental (see Chapter 8) | Children learn fine motor skills in a sequence.<br>They may experience a gap in their progression due to client factors (sensory, motor, cognitive), environment, or that occupational therapy practitioners can address (Howe et al., 2020; Llorens, 1982). | The progression of motor skills serves as a foundation for fine motor intervention. Progression generally follows:<br>• Gross to fine<br>• Proximal to distal<br>• Head to toe<br>• Unimanual to bimanual<br>• Simple to complex | Address fine motor skills for occupational performance<br>• Play-based activities, such as grasp rattle and catch ball.<br>• Self-care activities, such as bring spoon to mouth, wash face, put on clothing, button, and zip.<br>• Provide adaptive equipment, so child can engage in developmental activity (such as built-up handle). |
| Biomechanical (see Chapter 33) | Range of motion, strength, endurance, and pain interfere with child's fine motor skill performance leading to challenges in engaging in desired occupations. | Address strength, range of motion, endurance, and pain.<br>• Range of motion: Apply knowledge of kinesiology to support child's movement.<br>• Strength: Repetitions of movement with more weights leads to muscle strength.<br>• Endurance: Increase the time the child engages in the task (endurance).<br>• Pain: Address issues of pain before movement. | Provide postural support (such as supportive chair, positioning) for hand skills.<br>• Range of motion: Activities to illicit full range, such as painting (or applying shaving cream, reaching for objects on wall) from by extending arm above head to floor.<br>• Strength: Playing with toy truck adding sand or weights and rolling it a distance; Thera Putty games; resistive activities, such as building things with elastic and Popsicle sticks; crawling on floor; playing in sand.<br>• Endurance: Playing finger games (such as songs) for longer time; increasing number of repetitions; finger push-ups; engaging child in craft activity (such as pasting, gluing, cutting).<br>• Pain: Slow stretching, heat, warmth, joint protection strategies (follow the leader). |
| Contemporary motor control (see Chapter 29) | Movement is the result of the interaction between multiple systems, including child, environment, and the task itself. Children learn motor skills that are meaningful, whole, and performed in natural environment (with same objects).<br>Meaningful repetition within the natural environment promotes neuroplasticity. | | • Select activities that are meaningful to the child (engage the child in the selection process).<br>• Engage child in occupation, using the actual objects (such as feeding with their utensil, bowls, high chair).<br>• Scaffold movements so the child problem solves but is successful.<br>• Provide cues, feedback, and directions.<br>• Engage child in novel, creative, whole activities (such as coloring a picture, connecting dots, and completing a craft project).<br>• Allow children to reflect on their performance, make corrections, and plan. |

TABLE 30.6 **Frames of Reference for Occupational Therapy Intervention to Address Fine Motor Skills—cont'd**

| Frame of References | Principles | Description | Sample Activities |
|---|---|---|---|
| Sensory integration and processing (see Chapters 27 and 28) | Children use sensory information (visual, tactile, proprioception vestibular, kinesthesia, auditory) to respond motorically to environments. They use feedback (internal and external) to make an adaptive response. As they act upon the environment through repeatedly making an adaptive response, they develop improved neuronal connections (i.e., neuroplasticity). | • Children register sensory information, such as see, touch, hear, taste and sense position, balance, movement.<br>• They process the sensory information to apply meaning to it (for example, this object is something I would like).<br>• They respond to the feedback through an adaptive response (for example, pick up the toy). | Engage child in a variety of sensory experiences that require child to register, process, and respond. Activities should actively engage children and allow them to make choices.<br>• Visual discrimination activities: Find the like object; identify shapes.<br>• Tactile discrimination: Identify objects through touch; sort toys of different textures; engage in games with varied textures.<br>• Hear: Games to cue child to listen, such as Simon says; musical chairs; finger plays.<br>• Movement sense: Finger plays; finger puppet games; coloring on sandpaper (to provide additional proprioceptive input); drawing in sand; resistive hand games (such as those requiring play with elastics).<br>• Vestibular: Games involving whole body movements (such as swinging, rolling, and hopping) may support sensory processing and proximal control for hand skills. |

difficulties. Occupational therapy practitioners may address elements that make up fine motor skills (such as stability, strength, endurance, visual-motor integration, sensory processing, and motor planning). However, multiple elements interact when the child completes the skills within an occupation. Therefore, the practitioner creates opportunities for the child to complete multiple fine motor skills repeatedly during an occupation-based intervention session, which may include play-based activities as shown in Fig. 30.7.

Home programs and follow-up allow children to practice in multiple settings, providing them with necessary repetition. Occupational therapy practitioners carefully design home programs to ensure success. Home programs reinforce occupational therapy goals. For example, a child who is having difficulty with handwriting and is frustrated with school and feeling insecure may benefit from a home program that addresses hand strength and coordination to play on a keyboard, something that they enjoy but does not require the precision of handwriting. The practitioner in this situation provides the child with a simple melody and color-coats the keyboard. The child's home program includes that they learn melody for the next visit. This home program builds upon the child's motivation to play the keyboard while reinforcing repetitive finger movements of both hands, which they later use for handwriting. Occupational therapy practitioners use their skills at activity analysis to create home programs that support the child's skill development in meaningful ways. Practitioners also encourage children to reflect on their performance, so they can develop strategies for continued achievement and self-efficacy. Case Example 30.4, Maria, illustrates the use of an occupation-based intervention to address fine motor skills.

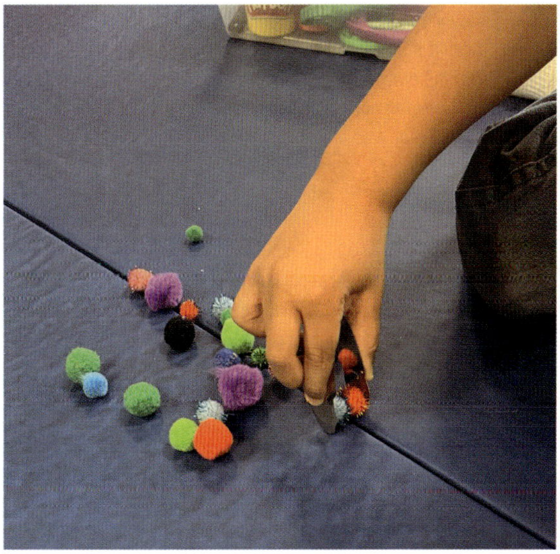

**Fig. 30.7** Occupational therapy intervention may include activities such as picking up colorful pom poms to encourage repetitive fine motor skills for play. This can be made into a game of feeding a puppet different types of berries and naming them based on the color of the pom poms.

## HANDWRITING

Handwriting is a form of communication where words are produced through written media. Penmanship is the art and skill of handwriting. Handwriting is a complex task that involves a variety

## CASE EXAMPLE 30.4 MARIA: OCCUPATION-BASED INTERVENTION TO ADDRESS FINE MOTOR SKILLS FOR PLAY AND FEEDING

Maria is a 2-year-old girl with a diagnosis of hemiplegia cerebral palsy. She presents with tightness and weakness in her right upper extremity but uses the extremity in almost all daily tasks. She did not meet the criteria for early intervention services. Therefore, Maria's parents sought services at an outpatient-based occupational therapy clinic.

**Evaluation:** The occupational therapist observed right upper extremity shoulder girdle weakness and increased muscle tone in her right arm and hand. The therapist observed poorly coordinated and limited fluidity of movements of the right upper extremity. Maria used palmar grasp patterns only with both the right and left hand. She used both her right and left hand equivalently during the evaluation.

While Maria engaged in many play activities expected for her age, at times she could not manipulate the toy as desired and showed signs of frustration by throwing toys or crying. Her parents reported that their main concern was that Maria was very messy when self-feeding and often frustrated during mealtimes. As a result, parents reported they frequently fed Maria. They planned on enrolling Maria in daycare but wanted her to be independent with feeding.

**Hypothesis and Intervention Plan:** The occupational therapist hypothesized that weakness in the right shoulder girdle and upper extremity contributed to poor accuracy in use of the arm (i.e., poor coordination and decreased fluidity). In addition, right upper extremity muscle tone (hypertonicity) contributed to difficulty with fluidity, coordination, and accuracy of motor movements. The occupational therapist designed interventions to address right upper extremity weakness and coordination to enhance Maria's ability to feed herself and play. Furthermore, the therapist reasoned that Maria would be less frustrated as she gained performance skills to do those things (such as feed herself and play with toys) that she wanted to do.

**Implementation of Plan:** The therapist engaged Maria in play activities that involved weight-bearing activities to build shoulder girdle strength. Maria enjoyed toys that made noises, so the occupational therapist created a small obstacle course that involved Maria rolling over a bolster, crawling through a tunnel, and crawling on her belly under an elevated surface to retrieve musical toys that she could play with along the way. To address strength in the right upper extremity, the practitioner engaged Maria in games involving resistance, such as pulling a toy with additional weights added and propelling herself prone on a scooter board that was on a rug (requiring she use more shoulder girdle muscle to move it forward).

To address Maria's grip strength and to allow Maria to be more successful with tool use so she would not be frustrated, the therapist scaffolded the activities. Maria used a raking pattern to pick up small items in her left and right hands. The therapist facilitated the next step (three jaw chuck pattern) by requiring Maria to approach items from the top. For example, the therapist placed finger puppets in nesting cups for Maria to retrieve. Maria loved animals and was excited to retrieve the animal finger puppets. The therapist helped Maria place them on her fingers and engaged in pretend play with the finger puppet animals (facilitating intrinsic finger strength and individuation). As needed, the therapist provided some stability at the wrist, but that faded as Maria became more successful with the task.

As Maria's shoulder stability and grasp improved, the therapist found activities to encourage a pincer grasp, such as playing with blocks and small food items. The occupational therapist encouraged the parents to provide Maria with finger foods to help her achieve finger skills and strengths (which would allow her to be successful while building her abilities to use utensils).

In therapy sessions, the therapist playfully engaged Maria in activities to encourage scooping and tool use (specifically using a spoon). For example, the therapist had Maria "feed" a puppet. At first, the puppet was very close to Maria so as not to require a lot of motor control. But as Maria's control over her extremities improved the therapist moved the puppet further away.

Finally, the occupational therapist directly addressed self-feeding and was happy to see Maria using her fingers and a spoon to feed herself. The mealtime was still messy, but she did not demonstrate any signs of frustration and completed the mealtime without assistance for feeding. Throughout the intervention process, the occupational therapist made sure to provide similar activities to parents to build into their home routine. Parents engaged in many of the same play tasks presented in the therapy session as part of their play routine. The therapist encouraged use of bilateral upper extremities while acknowledging that Maria would likely be left-handed and use her right upper extremity as an assist.

The therapist created occupation-based goals, engaged the child in multiple repetition of activities to address those goals in meaningful ways, and provided home programs to reinforce movements learned in therapy and to empower family members to support Maria's progress. The therapist encouraged the family to expect progress in the R UE while understanding that Maria would likely be left hand dominant.

of motor skills including grasp, strength, coordination, bimanual hand use, in-hand manipulation, separation of the sides of the hand, open web space, visual perception, visual-motor integration, and somatosensory processing. Children use handwriting to communicate, learn, and process information. However, approximately 10%–30% of school-age children with and without identified disabilities experience handwriting difficulties (Feder & Majnemer, 2007).

There are many potential causes for difficulty with handwriting as it is a complex task. Handwriting requires refined and sequential fine motor skill. It takes dexterity and coordination to produce letters and words. In addition, a child needs to hold information in their short-term memory before writing it down. Children with executive functioning difficulties and delays in fine motor skills may struggle with the complexity of holding the information they are writing and the motor execution for the letters in their mind. When that is coupled with motor planning difficulties, children may rely on cognition to produce the motor strokes. This complexity also provides a variety of avenues for intervention.

Grajo et al. (2020) found 19 studies examining handwriting conducted by occupational therapy clinicians and researchers. The four randomized control trials addressing component skills did not show evidence for an effect on handwriting legibility (addressing perception, kinesthesia, or motor skills), although there was moderate evidence for an effect of visual perception on handwriting speed. Strong evidence supports therapeutic practice over sensorimotor approaches or usual classroom activities for handwriting legibility. There is moderate evidence to support interventions to address handwriting legibility outcomes, including therapeutic practice, cognitive strategies such as self-evaluation techniques, and provision of performance feedback (Grajo et al., 2020). Isolated skills training to address prerequisite skills for handwriting does not translate to improved handwriting performance. Occupational therapy practitioners provide intervention to target handwriting through meaningful practice rather than rote copying. Addressing skills related to handwriting in isolation may improve those specific skills, but that does not necessarily translate to improved handwriting (Cahill & Beisbier, 2020). Writing during fun activities can enhance motivation for this difficult task (Box 30.2).

### BOX 30.2 Sample Handwriting Activities to Enhance Motivation

- Hide letters in a bag. Have a child reach with their hands into the bag using only touch to identify the letter. Once the letter is retrieved from the bag of the child, practice writing the letter or a word that starts with that letter.
- Use a scooter board to have a child navigate an area. Scatter letters or words at the child's reading level all around the treatment area. Have the child use the scooter board to navigate to a letter or word and practice writing it.
- Play games that involve asking questions such as 20 Questions, I Spy, or Headbanz. Instead of asking the question verbally, have the child write the question and response.
- Write letters to celebrities or characters of the movie that the child enjoys.
- Have a pen pal program in occupational therapy between different clients.
- Play preschool letter games but have the child write the letter and/or word that starts with the letter while playing the game.
- Spread out sight word cards or letters on the floor. Have a child retrieve the cards while swinging. Add an extra challenge to say a word or letter sound and have the child find that word/letter. Once retrieved, have the child write the letters, words, or use the words to generate sentences.

### TABLE 30.7 Selected Handwriting Curriculum-Based Programs

| Program | Description |
|---|---|
| Write Start (Case-Smith et al., 2011) | Integrated handwriting and writing program cotaught by occupational therapist and teachers using small group work, individualized support, peer and self-modeling, and frequent feedback |
| Handwriting Without Tears (Olsen, 2008; Olsen & Knapton, 2008) | Sensorimotor-based handwriting curriculum emphasizing stages of learning and play-based instruction for printing and cursive writing |
| Handwriting Without Tears – Get set for school (Olsen & Knapton, 2008) | Sensorimotor-based handwriting curriculum designed to teach preschool children prewriting skills necessary for kindergarten using music and movement and station teaching with multisensory tools to learn body awareness and fine motor skills |
| Fine motor and early writing Pre-K curriculum (see Donica, Goins & Wagne, 2013) | Handwriting readiness program using station teaching with adapted writing tools, workbooks, and sensory activities |

Adapted from Engel, C., Lillie, K., Zurawski, S., & Travers, B.G. (2018). Curriculum-based handwriting programs: A systematic review with effect sizes. *American Journal of Occupational Therapy, 72*, 7203205010.

Occupational therapy practitioners may design activities to address handwriting by using a specific program such as the examples provided in Table 30.7. Currently there is not sufficient research showing that any of the programs are superior to each other (Engel et al., 2018; Grajo et al., 2020). Research suggests completing handwriting programs within the general curriculum that are individualized for the child's strengths and challenges is effective (Cahill & Beisbier, 2020; Eddy et al., 2019; Grajo et al., 2020).

When beginning to teach handwriting, the occupational therapy practitioner begins by teaching the child to recognize their name and then write it, as this is meaningful to a child. The child should be taught to write their name using a capital first letter followed by lowercase letters. In writing, children practice lowercase letters more frequently, but when first teaching writing, it is best to learn upper- and lowercase letters after a child learns their name. Teaching letter sounds and phonemes while learning how to write letters reinforces the concepts that letters have meaning. Since writing is a form of communication, children benefit from reading out loud what they have written (Salameh-Matar et al., 2016). Children with reading difficulties may not be able to read the words they have written, which impacts the meaningfulness of handwriting. When addressing handwriting, occupational therapy practitioners match the level of written work to the child's reading level whenever possible.

To address the use of handwriting for academics and daily life activities, the practitioner addresses attention to written materials, details, formatting, and structure of handwriting. The practitioner may address speed and legibility of handwriting and fluency (ease of handwriting). The occupational therapy practitioner may address these skills or provide alternative ways for the child to complete written communication (such as keyboarding, dictating, or a combination of approaches). Case Example 30.5 Isaiah, shows how occupational therapy practitioners use all of these concepts in practice.

**Grasp of Writing Utensils.** There is a progression of grasps used on writing utensils. Children begin using writing utensils (crayons, markers, pencils, and pens) early and may initially use a palmar grasp to scribble. As skills become more refined, they may use a digital pronate grasp pattern. They may progress to a static four-finger grasp prior to a tripod grasp. Children using static grasps move their hand and arm as a unit. As muscle strength and dexterity increases, the child demonstrates a dynamic grasp, whereby their fingers move separately from the wrist and arm (Farris et al., 2022). Mature pencil grasps include the tripod grasp (Fig. 30.8) or lateral tripod, which has a thumb wrap; quadruped grasp or lateral quadruped (Fig. 30.9A and B) and the adapted tripod grasp (Fig. 30.9C) which positions the writing utensil between the index and middle finger. In these grasps, the forearm, wrist, and ulnar side of the hand are stable, while the radial side of the hand's distal joints (DIP, PIP, MCP) manipulate the pencil (Farris et al., 2022; Schwellnus et al., 2012).

Children who have weak hands may learn to compensate by holding pencils in ways that interfere with finger dexterity needed for writing. They may wrap their thumb around the pencil tightly and hold it closely in their palm with no web space. This pattern prevents movement of the distal interphalangeal (DIP) joint and results in difficulty writing. They may present with hyperextension of joints typically at DIP joint of the index finger or interphalangeal (IP) joint of thumb. This is a sign of laxity of joints, limited strength, and poor grading of force (proprioception) that can cause pain and stress to the joints. Children with shorter fingers hold the pencil with closed web space up until age 5. For children over 5 years of age, this interferes with moving the pencil due to decreased abduction of the thumb resulting in difficulty writing. To address this, occupational therapy practitioners may provide pencil grip adaptations such as those pictured in Fig. 30.10 or address grip strength during intervention. Box 30.3 provides some intervention activities to improve pencil grip.

Inefficient grasp patterns, such as those show in Fig. 30.11A–D, may impact a child's ability to produce legible handwriting in a timely manner as the grasp limits the motion of the pencil. It may also lead to joint pain with writing tasks (Burt & Benbow, 2008; McCleskey, 2008).

## CASE EXAMPLE 30.5 ISAIAH: ADDRESSING HANDWRITING CHALLENGES

Isaiah is an 8-year-old boy in the third grade who was referred to occupational therapy by his teacher. He has difficulty handwriting and only writes one- to two-word responses on open writing prompts. Isaiah was referred to special education services under the Individuals with Disabilities Education Improvement Act and the district's protocols. Isaiah also receives private occupational therapy services focusing on praxis using Ayres Sensory Integration.

**Occupational therapy evaluation:** The school-based therapist completed an occupational profile and examined Isaiah's handwriting performance by observing him in the classroom.

He reported that sometimes he gets frustrated when the teacher asks him to write and just does not do it because he does not want to write. Isaiah expressed he "hated writing." However, he also reported that he enjoys recess and playing kickball.

***Performance with handwriting:*** Isaiah was asked to write the alphabet from memory. He skipped some letters, indicated he did not know how to write other letters, and took more than 5 minutes to write the entire alphabet. When asked to copy a short sentence, his speed improved, but many letters were formed incorrectly. Isaiah used a right lateral pinch grasp on the pencil.

***Factors related to handwriting.***

- ***Strength:*** Isaiah demonstrated weak palmar grasp and had difficulty individualizing his fingers. He also demonstrated weak trunk and shoulder strength overall.
- ***Motor planning:*** Isaiah had difficulty generating the motor plan to produce letters. He had to think a lot about how letters are formed, which taxed his ability to hold information needed for writing.
- ***Visual perception kills:*** Isaiah demonstrated average visual perception skills.
- ***Visual-motor skills:*** Isaiah had difficulties with many visual-motor skills.

The therapist noted that Isaiah is having difficulty fulfilling his role as student due to his fine motor challenges and hypothesized that Isaiah's difficulty with motor planning may be to blame. The therapist worked with Isaiah individually for the first session to establish a rapport and identify specific goals that they would address in the classroom and at home. They created a **long-term goal** that: Isaiah will write three sentences addressing the in-class prompt within 15 minutes that are legible to the teacher. To address this goal, Isaiah participated in the following occupational therapy activities.

- Hand strengthening: The therapist provided a program (using sports photos to show that athletes frequently use strength programs) for Isaiah to use in the classroom and at home consisting of activities such as squeezing stress balls, clothes pins, pulling Velcro, and putty. These activities also helped him increase attention in the classroom.
- Pencil grip adaptations: The occupational therapist worked with Isaiah to trial various pencil grips. He found one he liked, and it helped him hold the pencil with an open web space, which improved his legibility and ease of writing.
- Motor planning: The occupational therapist recognized the motor planning was playing a role in Isaiah's ability to generate letters. The therapist worked with Isaiah to generate short sayings as they practiced the formation of each letter to help him remember how letters were generated. She built the handwriting practice into fun games such as writing clues or questions, playing word hide and seek, and doing Mad Libs.
- Scaffolding and meaningful practice: To support Isaiah's success, the therapist found out the weekly prompt in advance, so that they could work on sample responses before class. Once Isaiah achieved some success in writing and established strategies to complete the prompts, the therapist decreased the preparation and cueing. Isaiah began to look forward to the prompts when he read them aloud to his classmates, and they asked questions.
- The occupational therapist provided a handout to keep on Isaiah's desk with the short sayings next to each of the letters and phrases that he could use in his writing samples. As he continued to practice, Isaiah used the handout less. His writing became faster, and he began producing longer written responses.

**Prewriting Skills.** Prewriting skills require children to coordinate use of the eyes and hands to use a writing tool. They integrate a variety of skills, such as attention, visual-motor integration, body awareness, motor planning, and sensory processing, as they engage in exploratory play and handle objects with their hands. They figure out how objects fit together (e.g., stacking blocks), how to manipulate toys (e.g., rattles), and they begin to try out new ways of doing things (e.g., crawling behind an object). They play with paper, crayons, and pencils.

Table 30.8 provides an overview of the development of prewriting shapes (Ziviani & Wallen, 2006) which can guide occupational therapy intervention planning. At around 1 year, infants begin to scribble randomly. They progress from horizontal, to vertical, and finally to circular scribbles. Children first imitate prewriting strokes before they copy. Simple shapes come next with circle, cross, and square, in that order. Box 30.4 provides directions on how to teach a square as a tool to support prewriting skills. Right diagonal strokes are developed before left diagonal strokes, around the time a child is learning to produce a square. Diagonal strokes lead to production of an "x," followed by a triangle, and finally a diamond. In the United States, children are taught to form shapes and letters top to bottom and left to right. Circular scribbles and circular strokes occur in a counterclockwise direction, just as in the formulation of circular letters (i.e., "o," "a").

Different cultures may formulate letters and writing in different methods. For example, English language follows left to right

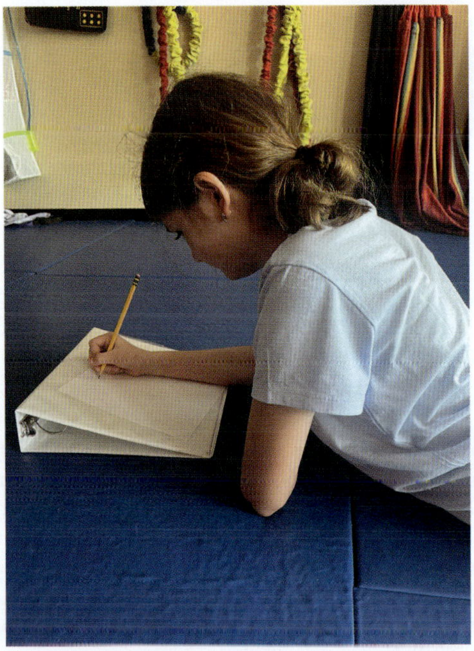

**Fig. 30.8** This girl writes using a tripod grasp with a thumb wrap with an open web space. Slant boards can be helpful in increasing wrist extension slightly to promote better finger flexion and pencil grasp.

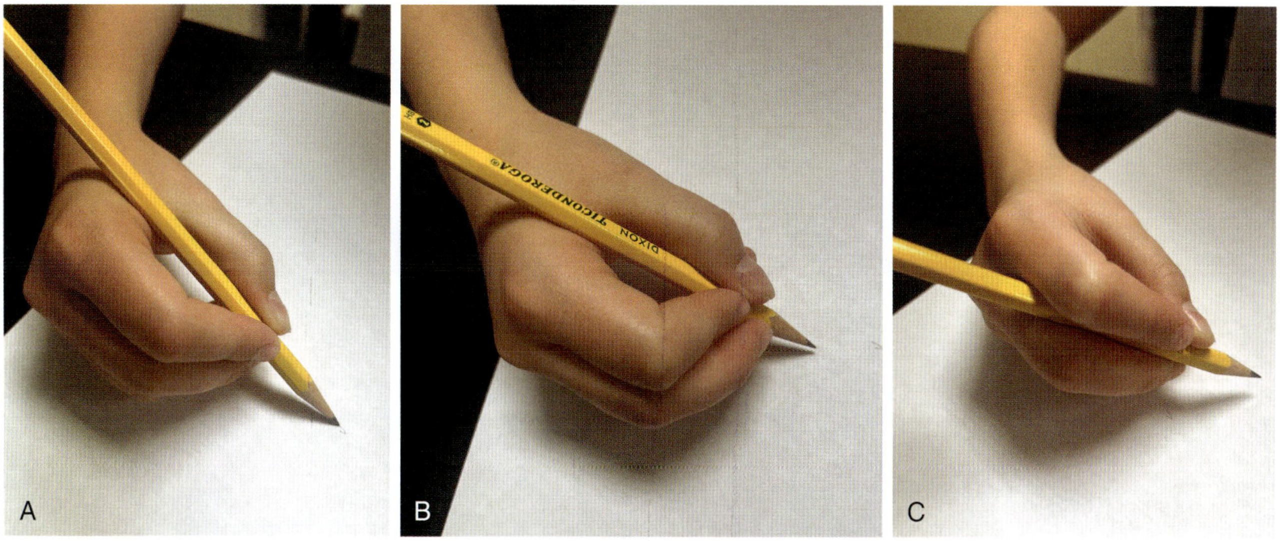


**Fig. 30.9** Efficient grasp patterns for handwriting.

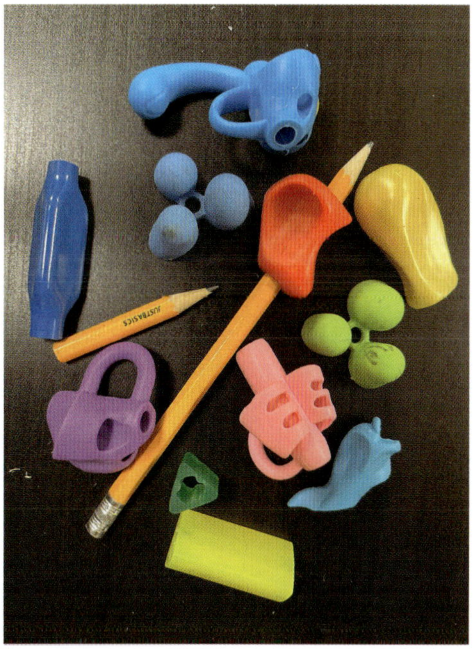

**Fig. 30.10** A variety of pencil grips exist to support children's hand positioning for writing. The grips provide stability and cues for how children should hold their pencil. They come in a variety of shapes, sizes, and colors to match children's needs.

for reading and writing, while the Arabic language and Hebrew both follow right to left. Repetitive practice of prewriting strokes is important. Children practice strokes in sequence first, before concerning themselves with the precision of the shape. For example, initially a circle may have a large overlap, but as the child develops more motor control, the ends meet more precisely to form a true circle. Using dots as visual cues can help children learn direction and precision of strokes. For example, when working on diagonal lines, providing dots at an angle for children to connect can help the child progress from a vertical to diagonal lines. The occupational therapy practitioner designs creative interventions using games and activities to make prewriting fun. Writing readiness may be improved with playful activities used in preschool classrooms (Martino & Lape, 2021).

**BOX 30.3 How to Improve Pencil Grasp**

- Address any underlying hand weakness through strengthening activities.
- Provide support at the forearm and wrist by having the child lie on their stomach (in prone position) to encourage a dynamic grasp.
- Writing on vertical surfaces (such as the chalkboard at school) promotes better pencil grip.
- Use tools with thicker handles, such as markers, built-up crayons, or pencil grips.
- Pencil grips come in a variety of designs and sizes to support children's grip. For example, a hair tie may be used as a pencil grip
- Playing with tongs may facilitate grasp patterns and use of radial side of hand.
- Holding a small item under ring and pinkie while grasping pencil supports a mature pencil grip.
- Shorter pencils (such as golf pencils) require children hold them in a three-jaw chuck grasp vs. a gross grasp.

## Keyboarding

Keyboarding has become an essential occupation to access computers for leisure activities as well as to produce written communication. Children use keyboarding skills to access the internet and other tools for academics and leisure. Keyboarding requires finger isolation and sequential finger movements. Over time, as children practice keyboarding, the movements become automatic, and the child "feels" the location of the keys (without relying on vision). This requires sensory processing and cognition. As with handwriting, children must be able to hold information in their mind to produce typed text. By sixth grade, children should be able to type around 17 words per minute (Morress et al., 2020).

There are many children's typing programs that make it fun for children to learn keyboarding. Keyboarding Without Tears is one specific keyboarding program used by occupational therapists (Donica et al., 2021). One benefit of keyboarding is that there are many shortcuts built into computer programs such as word prediction, spell check, and even dictation that can make the motor aspects of keyboarding quicker and easier for children.

## Scissor Skills

Cutting with scissors is also a complex activity. The use of the scissors as a tool requires a functional scissors grasp and the ability to judge

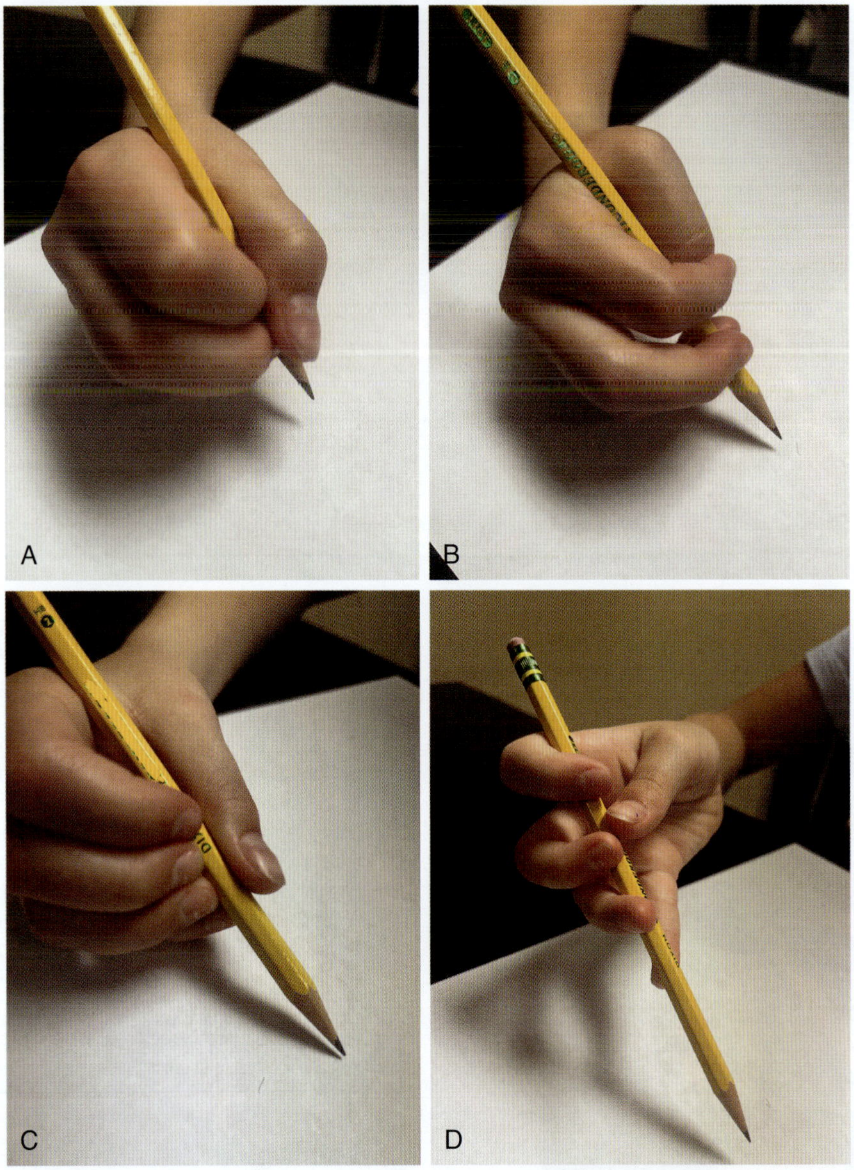


**Fig. 30.11** Ineffective grasp patterns for handwriting interfere with the child's ability to fluently move the pencil over the writing surface.

**BOX 30.4 How to Teach Making a Square**

Drawing a square directly relates to the formation of several letters, especially in block style print. Letters such as "E," "F," and "T" are generally formed in the same order of line production. Therefore, it is important to teach a square in the same progression as letters are formed.

Order of strokes to produce a square.

(1) Draw a line down.
(2) Bring pencil back to top of the line.
(3) Draw line left to right.
(4) Bring pencil to bottom of the first line.
(5) Draw line left to right.
(6) Bring pencil to the top of the second line.
(7) Draw line down to connect second and third lines.

Tip: Some children may have difficulty with the precision of generating sharp corners. Providing dots to have children connect can help provide a visual clue as to where to stop and start lines to produce sharp corners.

the force needed to close the scissors enough to cut, while not closing them so forcefully as to make them fall out of the paper. In addition, scissor skill requires the ability to separate the sides of the hand and use two hands together. The nondominant hand must be able to use wrist motion and in-hand manipulation to move, rotate, and reposition the paper for cutting with the dominant hand. And, to accurately cut a shape or line, visual-motor skills are required as well.

For effective scissor grasp, the child positions their thumb in the smaller hole with the middle finger in the larger hole and the index finger on the outside of the handle to stabilize the scissors. The lower handle rests on the DIP joining of the middle finger, and the wrist is positioned in an extended position. Immature scissor grasps may be the result of limited hand strength or wrist stability. Children with immature grasp may place two, three, or more fingers in the handle of the scissors; the wrist may be flexed rather than extended. When children hold scissors like this, they do not have adequate control of the scissors and tend to use larger muscles rather than the intrinsic muscles of the hand, preventing

**TABLE 30.8 Prewriting Shapes**

| Shape | Milestone | Example |
|---|---|---|
| Scribble | 1–2 years | 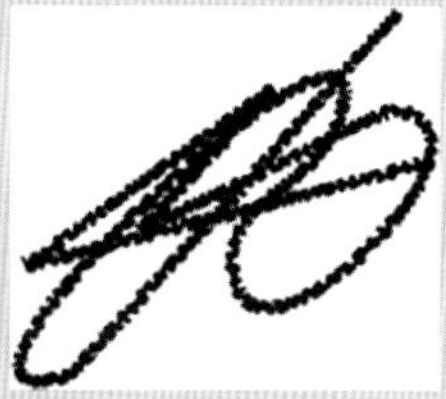 |
| Vertical line | 2–3 years |  |
| Horizontal line | 2–3 years |  |
| Circle | 3 years | 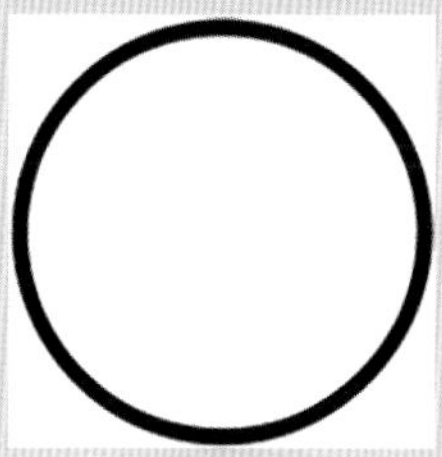 |
| Cross | 4 years | 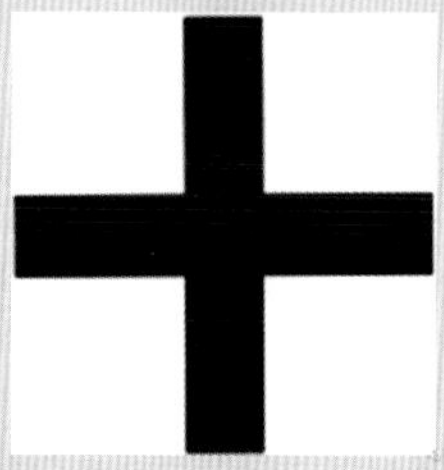 |
| Left diagonal | 4–4.5 years | 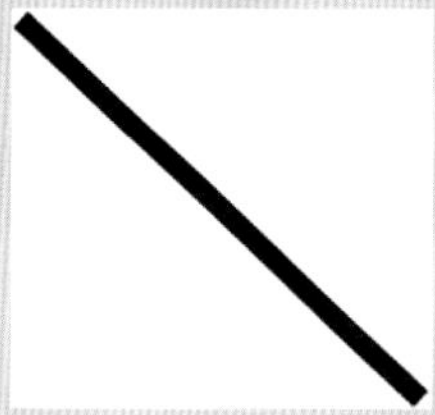 |
| Square | 4.5–5 years | 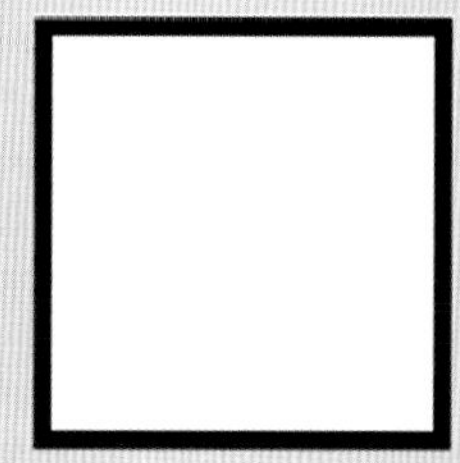 |
| Right diagonal | 4–5 years | 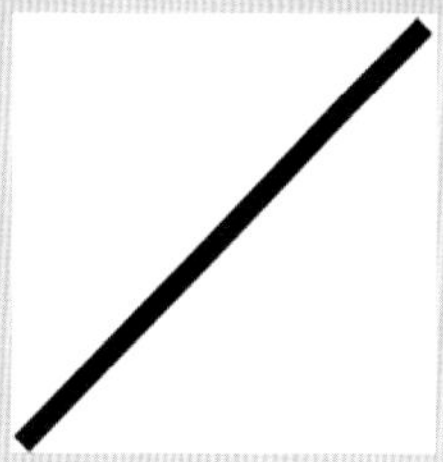 |

*Continued*

**TABLE 30.8 Prewriting Shapes—cont'd**

| Shape | Milestone | Example |
|---|---|---|
| "X" | 5 years | 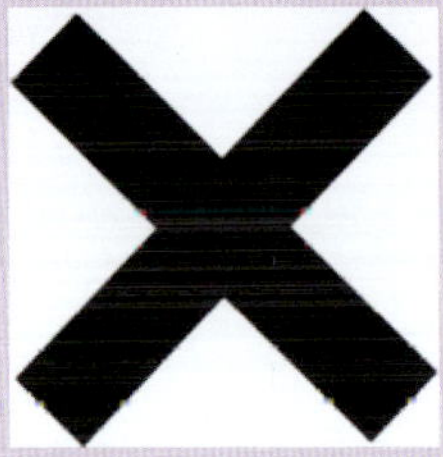 |
| Triangle | 5–5.5 years | 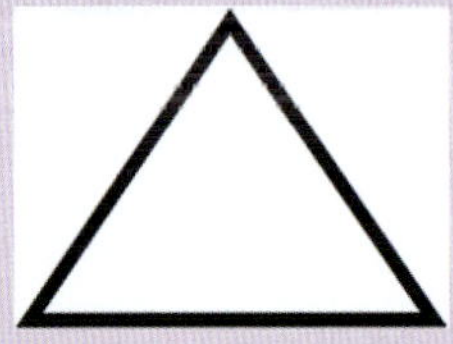 |

**BOX 30.5 Progression of Scissor Skills**

- Snipping
- Cutting a paper in two pieces
- Cutting a line
- Cutting a longer line
- Cutting curve
- Cutting circles
- Cutting squares and triangles
- Cutting more complex shapes

more refined and precise cutting skills (Meyers, 2006). In addition, a flexed wrist tips the scissors to the side, preventing the scissors blades from cutting. The external blade of the scissors should be on the outside when cutting so as not to block the view of the line that is to be cut. This requires using left-handed scissors when a child is cutting left-handed. The blades are opposite, so the cutting line is easily seen. Children start developing adequate hand skills for cutting around 3.5 years of age when two sides of the hand have developed, and intrinsic hand muscles are more refined. Box 30.5 describes the progression of scissor skills.

Children learn cutting first by snipping. Thicker paper can make it easier for children to be successful with snipping as it does not require as much control to hold in a stable position to cut. Thicker paper (such as card stock or construction paper) can also be used to increase hand strength of the preferred hand. Items other than paper may also be used to teach snipping as shown in Fig. 30.12. Playdough is an excellent way to teach beginning scissor skills as it provides increased feedback and prevents the scissors from sliding.

Once the child has mastered snipping, they can begin to cut a paper into two pieces. This requires manipulation of the paper with the nonpreferred hand and requires a child to snip and move the scissors up the paper. Starting with a ½″ strip of paper to snip pieces off and then progression to 1″, 1.5″, and 2″ allows a gradual progression of the number of successive snips needed to cut across the paper provided. Verbal cues can help a child to remember to close the scissors slowly and not close all the way. Some children benefit from learning to use the scissors as a puppet with the therapist, making them talk to each other, to practice the open and close motion with the cue to not close the mouth the whole way.

When ready to cut on a line, the practitioner can adapt the motor component by asking the child to cut along thick, short lines. Longer lines require more control to manipulate the paper and scissors in a coordinated manner with more bilateral coordination to move the hand (that is assisting) up the paper simultaneously with the cutting hand. Gradually lines are lengthened and thinned as the child gains skill. For some children, a fun way to work toward cutting on a line is to first cut within a maze line that is thick and mainly straight.

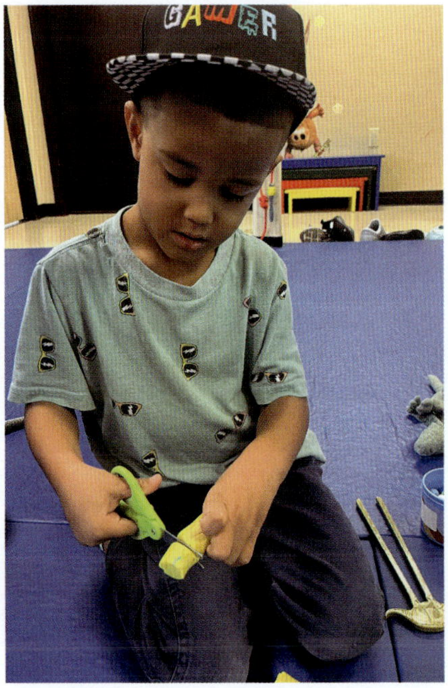

**Fig. 30.12** Cutting playdough with scissors provides resistance (which may improve hand strength) and provides sensory feedback to reinforce movements.

Cutting a circle is a skill that occurs prior to cutting a square, even though motorically the circle requires more bilateral coordination. The square requires more cognition to cut past the line before turning the paper. However, because of the increase in motor demands, some children with difficulties in bilateral coordination may exhibit mastery of cutting a square before cutting a circle. Children often have difficulty manipulating the circle shape with the nondominant hand. They may lift the cutting hand to cut up and over the circle rather than turning the circle shape while keeping their elbow by their side. Some children benefit from practicing first with wavy lines to gradually learn how to turn and reposition the paper before progressing to circles. Others benefit from cutting circles while in prone, propped on their elbows. This cues them to keep their arm and hand in one place and turn just the paper.

## SUMMARY

Occupational therapy practitioners frequently address children and youth's fine motor skills, so they can participate in daily occupations such as play, activities of daily, leisure, education, social participation, academic tasks, work, sleep and rest, and instrumental activities of daily living. They address the development of fine motor skills and the underlying factors influencing hand skills (such as stability, strength, endurance, range of motion) and processes (such as cognition, sensory processing, and visual-motor integration). Occupational therapy practitioners engage children and youth in repetitive occupation-based fine motor activities that are client-centered. They support children's strengths by promoting encouraging, problem-solving, and reflective sessions. Occupational therapy practitioners design creative activities to address fine motor performance, considering the child's strengths and challenges (motor, sensory, cognitive, and motivations), occupation (requirements, objects, and skills), and environment (culture, expectations, setting, and resources).

1. Occupational therapy practitioners are trained to analyze the motor, sensory, and cognitive factors that influence fine motor skills and use knowledge of the task or occupation in relation to the environment. They integrate knowledge of the sequence of fine motor development with the child's strengths and challenges, in combination with the cultural roles and expectations, to create intervention plans to support the child's occupational engagement.
2. Occupational therapy practitioners engage children in meaningful repetitions of fine motor tasks within their natural environment. Occupational therapy intervention is designed to empower children to see their own strengths. Therefore, in any occupational therapy intervention, practitioners encourage children to reflect on their performance and develop solutions.
3. Occupational therapy practitioners use occupation-based models of practice to structure their organization and to holistically examine the motor, social, cognitive, and environmental factors that influence fine motor skills for occupational performance. They analyze the factors influencing the child's fine motor skills (such as motor, sensory, and cognition), along with the environment and desired occupation. They examine the child's development to tailor activities specifically to the child. Practitioners create client-centered goals and engage children in meaningful activities to promote occupational performance. They scaffold activities, so the child challenges their abilities in many situations (e.g., home, school, community) to reinforce skills and performance.
4. Research suggests completing handwriting programs within the general curriculum that are individualized for the child's strengths and challenges is effective. Practitioners use a variety of frames of reference to address fine motor skills, including biomechanical, contemporary motor control, and motor learning, sensory integration, and developmental ones. The case examples provided illustrate how occupational therapy practitioners use these concepts in practice.

## REFERENCES


Alaniz, M. L., Galit, E., Necesito, C. I., & Rosario, E. R. (2015). Hand strength, handwriting, and functional skills in children with autism. *American Journal of Occupational Therapy, 69*. https://doi.org/10.5014/ajot.2015.016022. 6904220030.

Alhusaini, A. A., Melam, G. R., & Buragadda, S. (2016). Short-term sensorimotor-based intervention for handwriting performance in elementary school children. *Pediatrics International, 58*(11), 1118–1123. https://doi.org/10.1111/ped.13004.

American Occupational Therapy Association. (2020). Occupational therapy practice framework: Domain and process (4th ed.). *American Journal of Occupational Therapy, 74*(Suppl. 2). https://doi.org/10.5014/ajot.2020.74S2001. 7412410010.

Atakan, M. M., Li, Y., Koşar, Ş. N., Turnagöl, H. H., & Yan, X. (2021). Evidence-based effects of high-intensity interval training on exercise capacity and health: A review with historical perspective. *International Journal of Environmental Research and Public Health, 18*(13), 7201. https://doi.org/10.3390/ijerph18137201.

Axford, C., Joosten, A. V., & Harris, C. (2018). iPad applications that required a range of motor skills promoted motor coordination in children commencing primary school. *Australian Occupational Therapy Journal, 65*, 146–155. https://doi.org/10.1111/1440-1630.12450.

Burt, C., & Benbow, M. (2008). Children and handwriting ergonomics. In R. Lueder, & V. J. Berg Rice (Eds.), *Ergonomics for children: Designing products and places for toddlers and teens* (pp. 689–720). Taylor & Francis Group.

Cahill, C. M., & Beisbier, S. (2020). Occupational therapy practice guidelines for children and youth ages 5–21 years. *American Journal of Occupational Therapy, 74*(4). https://doi.org/10.5014/ajot.2020.744001. 7404397010p1–7404397010p48.

Caramia, S., Gill, A., Ohl, A., & Schelly, D. (2020). Brief report - fine motor activities in elementary school children: A replication study. *American Journal of Occupational Therapy, 74*. https://doi.org/10.5014/ajot.2020.035014. 7402345010.

Case-Smith, J., Holland, T., & Bishop, B. (2011). Effectiveness of an integration handwriting program for first grade students: A pilot study. *American Journal of Occupational Therapy, 65*, 670–678. https://doi.org/10.5014/ajot.2011.000984.

Center for Disease Control. (2022). *Milestone tracker*. https://www.cdc.gov/ncbddd/actearly/milestones-app.html.

Colangelo, C. A., & Shea, M. (2020). A biomechanical frame of reference to position children for function. In P. Kramer, J. Hinojosa, & T.-H. Howe (Eds.), *Frames of reference for pediatric occupational therapy* (4th ed.) (pp. 247–318). Wolters Kluwer.

Denton, P. L., Cope, S., & Moser, C. (2006). The effects of sensorimotor-based intervention versus therapeutic practice on improving handwriting performance in 6- to 11-year-old children. *American Journal of Occupational Therapy, 60*, 16–27. https://doi.org/10.5014/ajot.60.1.16.

Donica, D. K., Giroux, P., Kim, Y., & Branson, S. (2021). A comparison of two keyboarding instruction methods over 2 years for elementary students. *The Open Journal of Occupational Therapy, 9*(3), 1–13. https://doi.org/10.15453/2168-6408.1819.

Donica, D. K., Goins, A., & Wagner, L. (2013). Effectiveness of handwriting readiness programs on postural control, hand control, and letter and number formation in head start classrooms. *Journal of Occupational Therapy, Schools, & Early Intervention, 6*(2), 81–93. https://doi.org/10.1080/19411243.2013.810938.

Duncan, A. F., Bann, C. M., Maitre, N. L., Peralta-Carcelen, M., & Hintz, S. R. (2020). Hand function at 18-22 months is associated with school-age manual dexterity and motor performance in children born extremely premature. *The Journal of Pediatrics, 225*, 51–57. https://doi.org/10.1016/j.jpeds.2020.05.048.

Eddy, L. H., Wood, M. L., Shire, K. A., Bingham, D. D., Bonnick, E., Creaser, A., Mon-Williams, M., & Hill, L. J. B. (2019). A systematic review of randomized and case-controlled trials investigating the effectiveness of school-based motor skill interventions in 3- to 12-year-old children. *Child: Care, Health and Development, 45*, 773–790. https://doi.org/10.1111/cch.12712.

Engel, C., Lillie, K., Zurawski, S., & Travers, B. G. (2018). Curriculum-based handwriting programs: A systematic review with effect sizes.

*American Journal of Occupational Therapy*, *72*. https://doi.org/10.5014/ajot.2018.027110. 7203205010.

Farris, K. M., Fehrenbacher, R. E., Hayes, E. L., McEvoy, R., Smithg, A. P., & McCulloh, R. S. (2022). The relationship between muscle activation and handwriting quality with non-native grip styles. *Journal of Hand Therapy*, *35*, 558–568. https://doi.org/10.1016/j.jht.2021.03.004.

Feder, K. P., & Majnemer, A. (2007). Handwriting development, competency, and intervention. *Developmental Medicine and Child Neurology*, *49*, 312–317. https://doi.org/10.1111/j.1469-8749.2007.00312.x.

Grajo, L. C., Candler, C., & Sarafian, A. (2020). Interventions within the scope of occupational therapy to improve children's academic participation: A systematic review. *American Journal of Occupational Therapy*, *74*. https://doi.org/10.5014/ajot.2020.039016. 7402180030.

Howe, T. -H., Kramer, P., & Hinojose, J. (2020). Developmental perspective: Fundamentals of developmental theory. In P. Kramer, J. Hinojosa, & T. -H. Howe (Eds.), *Frames of reference for pediatric occupational therapy* (4th ed.) (pp. 20–28). Wolters Kluwer.

Howie, F. (2016). The wonders of messy play. *Every Child*, *22*(2), 30–31. https://doi.org/10.3316/ielapa.124243096575274.

Jackman, M., Lannin, N., Galea, C., Sakzewski, L., Miller, L., & Novak, L. (2020). What is the threshold does of upper limb training for children with cerebral palsy to improve function? A systematic review. *Australian Occupational Therapy Journal*, *67*, 269–280. https://doi.org/10.1111/1440-1630.12666.

Llorens, L. (1982). *Application of developmental theory for health and rehabilitation*. American Occupational Therapy Association.

Lust, C. A., & Donica, D. K. (2011). Effectiveness of a handwriting readiness program in head start: A two-group controlled trial. *American Journal of Occupational Therapy*, *65*, 560–568. https://doi.org/10.5014/ajot.2011.000612.

Mano, H., Fujiwara, S., & Haga, N. (2020). Effect of prostheses on children with congenital upper limb deficiencies. *Pediatric International*, *62*, 1039–1043. https://doi.org/10.1111/ped.14265.

Martino, E. M., & Lape, J. E. (2021). Occupational therapy in the preschool classroom - Promoting fine motor and visual motor skills for kindergarten readiness. *Journal of Occupational Therapy, Schools, & Early Intervention*, *14*(2), 134–152. https://doi.org/10.1080/19411243.2020.1822261.

McCleskey, J. (2008). *Development of a fine motor program for classrooms and for occupational therapy*. The Handwriting Clinic. https://www.thehandwritingclinic.com/CM/Brochures/Files/2019%20%20Developing%20a%20Fine%20Motor%20Program%20for%20Children.pdf.

McPhee, S. D. (1987). Functional hand evaluations: A review. *American Journal of Occupational Therapy*, *41*(3), 158–163. https://doi.org/10.5014/ajot.41.3.158.

Meyers, C. A. (2006). A fine motor program for preschoolers. In A. Henderson, & C. Pehoski (Eds.), *Hand function in the child: Foundations for remediation* (2nd ed.) (pp. 267–292). Mosby Elsevier.

Morress, C., Kula, S., Mangas, T., Schoen, K., & Surface, M. (2020). Keyboarding speed and accuracy norms of fifth- and sixth-grade students. *American Journal of Occupational Therapy*, *74*(4). https://doi.org/10.5014/ajot.2020.74S1-PO8114. 7411500058p1.

Naider-Steinhart, S., & Katz-Leurer, M. (2007). Analysis of proximal and distal muscle activity during handwriting tasks. *American Journal of Occupational Therapy*, *61*(4), 392–398. https://doi.org/10.5014/ajot.61.4.392.

Ohl, A. M., Graze, H., Weber, K., Kenny, S., Salvatore, C., & Wagreich, S. (2013). Effectiveness of a 10-week tier-1 response to intervention program in improving fine motor and visual–motor skills in general education kindergarten students. *American Journal of Occupational Therapy*, *67*, 507–514. https://doi.org/10.5014/ajot.2013.008110.

Olsen, J. Z. (2008). *Letters and numbers for me* (5th ed.). Handwriting Without Tears.

Olsen, J. Z., & Knapton, E. F. (2008). *Handwriting Without Tears kindergarten teacher's guide* (10th ed.). Handwriting Without Tears.

Prunty, M. M., Pratt, A., Raman, E., Simmons, L., & Steele-Bobat, F. (2020). Grip strength and pen pressure are not key contributors to handwriting difficulties in children with developmental coordination disorder. *British Journal of Occupational Therapy*, *83*(6), 387–396. https://doi.org/10.1177/0308022619885046.

Reed, C. L., & Ziat, M. (2018). *Haptic perception: From the skin to the brain. Ference module in neuroscience and biobehavioral psychology*. Elsevier.

Roley, S. S., Schaal, R. C., & Baltazar-Mori, A. (2020). Ayres sensory integration frame of reference. In P. Kramer, J. Hinojosa, & T. -H. Howe (Eds.), *Frames of reference for pediatric occupational therapy* (4th ed.) (pp. 87–158). Wolters Kluwer.

Rybski, M. (2012). Biomechanical intervention approach. In *Kinesiology for occupational therapy* (pp. 309–354). Slack Inc.

Sacrey, L., Arnold, B., Whishaw, I. Q., & Gonzalez, C. L. R. (2012). Precocious hand use preference in reach-to-eat behavior versus manual construction in 1- to 5- year-old children. *Developmental Psychobiology*, *55*(8), 902–911. https://doi.org/10.1002/dev.21083.

Salameh-Matar, A., Basel, N., & Weintraub, N. (2016). The relationship between linguistic skills, visual–motor functions, and handwriting performance at various developmental stages. *American Journal of Occupational Therapy*, *70*(4). https://doi.org/10.5014/ajot.2016.70S1-PO1042. (Suppl. 1), 7011505099p1.

Schneider, M., Myers, C., Morgan-Daniel, J., & Shectman, O. (2019). A scoping review of the relationship between grasp and handwriting performance in school-age children. *American Journal of Occupational Therapy*, *73*(4 Supp), Article 7311515335p1. https://doi.org/10.5014/ajot.2019.73S1-PO4018.

Schwellnus, H., Carnahan, H., Kushki, A., Polatajko, H., Missiuna, C., & Chau, T. (2012). Effect of pencil grasp on the speed and legibility of handwriting in children. *American Journal of Occupational Therapy*, *66*(6), 718–726. https://doi.org/10.5014/ajot.2012.004515.

Seminara, L., Gastaldo, P., Watt, S. J., Valyear, K. F., Zuher, F., & Mastrogiovanni, F. (2019). Active haptic perception in robots: A review. *Frontiers in Neurorobotics*, 13, Article 7311515335p1. https://doi.org/10.3389/fnbot.2019.00053.

Shumway-Cook, A., & Woollacott, M. H. (2017). *Motor control: Translating research into clinical practice* (5th ed.). Wolters Kluwer.

Stival, F., Michieletto, S., Cognolato, M., Enrico, P., Muller, H., & Atzori, M. (2019). A quantitative taxonomy of human grasp. *Journal of NeuroEngineering and Rehabilitation*, *16*(1), 1–17. https://doi.org/10.1186/s12984-019-0488-x.

Stricker, P. R., Faigenbaum, A. D., McCambridge, T. M., Council on Sport Medicine and Fitness, LaBella, C. R., Brooks, M. A., Canty, G., Diamond, A. B., Hennrikus, W., Logan, K., Moffatt, K., Nemeth, B. A., Pengel, K. B., Peterson, A. R (2020). Resistance training for children and adolescents. *Pediatrics*, *145*(6). E20201011. https://doi.org/10.1542/peds.2020-1011.

Wang, T., Howe, T., Hinojosa, J., & Weinberg, S. L. (2011). Relationship between postural control and fine motor skills in preterm infants at 6 and 12 months adjusted age. *American Journal of Occupational Therapy*, *65*(6), 695–701. https://doi.org/10.5014/ajot.2011.001503.

Ziviani, J. M., & Wallen, M. (2006). Development of graphomotor skills. In A. Henderson, & C. Pehoski (Eds.), *Hand function in the children: Foundations for remediation* (2nd ed.) (pp. 217–238). Elsevier.

31

# Vision and Visual Information Processing

*Mitchell Scheiman*

## GUIDING QUESTIONS

1. Why is it important for occupational therapy practitioners to screen for vision disorders?
2. What are the differences in models of vision among eye care professionals?
3. How do the differences in models of vision affect the examination of children with vision disorders?
4. What are the most prevalent vision problems in the pediatric populations seen by occupational therapy practitioners?
5. How can occupational therapy practitioners screen for visual efficiency and visual information processing challenges?
6. How can occupational therapy practitioners address vision challenges among children and youth?

## KEY TERMS

Accommodation
Accommodative amplitude
Astigmatism
Binocular vision
Convergence insufficiency
Hyperopia
Myopia
Refractive errors
Saccades
Strabismus
Vision therapy
Visual acuity
Visual analysis skills
Visual efficiency
Visual information processing
Visual integrity
Visual motor skills
Visual spatial skills

## THE IMPORTANCE OF UNDERSTANDING VISION FOR PEDIATRIC OCCUPATIONAL THERAPY PRACTITIONERS

Pediatric occupational therapy practitioners often provide service to children with autism, cerebral palsy, Down syndrome, intellectual disability, spina bifida, low birth weight syndrome, pervasive developmental delay, sensory integrative dysfunction, learning disabilities, and trauma. Studies have shown that children with these issues have a high prevalence of vision disorders (Anketell et al., 2015; Bakroon & Lakshminarayanan, 2016; Ciner et al., 1991; Coulter et al., 2015; Cregg et al., 2003; Fazzi et al., 2012; Hashemi et al., 2021; LoCascio, 1977; Makateb et al., 2020; Milne et al., 2009; Nandakumar et al., 2011; Satgunam et al., 2019; Scharre & Creedon, 1992; Scheiman, 1984, 1990; Simmons et al., 2009; Surman et al., 2006; Watt et al., 2015). Children with undetected and untreated vision problems may have difficulty participating in occupations such as reading, copying from the board, writing, playing, and sports, dressing, and grooming. Occupational therapy practitioners address visual challenges to improve children's ability to participate in meaningful activities for life satisfaction.

This chapter provides information on the complexity and importance of vision and how visual deficits can interfere with occupation. The chapter outlines models of vision, defines terms, and describes screening methods. The author examines the role of eye care professionals and occupational therapy practitioners in vision therapy. The chapter describes therapy techniques that can be used by occupational therapy practitioners to improve a child's visual skills for engagement in everyday occupations.

## MODELS OF VISION: BACKGROUND INFORMATION

When we think about vision and children, it is likely that one of the first images that come to mind is the school nurse performing a vision screening. This was our experience when we were children and again our experience with our own children. What is this ubiquitous school nurse vision screening designed to accomplish?

The child is asked to stand 20 ft from the traditional eye chart, cover one eye at a time, and call off the letters on the chart. This test, called visual acuity testing, is designed to detect vision problems that interfere with the ability to see small details at long distances. The primary vision disorder that causes blurred vision at long distances is *myopia* or nearsightedness. Children with this condition have excellent vision when reading but have difficulty seeing the board at school. The only other problems that would cause blurred vision at long distances are amblyopia (poor vision in one eye) or rare eye diseases like nystagmus, optic atrophy, and retinopathy of prematurity.

The important question to ask is: Why is the school nurse performing the vision screening? The answer is to identify children who are likely to have vision problems that could potentially interfere with academic performance. However, the primary test they use evaluates visual acuity, which detects myopia. Research shows that children with myopia tend to have higher intelligence and achievement test scores, better vocabularies, and better grades in school than unaffected children do (Grosvenor, 1970; Hirsch, 1959; Mutti et al., 2002; Williams et al., 2017). They are also more likely to pursue higher education (Cohn et al., 1988). Ironically, the school-based vision screening performed throughout the United States appears to identify all the children in school who are "at risk" for academic excellence! This is certainly not the way to spend limited educational funds devoted to vision screening. So where did we go wrong, and why is the school nurse spending so much time identifying the wrong children? The answer to these questions requires a discussion of "models of vision."

Currently in the United States, there are two primary models of vision that form the basis for the type of vision care provided to children and adults. The two models are described as the three-component model of vision and the one-component model of vision.

## THREE-COMPONENT MODEL OF VISION

The three-component model of vision includes the visual integrity, visual efficiency, and visual information processing outlined below and described in Table 31.1 and illustrated in Fig. 31.1.

### Component 1: Visual Integrity

The first part of the three-component model involves the ability to see clearly at all distances and deals with the optical system and eye health. Visual integrity includes visual acuity, refractive error, and eye health.

**Visual Acuity.** Visual acuity is a measure of the resolving power of the eye. An individual with 20/20 acuity has typical ability to see details at a distance. The numerator refers to the testing distance at which the child recognizes the stimulus, and the denominator refers to the distance at which the letter could be identified by a child with typical visual acuity. For example, 20/200 implies that a child with typical visual acuity could identify the letter presented at 200 ft.

**Refractive Error.** Refraction is the term used to describe the evaluation of the optical system of the eye. The refraction is the examination procedure used to determine if a child will benefit from glasses and the exact prescription that is appropriate. **Refractive error** refers to any disorder of refraction. When the optometrist performs the "refraction," they determine whether the individual is emmetropic (absence of refractive error), myopic (nearsighted), hyperopic (farsighted), or astigmatic. Myopia is a condition in which the length of the eye is too long, and a child has clear vision when reading but blurred vision when looking at a distance. Typically, myopia is easy to detect even without a vision examination because the child will simply say, "I cannot see the television," or "I cannot see the board." However, children with developmental disabilities and language problems may be unable to tell parents, teachers, and practitioners what is wrong. Case Example 31.1 illustrates this problem.

Hyperopia is a condition in which the length of the eye is too short, and a child has clear vision when looking at a distance but requires more effort to achieve clear vision when reading. This additional effort could cause eyestrain, blurred vision, and difficulty sustaining attention on a near task. In astigmatism, the length of the eye is not an issue. Rather, the curvature of the front of the eye is elliptical, instead of spherical, and the result is blurred vision at both far and near. All three conditions are easily treated with eyeglasses.

**Eye Health.** **Eye health** disorders can affect any part of the eye and its visual pathway. Fortunately, in the pediatric population, eye disease is quite rare. When eye disease is present, it may result in visual impairment. Visual impairment refers to a condition in which eye disease has caused permanent loss of tissue. Some eye diseases that occur in children are optic atrophy, nystagmus, retinopathy of prematurity, cortical visual impairment, and congenital cataracts. Children who are visually impaired have reduced visual acuity and are eligible to receive services from a teacher of the visually impaired in the school system.

### Component 2: Visual Efficiency

Visual efficiency refers to the effectiveness of the visual system to clearly, efficiently, and comfortably allow an individual to gather visual information at school and play (Scheiman, 2025). The various component skills of visual efficiency include the subcategories of accommodation, binocular vision, and ocular motility (i.e., eye movement).

**Accommodation (Focusing).** When an object is brought closer than 20 ft, a focusing adjustment must be made, or the object will appear blurred. This focusing adjustment is referred to as accommodation. Fig. 31.2 illustrates the front portion of the eye showing the lens and ciliary muscle.

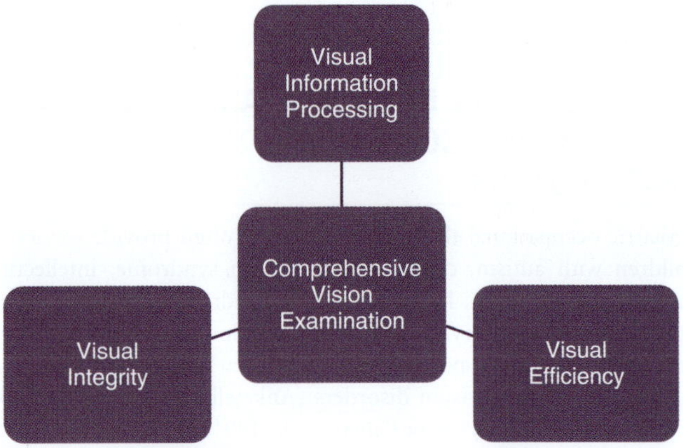


**Fig. 31.1** Three-component model of vision.

**TABLE 31.1 Three-Component Model of Vision**

| Component Name | Elements | Description |
|---|---|---|
| Visual integrity | Visual acuity | The ability to see fine detail |
| | Refractive error | The optical characteristics of the eye (myopia, hyperopia, and astigmatism) |
| | Eye health | Health of all components of the visual system from the eye to the brain |
| Visual efficiency | Accommodation | The ability to change focus form near to far objects |
| | Binocular vision | The ability to use both eyes in a coordinated manner |
| | Eye movements | The ability to maintain steady fixation on an object (fixation), to look form one object to another (saccades), and follow a moving object (pursuits) |
| Visual information processing | Visual spatial | The ability to understand right and left on one's own body and to project that awareness into space |
| | Visual analysis | The ability to analyze and interpret visual stimuli |
| | Visual motor integration | The ability to accurately reproduce a visual stimulus |

## CASE EXAMPLE 31.1

Peter, a 4-year-old child with autism, was referred to an optometrist for a vision examination by his occupational therapist. Peter was identified as a child with developmental delays very early in life, and recently the developmental pediatrician reached a diagnosis of autism. Peter has been receiving occupational therapy and speech-language services since the age of 2 years old through early intervention. Recently, his parents decided to seek the services of a private occupational therapist. This private practice occupational therapist performed an evaluation and was very concerned about a potential vision problem because Peter did not seem to look at objects when reaching for them, had poor visual attention, and appeared to get very close to objects when he did use his visual system.

The occupational therapist referred Peter to an optometrist for an examination. The results of this examination indicated that Peter has an unusually high degree of myopia (nearsightedness). The degree of myopia was so high that without glasses, Peter was unable to clearly see an object unless it was about 10 in from his eyes. The optometrist prescribed eyeglasses to be worn for all waking hours. The challenge was that Peter was also tactually defensive, and there was some doubt about whether Peter would wear the glasses. Fortunately, with the occupational therapist's help in dealing with the tactile defensiveness, Peter was able to adapt to the glasses in a week. Although this was only one of many problems for this child, the impact of the new glasses was significant, and the therapist noticed an immediate improvement in visually guided search behavior (visual attention). These improvements made other aspects of occupational and speech-language therapy progress more quickly.

This case illustrates a common problem in the care of children with developmental disabilities. The American Optometric Association (AOA Evidence-Based Optometry Guideline Development Group, 2017) recommends that for typically developing children, the first full eye examination should be at age 6 to 12 months. This should not be a screening at a pediatrician's office, but rather a comprehensive eye examination. The second comprehensive eye examination for the typically developing child should be at the age of 3 years. If this is the recommended schedule for the typically developing child, the importance of early vision care for the child with a development disability is even more important. Every child with a developmental disability should have a comprehensive vision examination as soon as such a disability is suspected. In this case, Peter likely needed eyeglasses even as a 6-month-old baby. Not knowing that high myopia was present from 4 years had a detrimental effect on his development, and this could have been avoided with early vision care.

When we look from far to near, the ciliary muscle contracts, and the lens changes shape, allowing us to focus on near objects. When we look from near to far, the ciliary muscle relaxes, and the shape of the lens returns to its resting state. **Accommodation** is the ability to change the focus of the eye so that objects at different distances can be seen clearly. Accommodative disorders are encountered in about 5% to 22.5% of children in the general population (Franco et al., 2021; Hussaindeen et al., 2016; Scheiman & Wick, 2019; Scheiman et al., 1996; Wajuihian & Hansraj, 2016a). Accommodative problems are more common in physically (LoCascio, 1977; Scheiman, 1984), intellectually (Watt et al., 2015), and developmentally delayed children (Chang et al., 2021; Scharre & Creedon, 1992; Simmons et al., 2009) and children who have had a cerebrovascular accident or traumatic brain injury (Master et al., 2016; Raghuram et al., 2019; Scheiman et al., 2021; Wiecek et al., 2021).

**Binocular Vision (Eye Teaming).** **Binocular vision** is the ability of the visual system to fuse or combine the information from the right and left eyes into one image. Other than refractive error, the most common vision problems encountered in clinical practice are binocular vision disorders. In a study of a clinical pediatric population, Scheiman et al. (1996) found that about 25% of children from 6 months to 18 years old had significant binocular vision disorders. Binocular vision problems are more common in physically, mentally, and developmentally delayed children, learning-disabled children, and children who have had a cerebrovascular accident or traumatic brain injury. There are two main types of binocular vision disorders: strabismic and nonstrabismic binocular disorders.

**Strabismus** is a condition in which the eyes are misaligned at least 1% of the time. It occurs in about 3% to 4% of the general population (McKean-Cowdin et al., 2013) and is often cosmetically obvious. Other terms used to describe strabismus include tropia, squint, cross-eyed, and wall-eyed. If the eyes tend to turn in, out, or up but this tendency is always controlled, the deviation is categorized as a nonstrabismic binocular vision disorder. Another frequently used term to describe this condition is phoria. When the eyes tend to drift inward, it is called esophoria, and when the eyes tend to drift outward, it is called exophoria. We become concerned about phoria when the tendency becomes moderate to large and the child's ability to compensate is inadequate.

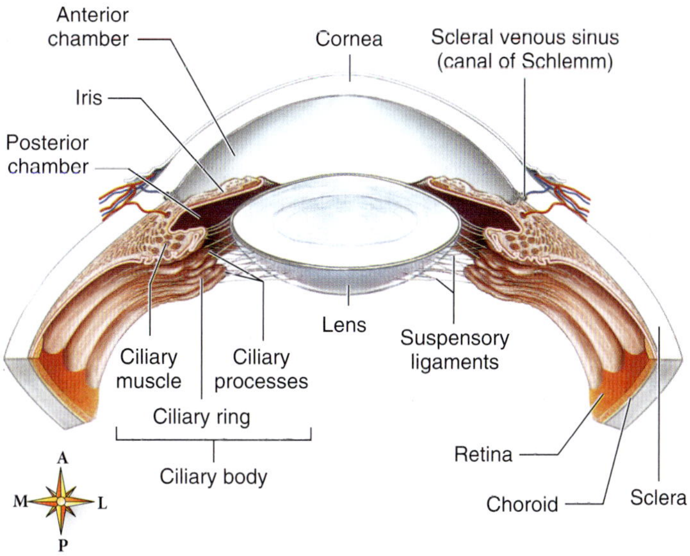


**Fig. 31.2** A diagram of the front portion of the eye showing the lens and ciliary muscle. (From Patton, K. T., & Thibodeau, G. A. (2013). *Anatomy & physiology* (8th ed.). Elsevier, p. 527.)

**Convergence insufficiency** is the most common nonstrabismic binocular vision disorder that occupational therapy practitioners encounter in children (Hussaindeen et al., 2016; Scheiman et al., 1996; Wajuihian & Hansraj, 2016b). It is a condition in which the eyes tend to drift outward during near work such as reading, while at a far distance the eyes work well together. This is one of the leading causes of eyestrain and discomfort. In the general population, convergence insufficiency is present in about 7% to 27% of the population (Carla et al., 2021; Hussaindeen et al., 2016; Ma et al., 2019; Nunes et al., 2019; Rouse et al., 1999; Wajuihian & Hansraj, 2016a, 2016b), while in the populations managed by occupational therapy practitioners the prevalence may be greater. Convergence insufficiency is also one of the most common vision problems that occurs after concussion in children (Master et al., 2016; Scheiman et al., 2021; Wiecek et al., 2021).

**Eye Movements.** There are three areas of eye movement function in which problems can occur: saccades, pursuits, and fixation. A **saccade** is an eye movement in which a child looks from one stationary object to another. The ideal saccade is a single eye movement that rapidly reaches and abruptly stops at the target of interest. *Pursuit* eye movements enable continuous clear vision of moving objects. This visual following reflex ideally produces eye movements that assure continuous foveal fixation of objects moving in space.

Eye movement disorders are an important diagnostic and management concern because of the effect such problems may have on occupations. For example, much of the emphasis of both researchers and clinicians has been on the relationship between eye movements and reading. During reading the two most important components of eye movements are saccades and fixations. Saccades take up approximately 10% of the reading time. The average saccade is about eight-to-nine-character spaces. Between the saccades, the eye is relatively still, in a fixational pause. For typical readers, the average duration of the fixation is 200 to 250 ms.

In early studies of the prevalence of eye movement disorders in elementary school-age children with learning and reading disabilities, 95% to 96% of the subjects had problems with eye movements such as saccades and pursuits (Hoffman, 1980; Sherman, 1973), and eye movement problems were the most prevalent vision disorder in the samples. Recently, eye movement issues have been used to predict dyslexia and have been associated with other neurodevelopmental disorders as well (Bilbao & Piñero, 2021a, 2021b; Prabha & Bhargavi, 2020; Ward & Kapoula, 2020).

Eye movement disorders can be divided into two distinct areas: saccadic and pursuit function. Saccades may be inaccurate, in two ways. The most common inaccuracy is a slight undershoot. In most cases the saccade is slightly short of the target, and the eye "glides" to alignment, but in more extreme cases, a second, smaller saccade is made to reach the target. A less common inaccuracy is an overshoot of the target. Saccadic dysfunction is a condition in which the accuracy and speed of saccadic eye movements are reduced relative to expected findings for the individual's age. Saccadic eye movement problems can lead to signs and symptoms such as loss of place when reading, difficulty copying from the board, and the need to use a guide when reading to avoid losing one's place. Problems in saccadic ability may be a primary factor interfering with a child's ability to read quickly, comfortably, and with adequate comprehension.

Pursuit dysfunction is a condition in which the individual is unable to accurately follow a moving object. Since pursuit eye movements are only involved when a target is moving, they are more difficult to relate to reading and school performance than saccades. However, pursuits may play a more significant role in occupations that require movement such as sports, games, bicycle riding, and activities in which the individual is moving, or the object of regard is moving.

### Component 3: Visual Information Processing Skills

Vision is more than just seeing clearly and comfortably. An individual must also be able to analyze, interpret, and make use of the incoming visual information to interact with the environment (Scheiman, 2025). This final aspect of the three-part model is visual information processing. **Visual information processing** refers to a group of visual cognitive skills used for extracting and organizing visual information from the environment and integrating this information with other sensory modalities and higher cognitive functions. Other terms such as visual perception, visual perceptual-motor, and visual processing may be used to describe similar skills. Visual information processing includes visual spatial, visual analysis, and **visual motor skills**. Occupational therapy practitioners frequently address visual processing skills to enable children and youth to engage in daily living, sports, play, and education.

**Visual Spatial Skills.** These allow a child to make judgments about the location of objects in visual space in reference to other objects and to the individual's own body. The terms *laterality* and *directionality* are also used when defining **visual spatial skills**. Laterality is the ability to understand right, left, front, back, up, and down on one's own body. Directionality is the ability of the child to project this awareness onto objects in their world.

**Visual Analysis Skills.** These skills contribute to the individual's ability to analyze and discriminate visually presented information, to determine the whole without seeing all of the parts, to identify more important features and ignore extraneous details, and to use visual imagery to recall past visual information (Scheiman, 2025). **Visual analysis skills** include the ability of the child to be aware of the distinctive features of visual forms, including shape, size, color, and orientation. Clinically, visual spatial dysfunction is subclassified into four categories: visual discrimination, visual figure ground, visual closure, and visual memory and visualization.

**Visual Motor Skills.** These skills refer to the child's ability to integrate visual information processing skills with fine and gross motor movement (e.g., copy designs, catching or kicking a ball) as well as executive functioning when completing novel tasks (Maurer & Roebers, 2021). Visual motor skills are a prerequisite for learning handwriting and keyboard skills and excelling in sports (Appelbaum & Erickson, 2016; Burris et al., 2020; Klein et al., 2011).

## ONE-COMPONENT MODEL OF VISION

The one-component model of vision, practiced by many eye care professionals, only includes an evaluation of visual integrity (i.e., visual acuity, refraction, and eye health). While the evaluation of *visual integrity* is an essential part of the vision examination, it is not sufficient to detect the vision problems that tend to be prevalent in the pediatric population. A natural question to ask is why a doctor would limit the vision examination to visual integrity and not evaluate all three components described above. The answer is often related to the nature of the professional education and training.

## THE EYE CARE PROFESSIONS

There are three primary providers in the eye care profession, sometimes referred to as the three "O's": opticianry, optometry, and ophthalmology. The differences between the three professions are significant and are related to the respective educational and clinical training programs for each profession (Table 31.2; Scheiman, 2025). The optician is the individual who helps a person select an appropriate eyeglass frame,

TABLE 31.2 **Eye Care Professions**

| Profession | Education/Clinical Training | VISUAL INTEGRITY Examination | VISUAL INTEGRITY Treatment | VISUAL EFFICIENCY Examination[a] | VISUAL EFFICIENCY Treatment | VISUAL PROCESSING Examination | VISUAL PROCESSING Vision Therapy |
|---|---|---|---|---|---|---|---|
| Optician | • Community college<br>• Technical schools<br>• Apprentice | X | X | X | X | X | X |
| Ophthalmologist | • 4 years college<br>• 4 years medical school<br>• Ophthalmology residency<br>• Fellowship | | • Lenses<br>• Prism<br>• Eye drops<br>• Surgery | • All will evaluate for strabismus<br>• Limited training for nonstrabismic, accommodative, and eye movement disorders | • Lenses<br>• Prism<br>• Eye drops<br>• Surgery<br>• No vision therapy | X• | X |
| Optometrist | • 4 years college<br>• 4 years optometry school<br>• Residency (15% complete a residency) | | • Lenses<br>• Prism<br>• Eye drops | • All trained<br>• Not all provide this service[a] | • All trained<br>• Not all provide this service[a] | • All trained<br>• Not all provide this service[a] | • All trained<br>• Not all provide this service[a] |

[a]To find an optometrist that follows the three-component model of vision, contact the American Academy of Optometry or COVD.

prepares the lenses based on the prescription, and then fits the frame to the person's face so that they are comfortable. The optician does not have the training to perform any clinical testing or treatment. The education and training of ophthalmologists (medical doctors) focuses on diagnosis and treatment of eye disease using medication and surgery. Thus, the emphasis is on the area defined above as "visual integrity." The areas of visual efficiency and visual processing problems are not emphasized in the training programs of the typical ophthalmologist.

The training and education of optometrists is quite different. Although optometrists are also educated to diagnose and treat eye disease, a significant portion of the educational program deals with the concept of vision and its relationship in play, school, work, and sports. The optometrist is taught to evaluate the visual system in a manner that allows diagnosis of visual conditions that can interfere with performance and affect quality of life. The educational curriculum for optometrists emphasizes the three-component model of vision.

With this background, one might think that the way to ensure that a child receives a comprehensive examination of visual integrity, efficiency, and processing would be to make sure the examination is performed by an optometrist. Unfortunately, it is not that simple, because while all optometrists receive this education, only a small percentage use this model of care in practice. Thus, a parent or an occupational therapy practitioner who wants to ensure that all aspects of vision are being evaluated must seek out an optometrist that practices with the three-component model of vision. Optometrists who offer this level of care often have completed additional residency training or have passed comprehensive examinations designed to assess their level of expertise in these areas. The two organizations that administer such examinations are the American Academy of Optometry (Binocular Vision, Perception, and Pediatric Optometry Section) and the College of Optometrists in Vision Development (COVD). Optometrists successfully completing the examination process for the American Academy of Optometry are called Diplomates in Binocular Vision, Perception, and Pediatric Optometry. Optometrists successfully completing the examination process for COVD are called Fellows of COVD (FCOVD).

These differences in educational experience and clinical training explain the experiences of practitioners relative to the eye care professions. Occupational therapy practitioners may experience frustration when attempting to help a child who they suspect may have a vision problem. For example, a practitioner may refer a child for an eye examination because of concern about tracking or focusing skills. Depending on the doctor to whom the child is referred, it would not be unusual for the child to be sent back with completely contradictory reports. Case Example 31.2 illustrates the importance of understanding each professional's role in vision.

This lack of uniformity in vision care is confusing to occupational therapy practitioners and to the public and may lead to a lack of identification and treatment of vision disorders that can interfere with occupation. The differences in approach between optometry and ophthalmology are important, and even within the optometric profession, philosophical differences may be significant. It is critical therefore that practitioners seeking meaningful information about a child's visual status make the referral to an eye care professional who has training and expertise in the areas of binocular vision, vision and learning, and vision therapy. This will require a referral to an optometrist who is either a Diplomate in Binocular Vision, Perception, and Pediatric Optometry (American Academy of Optometry, Diplomate in Binocular Vision, Perception, and Pediatric Optometry: https://aaopt.org/fellow-and-diplomate-directory/. Enter Binocular Vision, Perception, and Pediatric Optometry in the section entitled "Diplomate Section") or a Fellow in COVD (https://locate.covd.org/). The terms *behavioral optometrist* or *developmental optometrist* also may describe an optometrist with advanced expertise and training who would likely follow the three-component model of vision.

## PREVALENCE OF VISION PROBLEMS IN CHILDREN WITH TYPICAL DEVELOPMENT

Population-based studies remain the most valid way to determine the prevalence of a disease. While such studies exist for severe vision problems such as visual impairment and blindness, for the type of

## CASE EXAMPLE 31.2

Daniel, an 11-year-old child in sixth grade, has been complaining of difficulty with reading and working on a computer for almost 2 years. He complains of blurred vision and eyestrain after 10 to 15 minutes of reading. If he continues to read, the words start moving on the page, and ultimately, he begins to experience intermittent double vision and headaches. Because of these problems, he has not been able to complete homework assignments, his performance on written tests has deteriorated, and his overall school performance has changed from an A student to a C+ student.

His parents have been seeking answers for almost 2 years. First, in May of the fourth grade, they asked the school nurse to perform a vision screening even though he had passed the annual vision screening at school in October. The school nurse repeated the school vision screening and found perfect 20/20 vision in both eyes. School ended shortly thereafter, and most of Daniel's symptoms resolved over the summer. However, in the fall when he returned to school and started fifth grade, the problems recurred and became worse than the symptoms Daniel experienced in the fourth grade. In October, the parents brought Daniel to his pediatrician for an examination and advice. The pediatrician also performed a vision screening (visual acuity only) and found 20/20 vision in both eyes. Unable to find a medical basis for the visual symptoms and daily headaches, the pediatrician referred the child to a local pediatric ophthalmologist.

The pediatric ophthalmologist found that Daniel had a low degree of hyperopia (farsightedness) and 20/20 visual acuity in both eyes. She also found normal eye health and concluded that the symptoms Daniel was complaining about were not related to a vision problem. Because she could not find a basis for the daily headaches, she referred Daniel to a neurologist. By the time the parents were able to get an appointment with the neurologist it was already the end of February of Daniel's fifth grade experience. The neurologist was also unable to find an explanation and, to be conservative, ordered an MRI of the brain, which was also normal.

It was now April, and frustrated by this inability to find an answer that would help Daniel, his parents next turned to the family optometrist. The parents had been seeing this optometrist for about 10 years for their own eye care. The optometrist examined Daniel and confirmed that he had a low degree of hyperopia, 20/20 visual acuity in both eyes, and normal eye health. It was now almost the end of fifth grade, and Daniel continued to experience significant academic problems because of his inability to read comfortably for more than 10 minutes.

Daniel's parents began to look elsewhere for answers. A family member from another state told them that a friend's child recently had similar problems and had found an optometrist that practiced vision therapy. The therapy worked well for this child. After contacting these parents, they were given two websites to further explore the topic of vision therapy. The first was actually a Facebook page named "Vision Therapy Parents Unite." This Facebook page was developed by a parent who had a similar frustrating experience trying to find answers for their child. The second website provided was for the COVD, which provides educational and research information about vision therapy and learning-related vision problems along with a directory of optometrists who practice vision therapy.

With this new information, Daniel's parents found an optometrist in the area and scheduled an appointment. During the examination, the parents noticed that this optometrist performed many more and different examination procedures. The optometrist found that Daniel had a significant convergence insufficiency and accommodative insufficiency and recommended a 3-month period of vision therapy. Daniel had 1-hour weekly vision therapy sessions for about 14 weeks and had to practice some of the procedure he learned in the office at home (3 days a week for 15 minutes). He started experiencing better comfort about 6 to 8 weeks into the therapy program, and by 3 months, he was able to read comfortably for as long as necessary.

Unfortunately, this case study is not an unusual one, and many children and parents experience this long delay in finding a resolution to the vision problem. Daniel had to endure symptoms for almost 2 years and had to go through numerous unnecessary examinations. This case illustrates a number of important issues. First, the school vision screening has very little value and should not be relied on as an indication of whether a vision problem is present. Second, almost all pediatricians will refer only to a pediatric ophthalmologist who generally does not practice vision therapy. Finally, it illustrates the importance of determining the eye doctor's "model of vision" before scheduling an appointment. Before scheduling an appointment, parents should ask if the doctor will examine the areas of focusing, eye teaming, eye movements, and visual processing, and if a problem is found, whether the office offers vision therapy as a treatment option.

https://www.facebook.com/groups/VTparentsunite http://www.covd.org/

problems common in the pediatric population, most studies in the United States with school-age children have been clinic-based studies. The most common problems an optometrist is likely to encounter in children are accommodative and binocular vision disorders. In particular, nonstrabismic binocular vision problems, specifically convergence insufficiency and accommodative disorders, are quite common (Atowa et al., 2019; Hussaindeen et al., 2016; Jang & Park, 2015; Nunes et al., 2019; Scheiman et al., 1996). Thus, there is evidence that even in the typically developing pediatric population, visual efficiency problems are quite common in the United States and abroad.

## PREVALENCE OF VISION PROBLEMS IN CHILDREN WITH DISABILITIES

Many children with disabilities have undetected and untreated visual problems. They have a higher rate of vision disorders and should receive a comprehensive pediatric eye and vision examination (AOA Evidence-Based Optometry Guideline Development Group, 2017). Practice guidelines suggest "Early identification of specific visual deficits could lead to interventions to improve the educational and occupational achievement and quality of life for these high-risk children" (AOA Evidence-Based Optometry Guideline Development Group, 2017, p. 27).

Reviews document a high occurrence of visual difficulties in children with special needs (Bilbao & Piñero, 2021a, 2021b; Hussaindeen & Murali, 2020), including cerebral palsy (Heydarian et al., 2022), Down syndrome (Sun & Kraus, 2023), and autism (Little, 2018).

## PREVALENCE OF VISION PROBLEMS IN PEDIATRIC CONCUSSION

Pediatric concussion is increasingly common. Veliz et al. (2017) surveyed 13,088 adolescents (50.2% were female, 46.8% were white) with a mean age of 16 years. An estimated 19.5% of adolescents reported at least one diagnosed concussion in their lifetime; 14.0% reported one diagnosed concussion; and 5.5% reported being diagnosed with more than one concussion. In another study of 52,949 adolescents (Veliz et al., 2021) the lifetime prevalence of at least one self-reported concussion increased from 19.5% in 2016 to 24.6% in 2020. Another group of researchers (Haarbauer-Krupa et al., 2021) found a lifetime prevalence of concussion to be from 3.6% to 7.0% for children ages 3–17 years and from 6.5% to 18.3% for adolescents 13–17 years.

There are also increasing concerns that children may be particularly vulnerable to the consequences of concussion and may have more prolonged and complicated outcomes from a cognitive and developmental perspective (Halstead et al., 2018; Rotter & Kamat, 2019). In recent studies (Master et al., 2016; Scheiman et al., 2021), there was found a high prevalence of visual efficiency problems in children with concussion.

## VISION SCREENING FOR OCCUPATIONAL THERAPY PRACTITIONERS

There are many instruments and vision screening methods that have been suggested for the pediatric population. In most school systems in the United States, visual screening is performed at least once during the child's elementary school years and sometimes on an annual basis. Also, many pediatricians periodically perform a vision screening. However, the school and pediatrician-based vision screenings only examine visual acuity. Occupational therapy practitioners are also concerned with the child's visual efficiency and visual information processing as these skills influence occupational performance. This section describes screening techniques for the most frequently undetected vision problems, which are visual efficiency (binocular vision, accommodative, and eye movements) and visual information processing problems (visual spatial, visual analysis, and visual motor integration).

### Screening for Visual Efficiency Problems

One potential approach to deciding whether to administer a vision screening is to first administer a symptom questionnaire. The Convergence Insufficiency Symptom Survey (CISS; available at no cost) is a validated questionnaire for children 9 to 17 years of age that has been used in many clinical studies to identify children with visual symptoms (Borsting et al., 2003, Fig. 31.3). Although it was originally designed to identify children with convergence insufficiency who were

**Convergence Insufficiency Symptom Survey**

**Name** ____________________ **DATE** ___/___/___
**Instructions:** Read the following subject instructions and then each item exactly as written. If subject responds with "yes" - please qualify with frequency choices. **Do not give examples.**
**Subject instructions:** Please answer the following questions about how your eyes feel when reading or doing close work.

| | | Never | Infrequently | Sometimes | Fairly often | Always |
|---|---|---|---|---|---|---|
| 1. | Do your eyes feel tired when reading or doing close work? | 0 | 1 | 2 | 3 | 4 |
| 2. | Do your eyes feel uncomfortable when reading or doing close work? | 0 | 1 | 2 | 3 | 4 |
| 3. | Do you have headaches when reading or doing close work? | 0 | 1 | 2 | 3 | 4 |
| 4. | Do you feel sleepy when reading or doing close work? | 0 | 1 | 2 | 3 | 4 |
| 5. | Do you lose concentration when reading or doing close work? | 0 | 1 | 2 | 3 | 4 |
| 6. | Do you have trouble remembering what you have read? | 0 | 1 | 2 | 3 | 4 |
| 7. | Do you have double vision when reading or doing close work? | 0 | 1 | 2 | 3 | 4 |
| 8. | Do you see the words move, jump, swim or appear to float on the page when reading or doing close work? | 0 | 1 | 2 | 3 | 4 |
| 9. | Do you feel like you read slowly? | 0 | 1 | 2 | 3 | 4 |
| 10. | Do your eyes ever hurt when reading or doing close work? | 0 | 1 | 2 | 3 | 4 |
| 11. | Do your eyes ever feel sore when reading or doing close work? | 0 | 1 | 2 | 3 | 4 |
| 12. | Do you feel a "pulling" feeling around your eyes when reading or doing close work? | 0 | 1 | 2 | 3 | 4 |
| 13. | Do you notice the words blurring or coming in and out of focus when reading or doing close work? | 0 | 1 | 2 | 3 | 4 |
| 14. | Do you lose your place while reading or doing close work? | 0 | 1 | 2 | 3 | 4 |
| 15. | Do you have to re-read the same line of words when reading? | 0 | 1 | 2 | 3 | 4 |
| To | score, total the number of "X"s in each column | | | | | |
| Multiply by the column value | | x | x1 | x2 | x3 | x4 |
| Sum values | | | | | | |

CISS SCORE: ________________ CITT Study Group 2002

**Fig. 31.3** The Convergence Insufficiency Symptom Survey (CISS).

also symptomatic, it may be sensitive to other visual efficiency problems such as accommodative and eye movement disorders.

The questionnaire consists of 15 items that are read aloud to the child. The examiner reads the questions while the child views a card with the answers and is instructed to choose one of five possible answers (never, not too often, sometimes, fairly often, and always). Each response is scored as zero to four points, with four representing the highest frequency of symptom occurrence (i.e., always). The 15 item scores are summed to obtain the total CISS score. The lowest possible score (least symptoms) is zero and the highest is 60 (most symptomatic). Based on previous work (Borsting et al., 2003; Rouse et al., 1999), a CISS score of 16 or above suggests that a visual efficiency vision screening should be considered. It is important to understand that a high CISS score by itself should not be the basis for concluding that a vision problem is present. If based on the questionnaire the decision is made to do a vision screening, Table 31.3 summarizes recommended vision screening tests for visual efficiency, which include accommodation, binocular vision, and eye movement problems.

**Accommodation.** The most common accommodative problem in the pediatric population is accommodative insufficiency (Scheiman et al., 1996). The diagnosis of accommodative insufficiency is based on an assessment of accommodative amplitude. **Accommodative amplitude** refers to how much accommodative (focusing) ability an individual has available. The minimum acceptable accommodation amplitude for any child can be calculated using a formula: accommodative amplitude = 15 – 1/4(child's age). See Box 31.1 for an example of how this is calculated.

**Binocular Vision.** The most common binocular vision problem in the pediatric population is convergence insufficiency (Goering et al., 2024; Rouse et al., 1999). One of the key tests used to diagnose convergence insufficiency is the near point of convergence. In this test, the examiner moves an object toward the client's eyes and asks the client to try and maintain single vision for as long as possible. When the client reports double vision, the examiner records the distance from the eyes and refers to this measurement as the near point of convergence break. They then slowly move the target away from the client until they report single vision again. When the child reports single vision, the examiner records the distance from the child's eyes. This is the near point of convergence recovery finding. The expected finding for any child is to be able to maintain single vision to a distance less than 6 cm from the eyes. So, the break should be less than 6 cm and the recovery less than 9 cm. See online instructor resources for directions on measuring near point convergence.

**Eye Movements.** There are two distinct eye movements that should be evaluated in children: saccadic and pursuit eye movements. A saccade is an eye movement in which the child looks from one stationary object to another. Examples would be looking from the board to the desk, reading eye movements, and looking for an object in a desk.

There are two different tests that can be used for screening saccadic eye movements. The Developmental Eye Movement (DEM) test requires the child to rapidly call out numbers on a page (see Fig. 31.4 for DEM examples). The Northeastern State University College of Optometry Eye Movement Test (NSUCO) was developed at the Northeastern State University College of Optometry. It was designed as an inexpensive, low-tech, chairside technique that can be used with younger children who are unable to attend and concentrate for long enough periods of time to participate in more sophisticated eye movement testing using video recordings. Data are available showing that the test has acceptable test retest reliability (Maples, 1995). See Evolve site for directions on how to administer both tests.

**TABLE 31.3 Recommended Vision Screening Tests**

| Component to be Screened | Element to be Screened | Name of Test |
|---|---|---|
| Visual efficiency | Accommodation | • CISS<br>• Accommodative amplitude (near point rod) |
| | Binocular vision | • CISS<br>• Near point of convergence (near point rod) |
| | Eye movements | • CISS<br>• NSUCO eye movement test<br>• Developmental Eye Movement Test |
| Visual information processing | Visual spatial | • Garner reversal frequency test |
| | Visual analysis | • TVPS–4<br>• MFVPT |
| | Visual motor | • DTVMI |

*CISS*, Convergence Insufficiency Symptom Survey; *DTVMI*, Developmental Test of Visual Motor Integration; *NSUCO*, Northeastern State University College of Optometry Eye Movement Test; *TVPS–4*, Test of Visual Perceptual Skills, Fourth Edition.
Available from: (1) Gulden Ophthalmics, (2) Optometric Extension Program, and (3) Bernell Corporation.

**BOX 31.1 Measuring Amplitude of Accommodation**

**Example**: What would be the minimal acceptable accommodative amplitude for an 8-year-old child?

Calculation formula: accommodative amplitude = 15 – 1/4(age)
= 15 – 1/4(8)
= 15 – 2
= 13D

When referring to optics, the unit of measure is referred to as a diopter (D). So, the minimum accommodative amplitude for an 8-year-old child would be 13 diopters, or 13D.

The accommodative amplitude declines in all children as they develop, and this decline continues into adulthood. For example, based on the formula 15 – 1/4(age), a 4-year-old would be expected to have 14D, an 8-year-old 13D, a 12-year-old 12D, and a 16-year-old 11D of accommodation.

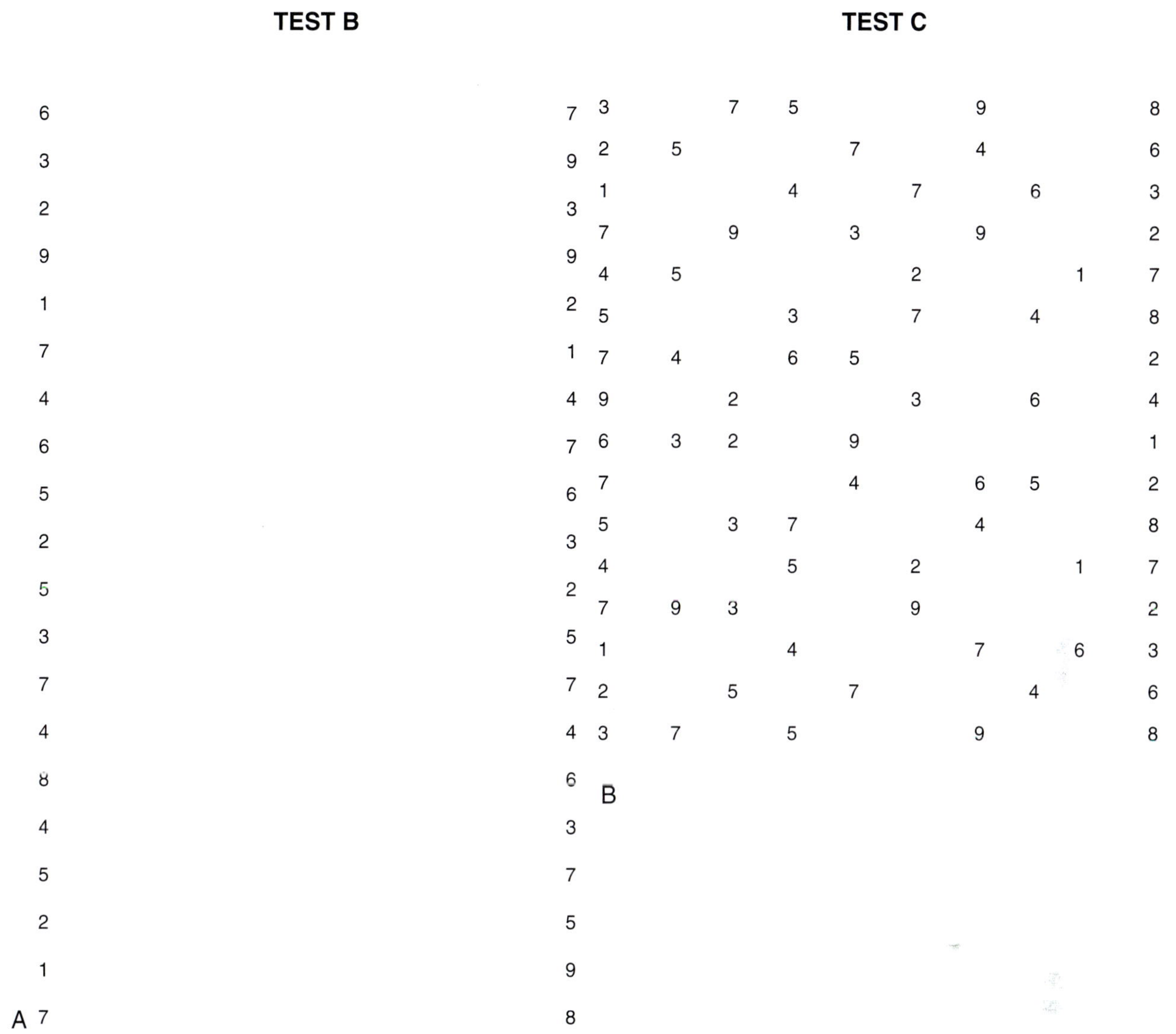


**Fig. 31.4** Developmental Eye Movement (DEM) test.

## Screening for Visual Information Processing Problems

Table 31.3 summarizes screening tests that may be used to evaluate visual information processing skills (i.e., visual spatial, visual analysis, and visual motor integration).

**Visual Spatial Skills.** The Gardner Reversal Frequent Test: Recognition Subtest evaluates the existence, nature, and frequency of occurrence of receptive letter and number reversals (reversals that the child can recognize). In this test, the child is asked to mark off those letters and numbers that are written backward or reversed. This test provides information about the child's development of normal internal and external spatial concepts.

This test is appropriate for children 5–15 years old. When administering this test, it is important to seat the child so that he or she cannot observe books and other written material that may provide information about letter and number orientation. This is an untimed test, and children who have difficulty in this area may become frustrated by this task and take excessively long periods of time to complete the test. When using this test as a screening, discontinue the test if it becomes clear after a short period of time that the child is struggling. See the test manual for testing procedures.

**Visual Analysis Skills.** The Test of Visual Perceptual Skills, Fourth Edition (TVPS–4) assesses seven aspects of visual analysis skills including visual discrimination, visual spatial relationships, visual form constancy, visual figure ground, visual closure, visual memory, and visual sequential memory.

Another popular test is the Motor Free Visual Perception Test (MVPT) that allows children to indicate responses without using motor skills. Refer to Appendix A for more information about these and other visual perceptual tests.

**Visual Motor Integration Skills.** The Developmental Test of Visual Motor Integration has well-developed normative data for ages 2 through 18 and can be used through adulthood as well. This test evaluates the child's ability to integrate visual information processing and fine motor skills by assessing their ability to accurately copy a visual stimulus. Refer to Appendix A for more information about this and other visual motor tests.

## VISUAL INTERVENTION

Occupational therapy practitioners must understand the treatment options that are available for refractive, visual efficiency, and visual information processing disorders. With this knowledge, they can be more effective as advocates for children and help parents decide when to seek vision care. The treatment options available for vision disorders include lenses, prism, occlusion, vision therapy, and surgery (see Table 31.4 for a list of treatment modalities and the areas they address).

### Eyeglasses

Refractive errors such as significant levels of myopia, hyperopia, and astigmatism are effectively treated with eyeglasses. Almost every child has some degree of refractive error. However, glasses are only prescribed when the degree of refractive error is outside the normal range and impacts in a negative way on occupation. Glasses can be prescribed for toddlers and infants when necessary. When children are older, eyeglasses can be replaced with contact lenses. Contact lenses are considered when the child is responsible enough to care for the lenses and has good hygiene habits.

Eyeglasses may also be prescribed for a child who has accommodative insufficiency (low amplitude of accommodation compared to the expected value). Children with accommodative insufficiency often complain of blurred vision, eyestrain, discomfort, and trouble concentrating when reading. Because the amplitude accommodation is low, the child will have blurry vision unless they use additional neuromuscular effort. However, this additional effort can cause the classic symptoms of eyestrain, fatigue, and trouble concentrating. One type of lens, called a "plus" lens or a "convex" lens, can help a child accommodate (focus) more effectively when looking at close objects. The problem with these lenses, however, is that they only help the child when looking at nearby objects. If the child tries to wear these glasses to see the board, their vision will be blurred. Thus, the child would have to remove the glasses for distance viewing. For a young child in elementary school, this can be problematic. The constant taking on and off the glasses may lead to broken frames, scratched lenses, and inconsistent use. Thus, in these situations, eye professionals typically prescribe eyeglasses with a bifocal lens, allowing the child to wear the glasses full time in school.

For children who have esophoria (eyes tend to drift inward), eyeglasses can often be helpful. The same lens that is prescribed for accommodative insufficiency (convex or plus lens) can be used to treat esophoria. To understand why this would work, one needs to understand a visual system reflex, referred to as the accommodative-convergence ratio, or AC/A ratio. When an individual looks from a far object to a near object, two things occur in unison. First the eyes must accommodate or focus from the distant object to the near object to achieve clear vision. The second thing that must occur is that the eyes must rotate in, or converge, to maintain one single image. The AC/A ratio is a reflex in which any accommodation response triggers a convergence response as well. So, when a child looks from far to near, the accommodative system adjusts and causes convergence to occur. Thus, if we place a plus lens in front of a child's eyes who has esophoria, because the child does not have to accommodate as much through the plus lens, less convergence occurs, which helps reduce the level of esophoria.

### Prism

Prism is a second treatment modality that can be used to treat binocular vision problems. Prism is considered the treatment of choice for vertical misalignment of the eyes. A prism bends or alters the direction of the light entering the eyes. Prism is not designed to eliminate the vertical deviation. Rather, it is a compensatory treatment approach. There is widespread consensus, as well as research support (London & Wick, 1987), that prism is an appropriate treatment for vertical misalignment of the eyes, and it has also been used to modify gait and posture in individuals with autism spectrum disorder (Errington et al., 2013; Suttle et al., 2015).

### Occlusion

The primary use of occlusion (patch) in children is to treat amblyopia. Amblyopia is a condition in which the visual acuity is less than 20/20 in one eye in spite of the fact that the eyes are healthy and the child is wearing glasses that correctly compensate for any refractive error. The loss of visual acuity is generally due to one of two causes. In some cases, the child develops a strabismus (crossed eye) before the age of 6 years; in such cases the brain experiences

**TABLE 31.4 Summary of Treatment Modalities**

| | Lenses | Prism | Occlusion | Vision Therapy | Eye Drops | Surgery |
|---|---|---|---|---|---|---|
| Refractive error | ✓ | | | | | |
| Amblyopia | ✓ | | ✓ | ✓ | ✓ | |
| Accommodation | ✓ | | | ✓ | | |
| Binocular vision–strabismus | ✓ | ✓ | ✓ | ✓ | ✓ | ✓ |
| Binocular vision–nonstrabismic | ✓ | ✓ | | ✓ | | |
| Eye movement | | | | ✓ | | |
| Visual information processing | | | | ✓ | | |

double vision, which is intolerable. If the condition is not detected and treated promptly, the brain adapts using a mechanism referred to as suppression. Suppression is a process in which the cells in the visual cortex show decreased responsivity to visual stimulation. Studies found physiologic and anatomic changes in the visual cortex cells associated with the amblyopic eye. As a result, when the child is asked to use that eye, the visual acuity is less than normal. The second cause of monocular amblyopia is a significant difference in the optics of the two eyes before the age of 6 years. For example, the right eye might have a low degree of hyperopia, while the left eye has a high degree of hyperopia. This condition is called anisometropia, and in such cases the brain favors the eye with the lower refractive error. The same adaptive process (suppression) described above for strabismus occurs in anisometropia, leading to amblyopia. Occlusion is effective for children with amblyopia of either etiology, and age should not be used as a variable to decide if treatment should be prescribed (AOA Evidence-Based Optometry Guideline Development Group, 2017; Chen et al., 2020; Papageorgiou et al., 2019; Park, 2019).

If a child has recent onset double vision due to the presence of strabismus (misaligned eyes), the first treatment attempts are always to restore alignment of the eyes using lenses, prism, or vision therapy. In some cases, surgery may be required. However, if none of these treatment options are effective for eliminating double vision, occlusion would be the remaining option. Occlusion, of course, is 100% effective for eliminating double vision. The problems are that the treatment is not satisfactory based on cosmesis, and the treatment is merely designed to eliminate symptoms, rather than to treat the underlying cause of the double vision.

### Vision Therapy

**Vision therapy** has been a treatment option for binocular vision, accommodative, and eye movement disorders since the 1920s and 1930s (Press, 2021). The treatment teaches the child how to use neuromuscular patterns of vision more effectively. Research has documented its effectiveness for convergence insufficiency, which is often associated with symptoms that interfere with everyday function such as frequent loss of place, loss of concentration, having to reread, reading slowly, trouble remembering what was read, sleepiness, blurred vision, diplopia, headaches, and/or eyestrain during reading or other near work (Barnhardt et al., 2012; Borsting et al., 2003; Carla et al., 2021; Davis et al., 2016; Hussaindeen et al., 2016; Letourneau & Ducic, 1988; Ma et al., 2019; Nunes et al., 2019; Rouse et al., 1999; Wajuihian & Hansraj, 2016b). The Convergence Insufficiency Treatment Trial Study Group (CITT Group) completed three multicenter, placebo-controlled RCTs evaluating the effectiveness of commonly prescribed treatments for children with symptomatic convergence insufficiency (CITT-ART Investigator Group, 2019b; Convergence Insufficiency Treatment Trial Investigator Group, 2008; Scheiman, Mitchell, et al., 2005) and demonstrated the effectiveness of office-based vision therapy for convergence insufficiency in children and young adults. A recent Cochrane systematic review of nonsurgical interventions for convergence insufficiency concluded that "office-based vision therapy is more effective than home-based convergence exercises or home-based computer vision therapy/orthoptics for children with symptomatic convergence insufficiency" (Scheiman et al., 2020). Another study of various home-based therapies, such as pencil push-ups and home-based therapy using computer software demonstrated that home-base therapy is no more effective than placebo treatment (Pediatric Eye Disease Investigator, 2016).

Vision therapy has been shown to be an effective treatment for accommodative problems (Chen et al., 2021; Scheiman et al., 2011) and is sometimes used in conjunction with lenses to achieve the best possible outcome (Scheiman & Wick, 2019). Lenses, prism, and surgery are not effective treatments for children with developmentally based eye movement problems; vision therapy is the treatment of choice. A number of studies have demonstrated the effectiveness of vision therapy for eye movement disorders (Dodick et al., 2017; Solan et al., 2003). Dodick et al. (2017) investigated the effect of in-school saccadic training on reading performance. In this crossover design, study participants were randomized into treatment and control groups, who then underwent 18 20-minute training sessions over five pre- and posttreatment reading assessments that included fluency, comprehension, and rapid number naming performance. The treatment group had significantly greater improvement than the control group in fluency and comprehension.

Similar to eye movements, lenses, prism, and surgery are not effective treatments for children with developmentally based visual information processing problems, and vision therapy is the treatment of choice. Several studies reported the effectiveness of vision therapy for visual information processing problems (Farr & Leibowitz, 1976; Seiderman, 1980; Solan et al., 2004; Tassinari & Eastland, 1997; Uttal et al., 2013). See Box 31.2 and Evolve site for more information on vision therapy.

**Vision Therapy and Occupation.** There is evidence that successful vision therapy leads to a decrease in symptoms, such as attention, reading, and visual function (Barnhardt et al., 2012). However a randomized clinical trial completed by the CITT-ART Investigator Group demonstrated that although there were significant gains in reading (CITT-ART Investigator Group, 2019a) and visual attention (CITT-ART Investigator Group, 2021) in both the vision therapy group and the control group, there was no significant difference between the two groups. These findings suggest that while successful treatment of convergence and accommodative problems leads to improved visual function and a reduction in symptoms, it will not by itself necessarily lead to improved reading performance. Thus, additional therapy such as reading remediation, speech-language, and occupational therapy may be necessary to achieve improvements in occupational performance.

## THE ROLE OF THE OCCUPATIONAL THERAPY PRACTITIONER IN VISION THERAPY

Vision therapy is considered part of the practice of optometry and is considered an appropriated treatment for accommodation, binocular vision, eye movements, visual information processing, and amblyopia. For some of these areas (i.e., eye movements and visual information processing), occupational therapy practitioners can comfortably participate in providing therapy within the context of occupation. However, occupational therapy practitioners should work with an optometrist when addressing binocular and accommodative disorders.

Occupational therapy practitioners are encouraged to work with an optometrist providing direct intervention to support children's progress and reinforce vision therapy while addressing the child's occupational performance goals. A child may make more progress if the practitioner reinforces their vision therapy during

**BOX 31.2 Vision Therapy**

Optometrists are taught to evaluate the visual system in a manner that allows diagnosis of visual conditions that can interfere with performance and quality of life. Optometrists and occupational therapy practitioners collaborate to support children and adolescents in improving their visual processing to participate in desired activities. Occupational therapy practitioners seeking to become more involved in vision therapy for eye movements and information processing may use a variety of screening tools and associated resources to intervene. See the Evolve Learning site for further description of vision therapy screening procedures and examples of intervention resources.

their sessions. It is important to understand that occupational therapy is not a substitute for optometric vision therapy. Rather, the techniques can be used by practitioners to supplement optometric vision therapy being performed in the optometric office (see Box 31.2). Before using any of these techniques, the child should have a vision examination by an optometrist that follows the three-component model of vision. Occupational therapy practitioners who address vision work very closely with the optometrist to coordinate techniques.

Occupational therapy practitioners may also perform vision therapy techniques while collaborating with an optometrist in a rehabilitation setting. A trend that is becoming more common is that optometrists are becoming more directly involved in the care of patients with acquired brain injury within rehabilitation hospitals. In most cases, the optometrist examines the patient within the hospital and prescribes appropriate treatment that may include lenses, prism, occlusion, and vision therapy. The vision therapy is carried out in the hospital by the occupational therapy practitioner, and progress is monitored by the optometrist (Scheiman, 2000). Case Example 31.3 describes the collaboration between an optometrist and occupational therapy practitioner.

Fessler et al. (2020) performed a qualitative study to investigate collaborative care between co-located occupational therapists and optometrists. Participants indicated that although barriers exist, exercising humility, upholding patient-centered focus, maintaining mutual respect, communicating frequently, and co-location were factors that enable collaboration. The authors concluded that the study results support the coordination of care, through optometry and occupational therapy collaboration, in the treatment of visual deficits in children.

## OCCUPATIONAL THERAPY INTERVENTION ADDRESSING VISUAL SKILLS FOR OCCUPATIONAL PERFORMANCE

Occupational therapy practitioners often work with children who have visual challenges. They provide a variety of intervention approaches to support children's engagement in meaningful daily occupations, such as school, play, activities of daily living, instrumental activities of daily living, leisure, work, and social participation (AOTA, 2020). As such, they frequently observe how visual challenges interfere with a child's ability to engage successfully in their occupations. They may notice infants who do not look at faces, pay visual attention to toys, scan the room to find objects or people, or reach for objects successfully. While occupational therapy practitioners do not address **visual integrity** (i.e., visual acuity, refractive error, eye health), they may make early referrals to appropriate eye professionals and may assist the family in following their plan of care. They may also teach children to take care of their glasses or contacts as part of self-care.

Occupational therapy practitioners do address issues of visual efficiency (i.e., accommodation, binocular vision, and eye movements) to support the child's ability to engage in a variety of play, academic, self-care, or social activities. In promoting a child's occupational performance, they reinforce vision through occupation. For example, with

**CASE EXAMPLE 31.3**

Molly, a 6-year-old child, was not doing well in first grade. She was having trouble with letter and number recognition; sight vocabulary; and reversing and transposing letters, numbers, and words; and she was unable to copy off the board quickly enough. She struggled in kindergarten with many of the same issues and at the end of the year had an evaluation by the school-based occupational therapist. The occupational therapist found fine motor issues, problems with her pencil grip, and visual perceptual problems in the areas of visual memory, visual discrimination, and visual motor integration. The school agreed to provide occupational therapy services twice a month for first grade.

The parents also brought Molly to a local optometrist who offered vision therapy as a service in her practice. This examination indicated that there was a moderate degree of hyperopia (farsightedness), problems with saccadic eye moments, directionality visual memory, visual form discrimination, and visual motor integration problems. The optometrist recommended eyeglasses to be worn full time to treat hyperopia. She also recommended weekly vision therapy sessions and suggested the therapy could take 6 to 9 months.

Molly's parents told the optometrist that Molly was already going to receive occupational therapy services, and they were not sure whether both vision therapy and occupational therapy were necessary. The optometrist reviewed the therapist's report, and there were some key differences in both the diagnosis and treatment approaches. First, the optometrist found significant eye movement and directionality problems that the occupational therapist had not found in her evaluation. Second, the optometrist felt that two 30-minute sessions of occupational therapy would not be sufficient to solve Molly's problem in a reasonable period of time. With the parents' permission, the optometrist contacted the occupational therapist, and after speaking, they agreed to collaborate in the care of Molly. The therapist added some saccadic eye movement procedures to her therapy and supplemented the therapy provided by the optometrist. The child had one vision therapy session once week at the optometrist's office and two 30-minute sessions of school-based occupational therapy.

This is an illustration of one way in which an optometrist and occupational therapist can collaborate in the care of a child with visual efficiency and visual information processing problems. While the occupational therapist concentrated on the school-related issues of letter, number, and word recognition and copying from the board, the optometrist therapy was designed to work on the skill level.

infants the practitioner may encourage reaching for a rattle as part of play and exploration. With an older child, the practitioner may address eye movement skills by engaging in activities such as "I spy" or word search games or games with ball skills. Games such as tetherball (Fig. 31.5A) or hoop games (Fig. 31.5B) or parachute games (Fig. 31.5C) are good ways for children to practice eye movement skills. They may engage children in games such as "Let's go Fishin" (See Fig. 31.6), tracking games on computers, *What's different between these two pictures?* type activities, and follow the light games. These activities allow children to fixate on an object, look from one object to another, and follow a moving object. The practitioner designs the activities so they are slightly challenging for the child's level. Table 31.5 provides examples of activities that address specific elements of vision.

As the child engages in the activity, the occupational therapy practitioner observes performance and grades and adapts activities as necessary. For example, the practitioner may reposition visual stimuli, use different colors or levels of contrast, slow down a moving object, or increase or decrease the size of the visual target. The practitioner may also need to decrease visual stimuli if the child has trouble being distracted.

Occupational therapy practitioners frequently address visual information processing skills (visual perceptual skills) to support a child's progress in school or at home. Therapy activities may require children to discriminate colors, shapes, sizes, and items through play or

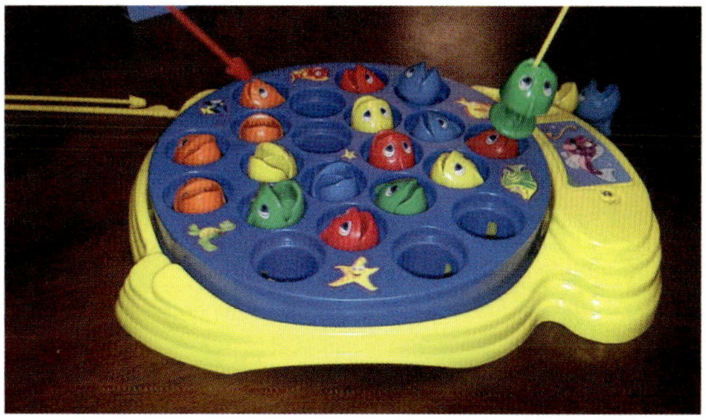

**Fig. 31.6** Occupational therapy practitioners engage children in games such as "Let's go Fishin" that promote visual tracking skills. The occupational therapy practitioner can modify the speed of the game to grade the visual motor skills required.

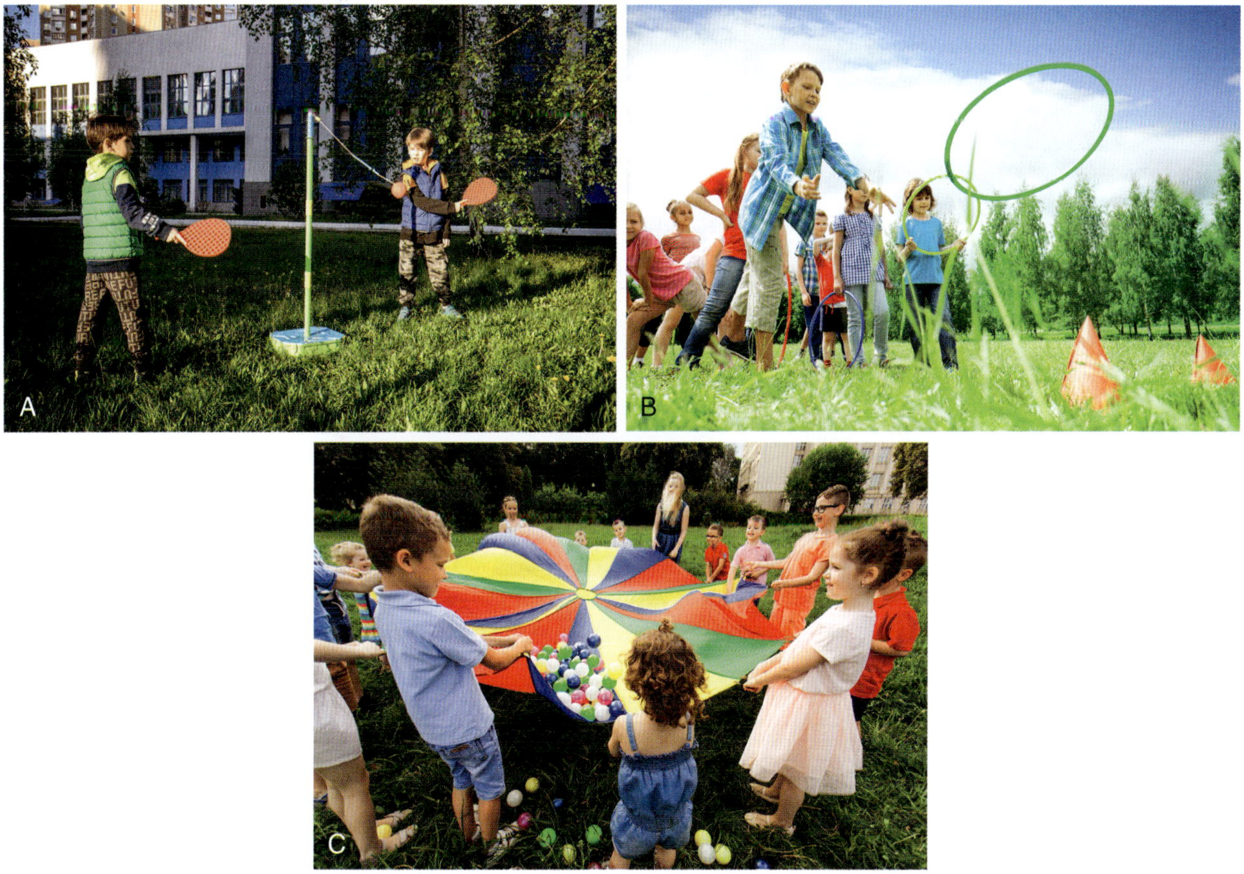

**Fig. 31.5** Occupational therapy practitioners promote children's eye movement through activities that require them to follow a moving object (ball). (A) Tetherball promotes visual motor integration as the child follows the ball and moves in accordance. (B) Playing games such as throwing the hoop over a target promotes visual tracking skills with bilateral upper extremity coordination. (C) Children practice visual tracking skills as they play parachute games.

**TABLE 31.5 Sample Activities That Occupational Therapy Practitioners May Use to Address Vision**

| Visual Skills | Occupational Therapy Games and Activities | Daily Use |
|---|---|---|
| Saccades | Games to follow the light<br>Catching bubbles<br>Find the specific letter (color or object) in a string | Reading, copying from board, shopping (scanning the products) |
| Pursuits | Hit the moving target (e.g., balloon volleyball)<br>Tracking games such as follow the rolling ball, roll the ball into a cup, find the object, throw an object to a target | Pursuits, reading, environmental awareness, playing sports (such as tetherball), scanning the room for objects, crossing the street (scanning the environment) |
| **Visual Information Processing** | | |
| Visual spatial skills | Differentiate between right and left sides, Simon says, dance games,<br>Games to understand position in space, such as right, left, up, down, over, under, in, out, on, below, obstacle courses, playing with figurines, building things | Body awareness, reading, writing, constructing, drawing, understanding distance and the relationship of objects to each other for organizing and using things |
| Visual analysis skills | **Discrimination:** Games to find differences in objects, Clue, I spy, identifying objects based on color, size, shape. | Selecting objects and items, such as toothbrush versus pencil, sorting coins, selecting dishes and utensils, choosing the correct key; identifying one's clothes or toys |
| | **Figure ground:** Finding objects in the background (such as hiding objects and having the child find them) | Figure ground is required in everyday tasks, such as finding a pencil on the desk, picking out clothes in drawers, finding an item |
| | **Visual closure:** dot to dot drawings, guess the picture (when you see only part of it), finish the shape, identify the partially hidden object | Making sense of objects that may be partially hidden, reading writing that is unclear, understanding pictures that may be missing parts; identifying signs and information from logos |
| | **Visual memory:** Playing games to remember items, such as name the items (after only viewing a short time); card games that require you to remember your cards; drawing or reproducing what you see; I spy games and matching games that require you to remember what you saw; remembering people's names or things about them | Grocery shopping, getting dressed, organizing one's materials for classes, finding needed items (remembering where you put things), identifying places that you have been, remembering people's faces and names |
| Visual motor integration | **Eye-hand coordination:** Games that require precision such as operation, card games, building with Legos, pick-up-sticks, Jenga, hitting a target (such as darts), dropping things into a container, picking up small objects, tossing bean bags to target | Daily fine motor tasks require you use your hands to manipulate items, such as Play-Doh, toys, dressing, zipping, holding, and bringing hand to mouth |
| | **Continuous motion:** Games that require the child to plan movement ahead of time, such as a paper task, where child puts a line following the trail without picking up the pencil | Activities that require the child to see and move at the same time, such as riding a bicycle, walking around the house, following others in line, writing on paper, getting dressed, combing hair, playing sports, or playing with friends |
| | **Complex spatial awareness:** Dance games, yoga poses, sports tasks (such as throwing a baseball), hopscotch, jump rope, building complex structures, creating arts projects | Sports, play, dance, and creating structures require complex spatial awareness, figuring out how things work (such as toy, everyday appliance) and how to fix objects (such as toy or small appliance); figuring out how to use tools (such as hammer, screwdriver); using writing utensils, scissors, and materials for education |

activities of daily living. The occupational therapy practitioner may engage children in activities to promote figure ground awareness, such as games to find objects around the room or *Where's Waldo?* type games. The ability to distinguish objects from the foreground is an important skill for daily activities, such as eating, dressing, meal management, household management (finding clothing), school functions such as finding supplies, locating objects within the classroom, and making sense of letters and numbers for reading. Practitioners may also work on discrimination of same and different through puzzles and simple matching games. Many of these types of activities can also be found in computer programs to promote repetition. See Evolve site for resources.

Children may benefit from practicing visual motor tasks as these skills are important for handwriting and copying from the board at school. They may learn by using blocks to reproduce patterns (see Fig. 31.7). Children can also practice tracing, completing mazes, drawing, or coloring. They can practice and gain skill with visual motor integration through gross motor activities as well, such as ball skill games (e.g., catching, kicking a moving ball, jumping over a bolster rolled toward the child) or obstacle courses where, for example, they must jump and land on specific targets or letters. Some children enjoy learning dance steps, whereby they reproduce movements based on what they see (either by someone demonstrating or in a picture sequence). The occupational therapy practitioner selects activities that are motivating to the child and at the child's level, so that they are challenged but also successful.

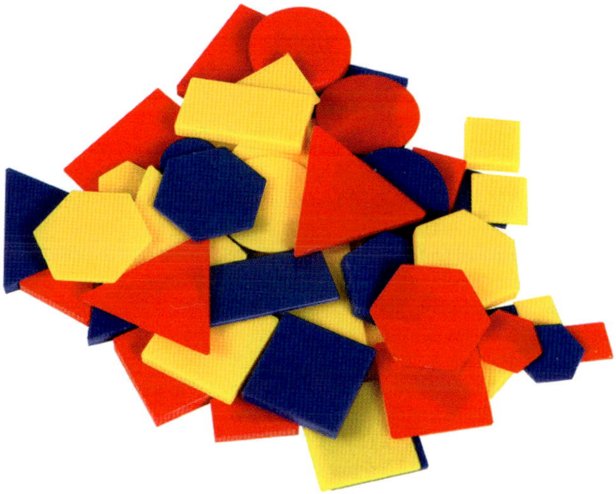

**Fig. 31.7** Engaging children in building with blocks, matching shapes, and sorting shapes (such as with attribute blocks) promotes visual spatial and visual analysis skills.

## SUMMARY

This chapter presents background information about vision problems in children and the potential roles occupational therapy practitioners play in the screening and intervention of these vision problems. This chapter presents a series of inexpensive and easy-to-learn screening methods for eye movement for accommodative, binocular vision, and visual information processing disorders.

1. Vision problems are prevalent in children typically seen by occupational therapy practitioners. If left undetected and untreated, these vision problems can create challenges in the child's ability to read, play, complete schoolwork, engage in daily living tasks, and participate in social events, sports, leisure, or work.
2. The two primary models that form the basis for the vision care include the three-component model of vision, which examines visual integrity, visual efficiency, and visual information processing skills, and the one-component model of vision, which only includes an evaluation of visual integrity. The *optician* is the individual who helps a person select an appropriate eyeglass frame, prepares the lenses based on the prescription, and then fits the frame to the person's face so that they can be comfortably worn. The optician does not have the training to perform any clinical testing or treatment. The education and training of *ophthalmologists* (medical doctors) have a strong focus on diagnosis and treatment of eye disease using medication and surgery. Thus, the emphasis is on the area defined above as "visual integrity." The areas of visual efficiency and visual processing problems are not emphasized in the training programs of the typical ophthalmologist. Optometrists are educated in concepts of vision and its relationship to performance in play, school, work, and sports. The optometrist is taught to evaluate the visual system in a manner that allows diagnosis of visual conditions that can interfere with performance and affect the quality of life.
3. The three-component model of vision examines visual integrity (i.e., ability to see clearly at distances, optical system, and eye health); visual efficiency (i.e., effectiveness of the visual system to see clearly, efficiently, and comfortably to gather information at school and play); and visual information processing skills (i.e., the ability to analyze, interpret, and use incoming visual information to interact with the environment). This model examines how the child uses visual information daily to complete such things as academics, play, and activities of daily living tasks. Whereas, the one-component model examines visual integrity alone.
4. Occupational therapy practitioners are most likely to see children with problems with accommodative, binocular vision, eye movement, and visual information processing problems and should be familiar with how to screen and address these problems.
5. Occupational therapy practitioners may screen for visual efficiency problems by using the CISS, accommodative amplitude (using near point rod), DEM, and the NSUCO. They may screen for visual information processing disorders using the TVPS–4; DTVMI, and clinical observations of child's performance in daily activities.
6. Occupational therapy practitioners can comfortably participate in providing therapy in the context of occupation for eye movement and visual information processing disorders. When it comes to binocular vision and accommodative disorders, occupational therapy practitioners should not attempt to work on these issues in isolation of an optometrist. A trend that is becoming more common is that optometrists are becoming more directly involved in the care of patients with acquired brain injury within rehabilitation hospitals. In most cases, the optometrist examines the patient within the hospital and prescribes appropriate treatment that may include lenses, prism, occlusion, and vision therapy. Vision therapy may be carried out in the hospital by the occupational therapy practitioner, and progress is monitored by the optometrist.

## REFERENCES


American Occupational Therapy Association. (2020). Occupational therapy practice framework: Domain and process (4th ed.). *American Journal of Occupational Therapy*, *74*(Suppl. 2), 7412410010.

Anketell, P. M., Saunders, K. J., Gallagher, S. M., Bailey, C., & Little, J. A. (2015). Brief report: Vision in children with autism spectrum disorder: What should clinicians expect? *Journal of Autism and Developmental Disorders*, *45*(9), 3041–3047.

AOA Evidence-Based Optometry Guideline Development Group. (2017). Comprehensive pediatric eye and vision examination. *©American Optometric Association*. http://aoa.uberflip.com/i/807465-cpg-pediatric-eye-and-vision-examination.

Atowa, U. C., Hansraj, R., & Wajuihian, S. O. (2019). Visual problems: A review of prevalence studies on visual impairment in school-age children. *International Journal of Ophthalmology*, *12*(6), 1037.

Appelbaum, L., & Erickson, G. (2016). Sport vision training: A review of the state-of-the-art in digital training techniques. *International Review of Sport and Exercise Psychology*, *11*, 160–189. https://api.semanticscholar.org/CorpusID:46950906.

Bakroon, A., & Lakshminarayanan, V. (2016). Visual function in autism spectrum disorders: A critical review. *Clinical and Experimental Optometry*, *99*(4), 297–308.

Barnhardt, C., Cotter, S. A., Mitchell, G. L., Scheiman, M., Kulp, M. T., & Group, C. S. (2012). Symptoms in children with convergence insufficiency: Before and after treatment. *Optometry and Vision Science*, *89*(10), 1512–1520.

Bilbao, C., & Piñero, D. P. (2021a). Distribution of visual and oculomotor alterations in a clinical population of children with and without neurodevelopmental disorders. *Brain Sciences*, *11*(3), 351.

Bilbao, C., & Piñero, D. P. (2021b). Objective and subjective evaluation of saccadic eye movements in healthy children and children with neurodevelopmental disorders: A pilot study. *Vision*, *5*(2), 28.

Borsting, E. J., Rouse, M. W., Mitchell, G. L., Scheiman, M., Cotter, S. A., Cooper, J., Kulp, M. T., London, R., & Convergence Insufficiency Treatment Trial Group. (2003). Validity and reliability of the revised convergence insufficiency symptom survey in children aged 9 to 18 years. *Optometry and Vision Science*, *80*(12), 832–838.

Burris, K., Liu, S., & Appelbaum, L. (2020). Visual-motor expertise in athletes: Insights from semiparametric modelling of 2317 athletes tested on the Nike SPARQ Sensory Station. *Journal of Sports Sciences*, *38*(3), 320–329.

Carla, S. C., Sara, B. F., Jm, C. R., & Catalina, P. A. (2021). Prevalence of convergence insufficiency among Spanish school children aged 6 to 14 years. *Journal of Optics*, *15*(4), 278–283.

Chang, M. Y., Doppee, D., Yu, F., Perez, C., Coleman, A. L., & Pineles, S. L. (2021). Prevalence of ophthalmologic diagnoses in children with autism spectrum disorder using the Optum dataset: A population-based study. *American Journal of Ophthalmology*, *221*, 147–153.

Chen, A. M., Roberts, T. L., Cotter, S. A., Kulp, M. T., Sinnott, L. T., Borsting, E. J., Tea, Y. C., Jones-Jordan, L. A., Hertle, R., Mitchell, G. L., Eugene Arnold, L., Chase, C., Scheiman, M. M., & CITT-ART Investigator Group. (2021). Effectiveness of vergence/accommodative therapy for accommodative dysfunction in children with convergence insufficiency. *Ophthalmic and Physiological Optics*, *41*(1), 21–32.

Chen, Y., He, Z., Mao, Y., Chen, H., Zhou, J., & Hess, R. F. (2020). Patching and suppression in amblyopia: One mechanism or two? *Frontiers in Neuroscience*, *13*, 1364.

Ciner, E. B., Macks, B., & Schanel-Klitsch, E. (1991). A cooperative demonstration project for early intervention vision services. *Occupational Therapy Practice*, *3*, 42–56.

CITT-ART Investigator Group. (2019a). Effect of vergence/accommodative therapy on reading in children with convergence insufficiency: A randomized clinical trial. *Optometry and Vision Science*, *96*(11), 836–849.

CITT-ART Investigator Group. (2019b). Treatment of symptomatic convergence insufficiency in children enrolled in the convergence insufficiency treatment trial-attention & reading trial: A randomized clinical trial. *Optometry and Vision Science*, *96*(11), 825–835.

CITT-ART Investigator Group. (2021). Effect of vergence/accommodative therapy on attention in children with convergence insufficiency: A randomized clinical trial. *Optometry and Vision Science*, *98*(3), 222–233.

Cohn, S. J., Cohn, C. M., & Jensen, A. R. (1988). Myopia and intelligence: A pleiotropic relationship? *Human Genetics*, *80*(1), 53–58.

Convergence Insufficiency Treatment Trial Investigator Group. (2008). A randomized clinical trial of treatments for symptomatic convergence insufficiency in children. *Archives of Ophthalmology*, *126*(10), 1336–1349.

Coulter, R. A., Bade, A., Tea, Y., Fecho, G., Amster, D., Jenewein, E., Rodena, J., Lyons, K. K., Mitchell, G. L., Quint, N., Dunbar, S., Ricamato, M., Trocchio, J., Kabat, B., Garcia, C., & Radik, I. (2015). Eye examination testability in children with autism and in typical peers. *Optometry and Vision Science*, *92*(1), 31–43.

Cregg, M., Woodhouse, J. M., Stewart, R. E., Pakeman, V. H., Bromham, N. R., Gunter, H. L., Trojanowska, L., Parker, M., & Fraser, W. I. (2003). Development of refractive error and strabismus in children with Down syndrome. *Investigative Ophthalmology and Visual Science*, *44*(3), 1023–1030.

Davis, A. L., Harvey, E. M., Twelker, J. D., Miller, J. M., Leonard-Green, T., & Campus, I. (2016). Convergence insufficiency, accommodative insufficiency, visual symptoms, and astigmatism in Tohono O'odham students. *Journal of Ophthalmology*, *2016*, 6963976.

Dodick, D., Starling, A. J., Wethe, J., Pang, Y., Messner, L. V., Smith, C., Master, C. L., Halker-Singh, R. B., Vargas, B. B., Bogle, J. M., Mandrekar, J., Talaber, A., & Leong, D. (2017). The effect of in-school saccadic training on reading fluency and comprehension in first and second grade students. *Journal of Child Neurology*, *32*(1), 104–111.

Errington, J. A., Menant, J. C., Suttle, C. M., Bruce, J., & Asper, L. J. (2013). The effects of vertical yoked prisms on gait. *Investigative Ophthalmology and Visual Science*, *54*(6), 3949–3956.

Farr, J. A., & Leibowitz, H. W. (1976). An experimental study of the efficacy of perceptual-motor training. *American Journal of Optometry and Physiological Optics*, *53*(9 Pt 1), 451–455.

Fazzi, E., Signorini, S. G., La Piana, R., Bertone, C., Misefari, W., Galli, J., Balottin, U., & Bianchi, P. E. (2012). Neuro-ophthalmological disorders in cerebral palsy: Ophthalmological, oculomotor, and visual aspects. *Developmental Medicine and Child Neurology*, *54*(8), 730–736.

Fessler, A., Kruemmling, B., & Scheiman, M. (2020). A worthwhile collaboration: Integrating optometry and occupational therapy in the treatment of children. *Vision Development and Rehabilitation*, *6*(3), 221–236.

Franco, S., Moreira, A., Fernandes, A., & Baptista, A. (2021). Accommodative and binocular vision dysfunctions in a Portuguese clinical population. *Journal of Optics*, *15*(4), 271–277.

Goering, M., Drennan, K. B., & Moshirfar, M. (2024). *Convergence insufficiency. StatPearls [Internet]*. StatPearls Publishing. https://www.ncbi.nim.nih.gov/books/NBK554390/.

Grosvenor, T. (1970). Refractive state, intelligence test scores, and academic ability. *American Journal of Optometry and Archives of American Academy of Optometry*, *47*(5), 355–361.

Haarbauer-Krupa, J., Lebrun-Harris, L. A., Black, L. I., Veliz, P., Daugherty, J., Desrocher, R., Schulenberg, J., Pilkey, D., & Breiding, M. (2021). Comparing prevalence estimates of concussion/head injury in U.S. children and adolescents in national surveys. *Annals of Epidemiology*, *54*, 11–20.

Halstead, M. E., Walter, K. D., Moffatt, K., LaBella, C. R., Brooks, M. A., Canty, G., & Stricker, P. R. (2018). Sport-related concussion in children and adolescents. *Pediatrics*, *142*(6), e20183074. https://doi.org/10.1542/peds.2018-3074.

Hashemi, H., Mehravaran, S., Asgari, S., & Dehghanian Nasrabadi, F. (2021). Refractive and vision status in Down syndrome: A comparative study. *Turkish Journal of Ophthalmology*, *51*(4), 199–205.

Heydarian, S., Abbasabadi, M. M., Khabazkhoob, M., Hoseini-Yazdi, H., & Gharib, M. (2022). *Vision abnormalities in children and young adults with cerebral palsy; A systematic review. Seminars in Ophthalmology* (Vol.37, No. 4, pp. 471–479). Taylor & Francis.

Hirsch, M. J. (1959). The relationship between refractive state of the eye and intelligence test scores. *American Journal of Optometry and Archives of American Academy of Optometry, 36*(1), 12–21.

Hoffman, L. G. (1980). Incidence of vision difficulties in children with learning disabilities. *Journal of the American Optometric Association, 51*, 447–451.

Hussaindeen, J. R., & Murali, A. (2020). Accommodative insufficiency: Prevalence, impact and treatment options. *Clinical Optometry, 12*, 135–149. https://doi.org/10.2147/OPTO.S224216. Article 32982529.

Hussaindeen, J. R., Rakshit, A., Singh, N. K., George, R., Swaminathan, M., Kapur, S., Scheiman, M., & Ramani, K. K. (2016). Prevalence of non-strabismic anomalies of binocular vision in Tamil Nadu: Report 2 of BAND study. *Clinical and Experimental Optometry, 100*(6), 642–648.

Jang, J. U., & Park, I. J. (2015). Prevalence of general binocular dysfunctions among rural school children in South Korea. *Taiwan Journal of Ophthalmology, 5*, 177–181.

Klein, S., Guiltner, V., Sollereder, P., & Cui, Y. (2011). Relationships between fine-motor, visual-motor, and visual perception scores and handwriting legibility and speed. *Physical and Occupational Therapy in Pediatrics, 31*(1), 103–114.

Letourneau, J. E., & Ducic, S. (1988). Prevalence of convergence insufficiency among elementary school children. *Canadian Journal of Optometry, 50*, 194–197.

Little, J. A. (2018). Vision in children with autism spectrum disorder: A critical review. *Clinical and Experimental Optometry, 101*(4), 504–513.

LoCascio, G. P. (1977). A study of vision in cerebral palsy. *American Journal of Optometry and Physiological Optics, 54*, 332–335.

London, R., & Wick, B. (1987). Vertical fixation disparity correction; effect on the horizontal forced vergence fixation disparity curve. *American Journal of Optometry and Physiological Optics, 64*, 653–656.

Ma, M. M., Long, W., She, Z., Li, W., Chen, X., Xie, L., Scheiman, M., Liu, Y., & Chen, X. (2019). Convergence insufficiency in Chinese high school students. *Clinical and Experimental Optometry, 102*(2), 166 171.

Makateb, A., Hashemi, H., Farahi, A., Mehravaran, S., Khabazkhoob, M., & Asgari, S. (2020). Ocular alignment, media, and eyelid disorders in Down syndrome. *Strabismus, 28*(1), 42.

Maples, W. C. (1995). *NSUCO oculomotor test. Optometric extension program.*

Master, C. L., Scheiman, M., Gallaway, M., Goodman, A., Robinson, R. L., Master, S. R., & Grady, M. F. (2016). Vision diagnoses are common after concussion in adolescents. *Clinical Pediatrics, 55*(3), 260–267.

Maurer, M. N., & Roebers, C. M. (2021). New insights into visual-motor integration exploring process measures during copying shapes. *Psychology of Sport and Exercise, 55*, 101954. https://doi.org/10.1016/j.psychsport.2021.101954.

McKean-Cowdin, R., Cotter, S. A., Tarczy-Hornoch, K., Wen, G., Kim, J., Borchert, M., Varma, R., & Multi-Ethnic Pediatric Eye Disease Study, G (2013). Prevalence of amblyopia or strabismus in Asian and non-hispanic white preschool children: Multi-ethnic pediatric eye disease study. *Ophthalmology, 120*(10), 2117–2124.

Milne, E., Griffiths, H., Buckley, D., & Scope, A. (2009). Vision in children and adolescents with autistic spectrum disorder: Evidence for reduced convergence. *Journal of Autism and Developmental Disorders, 39*(7), 965–975.

Mutti, D. O., Mitchell, G. L., Moeschberger, M. L., Jones, L. A., & Zadnik, K. (2002). Parental myopia, near work, school achievement, and children's refractive error. *Investigative Ophthalmology and Visual Science, 43*(12), 3633–3640.

Nandakumar, K., Evans, M. A., Briand, K., & Leat, S. J. (2011). Bifocals in Down syndrome study (BiDS): Analysis of video recorded sessions of literacy and visual perceptual skills. *Clinical and Experimental Optometry, 94*(6), 575–585.

Nunes, A. F., Monteiro, P. M. L., Ferreira, F. B. P., & Nunes, A. S. (2019). Convergence insufficiency and accommodative insufficiency in children. *BMC Ophthalmology, 19*(1), 58.

Papageorgiou, E., Asproudis, I., Maconachie, G., Tsironi, E. E., & Gottlob, I. (2019). The treatment of amblyopia: Current practice and emerging trends. *Graefe's Archive for Clinical and Experimental Ophthalmology, 257*, 1061–1078.

Park, S. H. (2019). Current management of childhood amblyopia. *Korean Journal of Ophthalmology, 33*(6), 557–568.

Pediatric Eye Disease Investigator, G. (2016). Home-based therapy for symptomatic convergence insufficiency in children: A randomized clinical trial. *Optometry and Vision Science, 93*(12), 1457–1465.

Prabha, A. J., & Bhargavi, R. (2020). Predictive model for dyslexia from fixations and saccadic eye movement events. *Computer Methods and Programs in Biomedicine, 195*, 105538.

Press, L. J. (2021). *Applied concepts in vision therapy 2.0. Optometric extension program foundation.*

Raghuram, A., Cotter, S. A., Gowrisankaran, S., Kanji, J., Howell, D. R., Meehan, W. P., 3rd, & Shah, A. S. (2019). Postconcussion: Receded near point of convergence is not diagnostic of convergence insufficiency. *American Journal of Ophthalmology, 206*, 235–244.

Rotter, J., & Kamat, D. (2019). Concussion in children. *Pediatric Annals, 48*(4), e182–e185.

Rouse, M. W., Borsting, E., Hyman, L., Hussein, M., Cotter, S., Flynn, M., Scheiman, M., Gallaway, M., De Land, P. N., & CIRS Group. (1999). Frequency of convergence insufficiency among fifth and sixth graders. *Optometry and Vision Science, 76*, 643–649.

Satgunam, P., Datta, S., & Sumalini, R. (2019). Near vision in individuals with Down syndrome: A vision screening study. *Eye, 33*(8), 1254–1260.

Scharre, J. E., & Creedon, M. P. (1992). Assessment of visual function in autistic children. *Optometry and Vision Science, 69*(6), 433–439.

Scheiman, M. (1990). In A. A. Rosenbloom, & M. W. Morgan (Eds.), *Assessment and management of the exceptional child.* JB Lippincott.

Scheiman, M. (1984). Optometric findings in children with cerebral palsy. *American Journal of Optometry and Physiological Optics, 61*, 321–327.

Scheiman, M. (2000). The eyes have it. *Advance for Directors in Rehab, 9*(10), 61–63.

Scheiman, M. (2025). *Understanding and managing visual deficits: A guide for occupational therapists* (4th ed.). Routledge.

Scheiman, M., Cotter, S., Kulp, M. T., Mitchell, G. L., Cooper, J., Gallaway, M., Hopkins, K. B., Bartuccio, M., Chung, I., & Convergence Insufficiency Treatment Trial Study Group (2011). Treatment of accommodative dysfunction in children: Results from a randomized clinical trial. *Optometry and Vision Science, 88*(11), 1343–1352.

Scheiman, M., Gallaway, M., Coulter, R., et al. (1996). Prevalence of vision and ocular disease conditions in a clinical pediatric population. *Journal of the American Optometric Association, 67*, 193–202.

Scheiman, M., Grady, M. F., Jenewein, E., Shoge, R., Podolak, O. E., Howell, D. H., & Master, C. L. (2021). Frequency of oculomotor disorders in adolescents 11 to 17 years of age with concussion, 4 to 12 weeks post injury. *Vision Research, 183*, 73–80.

Scheiman, M., Kulp, M. T., Cotter, S. A., Lawrenson, J. G., Wang, L., & Li, T. (2020). Interventions for convergence insufficiency: A network meta-analysis. *Cochrane Database of Systematic Reviews, 12*, CD006768.

Scheiman, M., Mitchell, G. L., Cotter, S., Cooper, J. C., Kulp, M. T., Rouse, M. W., Borsting, E., London, R., & CITT Study Group. (2005). A randomized trial of the effectiveness of treatments for convergence insufficiency in children. *Archives of Ophthalmology, 123*, 14–24.

Scheiman, M., & Wick, B. (2019). *Clinical management of binocular vision: Heterophoric, accommodative and eye movement disorders* (5th ed.). Lippincott, Williams and Wilkins.

Seiderman, A. S. (1980). Optometric vision therapy -- results of a demonstration project with a learning disabled population. *Journal of the American Optometric Association, 51*(5), 489–493.

Sherman, A. (1973). Relating vision disorder's to learning disability. *Journal of the American Optometric Association, 44*, 140–141.

Simmons, D. R., Robertson, A. E., McKay, L. S., Toal, E., McAleer, P., & Pollick, F. E. (2009). Vision in autism spectrum disorders. *Vision Research, 49*(22), 2705–2739.

Solan, H. A., Shelley-Tremblay, J., Ficarra, A., Silverman, M., & Larson, S. (2003). Effect of attention therapy on reading comprehension. *Journal of Learning Disabilities, 36*(6), 556–563.

Solan, H. A., Shelley-Tremblay, J., Hansen, P. C., Silverman, M. E., Larson, S., & Ficarra, A. (2004). M-cell deficit and reading disability: A preliminary study of the effects of temporal vision-processing therapy. *Optometry, 75*(10), 640–650.

Sun, F., & Kraus, C. L. (2023). The ophthalmic manifestations of Down syndrome. *Children, 10*(2), 341.

Surman, G., Bonellie, S., Chalmers, J., Colver, A., Dolk, H., Hemming, K., King, A., Kurinczuk, J. J., Parkes, J., & Platt, M. J. (2006). UKCP: A collaborative network of cerebral palsy registers in the United Kingdom. *Journal of Public Health, 28*(2), 148–156.

Suttle, C. M., Asper, L. J., Sturnieks, D., & Menant, J. (2015). Negligible impact on posture from 5-diopter vertical yoked prisms. *Investigative Ophthalmology & Visual Science, 56*(5), 2980–2984.

Tassinari, J. D., & Eastland, R. Q. (1997). Vision therapy for deficient visual-motor integration. *Journal of Optometric Vision Development, 28*, 214–226.

Uttal, D. H., Meadow, N. G., Tipton, E., Hand, L. L., Alden, A. R., Warren, C., & Newcombe, N. S. (2013). The malleability of spatial skills: A meta-analysis of training studies. *Psychological Bulletin, 139*(2), 352–402.

Veliz, P., McCabe, S. E., Eckner, J. T., & Schulenberg, J. E. (2017). Prevalence of concussion among US adolescents and correlated factors. *JAMA, 318*(12), 1180–1182.

Veliz, P., McCabe, S. E., Eckner, J. T., & Schulenberg, J. E. (2021). Trends in the prevalence of concussion reported by US adolescents, 2016-2020. *JAMA, 325*(17), 1789–1791.

Wajuihian, S. O., & Hansraj, R. (2016a). Accommodative anomalies in a sample of black high school students in South Africa. *Ophthalmic Epidemiology, 23*(5), 316–323.

Wajuihian, S. O., & Hansraj, R. (2016b). Vergence anomalies in a sample of high school students in South Africa. *Journal of Optics, 9*(4), 246–257.

Ward, L. M., & Kapoula, Z. (2020). Differential diagnosis of vergence and saccade disorders in dyslexia. *Scientific Reports, 10*(1), 22116.

Watt, T., Robertson, K., & Jacobs, R. J. (2015). Refractive error, binocular vision and accommodation of children with Down syndrome. *Clinical and Experimental Optometry, 98*(1), 3–11.

Wiecek, E. K., Roberts, T. L., Shah, A. S., & Raghuram, A. (2021). Vergence, accommodation, and visual tracking in children and adolescents evaluated in a multidisciplinary concussion clinic. *Vision Research, 184*, 30–36.

Williams, K. M., Hysi, P. G., Yonova-Doing, E., Mahroo, O. A., Snieder, H., & Hammond, C. J. (2017). Phenotypic and genotypic correlation between myopia and intelligence. *Scientific Reports, 7*, 45977.

## FURTHER READING

Scheiman, M. M., Hertle, R. W., Kraker, R. T., Beck, R. W., Birch, E. E., Felius, J., Holmes, J. M., Kundart, J., Morrison, D. G., Repka, M. X., Tamkins, S. M., & Pediatric Eye Disease Investigator, G. (2008). Patching vs atropine to treat amblyopia in children aged 7 to 12 years: A randomized trial. *Archives of Ophthalmology, 126*(12), 1634–1642.

32

# Interventions for Mobility

*Sandy Hanebrink and Jane Loscheider*

## GUIDING QUESTIONS

1. How does mobility influence a child's occupational performance?
2. What is the occupational therapy practitioner's role in mobility intervention?
3. What are some of the advantages/disadvantages of specific mobility devices and the associated parts?

## KEY TERMS

Assistive technology
Cocreation
Community mobility
Dependent mobility
Embodied cognition
Exoskeletons
Functional mobility
Learned helplessness
Object affordances
Strengths-based approach

## MOBILITY FOR OCCUPATIONAL PERFORMANCE

Mobility is fundamental to a child's overall development and engagement in daily occupations of education, social participation, activities of daily living, work, leisure, and play and is essential to quality of life. **Functional mobility** includes moving from one position or place to another (e.g., bed mobility, wheelchair mobility, and transfers [wheelchair, bed, car, tub or shower, toilet, or chair]), performing functional ambulation, and transporting objects (AOTA, 2020). **Community mobility** is defined as moving oneself in the community and using public or private transportation (e.g., driving or accessing buses, taxicabs, or other public transportation systems) (AOTA, 2020). Both are critical components of many aspects of occupation and participation. Therefore, the occupational therapy practitioner is a crucial member of the mobility team who must have a strong understanding of the importance of independent mobility and an awareness of the options available for providing it.

### Principles of Mobility

Mobility is important to a person's participation in meaningful activities. Infants, children, and adolescents move in a variety of ways and within numerous environments. Occupational therapy practitioners examine the many factors that influence movement while considering the individual, environment, and type of movement the person seeks to do. They engage children and families in a collaborative process to meet the child and family's needs. For example, one family who enjoyed camping was appreciative of the new electronic wheelchair that provided their teen with improved mobility within the community and school. However, they reported it was not useable when they went camping as a family. The occupational therapy practitioner acknowledged the unique situation and provided an alternative to meet this need. Understanding the principles of mobility from an occupational therapy perspective illustrates the breadth of services.

**Mobility Is Complex and Critical for Embodied Cognition.** In psychology and cognitive science research, the idea of *embodiment* or **embodied cognition** can be described as follows:

"Embodiment is the surprisingly radical hypothesis that the brain is not the sole cognitive resource we have available to us to solve problems. Our bodies and their perceptually guided motions through the world do much of the work required to achieve our goals, replacing the need for complex internal mental representations. This simple fact utterly changes our idea of what 'cognition' involves, and thus embodiment is not simply another factor acting on an otherwise disembodied cognitive processes" (Wilson & Golonka, 2013, p. 1).

In terms of occupational therapy, the ideas of embodied cognition reflect what practitioners have always known and done; that the body is an integrated part of problem-solving and that movement of the body is critical for learning.

Mobility is often categorized by gross motor milestones (see Chapter 8). Babies learn to roll, crawl, cruise, and walk in a relatively predictable sequence. Although this purely physical view of mobility is common, the embodied cognition view suggests mobility is more complex than this. Mobility stimulates cognition, visual-perceptual skills, safety awareness, vestibular processing, and social skills. Mobility and movement are ways to interact with the world, and development emerges from combined experiences of physical and social interactions (Adolph & Franchak, 2017). Movement is a catalyst for the interactions that drive cognition, language, and subsequent motor development (Smith & Gasser, 2005). The child works toward advancing motor skills while simultaneously integrating problem-solving, object exploration, and self-initiated movement for optimal performance (Harbourne & Berger, 2019). See Case Example 32.1 about embodied cognition.

It is easy to identify numerous segregated skills that are used during play. For example, in Case Example 32.1, the initial event was moving toward a distant ball, and the events were perpetuated because the baby could continue to move as the ball moved. Without independent mobility, the cascade of interactions that followed

### CASE EXAMPLE 32.1 THE INFLUENCE OF MOVEMENT

A mobile 8-month-old, who is an active crawler, moves across the room toward an interesting ball. He bumps the ball, causing it to roll, and then follows its course. He grabs at it several times before successfully picking it up, experiencing the ball's texture and physical properties while fine-tuning his grasp. He then may throw it, and his older sibling will retrieve it, rolling it back to him with a cascade of laughter. The two engage in a short-lived reciprocal game including vocal exchanges in addition to the physical ones with the ball. Movement and mobility play an integral role in this series of interactions. These types of interwoven activities are repeated in multiple contexts and variations throughout the baby's day and promote the child's overall development. Occupational therapy interventions to promote mobility in infants and young children support children moving on their own toward those toys and objects of interest to them. To help them feel the success of moving within the environment to act upon it (such as when getting a toy), the occupational therapy practitioner designs interventions that allow the child to move, such as on a scooter board (by propelling their hands), pumping the swing, or activating a switch (such as with a toy car). They may facilitate movement through physical guidance to promote skill development.

would not have occurred. These subsequent interactions were an intricate combination of motor, language, and cognition. Moving toward the ball involved the cognitive task of spatial mapping and laid the foundation for concepts such as near and far in addition to the physical movement (Clearfield, 2004). Picking up the desired ball included a combination of fine and gross motor skills necessary for reaching and grasping. This physical interaction taught the infant **object affordances** of a ball, including input on size, firmness, and texture. This tactile input then shapes motor planning and execution for subsequent hand-ball interactions (Lobo et al., 2014). As the 3-year-old brother enters the mix, the social component provides joint attention opportunities as the ball moves away, and the baby pays attention to both the location of the ball and his brother. Language skills abound as the children reference the ball and each other with reciprocal vocalizations.

These initial movements, when repeated in high doses by active infants and toddlers, provide a rich array of experiences that shape physical, cognitive, visual-perceptual, and social development. The baby's role in this process is a highly active one as independent movement allows the infant to cocreate. **Cocreation** is an infant's ability to participate in directing their experiences. This is evident as the baby's experiences lead to self-identified preferences that then guide the evolution of future interactions.

The literature emphasizes the critical role of mobility in all aspects of development. Language studies find that parents speak differently to children who are independently mobile (Clearfield, 2010). Independent mobility fosters cognitive development as infants better understand objects as they approach them and interact with them from multiple directions (Schwarzer et al., 2013).

**Mobility Is Important Throughout the Lifespan.** The integral role of movement does not end with the achievement of functional ambulation. Mobility continues to be a driving force for social interaction and for engagement in one's environment, beyond the mastery of the basic skills to move throughout the home and community. Children play with bikes, pogo sticks, skates, and skateboards, as well as participate in a variety of sports and general outdoor play. In many cases, these movement experiences involve a social component. Thus, mobility has a defining presence in how people develop and participate throughout infancy, childhood, and into adult life.

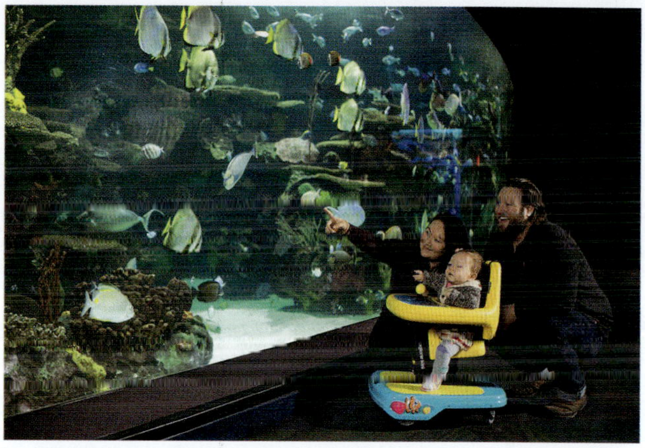

**Fig. 32.1** Infant in Explore Mini interacting with their parents while pointing at fish in a large aquarium. (Photo courtesy Permobil.)

**Immobility Has a Widespread Impact.** Children with disabilities may have impairments that result in motor delays, and while traditionally, there has been a strong prevalence of a "wait and see" attitude regarding missed early milestones, the delay or disruption of mobility has a profound effect on the number and type of interactions between a young child and their environment. This altered participation impacts opportunities to build cognition, language, and motor skills.

Immobility changes social interaction (Logan et al., 2016a; 2016b). When children move independently, they can use movement to initiate or terminate an interaction with a sibling, parent, or peer (Cheung et al., 2020). For example, they can move toward someone to play, stay with them, and then move away when finished with the interaction. Without independent mobility, a toddler must wait for a peer to come to them and for that peer to stay with them to interact. As the child increases in age, this social gap widens. Additionally, the presence of an adult caregiver to supplement mobility can shift the dynamics of peer-to-peer play (Fig. 32.1).

Furthermore, the lack of independent mobility lays a foundation for learned helplessness as a behavior. **Learned helplessness** refers to passivity and disengagement when presented with challenging tasks and an inability to persist in problem-solving behaviors (Rueger et al., 2021). Children who develop learned helplessness become unmotivated to explore and engage in new behaviors, waiting for someone to do things for them. They do not engage in novel activities and experiences. The consequences of delayed mobility extend beyond motor skills and can lead to anxiety, reluctance to accept challenging tasks, lower academic performance, and even depression (Rueger et al., 2021).

**Early Intervention for Independent Mobility Matters.** To prevent the issues described above, and promote development, early introduction of independent mobility options is important (Anderson et al., 2013; Bornstein et al., 2013; Currier et al., 2019; Feldner, 2019; Feldner et al., 2019). Therefore, Livingstone et al. (2020) suggest the introduction of mobility devices in children as young as 9 months. Early powered mobility provision may influence identity development and support perceptions of child competence (Feldner, 2019; Feldner et al., 2019).

**Moving Takes Time to Learn.** In a span of 1 hour, toddlers travel 2368 steps and fall at a rate of 17 times (Adolph et al., 2012). These statistics are an important benchmark to keep in mind with new

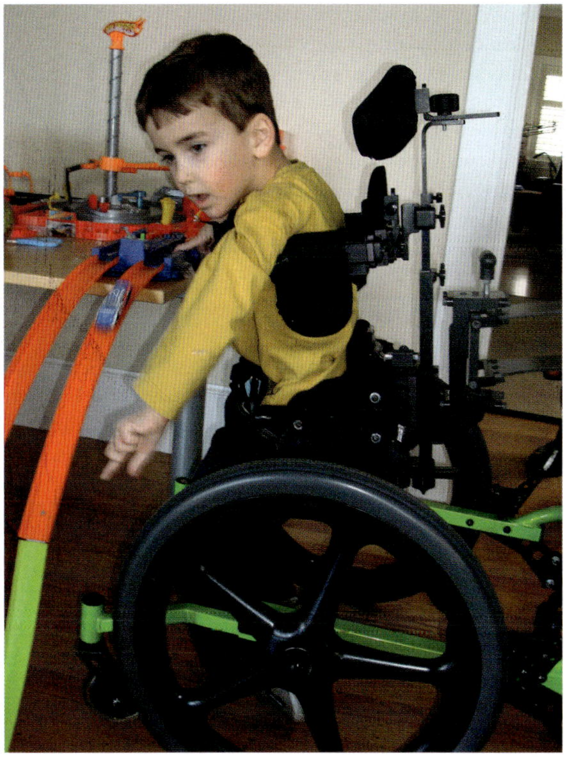

Fig. 32.2 Young boy stands playing with Hot Wheels cars and track in a posterior support wheeled stander that allows him to move himself to his activity of choice.

movers. Often, there is an expectation by both parents and clinicians that a child quickly shows mastery over mobility in a device with little opportunity for use. However, functional walking or crawling can take months to develop. Within that time, there is not only a high dose (time to practice) and high repetitions but also a high rate of failure or falls throughout the process. Frequent opportunities to use the device with opportunities to constantly "fall down" create a foundation for learning about movement.

**The Environment Matters.** Typically developing children have unlimited opportunities to engage with their environment. For example, a child may ride a bicycle, then a scooter, and then rollerblades. Children with mobility limitations require the same multimodal mobility options in all environments, all the time (Feldner et al., 2016). Movement experiences where a child can use a device to add social and physical interactions in a real-world context are ideal. An environment that can be safe and simultaneously allow a child to self-direct his movement provides the building blocks for successful use of the device, building self-efficacy (i.e., belief in one's abilities). Infants are motivated to move because of the interactions that movement affords them. "Training" in a large open empty space can be fun for a time but does not always provide the relationship between movement and purpose. Children become proficient with a variety of experiences where they use the mobility for participation (Fig. 32.2).

**Posture Matters.** Posture and task performance are interrelated (Harbourne & Kamm, 2015), and therefore, proper positioning is critical to successful upper extremity function, which leads to improved use of any mobility device. How an individual is positioned in a mobility device, whether it be standing or sitting, can influence several physiologic factors, including visual and motor performance (Fitzsimmons, 2014), postural control, ranges of movement, muscle tone (Nwaobi, 1987), endurance, comfort, respiration (Lin et al., 2006), energy conservation, and safe swallow (Alghadir et al., 2017). Optimal seating provides a stable place for the child's pelvis and spine, from which a range of movements for achieving functional tasks can occur. Seating is not static. Children assume many positions when engaging in desired occupations, including sitting, standing, moving, and rolling. Therefore, when designing mobility and positioning options, children should not be restrained with straps and harnesses but rather supported and provided with options.

## THE ROLE OF THE OCCUPATIONAL THERAPY PRACTITIONER IN MOBILITY INTERVENTION

The occupational therapy practitioner is an integral member of the mobility team. They always keep in mind the importance of occupation and the preferences of the family and child, as well as the results of the evaluation (see Chapter 9) when they make mobility recommendations. Occupational therapy practitioners on the mobility team collaborate regarding mobility recommendations and interventions, which requires preparing adequately and working with team members. Practitioners working on mobility teams engage in the following professional behaviors to address children and families' mobility needs:

- Remain current on the features and functions of mobility devices.
- Use professional reasoning to thoroughly understand the benefits and limitations of technology.
- Consider the properties of the equipment in relation to the child's unique situation, strengths, and challenges.
- Consider the needs both at the current time and in the future.
- Discuss options with children and family.
- Use information from team members, children, and family when making recommendations.
- Communicate clearly with children, family, and team members throughout the process.
- Problem solve with the child, family, and team members to find equipment that works in multiple settings.
- Ensure equipment has been trialed in multiple contexts (such as home, school, and community).
- Coach children and provide opportunities to practice using the equipment prior to purchasing it.
- Design activities to practice skills needed for independent mobility in a variety of settings.
- Train caregivers and children on the features and use of the device.
- Monitor the use of the equipment and make modifications as needed.
- Assist in finding funding, seek resources such as foundations, and write letters of medical necessity.
- Assure safe transportation while in the mobility device through education and consultation (see Box 32.1).

Case Example 32.2 illustrates this training process, and Box 32.2 provides an overview of intervention for mobility.

The occupational therapy practitioner uses a **strengths-based approach**, which is defined as an "approach to people that is primarily dependent upon positive attitudes about people's dignity, capacities, rights, uniqueness, and commonalities" (McCashen, 2005). A strengths-based approach allows children to see themselves at their best and to see their own value. In a strengths-based approach, deficits are not ignored, nor do practitioners ask individuals to ignore their pain or issues. This approach capitalizes on the child's strengths rather than focusing on deficits, to empower children and families to achieve goals such as independent mobility.

## BOX 32.1 Safe Transportation for Wheelchairs

Manufacturers of wheelchair mobility systems do not recommend using them as a seat in a motor vehicle. However, manufacturers now provide safer options for transporting a wheelchair with the child in it because of a voluntary American National Standards Institute (ANSI)/RESNA standard called WC-19 (ANSI/RESNA, 2000). Wheelchairs are considered WC-19 compliant if they have four accessible and identifiable points to secure the chair to the vehicle, as well as seating, a frame, and other components designed to allow better fit of a lap and shoulder belt, a manufacturer-disclosed rating, and a measure of wheelchair lateral stability when secured (RESNA, 2000). The standard requires wheelchairs to be dynamically crash tested at 30 mph and 20 *g* crash conditions, which are the same standards used to test child safety (Pin, 2007; ANSI/RESNA, 2000; RESNA, 2000).

The ANSI/RESNA WC-20 standards are for seating devices for use in motor vehicles (ANSI/RESNA, 2000; RESNA, 2000). One standard requires that all students being transported in a wheelchair on a bus must face forward. Wheelchairs that are transported in a side-facing position are more likely to deform and collapse in a crash, and the shoulder belt is ineffective (Shutrump et al., 2008). The lap belt must be snug and low on the pelvis and the shoulder belt positioned over the middle of the clavicle and across the sternum, where it connects to the pelvic belt over the hip. Any device such as an augmentative communication device or computer and lap tray must be removed and tied down separately.

The mobility team seeks the mobility device(s) that offers the best chance for independent mobility (Fig. 32-3A) and will allow children to play, interact, and explore with peers (Fig. 32.3B and C). All children need to participate in these activities. Providing a child with a device that allows them to be active improves their ability to play more appropriately with peers. In order to assist in making appropriate recommendations, the practitioner must be familiar with the variety of options for mobility that currently exist as well as those that are emerging or under development and will be available in the near future.

## EQUIPMENT TO IMPROVE MOBILITY

Occupational therapy practitioners working with children and families who have diverse needs familiarize themselves with equipment to understand the characteristics, operation, strengths, and limitations of equipment. Because each child has unique situations, goals, and environments, practitioners problem-solve with children, families, and team members to find equipment that will best meet the child's unique needs. Oftentimes, practitioners try out equipment, get feedback from children and families on equipment, and work with vendors to see options that may be available (for example, color choices, additional settings, and sizes). They become familiar with mobility equipment that is available for many settings (such as strollers, beach wheelchairs, and battery-operated adapted small toy cars).

## CASE EXAMPLE 32.2

Mateo is a 2-year-old boy with cerebral palsy (spastic quadriplegia with fluctuating muscle tone) and cortical visual impairment. He has a Gross Motor Function Classification System (GMFCS; Palisano et al., 1997) score of IV. Mateo is nonverbal, and he cannot sit unsupported. He presents with spastic movements and cannot reach a target with any accuracy. He cannot ambulate but can bear weight.

He uses a supported hands-free walker for standing and attempting steps. He cannot propel a manual wheelchair. When asked to, he will use all his force and cannot release the pressure from the switch. He requires a mobility system that will offer augmented mobility for exploration and provide opportunities for development and demonstration of interest and intent. He also needs an AAC (alternative augmentative communication) device.

### Equipment Trial

Mateo is being assessed for independent mobility. A primary consideration for the evaluation is his lack of experience with independent movement. Seating for support is critical for success for Mateo. If he is sitting unsupported, his trunk collapses, and his legs and arms extend.

Traditional access through a joystick is too difficult for him to manage. Because of the lack of fine motor control, he pushes the joystick to the end of the range and cannot release it. Since the joystick has 360 degrees of directional control, he struggles to push it in the direction he is trying to make it go. During the evaluation, proximity switches were used because he was unsuccessful in maintaining contact with the mechanical switch. He pushed too hard, causing his asymmetrical tonic neck reflex to engage, and he was unable to release the switch.

Mateo was assessed with a head array equipped with proximity sensors to allow the position of his head to make the chair move without force. A system was chosen so that the sensors could be unplugged and moved to other positions to allow him to manage the chair directions individually. This strategy speaks to his need to gain experience with independent movement. By being able to isolate the directions and position them wherever he can use them, Mateo is able to successfully experience mobility while still learning how to manage his body.

The power chair will need to have expandable electronics to support alternative drive controls such as a head array with proximity sensors. In addition, he needs to have an output module. This box will allow Mateo to use the same switches that he will drive with to control his communication device. This will be important so that he can independently move between talking and driving.

The display and all other controls will be mounted on the back of the chair. This allows Mateo to move physically close to an activity and engage directly without being distracted. His seating was flat and not contoured for the assessment. This allows the team to see his control. If he is over strapped or has deep contours, he is held into a position that is artificially imposed. Overcontrolling a child does not allow an occupational therapy practitioner to see how the child controls his/her body.

Mateo was evaluated in his classroom. The team taught Mateo using a series of single steps, so he could process one movement (touching a single pad to move in the right direction) and eventually progress to more complex and sophisticated movements. He moved his head easiest toward the right direction, so the occupational therapy practitioner started with a right turn only. This was achieved by unplugging the other two switches/directions, so the wheelchair could only make a right turn. This allowed Mateo to explore his environment in a safe manner without having to stop him for fear he would bump into obstacles. Mateo was successful at making the chair move and stop. Next the practitioner and Mateo went for a walk down the hallway. Unplugging the right switch and plugging the forward direction into the right pad allowed him to use his newly acquired experience and skill to successfully achieve this goal.

Mateo was placed in the hall near one of the walls. He was able to stop and go and enjoy and appreciate the artwork on the walls. Mateo stopped at an intersection. The occupational therapy practitioner asked him if he was interested in going down that hallway to look. He indicated that he did, so the practitioner plugged in the left switch that allowed him to turn left and explore that hallway. Taking it one step at a time allowed Mateo to be successful and move around the school.

Overall, Mateo demonstrated a clear understanding of the tasks presented. He successfully moved the chair and stopped when he intended. When coupled with activities that are meaningful and relevant to him, there is reason to believe that Mateo will be a successful driver. He was attentive to the task and demonstrated all the skills necessary to be successful.

**BOX 32.2 Occupational Therapy Intervention to Address Mobility**

- Training and practice in multiple contexts
- Coaching on mobility
- Promoting safety awareness
- Funding sources
- Physical assessment and interventions
- Environmental modifications
- Education: use of device, maintenance
- Follow-up: modifications or adjustments as needed
- Documentation
- Problem-solving technology solutions
- Addressing changes over time
- Knowledge of equipment and technology options (including emerging technology)
- Promoting mobility in multiple settings
- Exploring novel mobility experiences
- Enhancing social opportunities for children
- Advocating for access (such as ADA)

## Technology for Self-Initiated Movement and Mobility

To minimize the developmental implications from a lack of or a limited number and variety of experiences, infants and children may benefit from **assistive technology** for self-initiated movement using an approach that focuses mobility interventions on participation that involves family, friends, fitness, function, and fun (Rosenbaum & Gorter, 2012; Rosenbaum & Stewart, 2004). Assistive technology, whether low tech or high tech, can help bridge the gaps created by mobility delays and may help children feel more in control of events (Fig. 32.4A–C shows low-tech devices). For example, a child may begin to believe they influence the environment as they activate a toy using an adaptive switch. Chapter 34 provides information on assistive technology, and see Table 32.1. Box 32.3 describes the importance of using both low- and high-tech options to address mobility.

## Manual Wheelchairs

Manual wheelchairs are divided into two categories: dependent and independent mobility devices. Within those two categories, there are different types of equipment. Choosing the correct device for a child is important to maximizing function and independence. **Dependent mobility** devices include both wheelchairs and strollers and offer different benefits. A less complex wheelchair may be requested by a family to ease transportation of the device. While transportation is important, the child's positioning and support needs should be addressed first. Once those are addressed, transportation issues may be addressed.

**Medical Strollers.** There are different types of medical strollers manufactured. Strollers designed for the early intervention population are small, cosmetically pleasing, and provide positioning support (Fig. 32.5). Most have a manual tilt option and can "recline" if needed. They are not designed for children with high muscle tone, significant bony deformities, or pressure injuries. These chairs are planar and utilize foam padding and supports, so they cannot be customized for more complex children. However, they can be used with positioning supports such as lateral trunk supports, hip guides, pelvic supports, chest supports, and specialty head supports.

Strollers designed for older children are generally designed as secondary devices to a larger tilt-in-space wheelchair or to be used for ambulatory children who need assistance with mobility in the

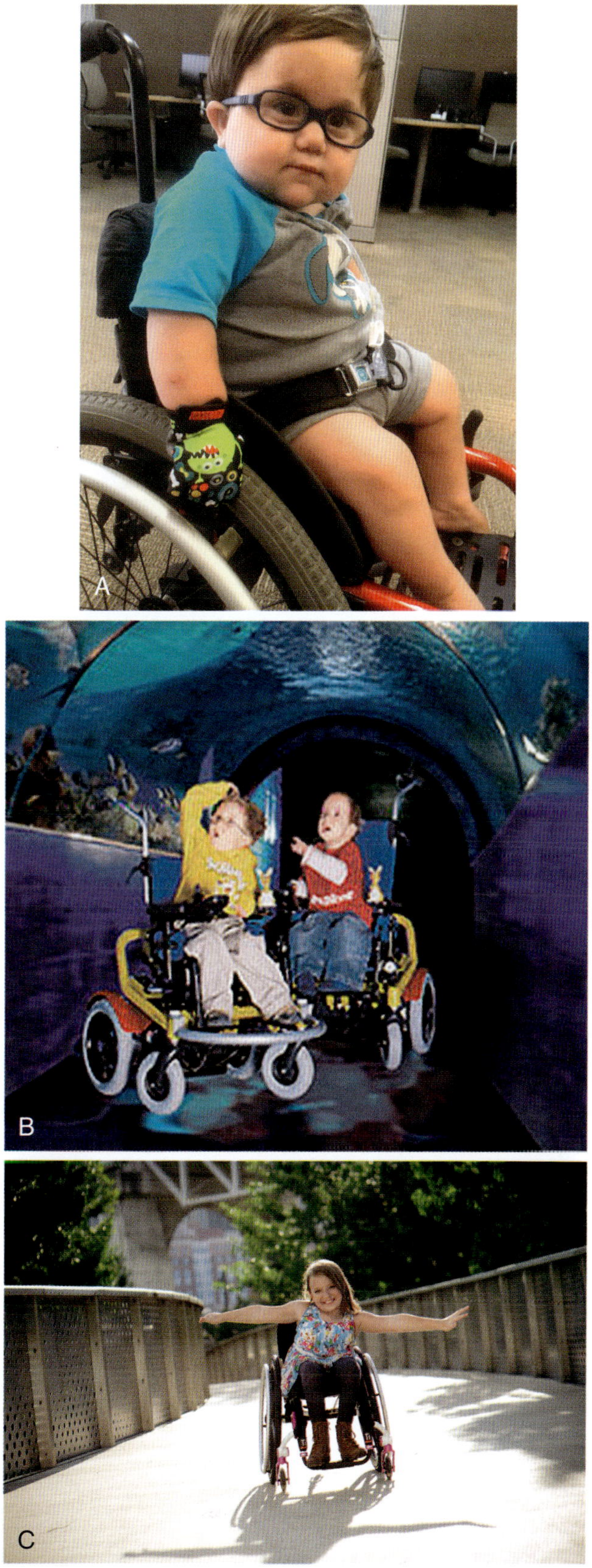


**Fig. 32.3** (A) Child in child-size wheelchair with long push cane for caregiver assistance. (B) Two children in power wheelchairs enjoying the aquarium. (C) Young girl in a child-size wheelchair playfully poising with arms outstretched as she rolls down a bridge slope along a city path.

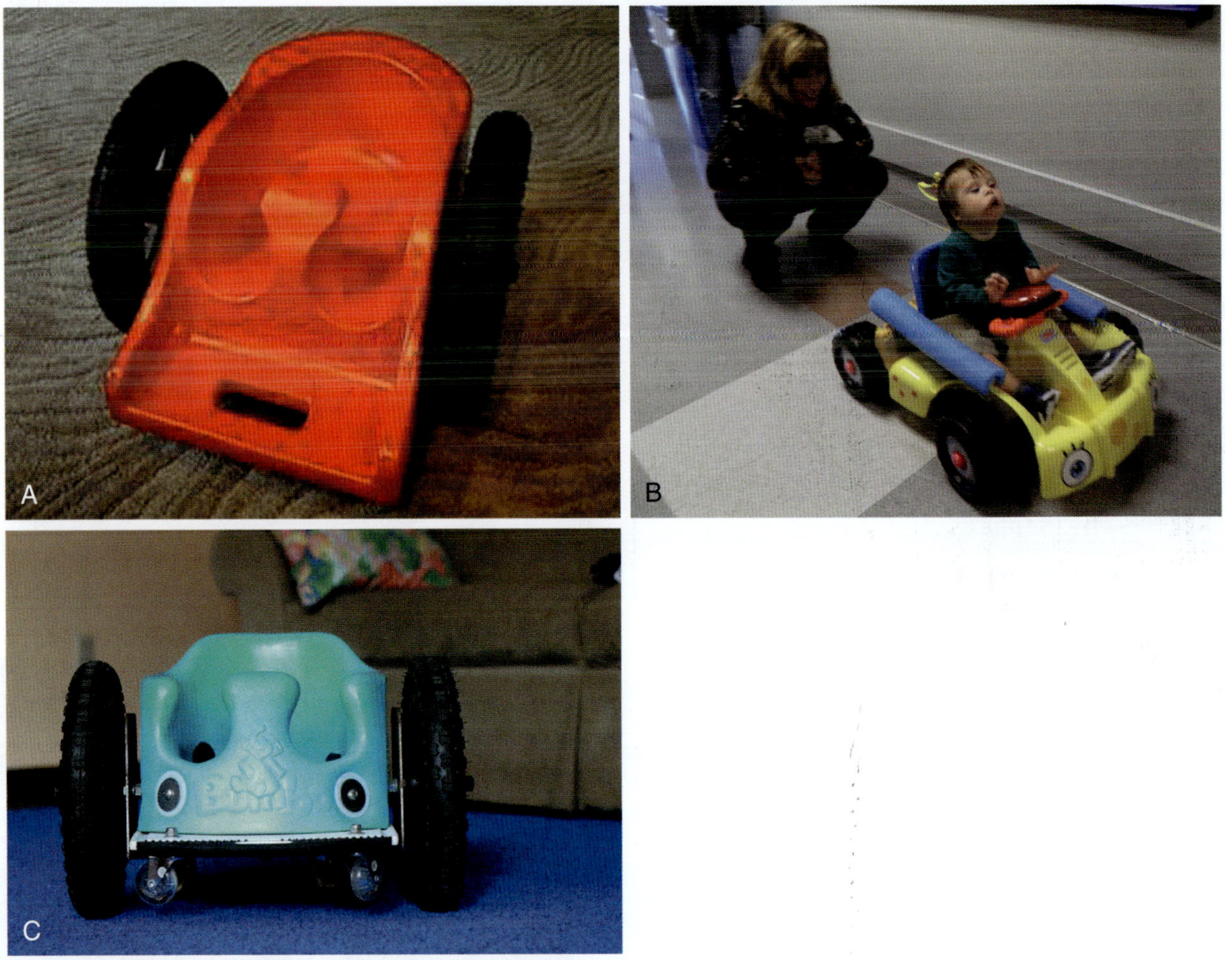


**Fig. 32.4** Low-technology mobility devices include (A) Zip Zap chair. (B) Go Baby Go car is a low-technology mobility option that allows a child to activate a switch to move. (C) Bumbo chair.

**TABLE 32.1 Low- and High-Technology Options for Mobility**

| Type of Technology | Examples |
|---|---|
| **Low Technology:** These are lightweight, general-use solutions that are designed for short-term usage. | • Walkers, crutches, and canes<br>• Direct to consumer mobility products such as the ZipZap chair (Fig. 32.4A)<br>• Go Baby Go (Huang & Galloway, 2012; Logan et al., 2016a) (Fig. 32.4B).<br>• Bumbo wheelchair uses a small manual wheelchair with a Bumbo chair as the seat (Fig. 32.4C) |
| **High Technology:** These are devices that address specific customized needs of client. Equipment is more durable and robust but is often more complex and costlier and may require accommodation for transportation and accessibility due to increased size and weight. | • Power wheelchairs<br>• Ultra-lightweight manual wheelchairs<br>• Exoskeletons |

**BOX 32.3 Importance of Combining Low- and High-Tech Options for Greater Participation and Access**

Combining low- and high-tech solutions allows for a greater variety of movement experiences (Feldner et al., 2016) and provides greater access to participate in a range of activities. For example, while a pediatric power wheelchair is durable with extensive battery life and may be a primary system for a large portion of a child's daily mobility, if that child is going to the park with a friend, the friend's family most likely will not have a wheelchair van to transport the child's chair. They may, however, have enough space to bring a modified ride-on car that has enough battery for the two friends to play and chase each other around the park for almost 2 hours.

Another example is the child who is highly functional in the classroom in a walker, as they can easily approach their peers and classroom activities. On the playground, however, the same walker does not allow them to keep up with their peers, and they easily fatigue as they try to navigate uneven surfaces. A different piece of equipment, such as a joystick-controlled power wheelchair or ultra lightweight wheelchair, affords them the same level of independence that they experience in the classroom.

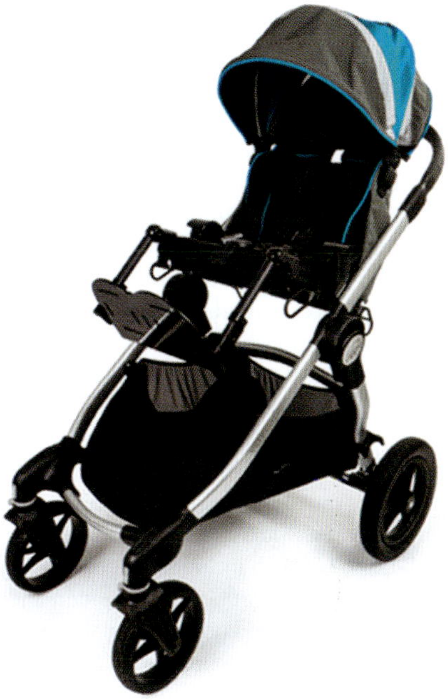

Fig. 32.5 Medical stroller with canopy and postural supports and adjustable footrest.

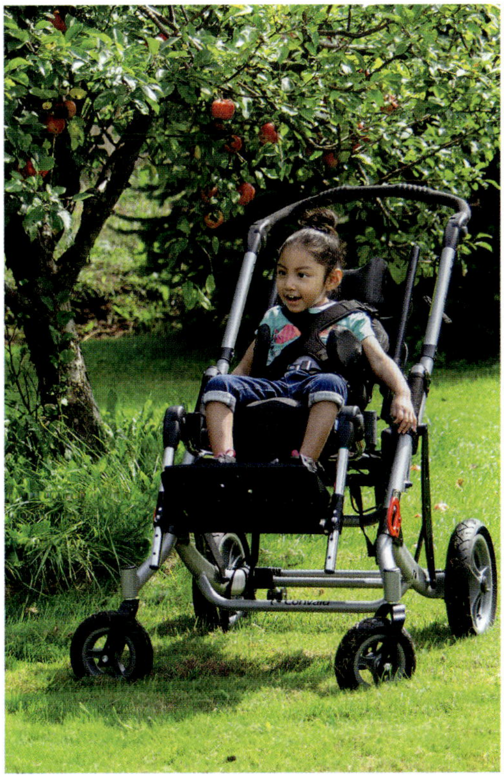

Fig. 32.6 Young girl using a Convaid stroller with a positioning belt and supports while out apple picking with her family. (Photo courtesy of Permobil.)

community (Fig. 32.6). Some children may be able to functionally walk in their home but need a mobility device in the community. These devices (similar to umbrella strollers) are made of stronger materials to withstand the weight of larger children. Most of these devices do not tilt and cannot accommodate bony deformities or pressure injuries, which is why they are not generally used as primary devices.

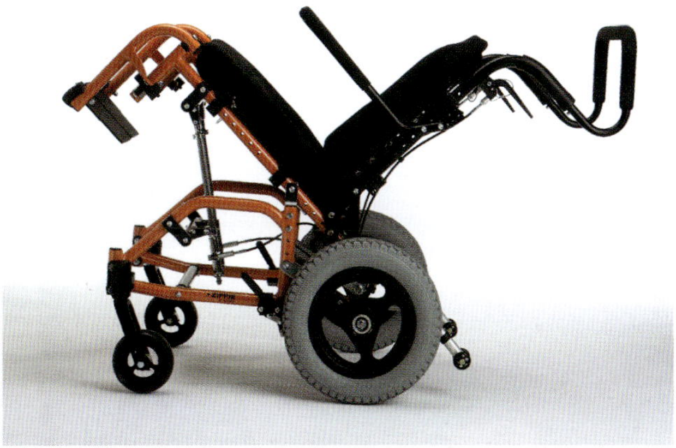

Fig. 32.7 Manual tilt wheelchair (missing needed headrest).

Some funding sources do not fund medical strollers beyond the early intervention sizes, since most children who utilize dependent mobility devices frequently require more support than is available in this style of device. In some states, payers do not fund secondary wheelchairs or equipment that will not be used in the home. The occupational therapy practitioner works with a durable medical equipment (DME) supplier to determine whether the equipment is available on a case-by-case basis. It is important for clinicians to understand other available funding resources to assist families in securing other mobility devices to support community engagement (such as Medicaid Waiver programs, Assistive Technology Act Programs, Shriners Hospitals, Easter Seals, or community organizations).

**Tilt-In-Space Wheelchairs.** Many children over the age of 3 who need dependent mobility devices require tilt-in-space wheelchairs that allow for 45–55 degrees of tilt. Practitioners teach families the importance of and how to fully tilt the wheelchair hourly for pressure relief to prevent development of pressure injuries. The tilt also aids in positioning the child during a transfer, as gravity assists by holding their bodies in the correct position as strapping and supports are attached. Additionally, it allows for a change in position throughout the day to assist with trunk and head control (Fig. 32.7). Specialty cushions, back supports, and headrests are designed to interface with tilt-in-space wheelchairs, which allow for customization to meet each child's needs and can be modified over time (Fig. 32.8).

**Self-Propelling Manual Wheelchairs.** Manual wheelchairs for mobility are divided into two categories: folding or rigid. *Folding* wheelchairs have a cross brace underneath that allows the wheelchair to be folded in half for transportation (Fig. 32.9A). Caregivers may choose folding frames for children because they perceive that they are easier to place into a vehicle and are more intuitive for others' assisting with transportation that are unfamiliar with wheelchair breakdown. *Rigid* wheelchairs have a rigid frame. The rigid frame can be broken down for transportation by folding the backrest onto the seat, or removing the backrest, and removing the wheels. Rigid frames are often lighter in weight and more durable; however, they may not have as much adjustability for growth (Fig. 32.9B). Table 32.2 provides information about important features of wheelchairs for children.

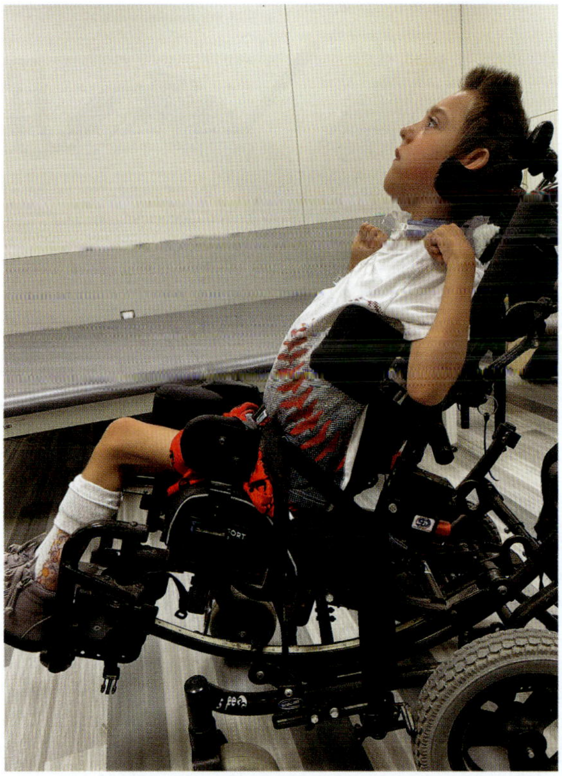

Fig. 32.8 Young boy in a manual tilt-in-space wheelchair with lateral trunk support, with headrest in approximately 25 degrees of tilt for improved posture and head support.

## Power Assist and Power Add-On Devices

Power assist devices provide greater access and independence for users (Fig. 32.10). Power assist wheels have built-in motors in each wheel or a motor on the back that drives the wheels. This technology adds significant weight, 20 lb or more, to the wheelchair and can make propulsion difficult. It can be difficult for some users to push straight as coordination of both upper extremities is necessary. The wheels can be removed for stowing the wheelchair in a vehicle. However, the process takes time, and the parts of the wheelchair are heavy.

The rear attaching device is a motor that can be added to a rigid-frame or folding-frame manual wheelchair (such as SmartDrive and Smoov). The power assist is activated by a smartwatch, Bluetooth, or manual switch, depending on the device, to allow for power-assisted mobility on demand. This device adds about 13 lb to the wheelchair. When not in use, the device is barely noticeable and does not restrict mobility (Fig. 32.11). The power assist device can also be added to wheelchairs, such as tilt-in-space devices, and the wired switch can be used by the care provider to aid in pushing. The Bluetooth switch includes a mobile app that enables the user to track distance and to aid in health promotion and prevention of injury, while providing the user and occupational therapy practitioner the ability to customize the device for optimal use.

Power add-on devices offer another option for manual wheelchair users who could benefit from power at times or where different environments make self-propulsion difficult or unattainable (Fig. 32.12). Power add-on devices are also appropriate for individuals with motor planning issues that make them unsuccessful with power assist devices (Fig. 32.13A and B). Power add-on devices may be appropriate for those who cannot always use power, such as if power cannot be used during the Sabbath, and there must be an option for manual mobility.

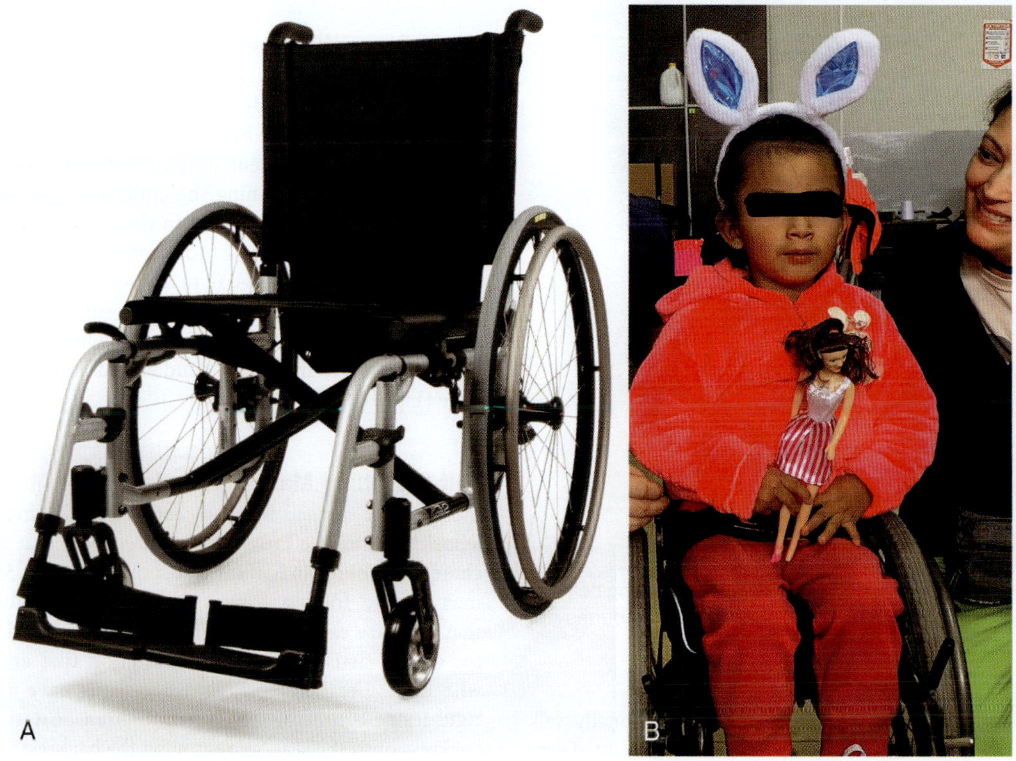

Fig. 32.9 (A) Standard folding wheelchair with upholstery seat and back, quick-release spoked wheels, swing away, removable leg rests, and push wheel locks available in child and adult sizes. (B) Little girl in a child-size wheelchair using pelvic positioning belt.

## TABLE 32.2 Important Features of Wheelchairs for Children and Youth

| Feature | Considerations | Importance |
|---|---|---|
| Chair setup | There are more than 13 measurements and specific features that need to be determined for all wheelchair setups (DiGiovine et al., 2012). Each feature needs to be individually chosen for the child based on their function, positioning, and needs. The center of gravity can be adjusted by the wheel placement with an ultra-lightweight wheelchair. The optimal wheel position is when the axle is in alignment with the child's shoulder, and with arms down, the axle touches their middle finger. | Better wheel position improves wheel contact, decreases the forces needed to propel, and decreases risk of upper extremity injury.<br>A more rearward center of gravity provides more stability in the chair to lessen the risk of the chair tipping over backward but can make wheelies difficult for navigating door thresholds and curbs. |
| Chair aesthetics | Pediatric wheelchairs are available in bright colors with different styles of wheels and other customizations to make the device personalized. Aesthetics and choice are important psychosocial considerations when selecting and designing the wheelchair. | When children feel good about themselves, they are more social, engaged, functional, and productive (Doubt & McColl, 2003).<br>The wheelchair is part of their overall appearance, and it should disappear underneath them as much as possible. When the wheelchair is properly adjusted to maximize function, the chair is not visible, and the child interacts with others without focusing on their wheelchair. |
| Chair weight | Pediatric ultra-lightweight aluminum rigid wheelchairs have similar adjustability and functionality to adult ultralight wheelchairs. These chairs weigh 12–16 lb compared to the more medical pediatric wheelchairs that have previously been available that weigh at least 25 lb. The manufacturer-published weight of the chair is just the chair itself, not the additional features added to the chair. As different features and positioning equipment are added to the chair, the heavier it becomes. Older children may be successful using manual wheelchairs made from lighter materials like titanium and carbon fiber. These chairs may provide tremor dampening (i.e., compensate for the child's tremors), which can improve the comfort of mobility across uneven surfaces. | For adults, heavier and larger wheelchairs increase the risk of injuries and limit overall function throughout the day (Ferrero et al., 2015). For a child who weighs 20–30 lb, having a chair that weighs almost the same as the child creates propulsion problems. Larger and less adjustable chairs are difficult to push and lead to decreased activity level, decreased function and participation, and weight gain. |
| Chair size | It is important to select a chair that will work for children as they grow.<br>Children with disabilities generally do not grow as fast as their age-matched peers. They tend to be 5%–10% shorter than their peers from age 2–8 years, and this difference increases by the year of age. They tend to grow more in length than they do in width (Krick et al., 1996). While practitioners order chairs to fit the child for a period of 5 years as the child grows, they must consider that children must use the chair daily. Therefore, ordering a wheelchair with a seat 3–5 in too wide is not recommended. | If the seat width is larger than necessary, the hand rims will be difficult to access in a manual wheelchair, placing the upper extremities in potentially injurious positions (Walter et al., 2002). This means that for 5 years, the child has to significantly abduct their shoulders to propel, which predisposes them to shoulder, elbow, and wrist injuries (Kirby et al., 1994)<br>It is also more difficult for children who must reach out to their wheels to propel the wheelchair, which limits their mobility, enjoyment, function, and independence. It is also important to note that hanging things on the back of the child's wheelchair adds weight and can offset the center of gravity adjustments. Pushing a heavier wheelchair puts unnecessary stress on the joints and can cause injuries, and added weight can cause the wheelchair to tip backward and is a safety risk. |

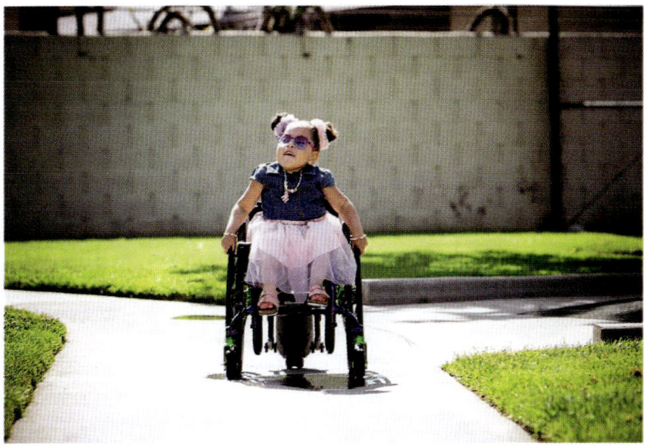

**Fig. 32.10** Young girl independently traveling down a sidewalk in her child-size wheelchair, using her SmartDrive. (Photo courtesy of Permobil.)

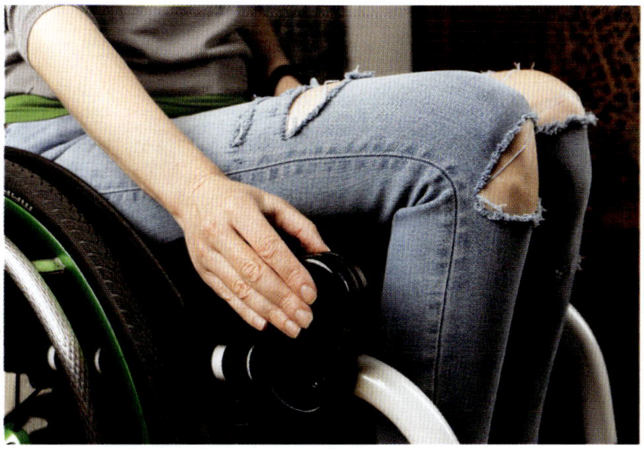

**Fig. 32.11** SmartDrive power assist installed on rigid-frame wheelchair with wired speed control dial mounted to frame near right thigh for easy access. (Photo courtesy of Permobil.)

## Power Wheelchairs

If a child cannot propel a wheelchair a functional distance at the same speed and efficiency as demonstrated by the average person walking, fatigues, and cannot functionally keep up with their peers, or has no experience or means of functional movement on their own, then the mobility team should consider power mobility. The advantages of a power wheelchair include increased speed capability, ease of maneuvering, better function on different surfaces, and less energy expenditure required for moving, particularly for long distances. Children who use a power wheelchair may also have a manual wheelchair for use in environments not accessible to a power wheelchair or when the power wheelchair is being repaired.

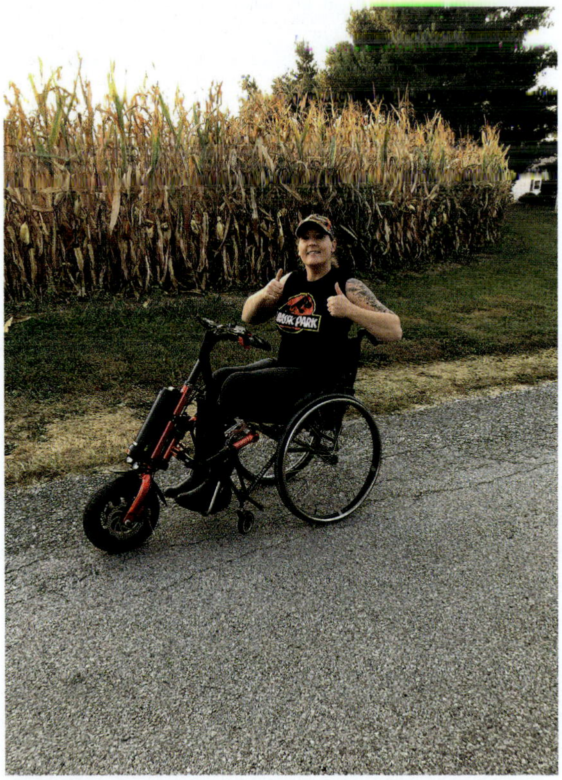

Fig. 32.12 Teen in manual wheelchair with Firelfy power add-on giving two thumbs up while trialing the device on a road in front of a cornfield. (Photo courtesy of Rio Mobility.)

Power wheelchairs are battery-operated motorized units the user drives by means of controls, such as a joystick, pneumatic sip-and-puff, proportional head controls, nonproportional head controls, proximity switches (i.e., switches that operate when the user moves close to them), multiple push switches, or eye gaze. Table 32.3 describes some of the switches that can be used for driving power wheelchairs.

Power wheelchairs are differentiated by the electronics, control systems, and placement of the drive wheel. The position of the drive wheel affects the maneuverability, stability, traction, and performance (e.g., speed, efficiency, obstacle climbing, and crossing side slope). Maneuverability depends on the wheelchair's turning radius. Fig. 32.14 shows the three types of wheelchair bases and describes the pros and cons of each. Occupational therapy practitioners consider drive wheel position when recommending mobility systems. They must consider the child's environment, while also considering how the equipment will be managed by caregivers. The practitioner works with the mobility team to make recommendations that can allow children to be independent. For example, it can make the difference in enabling a child to go into their bedroom or bathroom by themselves or getting into a bathroom stall to transfer to the toilet.

The speed and performance of the chair is set by programming the electronics. Wheelchairs may be adjusted regarding torque, tremor dampening, strength required to move the joystick, speed, acceleration, and tracking straight on slopes and uneven surfaces. Programming the chair requires a specialized programmer available through the DME supplier. Tracking may prove useful for children driving long distances in rural areas. Speed ranges from 4 to 7.5 miles per hour. The distance

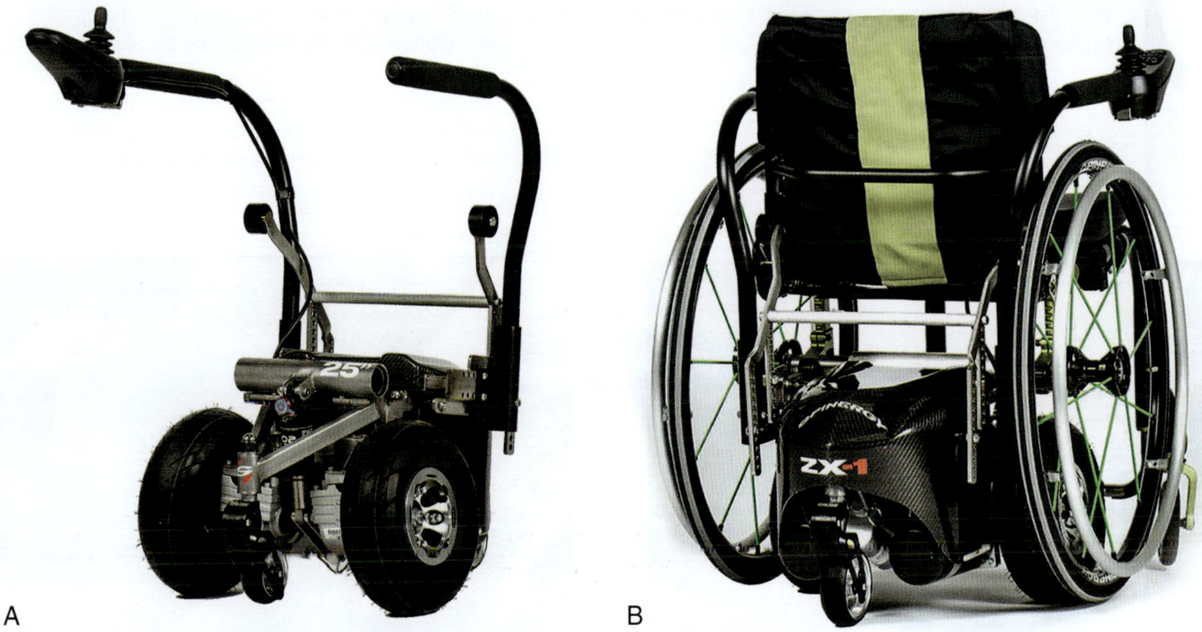


Fig. 32.13 (A) The ZX-1 is a power add-on device that converts virtually any manual wheelchair into a powered manual wheelchair. It requires no tools or assistance to attach and detach from the device. (B) The ZX-1 is attached to a manual wheelchair.

traveled on one battery charge ranges from 20 to 25 miles, depending on the state of the charge, quality of the batteries, and additional devices plugged into them.

There are several manufacturers of power wheelchairs, and each of the manufacturers have variations of powered mobility, wheel positions, seating, and powered seating options, with the most common being tilt, recline, and elevate (Fig. 32.15). Some have powered standing options, moving the seat down to the floor (Fig. 32.16A and B), anterior tilt, posterior tilt, and even lateral tilt (Fig. 32.17A–C). Recommendations depend on the child's medical needs for access like transfers, respiratory conditions, visual field orientation, circulation, or skin integrity, functional needs in their environments, and family preferences.

**TABLE 32.3 Description of Switches to Access Power**

| Switch | Description |
|---|---|
| Joystick | Long knob that moves in 360 directions<br>Comes in several sizes, which allows practitioner to select one that works best for child |
| Joystick knobs | Various styles, shapes, and sizes<br>T-shaped and U-shaped that can help users access power and drive wheelchair; the variety allows the practitioner to find the "right switch" for the child |
| Alternate control interfaces | Brackets to change position of switches, so that user can access switch as they are able |
| Proximity sensors | User gets close (or proximal) to the switch) |
| Fiber optic | Wave arm above it to operate |
| Sip and puff | User sips or puffs into tube to activate power |
| Eye gaze | Eye gazing on switch will activate it; requires minimal head movement and control |

It is important that the mobility team understand electronic navigation as this will be important for selecting the right wheelchair system that will last until another can be provided. Wheelchair manufacturers provide a choice of several models that are intended for joystick operation only. These are called nonexpendable electronics, and they cannot be modified to add extra seat functions, Augmentative and Alternative Communication (AAC) devices, or alternative drive controls. Models that include microprocessors are called expandable electronics. Power wheelchairs that have expandable electronics are capable of being changed and programmed to add features and functions.

When recommending a powered wheelchair, the mobility team considers a child's needs today and for up to the next 5 years. For instance, the access needs for a child with cerebral palsy will grow and change as the child gains experience. The child may develop better motor control and require different methods to control devices such as computer access, environmental controls, gaming, and other electronics, or an AAC device. Conversely, children experiencing limited strength or a decline in function may need different controls and expandable electronics.

Several features can be made available on power wheelchairs to increase a child's function. An attendant joystick mounted to the back of the wheelchair can be accessed by caregivers who need to drive the power wheelchair when accuracy is required, such as moving up a narrow ramp or when the child needs assistance (such as when tired or in a new environment). Many manufacturers provide USB and Bluetooth connections on wheelchairs or as part of the joystick. These features allow for plugging in mobile devices, communication devices, and environmental control units and provide opportunities for computer access, communication, and access and control of the user's environments.

Power wheelchairs do not typically fold for transport in a vehicle and weigh from 100 to 250+ lb. There are options for portable power wheelchairs; unfortunately, most of these are not reimbursed by insurance and have limited programming abilities and limited seating customizations or options. However, they are the solution for some, they do provide more options for transport as they either break down into a

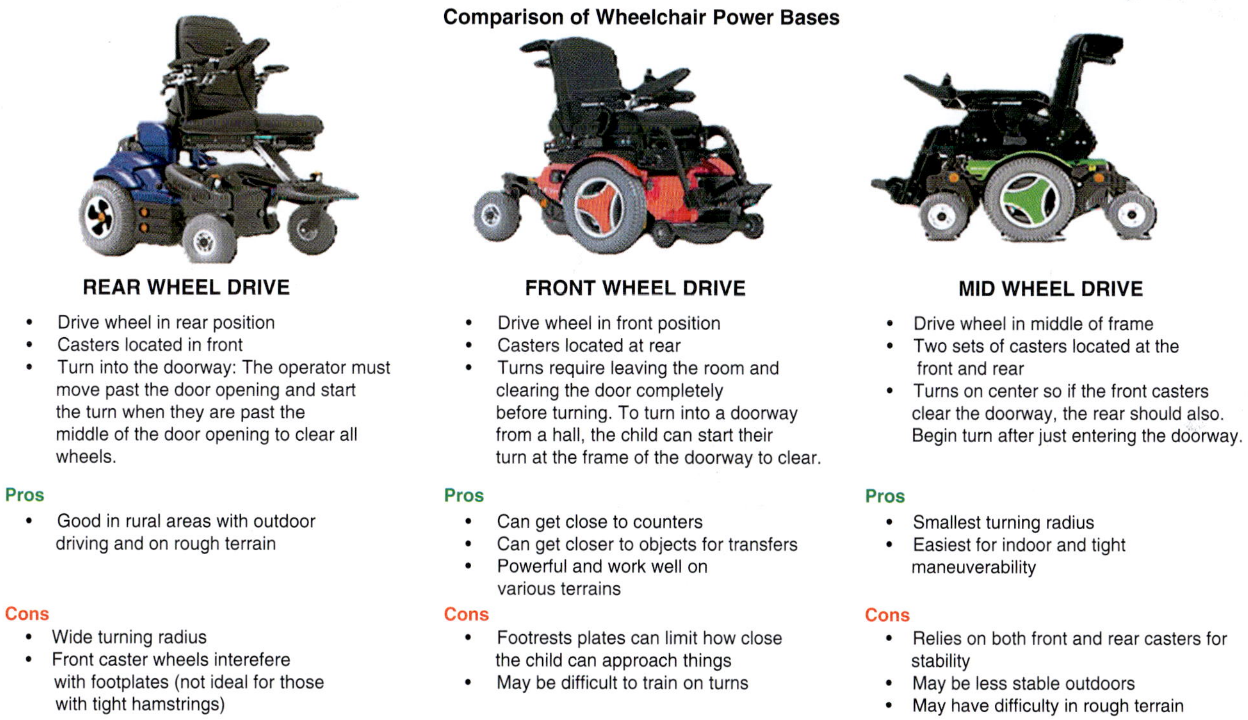


**Fig. 32.14** Side-by-side comparison of power wheelchair bases with pros and cons.

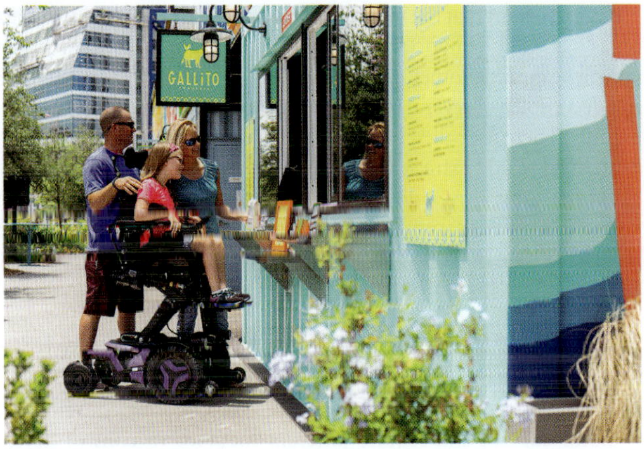


**Fig. 32.15** Young girl is with her family and is using a power seat elevator on a front wheel drive power wheelchair to order at a restaurant to-go window. (Photo courtesy of Permobil.)

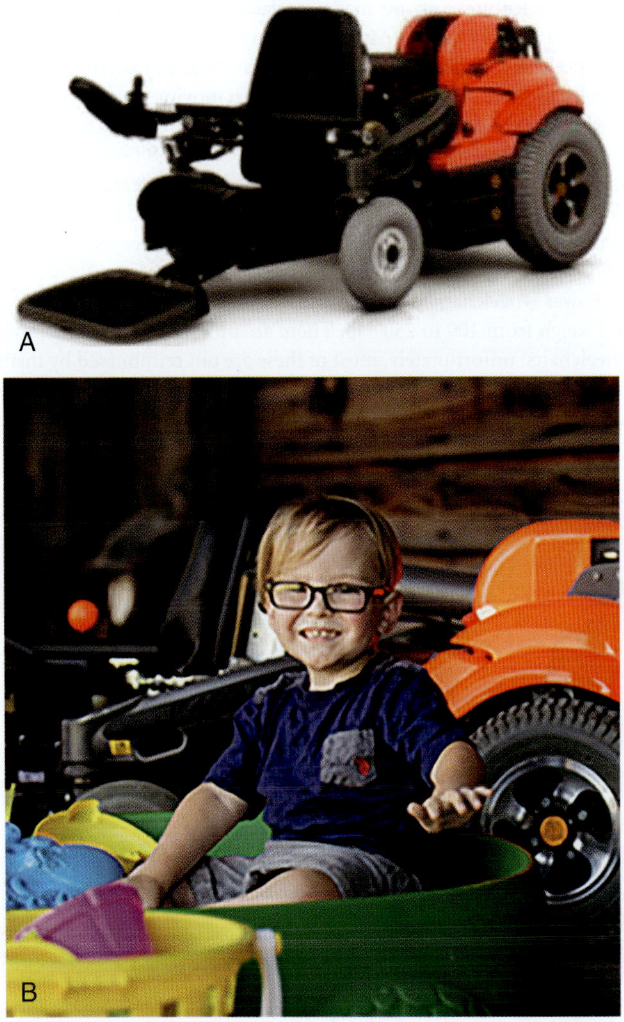

**Fig. 32.16** (A) The power wheelchair lower to floor feature allows children to play closer to floor. (B) Child who used power wheelchair lower to floor feature to transfer into sandbox to play. ((A) Courtesy of Permobil.)

few manageable parts or they fold, and the technology is evolving (Fig. 32.18). Accessible vans that have been modified with a lift or ramp are required for transporting the user and most power wheelchairs in a vehicle. If the child can be transferred to a car seat, a covered trailer or platform can be hitched to the back of a vehicle for transporting a power wheelchair. Power wheelchairs can be transported by the school bus or other public transportation.

## Mobility Scooters

Mobility scooters offer another option for powered mobility (Fig. 32.19). The child or youth who uses a scooter typically has good sitting balance, requires minimal adaptations for positioning, and understands and physically operates the tiller controls. Scooters require more room for maneuvering and therefore limit access to performing ADLs in most home environments.

## Standers

Anyone who cannot independently stand can benefit from the use of a stander (Paleg et al., 2013) if there are no contraindications for weight-bearing. For individuals who lack the strength to stand, a standing frame places them in a good position to stretch their lower extremity and trunk muscles for extended periods. This stretch can help maintain and improve lower extremity range of motion. See Box 32.4 for the important benefits of standing. Evidence suggests that children should stand at least 5 days a week for a minimum of 60 minutes to get the positive results of improved bone density (Thompson et al., 2000), contracture management, spasticity reduction, and lower urinary tract infection risk from standing (Goodwin et al., 2018; Paleg & Livingstone, 2015).

There are four main styles of standing systems: prone, supine, multipositional, and sit-to-stand. Within those types, there are dynamic and static standers. Additionally, there are standing systems that are integrated into both power and manual wheelchairs.

**Supine Versus Prone Versus Sit-To-Stand.** Supine standers are appropriate for medically fragile children and youth who have poor head control and those who have tracheostomies (Fig. 32.20A). Supine standers are the least stressful of all the types of standers because most of the weight is borne through the back rather than through the legs. This type of stander is easy for a family to use because the child is placed into the stander in supine. The more upright a child is positioned, the more weight-bearing they do through their legs.

Prone standers are used for children who are alert and interactive and who have fair to good head control (Fig. 32.20B). They can help improve head control if the caregiver closely supervises the child. A prone stander can facilitate weight-shifting because the child is leaning forward while in the stander. One problem with prone standers is that they can be difficult to position the child. This is because the child must be placed in the stander in a standing position. This can be a challenge for a parent who is alone and must hold the child in the correct position as the straps are adjusted and tightened.

For children who can benefit from a prone stander but still may not have the head control to use one for the needed amount of time, multipositional standers are needed. These standers allow the child to be positioned in supine and then moved into prone and back as is needed for head control. Newer models can do this in one motion without moving positioning equipment, which makes them easy for families to use.

Sit-to-stand standers work best for children who would use prone standers (Fig. 32.20C). This stander allows the individual to start in a sitting position, which is an easy position in which to secure the child. The other benefit of this type of stander is that some of these designs can be used in sitting for taking rest breaks. It can have an adjustable height and adjustable depth tray so that it can be used well in both positions.

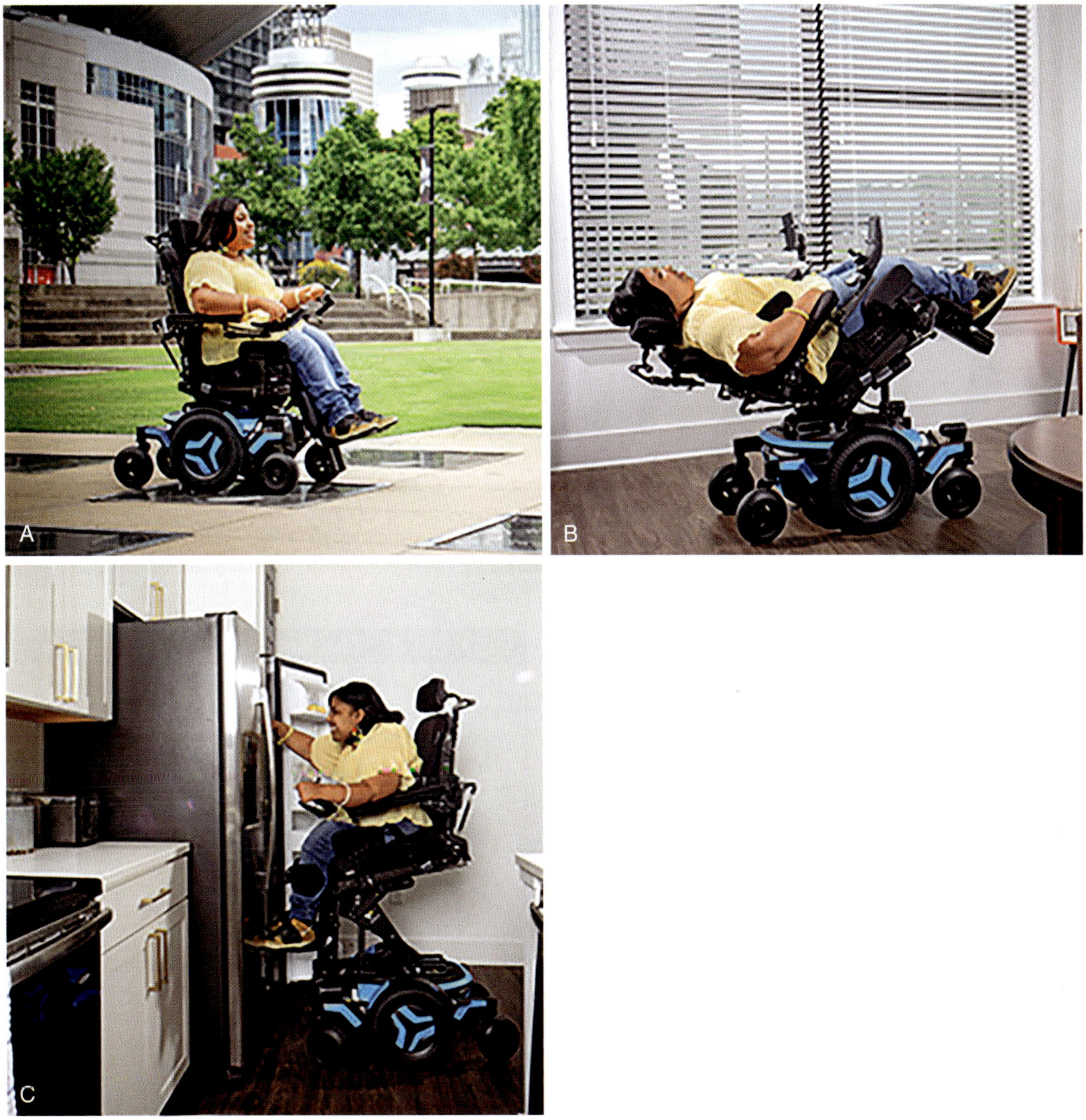


**Fig. 32.17** (A) Young adult crossing campus in a multifunction mid-wheel drive power wheelchair, (B) using posterior tilt and recline functions to take a break, and (C) using seat elevation and anterior tilt functions to reach the top shelf of the refrigerator. ((A–C) Courtesy of Permobil.)

**Dynamic, Static, or Mobile.** Static standers are the most prescribed type of stander. The child or youth is always fully supported, and the leg muscles are basically inactive. While most standers can be rolled from room to room by a caregiver, the person and the stander do not move.

Dynamic standers allow and encourage movement (Fig. 32.21A). The child weights and unweights their legs as well as flexes and extends their joints. Usually, this movement is obtained by grasping handles with the upper extremities like an elliptical trainer. These are usually referred to as gliders.

Mobile standers let the person move around their environment while in a standing position (Fig. 32.21B). They can be used in both the classroom and at home. They work well on level surfaces but not on playgrounds or on grass.

**Wheelchair Standers.** Power wheelchairs may have standers integrated into them. The benefit of these systems is that the person does not have to transfer out of the wheelchair to use the device, so they can use it more frequently. It also can assist the child to complete their activities of daily living and can increase their independence throughout the day (Fig. 32.22A). There are also manual wheelchairs with stander functions. Manual wheelchairs with stander functions are typically an additional piece of equipment like other standers as the extra weight impacts propulsion. This can

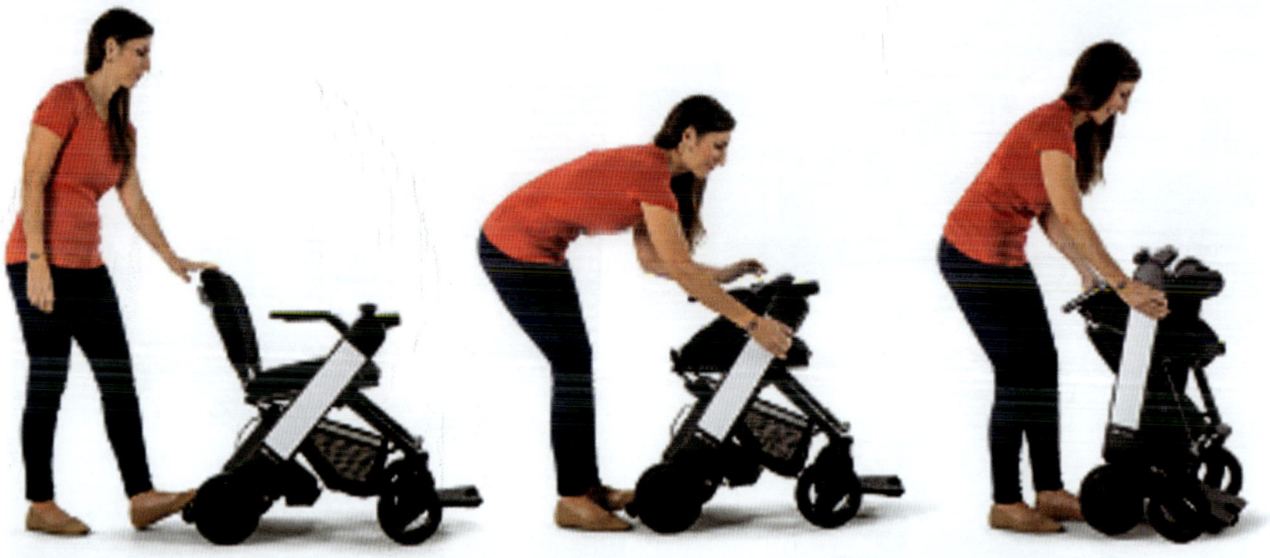

**Fig. 32.18** WHILL Model F lightweight folding power wheelchair is an example of portable power options. A female demonstrates folding the WHILL F in three steps. (1) Woman approaches the WHILL F from behind, (2) releases the frame lock and begins folding, and (3) stands holding the folded power wheelchair. (Courtesy of WHILL Inc.)

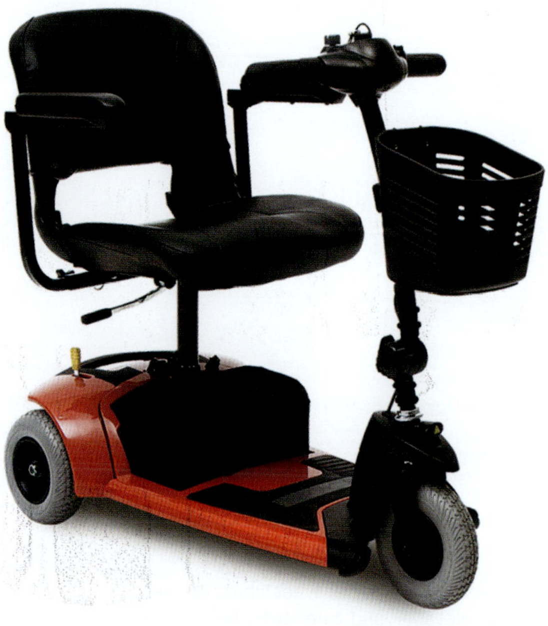

**Fig. 32.19** Three-wheel tiller controlled mobility scooter.

be excellent accommodation for classroom activities and science labs (Fig. 32.22B).

## Walkers

Children with the ability to pull to a standing position, maintain a grip on a handle, and steer with their arms may be able to use a handheld walker. These walkers are designed for use either in front of (anterior walker) or behind (reverse posture walker) the child (Fig. 32.23A and B). Children with mild to moderate cerebral palsy or lower levels of spina bifida with leg bracing most commonly use reverse posture walkers. Walkers can have two or four wheels and are available in various wheel sizes. The smaller the caster, the more difficult it is for use outdoors and over uneven surfaces. Posterior walkers are available with a feature in which the casters lock when the walker is pushed backward. This feature enables the child to stand and lean against the walker or the seat during rest periods. However, this feature makes maneuvering the walker more difficult because the child cannot move the walker in a reverse direction, which is needed when backing away and turning, without lifting it up to overcome the antirollback mechanism. Casters can be fixed rather than swiveled, which allows movement only in the forward direction, so the user must lift the walker to turn it. Swivel

### BOX 32.4 The Benefits of Standing

Standing provides children with a different view of their environment, which can be motivating and exciting. Along with psychological benefits, standing contributes to physical health and wellness. All children and youth benefit from time standing upright as indicated by the following important benefits:

- Decreases spasticity in children with cerebral palsy (Tremblay et al., 1990) and lessens spasticity in individuals with spinal cord injuries (Walter et al., 1999)
- Supports bone growth (Han et al., 2017; Henderson et al., 2004; Tosum, 2017; Whedon, 1982) and increases forming the acetabulum (Macias, 2005)
- May help prevent hip subluxation (Macias-Merlo et al., 2015a, 2015b, 2015c; Martinsson & Himmelmann, 2011)
- Improves bone mineral density (Han et al., 2017) and stabilizes the loss of bone mineral density in boys with Duchenne muscular dystrophy who have lost the ability to ambulate (Townsend et al., 2016); bone density is critical if the child is going to be able to use emerging technologies like exoskeletons and other walking technologies
- Reduces risk of pressure injuries (Delmore et al., 2019; Walter et al., 1999)
- Benefits people psychologically (Huston, 2001; Walter et al., 1999); people report improved quality of life when engaged in activities in standing; standing improves a person's self-esteem by allowing eye-to-eye conversations with peers; also, improves person's mood and decreases the risk of developing depression over time
- Improves motor function in children (Ahlborg et al., 2006; Netz et al., 2007).
- Facilitates emptying of the bladder, which can decrease the risk of urinary tract infections
- Improves circulatory, gastrointestinal, bowel control, and respiratory functions (Dunn et al., 1998; Edwards & Layne, 2007; Stuberg, 1992)

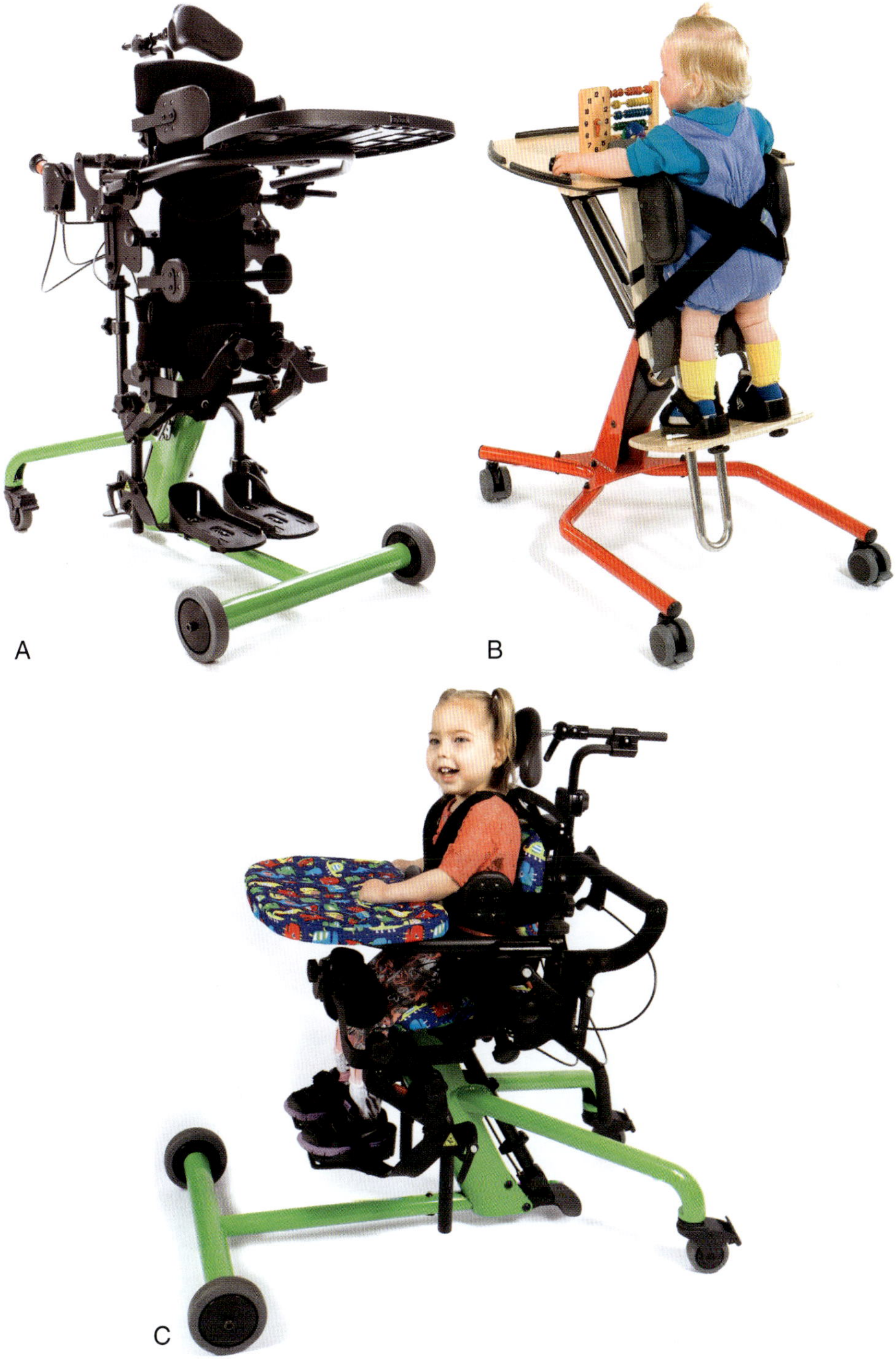

**Fig. 32.20** (A) Supine stander. (B) Toddler in Rifton prone stander playing with a wooden bead toy. (C) Young girl sitting in a sit-to-stand stander with multicolored tray, with lateral and head supports.

casters allow the child to turn the walker without lifting it, but this feature requires more postural control from the child to direct the walker. The advantage of handheld walkers is their convenient transportability. The disadvantage for some users is the fact that the hands are not free for performing tasks.

Gait trainers are designed for children who have some ability to move their legs reciprocally but need support at the pelvis, chest, and possibly the upper extremities and head (Fig. 32.24A and B). The gait trainer allows children to weight bear and engage in upright activity but does not train a child to walk. Occupational therapy practitioners are careful to discuss the purpose of the device with parents and children. In some cases, funding sources will pay for either a stander or a gait trainer, as both provide upright weight-bearing.

The child's team will make decisions regarding the type of gait trainer and support features based on the child's physical function and the environment. Selection of the appropriate features and adjustments to provide optimal positioning increases use of the device. For example, children who adduct or scissor their legs because of spasticity may propel the gait trainer more efficiently when sitting on a wider and longer padded seat as this reduces adduction and maintains leg alignment during ambulation. Adjustable posterior tilt, a feature that positions the child slightly behind vertical, may also assist a weak child in

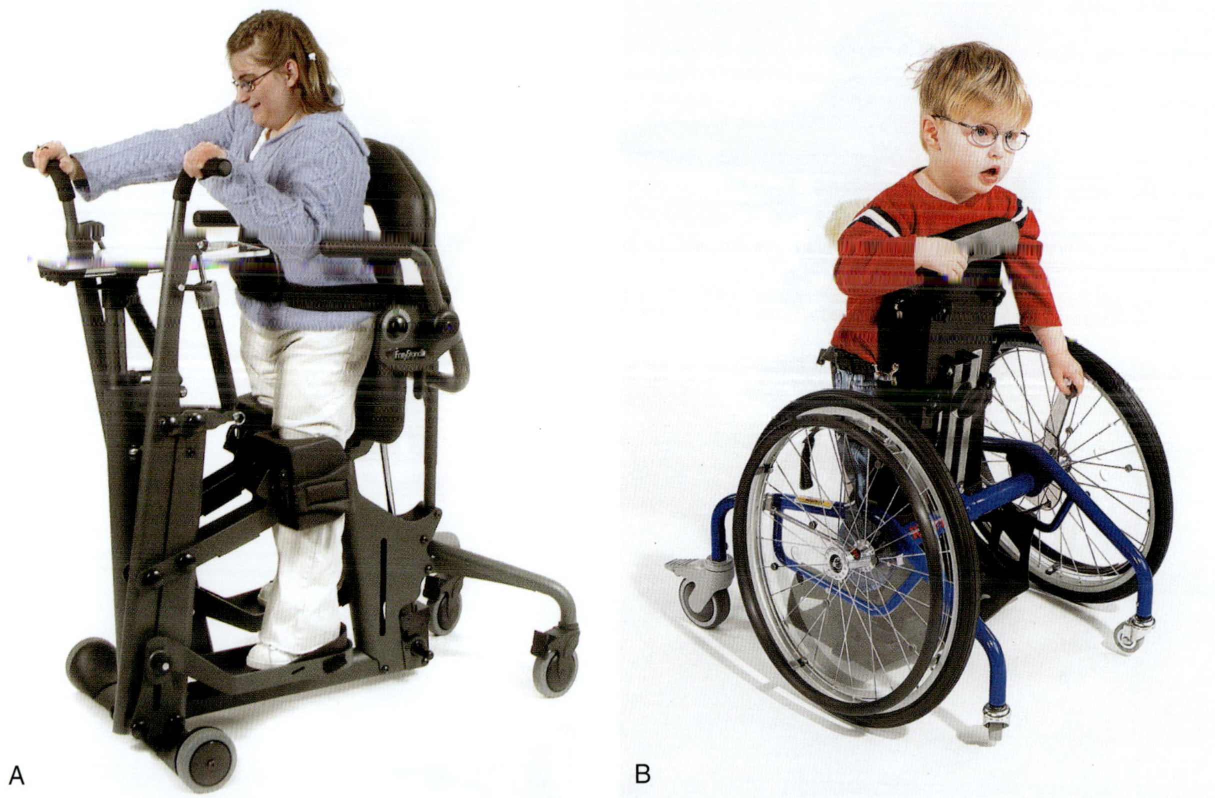

Fig. 32.21 (A) Girl using a dynamic, exercise glider stander. (B) Young boy using a Rabbit anterior support wheeled stander.

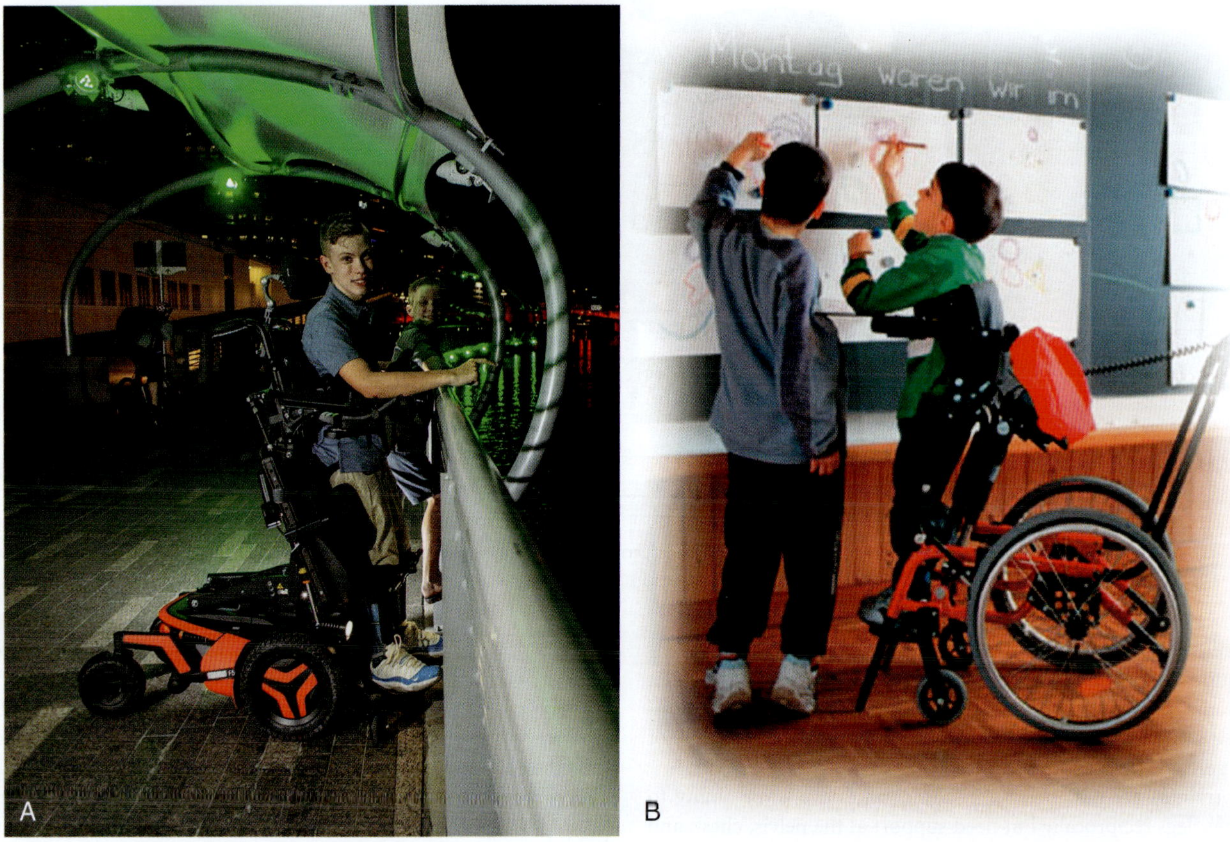


Fig. 32.22 (A) Teen using the standing feature of his power wheelchair, standing at the rail with his younger brother looking out across the night-lit waterway. (B) Boy stands next to his classmate as they write on papers hanging on the chalkboard while using a manual wheelchair with a stand feature. ((A) Courtesy of Permobil.)

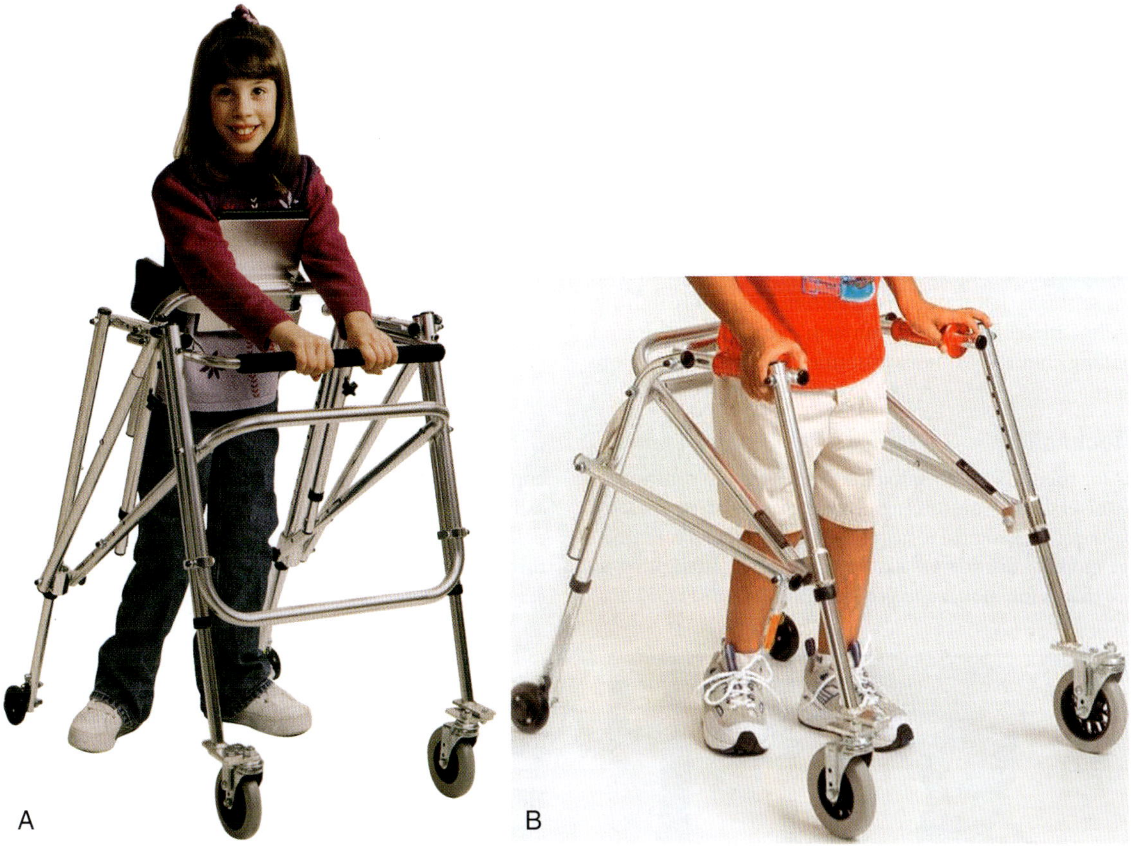

**Fig. 32.23** (A) Girl using an anterior walker with trunk support and horizontal grasp bar. (B) Youth using reverse posture walker without seat.

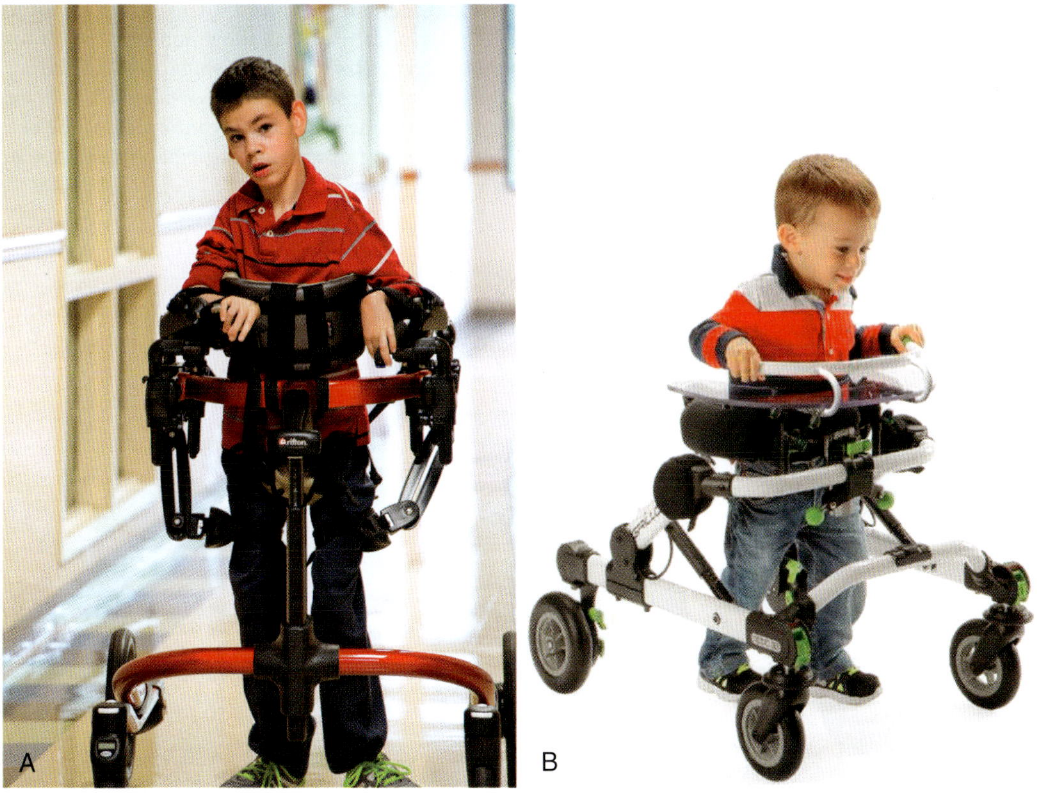

**Fig. 32.24** (A) Student uses gait trainer with arm supports to walk to class. (B) Toddler uses a gait trainer.

maintaining an upright trunk and head position. Children with spastic cerebral palsy may need to be tilted in a slightly forward lean position, which, along with a properly positioned pelvis (in neutral or anteriorly tilted position), assists in placing the feet behind the pelvis and trunk, thereby making it easier for the child to initiate movement in a forward direction. However, forward tilt can also make it more difficult for the child to keep the head upright if the child has limited head control.

Gait trainers provide children with the opportunity to explore their environment in an upright, hands-free position. Gait trainers generally have a large turning radius, which may limit their usefulness in indoor settings. Gait trainers with minimal hardware in front of the child allow the child to be within arm's reach of people and objects, providing children with opportunities to access and explore the environment.

## Emerging Technology

**Exoskeletons** for robotic assisted ambulation are here and continually emerging. A University of Houston engineer received funding to create a pediatric exoskeleton, designed to help children with spinal cord injuries and other mobility disorders walk. Researchers are attempting to create a device that is functional and grows with children (Fig. 32.25).

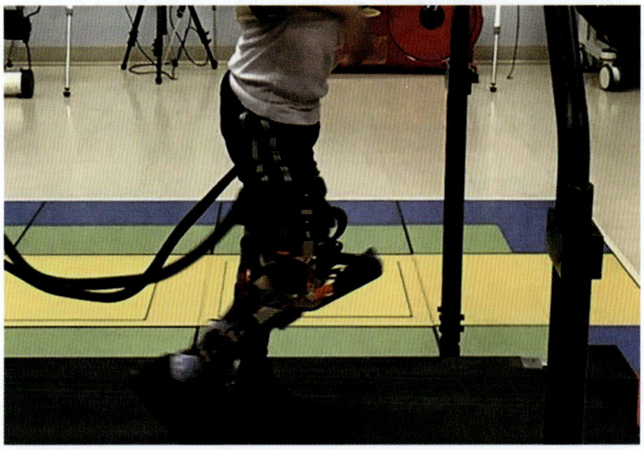

**Fig. 32.25** Youth using a clinical exoskeleton on a treadmill as part of NIH research.

There is much research and use of exoskeleton technology globally. A few exoskeletons now have approval for home use with many others having authorization for clinical use. The use of exoskeletons and other robotic orthosis and prosthetics continues to innovate.

Neurotechnologies, though around for a while, are emerging with implanted technologies that improve ambulation and upper extremity function for propulsion. Brain-computer interfaces are also seeing competition and research and development, as are artificial intelligence enabled neurotechnologies. Emerging technologies are an exciting opportunity for occupational therapy practitioners to contribute to cutting edge development to improve function and occupational performance for individuals with a variety of medical conditions.

Bluetooth technology, Wi-Fi, infrared, and z-wave are being integrated into joysticks to allow for computer access and control of other technologies. This creates increased opportunities to independently engage with environments and communicate and develop social skills. Mobile access can also be achieved through Bluetooth technologies and through USB ports, switch interface devices like Tecla, and through multifaceted environmental control units like the HouseMate (Fig. 32.26).

Wheelchair manufacturers work directly with emerging technologies to integrate options and plugin compatibility through the Environmental Control Unit or RCA controller or direct joystick ports. Technologies continue to evolve and allow access to all platforms like personal computers, Android, and iOS and to multiple devices at one time. Retail technologies like Amazon's Echo, Google Home, and Apple Home Kit with the growing number of environmental control modules including bed controls and door openers can all be accessed with built-in and add-on technologies or simply through the child's mobile phone, giving the child more independence and ability to develop skills like their peers. These companies are now committed to improving access for all users like the new Tap Alexa features that allow nonverbal users to control Amazon Alexa devices by typing or using icons and adding an AAC feature, making off the shelf technology useable by all. Occupational therapy practitioners should stay informed of the extra features available to ensure maximum participation and outcomes are afforded to their clients.

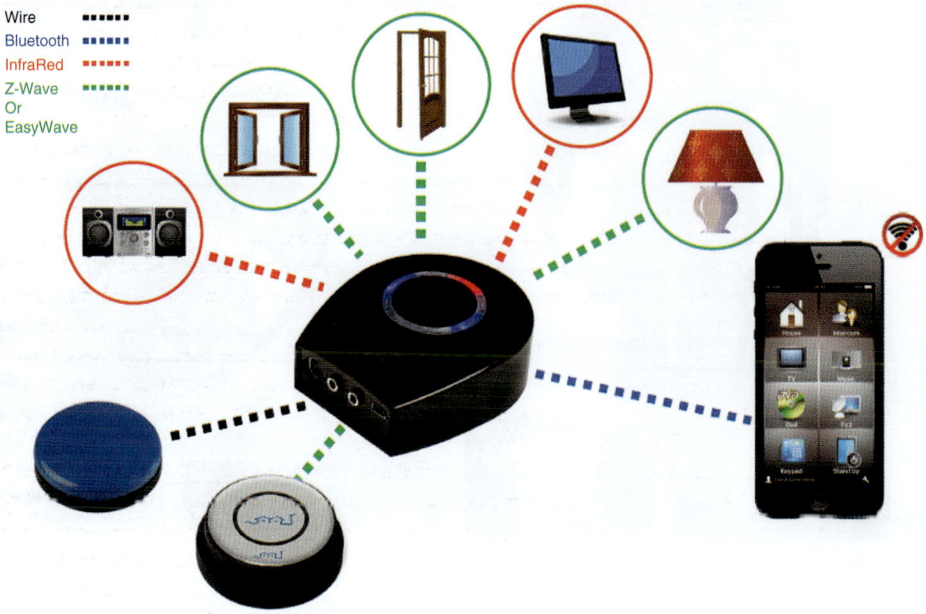


**Fig. 32.26** HouseMate environmental control.

### Sports and Recreation Mobility Technology

Sports and recreation equipment can play a major role in mobility, development, social skills, goal setting, confidence, and overall health and fitness. Children's main occupation is play. Adapted and specially designed sports and recreation equipment can help children engage in their play occupations. There are tricycles, recumbent cycles, handcycles, hand and foot cycles, racing chairs, companion joggers, gait trainers, gait racers, tennis wheelchairs, basketball wheelchairs, all terrain wheelchairs, beach wheelchairs, mono skis, sit skis, hockey sleds, and more (Fig. 32.27A–F) that allow children with disabilities to participate in sports and recreational activities. Helping to identify and recommend adapted and specialized equipment is key to meeting the child's goals. More information can be found through programs like US Paralympics, Challenged Athletes Foundation, Ambucs, Ainsley's Angels, and Disabled Sports USA.

## INTERVENTIONS FOR PRESSURE RELIEF

Pressure injuries are commonly experienced by full-time wheelchair users. A pressure injury is any localized injury to the skin and underlying tissue usually over a bony prominence caused by pressure or a combination of pressure and shear (Edsberg et al., 2016). Injuries can occur on any weight-bearing surface and are commonly seen on the pelvis (ischial tuberosities, sacrum, and coccyx). Pressure injuries can result in life-threatening conditions like sepsis and osteomyelitis when not managed properly. The best protection is appropriately fitted and sized equipment, along with education to the child, their family, and care providers about the importance and methods to perform pressure relief.

### Equipment for Pressure Relief: Cushions and Backs

There are thousands of cushions made of different materials fabricated for use in wheelchairs. Fig. 32.28 describes the pros and cons of the different types of cushions. The child's needs and the family dynamics as it relates to the care and management of equipment are considered when selecting a cushion. Some cushions may require frequent maintenance, while some are simpler to use. Cushions and backs can be prefabricated, adjustable, or custom-made. For most children, prefabricated equipment meets their needs. Pairing an anterior pelvic support, such as a pelvic positioning belt, with use of a positioning and skin protection cushion allows for improved posture and limits shifting and sliding on the cushion. If the child uses a manual wheelchair, the weight of all secondary supports needs consideration during the evaluation. For example, gel-based cushions are heavy compared to foam or air cushions. Children with significant deformities require adjustable or custom-made equipment.

Backrests can provide posterior or posterior-lateral support for the user. Fig. 32.29 illustrates the types of backs and describes their recommended use. The height of the back and need for lateral support are dependent on how much support the child needs in their sitting balance (this is determined in the mat assessment). If the child is propelling a manual wheelchair, the height of the back must be lower than their scapula to allow for upper movement through the chair, rather than the child losing their position or causing parts on the chair to break because of movement.

### Methods of Pressure Relief

Even with the best cushions and backs, children may develop pressure injuries if they do not use pressure redistribution techniques properly and at the correct intervals. Common techniques are a depression or push-up in the chair, a side or forward lean while seated, manual or power tilt, or a transition to a standing position. Fig. 32.30 shows a teen using a Smart Check valve to indicate if the cushion has the correct amount of air for optimal pressure relief.

## INTERVENTION FOR MOBILITY AND PROPULSION TRAINING

The occupational therapy practitioner will be involved with wheelchair training, which improves propulsion ability, safety, and functionality. Propelling a wheelchair can be performed using bilateral upper extremities, bilateral lower extremities, one arm and one leg, or with one arm. Determining how the child will propel the wheelchair depends on their physical abilities and setup of the chair. However, when a 2-year-old child starts propelling a wheelchair, they are not ready to learn to do wheelies, curbs, or stairs. As children age, they need to learn those skills to function in a world that is not wheelchair accessible (Sawatzky et al., 2012). Safety is a priority especially if training advanced skills like "popping a wheelie" or jumping a curb. When manual skills are taught, the practitioner should use a spotter belt or attach a transfer belt to the back frame to help prevent the chair from tipping backward. Fig. 32.31 shows a practitioner holding a transfer belt while a client safely practices wheelchair skills.

The Wheelchair Skills Program through Dalhousie University offers free online low-tech, high-impact, evidence-based resources for the assessment and training of the wheelchair skills of users of manual wheelchairs, powered wheelchairs, and motorized mobility scooters (https://wheelchairskillsprogram.ca).

Learning to operate a power mobility device takes time and patience, which is why training time varies for each child and should include the environments in which it will be used. Occupational therapy practitioners use graded activities to teach children to use a powered wheelchair by engaging the child in repetitive meaningful practice in the natural environment. Training with power mobility should begin in a large, open area that allows a child to safely explore and move. Training begins by helping the child want to move to an activity of interest. Often the practitioner starts with switches and in a familiar environment where the child feels comfortable and is motivated to explore the surroundings. The child can experience moving and stopping to learn how the power chair moves and what it feels like in a safe familiar place. See Case Example 32.3 illustrating this training. Children who practice daily in a natural environment are more successful in using a powered wheelchair than children who receive training once a week in a clinical setting. Fig. 32.32A–D shows a variety of repetitive meaningful activities that can be used to teach children to use a powered wheelchair.

When training, the practitioner keeps verbal directions short (one to three words at a time) and limits physical cueing to promote problem-solving and not confuse the child. If a child is trying to move toward an object, the practitioner provides cues regarding the desired outcome, such as, "Come closer," rather than provide specific commands, such as "Push the joystick left," or "Push the red switch and come over here." Positive feedback is more reinforcing, such as "That wall is really close. I got worried and stopped you. Let's back up and try it again," or "nice job getting that toy."

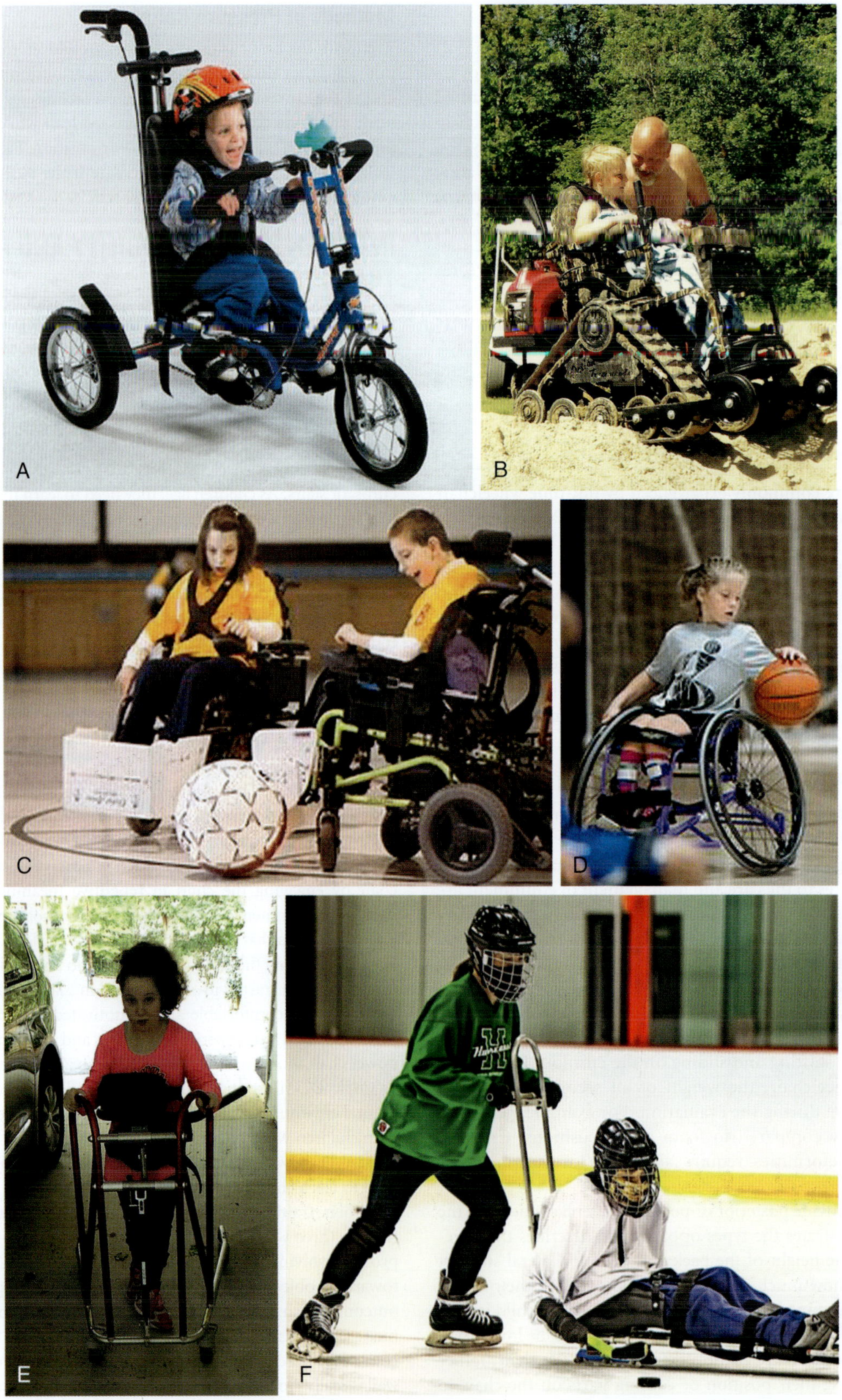

**Fig. 32.27** (A) Young child rides an adapted tricycle. (B) Boy using Trax all-terrain power wheelchair out mudding with his dad. (C) Two teammates go for the ball using their adapted power soccer wheelchairs. (D) Girl dribbles basketball while using her wheelchair basketball sports wheelchair. (E) Teen girl with cerebral palsy using the up and free gait trainer to exercise outside of her home. The gait trainer is adjustable, has a dynamic seat that moves as the user moves, and locks for transfers. (F) Disabled sled hockey player goes for the puck with his adapted hockey stick that is taped to his hand as an assistant pushes his sled.

### Types of Cushions

**General Use Foam Cushion**

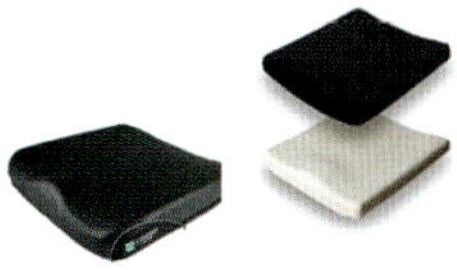

- Foam offers comfort, durability, and support.
- Usually 1–2 inches thick
- May be flat or slightly contoured

**Pros**
- Lightweight
- Inexpensive
- Variety of commercially available options

**Cons**
- Offers minimal support
- Requires clients to reposition themselves
- Tendency to trap heat near body
- Last average of 6-12 months

**Positioning & Skin Protection**

- At least 3 inches thick
- Goal is to redistribute pressure
- Includes honeycomb, gel, air, foam, or combination

**Gel Cushion**

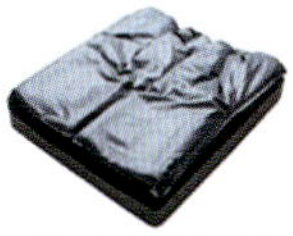

**Pros**
- Provides pelvic stability
- Conducts heat away from body
- Good shock absorption

**Cons**
- Requires moderate upkeep
- Gel must be kneaded daily before client sits on it
- Heavy–use caution with client who needs to propel a lighter manual wheelchair or those with shoulder pain who use a manual wheelchair

**Honeycomb Cushion**

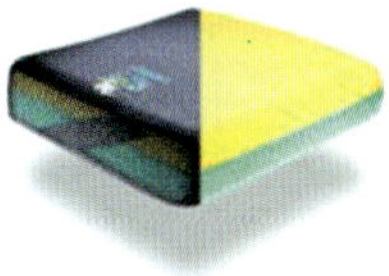

- Made of multiple cell layers that redistribute the pressure when pressure is applied.

**Pros**
- Antifungal and antibacterial
- Machine washable
- Allows air exchange–keeps moisture away from body

**Cons**
- Some clients feel it is too firm

**Air Cushion**

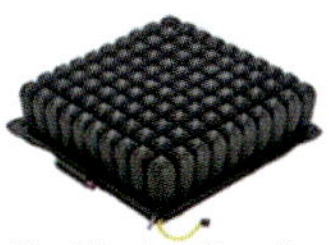

- Air filled cells allow excellent envelopment of ischial
- Pump features allow clients to inflate or release pressure as needed

**Pros**
- Most effective pressure redistribution cushion

**Cons**
- High maintenance
- Over-inflation leads to increased pressure over bony areas
- Under inflation leads to bottoming out (and no protection)
- Air alone is not sufficient

**Foam & Air Cushion**

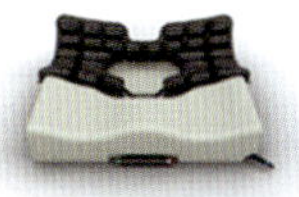

**Pros**
- Benefits of both foam and air

**Cons**
- Not customized

**Pressure Alternating Cushion**

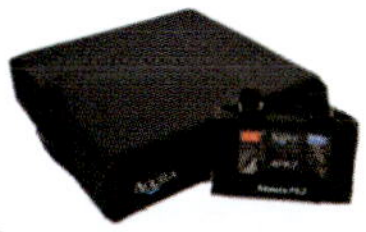

**Pros**
- Continuously adjust the pressure under the pelvis by inflating and deflating.

**Cons**
- Difficult to get insurance coverage for this cushion

**Custom Positioning**

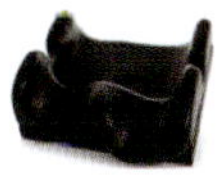

- Cushions made to fit an individual
- Used with clients that have postural asymmetries who require correction in the seating system.

**Pros**
- Provides excellent pressure redistribution
- Custom-made

**Cons**
- Expensive
- Requires monitoring as child grows

**Fig. 32.28** Description of types of cushions with pros and cons.

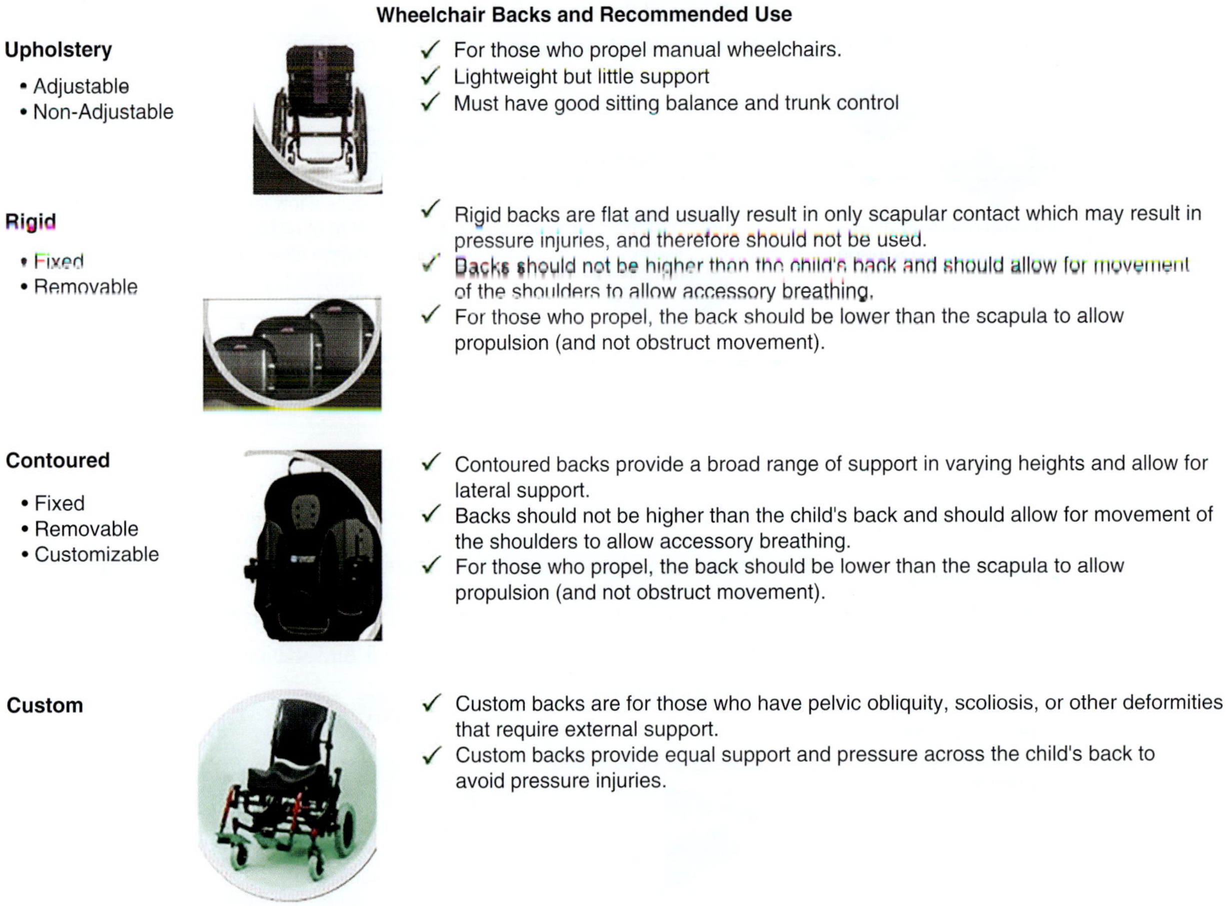
Wheelchair Backs and Recommended Use
Upholstery
• Adjustable
• Non-Adjustable
✓ For those who propel manual wheelchairs.
✓ Lightweight but little support
✓ Must have good sitting balance and trunk control
Rigid
• Fixed
• Removable
✓ Rigid backs are flat and usually result in only scapular contact which may result in pressure injuries, and therefore should not be used.
✓ Backs should not be higher than the child's back and should allow for movement of the shoulders to allow accessory breathing.
✓ For those who propel, the back should be lower than the scapula to allow propulsion (and not obstruct movement).
Contoured
• Fixed
• Removable
• Customizable
✓ Contoured backs provide a broad range of support in varying heights and allow for lateral support.
✓ Backs should not be higher than the child's back and should allow for movement of the shoulders to allow accessory breathing.
✓ For those who propel, the back should be lower than the scapula to allow propulsion (and not obstruct movement).
Custom
✓ Custom backs are for those who have pelvic obliquity, scoliosis, or other deformities that require external support.
✓ Custom backs provide equal support and pressure across the child's back to avoid pressure injuries.

**Fig. 32.29** Types of backs and recommendations for use.

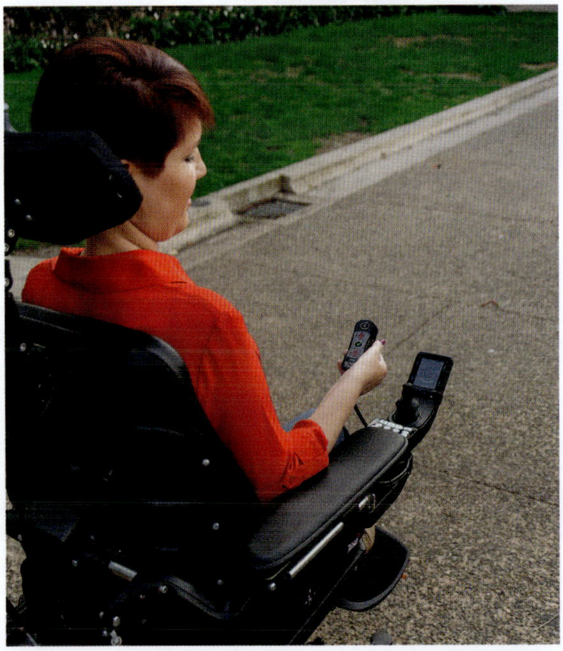

**Fig. 32.30** Some RoHO air cushions come with a Smart Check valve and notifications that indicate if the cushion has the correct amount of air for optimal pressure relief. Image is of woman in a power wheelchair, holding the Smart Check system. (Photo courtesy Permobil.)

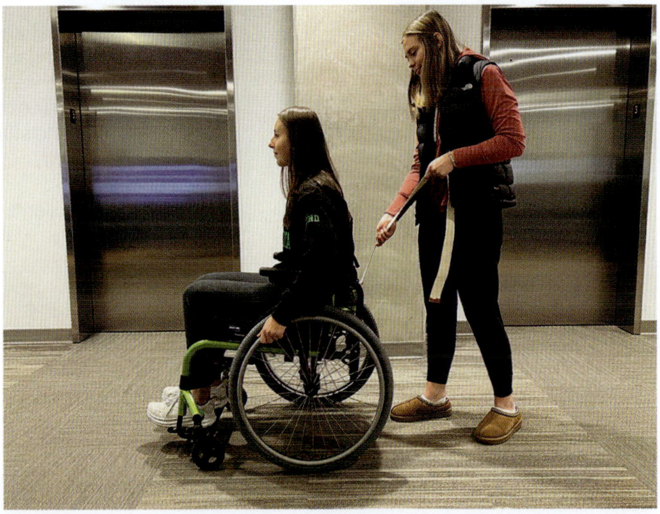

**Fig. 32.31** Wheelchair user propelling manual wheelchair with therapist holding a transfer belt while safely practicing wheelchair skills.

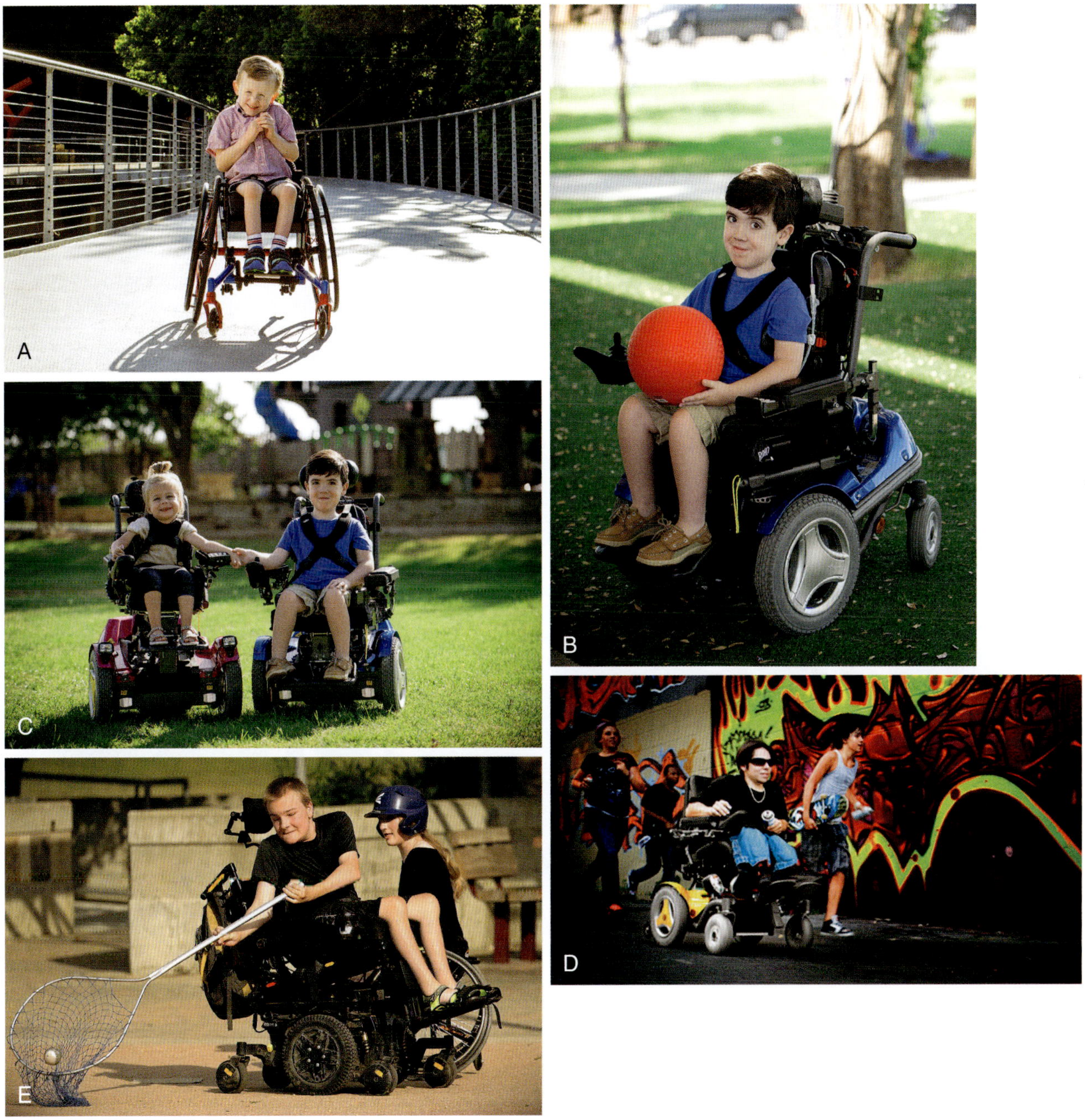

Fig. 32.32 (A) Child enjoys spending time outdoors. (B) Young boy in a power wheelchair is ready to join friends to play basketball. (C) Friends meet to play. (D) Teen with rear wheel drive power wheelchair races down city sidewalk with friends running beside and behind with graffiti wall background. (E) Teenage boy in mid-wheel drive power wheelchair playing softball, catches ball in fishing net. ((D) Courtesy of Permobil. (E) Photo Credit with permission: Nick Nelson/Grand Forks Herald.)

## Case Example 32.3

Jake is a 16-year-old youth with spastic diplegia cerebral palsy. He ambulates part-time (Gross Motor Function Classification System; GMFCS Level III) (Palisano et al., 1997) with quad canes and uses an ultralightweight manual wheelchair propeller. He is a junior in high school. At school, he leaves classes early and frequently arrives late due to his slow cadence in his chair. At home, Jake requires minimal assistance with his self-care primarily because his speed is slow. He is independent with his transfers. When he is in the community, he is unable to make it up his steep driveway independently, and though he can propel some on the sidewalks, his speed is ineffective outside of recreational mobility. The mobility team met with Jake and his parents for an evaluation for a new chair.

An interview was completed, and goals were set for improving Jake's independence, especially for community mobility as well as finding a system that would allow him to attend a full class period. Jake's plan is to go to college, so this system needs to be functional both in the high school as well as college settings. A mat assessment was completed and was significant for a posterior pelvic tilt, kyphotic posture, and decreased hamstring range of motion. Jake's lower extremities were more impaired than his upper extremities. When he moved his arms to propel his chair, his legs extended with increased quadricep recruitment.

Jake trialed a power chair and an ultralightweight manual wheelchair. He moved functionally for short distances with both, but only the power chair allowed him to meet his goals of efficiency and community mobility. However, Jake's parents were not in agreement with the power chair. They did not have the resources to purchase a van to transport the chair and were worried that he would not be able to travel with his sled hockey team if he used a power chair full-time.

Jake then trialed a power assist system on the ultralight manual wheelchair in the clinic; the trial was completely unsuccessful. His challenges with motor planning for new tasks were evident, and he was unable to safely control the system. However, the team recognized that Jake's issue was motor planning, rather than a lack of understanding, and decided a longer trial was indicated. A weekend trial was arranged with a demonstration unit from the manufacturer. After the trial period, Jake mastered control of the system, and he was able to functionally use it in his community and safely navigate up his driveway, and his parents were able to transport the system in their station wagon.

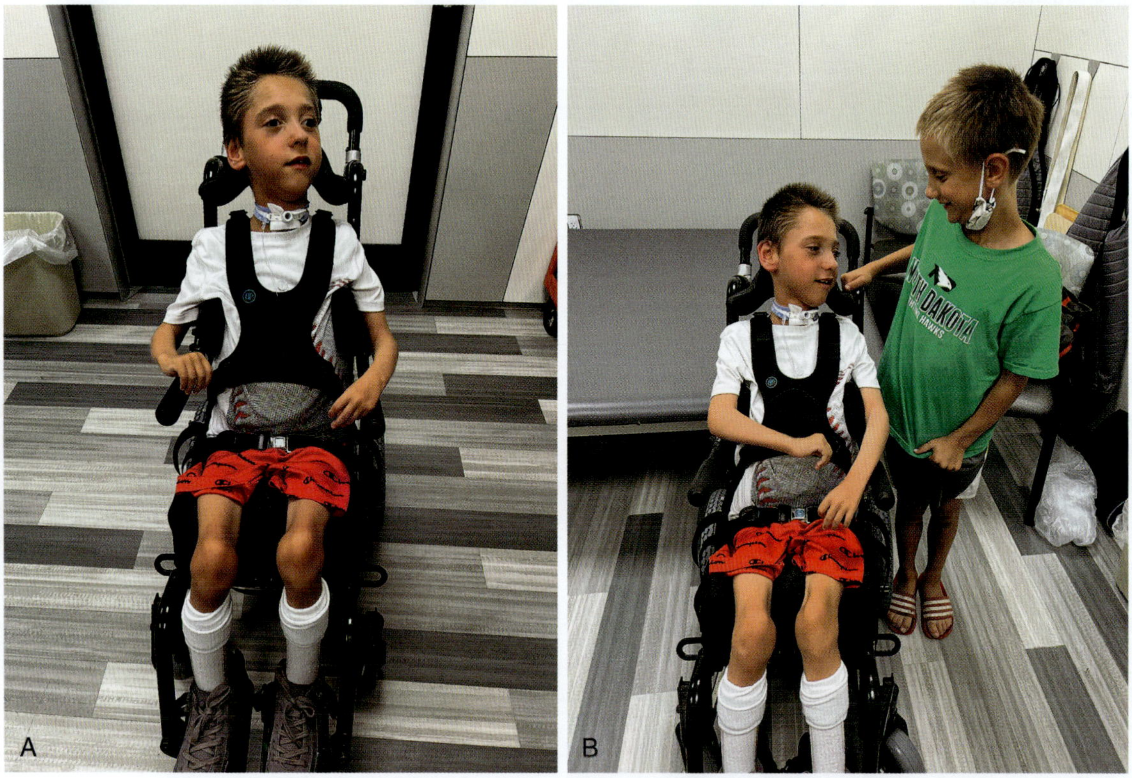

**Fig. 32.33** (A) Eli Wilcox, the ultimate teacher. (B) Eli with his twin brother.

## Acknowledgments

The authors acknowledge the prior edition contributions from Lauren Rosen, Lisa Rotelli, and Andrina Sabet.

This chapter is dedicated in memory of Eli Wilcox (Fig. 32.33A and B) and his family and the other clients who shared their experiences so that occupational therapy students and professionals can learn and serve future clients better. Our clients are the ultimate teachers. We are extremely grateful and Eli's legacy lives on through each of you and the clients who achieve their goals with mobility.

## SUMMARY

Independent mobility plays a role in cognitive, language, and social development. When mobility is severely delayed or restricted, emotional, cognitive, and psychosocial development are affected. Mobility devices provide young children with functional or transitional mobility. They allow children with physical disabilities greater opportunities to participate in occupations with peers. Occupational therapy intervention is a dynamic process between evaluation and intervention. Intervention includes practicing using the devices in a variety of environments, engaging the child and family in problem-solving, and adapting and modifying systems as the child grows and develops. The practitioner is responsible for ensuring that children with physical and cognitive disabilities receive opportunities for mobility at the earliest age possible to promote development, participation, and quality of life.

1. Self-initiated mobility allows young children with physical disabilities, including those with cognitive dysfunction, the opportunity to access and explore their surroundings, significantly contributing to visual spatial, sensory motor, social, emotional, and cognitive development. Mobility allows children and youth to engage in desired occupations and participate in activities with peers and family.
2. Occupational therapy intervention for mobility occurs once the team decides on the mobility device. The occupational therapy practitioner designs intervention to practice use of the device, encourage participation in a variety of activities, and measure the outcome. After trying out the equipment, the practitioner may suggest a new piece of equipment is necessary or adjustments need to be made to the current system. Practitioners providing intervention address the purpose or goals for using the device, environments in which the device will be used, features and adaptations that will meet the desired outcomes across environments, needs and concerns of the care providers and school personnel, options for transporting the device, and options for funding and acquiring the device(s).
3. Occupational therapy practitioners use knowledge of mobility devices to guide selection of devices and the associated parts. Consideration needs to be taken for weight of the device for transportation, weight of secondary supports for the child self-propelling their wheelchair, ease of maneuverability within all contexts, adjustability for accommodating growth, and funding resources to support the child in obtaining multiple devices for optimal occupational engagement. They become familiar the features and options within a variety of manual wheelchairs, medical strollers, tilt-in-space wheelchairs, self-propelling manual wheelchairs, power assist and power add-on devices, power wheelchairs, scooters, standers, wheelchair standers, walkers, sports and recreation mobility technology, and exoskeletons.

## REFERENCES

Adolph, K. E., Cole, W. G., Komati, M., Garciaguirre, J. S., Badaly, D., Lingeman, J. M., Chan, G. L., & Sotsky, R. B. (2012). How do you learn to walk? Thousands of steps and dozens of falls per day. *Psychological science, 23*(11), 1387–1394.

Adolph, K. E., & Franchak, J. M. (2017). The development of motor behavior. *Wiley Interdisciplinary Reviews: Cognitive Science, 8*, 1–2.

Ahlborg, L., Andersson, C., & Julin, P. (2006). Whole-body vibration training compared with resistance training: Effect on spasticity, muscle strength and motor performance in adults with cerebral palsy. *Journal of Rehabilitation Medicine, 38*(5), 302–308.

Alghadir, A. H., Zafar, H., Al-Eisa, E. S., & Iqbal, Z. A. (2017). Effect of posture on swallowing. *African Health Sciences, 17*(1), 133–137.

American National Standards Institute (ANSI)/Rehabilitation Engineering and Assistive Technology Society of North America (RESNA). (2000). *ANSI/RESNA WX 19: Wheelchairs used as seats in motor vehicles (Wheelchair Standard)*. Arlington, VA: RESNA. Retrieved from http://wc-transportation-safety.umtri.umich.edu/wts-standards/wc19-wheelchairs.

American Occupational Therapy Association. (2020). Occupational therapy practice framework: Domain and process (4th ed.). *American Journal of Occupational Therapy, 74*(Suppl. 2) Article 7412410010.

Anderson, D., Campos, J., Witherington, D., Dahl, A., Rivera, M., He, M., Uchiyama, I., & Barbu-Roth, M. (2013). The role of locomotion in psychological development. *Frontiers in Psychology, 4*, 440.

Bornstein, M. H., Hahn, C.-S., & Suwalsky, J. T. D. (2013). Physically developed and exploratory young infants contribute to their own long-term academic achievement. *Psychological Science, 24*(10), 1906–1917.

Cheung, W. C., Meadan, H., & Yang, H. W. (2020). Effects of powered mobility device interventions on social skills for children with disabilities: A systematic review. *Journal of Developmental and Physical Disabilities, 32*, 855–876.

Clearfield, M. W. (2010). Learning to walk changes infants social interactions. *Infant Behavior and Development, 34*, 15–25.

Clearfield, M. W. (2004). The role of crawling and walking experience in infant spatial memory. *Journal of Experimental Child Psychology, 89*, 2014–2041.

Currier, B. A., Jones, M. A., & DeGrace, B. W. (2019). Experiences of families with young power wheelchair users. *Journal of Early Intervention, 41*(2), 125–140.

Delmore, B., Deppisch, M., Sylvia, C., Luna-Anderson, C., & Nie, A. M. (2019). Pressure injuries in the pediatric population: A national pressure ulcer advisory panel white paper. *Advances in Skin & Wound Care, 32*(9), 394–408.

Digiovine, C., Rosen, L., Berner, T., Betz, K., Roesler, T., & Schmeler, M. (2012). *RESNA position on the application of ultralight wheelchairs.* RESNA. https://www.resna.org/Portals/0/Documents/Position%20Papers/UltraLightweightManualWheelchairs.pdf.

Doubt, L., & McColl, M. A. (2003). A secondary guy: Physically disabled teenagers in secondary schools. *Canadian Journal of Occupational Therapy, 70*(3), 139–151.

Dunn, R. B., Walter, J. S., Lucero, Y., Weaver, F., Langbein, E., Fehr, L., Johnson, P., & Riedy, L. (1998). Follow-up assessment of standing mobility device users. *Assistive Technology: The official journal of RESNA, 10*(2), 84–93.

Edsberg, L. E., Black, J. M., Goldberg, M., McNichol, L., Moore, L., & Sieggreen, M. (2016). Revised national pressure ulcer advisory panel pressure injury staging system: Revised pressure injury staging system. *J Wound Ostomy Continence Nurs, 43*(6), 585–597.

Edwards, L. C., & Layne, C. S. (2007). Effect of dynamic weight-bearing on neuromuscular activation after spinal cord injury. *American Journal of Physical Medicine and Rehabilitation, 86*(6), 499–506.

Feldner, H. A., Logan, S. W., & Galloway, J. C. (2019). Mobility in pictures: A participatory photovoice narrative study exploring powered mobility provision for children and families. *Disability and Rehabilitation: Assistive Technology, 14*(3), 301–311.

Feldner, H. A., Logan, S. W., & Galloway, J. C. (2016). Why the time is right for a radical paradigm shift in early powered mobility: The role of powered mobility technology devices, policy and stakeholders. *Disability and Rehabilitation: Assistive Technology, 11*(2), 89–102.

Feldner, H. (2019). Impacts of early powered mobility provision on disability identity: A case study. *Rehabilitation Psychology, 64*(2), 130.

Ferrero, G., Mijno, E., Actis, M. V., Zampa, A., Ratto, N., Arpaia, A., & Masse, A. (2015). Risk factors for shoulder pain in patients with spinal cord injury: A multicenter study. *Musculoskeletal Surgery, 99*(1), S53–S56.

Fitzsimmons, L. (2014). Positioning the head: Strategies to improve head control and posture. *Directions, 1*, 42–45. https://cdn.rifton.com/-/media/files/rifton/product-information/head-control-article-from-directions-publication.pdf?la=en&d=20201012T183246Z.

Goodwin, J., Colver, A., Basu, A., Crombie, S., Howel, D., Parr, J. R., McColl, E., Kolehmainen, N., Roberts, A., Lecouturier, J., Smith, J., Miller, K., & Cadwgan, J. (2018). Understanding frames: A UK survey of parents and professionals regarding the use of standing frames for children with cerebral palsy. *Child: Care, Health and Development, 44*(2), 195–202.

Han, E. Y., Choi, J. H., Kim, S. H., & Im, S. H. (2017). The effect of weight bearing on bone mineral density and bone growth in children with cerebral palsy. *Medicine (Baltimore), 96*(10), e5896.

Harbourne, R., & Kamm, K. (2015). Upper extremity function: What's posture got to do with it? *Journal of Hand Therapy, 28*(2), 106–113.

Harbourne, R. T., & Berger, S. E. (2019). Embodied cognition in practice: Exploring effects of a motor-based problem-solving intervention. *Physical Therapy, 99*(6), 786–796.

Henderson, R., Kiaralla, J., Abbas, A., & Stevenson, R. (2004). Predicting low bone density in children and young adults with quadriplegic cerebral palsy. *Developmental Mmedicine and Cchild Nneurology, 46*, 416–419.

Huang, H., & Galloway, J. C. (2012). Modified ride-on toy cars for early power mobility: A technical report. *Pediatric Physical Therapy, 24*(2), 149–154.

Huston, G. (2001). Use of prolonged standing for individuals with spinal cord injuries. *Physical Therapy, 81*(8), 1392–1399.

Kirby, R. L., Ackroyd-Stolarz, S. A., Brown, M. G., Kirkland, S. A., & MacLeod, D. A. (1994). Wheelchair-related accidents caused by tips and falls among noninstitutionalized users of manually propelled wheelchairs in Nova Scotia. *American Journal of Physical Medicine and Rehabilitation, 73*(5), 319–330.

Krick, J., Murphy-Miller, P., Zeger, S., & Weight, E. (1996). Pattern of growth in children with cerebral palsy. *Journal of the American Dietetic Association, 96*(7), 680–685.

Lin, F., Parthasarathy, S., Taylor, S. J., Pucci, D., Hendrix, R. W., & Makhsous, M. (2006). Effect of different sitting postures on lung capacity, expiratory flow, and lumbar lordosis. *Archives of Physical Medicine and Rehabilitation, 87*(4), 504–509.

Livingstone, R. W., Bone, J., & Field, D. A. (2020). Beginning power mobility: An exploration of factors associated with child use of early power mobility devices and parent device preference. *Journal of Rehabilitation and Assistive Technologies Engineering, 7* 2055668320926046.

Lobo, M. A., Kokkoni, E., de Campos, A. C., & Galloway, J. C. (2014). Not just playing around: Infants' behaviors with objects reflect ability, constraints, and object properties. *Infant Behavior and Development, 37*(3), 334–351.

Logan, S. W., Feldner, H. A., Galloway, J. C., & Huang, H.-H. (2016). Modified ride-on car use by children with complex medical needs. *Pediatric Physical Therapy, 28*, 100–107.

Logan, S. W., Ross, S. M., Schreiber, M. A., Feldner, H. A., Lobo, M. A., Catena, M. A., MacDonald, M., & Galloway, J. C. (2016). Why we move: Social mobility behaviors of non-disabled and disabled children across childcare contexts. *Frontiers in Public Health, 4*(4) Article 204.

Macias, L. M. (2005). The effects of the standing programs with abduction for children with spastic diplegia. *Pediatric Physical Therapy, 17*(1), 96.

Macias-Merlo, L., Bagur-Calafat, C., & Girabent-Farres, M. (2015). Standing programs to promote hip flexibility in children with spastic diplegic cerebral palsy. *Pediatric Physical Therapy, 27*, 243–249.

Macias-Merlo, L., Bagur-Calafat, C., Girabent-Farres, M., & Stuberg, W. (2015). Effects of the standing program with hip abduction on hip acetabular development in children with spastic diplegia cerebral palsy. *Disability & Rehabilitation, 38*(11), 1075–1081.

Macias-Merlo, L., et al. (2015). Standing programs to promote hip flexibility in children with spastic diplegic cerebral palsy. *Pediatric Physical Therapy, 27*, 243–249.

Martinsson, C., & Himmelmann, K. (2011). Effect of weight-bearing in abduction and extension on hip stability in children with cerebral palsy. *Pediatric Physical Therapy, 23*, 150–157.

McCashen, W. (2005). The strengths approach: A strengths-based resource for sharing power and creating change. *St. Lukes Innovative Resources.*

Netz, Y., Argov, E., Burstin, A., Brown, R., Heyman, S. N., Dunsky, A., & Alexander, N. B. (2007). Use of a device to support standing during a physical activity program to improve function of individuals with disabilities who reside in a nursing home. *Disability and Rehabilitation: Assistive Technology, 2*(1), 43–49. .

Nwaobi, O. (1987). Seating orientations and upper extremity function in children with cerebral palsy. *Physical Therapy, 67*(8), 1209–1212.

Paleg, G., & Livingstone, R. (2015). Systematic review and clinic recommendations for dosage of supported home-based standing programs for adults with stroke, spinal cord injury, and other neurologic conditions. *BMC Musculoskeletal Disorders, 16*, 1–16.

Paleg, G. S., Smith, B. A., & Glickman, L. B. (2013). Systematic review and evidence-based clinical recommendations for dosing of pediatric supported standing programs. *Pediatric Physical Therapy, 25*(3), 232–247. .

Palisano, R., Rosenbaum, P., Walter, S., Russell, D., Wood, E., & Galuppi, B. (1997). Development and reliability of a system to classify gross motor function in children with cerebral palsy. *Developmental Medicine and Child Neurology, 39*(4), 214–223. .

Pin, T. W. (2007). Effectiveness of static weight -bearing exercises in children with cerebral palsy. *Pediatric Physical Therapy, 19*(1), 62–73.

RESNA. (2000). *RESNA's position on wheelchairs used as seats in motor vehicles.* Retrieved from https://www.resna.org/Portals/0/Documents/Position%20Papers/RESNAPositiononWheelchairsUsedasSeatsinMotorVehicles.pdf.

Rosenbaum, P., & Gorter, J. W. (2012). The 'F-words' in childhood disability: I swear this is how we should think. *Child: Care, Health and Development, 38*(4), 457–463. .

Rosenbaum, P., & Stewart, D. (2004). The World Health Organization international classification of functioning, disability, and health: A model to guide clinical thinking, practice and research in the field of cerebral palsy. *Seminars in Pediatric Neurology, 11*(1), 5–10.

Rueger, S. Y., Cipra, A., Choe, H., Steggerda, J. C., Kirby, A. E., & Stone, L. B. (2021). Abbreviated assessment tool of learned helplessness and mastery orientation: The student behavior checklist—Brief. *Journal of Psychoeducational Assessment, 39*(6), 772–777. .

Sawatzky, B., Rushton, P. W., Denison, I., & McDonald, R. (2012). Wheelchair skills training programme for children: A pilot study. *Australian Occupational Therapy Journal, 59*(1), 2–9.

Schwarzer, G., Freitag, C., Schum, N., Horst, J. S., Schlesinger, M., & Perone, S. (2013). How crawling and manual object exploration are related to the mental rotation abilities of 9-month-old infants. *Frontiers in Psychology* (4), 97.

Shutrump, S. E., Manary, M. A., & Buning, M. E. (2008). Safe transportation for students who use wheelchairs on the school bus. *OT Practice, 13*(15), 8–12. https://www.researchgate.net/publication/288617753_Safe_transportation_for_students_who_use_wheelchairs_on_the_school_bus.

Smith, L., & Gasser, M. (2005). The development of embodied cognition: Six lessons from babies. *Artificial Life, 11*(1–2), 13–29.

Stuberg, W. A. (1992). Considerations related to weight-bearing programs in children with developmental disabilities. *Physical Therapy, 72*(1), 35–40.

Thompson, C. R., Figoni, S. F., Devocelle, H. A., Fifer-Moeller, T. M., Lockhart, T. L., & Lockhart, T. A. (2000). From the field. Effect of dynamic weight bearing on lower extremity bone mineral density in children with neuromuscular impairment. *Clinical Kinesiology, 54*(1), 13–18.

Tosum, A., Erisen Karaca, S., Unuvar, T., Yurekli, Y., Yenisey, C., & Omurlu, I. K. (2017). Bone mineral density and vitamin D status in children with epilepsy, cerebral palsy, and cerebral palsy with epilepsy. *Child's Nervous System: Child's Nervous System, 33*(1), 153–158. .

Townsend, E., et al. (2016). Supported standing in boys with Duchenne muscular dystrophy. *Pediatric Physical Therapy, 28*, 320–329.

Tremblay, F., Malouin, F., Richards, C. L., & Dumas, F. (1990). Effects of prolonged muscle stretch on reflex and voluntary muscle activations in children with spastic cerebral palsy. *Scandinavian Journal of Rehabilitation Medicine, 22*, 171–180.

Walter, J. S., Sacks, J., Othman, R., Rankin, A. Z., Nemchausky, B., Chintam, R., & Wheeler, J. S. (2002). A database of self-reported secondary medical problems among VA spinal cord injury patients: Its role in clinical care and management. *Journal of Rehabilitation Research and Development, 39*(1), 53–61.

Walter, J. S., Sola, P. G., Sacks, J., Lucero, Y., Langbein, E., & Weaver, F. (1999). Indications for a home standing program for individuals with spinal cord injury. *Journal of Spinal Cord Medicine, 22*(3), 152–158.

Whedon, G. D. (1982). Changes in weightlessness in calcium metabolism and in the musculoskeletal system. *Physiologist, 25*(6), S41–S44.

Wilson, A. D., & Golonka, S. (2013). Embodied cognition is not what you think it is. *Frontiers in Psychology, 4*, 58. https://doi.org/10.3389/fpsyg.2013.00058.

33

# Interventions for Hand Impairments in Children and Youth

*Jenny Marie Dorich and Karen Harpster*

*Man, through the use of his hands, as they are energized by mind and will, can influence the state of his own health.*

*–Mary Reilly.*

## GUIDING QUESTIONS

1. How do occupational therapy practitioners address hand challenges to promote occupational engagement in children and youth?
2. How do the principles and strategies of the biomechanical approach inform occupational therapy intervention to address hand challenges in children in youth?
3. What specific techniques do occupational therapy practitioners following a biomechanical approach use with children and youth who experience challenges in upper extremity functioning.

## KEY TERMS

Cryotherapy
Desensitization
Energy conservation technique
Joint protection strategies
Kinesiology tape
Mirror therapy
Physical agent modalities (PAMs)
Sensory reeducation
Serial casting
Static progressive orthoses

## OCCUPATIONAL THERAPY'S ROLE IN ADDRESSING HAND CHALLENGES

Hand function is essential to feeding, dressing, bathing, play, academics, and communication, and therefore, occupational therapy practitioners promote occupational participation for children who have hand impairments. The goal is to support the child's ability to engage in those things they find meaningful. When children have congenital differences of the hand or arm, upper extremity (UE) impairments from underlying disorders (such as cerebral palsy or rheumatoid arthritis), or injuries of the hand, they may require occupational therapy intervention to improve hand use. Practitioners examine multiple factors that influence hand movements and UE control and create intervention plans that are child centered. They consider the timing of the intervention, intensity of therapy services, and work with interprofessional team members. They collaborate with children and their families to address meaningful goals.

According to the American Society of Hand Therapists (ASHT), hand therapy is "the art and science of rehabilitation of the upper limb, which includes the hand, wrist, elbow, and shoulder girdle" (Keller et al., 2021). Traditionally, hand therapy practice has been most strongly grounded in the biomechanical model of practice (Burley et al., 2018). While practice continues to routinely apply biomechanical assessments and interventions, such as range of motion (ROM) measurements and exercises, in recent years occupational therapy practitioners of hand therapy have emphasized an increasing focus on the application of occupation-based interventions (Robinson et al., 2016).

Occupational therapy practitioners are most effective when they create interventions that are meaningful to the child, repeated often, include actual objects, and in the case of daily living skills, most resemble the actual activity in real life. Using an occupation-based model of practice provides the structure to organize one's assessment to inform the intervention plan and maintains a focus on occupation no matter the frame of reference chosen. A common frame of reference when working to improve hand function is the biomechanical frame of reference.

## BIOMECHANICAL FRAME OF REFERENCE AND OCCUPATIONAL THERAPY INTERVENTIONS

The biomechanical frame of reference focuses on the physical limitations that interfere with the child's ability to engage in occupations. Based on concepts from kinesiology, this frame of reference specifically addresses ROM, strength, endurance, and pain. When following a biomechanical frame of reference, the occupational therapist identifies how ROM, strength, endurance, and pain affect the child's ability to use their hands to engage in desired activities. The therapist creates an intervention plan to target the selected area that interferes with the child's engagement. However, an occupation-based intervention plan includes goals to address the child's use of their hands for daily activities, such as feeding, dressing, and playing. The therapist creates activities that are as close to the natural meaningful occupation as possible and use the same objects to provide the child with meaning and cues. Case 33.1 illustrates the use of an occupation-based model of practice (Model of Human Occupation) and the biomechanical

### CASE EXAMPLE 33.1 MODEL OF HUMAN OCCUPATION AND BIOMECHANICAL FRAME OF REFERENCE

Marque is a 7-year-old boy who has cerebral palsy (right hemiplegia) who was referred to the outpatient clinic for an evaluation of his hand function.

*Background information*: He is currently in the first grade and having difficulty completing a variety of activities due to limited use of his right upper extremity. His parents are concerned that his difficulties in hand functioning are interfering with his academics, play, and participation in self care. Marque has a younger 4-year-old sister. They live in a suburb. Both of his parents work. Marque spends time with his grandmother after school.

*Volition (Interests and Goals)*: Marque enjoys playing outdoors in the neighborhood and playing basketball with children his age. Although he cannot always keep up with them when they run, the children wait for him. Lately he feels frustrated that he cannot do everything he wants because his "right arm and hand get in the way." Marque reported he wanted to be able to (1) dress himself on his own (including pulling up his pants after going to the bathroom), (2) be a "better basketball player" (e.g., have strength to hold ball in both hands), (3) carry his tray (with both hands) at school, and (4) cut his food without help at school.

*Habituation (Habits and Roles)*: Marque is a first grade student who enjoys going to school. He is at grade level in reading, math, music, and gym. The teacher has noted that he gets frustrated during craft activities and writing and anxious about going to the bathroom. He has several friends who play with him at recess. He spends his afternoons at his grandmother's house, where the children play basketball in the neighborhood. He plays some with his 4-year-old sister. On the weekends, the family plays outside, go to community events, or watch movies together.

*Environment*: Marque lives in the suburbs near his grandmother. The family participates in community events often. The environment allows Marque to play outside (with minimal supervision). He lives in a single-family ranch-style home with his own bedroom. He receives physical and occupational therapy services at school.

*Physical observations*: Marque walks independently with a slight lean. He likes to do things on his own and is verbal about trying to figure out things. He has increased muscle tone in his right upper extremity and holds it in a flexed position (at elbow and wrist) and internally rotated at shoulder. His right hand is flexed, but he can release this upon request. He had limited active range of motion (elbow, wrist, and fingers) and decreased strength and sensation in his right upper extremity. His Manual Ability Classification is Level 2 (handles most objects with somewhat reduced quality of speed).

#### Assessment

- Marque has limited range of motion, strength and sensation in his right upper extremity interfering with his arm mobility, bilateral hands skills, and fine motor manipulation.

#### Intervention Plan

The occupational therapist created an intervention to address Marque's goals following the biomechanical frame of reference.

*Range of motion*: To increase the range of motion in his right upper extremity and reduce his hypertonicity, the occupational therapy practitioner began the session by asking Marque to stretch his right upper extremity gently, passively through the range and then bear weight with his hand open. The occupational therapist provided physical and verbal cues as needed. Once Marque could establish full passive range of motion in his right hand, the practitioner provided a variety of activities to promote grasp and release of clothing (for dressing and pulling his pants up).

*Strength*: The therapist engaged Marque in lifting tasks (to address his upper extremity strength for holding his tray and playing basketball). For example, the therapist asked him to lift an empty tray with both hands (as he would in school); after each successful lift, the practitioner added additional weight. They documented the weight so that Marque had a goal for the next session.

*Endurance*: Since the therapist wanted to end the strength training on a positive note, Marques practiced walking with the tray (with the weight he was able to successfully lift). In this activity, they measured the distance he was able to walk with the tray. After several rounds with the tray, the occupational therapist introduced a variety of weighted balls. In this activity to improve upper extremity strength and endurance, Marques picked up the lightest ball and attempted to make a basket. Once he successfully made the basket, he used a slightly heavier ball. Marques liked the activity. The last therapy activity was a sensory reeducation task that included identifying objects through touch.

They concluded the session by Marques reflecting on the session by identifying his perceived performance in the activities and how he may practice skills at home and school. They created ideas for the next session and reviewed home exercises to support Marques' intervention plan.

frame of reference. Range of motion, scarring from injury, strength, endurance, and pain may all have significant impacts on occupational performance.

## Improving Range of Motion

Range of motion refers to the distance that an extremity moves at a specific joint. For example, the ROM for elbow extension is 0–180. Limitations in ROM of the upper extremities may interfere with a child's ability to bring hands to mouth, reach for objects, play, engage in schoolwork, or participate in daily activities such as bathing and grooming. While assistive technology (e.g., reachers, extended handles) may allow children to compensate for limited ROM, the biomechanical approach provides additional strategies and techniques to address the limitations.

To enhance occupational performance, occupational therapy practitioners engage children in ROM activities that include the following.

- Active range of motion (AROM): the range of movements the child can do on their own
- Active-assistive range of motion (AAROM): the range that the child can complete with some support from the therapist
- Passive range of motion (PROM): ROM that the therapist can move the child's extremity (receiving no assistance from child)

Occupational therapy practitioners gently hold the joint when moving the child's extremity. They use knowledge of the specific post-surgical protocols that consider the structures injured or repaired and dictate which form of exercise is least stressful on the repair. For example, a commonly used protocol for children with flexor tendon repairs avoids AROM in the early rehabilitation phase while performing passive digit flexion exercises to preserve joint mobility (Skirven et al., 2021). Therapy for UE fractures begins with AROM and progresses to PROM when the referring physician indicates fracture healing can withstand the more aggressive force.

Young children rely on family member(s) to perform AAROM or PROM exercises. They respond best to structured play activities designed to achieve active movement within the desired plane. For example, a child who needs to work on shoulder flexion and elbow extension can perform finger painting on an easel. Toddlers and preschool children may enjoy singing songs that have associated movements (such as finger plays). School-age children may enjoy performing a set of specific exercises by following visual and/or written instruction or when the movement is part of play, leisure, self-care, or daily living. See Case 33.2 for a case describing occupational therapy intervention addressing ROM to promote development.

## CASE EXAMPLE 33.2 HAND THERAPY FOR AN INFANT WITH ARTHROGRYPOSIS

Kai is a 2-week-old male with arthrogryposis referred to occupational therapy to address his upper extremity range of motion limitations.

*Background information*: Kai has arthrogryposis, which is characterized by multiple joint contractures and muscle weakness and places him at risk for delays in using his upper extremities for holding bottle or breast, reaching for objects, and grasping items, and exploring his environment. He was born at 40 weeks gestation, weighing 7 pounds 6 ounces.

*Family*: Kai is the first-born child for his parents. Both parents work full-time but have arranged childcare with family members (who live nearby). His mother is taking 12 weeks maternity leave before returning to work; His father is taking 6 weeks paternity leave.

*Environment*: Kai lives in a 2-bedroom apartment home in the city. He has his own room, and toys, car seat, bath seat, and stroller. The parents have a baby monitor.

*Clinical Observations*: While in supine or being held in a semireclined position, Kai postured with both arms in full extension alongside his torso with his wrists in flexion and forearms pronated. His thumbs postured in 20 degrees of abduction, and his fingers rested in extension. He displayed minimal active movement of his upper extremities. Kai adducted his shoulders slightly. He partially flexed his fingers when reflexive grasp was evoked. He displayed limited active should flexion, did not flex his elbows, and did not fist his fingers into his hands (as is typically observed in newborns). Kai's parents expressed concern they would cause pain or harm to his joints if they positioned him in side-lying or prone positions.

Kai presented with bilateral passive range of motion as follows:

| Passive Range of Motion | Left Upper Extremity | Right Upper Extremity |
|---|---|---|
| Shoulder flexion to extension | 0–60 | 0–70 |
| Shoulder abduction to adduction | 0–60 | 0–60 |
| Shoulder external rotation | 0–30 | 0–40 |
| Elbow flexion to extension | 0–75 | 0–75 |
| Supination to pronation | −90 to −20 | −90 to −20 |
| Wrist flexion to extension | −90 to −50 | −90 to −40 |

*Interpretation of findings*: Kai exhibits limited passive range of motion (shoulder, wrist, elbow) and limited active range of motion in both left and right extremities. This places him at risk for contractures of elbow extension, wrist flexion, shoulder flexion, and shoulder external rotation. His limited active upper extremity movement interferes with his sensory exploration and fine motor development, including hands to mouth.

Kai would benefit from strategies to enhance positioning, range of motion, and development to promote fine and gross motor skills for daily activities (including self-soothing, holding bottle or breast, socialization, and play).

### Intervention Plan

The occupational therapist spent time explaining the characteristics of arthrogryposis and outlining strategies to promote Kai's development.

*Range of motion*: Kai's parents were trained on how to complete upper extremity passive range of motion for shoulder flexion, abduction and external rotation, elbow flexion, supination, wrist extension and composite digit flexion, and extension and thumb abduction. The therapist also demonstrated to the parents positioning and handling for dressing, feeding, bathing, and play.

Kai showed improvements in his passive range of motion at the 2-week follow-up. However, passive range of motion (PROM) in his right wrist remained less than neutral, so the practitioner fabricated a resting hand orthotic for his right upper extremity to be worn when sleeping. Three weeks later, 7-week-old Kai made gains in wrist extension, and his family opted to discontinue his night orthotic and continue with stretching. The practitioner provided them with playful activities to promote reaching and movement. Kai continued with monthly therapy appointments to update his home program for range of motion, fine motor development, bilateral upper extremity coordination, and to evaluate Kai's progress in meeting developmental milestones.

By 3 months of age Kai achieved bilateral passive shoulder range of motion within normal limits in all planes. He had full passive forearm rotation. His passive elbow flexion was to 80 on his right and 90 on his left, and he continued to display no active elbow flexion. His left passive wrist extension improved to neutral and his right to +5. He could bring his hands to midline and actively reach with bilateral hands in supine. He was reaching his gross motor milestones. His family was pleased with his progress and chose to continue with monthly therapy visits and range of motion exercises rather than upper extremity orthotics to address his limited passive motion in wrist extension and elbow flexion. They agreed that the home program fit their routines and habits.

***Blocking exercises*** are useful when the patient demonstrates difficulty with proximal interphalangeal (PIP) joint and/or distal interphalangeal (DIP) joint flexion and/or extension (Fig. 33.1). This type of exercise allows for more force to be transferred to the PIP and DIP joints to achieve greater active pull at the joint (Hays & Rozental, 2013). ***Static progressive stretches*** can be used when the referring physician clears the child for PROM (Fig. 33.2). Static progressive exercises are often the most effective for a child with joint or tendon tightness (Hardy, 2004).

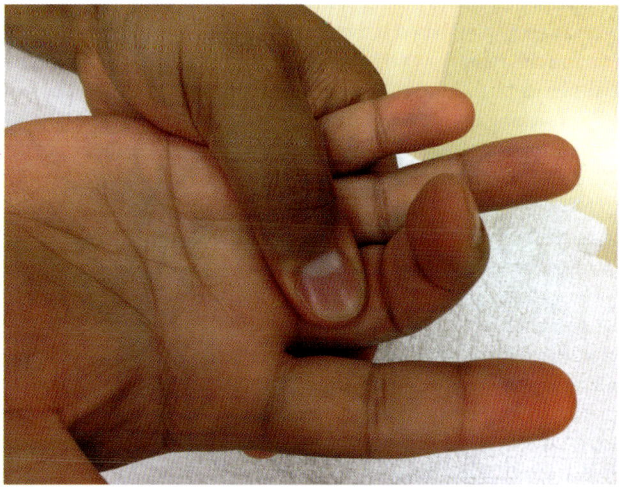

**Fig. 33.1** With a proximal interphalangeal (PIP) joint blocking exercise, the therapist supports the metacarpophalangeal in neutral extension while the child flexes the PIP joint.

## Improving Strength

To improve muscle strength, movements recruit new muscle fibers during a contraction, such that progressive/resistive activities cause hypertrophy (increase in size) and hyperplasia (increase in number) of muscle fibers (Grgic et al., 2022; Mukund & Subramaniam, 2020). Therefore, strength is developed by increasing the challenge to the muscle, such as when a person lifts a heavier weight or increases the number of repetitions.

The American Academy of Pediatrics recognizes the benefits and has guidelines for strength training for children and adolescents

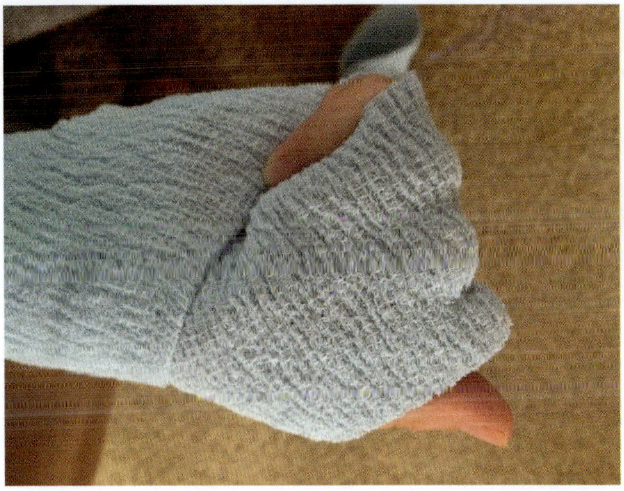

**Fig. 33.2** A flexion wrap is a static progressive exercise where the digit is wrapped into a light flexion stretch with Coban. After the child has become comfortable with the stretch, another wrap of tape is applied, pulling the digit into slightly more flexion.

(Stricker et al., 2020). When children engage in resistance training and gain strength they recruit more motor units to fire, but strength training does not result in hypertrophy until after puberty. Strength training programs for children should be closely supervised and modified according to the child's tolerance to avoid injury with strength training (Stricker et al., 2020).

Children must have a certain degree of hand strength to engage in daily activities. Occupational therapy practitioners grade strengthening programs from light to challenging. Children gain strength by increasing the number of repetitions of movements and also the level of resistance to the motion. They may also develop UE strength by engaging in weight-bearing activities, such as crawling on hands and knees during play. Occupational therapy practitioners create activities that encourage the child to hold, pull, grasp, or lift items that may be progressively more challenging (i.e., more weight). They also may improve hand strength by requiring the child to engage in more repetitions at a lighter weight, but until muscle fatigue. When engaging children in strengthening activities for the UEs, occupational therapy practitioners may address proximal control as this allows the child to have better UE control. They may provide external support (such as adapted seating) to work on hand skills despite limited proximal control.

A variety of play-based activities may be used to build hand strength in young children. For example, a 10-month-old recovering from brachial plexus birth injury (BPBI) can strengthen their shoulder muscles by reaching to throw a ball into a container placed above shoulder height or by engaging in play-based activities in quadruped. Children may enjoy playing with interlocking toys, Velcro toys, or clay, which can be used to strengthen pinch and grip. Infants with BPBI or hemiplegic cerebral palsy can strengthen the affected UE through crawling activities (Graessle, 2018).

Occupational therapy practitioners must be aware of precautions that prevent a child from engaging in a strengthening program. For example, children with a rheumatic disease in a stage of active joint inflammation should refrain from strengthening activities until the inflammation is resolved. Similarly, children recovering from surgery or UE injury need adequate healing time before engaging in resistive force to the arm and hand.

## Improving Endurance

Endurance refers to the sustained effort of muscles that is necessary for children to engage in desired occupations. When children have difficulty with endurance, they are unable to sustain the strength demands for a task over time, resulting in fatigue, pain and/or functional challenges. For example, school-age children must engage in handwriting tasks throughout the day, and they maintain upright position for sitting, while they pay attention for periods of time, where getting dressed requires standing endurance for 3–5 min and may include the endurance to complete buttoning of multiple buttons. Occupational therapy practitioners provide opportunities for the child to improve their muscular endurance and therefore their ability to continue activities over time, by providing opportunities to participate in activities that are motivating to the child for longer periods of time.

**BOX 33.1 Energy Conservation Techniques**

1. Plan ahead so less energy is used.
2. Plan for breaks or times of rest during the day. Take these breaks before you get tired.
3. Decide which tasks are more important and give yourself time to finish without rushing.
4. Alternate easy and hard tasks through the day.

Children experiencing fatigue, limiting activities, for example, those with systemic conditions such as juvenile idiopathic arthritis or Duchene muscular dystrophy, may benefit from learning **energy conservation techniques.** Although there is minimal research supporting energy conservation techniques in children, and little available with adults, it is a common technique used as part of larger packages of intervention (Bharati & Sahu, 2022; Ibrahim et al., 2023; Ip et al., 2006; Omura et al., 2022; Wingardh et al., 2020). See Box 33.1. The occupational therapy practitioner also observes how the child performs specific activities identified as difficult or contributing to fatigue. They educate the family and child on strategies used for energy conservation and develop a plan for applying the strategies at home.

## Reducing Pain

Pain may interfere with a child's ability to complete daily activities, play, and socially engage with others; therefore decreasing pain may enable children to engage in occupations. The biomechanical approach postulates that every pain has a source, and the intervention must be directed toward and influence the source of pain. Pain reduction is based on gate theory, where local stimulation of non-pain-mediated sensory afferents close the gate at the spinal cord level, thereby preventing further transmission of pain impulses (Mendell, 2014). The biomechanical approach provides physical modalities to address pain, including heat, ice massage, and cold packs.

Pain management is the first step toward helping a child with UE injury or joint inflammation to progress toward functional goals. If pain is present as is typical in most traumatic injuries or postsurgical cases, the occupational therapy practitioner provides intervention to minimize pain so that the child may be able to gain sufficient comfort to participate in therapy activities targeted at improving UE function. If the child still expresses pain in the session, the occupational therapy practitioner may need to consult with the referring physician or pain specialist.

**Joint Protection Strategies.** **Joint protection strategies** are techniques used to decrease pain caused by the amount of strain placed on a joint during a task or the amount of work a muscle group must perform to complete the task (Bobos et al., 2019; Dziedzic et al., 2015; Gavin et al., 2023). The occupational therapy practitioner explains the purpose and importance of joint protection strategies to children and their families. The practitioner determines which activities trigger pain for the child. They review the child's day and pattern of symptoms to determine the most beneficial strategies. They instruct the child and family on the strategies. They may provide written pictures or directions, practice techniques in therapy, answer questions, and follow up each week to evaluate the effectiveness of the strategies at reducing pain. Occupational therapy practitioners also address the pain through activity modifications and physical agent modalities.

**Activity Modifications.** **Activity modifications** are adaptations made to an activity to increase the child's ability to perform the activity or use a tool independently and without pain (Hill, 2016). The occupational therapy practitioner completes a task analysis to identify the most appropriate activity modification for the child. When using a biomechanical frame of reference, the practitioners examine the child's ROM, strength, endurance, and pain level when completing specific activities that are meaningful to the child and make up the child's desired occupations. The practitioner modifies the activities, so the child can complete them without pain. Examples of activity modifications include modified sports equipment or instruments, adapted writing utensils, assistive technology, and adaptive devices such as buttonhooks or pediatric-sized sock aids.

Activity modifications can be applied to limit pain that occurs or increases with specific activities. Occupational therapy practitioners carefully analyze the movement during a variety of activities and observe the child's pain level. They adjust the activity requirements to eliminate the child's pain. They may ask children to indicate their level of pain with a movement and adjust accordingly by changing the activity. They may change the activity demands by altering the ROM requirements, weight of objects, degree of motor precision, and time to complete activity. They may change the child's position and provide support to make the child more comfortable. For example, they can change the aggressiveness of passive stretching if they observe that the child is in pain. Activity modifications can occur during the intervention sessions. Addressing the child's pain during the intervention allows the child to fully engage in the session.

**Physical Agent Modalities.** A variety of physical agent modalities (PAMS) are available for pain management. The use of **PAMs** requires advanced knowledge of the techniques and precautions. Some states require advanced certification to use PAMs in practice. Occupational therapy practitioners use PAMs to prepare children for participation in the intervention session and promote occupational performance. Therefore, PAMs are part of the therapy session but used in conjunction with occupation-based activities.

PAMs refer to the use of a physical property, such as temperature, sound, or electricity, to achieve a specific therapeutic benefit (Bondoc & Feretti, 2018). PAMs are infrequently used in pediatric occupational therapy practice. Ultrasound in particular, a PAM that relies on the conversion of sound to produce a deep thermal heat, is not advised in children who are skeletally immature because it may harm growth plates in the bone (Baghdadi et al., 2022). The AOTA's Choosing Wisely Campaign (Gillen et al., 2019) has recommended that PAMs not be used in occupational therapy independently of occupation-based intervention, and there have been objections to the use of PAMs under the occupational therapy scope of practice (Brown, 2015). However, when PAMs are used, superficial thermal agents (such as heat and cold) and electrical modalities (such as neuromuscular electrical stimulation [NEMS] and transcutaneous electrical nerve stimulation [TENS]) are the most applied, and they should be considered preparatory methods.

Superficial thermal agents include both heat modalities and cryotherapy (i.e., the therapeutic application of cold). See Table 33.1 for an overview of superficial thermal agents.

Heat is typically used to achieve increased tissue extensibility to relieve pain. Heat modalities cannot be used in the presence of untreated infection or acute edema, immediately following vessel or nerve reconstruction, over newly placed skin grafts, or in regions of sensory impairment or malignancy (Skirven et al., 2021). Heat is usually applied at the start of a treatment session to prepare the tissue for therapeutic intervention.

Cryotherapy (ice massage) is most used when acute inflammation is present to relieve pain and tissue inflammation. It is contraindicated for use with children with Raynaud's disease, open wounds, acute vessel or nerve reconstruction, or sensory impairment (Skirven et al., 2021). Cryotherapy results in the tissue

**TABLE 33.1 Superficial Thermal Agents**

| Modality | Treatment Form | Description | Clinical Application |
|---|---|---|---|
| Moist heat | Heat | Delivers heat through the application of hot packs and multiple layers of toweling placed on a specific region of the upper extremity | Can be paired with a sustained stretch of a joint to achieve tissue elongation; can be replicated at home |
| Paraffin bath | Heat | Applies heat by child dipping his or her hand into heated paraffin wax | Can apply to the wrist and distal upper extremity; commonly used for pain management with arthritis |
| Fluidotherapy | Heat | A dry heat medium that is like a whirlpool; a fluidotherapy machine is filled with cellux (i.e., ground corn cobs that are like sand in texture); the fluidotherapy unit blows these particles around the extremity placed in the unit to deliver heat | The child may perform AROM during a fluidotherapy treatment; useful tool for desensitization |
| Ice packs | Cryotherapy | Delivers cold by placing ice packs on a specific region of the upper extremity | Can be replicated at home |
| Ice massage | Cryotherapy | A piece of ice is applied in a continuous pattern of movement (massage) directly over a specific region of the upper extremity | Particularly effective for tendonitis (Manias & Stasinopoulos, 2006) |

Adapted from Skirven, T. M., Osterman, A. L., Fedorczyk, J., & Amadio, P. C. (2011). Rehabilitation of the hand and upper extremity. (6th ed.). pp. 1495–1499). Elsevier; Skirven, T. M., Osterman, A. L., Fedorczyk, J., Amadio, P. C., Felder, S., & Shin, E. K. (2021). Rehabilitation of the hand and upper extremity (7th ed.). Elsevier Health Sciences.

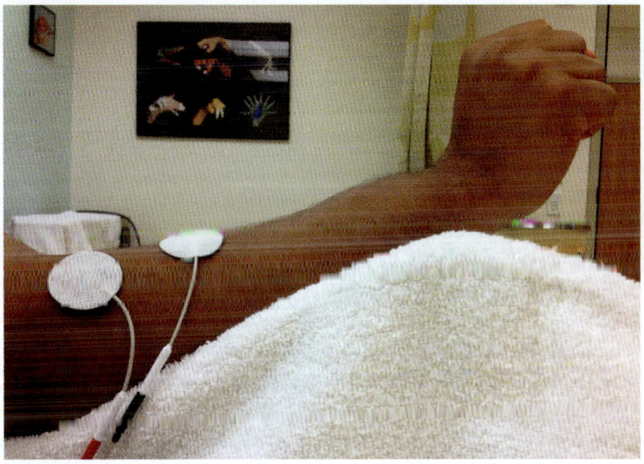

**Fig. 33.3** Neuromuscular electrical stimulation may be used to strengthen and retrain the wrist extensors (vs. the extensor digitorum communes [EDC]) to extend the wrist. The child keeps the fingers in a composite fist to prevent the EDC from extending the wrist.

contracting and the patient experiencing stiffness following application of the modality. As a result, cryotherapy is usually applied after the therapy session to alleviate or minimize tissue inflammation and pain.

**Electrotherapeutic PAMs** used with the pediatric population include neuromuscular electrical stimulation (NMES) and transcutaneous electrical nerve stimulation (TENS). NMES is most used to improve the recruitment of specific muscle groups, which results in improved active range of motion (AROM). Even when NMES does not result in improved AROM in the upper extremities, it has been found to result in muscle strength and hand function (Ou et al., 2023).

Children who have injury to the nerve at any level (spinal cord, brachial plexus, or peripheral nerve) or central nervous system damage that has resulted in abnormal muscle tone and movement patterns in the upper extremities (e.g., cerebral palsy; Ou et al., 2023) or spinal cord injury (SCI) (de Freitas, Szpoganicz, & Ilha, 2018) may benefit from NMES. When a child has sustained an injury to the nerve, the regrowth rate is 1 inch per month. As a result, significant atrophy occurs in the muscles innervated by the nerve distal to the site of injury. When an injured nerve begins to regenerate, the occupational therapy practitioner observes trace movements in the affected muscle or muscle groups. Once they observe signs of returning motor function, they may apply NMES to strengthen the atrophied muscles. NMES promotes muscle recruitment, and therefore it can be helpful in retraining specific muscle groups after an injury, fracture, or tendon transfer (Fig. 33.3).

Most children receiving pediatric hand therapy have pain that resolves as they are healing; however, some children are unable to engage in a therapy program or use their affected UE because of pain. When a child is having pain as a primary concern, TENS may be applied to the region of reported pain (Rastogi & McCarthy, 2018). TENS works through both central and peripheral nervous system mechanisms by activating the large diameter afferent nerve fibers, which then activate the central nervous system's inhibitory descending control to reduce pain (Vance et al., 2014).

## Provision of Orthoses

Orthoses are "external medical device(s) (such as a brace or splint) for supporting, immobilizing, or treating muscles, joints, or skeletal parts which are weak, ineffective, deformed, or injured" (Merriam-Webster, 2023). Occupational therapy practitioners use orthoses with children to (1) protect joints, (2) provide positioning for improved function, (3) prevent deformity, or (4) relieve pain. Orthoses may be prefabricated or custom-made and come in a variety of styles.

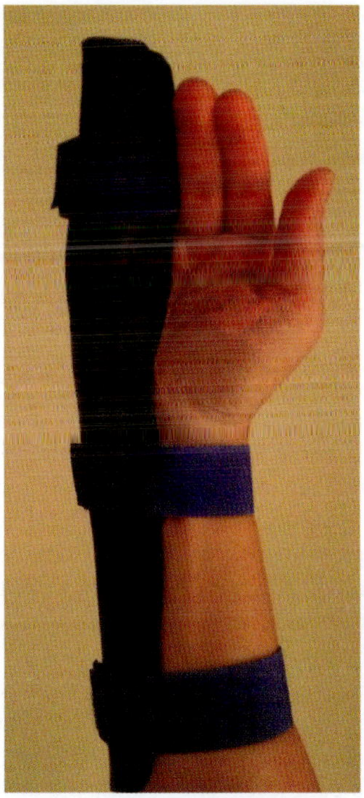

**Fig. 33.4** An ulnar gutter orthotic is an example of a protective orthosis. It is applied to protect a fracture of a digit or metacarpal in the ulnar two digits.

Orthoses may be used to protect or rest the hand or arm during acute phases of healing after an injury or UE surgery (Fig. 33.4). They provide pain relief and rest by supporting and positioning inflamed joints. For example, children with tendonitis in the UE (e.g., de Quervain tendonitis) or with a flare of arthritis symptoms in the arm or hand may benefit from an orthosis to rest the affected structures (e.g., joints/tendons) until their acute inflammation begins to resolve, which helps to provide pain relief.

Children who have conditions affecting their joint stability or joint mobility may be able to use their arms and hands more effectively when provided with an orthosis. For example, children with significant joint laxity leading to joint instability in the thumb may benefit from an orthosis that supports the first carpal metacarpal joint and thumb metacarpal phalangeal joints. The stability of the orthosis allows the child to stabilize the thumb against the other fingers for improved pinch grasp and radial grasp control (Fig. 33.5) (Ten Berge et al., 2012).

Additionally, orthoses designed for children who have limited active joint mobility or muscle spasticity can help prevent deformity. In this case, the orthosis serves to position the joints in the plane in which movement is limited or missing. For example, a child with a low radial nerve palsy may have no active wrist or metacarpal phalangeal extension of the digits and no active radial abduction of the thumb until the nerve regenerates. A radial nerve palsy orthosis can support the wrist in extension and provide dynamic support to the digits, holding them in extension while the hand is at rest and pulling them back into extension after active digit flexion. In this application the orthosis facilitates improved functional grasp and release with the affected hand and prevents flexion contractures until active movement is restored. Orthoses are used to improve ROM and correct deformity in cases of joint contracture or tendon tightness. Both static progressive orthoses and dynamic orthoses may be appropriate to improve ROM (Schwartz, 2012).

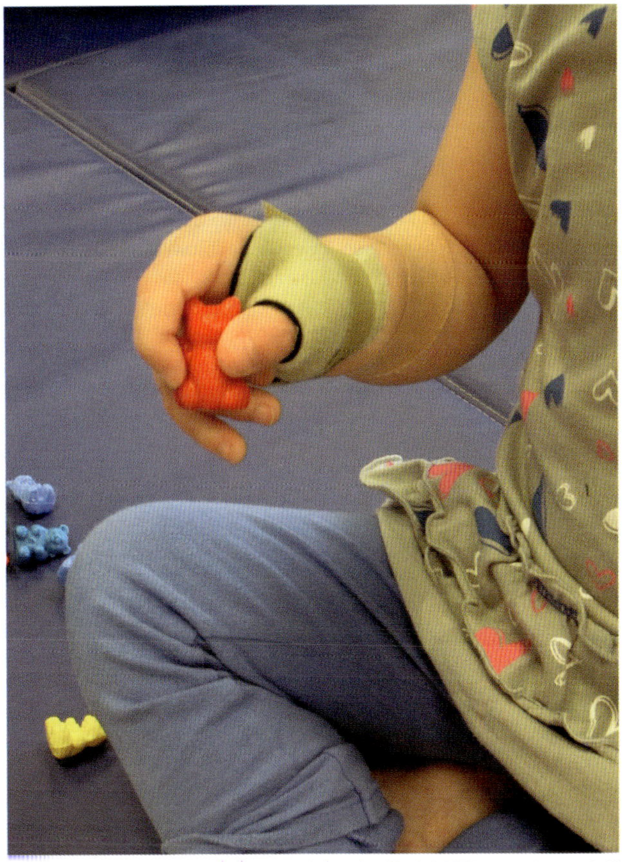

**Fig. 33.5** A McKie orthosis is one style of orthotic that provides stability to the metacarpophalangeal joint of the thumb for improved fine motor function.

**TABLE 33.2 The Types, Purposes, and Examples of a Selection of Orthoses**

| Type | Purpose | Example |
|---|---|---|
| Soft orthoses | To position, prevent contracture, provide joint support, decrease pain | Neoprene (Fig. 33.5) |
| Static orthoses | Prevent motion | Wrist and thumb spica |
| Static progressive orthoses | are used when mobility is limited by joint tightness with a soft end feel | Static progressive elbow extension orthosis (Fig. 33.6) |
| Dynamic orthoses | Apply a dynamic force to a joint, assist a child with a motion that is absent or very weak, and apply light sustained force to increase joint mobility | Orthosis that assists with MCP extension when a child has radial nerve palsy (Fig. 33.7) |

The styles of orthoses most used with children include soft orthoses, static orthoses (orthoses that prevent motion in the included joints), **static progressive orthoses** (orthoses that are serially modified to increase the joint angle), and dynamic orthotics with moveable components that apply a force to a specific joint(s) for moving that joint. Table 33.2 describes the types, purposes, and examples of a selection of orthoses. See Case Example 33.3 for an example of using orthoses as part of the occupational therapy intervention plan.

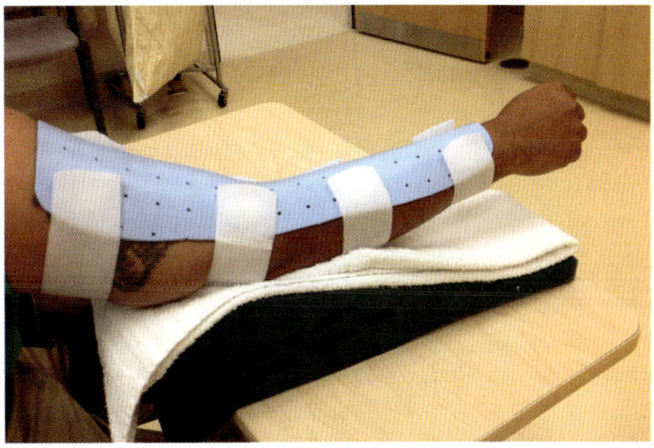

**Fig. 33.6** When a child has limited elbow extension, a static elbow extension orthotic can be used to improve range of motion. The orthosis is positioned at the child's end range of extension, and the child wears it when sleeping. The orthosis is readjusted for increased extension at future visits to gradually increase the stretch and the child's active elbow extension.

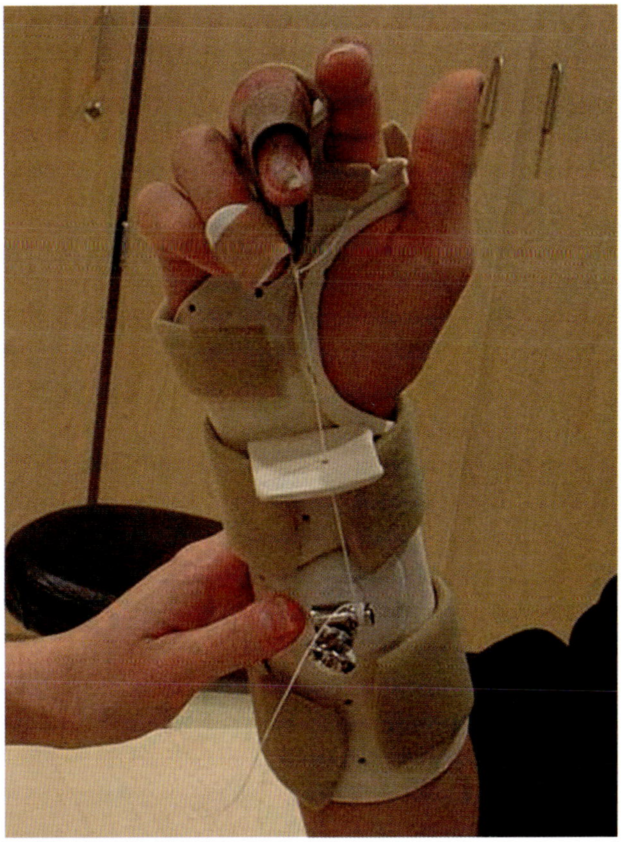

**Fig. 33.7** An example of a dynamic orthosis to increase proximal interphalangeal (PIP) joint flexion. The child turns the dial to gradually increase the PIP flexion stretch while wearing it.

## Casting

Occupational therapy practitioners fabricate casts to achieve specific treatment goals. **Serial casting** is used to increase joint mobility and tissue extensibility for improved ROM in the child's affected UE, typically when the child presents with joint tightness, atypical tone, or contracture (Durson et al., 2021; Schetzsle et al., 2023).

## CASE EXAMPLE 33.3 CANADIAN OCCUPATIONAL PERFORMANCE MEASURE (COPM) AND BIOMECHANICAL FRAME OF REFERENCE

Elio is a 15-year-old male with cerebral palsy with a right-sided hemiplegia. He is ambulatory and achieved a Manual Ability Classification System (MACS) level II (see table below).

Manual Ability Classification System and Mini-Manual Ability Classification System Levels

| | |
|---|---|
| Level 1 | Handles objects easily and successfully. At most limitations in the ease of performing manual tasks requiring speed and accuracy |
| Level 2 | Handles most objects, but with somewhat reduced quality and/or speed of achievement. May avoid some tasks or use alternative ways of performance |
| Level 3 | Handles objects with difficulty. Needs help to prepare and/or modify activities |
| Level 4 | Handles a limited selection of easily managed objects in adaptive situations. Requires continuous support |
| Level 5 | Does not handle objects and has severely limited ability to perform even simple actions. Requires total assistance |

MACS (ages 4–18 years) is from http://www.macs.nu/files/MACS%5identification%5chart%5eng.pdf. Mini-MACS (ages 1–4 years) is from http://www.macs.nu/files/Mini%2dMACS%5fEnglish%5f2016.pdf.

He participated in a variety of occupational therapy intervention sessions to maximize his right upper extremity function. He demonstrated awareness of his right upper extremity and attempted to use it as an active assist with bimanual activities; however, he had difficulty with grasp and wanted to improve function of his right arm for daily activities.

The occupational therapy practitioner wanted to understand Elio's goals, so the practitioner administered the Canadian Occupational Performance Measure (COPM), which allowed the child to identify their goals and measure their perceived performance and satisfaction. See findings in the chart below.

### CANADIAN OCCUPATIONAL PERFORMANCE MEASURE (COPM)

| | Performance | Satisfaction |
|---|---|---|
| Problem #1: Don deodorant under left arm | 1 | 3 |
| Problem #2: Hold bike handle with right hand | 2 | 1 |
| Problem #3: Hold right wrist straight | 2 | 3 |
| Problem #4: Wash with right hand in shower | 2 | 1 |
| Problem #5: Cut meat using both hands | 1 | 2 |
| Totals | 8 | 10 |

The COPM also provides total performance and satisfaction scores (the score divided by number of problems), which can be used to measure the child's progression in therapy. See chart below.

### CANADIAN OCCUPATIONAL PERFORMANCE MEASURE (COPM) TOTAL SCORES

| | Initial Score |
|---|---|
| Sum of performance scores | 8 |
| Number of problems | 5 |
| **Total performance score** | **1.6** |
| Sum of satisfaction scores | 10 |
| Number of problems | 5 |
| **Total satisfaction score** | **2** |

The occupational therapist evaluated Elio's abilities and noted that limitations with active extension of his right wrist impeded the effectiveness of his grasp. Furthermore, limitations in right active wrist extension contributed to his difficulty performing functional tasks specific to his COPM goals (such as putting on deodorant, holding bike handle, washing with his right hand, and cutting meat).

The hand surgeon determined Elio would benefit from a tendon transfer surgery to enhance his active wrist extension and functional grasp. Elio underwent surgery to transfer his extensor carpi ulnaris to his extensor carpi radialis longus and to release his flexor carpi ulnaris to allow for stronger wrist extension.

Two weeks following surgery, Elio began postoperative hand therapy. The occupational therapist positioned his wrist in a wrist cock-up orthotic in 15 degrees of extension for protection and instructed Elio on wrist extension A/PROM exercises to perform three times per day when not wearing the orthotic. The occupational therapist instructed him in scar management techniques. His therapy appointments occurred every 2 weeks. The following timeline provides a brief overview of Elio's occupational therapy intervention plan that uses an occupation-based model and a biomechanical frame of reference.

| Weeks Post Operation | Occupational Therapy Interventions |
|---|---|
| 2 weeks | Wrist extension A/PROM; scar management; wrist orthotic continual wear (off for home program only); review home program |
| 4 weeks | Wrist extension flexion AROM and grasp and release; wean from orthotic for light ADLS; continue at night and when out of the house |
| 6 weeks | Wrist extension AROM; extra soft putty for grip strengthening; functional activities for COPM goals; provide modified ways to complete goals for home |
| 8 weeks | Wrist extension AROM; putty for grip; 1-lb weight for wrist extension; functional activities for COPM goals; transition to night orthotic only; modify ways to complete goals for home if necessary (such as use of bath glove on right hand) |

Prior to surgery Elio could actively extend his right wrist to 15 degrees. He could not maintain it in extension and kept his wrist flexed throughout all functional activities. At his first therapy appointment 2 weeks following surgery, he could actively extend his wrist to 30 degrees. He completed a home program for range of motion and strengthening two times per day. The occupational therapist also modified activities, so Elio could follow his intervention plan but complete his goals. For example, at week 8, she provided him with a bath mitt for washing himself. He did not have to grip the towel but could achieve his goal within the parameters of his recovery. By 3 months post surgery, he could extend his right wrist to 45 degrees and had a right grip strength of 19 lbs. His progress on his COPM goals was as follows:

### CANADIAN OCCUPATIONAL PERFORMANCE MEASURE (COPM)

| | Performance | Satisfaction |
|---|---|---|
| Problem #1: Don deodorant under L arm | 6 | 6 |
| Problem #2: Hold bike handle with R | 7 | 10 |
| Problem #3: Hold R wrist straight | 8 | 7 |
| Problem #4: Wash with R hand in shower | 8 | 8 |
| Problem #5: Cut meat | 5 | 6 |
| Total | 34 | 37 |

### CANADIAN OCCUPATIONAL PERFORMANCE MEASURE (COPM) TOTAL SCORES

| | Reassessment Score |
|---|---|
| Sum of performance scores | 34 |
| Number of problems | 5 |
| **Total performance score** | **6.8** |
| Sum of satisfaction scores | 37 |
| Number of problems | 5 |
| **Total satisfaction score** | **7.4** |

Overall, Elio had a 5.2-point increase in his performance score compared to preoperative scores and a 7.2-point increase in his satisfaction score. He reported that he was using his right hand more in bimanual activities, and he could join his friends on bike rides.

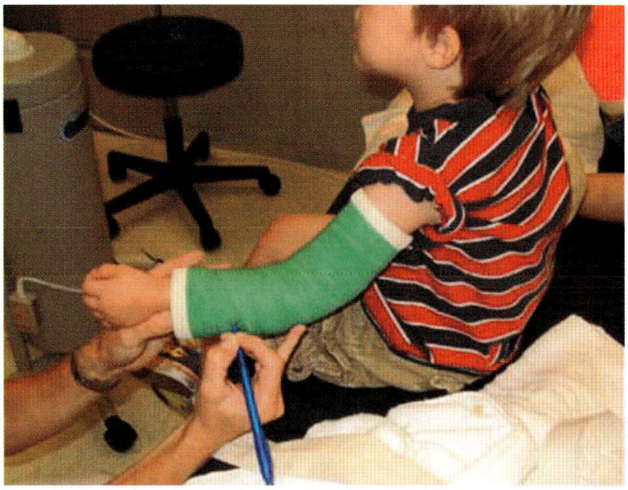

**Fig. 33.8** Serial cast for elbow extension. At each visit a new cast is applied in an increased extension stretch.

Serial casting (Fig. 33.8) is like static progressive orthoses in that a series of casts are applied, with each cast increasing the angle of the affected joint(s) to obtain the desired arc of movement. The serial cast is typically applied permanently until the child returns for the next cast to be applied. A serial cast can be formed as a bivalve cast that is removable in cases in which the child may require some time out of the cast.

Occupational therapy practitioners apply serial casting to increase UE movement following botulinum toxin or phenol injections and to decrease muscle spasticity in children who have movement limitations (Kumar et al., 2023; Leung et al., 2019; Mathevon et al., 2019).

## Kinesiology Tape

Kinesiology tape (KT) is used to facilitate or inhibit specific muscles or muscle groups to decrease pain, improve ROM, enhance muscle activation, or relax specific muscles. KT is elastic, waterproof tape (that was first used in sports therapy) and has more recently been applied in the practice of pediatric hand therapy. KT is latex-free and designed to allow skin to breathe. Taping provides gentle support and tactile cues to the muscles and can enhance lymphatic drainage and improve blood flow to decrease inflammation. Kinesiology taping improves the biomechanics of a joint, which results in more movement. For example, at the shoulder, multiple pieces of KT can be applied with tape in one region acting to inhibit specific muscles and another piece of tape placed to activate weakened muscles. The occupational therapy practitioner may use KT to improve shoulder and upper extremity kinematics, particularly for children who have joint hypermobility, hemiparesis, or shoulder pain (Fig. 33.9).

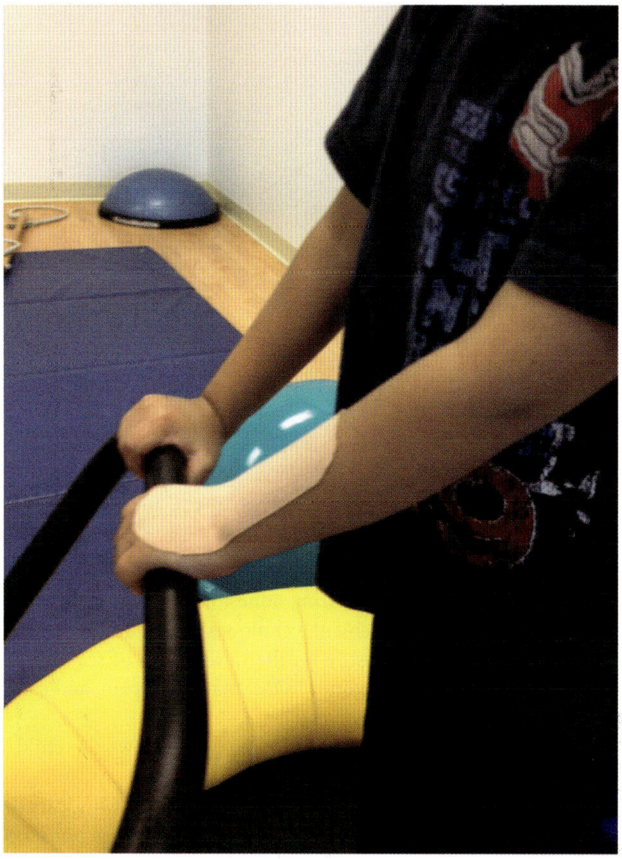

**Fig. 33.9** The child in this picture has hemiplegic cerebral palsy and weakness of the wrist extensors. The kinesiology tape is applied to facilitate the wrist extensors.

While some research shows that KT improves postural control, upper extremity, and hand function by providing stability and joint alignment (de Sire et al., 2022; García-Hernández, et al., 2019; Iosa, 2015; Karabay et al., 2016; Krause et al., 2021; Ramírez & de la Cruz, 2017; Rasti et al., 2017; Russo et al., 2018), other recent reviews and studies of KT suggest the benefits may be small or no better than other interventions (Ghozy et al., 2020; Hassan et al., 2020; Letafatkar et al., 2021; Russo et al., 2016). A recent survey of professionals who use KT reported the following contraindications: skin allergies, open wounds or lesions, rash or skin irritation, diabetes, active malignancy, and inability to communicate (Cheatham et al., 2021).

If based on the clinical presentation KT is an appropriate intervention, it may be cut in specific patterns and applied in a variety of ways to address specific goals. See online resources referring to how to apply tape to achieve specific outcomes desired. Children may wear KT for 3–5 days, and family members can be instructed on how to apply tape when it needs to be reapplied. Occupational therapy practitioners may apply a small test strip of tape on the child's skin to determine if the child has an adverse skin response to wearing the tape.

## Wound Care

Occupational therapy practitioners use knowledge about wound care when working with children after surgery or a traumatic UE injury. Trauma to the dermis such as abrasions in the arm or hand from shearing injuries results in lengthy wound healing through tissue granulation. Children who have skin grafts require an extended period for healing. The occupational therapy practitioner monitors the health and healing of the wounds and grafts and begins intervention when it is medically appropriate. For example, children may begin occupational therapy after surgery when pins or sutures are in place.

The practitioner consults with the referring physician regarding specific wound care strategies and provides the family education on wound care. The practitioner may also provide direct wound care such as dressing changes or debridement of loose eschar (e.g., scab formation). Skin graft precautions include avoiding shear force over new grafts, which can be caused by edema control garments or orthotics, and avoiding compression that could compromise blood flow to the graft.

## Scar Management

Scar management promotes movement by improving the tissue extensibility and limiting adhesions caused by scar tissue. The ability to move in a certain direction throughout a range is related to the integrity of the surrounding tissue. Therefore, preventing or reducing

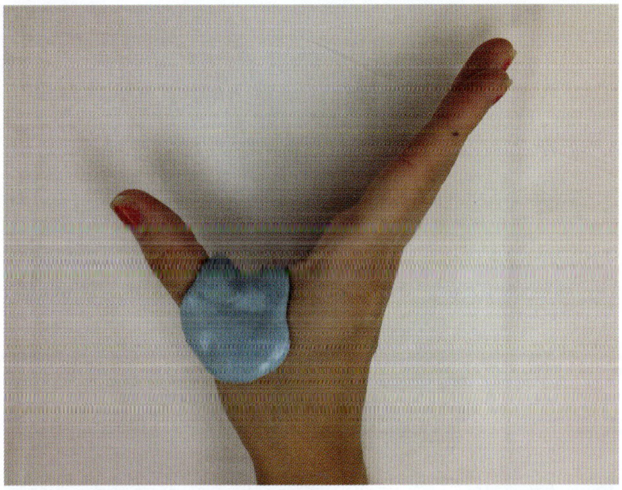

**Fig. 33.10** An example of an elastomer scar pad that a child wears when sleeping to improve scar pliability.

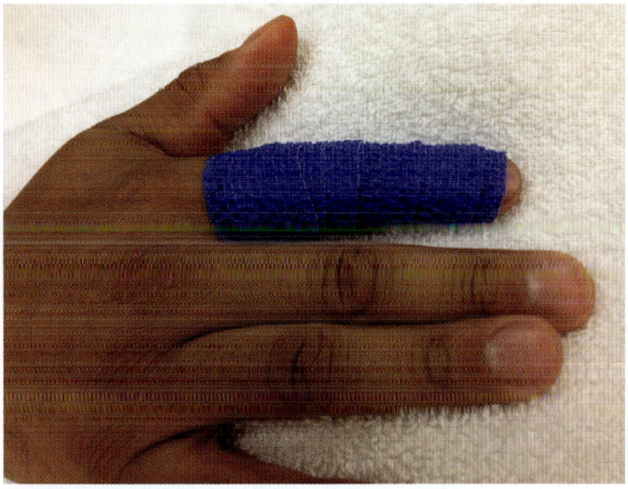

**Fig. 33.11** An example of a Coban wrap on the digit to decrease finger edema.

contractures as the result of scaring adhesions enhances movement and functioning. Scar management techniques include ROM exercises, massage, and providing pressure on the raised parts of scar to limit tissue adhesions. Scarring can limit ROM, may cause pain, and can be a cosmetic concern.

Once the postsurgical rehabilitation protocol allows the child to perform ROM in the joints affected by scarring, they can engage in ROM exercises to restore mobility. Scar massage is used with scars that limit AROM in a joint, lack pliability, are thick, extend the borders of the wound, or are a cosmetic concern. Scar massage is meant to help the scarred tissue move more like normal skin, which can be moved slightly in all directions. Scar massage is generally completed using any typical moisturizing lotion and gently rubbing the scar from the middle outward. Scar massage works in circular motions, up and down, and side to side, to improve skin flexibility and natural motion.

Pressure on scars is an effective strategy to improve tissue extensibility and cosmetics of scars (Sharp et al., 2016). Pressure can be applied for longer periods of time by using scar pads and compressive materials, which can be applied when the child is sleeping, so the UE is free for functional use during the day. Often, for small, minimally raised scars, compression with a soft material, such as neoprene donned under an orthotic, tape, or compressive wrap, is sufficient to promote healing (Yelvington et al., 2013). Occupational therapy practitioners use gel scar pads cut to cover the region of the scar or make a custom-molded scar pad from elastomer products in combination with an orthotic or compressive wrap to provide adequate compression (Monstrey et al., 2014). See Fig. 33.10 for an example of an elastomer scar pad. In cases of burns to the UE or skin grafts, custom-sized compression garments are necessary for optimal scar management (Berman et al., 2008; Téot et al., 2019). Compression garments are elastic clothing, specially made using elastomeric fibers and yarns that provide enough mechanical pressure and force on the skin to assist with reducing scarring (Xiong & Tao, 2018).

## Edema Control

Occupational therapy practitioners use edema control strategies to address swelling following surgery or an upper extremity injury. Edema control may also be used to manage pain that is associated with significant inflammation in the arm or hand. A variety of interventions are used for edema control in the UE, including active movement, compression, and positioning interventions (Priganc et al., 2020). Positioning a child's arm and hand resting above the heart may decrease edema. However, families with young children often report that this is a difficult strategy to implement with young children because of their high activity levels and resistance to prolonged periods of sitting. Occupational therapy practitioners also teach children and/or family members AROM exercises to reduce edema. Young children often respond best to performing the movements while engaging in play a few times throughout the day. For example, a variety of child songs accompanied by finger play can be used to promote UE ROM. Older children can be taught to avoid prolonged periods of full elbow extension of the affected UE until the edema begins to subside and, when cleared by the physician, to regularly perform AROM exercises.

When edema is moderate to severe or does not respond to positioning and AROM, the practitioner can use manual edema mobilization (Miller et al., 2017). **Manual edema mobilization** techniques (i.e., specific massage patterns that activate lymphatic drainage) may be used in cases of persistent edema (Priganc et al., 2020). The practitioner wraps Coban distal to proximal on a digit (Fig. 33.11) or applies compressive finger sleeves (available in sizes for larger children) to decrease digital edema. Compressive sleeves are available in graded sizes that can be donned over the wrist or proximal UE for edema control.

## Desensitization and Sensory Reeducation

Desensitization and sensory reeducation are two interventions occupational therapy practitioners use for children experiencing sensory impairments following peripheral injuries or trauma. Occupational therapy practitioners use desensitization strategies to reduce pain from touch and facilitate the child's use of the affected arm in everyday functional activities (Shah & Shinde, 2018). Hypersensitivity to touch can occur after an injury, especially if a nerve was involved. It may also occur spontaneously or after a minor injury, such as a sprain or strain to the wrist. A child with hypersensitivity to touch may experience pain in their UE when exposed to temperature, textures, and/or touch pressure. Graded exposure to touch and textures may allow a child to accept sensory input. Using play-based activities may increase a child's acceptance for desensitization activities (Fig. 33.12).

Sensory reeducation refers to a child's sensory return after a nerve injury. The occupational therapist exposes the UE to a variety of sensory activities to improve sensory discrimination (Antonopoulos et al., 2019). The occupational therapy practitioner can begin sensory reeducation when a child has a Semmes-Weinstein grade of monofilament 6.65 or better (Skirven et al., 2021). See Chapter 9 for an explanation of the Semmes-Weinstein test. The practitioner provides graded exposure to various items to increase the child's ability to differentiate between items through touch. For example, they may begin sensory reeducation

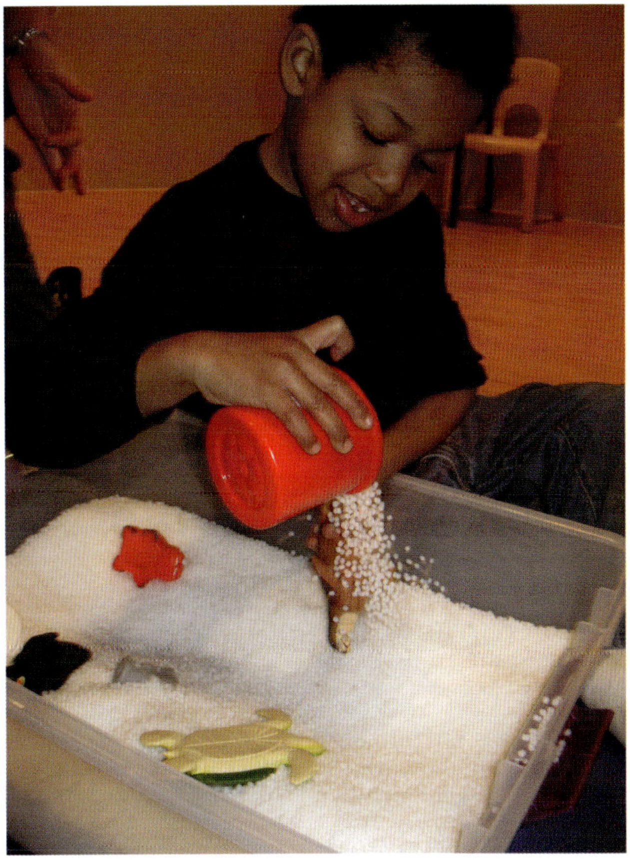

Fig. 33.12 Children who have hypersensitivity can perform grasp release of a sensory medium or find toys hidden in a sensory medium for desensitization of the extremity.

by engaging the child in activities where they feel and identify items with their eyes closed. The occupational therapy practitioner changes the textures and sensory properties of the items as the child progresses.

## Reducing Muscle Tone

Children may present with hypertonia (i.e., high muscle tone) in the affected upper extremity, interfering with their ROM, muscle strength, endurance, and subsequent ability to use their hands to participate in meaningful daily activities. Occupational therapy practitioners provide strategies to change muscle hypertonicity to help a child gain better control of movement in the upper extremity. The occupational therapy practitioner may use a variety of biomechanical strategies described above such as positioning, NMES, activity modification, and orthoses to address the effects of a child's hypertonicity.

Weight-bearing through the affected arm and hand can decrease muscle hypertonicity (Pin, 2007). Weight bearing may be used prior to engaging in manual activities. Children who have hypertonicity may benefit from manual activities that are calming, involve weight-bearing, allow them to work within their ROM, and are slow and predictable rather than quick and changing. NMES also may be used to reduce hypertonicity in specific muscle groups; however, reduction in hypertonicity is only seen during application of the NMES (Ozer et al., 2006). When OT intervention alone is insufficient to address the negative effects of hypertonicity, the OT may recommend the child consult with a rehabilitation medicine physician to discuss medical interventions to assist in controlling hypertonicity (Novak et al., 2020).

## Mirror Therapy

Mirror therapy (MT) is a therapeutic intervention first introduced in 1996 to decrease phantom limb pain in individuals with amputations (Ramachandran & Rogers-Ramachandran, 1996). In mirror therapy, a mirror is placed at midline so that it hides the affected upper extremity and the unaffected upper extremity is placed so that the child views the reflection of the unaffected upper extremity in the mirror. This positioning gives the child's brain the illusion that the affected upper extremity is functioning as well as the child's unaffected upper extremity. The mechanism at work is believed to be the mirror's effect on "learned paralysis." Learned paralysis occurs because of conflicts between the motor nerve's output and the sensory feedback. The brain sends a motor command but receives no visual or proprioceptive feedback from the motion. The mirror provides the false visual feedback that the limb is moving, restoring congruence between the inputs and outputs. This is believed to allow a child to unlearn the "learned paralysis" (Yeves-Lite et al., 2020).

Early research examined mirror therapy for reducing pain in phantom limbs and for improving neuromotor function in hemiparesis. More recently the effectiveness of mirror therapy as an intervention for children with brachial plexus birth injury and cerebral palsy has been evaluated. The available evidence for mirror therapy in children with cerebral palsy supports it as an effective intervention for addressing motor control (Novak et al., 2020). Additionally, mirror therapy is associated with better outcomes when combined with exercises or virtual reality (Barbin et al., 2016; Bruchez et al., 2016; Herrador Colmenero et al., 2018; Kara et al., 2020; Narimani et al., 2019; Park et al., 2016; Yeves-Lite et al., 2020).

## SUMMARY

Occupational therapy practitioners address hand and UE impairments in children and youth resulting from many possible conditions or injuries. They often use a biomechanical approach to address ROM, strength, endurance, and pain interfering with the child's ability to engage in meaningful activities. They provide intervention activities to promote occupational engagement that follow biomechanical principles, while simultaneously factoring in the child's goals, desires, and unique situations. In this way, occupational therapy practitioners create client-centered intervention plans that empower children and families to participate in home, school, and community. This chapter describes the use of an occupation-based perspective to apply the biomechanical frame of reference principles, strategies, and modalities for children who have UE impairments.

1. Occupational therapists addressing UE impairments in children consider many factors (i.e., child, occupation, and environment) that affect the child's engagement in meaningful activities. They use knowledge of the child's physical, social, cognitive, and communication skills and abilities, in addition to the child's interests, roles, habits, goals, and environmental resources and barriers to create meaningful intervention plans. They use knowledge of the child's medical history, condition, and current situation. The perspective from understanding a child's experience (gained from an occupation-based model of practice) informs intervention decisions and allows occupational therapy practitioners to provide a unique service to children and their families.
2. The biomechanical frame of reference addresses ROM, strength, endurance, and pain that interferes with hand functioning and the child's ability to engage in daily activities. Occupational therapy practitioners follow the guiding principles based on research evidence. Understanding the rationale for selecting specific techniques allows practitioners to problem solve and tailor the strategies and approaches to each child.

3. Occupational therapy practitioners use a variety of intervention strategies based on the biomechanical frame of reference to address ROM, strength, endurance, and pain for children with UE conditions. Occupational therapy sessions include engaging children in UE activities for occupational engagement, such as play, self-care (e.g., feeding, dressing, grooming), leisure, academics, and social participation. Occupational therapy practitioners may use PAMs, orthotics, casting, kinesiology taping, mirror therapy, and activity modifications as techniques to promote engagement. They may also support wound care, edema control, scar management, and pain management.

## REFERENCES


Antonopoulos, D. K., Mavrogenis, A. F., Megaloikonomos, P. D., Mitsiokapa, E., Georgoudis, G., Vottis, C. T., & Spyridonos, S. G. (2019). Similar 2-point discrimination and stereognosia but better locognosia at long term with an independent home-based sensory reeducation program vs no reeducation after low-median nerve transection and repair. *Journal of Hand Therapy*, *32*(3), 305–312.

Baghdadi, S., Harwood, K., Greenberg, E., Baldwin, K. D., & Lawrence, J. T. R. (2022). Effects of therapeutic ultrasound on growth plates: A systematic review. *Pediatric Physical Therapy*, *34*(1), 2–8.

Barbin, J., Seetha, V., Casillas, J.-M., Paysant, J., & Perennou, D. (2016). The effects of mirror therapy on pain and motor control of phantom limb in amputees: A systematic review. *Annals of Physical and Rehabilitation Medicine*, *59*(4), 270–275.

Berman, B., Viera, M. H., Amini, S., Huo, R., & Jones, I. S. (2008). Prevention and management of hypertrophic scars and keloids after burns in children. *Journal of Craniofacial Surgery*, *19*(4), 989–1006.

Bharati, B., & Sahu, K. S. (2022). Post-COVID-19 chronic fatigue and the role of energy conservation and work simplification techniques: An occupational therapy approach. *Indian Journal of Physiotherapy & Occupational Therapy Print-(ISSN 0973-5666) and Electronic–(ISSN 0973-5674)*, *16*(1), 1–5.

Bobos, P., Nazari, G., Szekeres, M., Lalone, E. A., Ferreira, L., & MacDermid, J. C. (2019). The effectiveness of joint-protection programs on pain, hand function, and grip strength levels in patients with hand arthritis: A systematic review and meta-analysis. *Journal of Hand Therapy*, *32*(2), 194–211.

Bondoc, S., & Feretti, A. M. (2018). Physical agents and mechanical modalities. *American Journal of Occupational Therapy*, *72*, 1–6.

Brown, T. (2015). Do physical agent modalities fit under an occupational therapy scope of practice? *British Journal of Occupational Therapy*, *78*(3) 143-143.

Bruchez, R., Jequier Gygax, M., Roches, S., Fluss, J., Jacquier, D., Ballabeni, P., … Newman, C. J. (2016). Mirror therapy in children with hemiparesis: A randomized observer–blinded trial. *Developmental Medicine and Child Neurology*, *58*(9), 970–978.

Burley, S., Di Tommaso, A., Cox, R., & Molineux, M. (2018). An occupational perspective in hand therapy: A scoping review. *British Journal of Occupational Therapy*, *81*(6), 299–318.

Cheatham, S. W., Baker, R. T., & Abdenour, T. E. (2021). Kinesiology tape: A descriptive survey of healthcare professionals in the United States. *International Journal of Sports Physical Therapy*, *16*(3), 778.

de Freitas, G. R., Szpoganicz, C., & Ilha, J. (2018). Does neuromuscular electrical stimulation therapy increase voluntary muscle strength after spinal cord injury? A systematic review. *Topics in Spinal Cord Injury Rehabilitation*, *24*(1), 6–17.

de Sire, A., Curci, C., Ferrara, M., Losco, L., Spalek, R., Cisari, C., Invernizzi, M., & Solaro, C. (2022). Efficacy of kinesio taping on hand functioning in patients with mild carpal tunnel syndrome. A double-blind randomized controlled trial. *Journal of Hand Therapy*, *35*(4), 605–612.

Dursun, N., Gokbel, T., Akarsu, M., Bonikowski, M., Pyrzanowska, W., & Dursun, E. (2021). Intermittent serial casting for wrist flexion deformity in children with spastic cerebral palsy: A randomized controlled trial. *Developmental Medicine and Child Neurology*, *63*(6), 743–747.

Dziedzic, K., Nicholls, E., Hill, S., Hammond, A., Handy, J., Thomas, E., & Hay, E. (2015). Self-management approaches for osteoarthritis in the hand: A 2×2 factorial randomised trial. *Annals of the Rheumatic Diseases*, *74*(1), 108–118.

García Hernández, N., Corona-Cortés, J., García-Fuentes, L., González-Santibañez, R. D., & Parra-Vega, V. (2019). Biomechanical and functional effects of shoulder kinesio taping® on cerebral palsy children interacting with virtual objects. *Computer Methods in Biomechanics and Biomedical Engineering*, *22*(6), 676–684.

Gavin, J. P., Rossiter, L., Adams, J., Fenerty, V., Leese, J., Hammond, A., & Backman, C. (2023). The role of occupational therapy for the self-management of rheumatoid arthritis: A mixed methods systematic review. *Rheumatology*, *62*(Suppl_2), 104–145.

Ghozy, S., Dung, N. M., Morra, M. E., Morsy, S., Elsayed, G. G., Tran, L., & Huy, N. T. (2020). Efficacy of kinesio taping in treatment of shoulder pain and disability: A systematic review and meta-analysis of randomised controlled trials. *Physiotherapy*, *107*, 176–188.

Gillen, G., Hunter, E. G., Lieberman, D., & Stutzbach, M. (2019). AOTA's top 5 choosing wisely® recommendations. *American Journal of Occupational Therapy*, *73*(2), p1–p9.

Graessle, E. (2018). Infant crawling orthosis and home program to strengthen a neurologically impaired upper extremity. *Journal of Hand Therapy*, *31*(3), 411–415.

Grgic, J., Schoenfeld, B. J., Orazem, J., & Sabol, F. (2022). Effects of resistance training performed to repetition failure or non-failure on muscular strength and hypertrophy: A systematic review and meta-analysis. *Journal of Sport and Health Science*, *11*(2), 202–211.

Hardy, M. A. (2004). Principles of metacarpal and phalangeal fracture management: A review of rehabilitation concepts. *Journal of Orthopaedic & Sports Physical Therapy*, *34*(12), 781–799.

Hassan, B. S., Abbass, M. E., & Elshennawy, S. (2020). Systematic review of the effectiveness of Kinesio taping for children with brachial plexus injury. *Physiotherapy Research International*, *25*(1), e1794.

Hays, P. L., & Rozental, T. D. (2013). Rehabilitative strategies following hand fractures. *Hand Clinics*, *29*(4), 585–600.

Herrador Colmenero, L., Perez Marmol, J. M., Martí-García, C., Querol Zaldivar, M. d. l. Á., Tapia Haro, R. M., Castro Sánchez, A. M., & Aguilar-Ferrándiz, M. E. (2018). Effectiveness of mirror therapy, motor imagery, and virtual feedback on phantom limb pain following amputation: A systematic review. *Prosthetics and Orthotics International*, *42*(3), 288–298.

Hill, W. (2016). The role of occupational therapy in pain management. *Anaesthesia and Intensive Care Medicine*, *17*(9), 451–453.

Ibrahim, M. B., Labib, M. A., Moussa, H. H., Taha, T. S. E. D., & AboAli, S. E. M. (2023). Efficacy of energy conservation techniques on pulmonary functions in children with cystic fibrosis. *Journal of Pharmaceutical Negative Results*, 315–320. https://doi.org/10.47750/pnr.2023.14.S01.34.

Iosa, M. (2015). The application of Kinesio Taping in children with cerebral palsy. *Developmental Medicine and Child Neurology*, *57*(1), 11–12.

Ip, W. M., Woo, J., Yue, S. Y., Kwan, M., Sum, S. M., Kwok, T., & Hui, S. S. (2006). Evaluation of the effect of energy conservation techniques in the performance of activity of daily living tasks. *Clinical Rehabilitation*, *20*(3), 254–261.

Kara, O. K., Yardimci, B. N., Sahin, S., Orhan, C., Livanelioglu, A., & Soylu, A. R. (2020). Combined effects of mirror therapy and exercises on the upper extremities in children with unilateral cerebral palsy: A randomized controlled trial. *Developmental Neurorehabilitation*, *23*(4), 253–264.

Karabay, İ., Doğan, A., Ekiz, T., Köseoğlu, B. F., & Ersöz, M. (2016). Training postural control and sitting in children with cerebral palsy: Kinesio taping vs. neuromuscular electrical stimulation. *Complementary Therapies in Clinical Practice*, *24*, 67–72.

Keller, J. L., Henderson, J. P., Landrieu, K. W., Dimick, M. P., & Walsh, J. M. (2021). The 2019 practice analysis of hand therapy and the use of orthoses by certified hand therapists. *Journal of Hand Therapy*, *35*(4), 628–640.

Krause, D., Roll, S. C., Javaherian-Dysinger, H., & Daher, N. (2021). Comparative efficacy of the dorsal application of kinesio tape and splinting for carpal tunnel syndrome: A randomized controlled trial. *Journal of Hand Therapy*, *34*(3), 351–361.

Kumar, D., Kumar, R., Mudgal, S. K., Ranjan, P., & Kumar, S. (2023). The effects of botulinum toxin and casting in spastic children with cerebral palsy: A systematic review and meta-analysis. *Cureus*, *15*(3),e36851. https://doi.org/10.7759/cureus.36851.

Letafatkar, A., Rabiei, P., Kazempour, S., & Alaei-Parapari, S. (2021). Comparing the effects of no intervention with therapeutic exercise, and exercise with additional Kinesio tape in patients with shoulder impingement syndrome. A three-arm randomized controlled trial. *Clinical Rehabilitation*, *35*(4), 558–567.

Leung, J., King, C., & Fereday, S. (2019). Effectiveness of a programme comprising serial casting, botulinum toxin, splinting and motor training for contracture management: A randomized controlled trial. *Clinical Rehabilitation*, *33*(6), 1035–1044.

Mathevon, L., Bonan, I., Barnais, J.-L., Boyer, F., & Dinomais, M. (2019). Adjunct therapies to improve outcomes after botulinum toxin injection in children: A systematic review. *Annals of Physical and Rehabilitation Medicine*, *62*(4), 283–290.

Mendell, L. M. (2014). Constructing and deconstructing the gate theory of pain. *Pain®*, *155*(2), 210–216.

Miller, L. K., Jerosch-Herold, C., & Shepstone, L. (2017). Effectiveness of edema management techniques for subacute hand edema: A systematic review. *Journal of Hand Therapy*, *30*(4), 432–446.

Monstrey, S., Middelkoop, E., Vranckx, J. J., Bassetto, F., Ziegler, U. E., Meaume, S., & Teot, L. (2014). Updated scar management practical guidelines: Non-invasive and invasive measures. *J Plast Reconstr Aesthet Surg*, *67*(8), 1017–1025.

Mukund, K., & Subramaniam, S. (2020). Skeletal muscle: A review of molecular structure and function, in health and disease. *Wiley Interdisciplinary Reviews. Systems Biology and Medicine*, *12*(1), e1462. https://doi.org/10.1002/wsbm.1462.

Narimani, A., Kalantari, M., Dalvand, H., & Tabatabaee, S. M. (2019). Effect of mirror therapy on dexterity and hand grasp in children aged 9-14 Years with hemiplegic cerebral palsy. *Iranian Journal of Child Neurology*, *13*(4), 135.

Novak, I., Morgan, C., Fahey, M., Finch-Edmondson, M., Galea, C., Hines, A., ... Badawi, N. (2020). State of the evidence traffic lights 2019: Systematic review of interventions for preventing and treating children with cerebral palsy. *Current Neurology and Neuroscience Reports*, *20*(3), 1–21. https://doi.org/10.1007/s11910-020-1022-z.

Ou, C.-H., Shiue, C.-C., Kuan, Y.-C., Liou, T.-H., Chen, H.-C., & Kuo, T.-J. (2023). Neuromuscular electrical stimulation of upper limbs in patients with cerebral palsy: A systematic review and meta analysis of randomized controlled trials. *American Journal of Physical Medicine & Rehabilitation*, *102*(2), 151–158.

Ozer, K., Chesher, S. P., & Scheker, L. R. (2006). Neuromuscular electrical stimulation and dynamic bracing for the management of upper–extremity spasticity in children with cerebral palsy. *Developmental Medicine and Child Neurology*, *48*(7), 559–563.

Park, E. J., Baek, S. H., & Park, S. (2016). Systematic review of the effects of mirror therapy in children with cerebral palsy. *Journal of Physical Therapy Science*, *28*(11), 3227–3231.

Pin, T. W. (2007). Effectiveness of static weight-bearing exercises in children with cerebral palsy. *Pediatric Physical Therapy*, *19*(1), 62–73.

Priganc, V., Walter, J. R., & Sublett, S. H. (2020). Edema assessment and management practice patterns among hand therapists: Survey research. *Journal of Hand Therapy*, *33*(3), 378–385.

Ramírez, J. O., & de la Cruz, S. P. (2017). Therapeutic effects of kinesio taping in children with cerebral palsy: A systematic review. *Archivos Argentinos de Pediatria*, *115*(6), e356–e361.

Ramachandran, V. S., & Rogers-Ramachandran, D. C. (1996). Synaesthesia in phantom limbs induced with mirrors. *Proceedings of the Royal Society of London*, *263*, 377–386.

Rasti, Z. A., Shamsoddini, A., Dalvand, H., & Labaf, S. (2017). The effect of kinesio taping on handgrip and active range of motion of hand in children with cerebral palsy. *Iranian Journal of Child Neurology*, *11*(4), 43.

Rastogi, S., & McCarthy, K. (2018). Complex pain in children and young people; part 2: Management. *BJA Education*, *18*(3), 82.

Robinson, L. S., Brown, T., & O'Brien, L. (2016). Embracing an occupational perspective: Occupation-based interventions in hand therapy practice. *Australian Occupational Therapy Journal*, *63*(4), 293–296.

Russo, S. A., Rodriguez, L. M., Kozin, S. H., Zlotolow, D. A., Chafetz, R. S., Killelea, C. M., & Richards, J. G. (2016). Therapeutic taping for scapular stabilization in children with brachial plexus birth palsy. *American Journal of Occupational Therapy*, *70*(5), p1–p11.

Russo, S. A., Zlotolow, D. A., Chafetz, R. S., Rodriguez, L. M., Kelly, D., Linamen, H., & Kozin, S. H. (2018). Efficacy of 3 therapeutic taping configurations for children with brachial plexus birth palsy. *Journal of Hand Therapy*, *31*(3), 357–370.

Schetzsle, S., Lin, W. W. C., Purushothaman, P., Ding, J., Kwan, P., & Tredget, E. E. (2023). Serial casting as an effective method for burn scar contracture rehabilitation: A case series. *Journal of Burn Care and Research*, *44*(5), 1062–1072.

Schwartz, D. A. (2012). Static progressive orthoses for the upper extremity: A comprehensive literature review. *Hand*, *7*(1), 10–17.

Shah, P. S., & Shinde, S. B. (2018). Effect of desensitization methods during the early mobilization phase in post-fracture conditions of upper extremity. *Asian Jjournal of Pharmaceutical and Clinical Research*, 93–96.

Sharp, P. A., Pan, B., Yakuboff, K. P., & Rothchild, D. (2016). Development of a best evidence statement for the use of pressure therapy for management of hypertrophic scarring. *Journal of Burn Care and Research*, *37*(4), 255–264.

Skirven, T. M., Osterman, A. L., Fedorczyk, J., Amadio, P. C., Felder, S., & Shin, E. K. (2021). *Rehabilitation of the hand and upper extremity* (7th ed.). Elsevier Health Sciences.

Skirven, T. M., Osterman, A. L., Fedorczyk, J., & Amadio, P. C. (2011). *Rehabilitation of the hand and upper extremity* (6th ed.) (pp. 1495–1499). Elsevier.

Stricker, P. R., Faigenbaum, A. D., McCambridge, T. M., LaBella, C. R., Brooks, M. A., Canty, G., ... Peterson, A. R. (2020). Resistance training for children and adolescents. *Pediatrics*, *145*(6),e20201011.

Téot, L., Masanovic, M. G., & Faure-Chazelles, C. (2019). Compression for managing scars. In *Compression and chronic wound management* (pp. 205–214). Springer.

Ten Berge, S. R., Boonstra, A. M., Dijkstra, P. U., Hadders-Algra, M., Haga, N., & Maathuis, C. G. (2012). A systematic evaluation of the effect of thumb opponens splints on hand function in children with unilateral spastic cerebral palsy. *Clinical Rehabilitation*, *26*(4), 362–371. https://doi.org/10.1177/0269215511411936.

Vance, C. G., Dailey, D. L., Rakel, B. A., & Sluka, K. A. (2014). Using TENS for pain control: The state of the evidence. *Pain Management*, *4*(3), 197–209. https://doi.org/10.2217/pmt.14.13.

Wingårdh, A. S. L., Göransson, C., Larsson, S., Slinde, F., & Vanfleteren, L. E. (2020). Effectiveness of energy conservation techniques in patients with COPD. *Respiration*, *99*(5), 409–416.

Xiong, Y., & Tao, X. (2018). Compression garments for medical therapy and sports. *Polymers*, *10*(6), 663. https://doi.org/10.3390/polym10060663.

Yelvington, M., Brown, S., Castro, M. M., & Nick, T. G. (2013). The use of neoprene as a scar management modality. *Burns*, *39*(5), 866–875.

Yeves-Lite, A., Zuil-Escobar, J. C., Martínez-Cepa, C., Romay-Barrero, H., Ferri-Morales, A., & Palomo-Carrión, R. (2020). Conventional and virtual reality mirror therapies in upper obstetric brachial palsy: A randomized pilot study. *Journal of Clinical Medicine*, *9*(9), 3021.

# 34

# Assistive Technology Interventions to Promote Occupational Performance

*Judith Weenink Schoonover and Elisa Wern*

*"Not every child has an equal talent or an equal ability or equal motivation,*
*but children have the equal right to develop their talent, their ability, and their motivation."*

*John F. Kennedy.*

## GUIDING QUESTIONS

1. How can assistive technology (AT) enhance childhood occupations?
2. What factors influence AT services and outcomes?
3. What frameworks guide decisions about AT selection?
4. What are examples of lite to high technology AT solutions?

## KEY TERMS

Accessibility
Assistive technology (AT)
Alternate and augmentative communication (AAC)
Ergonomics
Operating system
Self-determination
Transition plan
Universal design
Universal Design for Learning (UDL)

## INTRODUCTION TO ASSISTIVE TECHNOLOGY

Assistive technology (AT) is legally defined by The Assistive Technology Act of 2004 (PL 108–364) as "any item, piece of equipment, or product system whether acquired commercially, off the shelf, modified, or customized that is used to increase, maintain, or improve functional capabilities of individuals with disabilities." Besides devices, AT may also refer to structural changes that help individuals engage in meaningful activities in different environments (AOTA, 2016). The World Health Organization (2018)

> *"Assistive technology enables people to live healthy, productive, independent, and dignified lives, and to participate in education, the labor market, and civic life. Assistive technology reduces the need for formal health and support services, long-term care, and the work of caregivers" (p. 1). describes the impact of AT as follows:*

AT is a broad term that encompasses devices ranging from lite or no technology to high technology. Low-tech (lite technology) devices (e.g., pencil-and-paper communication boards and built-up foam handles) are inexpensive, simple to make, and easy to obtain. High-tech devices (e.g., power wheelchairs, dynamic screen devices with voice output, and specialized computer software and peripherals) are generally expensive, more difficult to make, and may take longer to obtain. Mid-tech devices fall somewhere in between and may consist of handmade or commercially available items.

Occupational therapy practitioners use AT devices (also called adaptive equipment), such as reachers, buttonhooks, and pencil grips, to promote functional independence in children and youth. Judiciously selected AT affords children with creative solutions, offering them greater independence and opportunities for participation at home, at school, in the workforce, in the community, and in society. Case Example 34.1 shows lite technology used to support an infant's development.

AT can unlock a child's potential and optimize performance throughout the life span and across contexts and allow children and adolescents to assume or regain valued life roles, bridging the gap between what children *want* to do and what they *can* do to participate in activities that

### CASE EXAMPLE 34.1 SARI

Sari is an 8-month-old infant who is recovering from cardiac surgery. Sari has poor endurance and limited upper extremity strength. The occupational therapist showed Sari's parents how to place her in a semireclined position using a small wedge. This positioned Sari with her arms forward so that she could reach for objects more easily. Sari was not able to hold a typical rattle since it was too heavy for her. The occupational therapist found a lightweight rattle that Sari was able to hold and shake. Additionally, a 3D printed universal cuff was made to assist with her grasp, so that she could engage and hold it without having to maintain a tight whole-hand grasp. Sari's parents were encouraged when they observed her engage in typical infant behaviors. These simple adaptations allowed Sari to engage in play and begin to develop endurance and strength as is needed after cardiac surgery. This is an example of using assistive technology (positioning device, adapted rattle, and 3D printed cuff) in occupational therapy intervention.

## CASE EXAMPLE 34.2 JEREMY

Jeremy is a 2-year-old boy with Down syndrome. His family wants to provide every opportunity for him to develop cognitive skills. They plan for him to attend general education classrooms as he gets older. They were recently at a conference and heard about tablet technologies as tools for supporting learning and educational performance for some children with Down syndrome. They asked the early intervention team to recommend a tablet and apps to use with Jeremy.

- Would you recommend a tablet for 2-year-old Jeremy? If so, what criterion would you use to determine which apps to recommend?

### Assistive Technology (AT) Recommendations

The team used the SETT framework (Fig. 34.1) to guide the team in determining what technology might best work with Jeremy. They evaluated Jeremy's cognitive, motor, perceptual, and sensory abilities to develop a sense of his strengths and challenges.

The team questioned if he needed a tablet to support learning and educational performance, or if it might enhance his occupational performance. While tablet technologies are appealing to all children, offering a multisensory experience, it is important to match the features of the tablet and any app selected to the needs of the individual. Choosing an app that is "good for children with Down syndrome" may not be the best approach.

Since Jeremy's parents sought information from the team about use of a tablet, they may be more likely to follow through on use of the tablet and any recommended apps. Depending on Jeremy's needs, interests, and abilities, other tools and strategies could be used in addition to or instead of a tablet. Finding a balance between time spent using the tablet versus other developmentally appropriate experiences is important for Jeremey's overall health and well-being. The team decided to begin by introducing some apps to improve Jeremey's communication and picture identification during intervention sessions on a trial basis. This would allow the team to better determine Jeremy's learning needs before recommending the family purchase a tablet.

are meaningful. AT can serve a variety of needs and can be part of the educational, habilitative, and/or rehabilitative process.

AT service is comprehensive and includes (1) evaluating needs and current abilities for AT; (2) acquiring AT; (3) selecting, designing, repairing, and fabricating AT; (4) collaborating and coordinating services with other therapies; and (5) training both individuals with disabilities and those working with them to use the technologies effectively (AT Act, 2004). In Case Example 34.2, the occupational therapy practitioner provided AT services in the form of assessing the need for AT intervention, acquiring AT, and training Jeremy's parents how to use the AT so he could engage in typical childhood occupations.

AT assessment and intervention occur in many practice settings (see Table 34.1), but one of the most common is the public school. According to statistics published by the National Center for Education Statistics (2022), an estimated 7.2 million, or 15% of all children and youth ages 3–21 receive special education services. The Individuals with Disabilities Education Improvement Act (IDEA, 2004; PL 108–446) views AT services as a means of providing a free and appropriate public education. IDEA 2004 requires that Individualized Education Program (IEP) and Individualized Family Service Plan (IFSP) teams consider a child's need for AT devices and services at least annually during the development of the IEP or IFSP. If it is determined during the required yearly consideration that AT is necessary for the student to receive a free and appropriate education in the least restrictive environment, the school district is responsible for providing it.

AT devices and services can help a student improve, increase, maintain, or substitute performance of functional skills (e.g., self-help, mobility, or communication) to access curriculum (e.g., multimedia) and become a more efficient learner (e.g., pencil grips and raised lined paper to improve writing legibility) or compensate for lack of skills (e.g., word prediction software to assist with spelling or reduce keystrokes) (O'Brien et al., 2016; Watson et al., 2010). In more recent times, children have utilized AT to participate in online and virtual classrooms, which enables them to successfully complete their academic tasks.

**TABLE 34.1 Assistive Technology Service provided to Children and Youth in a Variety of Practice Settings**

| Practice Setting | Assistive Technology (AT) Services |
|---|---|
| Hospital or medical center | Primary role is evaluation that is typically provided on an outpatient basis for a series of assessments (one to two visits); may require an inpatient stay of 2–3 weeks<br>Referrals and recommendations made directly to agencies or third-party payers<br>Limited access to child for follow-up and training; limited opportunities to consult with parents and teachers<br>May provide direct treatment, particularly for children under the age of 3 years or those who have an acquired disability (e.g., spinal cord injury) |
| Regional center | Developed in response to legislation, funded by the Department of Education or other agencies for individuals with disabilities<br>Often has AT lending library for borrowing equipment on a short-term basis<br>Team has broad-based experience with various diagnoses, resources for obtaining equipment, types of AT, and adapted methods of use<br>Also involved in advocacy, consumer awareness, and focus groups<br>Limited follow-up care and minimal input into training the child, family, and educational team |
| Public school | Most children receive AT services at a school<br>Daily problem-solving related to AT use can occur, and child receives support in the natural environment in which AT is to be used<br>School-based team has easy access to child and understands educational curriculum but may lack expertise or experience with more complex AT systems |
| Teletherapy/virtual setting | Provided via video conferencing technology that is HIPAA compliant, allowing both video and audio interaction<br>Allows intervention to happen in the child's natural environment<br>Provide in-the-moment support for child's routines<br>May have technology or internet issues that interrupt service |
| Home and community setting | May provide direct treatment, especially for children under the age of 3 years<br>Direct training available to child and family<br>Problem-solving related to AT use can occur, and child receives support in the natural environment in which AT is to be used<br>Can provide carryover to other practice settings such as school or work<br>May have limited opportunities to consult with others |

AT can also be instrumental in helping young children with disabilities learn valuable skills such as social skills (e.g., sharing and taking turns), communication skills, fine and gross motor skills, self-confidence, and independence (Budai & Neuland, 2015; Watson et al., 2010; Zachry & Mitchell, 2012). The use of AT can create novel opportunities for children to explore, interact, and function in their environments. Early access to tools that enable participation and completion of tasks helps to develop skills that are essential for life-long positive outcomes.

*Self-determination* refers to making one's own choices and decisions regarding one's actions and quality of life (D'Arrigo et al., 2017). Self-determination includes self-efficacy (one's belief in their ability to perform and expectation of success) and self-advocacy (one's ability to voice opinions and assert themselves). *Self-efficacy* includes personal beliefs about whether a behavior will lead to a specific consequence (being able to determine if one's goals are realistic) (Lee & Kielhofner, 2017). *Self-advocacy* refers to the ability to communicate, make decisions for oneself, and voice one's rights, particularly when those rights have been violated or diminished.

AT devices help children develop and practice self-determination behaviors by providing them with opportunities to accomplish tasks independently, or with less assistance (e.g., using a spoon with a built-up handle to self-feed, using word prediction to compose on a tablet, or using a communication system to express themselves). Successfully performing activities such as dressing "on their own" with the help of a tool (rather than a person) provides children with a sense of accomplishment and empowers them.

Children with disabilities may perceive that they have little control over outcomes within their environments, which can result in learned helplessness, especially if another person or group of persons provides services on their behalf (e.g., speaking for them or moving them without being directed by the child). Learned helplessness can become a secondary disability whereby children exhibit low self-determination leading to low volition to interact and perform daily activities. They may demonstrate a lack of initiation or curiosity, noncompliance, resistance, or an inability to problem solve or cope with events around them. Introducing AT early provides opportunities to complete daily activities more independently and learn that they have some control over the environment, leading to a positive sense of self-determination and self-efficacy (Dunst et al., 2013; Livingstone & Paleg, 2013).

**BOX 34.1 Factors That Affect Assistive Technology (AT) Delivery**

| Factor | Description of Considerations for AT Services |
|---|---|
| Social | • People interacting with child<br>• Environments in which the child spends time<br>• Communication skills and needs<br>• Style of expressing emotions<br>• Sources of social support<br>• Body language |
| Spiritual | • Sense of control over things that happen<br>• Beliefs about causality<br>• Typical or preferred coping strategies<br>• View of inner workings of body<br>• View of health and wellness<br>• Sense of one's purpose within family, community, and society |
| Cultural | • Degree of importance attributed to independence<br>• Values regarding health and wellness<br>• Use of time<br>• Sense of personal space<br>• Values regarding finances<br>• Importance of physical appearance<br>• Roles within family and society<br>• Adherence to traditions (family, culture, and history)<br>• Acceptable amount of assistance from others<br>• View of healthcare |
| Family | • Roles assumed by family members<br>• Balance of work and play<br>• Members (immediate, extended, and relatives)<br>• Makeup of family and where child fits in<br>• Family dynamics<br>• Support and resources<br>• Position within family |

From O'Rourke, P., Ekins, R., Timmins, B., Timmins, F., Long, S., & Coyle, E. (2013). Crucial design issues for special access technology: A Delphi study. *Disability and Rehabilitation: Assistive Technology.*

## ASSISTIVE TECHNOLOGY TO ENHANCE OCCUPATIONAL PARTICIPATION

Following the comprehensive occupational therapy evaluation or the more specialized AT assessment (see Chapter 9), one of the first steps in providing AT intervention is obtaining the recommended device(s). Occupational therapy practitioners and teams consider social, spiritual, cultural, and family circumstances when evaluating the child's assistive technology needs. Box 34.1 provides a description of some of the considerations that affect each factor. Occupational therapy practitioners may use a variety of frameworks to evaluate and design intervention using AT. Table 34.2 summarizes several of these frameworks, and Fig. 34.1 provides questions based on the SETT framework that practitioners consider when evaluating and creating intervention regarding AT use.

### Device Procurement and Funding

Occupational therapy practitioners working with children and youth requiring AT are often involved in helping procure the appropriate devices. They may provide the data and documentation for funding. Funding can come from various sources, including Medicaid, grants, private insurance, nonprofit agencies (such as United Cerebral Palsy), private foundations, schools, and individuals. In some states, funds to purchase AT devices are available through the Department of Developmental Disabilities, the Department of Health, or the Department of Social Services. The state's vocational rehabilitation agency may also assist with funding devices for students as they enter high school and transition to work and career sites. In addition, the team can consider alternative sources of funding, such as community service organizations, equipment loan programs, used and recycled equipment, and technical assistance programs. Occupational therapy practitioners may pursue creative funding options or reuse programs (such as the Pass It on Center National Assistive Technology Device Reutilization Coordination and Technical Assistance Center at https://pioc.gatech.edu/).

Funding of AT in school districts raises unique issues. IDEA provides funding that can be used for AT devices and to pay for the personnel that provide AT services. Federal law requires that districts ensure that AT devices and/or services are available to special education students who need them as part of their special education and/

**TABLE 34.2 Frameworks and Guides for AT Decision-Making**

| FRAMEWORKS AND GUIDES FOR ASSISTIVE TECHNOLOGY | | | |
|---|---|---|---|
| **HAAT (Human, Activity, Assistive Technology)** | **SETT (Student, Environments, Tasks, Tools)** | **MPT (Matching Person and Technology)** | **WATI (Wisconsin Assistive Technology Initiative)** |
| Dynamic and interactive model in which three factors (the human, activity, and AT) form a collective whole that is placed within the context of participation (Cook et al., 2020). Participation includes the physical context: the natural and built surroundings and physical parameters; the social context: relationships and interactions with others; the cultural context: child and family's beliefs, values, and customs; and the institutional context: broader social and cultural contexts that provide a legislative and moral behavioral framework. The human component includes physical, cognitive, and emotional elements of the person. Activities are divided broadly into daily living, work, and play and leisure. AT refers to a device and/or service provided as an extrinsic enabler (e.g., positioning supports, communication systems, academic and learning aids, environmental control units, and computer access technologies). | Developed for school settings to enable educational teams to use sound decision-making that promotes collaboration, communication, sharing of knowledge and perspectives, and flexibility. SETT encourages teams to discuss the student's needs and strengths, the environments in which the student is expected to perform, and the tasks they need to or want to accomplish. The goals of these discussions should be to determine student-centered, environmentally specific, and task-focused systems of tools to support the student's participation in curricular and extracurricular activities throughout the school day. SETT includes a series of questions designed to guide discussion, evaluation, and intervention. Teams may choose to use some or all questions, depending on the needs of the student. SETT documents can be found at https://www.joyzabala.com/links-resources. | Assessment process designed to match a person with the most appropriate AT (Institute for Matching Person and Technology, 2015). This process considers the milieu-environment and psychosocial in which the technology is being used (e.g., the technology may differ if the child is using a tablet in a busy classroom or at home in a quiet setting). The fit between the technology and the child's person factors—personality, temperament, and preferences—is examined, so the person can use technology without frustration. For example, a student may want to read from a paper-based document to "fit in with peers" even if they are more successful with text-to-speech on a tablet. Technology features and functions are considered to ensure the best fit between the person and technology. Learn more about the MPT at https://sites.google.com/view/matchingpersontechnology/menu/assessment-process. | Based on the SETT framework, the Wisconsin Assistive Technology Initiative (WATI) assessment package was designed to provide training and specific strategies to build the capacity for school districts to provide AT services. The assessment and consideration forms include forms for teams to document sensory, motor, and cognitive abilities and needs of the student; a checklist of environmental considerations; and a format to analyze the tasks that are difficult for the student (WATI, 2017). Teams use these forms to determine the technology intervention and needs, brainstorm solutions, and to prioritize and develop intervention plans. Find WATI materials at http://www.wati.org/. |

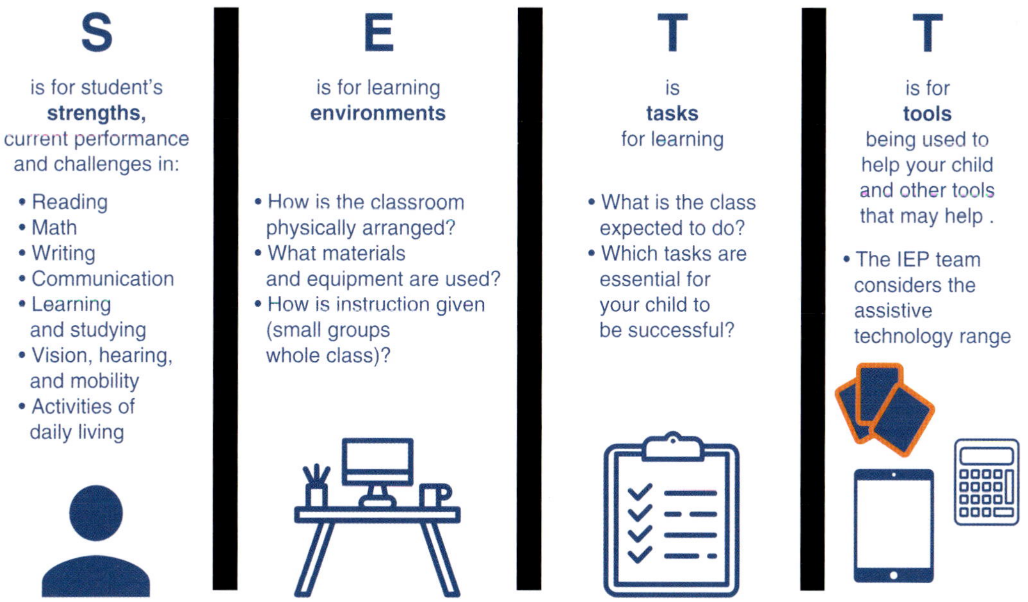


**Fig. 34.1** SETT framework. (Adapted from Hollingshead, A., Zabala, J., & Carson, J. (2021). SETT Framework and AT Evaluation. *Council for Exception Children.* https://exceptionalchildren.org/blog/sett-framework-and-evaluating-assistive-technology-remotely)

or related services or the supplemental aids and services used to assist students in being placed in the least restrictive environment (34 C.F.R. Sec. 300.105.).

Public or private insurance can be applied to obtain AT devices and services when they are determined to be medically necessary. The use of these funds must be voluntary on the part of the parents and with their written consent. School districts can also work with community service organizations or associations (e.g., the Muscular Dystrophy Association) to purchase AT devices. If the AT device is purchased with the parents' funds or insurance, then the device belongs to the child and family. However, if the school district purchases the device, the school district owns the device (ATIA Funding Guide, 2017).

## Implementing the Assistive Technology Plan

Once the AT system arrives, it may be up to the occupational therapy practitioner or team to put the system together, test the system, and begin training. Some companies provide representatives who help with the process, and others have videos that come with the system. Technology support may be available through help desks, discussion boards, and YouTube videos. The "service" aspect of AT includes training and assisting the child and family and/or school personnel and engaging in problem-solving to get the AT device working properly. This may require that practitioners use the device within their treatment sessions.

An AT implementation plan includes a description of the person(s) responsible, conditions of use, frequency of use, and duration of use. The plan considers the tasks and contexts in which the AT will be used. For example, if a student requires a voice output communication system, it should be readily available throughout their day (e.g., at lunch or recess to socialize, during instruction to ask or answer questions, during independent work to indicate needs and wants, and at home to interact with their family).

Time must be spent training and practicing within the child's natural environments (e.g., school, home, community) so that the family and other professionals integrate use of the device into the child's everyday activities. When AT is included in IEPs, school districts develop the goals describing the outcome (e.g., child will compose a paragraph of five or more sentences in three out of four opportunities) and list the AT (e.g., word prediction, voice dictation) under the accommodations. In this case, the goal states what the student will do and the accommodation states what the student requires to meet the goal. Periodic review of the plan helps avoid the potential discontinuance of recommended AT devices and services.

## Interprofessional Collaboration

Successful implementation of AT requires a cohesive and effective team with a shared vision. Interprofessional collaboration is linked to high-quality care and informs intervention plans (Cooper-Duffy & Eaker, 2017). Team member input is critical to making decisions regarding AT because devices are used across environments and address multiple performance goals that cross professional boundaries. The effectiveness of AT increases when staff work as a team and time is provided for them to communicate (Ogletree et al., 2017).

## Measuring Progress and Outcomes

Data collection is critical to measuring outcomes to evaluate the effectiveness of the selected AT, support its continued use, or justify the need for follow-up assessment. Data collection should be simple and straightforward, so whoever is collecting it (including family) understands and collects it with fidelity. Box 34.2 provides sample goals and associated outcome measurements that may be used in practice. The outcomes measured specify how the device is accessed and used. For example, when designing a data sheet for switch use, one considers which part of the body will be used to activate the switch, how much wait time will be allowed before a prompt is given, the type of prompt to be given (e.g., visual, verbal, touch), and what constitutes success for the given task (e.g., single switch activation, activation or deactivation of an electronic device, holding a switch for a specified amount of time). See Chapter 10 for information on outcomes data. Often data collected on targeted goals and objectives are dependent on the service settings in which the device is used. Possible factors to measure include changes in the child's performance or level of function, level of participation, how often the device is used and under what circumstances, overall consumer satisfaction, goal achievement, quality of life, and cost analysis/savings.

### BOX 34.2 Intervention Goals Embedding Assistive Technology (AT) and Associated Outcome Measurements

| Goals | Outcome Measurement |
|---|---|
| Given extended time and access to scheduling assistive technology, learner will complete assignments and turn in, with no more than two verbal cues from an adult, four out of five days per school week. | Teacher keeps records of homework completion as well as student checklist for daily homework completed by the learner. |
| Given access to language AAC device, learner will initiate a social conversation with a peer, with minimal verbal cues/encouragement, that lasts at least two to three exchanges, during centers or free play activities. | Therapist or staff observes during centers/free play activities and tracks information using a data sheet with back up data available from AAC device data collection. |
| Learner will open and close adaptive mealtime containers independently at breakfast and lunch daily, given fading verbal cues only. | Teacher or aide observes the child daily and notes if they can open and close adapted containers. They document any containers that are difficult to open, so therapists can modify or adapt. |
| Given computer access and word prediction software and task checklists, learner will complete writing assignments, including saving and submitting to their teacher, with verbal reminders, in three of four observed opportunities. | Therapist observes during writing activities and documents assistance needed and writing produced. Data from the document and use of word prediction can also be used to gauge progress. |

## Follow-Up Plan

Within private practice settings, once the child and family have a basic understanding of the AT system and use it independently, the child may be discharged from direct services. Discharge from a regular routine of intervention includes a follow-up plan. Follow-up can occur in several ways, from a telephone call to an extended clinic visit or simple review and analysis of data collected. The type of follow-up and when it should occur depends on the complexity of the system and the skills of the child, family, and other professionals working with the child. Effective service delivery includes a predetermined schedule for follow-up (e.g., at intervals of 6 months). Problems and delays in service can be prevented with planned periodic review. Within the school setting, a learner may transition to consultative services with ongoing follow-up and monitoring so that as the child's needs change, the tools can be updated or adjusted to continue to support the child. This could also include collaboration with private practitioners to support the student across environments.

### Assistive Technology Discontinuance or Abandonment

Despite the many promises of technology, one-third or more of individuals discontinue use of their AT devices when a device fails to live up to its promise of potential, freedom, and independence (Cook & Knue, 2010). The primary reason for abandonment is failure to consider the user's preferences, ideas, and desires (Cook & Knue, 2010). Abandonment often signifies a mismatch between the user and the device. Cruz et al. (2016) found that AT was not being used because of distrust in its benefits, aesthetic issues, need of more reliable devices, nonacceptance of disability, low-quality products, inadequate social support in the user's environment, architectural barriers, and inappropriate instruction and training for device acquisition.

The following barriers limit AT use in schools (Alharbi, 2016):

- lack of staff training and support
- negative staff attitudes
- inadequate assessment and planning processes
- insufficient funding
- difficulties with procuring and managing equipment
- time constraints

When service providers have insight into why technology is discontinued, they do a better job of updating, revising, and improving AT services for children and family members, which results in more consistent use of technology.

### Quality Assurance

In addition to measuring individual outcomes, teams conduct quality assurance studies to evaluate the services that they provide. The Quality Indicators for Assistive Technology (QIATs) (QIAT Consortium, 2015) are used in school settings to support the development and delivery of AT services. Use of these indicators as guidelines supports outcomes for the child, the family, the classroom, and the educational setting.

### Transition Planning

As children with disabilities transition from preschool to elementary school to high school, and into early adulthood, they may need assistance transitioning and accessing technology to participate in each of these new environments. Critical information, as well as competencies, can be lost if positioning, teaching methodologies, and information regarding specialized technology are not passed along from one stage and setting to the next. **Transition plans** address the AT needs of the user, including roles and training needs of team members, subsequent steps in AT use, and follow-up after transition takes place (QIAT, 2015). Box 34.3 lists the responsibilities for effective transition plans.

**BOX 34.3 Responsibilities of Effective Transition Plans for Assistive Technology (AT) Users**

- Address the AT needs of the student, including roles and training needs of team members, subsequent steps in AT use, and follow-up after transition takes place.
- Empower the student using AT to participate in the transition planning at a level appropriate to age and ability.
- Recognize advocacy, as related to AT use, as critical to the plan's success.
- Identify the AT requirements in the receiving environment.
- Proceed according to an individualized timeline.
- Address specific equipment, training, and funding issues such as transfer or acquisition of AT, manuals, and support documents.

From Quality Indicators for Assistive Technology (QIAT) Consortium. (2015). Guiding the provision of quality assistive technology services. https://www.qiat.org/indicators.html

## IMPORTANT FUNCTIONS AND OUTCOMES OF APPROPRIATE ASSISTIVE TECHNOLOGY

AT plays an essential role in providing children and youth access to meaningful occupations, positioning for comfort and occupational engagement, and support for life skills such as communication with others, leading to positive quality of life. AT allows children and youth to engage in a variety of occupations within their home, school, and community.

### AT Provides Greater Access

AT can be used by children and youth to provide them physical access to schools, homes, and community buildings. For example, curb cuts, ramps, railings, and door openers allow children with disabilities to navigate inside and outside of buildings safely. Technology may include labeling key areas with pictures, text, and braille. Children and youth of varying sizes or those who use wheelchairs may require accommodations to access restrooms, water fountains, or elevators.

Occupational therapy practitioners may arrange resources or modify the environment for **accessibility** (i.e., means of entering a place or engaging in event) and participation. They may modify environments or provide children with alternative ways to engage. Practitioners also advocate for access to spaces and environments for all children and youth. They may create spaces that include children and youth with and without disabilities. For example, seating and playground modifications can enhance safe mobility and participation in recreational activities (Miller et al., 2017; Moore & Lynch, 2015; Soltani et al., 2012). Occupational therapy practitioners may also be involved in adapting parks, ballparks, water sports, and skiing so that children and youth with disabilities may participate. Bus modifications for entry and exit and safe seating can help with transportation to and from school or community and school-related activities including field trips, sports, and recreation activities (see Chapter 17). Providing children and youth access to events, community, and buildings promotes social participation and allows children to engage in meaningful occupations.

#### Using Computers, Tablets, and Phones for Greater Access.

Children and youth use personal computers, tablets, and phones at school, home, social, and work settings. These are flexible, motivating, and powerful instructional tools that facilitate individualized teaching and learning. Computers with or without specialized software provide multiple means of communicating, playing, exploring,

## CASE EXAMPLE 34.3 LINNEA

Linnea is a third-grade student with spinal muscular atrophy. She is fully included in her neighborhood school with support from related services as needed. Recently, she complained to her parents and therapists that her hand gets tired when writing and that her handwriting looks "sloppy." Her teacher also noticed that Linnea is irritable and lacks concentration during class. Linnea, her family, and therapists discussed using computers for written communication in the past, but Linnea and her family were reluctant to explore this because she did not want to "look different." Linnea had experience with computers since kindergarten. Her class goes to the computer lab three times a week, and she learned basic keyboarding skills in second grade. Her classroom has two desktop computers, two Chromebooks, and four tablets that students use for drills, practice, and special projects.

1. How would you address written language requirements in the context of Linnea's classroom using a UDL approach?
2. Would you come to a different conclusion if Linnea was in high school?
3. What environmental factors might you consider?

### Assistive Technology (AT) Recommendations

Linnea's situation challenges the occupational therapy practitioner to collaborate as a part of the educational team to come up with several solutions to address her challenges in writing:

- Provide modeling and whole classroom instruction on use of the current technology in the classroom so that all students are familiar with use of the desktop computers, Chrome books, and tablets as options for completing written language assignments.
- Explore word prediction software to cut down on keystrokes, reduce fatigue, and support spelling.
- Determine alternatives to written language expression to convey information such as photography, PowerPoint presentations, voice recording, or art.

### Response to Questions

1. The occupational therapist and teacher created a rotation system in the classroom so that the tools were readily available to all children for use during language arts so that Linnea did not "look different" than her peers. While voice typing (speech recognition) is a potential alternative, it is important to assess Linnea's voice volume and intelligibility, her ability to organize and verbalize her thoughts, her understanding of punctuation, and her ability to navigate and edit a dictated document.
2. If Linnea were in high school, voice typing would likely be more commonplace, as many students use personal devices, including their phones, throughout the school day to dictate texts, record assignments, and so on, and her concern for "looking different" might be lessened. Linnea's ability to organize and verbalize her thoughts, her understanding of punctuation, and her ability to navigate and edit a dictated document would also be more skilled than that of a third grader.
3. Environmental factors might include whether Linnea needs to leave the classroom to successfully use voice dictation. Depending on the device used, accuracy of voice dictation can be impacted by ambient noise or other voices within the classroom.

self-expression, interacting with the environment, learning cause and effect, and completing school- and work-related tasks. Most children have some exposure to a computer system, tablet, or phone by the time they enter school. At home, digital devices might be used for recreation, entertainment, communication, work, and study. Social connections with others can be formed through email, instant messaging, and social networking sites (Schultz, 2013).

Digital devices may motivate children to learn and develop a large repertoire of skills and they allow practice and repetition (see Case Example 34.3). They provide simulations that some cannot otherwise

**TABLE 34.3 Benefits of Computers and Tablets**

| Benefit | Examples |
|---|---|
| Allows child to be in control | Use child-directed software<br>Allow child to move at his or her own pace<br>Accessible to children with limited motor control<br>Use two-switch step scanning for simple cognitive interface |
| Engages the child cognitively | Use two-switch software whereby each switch has a distinct function<br>Provide trial-and-error learning<br>Provide logical consequences to the child's efforts<br>Use of patterns and use of surprise<br>Provide experiences with familiar objects and tasks<br>Allow for active versus passive learning |
| Provides opportunities for choice making | Sustain attention: increase opportunity for control and cognitive engagement<br>Further expand awareness of consequences<br>Provide error-free learning environment |
| Provides language immersion | Provide voice-output feedback describing child's actions<br>Use simple but functional language<br>Provide opportunities for sound play<br>Offer predictable repeated lines with periodic surprise lines to go along with the action<br>Relate three-dimensional experiences with objects and toys to two-dimensional screen |
| Provides opportunities for joint attention and shared interaction | Give opportunity for adult-child interaction<br>Encourage pointing, showing, and shared enjoyment<br>Provide opportunity for the child to take the lead and the adult to follow along and support<br>Provide opportunities for child-child interaction |
| Facilitates communicative interaction | Allow the child to express ideas<br>Provide voice-output and visual information that may be used to communicate to someone else |
| Provides multisensory feedback with consistency and repetition of language and cognitive concepts | Allow virtual manipulation of objects to develop cognitive skills<br>Provide immediate feedback to child<br>Allow child to control repetition as desired<br>Reinforce emerging literacy skills<br>Reinforce emerging mathematical skills or sequence, numbers, and patterns within a play context (not adult directed) |
| Ensures cognitive simplicity | Present concepts in small steps<br>Help child maintain attention by providing immediate success<br>Help child stay out of a random "guessing mode" or "trying to please mode," which could lead to inaccurate or confusing consequences |

From United States Department of Education & United States Department of Health and Human Services. (2016). *Early learning and educational technology brief.* https://tech.ed.gov/earlylearning/

experience and are part of mainstream technology, removing the social stigma of looking "different." A variety of customizable software and devices are available to support a user's needs. Table 34.3 outlines the benefits of computer use for children.

***Digital Devices in the Educational Setting.*** At school, children typically use word processing programs, the internet, e-mail, and virtual classrooms in aspects of their education. Software programs, websites, and apps cover most academic subjects as well as recreational and competitive activities. The multimedia features of digital devices can support learning rules, turn-taking, and social skills. Math software, apps, and websites include features such as virtual manipulatives or drills; creative writing software has recording features, sound, graphics, and animations; and keyboarding software teaches typing. Software and website designers continue to add features that make their products and sites accessible for a range of abilities.

Digital devices and software can help develop literacy or strengthen skills through games, screen readers, and online books. "Virtual field trips" make it possible to visit and explore environments that might otherwise be inaccessible. Multimedia simulations can provide preparation for social situations, academic tasks, prevocational training, and driver education. For children who are unable to recognize print in traditional formats, modifications to access the same text as that for their peers can decrease their dependence on the support of others in the environment to read or write for them.

Children who find it challenging to produce art products or written work, because of motor, emotional, or attention difficulties, can generate digital artwork or text that is neat and uniform in appearance. Producing accurate, legible, or attractive work may increase self-esteem and self-expression and decrease frustration. As with any tool, the child must be aware of its features and trained in its applications and maintenance to receive full benefits.

Various types of devices (e.g., Macs, Chromebooks, tablets, phones, or personal computers [PCs]) are available in home, school, clinic, and work settings. Before recommending the purchase of software programs or adapted devices for access, the memory and technology of the system must be evaluated to determine its compatibility with the program. Many software programs are both PC and Mac compatible. Occupational therapy practitioners should possess the ability to operate the major computing systems used in public schools, troubleshoot system problems, establish networks using telecommunications systems, operate general application programs, apply teacher utility tools, and provide computer-based instruction.

iPads and Android tablets offer a lightweight, portable, versatile, and socially acceptable solution for many children and adolescents. They have a relatively long battery life, are affordable, connect to the internet, can take pictures, display multimedia, and support apps to meet academic and social needs. The touch screen allows younger students or those who do not have the motor skills to use a typical computer, keyboard, or mouse.

iPads and Android tablets have built-in accessibility features to support vision, hearing, motor skills, learning, and literacy differences. On the iOS platform, these include Assistive Touch, Switch Control, Touch Accommodations, Support for third-party keyboards, and Siri. Accessibility settings that allow users to increase the size of the default font, use zoom mode to view the screen, use speech-to-text features, and see subtitles and captioning. On iOS, the Assistive Touch setting allows custom gestures to be created and normal gestures to be executed through a menu system displayed on the screen. Bluetooth extends the potential for adding external devices such as accessible keyboards, switches, and joysticks.

***Software and Apps.*** Careful decisions must be made to find programs and apps that match a child's interests and skills. Software programs or apps may require that the user make specific, discrete responses to visual, auditory, or tactile stimuli. Programs and operating systems can be adjusted in terms of sound, touch sensitivity, visual display, and response time. The user must be able to attend briefly and have the interest and motivation to engage in the activity. Computer activities and programs, including public domain software, online activities, and apps, can be used to teach basic skills, such as object permanence, sustained attention, cause-and-effect relationships, discrimination, matching, and directionality. The occupational therapy practitioner decides how to customize the video and audio display to meet the students' unique needs. A large variety of software, online activities, and apps are available to promote children's functional independence in life roles.

**Switches as Access Method.** For children with complex neurological diagnoses, switches are often the earliest introduced AT devices. Switches are alternative "buttons" accessed via some form of physical response, and once activated, they send a command or series of keystrokes to the device that they are connected to. Control of the environment via switches can promote independence, which may become a foundational skill for future AT systems. Simple devices that provide sensory input (e.g., fans, vibrators, music, lights) can engage, alert, and motivate. For all switches, it is important to ensure that it is clear to the user what will occur when the switch is activated. This can be accomplished through placing an object or picture icon on the switch.

Often toys or short recorded messages are controlled through a single switch, typically a touch switch that requires a press and release (Fig. 34.2A and B). However, some children may not have the physical skills to press or pull against resistance and may use a switch that is activated through light touch, movement in the proximity of the switch, vocalization, sip or puff, or eye blink. Fig. 34.3A and B use light touch or a pull switch to activate. Switches can be mounted so that the position can be easily adjusted to improve access. Switches can also be plugged into an environmental control unit (ECU). Environmental control units extend the use of a switch to include turning appliances plugged into the ECU on and off. Switches are considered an access tool, connecting users with other actions. In addition to toys and appliances, there are many resources available online that can be activated with switches to motivate and teach. Burkhart (2018) shares a switch progression plan that can be referred to when designing interventions in this area.

***Switch Use with Computers and Tablets.*** Switches can be used to access a computer, camera, or a tablet. Once a switch is chosen, interfacing it with a device allows the user to control multiple settings. Positioning the switch and device may require the use of mounts to put each in the optimal position for access, as illustrated in Fig. 34.4. More complex switch systems use indirect selection, such as scanning, which requires several steps. Occupational and physical therapists collaborate to develop appropriate positioning to enable efficient movement for engagement in daily activities.

When deciding on a switch-driven system, the team considers both motor and cognitive requirements. The placement of the switch (e.g., a head switch versus a switch that is activated by another body part) may change the cognitive requirements and affect a child's accuracy. A single (or dual) switch can be used to run systems such as scanning (Burkhart, 2018). For some learners, using two switches can be most effective. If one- or two-switch scanning is not effective and efficient due to the child's motor coordination issues, other options such as eye gaze control and voice command control can be considered.

## Positioning

**Positioning** includes physical positioning for comfort, function, and work; location of the child within the environment; and location of supports in relationship to the child. Seating, positioning, and mobility

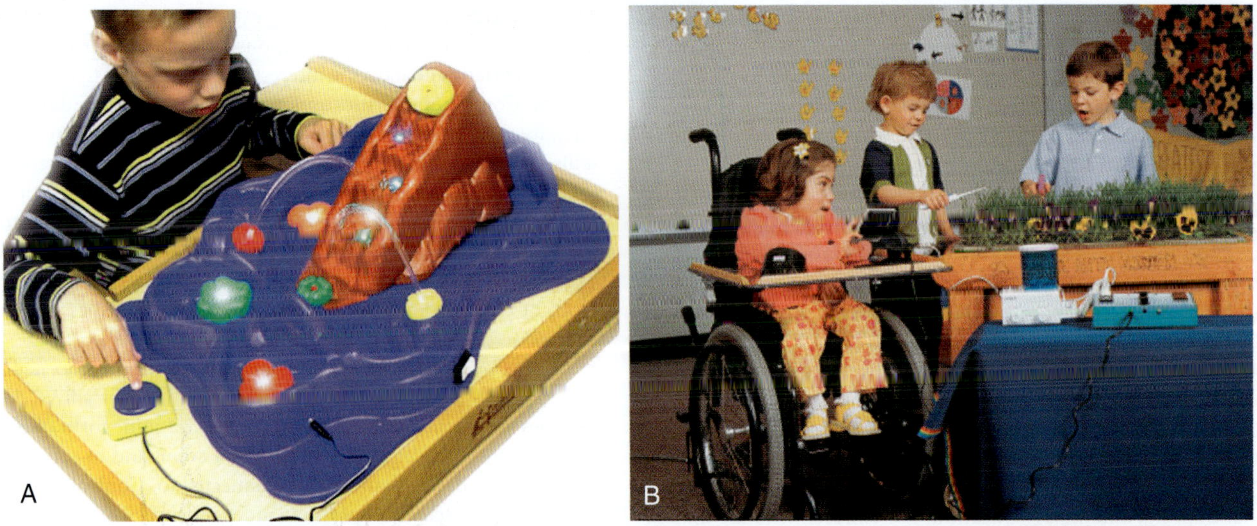

**Fig. 34.2** (A) The child uses the switch to play with the water toy. (B) The child uses the switch to participate in a gardening activity with peers. ((A) Photo courtesy Ablenet; (B) Photo courtesy Enabling Devices.)

devices are often the foundation for successful use of AT, and they may be used to improve body stability, provide proximal trunk and head support, and allow for exploration of the environment (see Chapter 32).

Ergonomics refers to designing and arranging things so that people interact with them efficiently and safely (Ergonomics, n.d.). Spending hours at a time in front of a variety of screens (e.g., computers, tablets, phones, televisions) puts everyone at high risk for wrist, neck, and back problems. If children, or those advocating on their behalf, learn at an early age how to adjust a workstation, they may make similar adjustments later in life. These habits and skills can be established as early as preschool years. Fig. 34.5 outlines reminders for practitioners when considering ergonomics and positioning.

Positioning should never be static in nature (refer to Chapter 32). Since standard furniture may not be adjustable to fit everyone comfortably, customized seating and positioning ranging from low-tech adaptations to specifically purchased items allow users to work in neutral, relaxed positions that consider energy conservation and maximize productivity while protecting health and minimizing the risk of injury (Fig. 34.6A and B).

## Supporting Life Skills

There is a continuum of AT options to address life skills such as communication, mobility self-help, play and leisure, academics, and work. These include adapted tools for feeding (i.e., built-up utensils, cut-out cups, suctioned bowls), dressing (i.e., buttonhooks, reachers, adapted clothing), bathing (i.e., bath seats, bath mitts with soap, shower chairs), toileting (i.e., potty seats, diapers, pull-ups), interacting with musical instruments, art activities, and sports and recreation (i.e., Velcro baseball mitt, adapted skis, skating walkers, adapted paint brush, slanted easels). Some modifications to assist with viewing, understanding, holding, and manipulating materials can be created from everyday materials as illustrated in Fig. 34.7A–C while more complex ones can be purchased (Schoonover & Schwind, 2017).

## Improving Communication

The purpose of communication is to express wants and needs, exchange, and share. The Committee for the Communication Needs of Persons with Severe Disabilities (NJC) created the Communication Bill of Rights, which describes basic communication rights that should be afforded to all persons (see https://www.asha.org/njc/communication-bill-of-rights/). Children with disabilities may present with a range of difficulties related to receptive and expressive language. **Alternative and augmentative communication (AAC)** is voice output and communication support, often aided by technology, that should be used in addition to vocal speech, or in place of it if it is not available due to medical diagnoses. An AAC system uses a combination of all the methods of communication available to a child. This can include residual speech, vocalizations, gestures, and communicative behaviors. Children and youth with complex communication needs who do not gain successful access to AAC are at high risk for abuse, crime, unemployment, and limited social networks (RERC, 2019). Chris Klein, an adult AAC user shares that, "the goal of AAC should be to say anything that you want to say. It isn't about telling a person what you need and/or want. It's about becoming an effective communicator, so you can build relationships." (Klein, 2017). Occupational therapy professionals play a key role in enabling this critical relationship building, through therapy interventions.

AAC supports the development of language and emerging literacy skills, enhances participation in educational settings, facilitates friendships, and supports interactions with family members and people in the greater community (Cook et al., 2020). Some families may be hesitant to start using AAC, because they think it will interfere with their child's speech development. However, researchers report that early use of AAC enhances language and communication (Smith et al., 2016). Since communication impacts the entire family, a family-centered approach is required to make certain AAC is part of the child and family's daily experience. Box 34.4 provides strategies to facilitate communication with children.

Members of the team bring different levels of expertise to share; for example, child, siblings, and parents understand the child's daily communication needs and routines; teachers understand literacy and instruction; speech-language pathologists are experts in language development; and occupational and physical therapists provide services related to positioning, accessing, and physically using the AAC system. For these reasons, it is imperative to use a collaborative team approach when evaluating, designing, and implementing AAC systems.

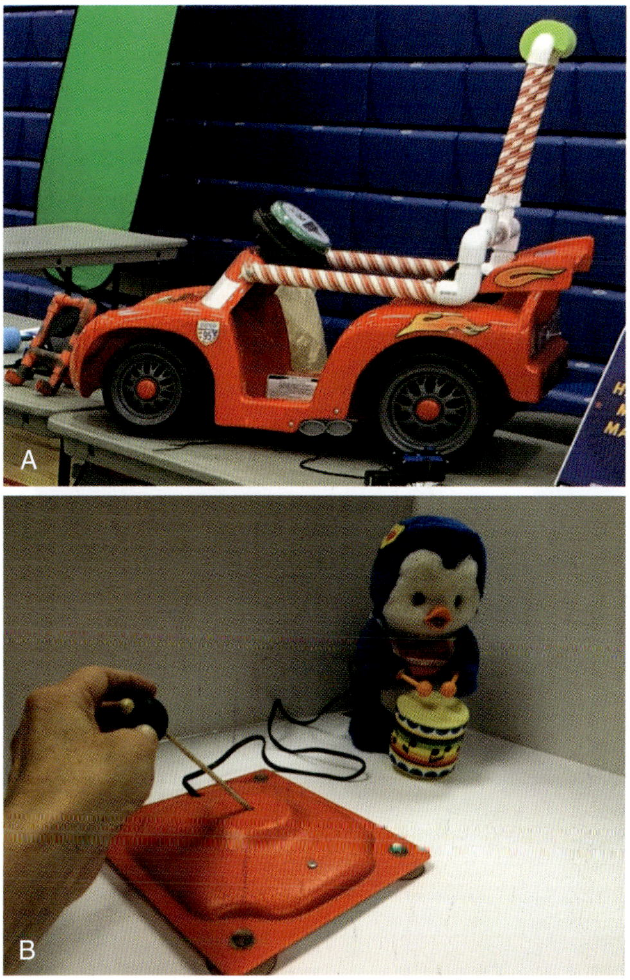

Fig. 34.3 (A) An example of a light touch switch used to activate an adapted battery-operated ride-on car. (B) An example of a pull switch that activates the toy. (Photos courtesy Judith Schoonover and Elisa Wern.)

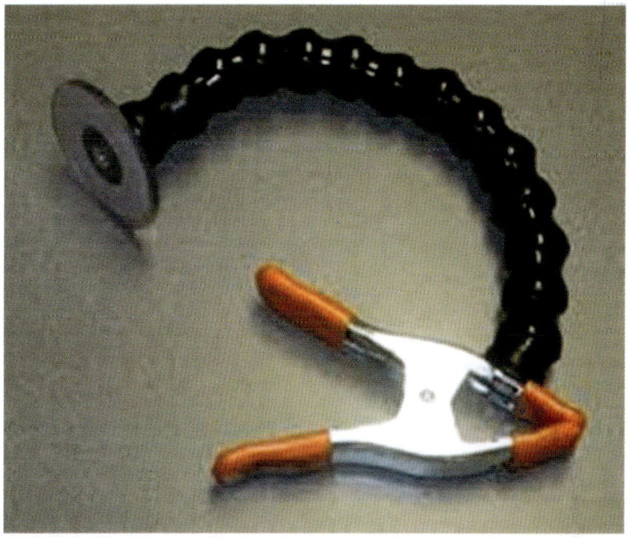

Fig. 34.4 This adjustable mount allows practitioners to position switches so that children can easily access them. (Photo courtesy Elisa Wern.)

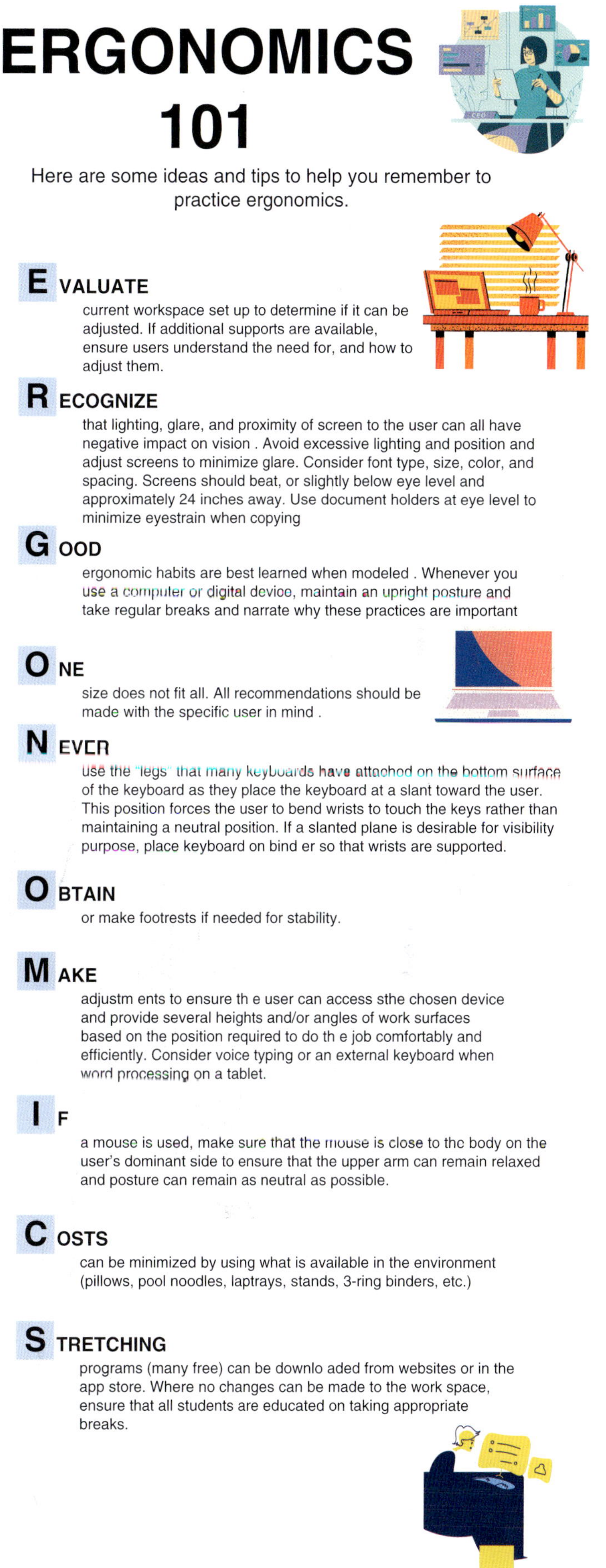

# ERGONOMICS 101

Here are some ideas and tips to help you remember to practice ergonomics.

**E VALUATE**
current workspace set up to determine if it can be adjusted. If additional supports are available, ensure users understand the need for, and how to adjust them.

**R ECOGNIZE**
that lighting, glare, and proximity of screen to the user can all have negative impact on vision . Avoid excessive lighting and position and adjust screens to minimize glare. Consider font type, size, color, and spacing. Screens should beat, or slightly below eye level and approximately 24 inches away. Use document holders at eye level to minimize eyestrain when copying

**G OOD**
ergonomic habits are best learned when modeled . Whenever you use a computer or digital device, maintain an upright posture and take regular breaks and narrate why these practices are important

**O NE**
size does not fit all. All recommendations should be made with the specific user in mind .

**N EVER**
use the "legs" that many keyboards have attached on the bottom surface of the keyboard as they place the keyboard at a slant toward the user. This position forces the user to bend wrists to touch the keys rather than maintaining a neutral position. If a slanted plane is desirable for visibility purpose, place keyboard on bind er so that wrists are supported.

**O BTAIN**
or make footrests if needed for stability.

**M AKE**
adjustm ents to ensure th e user can access sthe chosen device and provide several heights and/or angles of work surfaces based on the position required to do th e job comfortably and efficiently. Consider voice typing or an external keyboard when word processing on a tablet.

**I F**
a mouse is used, make sure that the mouse is close to the body on the user's dominant side to ensure that the upper arm can remain relaxed and posture can remain as neutral as possible.

**C OSTS**
can be minimized by using what is available in the environment (pillows, pool noodles, laptrays, stands, 3-ring binders, etc.)

**S TRETCHING**
programs (many free) can be downlo aded from websites or in the app store. Where no changes can be made to the work space, ensure that all students are educated on taking appropriate breaks.

Fig. 34.5 Ergonomics considerations for therapists. (Reproduced from Schoonover, J., & Wern, E. (October 2020). *Working comfortably in the digital age: Ergonomics for educators*. New Jersey AT Summit.)

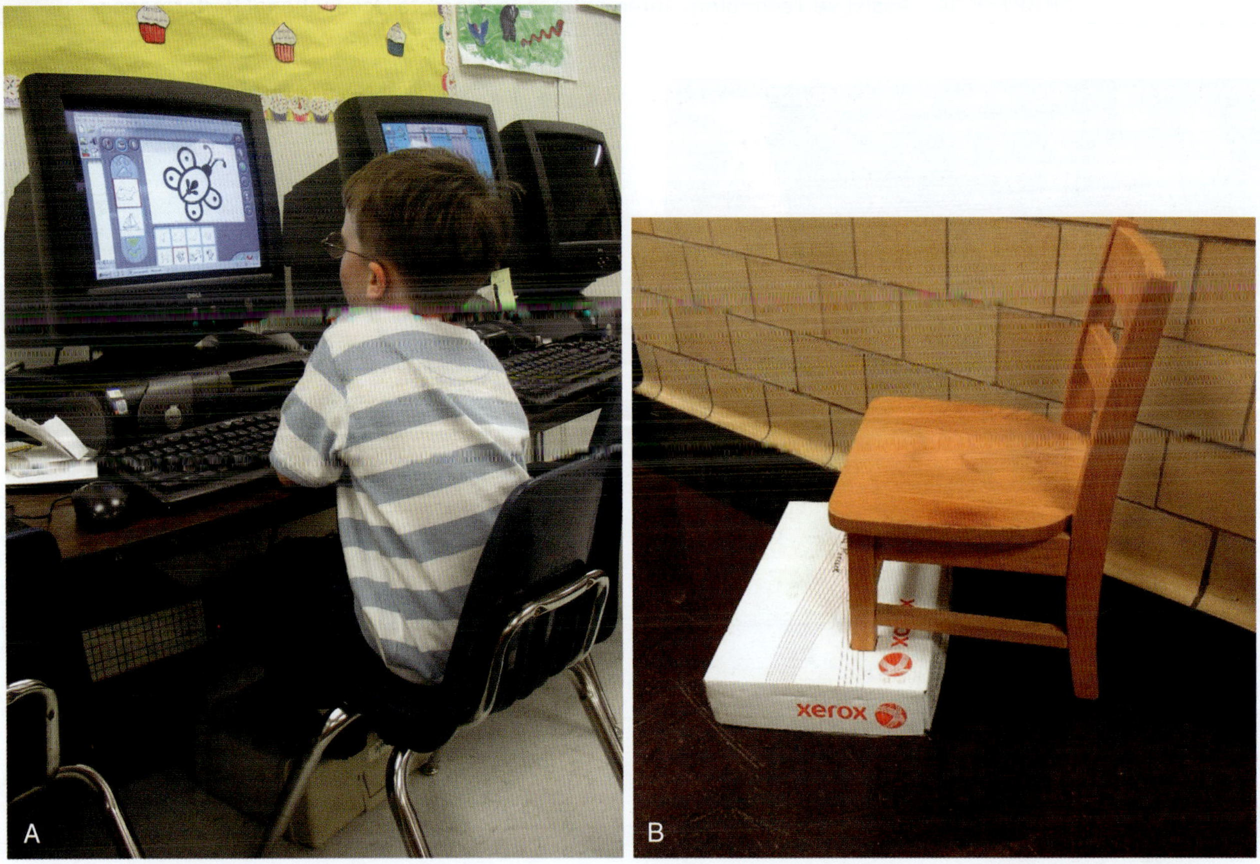


**Fig. 34.6** (A) One size does not fit all. It is important to adjust learning environments to promote health and productivity. (B) Adaptations can be made with items available in the environment or through the purchase of specific positioning equipment. (Photos courtesy Judith Schoonover.)

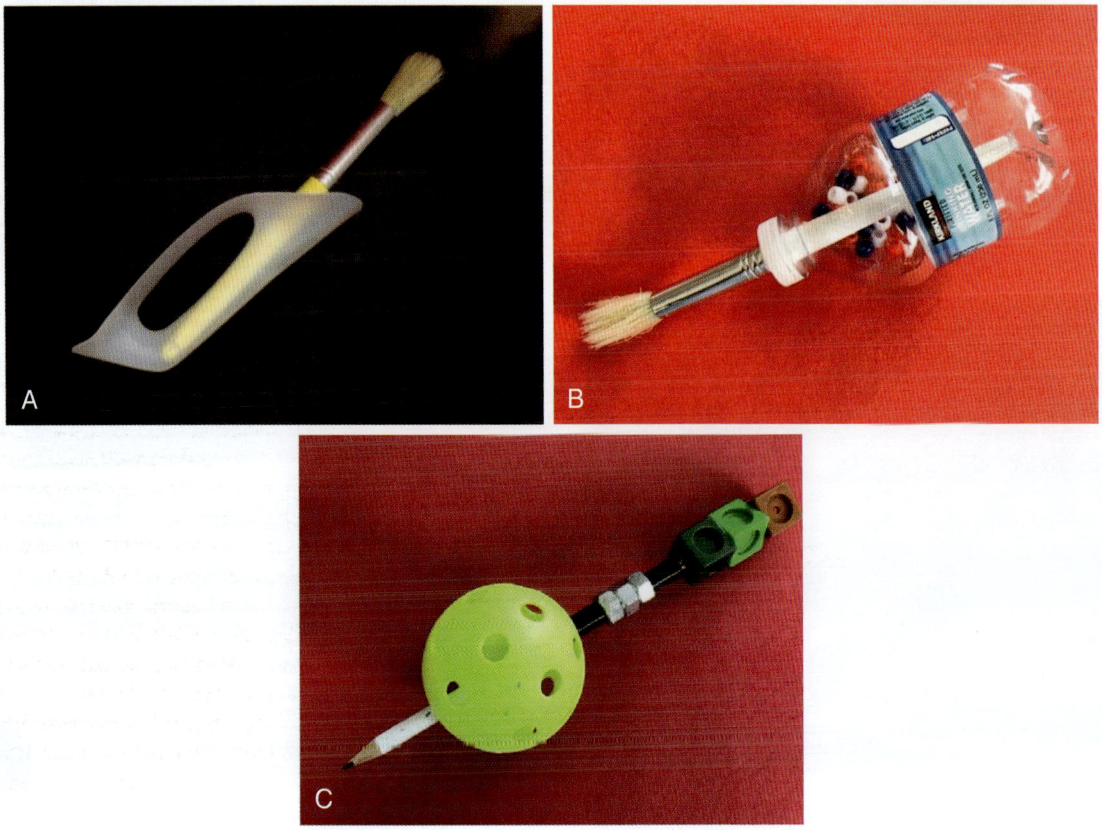


**Fig. 34.7** Simple art tools created from easily found materials to provide access to art activities. (A) Milk jug handle. (B) "Noisy" with easy to grasp water bottle handle. (C) Hex-nut-weighted pencil with a wiffle ball handle and fidgets on the end. (Photos courtesy Judith Schoonover.)

## BOX 34.4 Strategies to Facilitate Communication

1. Structure the environment to foster interaction.
   - Create a comfortable environment and child-friendly setting.
   - Limit distractions.
2. Attend to the child. Develop a therapeutic relationship.
   - Sit at eye level with the child.
   - Make eye contact.
   - Show interest in the child and his/her activities.
3. Provide meaningful opportunities for communication.
   - Develop rapport with child.
   - Find out the child's interests.
   - Engage the child in fun activities.
4. Have realistic expectations for the child.
   - Introduce yourself and let the child know the purpose of interaction.
   - Allow the child to ask questions.
   - Keep directions simple and allow for processing time.
5. Provide appropriate language input.
   - Speak at the child's level, paying attention to the child's age and interests.
   - Get the child's attention before speaking.
   - Keep directions short.
   - Allow the child to respond.
6. Avoid yes/no questions and "test" questions.
   - Ask open-ended questions.
   - Follow the child's lead.
   - Allow the conversation to flow.
   - Respond to the child's comments and questions.
7. Pace the interaction. Give the student time to communicate. WAIT.
   - Allow for time for the child to respond.
   - Listen carefully to the child's responses and acknowledge that you heard them.
8. Follow the child's lead. Respond to a child's attempts to communicate.
   - You might want to see how the family is communicating with the child for tips on how to read the child's communication.
   - Clarify if you do not understand, and be very patient.
   - Allow the child to make some decisions.
   - Collaborate with family.
9. Provide models for the child's expressive modes of communication. Coach the child as needed.
   - Smile or laugh to express pleasure; look at the child directly when listening; nod to let the child know you are listening and understand.
   - Patiently ask the child to repeat answers or allow for another mode of response if things are not clear.
   - Use hand gestures and facial expressions to communicate more clearly.
10. Prompt if necessary. Remember to fade out prompts to natural cues. Enjoy communication.
    - Ask simple open-ended questions.
    - Provide prompts with pictures or objects if needed.
    - Provide child with options (such as lists) but fade out over time.
    - Provide a child with opportunities to express emotions (even if the child only points to pictures showing how he/she feels). Provide time to process a child's feelings.
11. Engage family in the evaluation and intervention session early and often
    - Ask the family to show you how they communicate and engage the child.
    - Use cues from family's styles regarding what works well.
    - Allow family to try out new things.
    - Act as a coach to enable family to succeed.
    - When things are difficult, step in and support family and child.
    - Collaborate with family and child throughout the session.
    - Problem solve with family and child.
    - Ask how strategies or technology worked and listen to responses.
    - Be honest with the family and child.
    - Follow-up and seek out resources.

**Types of Alternative and Augmentative Communication Devices.** Children may use a combination of aided and unaided communication and low- and high-tech devices. Fig. 34.8 provides a depiction of how AAC may be organized. Picture-based systems are used increasingly with children with complex communication needs. They come in a variety of styles and devices as illustrated in Fig. 34.9A–E. It is important that all team members approach communication from the perspective that there are no prerequisites for communication. As stated by Mirenda (1993):

"… breathing is the only prerequisite that is relevant to communication. Breathing equals life, and life equals communication. It is that simple. We realize that everyone can communicate, and, in fact, everyone does communicate in some way, somehow, if there is something important to say. In other words, communication is neither a right nor something that has to be learned—it is an inevitability: people cannot not communicate."

The Picture Exchange Communication System (PECS) is a formalized approach of AAC that may be used with individuals with a variety of communicative, cognitive, and physical difficulties, including preschoolers, adolescents, and adults who have little or no verbal ability. Practitioners follow the process outlined in the approach (i.e., fidelity) and use PECS to enable growth of communicative intent. Current research supports providing access to core vocabulary over single fringe words.

Visual representation such as objects, photographs, realistic drawings, line drawings, and written words can be used to increase understanding, communication, and social connectedness and can take many forms depending on the environment and the circumstances under which they are used. Visual supports can be a part of a designed AAC system, but they are not a communication system alone. They help to guide a communicator in knowing what expectations are present, what to expect in a routine or schedule, and how many parts of a task remain. Visual support can also be used during reading and writing activities and may help students with disabilities complete tasks more independently (Cohen & Demchak, 2018).

Tangible symbols, pictures, or true objects are often used to support expressive language with communicators that have a visual diagnosis. Using objects with meaning to the communicator can assist in requesting assistance, expressing preferences, and answering questions. For example, a piece of chain can represent a swing on the playground, and a user can access it tactilely using their hands and hand it to a communication partner to request a turn swinging. For example, the Standardized Tactile Augmentative Communication Symbols Kit (STACS) contains materials to construct a standardized vocabulary system for a learner who is deaf/blind.

Electronic communication aids or devices are generally considered high-tech and include speech-generating devices (SGDs),

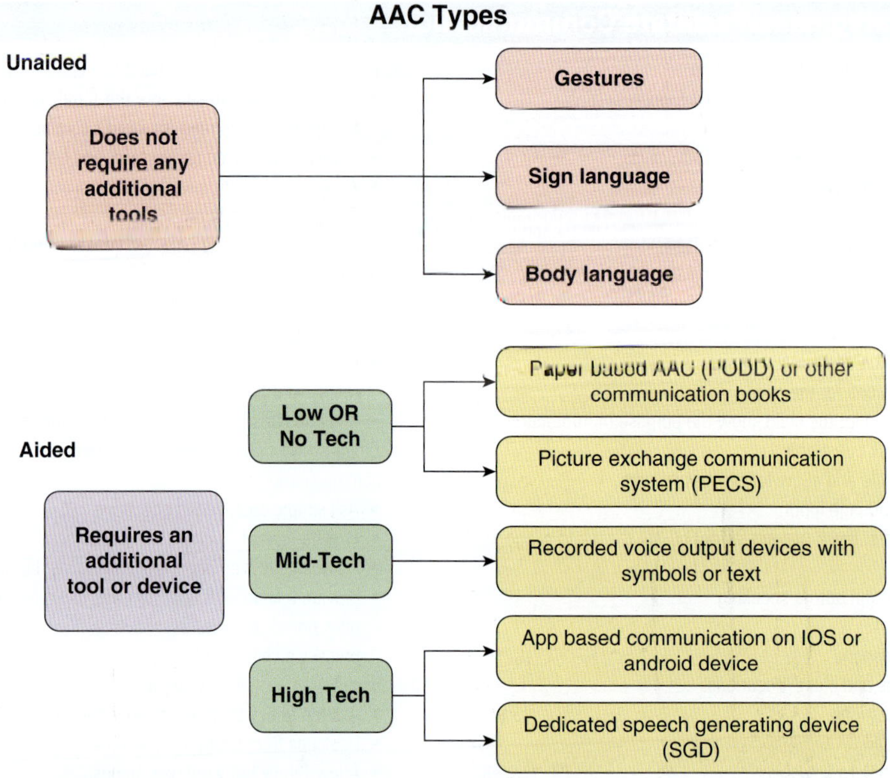


**Fig. 34.8** Unaided and aided types of AAC devices. (Photo courtesy of Elisa Wern.)

talking frames, cell or smart phones, tablets, or computers. Speech generating devices may produce digitized or synthesized speech output (Cook et al., 2020). *Digitized speech* records a person's actual voice. *Synthesized speech* is generated electronically but has the advantage of text-to-speech capabilities. The intelligibility of synthesized speech can vary depending on the type of system and the voice chosen.

High-tech electronic communication aids generally are computer-based or dedicated systems. *Computer-based communication* systems use specialized software and other modifications but can also carry out other functions such as environmental control. Computer-based systems can be mounted or may be portable. Dedicated systems operate primarily as communication devices, such as the one shown in Fig. 34.10, and include hardware and software features specifically designed for communication purposes. These systems are available in various sizes and weights and provide auditory, visual, or printed output. These devices are programmed with individualized pages. Each page can provide as few as two and as many as 128 or more choices to the child.

**Ethical and Cultural Considerations.** When making decisions related to AAC, practitioners are mindful of cultural and ethical considerations. The images or icons used should reflect the ethnicity of the user, so that they can see themselves represented within their system. Representation of voices is also considered (e.g., Tamira, the first Adult African American English voice). Those assisting the user in customizing voices also consider religious traditions, sexual orientation, and preferred pronouns. Personal core or fringe vocabulary should be added to address the communicator's preferences, as well as other things and people who are important to them. This can include people in their family, their classroom, and desired foods and drinks. Occupational therapy practitioners can assist by taking language samples during therapy and encouraging family members and users to advocate that needed vocabulary be available. Occupational therapy practitioners consider and support the user's potential sensory challenges, when selecting AAC. Gregory and Wern (2023) discuss the need to adjust for tactile, visual, and auditory processing, as well as ensuring the needed vocabulary is available in the device to advocate for vestibular, proprioception, or interoception needs.

**Selecting an Alternative and Augmentative Communication System.** Current best practice supports providing a AAC system with a grid size as large as the child can see with moderate accuracy. Current research supports opening up access to core vocabulary and modeling through aided language stimulation (Sennott et al., 2016) or structured programs (Senner et al., 2019), where parents and other team members utilize partner-augmentative input to assist the user in learning their communication system. All team members seek to determine the right device for the individual (not make the user fit the device).

One important factor to consider when selecting the AAC system is the user's understanding of symbolic representation. The focus when selecting the AAC system is on ensuring the child has the motor planning, skills, and abilities to produce a desired message. The symbols can be changed as the child learns them. Access to the alphabet within a communication device is important so that spontaneous, novel utterance generation can occur, as it is impossible to program every possible word into a device (Hill, 2014). Communication systems include the voice output device as well as paper-based AAC replications that can be used if there are technical difficulties, or the device is unavailable.

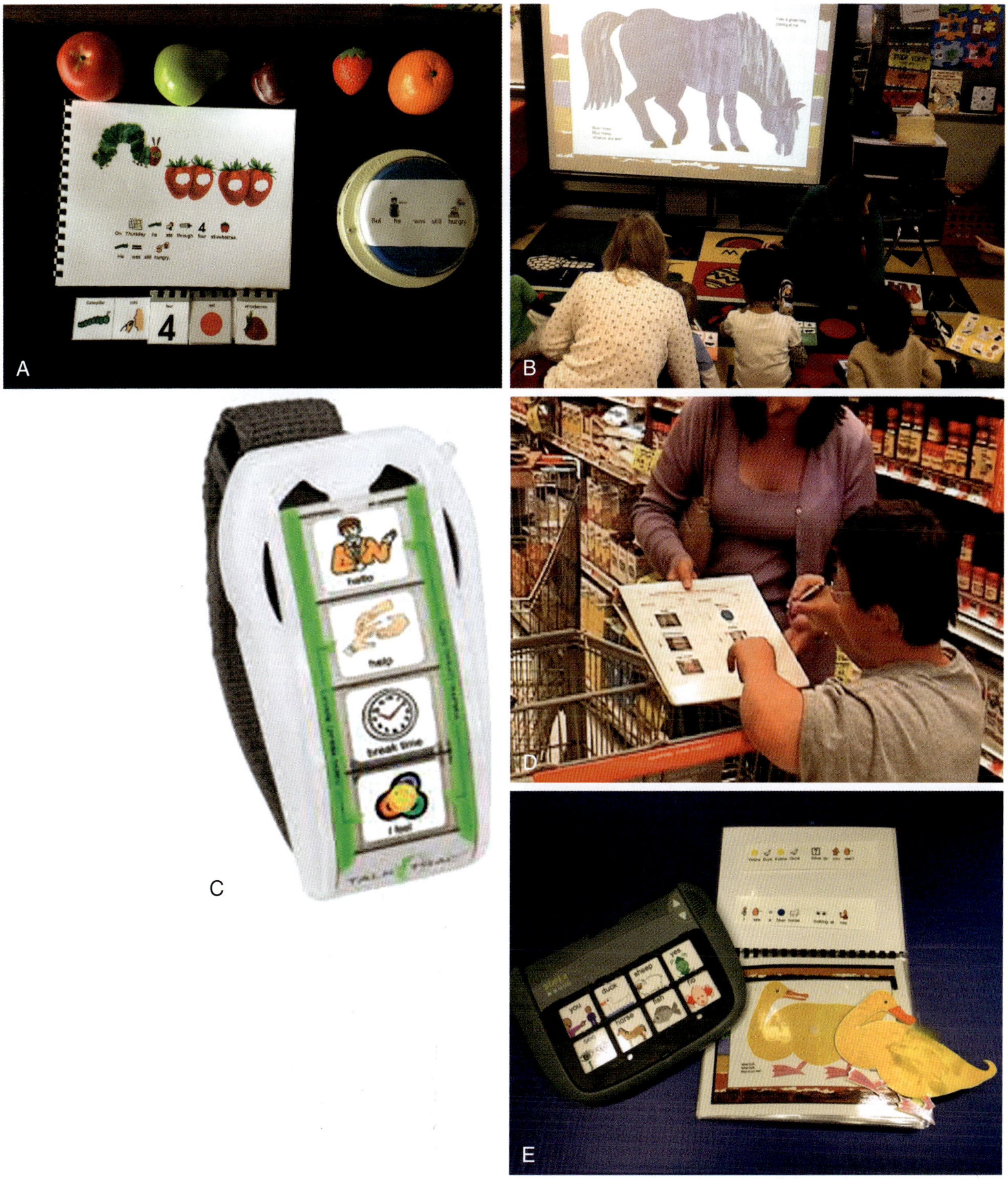


**Fig. 34.9** AAC devices. (A) BIGMack communication devise used in conjunction with an adapted book activity. (B) Using a continuum of communication support to participate in story time. (C) Talk trac communication device. (D) Using symbols while shopping to help the user remember. (E) Supertalker to retell story. (Photos courtesy Judith Schoonover.)

Devices may be accessed through use of a keyboard, joystick, mouse, or alternative pointing devices (Cook et al., 2020). Selections can be made directly by pointing or touching or via an indirect method such as auditory or visual scanning, directed scanning, or coded access. For faster communication than the rate of keying in text, encoding (or symbol) systems are used that employ sequenced multiple-meaning icons to retrieve words, phrases, or sentences. Many communication systems incorporate word prediction programs to reduce needed keystrokes to produce a message. In addition to the input method, AAC devices use two visual display types (screens). A dynamic communication display offers thousands of graphics (some that are electronically animated) and text options. The display changes based on the choices of the user. They are often accessed via a touch screen. Dynamic displays, such as the one in Fig. 34.10, are helpful for children who may have difficulties with memory, but they require a high level of visual attention, constant decision-making, and mastery of object permanence. The second type, visual scene displays, offers "hot spots" that are contextually embedded within graphics that provide more meaningful and individualized interactive displays.

**Training in Alternative and Augmented Communication Devices.** Once a device has been obtained, the team programs the device and trains the child and communication partners. The team, child, and family collaborate to identify vocabulary that includes conversational messages (greetings, information sharing, and requests),

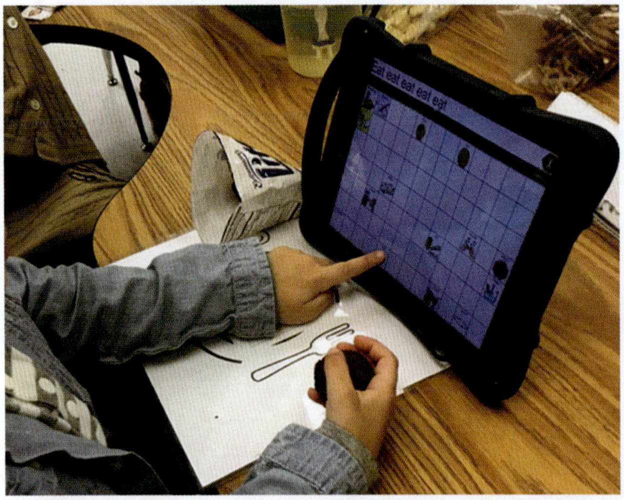

Fig. 34.10 Example of a dedicated, dynamic display augmentative and alternative communication device. (Photo courtesy of Judith Schoonover.)

core vocabulary (for literate or preliterate children to encourage language and cognitive development), and fringe vocabulary (unique to the child's activities, preferences, family, environments, and favorite expressions; Cook et al., 2020). The user is taught specific functions of communication, such as requesting; rejecting/protesting; gaining attention; engaging in greetings, farewells, and other social niceties; commenting; achieving social closeness; asking for information; and confirming/denying (Light & McNaughton, 2014). Fig. 34.11 describes the areas of communication competence, which can be used to establish goals for children and help teams address communication assessment and intervention.

## Improving Engagement in Leisure

Assistive technology can support engagement in leisure activities, which reduces social stigma, increases social interaction opportunities, improves overall self-confidence, enhances positive self-esteem. Leisure activities may include reading a book, playing a board game, or engaging in adaptive sports.

Adaptive gaming for popular gaming systems enables those with neurological diagnoses or limb differences to use controllers (e.g., eye gaze, switches) so that they can play alongside their siblings and friends. Occupational therapy practitioners can partner with organizations such as Able Gamers (https://ablegamers.org/), ATMakers.org (https://atmakers.org), or GRIP UF (https://www.bme.ufl.edu/labs/grip/) to provide gaming systems that children can access and use. Often these adaptations involve customizing and 3D printing pieces that are individualized to the user. Video game activities and virtual reality technologies can benefit children with disabilities by increasing reaction time, practicing real-world situations, and improving social interaction with peers (Jiménez et al., 2015).

## Improving Daily Living

Electronic aids to daily living, also referred to as environmental control units (ECUs), allow the children to interact with and manipulate

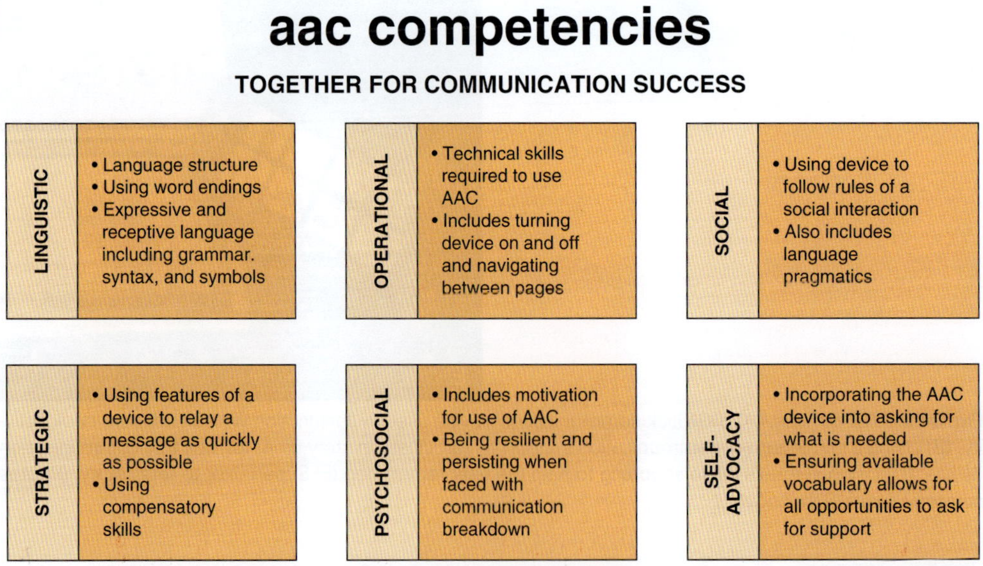


**Fig. 34.11** Areas of communicative competence. (Created by and image courtesy of Elisa Wern. References: Light, J., & McNaughton, D. (2014). Communicative competence for individuals who require augmentative and alternative communication: A new definition for a new era of communication? *Augmentative and Alternative Communication, 30*, 1–18.
Light, J. (2003). Shattering the silence: Development of communicative competence by individuals who use AAC. In J. C. Light, D. R. Beukelman, & J. Reichle (Eds.). *Communicative competence for individuals who use AAC: From research to effective practice* (pp. 3–38). Paul H. Brookes.)

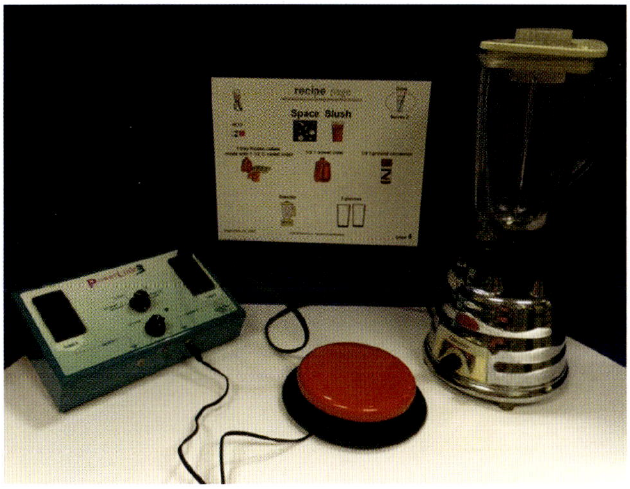


**Fig. 34.12** Visual recipe, Powerlink, switch, and blender set up for cooking activity. (Photo courtesy Judith Schoonover.)

one or more electronic appliances, such as a television, radio, CD player, lights, telephone, or fan, using voice activation, switch access, computer interface, or adaptations such as X-10 units. X-10 units are transmitters and receivers that allow compatible products to interact with each other using the existing electrical wiring. App-based systems incorporating Apple Homekit and Alexa can also serve as electronic aids to daily living. The system should be easy to assemble, learn to use, and maintain. Electronic aids to daily living can be integrated into a computer system, tablet, smartphone, or stand-alone systems. Some systems have a discrete control interface (an electronic device is turned either on or off, such as a light, fan, or television), and others are capable of continuous control interface (devices that operate in successively greater or smaller degrees of control). Lowering and raising the volume on a television and dimming a light are examples of continuous control. A common electronic aid to daily living setup used with children is shown in Fig. 34.12. In recent years, AT users and advocates found ways of using mainstream "smart devices" such as the Amazon Echo as a voice controlled personal assistant to answer questions, play music, read, check schedule, control smart home devices, and more.

## CHANGING THE LANDSCAPE IN EDUCATION: PLANNING FOR EVERY STUDENT

AT and knowledge of students' unique learning styles led to a framework to best address every student's education. Teams evaluate children and create learning environments and support to enable all students to achieve, using principles of Universal Design for Learning (UDL). For example, there are many solutions that occupational therapy practitioners can use to help student access their computers for learning (Table 34.4).

### Universal Design for Learning

Ron Mace used the term **universal design** (UD) to describe the concept of making all products and the built environment physically pleasing and useable to the greatest extent possible by everyone, regardless of their age, ability, or status in life. His work on accessible design was instrumental in the passage of national legislation prohibiting discrimination against people with disabilities, the Fair Housing Amendments Act of 1988, and the Americans with Disabilities Act of 1990 (Americans with Disability Act of 1990). The principles of universal design are outlined in Box 34.5.

According to the Center for Universal Design, "the intent of UD is to simplify life for everyone by making products, communications, and the built environment more useable by as many people as possible at little or no extra cost" (Center for Universal Design, 1997). UD is a proactive approach that eliminates many barriers but does not replace the need for individualized AT. Although typical furnishings, toys, and instructional materials found in homes and classrooms may meet the needs of many, items that are easier to grip, hold, manipulate, visualize, figure out, or use in some other way may be required for others.

Based on the principles of universal design, **Universal Design for Learning (UDL)** is a framework for educational reform that focuses on providing curriculum and materials to support learners with diverse needs in schools (see Chapter 15). The principles of UDL assume that students with a variety of skills and needs will be participants in learning and that the goals, curriculum, instructional materials, and assessments need to proactively anticipate and address this diversity through alternatives, options, and adaptations. Universal design for learning (UDL) emphasizes change in the educational environment in which instructional design meets diverse learning styles and needs.

### Instructional Technology

Technology provides dynamic and continuously changing tools that influence the way children and youth learn, work, play, and socialize. Technology also plays a significant role in the way educators present information and how students respond (U.S. Department of Education, 2016). Children with learning or physical challenges may rely on technology in the classroom. In these situations, technology is considered *assistive*. For example, students with disabilities might *need* to use calculators or word processors to participate in math or writing activities. Common classroom tools may be considered as AT and may be a required service in the Individualized Education Program (IEP); therefore, it is important to consider how important the tool is to the student's learning and participation.

Universal design principles have extended to computer technologies. Embedded accessibility features are on most computers, tablets, and smartphones. These "off-the-shelf" tools allow users to customize their device based on their preferences or individual needs and allow children with disabilities greater access to the digital world (Koch, 2017). See Table 34.5 for features available in computer systems that support a variety of accessibility needs. Occupational therapy practitioners use knowledge of the accessibility features of computer and tablet operating systems and network software; an awareness of the attributes available in instructional tools such as overhead projectors, interactive whiteboards, digital cameras, and tablet computing; and an ability to use the internet and programs, software, or apps to connect with others electronically, to support children and youth.

## SUPPORTING LEARNERS' EDUCATION

Occupational therapy practitioners support children's education in school environments by providing direct intervention to address skill challenges (such as occupational therapy sessions to increase fine motor skills); providing children with accommodations to focus on their strengths through AT; providing alternative ways of doing academic work through AT; and addressing mobility and social participation in school. Occupational therapy practitioners use a variety of AT to address reading, writing, spelling, communication, math, and executive functioning. Table 34.6 describes a variety of technology to support learning.

## TABLE 34.4 Solutions for Computer Access

| Access Concerns | Potential Solutions |
|---|---|
| Difficulty pressing one or more keys or accessing the keyboard | Change height of table or chair<br>Change position of keyboard<br>Change sensitivity of key or active delayed acceptance<br>Direct (expanded) and indirect (letter scanning or switch) selection<br>Keyboard adaptations (color-coded, alphabetic, or key guards)<br>Use an expanded keyboard with larger keys<br>Use a stylus, mouth stick, or head stick<br>Change size of letters or use an ergonomic layout keyboard<br>Direct (expanded) and indirect (letter scanning or switch) selection<br>Alternative keyboards (membrane/touch, miniature, chord, or on-screen)<br>Other types of input systems used with children include **eye-gaze systems**, braille, touch-free switch, and a tongue-touch keypad. Once the user activates the keys, a signal is sent to an interface box connected to the computer, and then the command or key is entered into the system |
| Tendency to produce multiple characters rather than one | Change height of table or chair<br>Change position of keyboard<br>Change sensitivity of key or active delayed acceptance<br>Deactivate auto-repeat |
| Difficulty holding down more than one key simultaneously | Use sticky keys feature or utility<br>Use a mechanical key latch |
| Ability to use only one hand | Teach student to use one-handed typing techniques for standard keyboard<br>Use a chord keyboard<br>Reconfigure the keyboard to use one-handed pattern<br>Use on-screen keyboard and mouse for typing |
| Difficulty with the standard mouse | Use a trackball<br>Use a trackpad<br>Create a mouse track template<br>Use MouseKeys feature of operating system<br>Mouse emulators (devices that simulate mouse movement and selection, including arrow keys, touch pads, trackballs, head pointers, interactive whiteboards, and touch windows and screens) |
| Slow or inefficient input | Increase keyboarding practice so that motor patterns are more automatic<br>Set up templates for standard formats<br>Use macros and abbreviation expansion for repeated words and phrases<br>Use word prediction software programs<br>Voice recognition (the computer or tablet recognizes and translates voice sounds into text or commands) |
| Drooling | Use a keyboard cover (Safe Skin)<br>Use alternative keyboards that are not moisture sensitive |
| Difficulty seeing the screen or highlights | Ensure that the monitor is not facing a window or that the blinds are drawn<br>Use an antiglare filter<br>Reduce glare by turning down overhead lights<br>Change size of font<br>Change font (serif fonts are better for reading; OpenDyslexic and Lexend fonts are designed to be more widely accessible; sans serif fonts are better for letter recognition)<br>Change attributes of font (bold)<br>Change color of background or text for greater contrast; use high contrast within accessibility features or as a browser extension<br>Set screen to monochrome<br>Use a large screen or lower screen resolution<br>Use a screen magnifier (hardware or software) |
| Difficulty reading text | Ensure that the monitor is not facing a window or that the blinds are drawn<br>Use an antiglare filter<br>Reduce glare by turning down overhead lights<br>Change size of font<br>Change font (serif fonts are better for reading text; sans serif fonts are better for letter recognition)<br>Change attributes of font (bold)<br>Change color of background or text for greater contrast<br>Set screen to monochrome<br>Use a large screen or lower screen resolution<br>Use a screen magnifier (hardware or software)<br>Use a voice output tool (screen reader) |

TABLE 34.4 **Solutions for Computer Access—cont'd**

| Access Concerns | Potential Solutions |
|---|---|
| Tendency to be distracted by sound | Turn off sound features of application<br>Turn down volume from system control panel |
| Difficulty hearing feedback | Use hearing protectors or noise-canceling ear protectors<br>Turn up volume (can use headphones)<br>Use amplified speakers |
| Difficulty finding correct key on the keyboard | Use stickers or enlarged key letters to highlight correct keys<br>Increase size or contrast of keyboard caps<br>Use color coding for "landmark" keys<br>Use LearningBoard (Chester Creek); or mini-sized keyboards (for younger students)<br>Mask nonapplicable keys during instruction |
| Difficulty shifting between information on the screen, the keyboard, and the desktop | Use document clip to suspend printed page next to monitor<br>Change position of keyboard<br>Change position of monitor<br>Use a touch screen and on-screen keyboard |
| Difficulty remembering keyboard functions | Develop a "cheat sheet" of keyboard shortcuts to keep within user's line of vision/attached to monitor<br>Develop keyboard mnemonics to aid memory of keyboard functions |
| Limited motivation | Recheck student goals to ensure student involvement in goal-making process<br>Try a different software program to address goal<br>Change the purpose for which the computer is being used<br>Change the access method<br>Decrease the amount of time on the computer<br>Level the activity to the student's skills (up or down) |

Adapted from Koch, K. (2017). Stay in the box! Embedded assistive technology improves access for students with disabilities. *Education Sciences, 7*(4), 82.

BOX 34.5 **Principles of Universal Design**

**Principle One: Equitable Use**
The design is useful and marketable to people with diverse abilities.

**Principle Two: Flexibility in Use**
The design accommodates a wide range of individual preferences and abilities.

**Principle Three: Simple and Intuitive Use**
Use of the design is easy to understand, regardless of the user's experience, knowledge, language skills, or current concentration level.

**Principle Four: Perceptible Information**
The design communicates necessary information effectively to the user, regardless of ambient conditions or the user's sensory abilities.

**Principle Five: Tolerance for Error**
The design minimizes hazards and the adverse consequences of accidental or unintended actions.

**Principle Six: Low Physical Effort**
The design can be used efficiently and comfortably and with a minimum of fatigue.

**Principle Seven: Size and Space for Approach and Use**
Appropriate size and space are provided for approach, reach, manipulation, and use regardless of the user's body size, posture, or mobility.

Connell, B. R., et al. (1997). *The principles of universal design, version 2.0.* North Carolina State University. http://www.ncsu.edu/ncsu/design/cud/about_ud/udprinciples.htm

## Literacy Skills

Literacy skills include the processes of reading, writing, and spelling as forms of communication. Reading is the process of constructing meaning from written text, and writing is the process of composing meaningful text. AT can help children with disabilities acquire language skills by learning to attend to words and enhancing their interest in listening to stories. *Comprehensive literacy* refers to using reading, writing, and spelling skills to accomplish daily tasks in the home school, community, and work settings (Erickson & Koppenhaver, 2020). A variety of software, text readers, apps, and electronic books are available to support children's literacy. An essential element related to the effectiveness of technology in supporting literacy is its interactive quality, which allows children to get involved with the content as they manipulate the media, like a parent reading to a child and involving them in the book by turning the pages, looking at pictures, and asking questions. Technology can be customized to the child's interests. It is important to start literacy early for all children.

### Reading Skills

For children with physical, visual, communication, or cognitive delays, traditional books may restrict their abilities to interact with and enjoy books. Adapting books can make them easier to manipulate (turning pages or holding) and text easier to read (simplified or changed) and remember. The original story or subject is maintained but may contain modified language, clear visual representations, and manageable page layouts. Adapted books can be created with props (such as toys, puppets), paper, or digital using software programs or apps. Adapted books can be used by themselves or with additional AT ranging from do it yourself page "fluffers" and easels to switches, voice output communication aids, braille or large print materials, communication systems, or adapted props. Copyright laws allow the creation and use of books in an alternate format solely to make the book accessible to persons with disabilities. A copy of the original book is required when using an adapted book. Books can be adapted to provide physical access to text by:

- Creating space between pages with page "fluffers" (foam, weather stripping, sponges, giant paper clips, or clothespins)

**TABLE 34.5 Accessibility Features in Operating Systems, Browsers, Software, Apps, and Websites**

| ACCESSIBILITY FEATURES IN OPERATING SYSTEMS, BROWSERS, SOFTWARE, APPS, AND WEBSITES | | |
|---|---|---|
| **Area of Concern** | **Design Feature** | **Beneficiary** |
| Reading/vision | Physical characteristics of text can be altered including adding braille; screen narration; adjustments for light and color sensitivity with color control; personalized cursor size and color, font, text size, and color; and screen magnification and zoom | Students with low vision; those who need to adjust the text due to glare or fatigue |
| | Altering the spacing between characters, words, lines of text, and increasing the size of margins | Students experiencing difficulty with visual tracking or visual perception |
| | Text can be scaffolded to accommodate interests and reading abilities by adding pictures; online text summarizing tools (e.g., TextCompactor); online text simplification sites (e.g., ReWordify); or electronic dictionaries with or without speech support | Students who lack background knowledge; struggling readers; students with focus or cognitive differences |
| | The reading view on some webpages can be simplified to reduce distraction | Students experiencing difficulty with focus |
| Listening | Audio support including screen narration, text-to-speech, and closed captioning | Students with low decoding skills or poor fluency; auditory reinforcement and auditory learners |
| Writing | Word prediction; graphic organizers; record features; speech to text; spelling and grammar check; readability; thesaurus, SmartArt, shapes, and diagrams; voice notes | Students who struggle with writing or composing |
| Mobility | On-screen keyboard; touch pad settings; sticky keys; voice control; navigate screen apps with eyes; speech to text | Students with mobility issues are provided with alternatives to holding and transporting books and manipulating pages, as well as using keyboard or controlling action on screen |
| | AutoCorrect and AutoText | Students who struggle with motor aspect of word processing, or spelling |
| Executive function | Digital organizers; timers; highlighters; sticky notes; calendars; alarms | Students who struggle with focus, memory, organization, and task completion |

Adapted from Edyburn, D. L., & Edyburn, K. D. (2012). Tools for creating accessible, tiered, and multilingual web-based curricula. *Intervention in School and Clinic, 47*(4), 199–205. https://www.researchgate.net

**TABLE 34.6 Assistive Technology Supports for the Learning Process**

| **Curriculum Area** | **Description of Types of Support** |
|---|---|
| Reading | Text to speech, audio books, digital text with adjustable reading levels; access tools (page fluffers, slant boards, color overlays, or reading windows); using digital text with tracking and voice output |
| Writing | Adaptive writing tools (pencil grips, large barrel or weighted writing tools, and raised line paper or graph paper); word prediction software; spelling and grammar checkers and speech to text/voice recognition; guided notes/note shells; outline templates and brainstorming models |
| Math | Tools for production of numbers (number line/ruler; visual support for writing numbers correctly); TouchMath https://www.touchmath.com/ (multisensory teaching approach that links manipulation with memorization of math facts) |
| | Enlarged or masked math worksheets; reduce visual clutter and provide additional space for showing work; graph or grid paper that supports alignment of problems |
| | Alternative response methods (number stamps, stamps for drawing graphs, clocks, and number lines); specialized calculator: talking, large key, or computer-based on-screen calculators; money, tactile, or braille based, or talking scientific and graphing, including emulators) |
| Executive functioning | Schedules (visual, text, app/computer-based calendars, and timers); organizational supports (color coding, sticky notes, labels, and highlighters); smart watches and apps for reminders; checklist creators/online flashcards (http://pblchecklist.4teachers.org/checklist.shtml; Quizlet/Quizizz) |

- Using book holders for stabilization (recipe book holders, card holders, acrylic display frames, or easels) or reproducing them so that they can be listened to or viewed with technology
- Using e-books that combine reading, writing, listening, and speaking and provide a multisensory approach with related pictures, sound, and video and appeal to different learning styles

The ability to read is essential for many daily life activities and participation in home, school, work, and community activities. For example, reading contributes to play and leisure, academics and world knowledge, communication and social awareness, following directions and schedules, shopping and meal preparation, and work-related tasks.

Print materials can be designed or transformed with support embedded to ensure that all learners have access to information using common software features. Students can also be taught to alter the amount, cognitive challenge, and appearance of digital text (Norton-Darr & Schoonover, 2012). Other accommodations for reading disabilities include the use of commercially available talking photo albums, specific reading software, apps, e-books, audio recordings, screen readers, and multimedia.

Although trends in education are changing and more school districts use digital resources, many districts continue to use printed books and worksheets. Some students may have difficulty accessing printed materials, such as those with low vision or blindness or those with physical challenges who are unable to hold a book or turn pages. Occupational therapy practitioners help children access the materials they need for education.

## Writing Skills

Handwriting is the most common reason for referrals to occupational therapy in school-based practice; therefore, occupational therapy practitioners frequently enhance writing skills with no-tech or low-tech aids and devices. See Chapter 30 for more information on handwriting intervention. Using tools that are intuitive may mean borrowing or adapting tools that already exist in the classroom (Fig. 34.13).

Occupational therapy practitioners may teach keyboarding as an alternative to handwriting, but they also examine the accessibility features of computer operating systems to enhance the child's ability to write, organize, and connect with others. Concept-mapping software allows the user to conceptualize information graphically using a combination of pictures and/or text. It is helpful for planning, organizing, and drafting and frequently offers templates for getting started.

Software products and apps allow the child to complete a written assignment with visual and/or auditory feedback. Word prediction and word completion can reduce the number of keystrokes necessary and increase overall speed (Cook et al., 2020). After a child types the first few letters of a word, the program attempts to predict whole words and presents a list of choices for the child to scan and select (Fig. 34.14). Many word prediction programs include customizable dictionaries that suggest alternative word selections to improve the quality of a child's written work. These features support spelling for children who have good word recognition skills. Spell-checking programs are helpful editing tools, specifically when integrated into a word processing program. A traditional digital or picture dictionary or thesaurus may help children who have word retrieval deficits.

Most text-to-speech applications feature highlighting functions providing audio as well as visual support. Users with writing disabilities can also access contents of web pages, e-mail, e-books, or printed documents when paired with digital speech output, which is available in many applications.

While universally accessible options work for most students, some require more specific voice typing software with added features such as complete control of the entire computer or voice recognition that is specifically trained to the user. This allows individuals with intelligible speech to express themselves, even when writing is problematic (Cochrane & Key, 2020).

## Math Skills

Mathematics is a part of a typical school curriculum and is considered a functional life skill. Mathematical concepts include sorting, identifying attributes (color, shape, size, and patterns), counting, sequencing, graphing, and understanding and manipulating numbers. Ideally, children engage in numerous opportunities to use and manipulate concrete objects to count, sort, compare, and combine to reinforce concepts of same/different and greater than/less than/equal to. Additional support (e.g., grippers, nonskid materials), access to a calculator, or alternatives to hands-on manipulation such as "virtual manipulation" allow active participation in math exploration for all.

Concepts related to fractions, multiplication, and division can be illustrated with animation and sound. Apps allow students to take a picture of math problems and see them solved virtually and graphed if

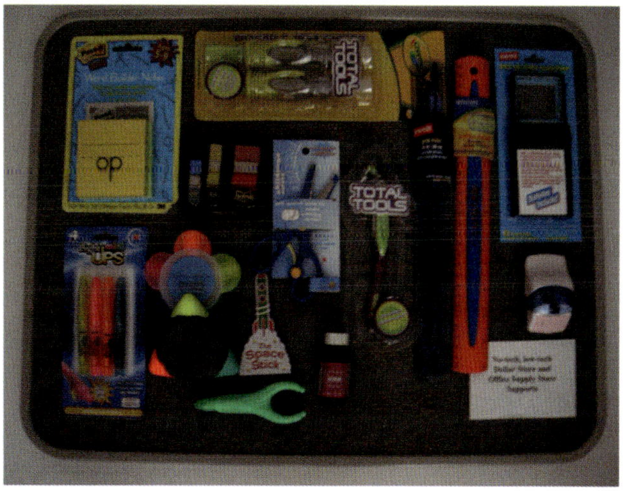


Fig. 34.13 Examples of readily available, universally designed low-tech tools. (Photo courtesy Judith Schoonover.)

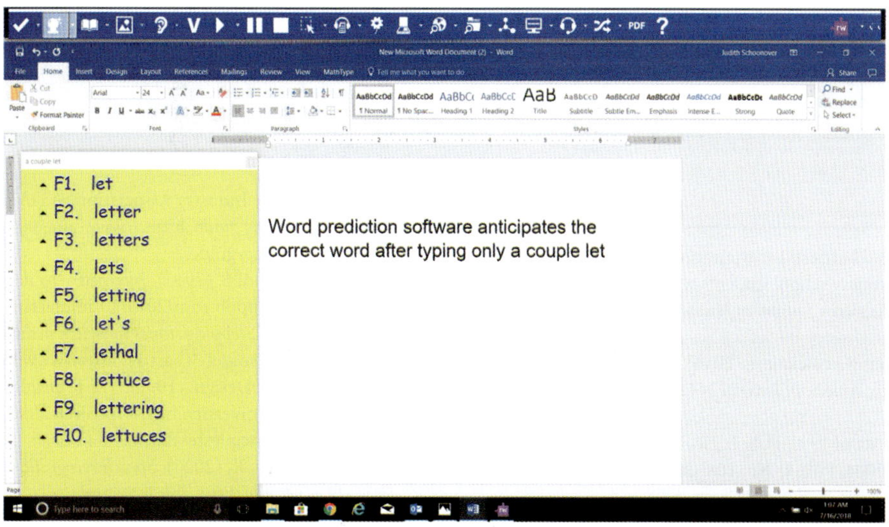


Fig. 34.14 Example of word prediction software. (Photo courtesy Elisa Wern.)

needed. For students who struggle with remembering steps for completion of math problems, this support can be used to reinforce instruction.

### Executive Functioning Skills

Assistive technology can reduce barriers associated with cognitive skills such as focus, memory, organization, and task completion. A continuum of tools from paper-based sticky notes and checklists to digital reminders such as visual schedules, steps to a routine/task, or a list of behavioral expectations can be used to remind students of necessary components of specific tasks. For nonreaders, graphic or pictorial representation of concepts might be used as visual reminders. Digital personal reminders such as watches with programmable timers may assist children with schedules. Smart technologies allow users to set alarms, refer to a calendar, break tasks down into manageable increments, or be reminded to engage in deep breathing and relaxation exercises. Digital organizers assist in organization and self-regulation by providing self-directed electronic task management support for vocational and nonvocational activities (Gentry et al., 2010).

Personal tablet devices, smartwatches with alarm and messaging features, and mobile devices, including cell phones with reminder features, may help children with executive functioning difficulties. Devices that have touch screens allow a person to input, save, and retrieve information in whatever setting they find themselves. These devices offer a portable solution for keeping track of assignments, appointments, reminders, and contact information, as well as to deliver prompts or access preferred stimuli, and they may include microphones, forward- and backward-facing cameras, and touch screen capabilities. Pictures and videos can be used to provide social cues, step-by-step directions, and more. Personal calendars and daily planners can be used to manage time and complete tasks. Global positioning system receivers can help children and youth navigate independently and safely within the community. The multiple function capabilities of mobile device platforms may permit a consolidation of devices.

Apps, software, and free internet sites can help organize daily and monthly activities. Online tutorials and apps can deliver training that can be repeated many times. It is important to consider the limitations of mobile devices, including the need for technical competencies to use them independently, and the possibility of disruption from damage, malfunction, or theft.

Not all cognitive supports are high-tech in nature. Structuring the environment can also enhance performance. For example, shields or color codes on equipment can help with focus and sequencing; using carrels around work areas can reduce visual distractions; and earphones can help block out sound distractions. Other simple solutions include portable timers, alarm clocks, social scripts, and watches with alarms.

## SUMMARY

Assistive technology (AT) devices and services help children and youth with disabilities participate in everyday activities and learning. Occupational therapy practitioners are integral members of AT teams to determine the right fit between the technology and the child's needs.

1. AT helps children and youth engage in those things that they find meaningful. It allows children to develop skills, self-determination, and competence. Technology can enable children to engage independently in play, activities of daily living, instrumental activities of daily living, education, and work. Children who use AT early in life have the advantage of developing with and using it to benefit them throughout their lives. AT allows children to be active participants in childhood occupations, which promotes learning, engagement, and self-efficacy.
2. Many factors influence AT service decisions and outcomes. Best practices consider the child, family, culture, the environments in which the child performs, and the child's desired occupations. The team uses knowledge of the child's strengths, abilities, and challenges to find suitable technology. They consider the durability of technology, size, user preferences, maintenance needs, and the setting in which the device will be used when recommending AT. Importantly, the team along determines how the technology will help the child participate more fully in school, play, home, and community activities.
3. Team members collaborate by sharing their expertise and listening to each other, the child, and the family to understand how AT can best enable the child to engage in everyday activities. Selecting AT involves many factors and information from team members (including child and family), which is essential for continued use and success of the devices. Several frameworks and assessment guides have been developed to evaluate the need, selection, and outcomes of AT. These decision-making tools include human, activity, assistive technology (HAAT), student, environments, tasks, tools (SETT), matching, person, technology (MPT), and the Wisconsin Assistive Technology Initiative (WATI) assessment package (see Table 34.2).
4. AT ranges from lite- or no-tech (e.g., reachers, built-up handles, adapted utensils, Velcro closures) to high-tech (e.g., computer systems, augmentative communication devices, powered wheelchairs, ECUs).

## REFERENCES

Alharbi, S. (2016). Benefits and barriers: Incorporating assistive technology in an inclusive setting for primary school students with learning disabilities in language arts. *American Research Journal of Humanities and Social Sciences, 2*, 1–11.

American Occupational Therapy Association. (2016). Assistive technology and occupational performance. *American Journal of Occupational Therapy, 70* 7012410030.

Americans With Disabilities Act of 1990, Pub. L. No. 101–336.

Assistive Technology Act of 2004, Pub. L. No. 108–364, 29 U.S.C., 2001 et seq.

Assistive Technology Industry Association (ATIA). (2017). *Assistive technology funding guide*. https://www.atia.org/at-resources/what-is-at/resources-funding-guide.

Budai, M., & Neuland, E. (2015). *Interactive by design*. Rehab Management. http://www.rehabpub.com/2015/10/interactive-design/.

Burkhart, L. (2018). *Stepping stones to switch access. Perspectives of the ASHA Special Interest Groups*, 3(part 1). http://www.lburkhart.com.

Center for Universal Design. (1997). *The principles of universal design*. North Carolina State University. https://projects.ncsu.edu/ncsu/design/cud/about_ud/udprinciplestext.htm.

Cochrane, D., & Key, K. (2020). *Speech recognition as AT for writing: A guide for K-12 education*. http://bit.ly/srguide/.

Cohen, A., & Demchak, M. (2018). Use of visual supports to increase task independence in students with severe disabilities in inclusive educational settings. *Education and Training in Autism and Developmental Disabilities, 53*(1), 84–99.

Connell, B. R., et al. (1997). *The principles of universal design, version 2.0.* Raleigh, NC: North Carolina State University. http://www.ncsu.edu/ncsu/design/cud/about_ud/udprinciples.htm.

Cook, A. M., Polgar, J. M., & Encarnação, P. (Eds.). (2020). *Assistive technologies: Principles and practice* (5th ed.). St. Louis: Elsevier Mosby.

Cook, D., & Knue, A. (2010). *What you need to know about assistive technology.* Center on Technology and Disability Studies at CHDD, University of Washington. http://depts.washington.edu/healthtr/documents/assistivetech.pdf.

Cooper-Duffy, K., & Eaker, K. (2017). Effective team practices: Interprofessional contributions to communication issues with a parent's perspective. *American Journal of Speech-Language Pathology, 26*(2), 181–192.

Cruz, D. M. C., Emmel, M. L. G., Manzini, M. F., & Braga Mendes, P. V. (2016). Assistive technology accessibility and abandonment: Challenges for occupational therapists. *The Open Journal of Occupational Therapy, 4*(1) Article 10.

D'Arrigo, R., Ziviani, J., Poulsen, A., Copley, J., & King, G. (2017). Child and parent engagement in therapy. What is the key? *Australian Occupational Therapy Journal, 64*, 340–343.

Dunst, C. J., Trivette, C. M., Hamby, D. W., & Simkus, A. (2013). Systematic review of studies promoting the use of assistive technology devices by young children with disabilities. *Practical Evaluation Reports, 5*(1), 1–32.

Edyburn, D. L., & Edyburn, K. D. (2012). Tools for creating accessible, tiered, and multilingual web-based curricula. *Intervention in School and Clinic, 47*(4), 199–205. https://www.researchgate.net.

Ergonomics (n.d.). *Merriam-Webster's online dictionary.* www.merriam-webster.com/dictionary/ergonomics

Erickson, K. A., & Koppenhaver, D. A. (2020). *Comprehensive literacy for all: Teaching students with significant disabilities to read & write.* Baltimore, MD: Brookes.

Fair Housing Act (1988) U.S. Pub. L. 90–284, title VIII, § 804, Sept. 13, 1988, 102 Stat 1636.

Gentry, T., Wallace, J., Kvarfordt, C., & Lynch, K. B. (2010). Personal digital assistants as cognitive aids for high school students with autism: Results from a community-based trial. *Journal of Vocational Rehabilitation, 32*(2), 101–107.

Gregory, S., & Wern, E. (2023). AAC for individuals with sensory integration challenges. In N. Hall, J. Juengling-Sudkamp, M. L. Gutmann, & E. R. Cohn (Eds.), *Fundamentals of AAC: A case based approach to enhancing communication* (pp. 353–367). Plural Publishing. https://lccn.loc.gov/2021055247.

Hill, K. (2014). *Achieving success in AAC: Assessment and intervention.* AAC Institute. http://aacinstitute.org/wp-content/uploads/2014/12/Achieving-Success-In-AAC.pdf.

Individuals with Disabilities Education Act (IDEA) of 2004 (P.L. 108–446). https://sites.ed.gov/idea/.

Institute for Matching Person and Technology. (2015). *Matching person and technology (MPT) assessment process.* http://www.matchingpersonandtechnology.com/mptdesc.html.

Jiménez, M., Pulina, F., Lanfranchi, S., & Jiménez, R. (2015). Video games and Intellectual disabilities: A literature review -IRCCS life span and disability. *Life Span and Disability, 2*, 147–165.

Klein, C. (2017). Communication and developing relationships for people who use augmentative and alternative communication. *Assistive Technology Outcomes and Benefits, 11*(Summer 2017), 58–65.

Koch, K. (2017). Stay in the box! Embedded assistive technology improves access for students with disabilities. *Education Sciences, 7*(4), 82.

Lee, S. W., & Kielhofner, G. (2017). Volition. In R. Taylor (Ed.), *Kielhofner's model of human occupation* (5th ed.) (pp. 38–56). Philadelphia: Wolters Kluwer.

Light, J., & McNaughton, D. (2014). Communicative competence for individuals who require augmentative and alternative communication: A new definition for a new era of communication? *Augmentative and Alternative Communication, 30*, 1–18.

Livingstone, R., & Paleg, G. (2013). Practice considerations for the introduction and use of power mobility for children. *Developmental Medicine and Child Neurology, 56*(3), 210–221.

Miller, L. J., et al. (2017). Play in natural environments: A pilot study quantifying the behavior of children on playground equipment. *Journal of Occupational Therapy, Schools, & Early Intervention, 10*(3), 213–231.

Mirenda, P. (1993). Bonding the uncertain mosaic. *Augmentative and Alternative Communication, 9*(1), 3–9.

Moore, A., & Lynch, H. (2015). Accessibility and usability of playground environments for children under 12: A scoping review. *Scandinavian Journal of Occupational Therapy, 22*(5), 331–344.

National Center for Education Statistics. (2022). *Students with disabilities.* Condition of Education. U.S. Department of Education, Institute of Education Sciences. https://nces.ed.gov/programs/coe/indicator/cgg.

Norton-Darr, S., & Schoonover, J. (2012). Spreading "the word" about cognitive rescaling as a tool for inclusion. *Closing the Gap*, 7–13. http://technoranger.acpsmd.org/Publish/articles/Cognitive%20Rescaling%20as%20a%20Tool%20for%20Inclusion.pdf.

O'Rourke, P., Ekins, R., Timmins, B., Timmins, F., Long, S., & Coyle, E. (July 2013). Crucial design issues for special access technology: A Delphi study. *Disability and Rehabilitation: Assistive Technology.* http://informahealthcare.com/journal/idt.

O'Brien, A., Schlosser, R. W., Shane, H. C., Abramson, J., Allen, A. A., Flynn, S., Yu, C., et al. (2016). Brief report: Just-in-time visual supports to children with autism via the Apple Watch®: A pilot feasibility study. *Journal of Autism and Developmental Disorders, 46*(12), 3818–3823.

Ogletree, B. T., Brady, N., Bruce, S., Dean, E., Romski, M., Sylvester, L., et al. (2017). Mary's case: An illustration of interprofessional collaborative practice for a child with severe disabilities. *American Journal of Speech-Language Pathology, 26*(2), 217–226.

Quality Indicators for Assistive Technology (QIAT) Consortium. (2015). *Guiding the provision of quality assistive technology services.* https://www.qiat.org/indicators.html.

Schoonover, J., & Schwind, D. B. (2017). Grant's ART toolbox: Adapted repurposed tools. *OT Practice, 22*(9), 12–13 8–10.

Schultz, S. (2013). *Social media as a communication tool for individuals with disabilities living in rural settings.* Education Faculty Publications, 40. http://fisherpub.sjfc.edu/education_facpub/40/.

Senner, J. E., Post, K. A., Baud, M. R., Patterson, B., Bolin, B., Lopez, J., & Williams, E. (2019). Effects of parent instruction in partner-augmented input on parent and child speech generating device use. *Technology and Disability, 31*(1–2), 27–38.

Sennot, S. C., Light, J. C., & McNaughton, D. (2016). AAC modeling intervention research review. *Research and Practice for Persons with Severe Disabilities, 41*, 101–115.

Smith, A. L., Barton-Hulsey, A., & Nwosu, N. (2016). AAC and families: Dispelling myths and empowering parents. *Perspectives of the ASHA Special Interest Groups, 1*(12), 10–20.

Soltani, S. H. K., Abbas, M. Y., & Awang, M. B. (2012). Disabled children in public playgrounds: A pilot study. *Procedia—Social and Behavioral Sciences, 36*, 670–676.

The Rehabilitation Engineering Research Center on Augmentative and Alternative Communication. (2019). The urgent need for augmentative and alternative communication research, technology development, training, and services to support individuals with complex communication needs: RERC on AAC white paper. https://rercaac.psu.edu/free-eprints-available/.

United States Department of Education and United States Department of Health and Human Services. (2016). *Early learning and educational technology brief.* https://tech.ed.gov/earlylearning/.

WATI Development Team. (2017). *Assistive technology assessment and consideration forms.* http://www.wati.org/free-publications/assistive-technology-consideration-to-assessment/.

Watson, A. H., Ito, M., Smith, R. O., & Andersen, L. T. (2010). Effect of assistive technology in a public-school setting. *American Journal of Occupational Therapy, 64*, 18–29.

World Health Organization. (May 18, 2018). *Fact sheet: Assistive technology.* http://www.who.int/en/news-room/fact-sheets/detail/assistive-technology.

Zachry, A. H., & Mitchell, A. W. (2012). Goal-directed actions and early experience with crawling. *OTJR: Occupation, Participation and Health, 32*(2), 48–55.

# 35

# Case Studies to Illustrate Professional Reasoning in Pediatric Practice*

*Jarrett Wolske and Jane Clifford O'Brien*

## GUIDING QUESTIONS

1. How do occupational therapy practitioners use knowledge from conceptual practice models to inform professional reasoning?
2. How do types of professional reasoning inform the occupational therapy process?
3. What are examples of person, occupation, and environmental factors based on cases that influence professional reasoning?
4. How does analysis of case studies support professional reasoning?

## KEY TERMS

Conditional reasoning
Ethical reasoning
Interactive reasoning
Metacognition
Narrative reasoning
Pragmatic reasoning
Procedural reasoning
Professional reasoning
Scientific reasoning

## PROFESSIONAL REASONING PROCESS

Occupational therapy practitioners working with children and youth practice in multifaceted, dynamic, and evolving settings, such as homes, clinics, schools, hospitals, and privately owned areas of practice. They encounter children and youth with a variety of needs, hopes, concerns, cultures, narratives, and environmental circumstances. In each therapeutic encounter, occupational therapy practitioners juggle the demands of the client and their broader social environment, practice setting, reimbursement sources, documentation standards, caregivers, and teams (e.g., medical, rehabilitation, educational). Admittedly, the variety of possibilities involved in occupational therapy practice can appear dizzying.

The professional reasoning process involves integrating information from multiple sources to make decisions, assess children's skills and abilities, prioritize goals, create intervention plans, implement plans, and reflect upon the process (O'Brien et al., 2023). The steps to the professional reasoning process are illustrated in Fig. 35.1. As practitioners work through the process, they use various types of reasoning, including conditional, ethical, interactive, narrative, pragmatic, and scientific reasoning (Patnaude, 2023). Table 35.1 describes each type of reasoning.

When occupational therapy practitioners engage in professional reasoning, they engage in metacognition. **Metacognition** refers to thinking about one's own thinking. Practitioners use metacognition when they provide their rationale for their decisions, reflect upon their problem-solving regarding their practice, consider alternative approaches, and select models of practice and intervention strategies for clients (Patnaude, 2023). Wong and Fisher (2015) proposed a way of unifying professional reasoning while using conceptual practice models so that practitioners could utilize the best available evidence and research while maintaining an occupation-based focus in practice. Practitioners seek to understand clients universally using occupation-based models and seek to understand performance patterns, factors, and deficits through frames of reference. Thus, practitioners have a micro and macro perspective of the clients they are working with (Patnaude & O'Brien, 2023).

To showcase this process, the chapter is composed of many case examples. Case examples assist with learning professional reasoning in context (Kassier, 2010), which facilitates the development of problem-solving skills (Allen & Toth-Cohen, 2019). Case examples also allow practitioners to utilize metacognitive strategies to strengthen practice decisions.

This chapter provides a variety of cases representing ages, settings, diagnoses, and life experiences to illustrate the professional reasoning process through assessment, intervention planning, and outcomes measurement. The cases show snapshots of the therapy process to illustrate the types of reasoning, present multiple viewpoints, and to emphasize the complexity of occupational therapy practice. Some cases are told from the practitioner's viewpoint, while others are told from the client's lived experience. The authors emphasize key aspects of each case including aspects of professional reasoning. Table 35.2 details the cases and factors emphasized by each case in this chapter.

## NEONATAL INTENSIVE CARE UNIT SETTING

The NICU setting is typically not considered entry level practice; however, this case is included here to provide an example of a practitioner's reasoning integrally aligned with family needs during a very stressful family time. Occupational therapy practitioners who work in the NICU receive advanced training and seek out mentors to meet the needs of infants and their families.

*With contributions from Patty Coker-Bolt, Kristen Mollineau, Lynthea Reefe, Teressa Reidy, Virginia Spielman, and Mikkel Wilson.

Blaise was born at 27 weeks gestation by emergency C-section for significant fetal distress after his mother experienced preeclampsia. He required intubation and high-frequency oscillating ventilator support and remained intubated for 10 days to support his immature lungs.

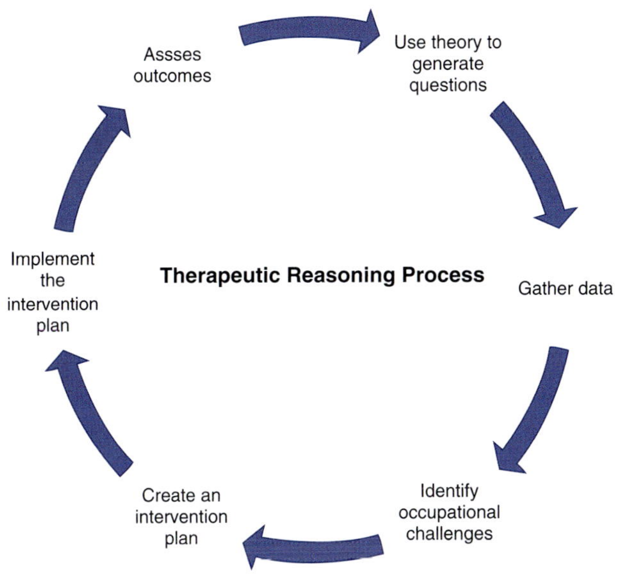


**Fig. 35.1** Therapeutic reasoning process. (Based on O'Brien et al., 2023, p. 8.)

Blaise's parents took turns staying with him. They lived 2 hours from the hospital and had two older children (2 and 4 years old). Blaise remained in the NICU for 30 days before going home with his parents. Blaise had difficulty with suck-swallow-breathing. He received intra-oral feedings.

The occupational therapist working in the NICU collaborated with nursing staff and arranged to be present during feeding attempts. The therapist provided support to the parents and suggestions to promote feeding (e.g., positioning, limiting stimuli, holding cheeks to prevent some suction). They tried different nipples and mom expressed breast-milk in a bottle. They discussed conserving the infant's energy for feeding and increasing the time gradually as the infant was able.

The therapist also acknowledged the parents' stress and provided support and positive reinforcement. The therapist encouraged the parents to hold, rock, and interact with Blaise. To help the family enjoy Blaise, the therapist suggested the children color cards for him, and they took pictures of the family to place in Blaise's room. The therapist also reminded the mother of the importance of caring for herself, and they created a plan for getting her help at home (at least at the beginning).

They discussed their concerns with feeding and his future development. The practitioner provided information on resources close to them and reinforced that Blaise may benefit from occupational therapy on discharge. Blaise had good days and bad days, as did the parents, and the occupational therapist and team acknowledged these days and worked together to build the family's level of competence in caring for their infant.

**TABLE 35.1 Types of Therapeutic Reasoning**

| Type | Description | Example |
|---|---|---|
| Conditional reasoning | Understanding the child's strengths and challenges by synthesizing information from many sources (such as knowledge of child's diagnoses, roles, habits, interactive style and preferences, ethics and politics, family history, and environmental resources). Ability to think about what the future might hold and reasoning with respect to future concerns | Practitioners create an intervention plan using information from family, teacher, and child along with setting policies and procedures, assessment data, clinical experience, and current research. Practitioner creates goals that are client-centered and suitable to the family, setting, and child's strengths and challenges. |
| Ethical reasoning | Following the AOTA Code of Ethics (2020), and state and federal laws, facility policies, and procedures (Grajo & Rushanan, 2021) when thinking through what needs to be done in relation to what should be done (Boyt-Schell, 2019) | Practitioner advocates for resources and services for children and their families (justice); collaborates with families to meet their needs (beneficence); respects parents' decision (autonomy); and documents services honestly (veracity). |
| Interactive reasoning | Examining therapeutic communication and interactions as one engages with children and families | Practitioner provides positive verbal to encourage child to keep going. The child struggles but completes the task and smiles proudly. The practitioner makes a note that when provided support (physical or emotional), the child enjoys challenges. |
| Narrative reasoning | Using information or perspective from the client's story or lived experience to make decisions | Practitioner creates opportunities for a child to complete projects with peers for a child who "feels left out in school, because he is not able to do the same things they do. |
| Pragmatic reasoning | Considering the situation at present when making decisions, such as payor, referral source, resources, costs, environment, and duration of services | Practitioner creates intervention goals considering that the child is receiving services in an inpatient acute care hospital setting. |
| Procedural reasoning (may also be considered part of scientific reasoning) | Refers to making decisions based on a protocol or set of steps or processes | Practitioner followed the administration steps according to the test manual.<br>Practitioner created goals with the client as part of departmental policy. |
| Scientific reasoning | Seek to understand client's condition, cause, symptoms, progression of condition, and its effects on occupational performance (Boyt-Schell, 2019) | Practitioner hypothesizes that the progression of the child's condition will interfere with their ability to complete daily tasks. |

Base on Patnaude, M.E., (2023). Student success: Therapeutic reasoning process. In Jane O'Brien, M. E. Patnaude, & T. Garcia Reidy (Eds.), Therapeutic reasoning in occupational therapy (pp. 1–17). Elsevier.

**TABLE 35.2 Case Example Matrix**

| Name | Age | Setting | Diagnosis or Occupational Challenge | Conceptual Practice Model and Frame(s) of Reference |
|---|---|---|---|---|
| Blasie | 27 weeks gestation | Neonatal intensive care unit and early intervention | Prematurity | Medical model |
| Connor | 3 years old | Transition from early intervention to outpatient pediatric clinic | Cerebral palsy | Motor control and motor learning |
| Julian | 4 years old | Outpatient pediatric clinic | Mixed expressive and receptive communication delay | Person environment occupation performance model |
| Laura | 6 years old | School | Somatodyspraxia | Model of Human Occupation; Ayres Sensory integration; social and behavioral approaches |
| Kevin | 7 years old | Outpatient pediatric clinic | Duchenne muscular dystrophy | Model of Human Occupation; biomechanical; Intentional Relationship Model |
| Juana | 13 years old | Secondary school therapy group | Attention-deficit hyperactivity disorder | Occupational analysis and group processes; social behavioral approach |
| Alessio | 16 years old | Inpatient hospital setting | Cancer | Model of Human Occupation; biomechanical |
| Miriam | Transition aged | Secondary to postsecondary transition | Postsecondary transition challenges (secondary COVID-19 pandemic) | Person-environment-occupation (PEO) |

### Synopsis of Professional Reasoning

Occupational therapy practitioners working in a hospital setting often use **scientific reasoning** to understand the child's medical conditions and health status. For example, Blaise's condition (prematurity and fetal distress) may result in an immature nervous system, which impacts many aspects of occupational performance. He is at risk for physical (e.g., muscle tone challenges) and developmental delays (including cognitive, motor, social, communication, and sensory). Blaise will benefit from early intervention to address his developmental milestones, with specific consideration for feeding and eating issues.

Occupational therapy practitioners seek to understand the child's situation beyond the scientific level to support the family and his goals. They use **narrative reasoning** to understand the family's situation such as beliefs, values, goals, expectations, culture, and routines. Practitioners discuss children's progress, listen to family concerns, and allow the parents to describe their perspectives, feelings, and stresses. For example, Blaise's parents experienced stress as parents with three young children. The therapist supports parents and empowers family members by addressing their concerns and finding resources for them (for example, support groups, extra help, resources for children) as needed. They may explain things to family as needed. The therapist often used **interactive reasoning** to read the parents' and child's cues during intervention. For example, the therapist noted one day the parents' facial expressions when discussing the infant's progress. Together they discussed their feelings and realized the parents were overwhelmed with bringing the infant home who was not an "easy feeder." The therapist readjusted the intervention plan and suggested they meet the therapist who would be following up with them at home prior to discharge for a consultation. The parents were reassured that the follow-up would be scheduled and that the two therapists would discuss the care plan (so that they would not have to do that). The therapist used **ethical reasoning** to determine how to ensure the parents felt comfortable feeding their infant at home and getting the resources at home (beneficence). The therapist considered the privacy and confidentiality issues associated with having another therapist consult with them. The therapist will have the family complete the necessary forms prior to the meeting. The therapist will ask the parents again if they want this meeting (autonomy).

The occupational therapy practitioner working in the NICU uses **conditional reasoning** to create an intervention plan that considers the child's condition, age, and stage of development, family situation, setting specific guidelines, along with applying principles from the biomechanical frame of reference (regarding endurance for feeding and physical activity) to support an infant's occupation (e.g., feeding/eating, play, exploration, social interactions, and behaviors). The therapist provides the family with suggestions to promote development and allow them to feel comfortable with their newborn. The practitioner allows the family to express their stress related to the hospitalizations. As part of the professional reasoning process, the practitioner reviews each intervention session to reflect upon both the child's engagement, family questions and concerns, and their ability to meet their infant's and family's needs.

## EARLY INTERVENTION SETTING AND OUTPATIENT CARE

Contributed by Teressa Reidy, MS, OTR/L, and Patty Coker-Bolt, PhD, OTR/L, FNAP, FAOTA.

Connor, who is 2 years and 11 months old, has left-sided hemiplegic cerebral palsy. He has received early intervention occupational therapy services weekly since 9 months of age, and he will transition to an outpatient clinic when he turns 3 years and no longer qualifies for early intervention services. Connor continues to struggle with managing lower body dressing and transporting large toys from place to place. Connor recently started preschool, and his teacher reports that he has difficulty holding the paper with his left hand while grasping a marker with his right-dominant hand. He needs maximum assistance to don his jacket, and minimal assistance to doff it. This upsets Connor because he loves playground time with his peers. Connor enjoys active, outdoor play; he climbs in an adaptive way using his right hand.

The occupational therapy practitioner working in early intervention recommended Connor participate in an outpatient pediatric

**BOX 35.1 Constraint-induced movement therapy principles**

- Limitations in hand and arm activities prevent children from engaging in meaningful occupations.
- Restricting use of the unaffected limb encourages children to use their affected limb.
- Therapy involves massed, repetitive, and structured (scaffolded to promote success) practice of the affected arm and hand to promote movement through brain plasticity.
- Promoting problem-solving and practice with the affected arm and hand use in everyday situations reinforces motor learning.
- Intensive activity with the affected limb results in brain changes due to neuroplasticity (e.g., cortical reorganization, dendrite branching, redundancy learned, and improved synapsis).

course of *Constraint Induced Movement Therapy (CIMT)* to improve his left-hand grip and left upper body strength. CIMT is a widely used, evidenced-based intervention to address functional deficits of the upper extremity in children with hemiplegia (Chiu & Ada, 2016; DeLuca et al., 2017; Ramey et al., 2021). Box 35.1 provides a brief description of CIMT principles.

Connor's family enrolled him in a 4-week intensive CIMT program. The occupational therapist assessed Connor's skills at admission and discharge with the Quality of Upper Extremity Skills Test (QUEST) to measure hand function (DeMatteo et al., 1992) and the Canadian Occupational Performance measure (COPM) to measure performance satisfaction (Law et al., 1998). The therapist collaborated with Connor's father, and they created the following goals:

1. Connor will push both arms through the sleeves of a long sleeve shirt or jacket with minimal assistance from therapist or caregiver 100% of trials over 3 consecutive days.
2. Connor will pull up sweatpants from his knees to his waist after toileting with minimal assistance from therapist or caregiver 80% of trials over 3 consecutive days.

## Intervention Plan

The CIMT program consisted of task-specific practice for 3 hours a day, 5 days a week, for 4 consecutive weeks. The last 3 days of this program focused on bimanual activities that incorporated the new movements of Connor's left arm and hand into everyday tasks. This intensive program provided a total of 60 hours of therapy. During the CIMT program, Connor wore a cast on his strong, right upper extremity for 24 hours a day. He engaged in activities using his upper left extremity. The occupational therapy practitioner designed motivating and fun activities, tailored to Connor's interests, such as carrying a bucket loaded with toy cars and picking up the toy cars and putting them on a racetrack repeatedly.

His activity progressed incrementally as he mastered new tasks and gained new movement in his left upper extremity. For example, during the first week of the program, Connor put a car into a wide bucket on the floor, repeatedly, up to 30 times playing with different size and shape cars. The next week, Connor was able to release the cars onto a racetrack at eye level. During the third week, he was able to place the cars on a track above eye level with greater than 90 degrees of left shoulder flexion. The therapist started incorporating imaginary play activities, such as having Connor push his affected arm through dress-up clothes. These activities helped Connor generalize his new skills to engage in activities of daily living.

Prior to discharge the occupational therapy practitioner provided a comprehensive "transfer plan" that included home activities embedded into Connor's self-care and play routine. This ensured that Connor continued to use his newly developed movement in his left arm and hand skills in everyday activities.

The occupational therapy practitioner followed up a week later with a telehealth session to observe Connor's functioning in his home environment. The practitioner observed Connor use both hands together to put on his coat and play catch with his father. The therapist provided coaching and positive feedback as needed. Connor's father reported that they noticed that Connor spontaneously used his left hand when climbing the stairs to the slide and used both hands on the playground equipment more consistently. They noted Connor was less frustrated at school when preparing for recess.

## Synopsis of Professional Reasoning

Connor's occupational therapy practitioners followed motor control and motor learning principles (Chapter 29) to guide Connor's therapy. They used scientific reasoning as they determined that his diagnosis of hemiplegia and his age and level of functioning would make him a good candidate for CIMT. The practitioner engaged in **procedural reasoning** by following the protocol guidelines, documenting Connor's performance, and creating the intervention plan. This required they use conditional reasoning to integrate Connor's strengths (such as his love of cars and trucks, personal style, and ability to play) and challenges (such as limited use left hand, frustration when he is not able to do things), goals, in combination with the CIMT protocol, setting, family expectations, and team.

During the intervention sessions, the practitioner used interactive reasoning as they watched Connor and adjusted, encouraged, and cued him as needed so he would not become frustrated but would challenge his abilities. The practitioner played with Connor and was mindful of their therapeutic interactions, reflecting on their mode use as described in the Intentional Relationship Model (Taylor, 2020, Chapter 3).

The practitioner used ethical reasoning as a foundation for the intervention sessions. The practitioner was honest throughout the intervention session about the child's progress and the effectiveness of the intervention, answered questions truthfully, and documented correctly (veracity). The practitioner respected the family's right to miss a session (autonomy) and did not treat them differently for missing (justice). The practitioner continued to provide intervention to address the child's challenges using the CIMT protocol and in a fun and motivating way that supported the child's self-efficacy (beneficence).

Throughout the occupational therapy process, the practitioners reflected on the CIMT protocol, motor control and motor learning strategies, and their therapeutic use of self. They used **metacognition** to consider what was working, things that could be enhanced, and areas they could learn more about to benefit the child.

# OUTPATIENT SETTING

When Julian was 2 years old, his parents noticed that he did not communicate like his peers. Julian met or exceeded expected gross and fine motor milestones, and the pediatrician noted that children achieve milestones at different stages. The pediatrician advised the parents to wait a few months. However, Julian was referred to a speech-language pathologist (SLP) a few months later where he received a diagnosis of mixed expressive and receptive language delays. After a year of speech-language service, Julian was more expressive with both verbal and nonverbal communication. However, the speech language pathologist noted he had trouble with transitions, where he would throw, kick, or flail his arms and legs when it was time to leave or complete a task. He was referred to occupational therapy services to identify possible causes of these behaviors.

Julian was scheduled for an occupational therapy evaluation. Grady, a fieldwork student, conducted the initial evaluation with oversight from his fieldwork coordinator. Grady decided to use the Person-Environment-Occupation-Performance Model (PEOP) to frame the assessment and intervention planning. Grady created questions generated from the model to obtain an occupational narrative. He decided to gather information by interviewing the parents and observing Julian and conducting a standardized assessment to determine his gross and fine motor skill levels.

### Observations and Findings

Grady gathered information from the parents and clinical observations. Julian is a 4-year-old boy who lives with his parents in a third floor apartment in the Midwestern United States. His parents reported no complication during pregnancy and delivery. A recent physical examination found no visual or hearing difficulties. Julian is within the expected range for weight and height. Julian's mother stated, "Julian loves to play with toys, bath time, and water play. But we struggle to interact with him. He wants to do things when and how he wants it."

Grady was not able to conduct a standardized assessment. Julian did not follow simple 2-step directions and refused items that he did not want to do. Grady made the following behavioral observations:

- Julian responded 50% of the time when his name was called. Julian smiled with his parents. He made intermittent eye contact and did not smile at Grady. For example, he did not play catch with Grady, but he did with his parents.
- Julian eloped three times from the occupational therapy room into the therapy gym, which contained a slide, ball pit, and swings. After the third time, Grady conducted the rest of the evaluation in the therapy gym.
- Julian jumped on two feet and loved the feeling of jumping into the ball pit. He splashed around the ball pit as if it was water, and threw, with one hand, toys out of the ball pit.
- Julian struggled to leave the session despite prompts and a transition toy. Julian cried and knocked games off the shelf. His father picked up Julian and took him outside of the clinic.
- Julian has difficulty with expressive and receptive language skills but responds to familiar people.
- He does not make eye contact with unfamiliar people and has trouble with transitions.

### Interpretation

Grady hypothesized that Julian's difficulties with communication (expressive and receptive language skills) interfere with transitions and play behaviors. Grady further hypothesized that Julian may be uncomfortable around new people (as evidenced by his lack of eye contact) because he has difficulty communicating. Grady also noted Julian calmed to sensory input such as jumping and will examine this further during the next session.

### Synopsis of Professional Reasoning

The occupational therapy practitioner used the PEOP model to obtain a holistic perspective on the factors related to the child, occupation, and environment that influence Julian's occupational performance. Grady had to quickly change his plans during the evaluation when Julian refused to complete the assessments of follow simple directions. This requires the practitioner to use flexible thinking in real time and change one's plan, which relies on quickly analyzing the situation, reading the child's cues.

After the evaluation, Grady used **conditional reasoning** to put all the information together and create a plan that would specifically work for Julian and his family within the school and home environment. For example, Grady observed Julian make eye contact with his mother and play a game of catch. This provided evidence that Julian has this ability, which Grady can use to facilitate play with peers at school.

As Grady reflected on the assessment, he realized that he needed to be conscious of his decisions during intervention upcoming sessions. He will have to carefully use **interactive reasoning** to time turn taking and social play so that Julian does not become frustrated, overwhelmed, and flee to another room.

Grady plans to search for information and strategies from developmental, social, and behavioral approaches to use in the intervention session. His goal for the next session is to examine Julian's sensory needs to identify those activities that are enjoyable for Julian. He will engage Julian in novel, interesting, and challenging activities (providing cues as needed, but allowing Julian to problem solve as well), paying attention to verbal and nonverbal cues regarding how to interact.

## SCHOOL SETTING

Contributed by Virginia Spielmann PhD, OTR/L.

Six-year-old Laura started Kindergarten 10 weeks ago. In the first 3 weeks of school, Laura was asked to stand by the teacher's desk, and this quickly escalated to standing outside the classroom. Her teacher explained that her attention-seeking behaviors disrupted the learning of the other students. After being sent to the principal's office for the third time, a parent meeting was held. The team felt that Laura's enthusiasm about learning and school, and classroom membership, did not match her current behaviors. She was referred for an occupational therapy assessment to identify supports and barriers to classroom participation.

Laura's parents reported that she met her developmental milestones (including speech and language) "on time." She started crawling around 11 months, and she "enjoyed making people laugh by crawling from a seated position with one arm in a kind of step-scoot." This stage passed quickly as Laura went straight to cruising around the furniture before walking independently at around 19 months. Her parents described her as a cheerful child with a winning smile. The preschool teachers reported that she had many friends and was well liked by teachers.

### Occupational Profile

Laura lives at home with both parents, Abuela (grandmother), and three older sisters. The family speaks English and Spanish at home. She was excited to attend the same school as her sisters and enthusiastic about learning. Laura, her sisters, and mother walk to school together each morning. Laura enjoys swimming in the small pool shared by their rental community and visiting splash pads. Laura loves everything related to horses. Her father works full time, and her mother, a nurse practitioner, intends to return to work soon.

### Gathering Information and Assessment

Table 35.3 outlines the methods used to assess Laura's performance. While gathering the initial data, Laura's occupational therapist began to hypothesize that sensory integration and processing may be influencing Laura's occupational performance. The occupational therapist proceeded to gather further information about sensory integration and processing differences and their connection to function within the academic setting. Therefore, as part of the evaluation process, the occupational therapist also completed:

- Structured Observations of Sensory Integration-Motor (SOSI-M) and the Comprehensive Observations of Proprioception (COP-R) (Blanche et al., 2021)

**TABLE 35.3 Summary of Laura's Assessment Findings**

| Method | Summary of Findings |
|---|---|
| Teacher interview<br>Abbreviated Short Child Occupational Profile (SCOPE) (Bowyer et al., 2008) | • Class comedian<br>• Often seems to seek approval from teacher<br>• Knocks over other children's belongings<br>• Only gets upset once she has been sent into hallway<br>• Often seems surprised when she moves down the reward chart and loses privileges<br>• Requires multiple cues and substantial assistance during transition times<br>• Requires occasional cueing and redirection during transitions<br>• Spontaneously initiates and maintains conversations with peers and adults<br>• Demonstrates some ability to maintain relationships<br>• Is rarely able to make a plan and requires significant cues to follow through with a plan<br>• Exhibits uncoordinated movement through some fine and gross motor activities |

- Parent report measure: Sensory Processing Measure – 2 (SPM–2) (Parham et al., 2021)

In reporting the evaluation findings, the occupational therapist used impact statements to connect client factors to occupational outcomes of function and participation.

**Impact of Challenges With Motor Planning on Observable Behaviors and Classroom Citizenship.** Laura's ability to organize her body, plan, sequence movement, and execute a motor plan is not at age expectation. These sensory processes support movement, learning, and play at a subconscious and automatic level. Laura, however, must exert a considerable amount of attention and conscious thought to be successful in daily activities. When a motor task is new or complex (in Laura's case involving more than three steps), she tends to become dysregulated (i.e., inability to control one's emotional response), and her body moves into a state of high arousal (i.e., behaviors where child has difficulty focusing, concentrating, or attending). At this point, she may exhibit behaviors, such as impulsivity and silliness (e.g., goofing or clowning around). While Laura is eager to engage in classroom activities, please her teacher, and be liked, she uses laughter as a useful strategy for distracting others from her motor challenges.

**Impact of Challenges With Sequencing Tasks on Engagement in Classroom Learning Activities.** Laura is not yet able to remember multiple steps to complete a task successfully. She either relies on step-by-step demonstration (which she can do with her sisters or friends) or does her best with what she does remember, leading to poor and incomplete work. Laura also has difficulty visualizing other ways that things might be done. For example, she struggles to problem solve when an activity does not go as planned. She often becomes overwhelmed by the cognitive effort she uses to compensate for body-based planning and sequencing challenges. Laura's has difficulty with tactile discrimination (i.e., making sense of what she touches). For example, she had difficulty organizing objects that are in a lidded container, pot, or zipped-up case. Laura's strategy for managing many small items (i.e., markers, pencils, crayons, etc.) consists of tipping them out and spreading them across the floor or surface until she can locate and pick up the needed item with ease. Laura's difficulty with motor planning, sequencing, and tactile discrimination influences her grasp development and general tool use. She holds markers and crayons with a palmar grasp.

**Impact of Challenges With Generating Ideas for Action on Recess Behaviors.** Laura has a small repertoire of play ideas for open-ended or free play; these tend to involve cause and effect play (knocking things over), chasing, and pretending to be a horse. She struggles to play in novel ways and incorporate the ideas of others. However, as a very social and outgoing child, she aptly recruits her classmates into her style of play rather than being left out.

### Evaluation Summary

Laura is an outgoing and enthusiastic 6-year-old who is excited about school and wants to be an active member of her classroom community. She struggles with creating and executing a motor plan, especially as it increases in complexity and novelty. These performance patterns are particularly mismatched to the activities and environmental challenges of recess and physical education.

### Goals

The occupational therapist used goal attainment scaling to set goals in collaboration with the individualized education plan (IEP) team and family. Laura's goals, listed in Table 35.4, were set with a plan to review in 12 weeks.

### Synopsis of Professional Reasoning

The occupational therapist began the evaluation using an occupation-centered model of practice, Model of Human Occupation (MOHO), which examined interaction between person elements (volition, habituation, and performance capacity) and the environment. The therapist used **conditional reasoning** to synthesize the information to create an intervention plan. During the evaluation the therapist became aware that Laura experienced occupational performance challenges related to recess and school, although she was motivated to engage with others and participate in school activities. According to MOHO, the discrepancy between Laura's ability to do those things that she wanted to do results in frustration and decreased self-efficacy, which may interfere with her occupational identity.

The therapist identified Laura's strengths as her desire to engage socially and participate in school. Furthermore, the therapist hypothesized that challenges in sensory-based motor planning caused her to "act out" at school. The therapist supported this hypothesis by observing Laura's challenges in vestibular (e.g., balance), proprioception (e.g., sense of muscles and joints), and tactile discrimination (e.g., ability to identify objects with touch), which all contribute to motor planning.

The therapist used **pragmatic reasoning** to make the referral to an outpatient therapist to address sensory integration challenges directly, as occupational therapy practitioners working in school systems address school-based challenges. The school-based therapist used social and behavioral approaches to engage Laura in activities to strengthen her ability to organize her movements, engage with others, and express herself in the classroom. She created intervention to teach Laura new skills (such as communication and negotiation) and provided strategies to help Laura organize her classroom materials, follow directions, and play with peers. The therapists used a variety of activities that allowed Laura to develop skills and feel successful, contributing to feelings of self-efficacy and leading to occupational identity.

**TABLE 35.4 Laura's Goal Attainment Scaled Goals**

| −2 | −1 | 0 | 1 | 2 |
|---|---|---|---|---|
| Laura struggles to manage and organize writing/art supplies, and containers/ fastener. She tends to dump items all over the desk and floor due to poor tactile discrimination. | In the writing center, Laura will be able to identify writing/art supplies with three attempts. | In the writing center, Laura will be able to identify writing/art supplies with two attempts. | In the writing center, Laura will be able to identify writing/art supplies with one attempt. | In the writing center, Laura will be able to independently identify writing/art supplies. |
| When Laura becomes dysregulated, she acts "impulsive and goofy" per teacher report. | Laura will identify when she is becoming dysregulated with direct questioning from the teacher. | Laura will identify when she is becoming dysregulated and attempt to use a sensory strategy with verbal prompts from the teacher. | Laura will identify when she is becoming dysregulated and attempt to use a sensory strategy. | Laura will identify when she is becoming dysregulated and successfully use a sensory strategy. |
| Laura is unable to process and retain multistep spoken instructions. She tends to jump ahead leading to incomplete and inaccurate work products. | During literacy center activities with verbal prompts and a visual schedule, Laura will be able to complete a two-step task successfully. | During literacy center activities with verbal prompts Laura will be able to complete a two-step task successfully. | During literacy center activities Laura will be able to complete a two-step task independently. | During literacy center activities with verbal prompts and a visual schedule, Laura will be able to complete a three-step task successfully. |
| Laura has a limited repertoire of play and relies on one or two familiar ideas for play (i.e., horses, chase, etc.) | During recess Laura will explore a new idea in play (construction play, motor, pretend, role play etc.) one time per week. | During recess Laura will explore a new idea in play (construction play, motor, pretend, role play etc.) two times per week. | During recess Laura will explore a new idea in play (construction play, motor, pretend, role play etc.) three times per week. | During recess Laura will explore a new idea in play (construction play, motor, pretend, role play etc.) four times per week. |

## SCHOOL SETTING

Contributed by Mikkel Wilson, Kristen Mollineau, and Lynthea Reefe.

Kevin is a school-aged child who was referred to occupational therapy services secondary to functional limitations caused by his diagnosis of Duchenne muscular dystrophy (DMD). Kevin can independently complete most self-care activities; however, he struggles with timing, pacing, and energy conservation in carrying out those activities. Kevin has a supportive home and school environment in which his family and friends strive to provide him with the right support to complete his daily occupations. Kevin's lower muscle tone and limited range of motion affect his ability to ambulate for long periods without fatigue. Despite his outgoing personality, superior social skills, and competency with age-related assistive technology at home, Kevin struggles with self-confidence and interacting with unfamiliar people. Kevin's father hopes that occupational therapy will assist Kevin with his self-confidence and self-acceptance in relation to his ability to complete daily tasks, to learn energy conservation techniques, to improve his ambulation, and to decrease his fatigue during self-care activities. Kevin was assessed by Mindy, a pediatric occupational therapist, and her fieldwork student Noemi. Noemi utilized the MOHO to structure her therapeutic reasoning during the evaluation. Results were organized based on MOHO elements (Taylor et al., 2024).

### Volition

Kevin's father indicated that Kevin experiences low self-confidence, as exhibited by his desire to be lifted and carried when meeting new people or in unfamiliar environments and his unwillingness to speak about his diagnosis.

Since Kevin's father was monopolizing the evaluation, Noemi wanted to learn more about Kevin from Kevin's perspective. Kevin shyly stated that he enjoys playing with the tablet and his parents' cellphone. On the weekend, he enjoys spending time with his older brother watching movies, swimming, and roughhousing.

### Habituation

While Kevin did not use this terminology, Noemi noted that Kevin participates in the student, brother, friend, and religious participant roles. Related to those roles, Kevin attends a public school with his older brother. A typical weekend for Kevin, includes waking up to some tablet time, watching YouTube videos, swimming in the pool, and attending Sunday services and religious education classes at the local Anglican church.

### Performance Capacity

Kevin does not like to discuss his diagnosis, nor how it impacts him in his daily life. Observationally, Kevin performs the actions of independently donning and doffing a shirt and manipulating his lunch box and containers to access food. He is also able to utilize utensils. He struggles with manipulating containers that have twist-on tops. Kevin is unable to thoroughly wash and dry his body and face, don socks, and tie his shoes. He experiences challenges with community mobility and is only able to walk for about 2 minutes at a time before becoming fatigued. In the pool, Kevin typically lies on a floating device.

### Environment

Kevin has a supportive social environment with his family. His parents actively seek medical and therapeutic interventions to support him. Kevin's home is a one-story ranch. His school environment has also made accommodations by keeping his classroom on the ground floor. His brother carries his bag into school so that he does not get too tired while walking to class.

### Interpretation

Noemi hypothesized that Kevin may struggle with learned helplessness (i.e., dependence upon others even when they are able to participate on their own). He engages in physically demanding activities with his brother and friends but not with his parents. Additionally, Kevin's family may enable some of the behaviors as indicated by his father speaking for Kevin, rather than encouraging Kevin to speak. Related to performance capacity, Noemi was unable to obtain information about Kevin's lived experience with DMD from his perspective.

### Plan

The occupational therapy plan focused on improving Kevin's independence in self through energy conservation strategies and fostering self-confidence and self-efficacy. As Kevin gains confidence and competence by independently completing his self-care tasks, he will become able to complete a variety of tasks in numerous situations, resulting in occupational adaptation and a sense of occupational identity. Table 35.5 outlines Kevin's intervention plan.

### Synopsis of Professional Reasoning

Noemi and Mindy utilized the Model of Human Occupation (MOHO) to structure their professional reasoning. Noemi examined the child's volition, habituation, performance capacity, and environment to understand Keven's strengths and challenges and to create an intervention plan. Using this model allowed the therapist to use a strengths-based approach to address Kevin's occupational performance. They examined the interactions between the systems and created goals to enable Kevin to succeed, develop competence leading to self-efficacy, occupational identity, and eventually occupational adaptation. The intervention plan included targeting Kevin's performance capacity in terms of endurance using a biomechanical frame of reference. The practitioner engages Kevin in repeated meaningful activities designed to conserve energy so he could engage in the activity for longer periods of time. They also used the principle of MOHO that a change in any one element (i.e., performance capacity) would result in changes in other systems (O'Brien & Wolske, 2024), such as volition, resulting in the child being more engaged in doing his routines, play, and gaining a sense of purpose through doing.

As the therapists guided Kevin by providing cues, coaching, validating, and providing physical assistance, they were mindful of their interactions. They used **interactive reasoning** during the sessions by considering their mode as cited in the Intentional Relationship Model (Taylor, 2020). They reflected throughout the intervention process on their approaches, activities, and guidance. They used **conditional reasoning** throughout the process to consider multiple aspects of Kevin's story, performance, resources, and theory.

## SCHOOL SETTING

Juana is a seventh-grade girl who takes part in a 10-person social and executive functioning skills group at her middle school. The group is facilitated by Sade, the speech-language pathologist, and Eleonora, a certified occupational therapy assistant, who both recognized that they had many of the same students on their caseloads who had mental health and executive functioning needs. The goal of the group is to facilitate executive functioning skills (e.g., planning and organization), social skills (e.g., expressive communication, negotiating, problem-solving), and a sense of belonging (e.g., teamwork, friendships, peer support) through participation in activities and occupations.

Sade and Eleonora considered various aspects of group structure, climate, and styles of leadership when creating the group (Lambdin-Pattavina, 2021). The group was organized with a democratic style, so that Sade and Eleonora served as group facilitators, and the students had input in the group norms and expectations. The group met twice a month for 30 minutes in a classroom within the school building.

**TABLE 35.5 Kevin's Occupational Therapy Plan**

| Short-Term Goal Areas | Frame of Reference Used to Address Goals | Intervention Approaches/Methods |
|---|---|---|
| Increase independence in self-care activities while considering energy conservation strategies. | Biomechanical | Principles of energy conservation: Use proximal over distal control as possible; take frequent pauses during activity; sit when possible. Prioritize activities throughout the day (compensate or use adaptive equipment to make other tasks easier). The practitioner will provide education, a visual schedule to remind the child, and practice strategies in sessions. |
| | Intentional Relationship Model (Taylor, 2020) | In the therapeutic setting, corrective modifications to the environment will be offered to the client while performing self-care tasks. The practitioner will use instructing and encouraging modes to encourage the client to complete the task. |
| Foster self-confidence, self-efficacy, and occupational identity. | Model of Human Occupation (Taylor et al., 2024) | Engage the child's volition through meaningful activities to promote a sense of achievement such as the use of meaningful social stories. |
| | Intentional Relationship Model (Taylor, 2020) | The child's competitive nature will be used in the sessions to motivate and challenge him so he feels a sense of accomplishment. The practitioner will use collaborating and problem-solving modes to promote the child's confidence and belief in his abilities, while also using empathizing mode to support the child's engagement in difficult tasks. |

**Sample Group Session.** During a group session, Juana suggests eagerly to the group "Spring break will start in a few weeks; maybe we can help decorate the school to celebrate?" The group votes and decides that their goal for the next month is to decorate the school for spring break. They brainstorm for 15 minutes about all the tasks and activities they need to complete (with guidance from Sade and Eleonora). The group created the following list:

- Obtain administrative approval.
- Determine materials.
- Determine how materials will be obtained, and with what funding.
- Create a budget for decorations.
- Raise funds for the decorations.
- Order the materials.
- Plan a day and time to decorate.

Since this was Juana's idea, she was selected to lead the group. The therapists guided Juana on how to motivate members, including everyone, and how to keep the activity fun. They praised her efforts. Juana was proud of the decorations and her role, and she thanked the group for all their work. As the group reflected on the project, many members expressed how nice it felt to give back to the school and even praised individual members' artwork. They agreed they would like to do something like this again, perhaps for Valentine's Day.

### Synopsis of Professional Reasoning

The school-based team utilized group processes to create and implement a group-based intervention plan. This occurred because two practitioners identified the commonalities of the occupational challenges they saw among their respective caseloads. Through the group process, the students gained executive functioning skills and a sense of belonging important for mental health through occupation-based tasks (such as decorating the school).

The therapists used professional reasoning skills during the planning, implementation, and assessment stages of the group. They identified the purpose of the group and selected members that would fit the purpose (to promote sense of belonging, social participation, and mental health needs of children in school). They used procedural reasoning to design the format, structure, and expectations of the group. They employed pragmatic reasoning when deciding it would meet twice a week for 30 minutes due to classroom schedules. They also considered the room, budget for supplies, and expectations of members based on schedules. During the group sessions, the therapists used **conditional reasoning** to promote each member's goals in different ways and in relation to other members and the circumstances of the day. They adjusted expectations as needed and used **interactive reasoning** to make decisions about how to address topics, moods, or statements. As the group gained a sense of unity, belongingness, and emotional safety, the therapists provided coaching on coping strategies and addressed more sensitive topics (while still following school procedures to inform parents as needed). The therapists found they also engaged in interactive reasoning to read each other and determine when to intervene or step back. They reflected after each session to make decisions about the next week, plan activities, and reassess the member's goals.

## HOSPITAL SETTING

"I just want to enjoy life. I want to enjoy it with no regrets," I told my cousin over the phone. The silence for his reply feels like an eternity. We continued to chat about my cancer symptoms. After pouring my heart out to him for the past 10 minutes about my cancer-based worries, all he can respond with is, "Well, at least you are sporting a sweet haircut!" I know he's trying to help, but I feel self-conscious about how the chemotherapy has impacted my body. I quickly return, "You promise that you will shave your head too?" "I promise," he replies.

I glance at myself in the mirror—after a few weeks of treatment, I decided to shave my hair because it was falling out in clumps. The doctors warned me of this. As I lie back in my hospital bed, the images of the past few months swirl around me as if I stuck my head into a beehive. I feel the intensity of the worry and despair bubbling up to the surface. I feel like I have been condemned to a sanitized prison sentence of a hospital. I keep hearing the word "cancer" in my head. For a few weeks, I had a throat infection. The doctor initially brushed off the concern. But then a tiredness washed over me like I had never experienced before. I was bruising easily, and my skin grew pale. One night, I woke up in night sweats with a raging fever. Not long after a rush to the hospital, I was diagnosed with acute myeloid leukemia.

I don't know if I will ever participate in my high school graduation, let alone go to prom, obtain my driver's license, have a girlfriend, or play sports with my friends again. I want to see my mom and dad. I want to tease my sister. I want to taste my grandmother's cooking. All my family annoyances seem trivial now. As the feelings wash over me, and tears swell in the bottom of my eyes, a knock at the door diverts my attention.

"Oh, it's you again. "Why are you always so happy?" I bemoan. "Because I get to work with all of my wonderful patients," Veronica, my occupational therapist, says as she bounces into the hospital room. I try to choke down my scoff.

"How has your day been?" Veronica asks. I ponder to myself. Well, I have been having a hard time swallowing food and liquid due to the mouth sores that have developed from the chemotherapy. Except, I don't even want to eat food because I'm nauseous. My muscle mass is gone. I can barely get up from this bed. And on top of that, I fall asleep randomly.

"Eh," I respond. Veronica begins to say something, but I ignore her and watch highlights of the football game on TV. As she drones on, I hear her say something of interest.

"What?" I ask. Veronica explains that she sees I frequently watch sports on TV, so she figured that we could start our session by throwing around a football. As we throw the football back and forth, Veronica encourages me to sit at the edge of the bed with the best posture that I can. My back feels stiff, but I think I am doing a good job. I tell Veronica, "Now, if only we can go outside" as I look toward the window. Veronica explains that we cannot go outside due to my compromised immune system. That was all I needed to hear so that I could ignore her again.

Meanwhile Angelica, my nurse, walks into the room and says dryly, "The OTs have an interesting job. Just don't hit any of the equipment with that football, Veronica. I have to note his vitals. Blood pressure is 130/78, heart rate is 75, and oxygen is 98%, not bad." I like Angelica. She's sarcastic, and blunt, like me. Meanwhile, Veronica is over here living her best life treating kids in the cancer ward.

### Synopsis of Professional Reasoning

Implicitly, it appears that Veronica utilized aspects of Model of Human Occupation (MOHO), such as volition, to try and utilize Alessio's interest to participate in therapy. Veronica also utilized aspects of the biomechanical frame of reference to work on Alessio's sitting tolerance and general strength and endurance. However, Veronica seemed to lack the insight into understanding how her own therapeutic use of self influenced Alessio. Veronica can learn more about her choices to become an even more effective practitioner by engaging in metacognitive activities, such as reflecting on the session and her reasoning, discussing with peers, reading more on MOHO, and thinking about Alessio's responses, goals, and situation.

Veronica used scientific reasoning as she used knowledge of Alessio's condition and biomechanical principles to create a plan. However, she did not use conditional reasoning to synthesize information about his story (narrative reasoning) and the pragmatic resources available (such as walking to the cafeteria, listening to sounds, looking outside, opening a window) or interactive reasoning

TABLE 35.6 **Summary of Accompany Program Evaluation**

| Person (Clients Served) | Environment (Supports and Barriers) | Occupation (Tasks Associated With Social Participation and Education) |
|---|---|---|
| 18–21 years old<br>The most prominent diagnosis is autism spectrum disorder.<br>Have an individualized education plan (IEP).<br>Seek an associate degree or certificate program in the postsecondary setting.<br>Some students also hold a part-time job, participate in community or church activities, and act as caregivers.<br>Skills and abilities to participate in academic work with accommodations (as determined in IEP). | Students attend the postsecondary institution, rather than the high school setting.<br>Students have different routines, class schedules, and modes with which they take courses.<br>Each postsecondary institution has different modes of classes (e.g., online self-pace, blended, and in-person).<br>Each postsecondary institution offers numerous days and times in which classes can be taken.<br>The social environment differs at each postsecondary institution including what services, organizations, clubs, and activities are offered.<br>Student support services are present through the Accompany program (and institution services, such as computer technology, writing support, and faculty office hours). | Navigating the postsecondary education system<br>Obtaining the college student role<br>Participating in classes by engaging in work and asking questions<br>Community mobility and transportation to and from the program and postsecondary institution varies depending on where the student lives<br>Social interaction and participation in class and in social events on campus and after classes<br>Time management to get work done on time and manage online work<br>Self-advocacy with instructors and staff regarding rights and accommodations |

within her intervention session. Veronica attempted to use interactive reasoning by using humor and knowledge of his interests. However, despite Alessio ignoring her attempts, she continues to press on with her treatment, without integrating what she has learned about him.

Veronica could have used more narrative reasoning paired with the MOHO to gauge Alessio's interest and volitional desires to go outside. Alessio is also very aware of his lived body and the changes his body has undergone as a result of his cancer diagnosis, as noted by his internal dialog. Had Veronica built more of a trusting rapport, and matched his emotional state, Alessio may have been more open to discussing his thoughts, feelings, frustrations, and views of his own performance capacities with Veronica. Thus, she would be able to provide future interventions that are more meaningful and targeted to his needs.

## HIGH SCHOOL SETTING AND TRANSITION PLANNING

Miriam is an occupational therapist who works as a consultant in private practice. Miriam was recently contacted by a transition program, Accompany, to help them establish goals and metrics for their program. Accompany is a school-based transition program for students leaving high school. The program's mission is to assist students aged 18 to 21 years in obtaining the skills necessary for postsecondary pursuits. The Accompany program frequently collaborates with local agencies and postsecondary 2-year institutions. In recent years due to the COVID-19 pandemic, students have struggled both with participating in the program and meeting their postsecondary goals. Some students failed classes they took at the postsecondary institutions, leading to participant and familial dissatisfaction. As a result, the principal of the school and the transition coordinator want to re-envision the Accompany program to best serve students after the pandemic.

Miriam utilized the Person-Environment-Occupation-Performance (PEOP) (Law et al., 1996) model to better understand the needs of the Accompany Program. Using PEOP provided a structure to examine the fit between the person, environment, and occupation to understand the occupational performance of clients (Law et al., 1996). Miriam completed three separate visits to obtain the information she needed to create relevant and meaningful program goals and metrics. Miriam visited a high school and two local community colleges, interviewed current students and alumni of the Accompany program, and spoke with faculty and staff. Table 35.6 summarizes her findings.

Miriam considered the student and the environment (i.e., postsecondary institute) in combination with the occupations the students must engage in (i.e., education, social participation). The Accompany program can support students' occupational performance by providing one-on-one support, resources, and referrals to support services on campus.

Miriam explained that one-on-one support with coaching was necessary to ensure that the program maintained a student-centered approach. The person, environment, and occupation vary from each student and institution. Miriam recommended that the best place to start is to focus on addressing the need to navigate the postsecondary environment. Additionally, students need to learn to seek out appropriate support and communicate their needs over time.

### Synopsis of Professional Reasoning

Miriam gathered comprehensive data from stakeholders through discussion and observation and organized her findings and observations using the PEOP model. She examined the findings and explored the interactions between multiple systems to create goals for the Accompany program. She used **conditional reasoning** to synthesize the information from multiple sources, while considering the missions of the program, high schools, and students' needs. She considered resources (e.g., personnel, financial, physical) and factored in the individual students' needs. Consulting regarding program analysis requires advance reasoning skills to interview stakeholders (paying attention to verbal and nonverbal communication using **interactive reasoning**). It requires knowledge of the educational system and factors influencing enrollment, as well as knowledge of the students' needs. **Narrative reasoning** often adds to the quality of the data used to inform decisions by providing stories from stakeholders. It also involves **pragmatic reasoning,** where the consultant examines available resources (e.g., transportation, building, type of classes offered, services available, funding sources). **Ethical reasoning** requires the consultant to be truthful, honest, and provide quality assessment and recommendations. It requires the consultant to understand laws and regulations when making recommendations.

Miriam used metacognition skills as she reflected upon the data she received from observations and discussions to create recommendations based on current resources and students' needs. She synthesized information from reliable sources and used knowledge from occupational therapy and educational research to support her recommendations.

## CONCLUSION

This chapter provided case studies that spanned various settings, situations, and experiences in pediatric occupational therapy practice to illustrate the professional reasoning process. Occupational therapy practitioners engage in professional reasoning (also referred to as clinical reasoning and therapeutic reasoning) at every step of the occupational therapy process. Reflecting on one's reasoning is essential for best practice. Using case examples provides a tool to examine one's reasoning and can enhance practitioners' understanding of the process. Occupational therapy practitioners can continue to develop professional reasoning as they critically reflect and engage in professional reasoning.

1. Conceptual practice models (including occupation-centered models of practice and frames of reference) provide theory, principles, strategies, and techniques to inform practice decisions. Occupational therapy practitioners use knowledge of the client, setting, and clinical experience to select evaluation methods, create goals and intervention plans, implement plans, and reassess to measure outcomes. By using professional reasoning along with knowledge of conceptual practice models that are developed based on theory and research evidence, practitioners can tailor practice approaches, strategies, and techniques to individual clients.
2. The types of professional reasoning include conditional, ethical, interactive, narrative, pragmatic, procedural, and scientific types. Each type of reasoning informs occupational therapy practice decisions. Since occupational therapy practitioners work with a variety of children and their families, and address everyday activities, they engage in complex reasoning involving multiple types. Understanding the types of reasoning allows practitioners to explore their thought process more effectively to benefit children and families.
3. The case examples provided in this chapter highlight a variety of person factors, including age, condition, physical, sensory, cognitive, and social emotional ones. The case examples address occupations including self-care, school, social participation, work, play, leisure, and community involvement. Furthermore, occupational therapy practitioners consider the environment (e.g., physical, social, and attitudinal) when creating goals and designing intervention. The cases provided illustrate how decisions may be influenced by family, work setting, home, and community.
4. Analyzing case examples allows practitioners to examine concepts that reflect occupational therapy practice. Engaging in problem-solving, information gathering, and examination of the process, principles, and concepts through case analysis provides practice in a relaxed setting to support learning. It allows readers to think through things, revisit content, and make decisions based on available information. The case examples provided are based on actual clients to allow readers to reflect, gain new knowledge, and apply concepts for use in practice. Readers may want to re-read selected chapters to gain new insights and apply knowledge to case examples. For example, readers may apply the same case using a different occupation-centered frame of reference. It may be beneficial to discuss your thought process and questions you have regarding the cases with peers, to stimulate ongoing professional reasoning development. Appendix B lists all the case studies that are present throughout this textbook, so that you may access other case examples to develop professional reasoning for practice.

## REFERENCES


Allen, D. D., & Toth-Cohen, S. (2019). Use of case studies to promote critical thinking in occupational therapy students. *Journal of Occupational Therapy Education, 3*(3), 1–18.

Blanche, E. I., Reinoso, G., & Kiefer, D. B. (2021). *Structured observations of sensory integration-motor*. Academic Therapy Publications.

Bowyer, P., Kramer, J., Ploszaj, A., Ross, M., Schwartz, O., Kielhofner, G., & Kramer, K. (2008). *The Short Child Occupational Profile (SCOPE) (version 2.2)*. Model of Human Occupation Clearinghouse, Department of Occupational Therapy, University of Illinois at Chicago.

Boyt-Schell, B. A. (2019). Professional reasoning in practice. In B. A. B. Schell, & G. Gillen (Eds.), *Willard and Spackman's occupational therapy* (13th ed.) (pp. 482–497). Wolters Kluwer.

Chiu, H.-C., & Ada, L. (2016). Constraint-induced movement therapy improves upper limb activity and participation in hemiplegic cerebral palsy: A systematic review. *Journal of Physiotherapy, 62*, 130–137.

DeLuca, S. C., Trucks, M. R., Wallace, D. A., & Ramey, S. L. (2017). Practice-based evidence from a clinical cohort that received pediatric constraint-induced movement therapy. *Journal of Pediatric Rehabilitation Medicine, 10*, 37–46.

DeMatteo, C., Law, M., Russel, D., Pollock, N., Rosenbaum, P., & Walter, S. (1992). *QUEST: Quality of upper extremity skills test*. McMaster University, CanChild Centre for Childhood Disability Research.

Grajo, L., & Rushanan, S. (2021). Ethical decision-making in occupational therapy practice. In J. O'Brien, & J. Solomon (Eds.), *Occupational analysis and group process* (2nd ed.) (p. 173). Elsevier.

Kassier, J. P. (2010). Teaching clinical reasoning: Case-based and coached. *Academic Medicine, 85*(7), 1118–1124.

Lambdin-Pattavina. (2021). Managing and facilitating groups. In J. C. O'Brien, & J. Solomon (Eds.), *Occupational analysis and group process* (2nd ed.) (pp. 62–75). Elsevier.

Law, M. C., Baptiste, S., Carswell, A., McColl, M. A., Polatajko, H., & Pollock, N. (1998). *Canadian occupational performance measure: COPM*. CAOT Publ. ACE.

Law, M., Cooper, B., Strong, S., Stewart, D., Rigby, P., & Letts, L. (1996). The person-environment-occupation model: A transactive approach to occupational performance. *Canadian Journal of Occupational Therapy, 63*(1), 9–23.

O'Brien, J. C., Patnaude, M. E., & Garcia Reidy, T. (2023). *Therapeutic reasoning in occupational therapy: How to develop critical thinking for practice*. Elsevier.

O'Brien, J. C., & Wolske, J. (2024). Examining the dynamics of human occupation. In R. Taylor, P. Bowyer, & G. Fisher (Eds.), *Kielhofner's model of human occupation: Theory and application* (6th ed.) (pp. 23–40). Wolters Kluwer Health.

Parham, L. D., Ecker, C. L., Kuhaneck, H., Henry, D. A., & Glennon, T. J. (2021). *Sensory processing measure SPM-2* (2nd ed.). Western Psychological Services.

Patnaude, M. E., & O'Brien, J. C. (2023). Occupation as the foundation for therapeutic reasoning. In J. C. O'Brien, M. E. Patnaude, & T. Garcia Reidy (Eds.), *Therapeutic reasoning in occupational therapy* (pp. 18–49). Elsevier.

Patnaude, M. E. (2023). Student success: Therapeutic reasoning process. In J. C. O'Brien, M. E. Patnaude, & T. Garcia Reidy (Eds.), *Therapeutic reasoning in occupational therapy* (pp. 1–17). Elsevier.

Ramey, S. L., DeLuca, S. C., Stevenson, R. D., Conaway, M., Darragh, A. R., Lo, W., & CHAMP. (2021). Constraint-induced movement therapy for cerebral palsy: A randomized trial. *Pediatrics, 148*(5), e2020033878.

Taylor, R., Bowyer, P., & Fisher, G. (2024). *Kielhofner's model of human occupation: Theory and application* (6th ed.). Wolters Kluwer Health.

Taylor, R. R. (2020). *The intentional relationship: Occupational therapy and use of self.* FA Davis.

Wong, S. R., & Fisher, G. (2015). Comparing and using occupation-focused models. *Occupational Therapy in Health Care, 29*(3), 297–315.

# APPENDIX A

# Pediatric Assessments

## KEY TO ABBREVIATIONS

ADL = activities of daily living
IADL = instrumental activities of daily living
Telehealth = assessments that can be used via telehealth

*Age range is reported in years. If a partial year is reported it will be indicated by the number of months after the decimal, so 3.11 = 3 years and 11 months and .8 = 8 months.

For more information: Some of the links provide access to assessments, other links may require practitioners register to receive assessments, others may require purchase.

| Assessment | Authors | Age Range* | Type | Areas Assessed |
|---|---|---|---|---|
| Activity Scale for Kids (ASK) | Young, Yoshida, Williams, & Wright (2016) | 5–15 | • Interview format/or observational checklist<br>• Questionnaire | • ADL<br>• Gross motor/mobility<br>• Play/leisure<br>• There are two scales (performance and capability) |
| For more information: https://eprovide.mapi-trust.org/instruments/activities-scale-for-kids-c-capability | | | | |
| Adaptive Behavior Assessment System-3 (ABAS-3) | Harrison & Oakland (2015) | 0–89 | • Standardized norm referenced<br>• Questionnaire<br>• Telehealth | • ADL<br>• IADL |
| For more information: https://www.wpspublish.com/abas-3-adaptive-behavior-assessment-system-third-edition | | | | |
| Adolescent and Young Adult Activity Card Sort (AYA-ACS) | Berg, McCollum, Cho, & Jason (2015) | 18–25 | • Interview format or observational checklist<br>• Not standardized | • IADL<br>• Play/leisure<br>• Social participation or social skills<br>• Work/transition |
| For more information: https://pubmed.ncbi.nlm.gov/27505902 | | | | |
| Affect in Play Scale (APS) and Affect in Play Scale—Preschool Version (APS-P) | Russ, Niec, & Kaugars (2000)<br>Kaugars & Russ (2009) | 6–10 | • Standardized, criterion referenced | • Play/leisure |
| For more information: https://psycnet.apa.org/record/2001-01062-026 and https://www.tandfonline.com/doi/abs/10.1080/10409280802545388?journalCode=heed20 | | | | |
| Ages and Stages Questionnaire | Squires & Bricker | .1–5.6 | • Developmental screening<br>• Questionnaire<br>• Screening tool<br>• Standardized, norm referenced<br>• Telehealth | • Developmental |

*Continued*

| Assessment | Authors | Age Range* | Type | Areas Assessed |
|---|---|---|---|---|
| For more information: https://agesandstages.com/ | | | | |
| AIR Self Determination Scale | American Institutes for Research (1994) | School age | • Questionnaire | • Behavioral/social emotional<br>• Cognitive<br>• Mental health |
| For more information: https://www.ou.edu/education/zarrow/resources/assessments and https://www.ou.edu/zarrow/AIR%20User%20Guide.pdf (available for free) | | | | |
| Alberta Infant Motor Scale (2nd ed.) | Piper & Darrah | 0–1.6 | • Developmental screening<br>• Standardized, norm referenced | • Fine motor<br>• Gross motor/mobility |
| For more information: https://www.us.elsevierhealth.com/alberta-infant-motor-scale-score-sheets-aims-9780323798426.html | | | | |
| ARC Self-Determination Scale | Wehmeyer & Kelchner (1995) | All school age | • Questionnaire<br>• Standardized, norm referenced | • Behavioral/social emotional<br>• Mental health (autonomy, self-regulation, psychological empowerment, and self-realization) |
| For more information: https://www.ou.edu/education/zarrow/resources/assessments (available for free) | | | | |
| Assessment of Communication and Interaction Skills (ACIS) | Forsyth, Salamy, Simon, & Kielhofner (1998) | 4 + | • Observational assessment<br>• Not standardized | • Social participation or social skills<br>• Interaction skills |
| For more information: https://moho-irm.uic.edu/productDetails.aspx?aid=1#:~:text=The%20ACIS%20is%20an%20observational,aspects%20of%20communication%20and%20interaction | | | | |
| Assessment of Functional Living Skills (AFLS) | Partington & Mueller (2012) | 2+ | • Interview format or observational checklist<br>• Questionnaire | • ADL<br>• IADL<br>• Social participation or social skills<br>• Work/transition |
| For more information: https://www.wpspublish.com/afls-assessment-of-functional-living-skills | | | | |
| Assessment of Motor and Process Skills | Fisher & Center for Innovative OT Solutions | All | • Standardized, criterion referenced | • ADL<br>• IADL<br>• Other: underlying motor and process performing skills |
| For more information: https://www.innovativeotsolutions.com/resource/amps-documents/ | | | | |
| Basic Behavior Assessment System for Children (BASC-3) | Reynolds & Kamphaus (2015) | 2–21.11 | • Standardized, norm referenced<br>• Telehealth | • Behavioral/social emotional |
| For more information: https://www.pearsonassessments.com/store/usassessments/en/Store/Professional-Assessments/Behavior/Comprehensive/Behavior-Assessment-System-for-Children-%7C-Third-Edition-/p/100001402.html | | | | |
| Battelle Developmental Inventory-3 (BDI-3) | Newborg (2020) | 0–7.11 | • Developmental screening<br>• Screening tool<br>• Standardized, norm referenced | • ADL<br>• Behavioral/social emotional<br>• Cognitive<br>• Feeding<br>• Fine motor Gross motor/mobility<br>• Play/leisure |
| For more information: https://riversideinsights.com/battelle_3e | | | | |
| Bayley Scales of Infant & Toddler Development (4th ed.) (Bayley—4) | Bayley & Aylward (2019) | .1–3.6 | • Developmental screening<br>• Standardized, norm referenced<br>• Telehealth | • ADL<br>• Behavioral/social emotional<br>• Cognitive<br>• Feeding<br>• Fine motor<br>• Gross motor/mobility<br>• Play/leisure |

| Assessment | Authors | Age Range* | Type | Areas Assessed |
|---|---|---|---|---|
| For more information: https://www.pearsonassessments.com/store/usassessments/en/Store/Professional-Assessments/Cognition-%26-Neuro/Bayley-Scales-of-Infant-and-Toddler-Development-%7C-Fourth-Edition/p/100001996.html | | | | |
| Beery-Buktenica Developmental Test of Visual Motor Integration (6th ed.) (Beery VMI) | Beery, Buktenica, & Beery (2010) | 2–99.11 | • Standardized, norm referenced<br>• Telehealth | • Fine motor<br>• Visual motor<br>• Visual perceptual |
| For more information: https://www.pearsonassessments.com/store/usassessments/en/Store/Professional-Assessments/Academic-Learning/Brief/Beery-Buktenica-Developmental-Test-of-Visual-Motor-Integration-%7C-Sixth-Edition/p/100000663.html | | | | |
| Behavioral Assessment of Baby's Emotional and Social Style (BABES) | Finello & Poulsen (2018) | 0–3 | • Interview format/or observational checklist<br>• Questionnaire<br>• Screening tool | • Behavioral/social emotional<br>• Sleep |
| For more information: https://www.wested.org/resources/babes-toolkit/ | | | | |
| Behavioral Assessment of the Dysexecutive Syndrome in Children (BADS-C) | Emslie, Wilson, Burden, Nimmo-Smith, & Wilson | 8–16 | • Standardized, norm referenced | • Cognitive |
| For more information: https://www.pearsonassessments.com/store/usassessments/en/Store/Professional-Assessments/Cognition-%26-Neuro/Behavioural-Assessment-of-the-Dysexecutive-Syndrome-in-Children/p/100000707.html | | | | |
| Behavioral Pediatrics Feeding Assessment Scale (BPFAS) | Crist & Napier-Phillips (2001) | .9–7 | • Questionnaire | • ADL<br>• Feeding behaviors |
| For more information: https://pubmed.ncbi.nlm.nih.gov/11718230/ and https://scholarworks.gsu.edu/cgi/viewcontent.cgi?article=1034&context=nutrition_theses | | | | |
| Behavior Rating Inventory of Executive Function-2 (BRIEF-2) | Gioia, Isquith, Guy, & Kenworthy (2015) | 5–18 | • Standardized, norm referenced<br>• Telehealth | • Behavioral/social emotional<br>• Cognitive |
| For more information: https://www.parinc.com/products/BRIEF-2 | | | | |
| Behavior Rating Inventory of Executive Function—Preschool Version (BRIEF-P) | Gioia, Espy, & Isquith (2003) | 2–5.11 | • Standardized, norm referenced | • Behavioral/social emotional<br>• Cognitive |
| For more information: https://www.parinc.com/Products/Pkey/26 | | | | |
| Brief Infant Toddler Social Emotional Assessment (BITSEA) | Briggs-Gowan, Irwin, Wachtel, & Cicchetti (2004) | 1–3 | • Screening tool | • Behavioral/social emotional |
| For more information: https://eprovide.mapi-trust.org/instruments/brief-infant-toddler-social-emotional-assessment | | | | |
| Brigance Curriculum based assessments and resources (2nd ed.) | Brigance (1970) | 0–7 | • Standardized, criterion referenced<br>• Standardized, norm referenced | • Cognitive<br>• School readiness assessments<br>• Educational resources |
| For more information: https://www.curriculumassociates.com/programs/brigance | | | | |
| Bruininks-Oseretsky Test of Motor Proficiency (3rd ed.) (BOT-3) | Bruininks & Bruininks (2024) | 4–25.11 | • Standardized, norm referenced | • Fine motor<br>• Gross motor/mobility<br>• Visual motor<br>• Visual perceptual |

*Continued*

| Assessment | Authors | Age Range* | Type | Areas Assessed |
|---|---|---|---|---|
| For more information: https://www.pearsonassessments.com/store/usassessments/en/Store/Professional-Assessments/Motor-Sensory/Bruininks-Oseretsky-Test-of-Motor-Proficiency-%7C-Second-Edition/p/100000648.html | | | | |
| Canadian Occupational Performance Measure (5th ed.) (COPM) | Law, Baptiste, Carswell, McColl, Polatajko, & Pollock (2014) | 7+ | • Interview format/or observational checklist | • ADL<br>• IADL<br>• Play/leisure<br>• Social participation or social skills<br>• Other: rates performance and satisfaction |
| For more information: http://www.thecopm.ca/ | | | | |
| Carolina Curriculum for Infant/toddlers with Special Needs (3rd ed.) (CCITSN) | CCITSN: Johnson-Martin, Attermeier, & Hacker (2004) | 0–3 | • Standardized, criterion referenced | • Behavioral/social emotional<br>• Cognition<br>• Fine motor<br>• Gross motor/mobility<br>• Social participation or social skills<br>• Other: communication |
| Carolina Curriculum for Preschoolers with Special Needs (2nd ed.) (CCPSN) | CCPSN: Johnson-Martin, Hacker, & Attermeier (2004) | 2–5 | | |
| For more information: https://brookespublishing.com/product/the-carolina-curriculum/ | | | | |
| Casey Life Skills (CLS) | Casey Life Program (2021) | 14–21 | • Interview format/or observational checklist<br>• Standardized, criterion referenced | • ADL<br>• IADL<br>• Social relationships and civic engagement<br>• Work and study habits<br>• Other: developed to support youth in foster care<br>• Navigating the child welfare system |
| For more information: https://www.casey.org/casey-life-skills/ | | | | |
| Child-initiated Pretend Play Assessment (2nd ed.) (ChIPPA-2) | Stagnitti (2020) | 3–7.11 | • Standardized, norm referenced | • Play/leisure |
| For more information: https://www.learntoplayevents.com/product/child-initiated-pretend-play-assessment-2-chippa-2-kit/ | | | | |
| Child Occupational Self-Assessment (Version 2.2) (COSA) | Kramer, ten Velden, Kafkes, Basu, Federico, & Kielhofner (2014) | 7–17 | • Not standardized<br>• Questionnaire | • ADL<br>• IADL<br>• Play/leisure<br>• Social participation or social skills<br>• Measures child's perceived self-efficacy and what they value (importance) |
| For more information: https://moho-irm.uic.edu/productDetails.aspx?aid=3 | | | | |
| Children's Assessment of Participation and Enjoyment (CAPE) and Preference for Activities of Children (PAC) | King, Law, King. Hurley, Hanna, Kertoy, Rosenbaum, & Young (2004) | 6–21 | • Interview format or observational checklist<br>• Questionnaire | • Play/leisure<br>• Social participation or social skills<br>• CAPE measures diversity, intensity and enjoyment<br>• PAC measures preferences for activities |
| For more information: https://www.canchild.ca/en/resources/43-measures-of-participation-cape-pac | | | | |
| Children Helping Out: Responsibilities, Expectations, and Supports (CHORES) | Dunn, Magalhaes, & Mancini (2014) | 6–14 | • Interview format or observational checklist<br>• Questionnaire | • ADL<br>• IADL |

| Assessment | Authors | Age Range* | Type | Areas Assessed |
|---|---|---|---|---|
| For more information: https://research.aota.org/ajot/article/68/3/286/5882/Internal-Structure-of-the-Children-Helping-Out | | | | |
| Children's Participation Questionnaire (CPQ) | Rosenberg, Jarus, & Bart (2010) | 4–6 | • Questionnaire | • IADL<br>• Play/leisure<br>• Social participation or social skills |
| For more information: https://www.tandfonline.com/doi/full/10.3109/09638281003611086 | | | | |
| Choosing Options and Accommodations for Children (3rd ed.) (COACH-3) | Giangreco, Cloninger, & Iverson (2011) | 3–21 | • Interview format or observational checklist<br>• Questionnaire | • ADL<br>• IADL<br>• Social participation or social skills<br>• Work/transition<br>• Tool to assist with educational planning and goals |
| For more information: https://products.brookespublishing.com/Choosing-Outcomes-and-Accommodations-for-Children-COACH-P463.aspx | | | | |
| Clinical Observations of Motor and Postural Skills (2nd ed.) (COMPS) | Wilson, Kaplan, Pollock, & Law (2000) | 5–15 | • Observational checklist<br>• Not standardized | • Gross motor/mobility<br>• Sensory processing/sensory integration |
| For more information: https://www.southpaw.com/clinical-observations-of-motor-and-postural-skills-comps-2nd-edition/ | | | | |
| Denver II Developmental Screening Test (Denver-II) | Frankenburg, Dodds, Archer, Bresnick, Maschka, Edelman, & Shapiro (1992) | 0–6 | • Developmental screening<br>• Screening tool<br>• Standardized, norm referenced | • ADL<br>• Fine motor<br>• Gross motor/mobility<br>• Language<br>• Social participation or social skills |
| For more information: https://www.hogrefe.com/uk/shop/denver-ii-developmental-screening-test.html | | | | |
| Detailed Assessment of Speed of Handwriting (2nd ed.) (DASH-2) | Barnett, Henderson, & Scheib (2024) | 9–16 | • Standardized, norm referenced<br>• Telehealth | • Handwriting |
| For more information: https://www.pearsonassessments.com/store/usassessments/en/Store/Professional-Assessments/Motor-Sensory/Detailed-Assessment-of-Speed-of-Handwriting/p/100000775.html | | | | |
| Developmental Assessment for Students with Severe Disabilities (3rd ed.) (DASH-3) | Dykes & Mruzek (2015) | .6–adult | • Developmental screening<br>• Interview format/or observational checklist<br>• Questionnaire<br>• Standardized, criterion referenced | • ADL<br>• Behavioral/Social emotional<br>• Cognitive<br>• Gross motor/mobility<br>• IADL<br>• Sensory processing/sensory integration<br>• Social participation or social skills |
| For more information: https://www.wpspublish.com/dash-3-developmental-assessment-for-individuals-with-severe-disabilities-third-edition | | | | |
| Developmental Play Assessment for Practitioners (DPA-P) | Lifter, Mason, Cannarella, & Cameron (2022) | .8–5 | • Interview format/or observational checklist<br>• Not standardized<br>• Questionnaire | • Play/leisure |
| For more information: https://www.routledge.com/Developmental-Play-Assessment-for-Practitioners-DPA-P-Guidebook-and-Training/Lifter-Mason-Cannarella-Cameron/p/book/9780367553593 https://www.northeastern.edu/projectplay/about/ | | | | |

Continued

| Assessment | Authors | Age Range* | Type | Areas Assessed |
|---|---|---|---|---|
| Developmental Profile (4th ed.) (DP-4)<br>For more information:<br>https://www.wpspublish.com/dp-4-developmental-profile-4.html | Alpern (2020) | 0–21.11 | • Developmental screening<br>• Interview format/or observational checklist<br>• Questionnaire<br>• Standardized, norm referenced<br>• Telehealth | • ADL<br>• Behavioral/social emotional<br>• Cognitive<br>• Fine motor<br>• Gross motor/mobility<br>• Social participation or social skills |
| Developmental Test of Visual Perception (3rd ed.) (DTVP – 3)<br>For more information:<br>https://www.pearsonassessments.com/store/usassessments/en/Store/Professional-Assessments/Motor-Sensory/Developmental-Test-of-Visual-Perception-%7C-Third-Edition/p/100000779.html | Hammill, Pearson, & Voress (2013) | 4–12.11 | • Standardized, norm referenced | • Visual motor integration (copying, eye hand coordination)<br>• Visual perception (figure ground, visual closure, form constancy) |
| Devereux Student Strengths Assessment (DESSA System)<br>For more information:<br>https://apertureed.com/ | Devereux Foundation | K–8th grade | • Standardized, norm referenced | • Educational assessments and program<br>• Resilience skills<br>• Behavioral/social emotional<br>• Social participation or social skills |
| Disabilities of the Arm, Shoulder and Hand (3rd ed.) (DASH)<br>Also available: QuickDash (shorter version)<br>For more information:<br>https://dash.iwh.on.ca/about-dash | Kennedy, Beaton Solway, McConnell, & Bombardier (2011) | 18–65 | • Interview format/or observational checklist<br>• Questionnaire | • Fine motor<br>• Gross motor/mobility |
| Early Coping Inventory (ECI)<br>For more information:<br>https://stsme.com/prod/ECI/ | Zeitlin, Williamson, & Szczepanski (1988) | .4–3 | • Interview format/or observational checklist<br>• Not standardized | • Behavioral/social emotional<br>• Mental health: coping-related, reactive, and self-initiation behaviors<br>• Sensory processing/sensory integration |
| Early Feeding Skills (EFS)<br>For more information:<br>https://feedingflockteam.org/tool/early-feeding-skills-efs | Thoyre, Shaker, & Pridham (2005) | Preterm infants | • Observational checklist<br>• Not standardized | • Feeding |
| Early Learning Accomplishment Profile (E-LAP)<br>For more information:<br>https://www.kaplanco.com/product/13649/early-learning-accomplishment-profile-e-lap-kit?c=17%7CEA1035 | Glover, Preminger, & Sanford (2004) | 0–3 | • Standardized, criterion referenced | • ADL<br>• Cognitive<br>• Fine motor<br>• Gross motor/mobility<br>• Language<br>• Social emotional |
| Evaluation in Ayres Sensory Integration (EASI)<br>For more information:<br>https://www.cl-asi.org/easi | Mailloux, Parham, Roley, Ruzzano, & Schaaf (2018) | 3–12 | • Standardized, norm referenced | • Sensory processing/sensory integration |
| Evaluation Tool of Children's Handwriting (ETCH) | Amundson (1995) | Grades 1–6 | • Standardized, criterion referenced | • Handwriting |

| Assessment | Authors | Age Range* | Type | Areas Assessed |
|---|---|---|---|---|
| For more information:<br>https://www.therapro.com/Evaluations/Handwriting-Assessments/Evaluation-Tool-of-Childrens-Handwriting-ETCH.html | | | | |
| Family-Centered Care Assessment for Families (FCCA-F)<br>For more information:<br>https://familyvoices.org/fcca/ | Family Voices (2014) | Families | • Questionnaire | • Other: Designed to support family centered care and family engagement<br>• Engages family in process and goal setting |
| First Year Inventory (FYI)<br>For more information:<br>https://www.med.unc.edu/healthsciences/pearls/research/first-year-inventory-fyi-development/ | Baranek, Watson, Crais, & Reznick (2003) | 1 | • Questionnaire<br>• Screening tool<br>• Standardized, norm referenced | • Sensory regulation<br>• Social communication |
| Functional Emotional Assessment Scale (FEAS)<br>For more information:<br>https://www.icdl.com/research/functional-emotional-assessment-scale | Greenspan, DeGangi, & Wieder (2001) | .7–4 | • Standardized, criterion referenced | • Behavioral/social emotional<br>• Functional emotional capacity<br>• Self-regulation<br>• Social participation or social skills |
| Goal Oriented Assessment of Life Skills (GOALS)<br>For more information:<br>https://www.wpspublish.com/goal-goal-oriented-assessment-of-lifeskills.html | Miller, Oakland, & Herzberg (2013) | 7–17 | • Standardized, norm referenced | • Fine motor<br>• Gross motor/mobility |
| Great Recess Framework–Observational Tool (GRF-OT)<br>For more information:<br>https://www.playworks.org/resources/great-recess-framework/ | Massey, Stellino, Mullen, Claassen, & Wilkinson (2018) | Elementary | • Observational checklist | • Play/leisure<br>• Safety, structure, behavior, adult supervision |
| Gross Motor Function Measure (GMFM)<br>For more information:<br>https://canchild.ca/en/resources/44-gross-motor-function-measure-gmfm | Russell, Rosenbaum, Wright, & Avery (2002) | .5–16 | • Interview format/or observational checklist<br>• Standardized, criterion referenced | • Gross motor/mobility |
| Handwriting without Tears: The Print tool Evaluation and Remediation<br>For more information:<br>https://shopping.lwtears.com/LWTstore/s/product/the-print-tool-evaluation-remediation-package/01t4V000007a2pxQAA | Olsen, & Knapton (2004) | Grades preK–5th | • Observational checklist<br>• Not standardized | • Handwriting |
| Hawaii Early Learning Profile (HELP)<br>For more information:<br>https://shineearly.store/products/help-strands-0-3 and https://shineearly.store/products/help-3-6-assessment-strands-2nd-ed | HELP 0–3<br>Warshaw (2006)<br>HELP 3–6<br>Teaford, Wheat, & Baker (2010) | 0–6 | • Developmental screening<br>• Standardized, criterion referenced | • ADL<br>• Behavioral/social emotional<br>• Cognitive<br>• Fine motor<br>• Gross motor/mobility<br>• Play/leisure<br>• Social participation or social skills |
| Here's How I Write (HHIW) | Goldstand, Gavir, Cermak, & Bissell (2014) | Grades 2–5 | • Standardized, criterion referenced | • Handwriting |

*Continued*

| Assessment | Authors | Age Range* | Type | Areas Assessed |
|---|---|---|---|---|
| For more information: https://www.therapro.com/Heres-How-I-Write-A-Childs-Self-Assessment-and-Goal-Setting-Tool-Improving-Handwriting_2.html | | | | |
| Home Observation for Measurement of the Environment-SF (HOME SF) | Caldwell & Bradley (2003) | 0–15 | • Interview format/or observational checklist<br>• Not standardized | • Quality and quantity of support, structure, and stimulation available to child in home |
| For more information: https://edinstruments.org/instruments/home-observation-measurement-environment-short-form-home-sf | | | | |
| Infant Neurological International Battery (Infanib) | Ellison, Horn, & Browning (1985) | .1–1.6 | • Developmental screening<br>• Screening tool | • Gross motor/mobility |
| For more information: https://pubmed.ncbi.nlm.nih.gov/2412245/ and https://www.physio-pedia.com/Infant_Neurological_International_Battery_(INFANIB) | | | | |
| Infant-Toddler Developmental Assessment (2nd ed.) (IDA-2) | Provence, Erickson, Vater, Pruett, Rosinia, & Palmeri (2016) | 0–3 | • Developmental screening<br>• Interview format/or observational checklist<br>• Questionnaire<br>• Standardized, criterion referenced | • ADL<br>• Behavioral/social emotional<br>• Fine motor<br>• Gross motor/mobility<br>• Language/communication<br>• Social participation or social skills |
| For more information: https://ida2.org/ | | | | |
| Infant/Toddler Social and Emotional Assessment (ITSEA) | Briggs-Gowan & Carter (1998) | 1–3 | • Questionnaire | • Behavioral/social emotional<br>• Social participation or social skills |
| For more information: https://eprovide.mapi-trust.org/instruments/infant-toddler-social-emotional-assessment | | | | |
| Jebsen-Taylor Hand Function Test (JTHFT) | Jebsen, Taylor, Trieschmann, Trotter, & Howard (1969) | 5+ | • Observational checklist | • Fine motor |
| For more information: https://www.prohealthcareproducts.com/jebsen-taylor-test-of-hand-function/ | | | | |
| Knox Preschool Play Scale (KPPS) | Knox | 0–6 | • Observational checklist<br>• Not standardized | • Behavioral/social emotional<br>• Cognitive<br>• Fine motor<br>• Gross motor/mobility<br>• Play/leisure<br>• Social participation or social skills |
| For more information: Knox, S. (2005). Play. In J. Case-Smith (Ed.), *Occupational therapy for children* (5th ed., pp. 571–586). St. Louis, MO: Mosby. Or Parham, L. D. & Fazio, L. S. (2008). *Play in occupational therapy for children.* St. Louis, MO: Mosby Elsevier. | | | | |
| Learning Accomplishment Profile (3rd ed.) (LAP-3) | Hardin & Peisner-Feinberg (2004) | 3–6 | • Interview format/or observational checklist<br>• Standardized, criterion referenced<br>• Telehealth | • Behavioral/social emotional<br>• Cognitive<br>• Fine motor<br>• Gross motor/mobility<br>• Handwriting – Prewriting<br>• Language |
| For more information: https://www.kaplanco.com/shop/assessments-and-evaluations/learning-accomplishment-profilelap | | | | |
| Life Habits (4th ed.) (Life-H 4.0) | Fougeyrollas, Noreau, & LePage (2014) | 5–13 | • Interview format<br>• Questionnaire | • Communication<br>• Education<br>• Gross motor/mobility<br>• Play/leisure/recreation<br>• Social emotional and participation |

| Assessment | Authors | Age Range* | Type | Areas Assessed |
|---|---|---|---|---|
| For more information: https://ripph.qc.ca/wp-content/uploads/2018/05/5-13_ans_MHAVIE_4_0_90_items_ang_final_juin_2016-SPECIMEN-taille-reduite-protege.pdf | | | | |
| Life Participation for Parents (LPP) | Fingerhut (2005) | Parent | • Not standardized<br>• Questionnaire | • Tool to understand family satisfaction and sense of efficacy |
| For more information: https://veipd.org/earlyintervention/wp-content/uploads/2012/12/Life-Participation-for-Parents-and-description.pdf | | | | |
| Life Skills Inventory (LSI) | Washington State Department of Social and Health Services (2022) | Young adult | • Not standardized<br>• Questionnaire | • IADL (money management and consumer awareness, food management, personal appearance and hygiene, health, housekeeping, housing, transportation)<br>• Work/transition (educational planning, job seeking skills, job maintenance skills)<br>• Knowledge of community resources, emergency and safety skills.<br>• Interpersonal skills, legal issues, and pregnancy (parenting and childcare) |
| For more information: https://embracefamilies.org/wp-content/uploads/2022/06/Life-Skills-Washington-State-Assessment-Tool-5.27.22-fillable.pdf | | | | |
| Measure of Environmental Qualities of Activity Settings (MEQAS) | King, Rigby, Batorowicz, McMain-Klein, Petrenchik, Thompson, & Gibson (2014) | Youth | • Observational checklist | • Qualities and affordances of physical and social environment in an activity setting |
| For more information: https://hollandbloorview.ca/research-education/bloorview-research-institute/outcome-measures/measure-environmental-qualities-2 | | | | |
| Measure of Processes of Care (MPOC) | King, Rosenbaum, & King (1995) | Parents of children 0–17 | • Questionnaire<br>• Telehealth | • Parents' perceptions of the care they and their children receive in rehabilitation<br>• Assesses family-centered behaviors of health care providers |
| For more information: https://canchild.ca/en/shop/1-mpoc-20 and https://www.canchild.ca/en/resources/47-measure-of-processes-of-care#:~:text=The%20purpose%20of%20the%20Measure,behaviours%20of%20health%20care%20providers | | | | |
| Miller Function and Participation Scales (M-FUN) | Miller (2006) | 2.0–7.11 | • Standardized, norm referenced | • Cognitive<br>• Fine motor<br>• Gross motor/mobility<br>• Visual motor<br>• Visual perception<br>• Social participation or social skills |
| For more information: https://www.pearsonassessments.com/store/usassessments/en/Store/Professional-Assessments/Developmental-Early-Childhood/Miller-Function-and-Participation-Scales/p/100000557.html | | | | |
| Minnesota Handwriting Assessment | Reisman (1999) | Grades 1 and 2 | • Standardized, norm referenced | • Handwriting |
| For more information: https://www.pearsonassessments.com/store/usassessments/en/Store/Professional-Assessments/Motor-Sensory/Minnesota-Handwriting-Assessment/p/100000275.html | | | | |
| Motivation Assessment Scale (MAS) | Durand, & Crimmins (1992) | Not reported | • Interview format/or observational checklist<br>• Not standardized | • Behavioral/social emotional<br>• Assesses person's motivations |

Continued

| Assessment | Authors | Age Range* | Type | Areas Assessed |
|---|---|---|---|---|
| For more information: https://store.monacoassociates.com/motivation-assessment-scale.aspx and https://elearning.aba-onv.eu/pluginfile.php/72/mod_resource/content/0/Motivation_Assessment_Scale_II-1_5B2_5D%20-%20Test%20version.pdf | | | | |
| Motor Free Visual Perception Test (4th ed.) (MVPT-4) | Colarusso & Hammill (2015) | 4–80 | • Standardized, norm referenced | • Visual perception (visual discrimination, spatial relationships visual memory, visual closure, figure ground) |
| For more information: https://www.proedinc.com/Products/14716/motorfree-visual-perception-testfourth-edition-mvpt4.aspx | | | | |
| Movement Assessment Battery for Children (3rd ed.) (MABC-3) | Henderson, Sugden, & Barnett (2023) | 3–25 | • Standardized, norm referenced<br>• Telehealth | • Fine motor<br>• Gross motor/mobility |
| For more information: https://www.pearsonassessments.com/store/usassessments/en/Store/Professional-Assessments/Motor-Sensory/Movement-Assessment-Battery-for-Children%2C-Third-Edition/p/P100051002.html | | | | |
| Mullen Scales of Early Learning (MSEL) | Mullen (1995) | 0–5.8 | • Developmental screening<br>• Standardized, norm referenced | • Fine motor<br>• Gross motor/mobility<br>• Visual perception<br>• Expressive language<br>• Receptive language |
| For more information: https://www.pearsonassessments.com/store/usassessments/en/Store/Professional-Assessments/Developmental-Early-Childhood/Mullen-Scales-of-Early-Learning/p/100000306.html | | | | |
| My Child's Play (MCP) | Schneider & Rosenblum (2014) | 3–9 | • Questionnaire | • Play/leisure |
| For more information: https://chap.haifa.ac.il/wp-content/uploads/2023/11/MCP-english.pdf | | | | |
| Neonatal Behavioral Assessment Scale (4th ed.) | Brazelton Nugent (2011) | Infant | • Developmental screening<br>• Interview format/or observational checklist | • Behavioral/social emotional<br>• Gross motor/mobility |
| For more information: https://www.newbornbehaviorinternational.org/nbas-1<br>Brazelton, T. B. & Nugent, J. K. (2011). *The Neonatal Behavioral Assessment Scale.* MacKeith Press, Cambridge. | | | | |
| Nine-Hole Peg Test (NHPT) | Mathiowetz, Weber, Kashman, & Volland (1985) | 4–19 | • Standardized, norm referenced | • Fine motor |
| For more information: https://www.sralab.org/rehabilitation-measures/nine-hole-peg-test | | | | |
| Occupational Performance Inventory of Sexuality and Intimacy (OPISI) | Walker (2020) | 13–15 | • Questionnaire | • Sexuality |
| For more information: https://uindy.edu/health-sciences/ot/opisi | | | | |
| Occupational Self-Assessment (OSA) | Baron, Kielhofner, Iyenger, Goldhammer, & Wolenski (2006) | Teens–Adult | • Questionnaire | • ADL<br>• IADL<br>• Person's value for the occupation and perceived competence (self-efficacy) |
| For more information: https://moho-irm.uic.edu/productDetails.aspx?aid=2 | | | | |
| Occupational Therapy Functional Assessment Compilation Tool and School (OT FACT) | Rehabilitation Research Design & Disability (R2D2) Center, University of Wisconsin, Milwaukee | All | • Interview format/or observational checklist<br>• Not standardized<br>• Questionnaire | • ADL<br>• IADL<br>• Behavioral/social emotional<br>• Cognitive<br>• Fine motor<br>• Gross motor/mobility |

| Assessment | Authors | Age Range* | Type | Areas Assessed |
|---|---|---|---|---|
| For more information: https://uwm.edu/r2d2/projects/ot-fact/about-ot-fact/ | | | | |
| Occupational Therapy Psychosocial Assessment of Learning (OT PAL) | Townsend, Carey, Hollins, Helfrich, Blondis, Hoffman, Collins, Knudson, & Blackwell (1999) | 6–12 | • Interview format/or observational checklist | • Behavioral/social emotional<br>• Mental health<br>• Evaluates student's volition (the ability to make choices), habituation (roles and routines), and environmental fit within the classroom setting. |
| For more information: https://moho-irm.uic.edu/productDetails.aspx?aid=33#:~:text=OT%20PAL&text=This%20assessment%20uses%20observation%20and,assessment%20and%20data%20summary%20forms | | | | |
| Parent/Caregiver's Support of Children's Playfulness (PC-SCP) | Waldman-Levi, A. & Bundy, A. (2023). Parent/caregiver support of children's playfulness (PC-SCP). American Occupational Therapy Association. | Parents of children .6–6 years | • Interview format/or observational checklist | • Play/leisure<br>• Assess parents' or other caregivers' support of children's playfulness. |
| For more information: https://www.tandfonline.com/doi/abs/10.1080/0164212X.2015.1116420 | | | | |
| Parent Child Relationship Inventory (PCRI) | Gerard (1994) | Parents of children 3–13 | • Questionnaire – self-report<br>• Standardized, norm referenced | • Parenting skills and attitudes toward parenting<br>• Measures parental support, satisfaction, involvement, communication, limit setting, autonomy, and role orientation |
| For more information: https://www.wpspublish.com/pcri-parent-child-relationship-inventory | | | | |
| Parenting Interactions with Children: Checklist of Observations Linked to Outcomes (PICCOLO) | Roggman, Cook, Innocenti, Norman, Anderson, & Christiansen (2013) | Parents of children 0–3.11 | • Observational checklist | • Quality of parent–child interactions |
| For more information: https://brookespublishing.com/product/piccolo/ | | | | |
| Parenting Relationship Questionnaire (PRQ) | Kamphaus, & Reynolds (2015) | Parents of children 2–21 | • Questionnaire<br>• Standardized, norm referenced<br>• Telehealth | • Measures parental perspective<br>• Includes measures of attachment, communication, discipline practices, involvement, parenting confidence, satisfaction with school, and relational frustration. |
| For more information: https://www.pearsonassessments.com/store/usassessments/en/Store/Professional-Assessments/Behavior/BASC-3-Parenting-Relationship-Questionnaire/p/100001502.html?tab=overview | | | | |
| Parenting Stress Index (4th ed.) (PSI-4) | Abidin (2012) | Parents of children 0–12 | • Questionnaire<br>• Standardized, norm referenced | • Assesses at risk behaviors and/or stress in child and parent relationship |
| For more information: https://www.parinc.com/product/groups/psi-assessments | | | | |
| Participation and Environment Measure for Children and Youth (PEM-CY) | Coster, Law, & Bedell (2011) | 5–17 | • Questionnaire | • IADL<br>• Other: perceived impact of environment on participation |
| Young Children's Participation and Environment Measure (YC-PEM) | Khetani, Coster, Law, & Bedell (2013) | 0–5 | | |

*Continued*

| Assessment | Authors | Age Range* | Type | Areas Assessed |
|---|---|---|---|---|
| For more information: https://canchild.ca/en/shop/2-pem-cy-participation-and-environment-measure-children-and-youth | | | | |
| Peabody Developmental Motor Scales (3rd ed.) (PDMS-3) | Folio & Fewell (2023) | 0–5.11 | • Developmental screening<br>• Standardized, criterion referenced<br>• Standardized, norm referenced | • Fine motor<br>• Gross motor/mobility<br>• Visual motor<br>• Visual perception |
| For more information: https://www.proedinc.com/Products/15065/pdms3-peabody-developmental-motor-scalesthird-edition-complete-kit.aspx | | | | |
| Pediatric Activity Card Sort (PAC3) | Mandich, Polatajko, Miller, & Baum (2004) | 6–12 | • Interview format/or observational checklist<br>• Questionnaire | • Occupational engagement and participation<br>• Play/leisure<br>• Social participation |
| For more information: https://caot.ca/client/product2/12/item.html | | | | |
| Pediatric Balance Scale (PBS-2) | Franjoine & Darr (2022) | 2–13 | • Observational checklist | • Gross motor/mobility (balance) |
| For more information: PBS+2+Administration+Directions_June+2024.pdf | | | | |
| Pediatric Evaluation of Disability Inventory—Computer Adaptive Test (PEDI-CAT) | Haley, Coster, Dumas, Fragala-Pinkham, & Moed (2020) | .6–21 | • Standardized, norm referenced<br>• Questionnaire (electronic) | • ADL<br>• Caregiver responsibility<br>• Cognitive<br>• Gross motor/mobility<br>• Social participation or social skills |
| For more information: https://www.pearsonassessments.com/store/usassessments/en/Store/Professional-Assessments/Behavior/Pediatric-Evaluation-of-Disability-Inventory-Computer-Adaptive-Test/p/100002037.html?tab=product-details | | | | |
| Pediatric Interest Profiles (PIP)<br>Includes Kids, Pre-teen and Adolescent versions | Henry (2000) | 6–21 | • Not standardized | • Play/leisure<br>• Social participation or social skills |
| For more information: https://moho-irm.uic.edu/productDetails.aspx?aid=43 | | | | |
| Pediatric Outcomes Data Collection Instrument (PODCI) | Daltroy, Goldberg, Liang, & Fossel (1998) | 2–10 | • Interview format/or observational checklist | • Fine motor<br>• Gross motor/mobility<br>• Play/leisure<br>• Other |
| For more information: https://eprovide.mapi-trust.org/instruments/pediatric-outcomes-data-collection-instrument-parent - coas_member_access_content | | | | |
| Pediatric Volitional Questionnaire (PVQ) | Basu, Kafkes, Schatz, Kiraly, & Kielhofner (2008) | 2–7 | • observational checklist | • Exploration<br>• Competency<br>• Achievement |
| For more information: https://moho-irm.uic.edu/productDetails.aspx?aid=7 | | | | |
| Perceived Efficacy and Goal Setting System (2nd ed.) (PEGS) | Pollock & Missiuna (2015) | 5–9 | • Interview format/or observational checklist<br>• Questionnaire | • Self-determination<br>• Self-efficacy<br>• Goal setting |
| For more information: https://www.canchild.ca/en/resources/48-perceived-efficacy-and-goal-setting-pegs | | | | |
| Performance Assessment of Self-Care Skills (PASS) | Rogers, Holm, & Chisholm (2016) | Adolescent+ | • Observational checklist<br>• Standardized, criterion referenced | • ADL<br>• Cognition<br>• Functional mobility<br>• IADL |

| Assessment | Authors | Age Range* | Type | Areas Assessed |
|---|---|---|---|---|
| For more information: https://www.shrs.pitt.edu/ot/about/performance-assessment-self-care-skills-pass | | | | |
| Piers-Harris Self Concept Scale (3rd ed.) (Piers-Harris 3) | Piers, Shemmassian, & Herzberg (2018) | 6–12 | • Questionnaire<br>• Standardized, norm referenced | • Self-concept |
| For more information: https://www.wpspublish.com/piers-harris-3-piers-harris-self-concept-scale-third-edition.html | | | | |
| Play In Early Childhood Evaluation System (PIECES) | Kelly-Vance & Ryalls (2005) | .9–5 | • Observational checklist<br>• Not standardized | • Play/leisure |
| For more information: Kelly-Vance, L., & Ryalls, B. O. (2005). A systematic, reliable approach to play assessment in preschoolers. *School Psychology International*, 26(4), 398–412. https://doi.org/10.1177/0143034305059017 | | | | |
| Play Space Assessment | Head Start | 3–5 | • Observational checklist | • Assesses play space environments |
| For more information: https://eclkc.ohs.acf.hhs.gov/learning-environments/article/play-space-assessment-preschool | | | | |
| Playable Space Quality Assessment Tool (5th ed.) | Play England (2016) | All | • Interview format/or observational checklist<br>• Not standardized | • Play spaces<br>• Tool to engage others (children, parents, community, government) in creating and designing play spaces |
| For more information: https://www.playengland.org.uk/quality-in-play | | | | |
| Posture and Fine Motor Assessment of Infants (PFMAI) | Case-Smith & Bigsby (2000) | .2–1 | • Developmental screening tool<br>• Interview format/or observational checklist | • Gross motor/mobility<br>• Fine motor |
| For more information: https://pubmed.ncbi.nlm.nih.gov/1621795/ and https://psycnet.apa.org/doiLanding?doi=10.1037%2Ft15151-000 | | | | |
| Preschool Activity Card Sort | Berg & LaVasser (2006) | 3–6 | • Interview format/or observational checklist<br>• Questionnaire | • ADL<br>• Education<br>• Gross motor/mobility<br>• Play/leisure<br>• Social participation |
| For more information: https://journals.sagepub.com/doi/10.1177/153944920602600404 | | | | |
| Preschool Outdoor Environment Measurement Scale (POEMS) | DeBord, Hestenes, Moore, Cosco, & McGinnis (2005) | | • Interview format and Observational checklist<br>• Not standardized | • Play/leisure<br>• Assesses the quality of outdoor environment for play |
| For more information: https://www.kaplanco.com/product/39502/preschool-outdoor-environment-measurement-scale-poems?c=29%7COL1030 | | | | |
| Preschool Visual Motor Integration Assessment (PVMIA) | Deitchman & Puttkammer (2001) | 3.6–5.6 | • Standardized, norm referenced | • Visual motor<br>• Visual perception |
| For more information: https://www.therapro.com/Preschool-Visual-Motor-Integration-Assessment-PVMIA_9.html | | | | |
| Quality of Upper Extremity Skills Test (QUEST) | DeMatteo, Law, Russell, Pollack, Rosenbaum, & Walter (1992) | .8–8 | • Observational checklist | • Upper extremity function (dissociation, grasp, protective extension, weight bearing) |

*Continued*

| Assessment | Authors | Age Range* | Type | Areas Assessed |
|---|---|---|---|---|
| For more information:<br>https://canchild.ca/en/resources/49-quality-of-upper-extremity-skills-test-quest | | | | |
| Refreshing Recess Environmental Analysis | Bazyk (2021) | K–12 grade | • Observational checklist<br>• Not standardized | • Play/leisure<br>• Assesses school recess environment |
| For more information:<br>http://s3.us-east-2.amazonaws.com/s3.everymomentcounts.com/wp-content/uploads/2021/03/01192800/RR_EnvironmentalAnalysis_FINAL_fillable_3-1-21.pdf | | | | |
| Roll Evaluation of Activities of Life (REAL) | Roll & Roll (2013) | 2–18.11 | • Interview and observational checklist<br>• Screening tool<br>• Standardized, norm referenced | • ADL<br>• IADL<br>• Other: Parent rates child's skills |
| For more information:<br>https://www.pearsonassessments.com/store/usassessments/en/Store/Professional-Assessments/Behavior/Adaptive/The-Roll-Evaluation-of-Activities-of-Life/p/100000762.html | | | | |
| Schoodles Pediatric Fine Motor Assessment (3rd ed.) | Frank & Wing (2014) | 3+ | • Observational checklist<br>• Not standardized<br>• Telehealth | • Classroom skills<br>• Fine motor<br>• Handwriting<br>• Supporting skills<br>• Visual motor |
| For more information:<br>https://schoodles.com/ | | | | |
| School Assessment of Motor and Process Skills (School AMPS) | Fisher, Bryze, Hume, & Griswold | 3–15 | • Observational checklist | • ADL<br>• Cognitive (attention, working memory, executive functioning, reasoning, problem solving, insight, processing speed)<br>• Fine motor<br>• Gross motor/mobility (balance, vestibular coordination, gait)<br>• Occupational Performance |
| For more information:<br>https://www.innovativeotsolutions.com/wp-content/uploads/2019/05/School-AMPS-rationale-1.pdf | | | | |
| School Function Assessment (SFA) | Coster, Deeney, Haltiwanger, & Haley (1998) | K–6th grade | • Interview format/or observational checklist<br>• Questionnaire<br>• Standardized, criterion referenced | • Behavioral/social emotional<br>• Fine motor<br>• Gross motor/mobility<br>• Handwriting<br>• Social participation or social skills<br>• Other |
| For more information:<br>https://www.pearsonassessments.com/store/usassessments/en/Store/Professional-Assessments/Behavior/Adaptive/School-Function-Assessment/p/100000547.html | | | | |
| School Function Assessment, AT Supplement (SFA-AT) | Silverman, Stratman, Grogan, & Smith (2003) | K–6th grade | • Interview format/or observational checklist | • Assistive technology<br>• Social participation or social skills |
| For more information:<br>https://uwm.edu/r2d2/projects/oats/sfa-at-project-oats-version/#:~:text=School%20Function%20Assessment%20Assistive%20Technology%20Supplement%20(SFA%2DAT),-Michelle%20Silverman%20M.S.&text=The%20SFA%2DAT%20is%20based,tasks%20covered%20in%20the%20SFA | | | | |
| School Motivation and Learning Strategies Inventory (SMALSI) | Stroud & Reynolds (2014) | 8–18<br>College: Freshman to graduate level | • Standardized, norm referenced | • Assess and target learning strategies that affect school performance (e.g., study strategies, note taking, listening, reading comprehension) |

| Assessment | Authors | Age Range* | Type | Areas Assessed |
|---|---|---|---|---|
| For more information: https://www.wpspublish.com/smalsi-school-motivation-and-learning-strategies-inventory | | | | |
| School Setting Interview (SSI) | Hemmingsson, Egilson, Hoffman, & Kielhofner (2005) | School-aged children | • Semi-structured interview<br>• Not standardized | • Assess school-environment-fit<br>• Includes child's participation in classroom, playground, gymnasium, corridors, field trips, and social events. |
| For more information: https://moho-irm.uic.edu/productDetails.aspx?aid=10 | | | | |
| Sensory Integration Inventory: Revised for Individuals with Developmental Disabilities (SII-R) | Reisman & Hanschu (1992) | All | • Not standardized<br>• Screening tool | • Sensory processing/sensory integration |
| For more information: https://www.therapro.com/Evaluations/Sensory-Processing-Assessments/Sensory-Integration-Inventory-Revised-for-Individuals-with-Developmental-Disabilities.html | | | | |
| Sensory Integration and Praxis Tests (SIPT) | Ayres (1989) | 4–9 | • Standardized, norm referenced | • Sensory processing/sensory integration |
| For more information: https://www.wpspublish.com/sipt-sensory-integration-and-praxis-tests | | | | |
| Sensory Processing Measure (2nd ed.) (SPM-2) | Parham, Ecker, Kuhaneck, Henry, & Glennon (2021) | Infant through adult | • Questionnaire<br>• Standardized, norm referenced<br>• Telehealth | • Gross motor/mobility<br>• Play/leisure<br>• Sensory processing/sensory integration<br>• Social participation or social skills |
| For more information: https://www.wpspublish.com/spm-2 | | | | |
| Sensory Profile-2 | Dunn (2014) | 0–15 | • Questionnaire<br>• Standardized, criterion referenced | • Behavioral/social emotional<br>• Sensory processing/sensory integration |
| For more information: https://www.pearsonassessments.com/store/usassessments/en/Store/Professional-Assessments/Motor-Sensory/Sensory-Profile-2/p/100000822.html | | | | |
| Sexuality Behavior Scale (SBS) | Stokes & Kaur (2005) | Adults (caregivers) who have children with autism | • Questionnaire | • Sexuality (e.g., social behaviors, privacy, sexual education, sexual behaviors, parent concerns) |
| For more information: https://psycnet.apa.org/doiLanding?doi=10.1037%2Ft18506-000 | | | | |
| Short Child Occupational Profile (SCOPE) | Bowyer, Kramer, Ploszaj, Ross, Schwartz, Kielhofner & Kramer (2008) | 0–21 | • Interview format/or observational checklist<br>• Not standardized | • Assesses child's volition (motivations, self-efficacy, values), habits and roles, performance capacity (perceived competence) and environment. |
| For more information: https://moho-irm.uic.edu/productDetails.aspx?aid=9 | | | | |
| Social Profile – Child Version | Donohue (2022) | 1.6–adult | • Standardized, criterion referenced | • Behavioral/social emotional<br>• Social participation or social skills |
| For more information: https://library.aota.org/1snc2cq/ | | | | |
| Social Responsiveness Scale (2nd ed.) (SRS-2) | Constantino (2012) | 2.6–adult | • Standardized, norm referenced | • Social participation or social skills |

Continued

| Assessment | Authors | Age Range* | Type | Areas Assessed |
|---|---|---|---|---|
| For more information: https://www.wpspublish.com/srs-2-social-responsiveness-scale-second-edition?utm_term=&utm_campaign=Search+%7C+Development+%26+Adaptive+Behavior&utm_source=adwords&utm_medium=ppc&hsa_net=adwords&hsa_tgt=aud-1456304315200:dsa-437115340933&hsa_ad=453117550270&hsa_acc=6243382947&hsa_grp=84191084381&hsa_mt=&hsa_cam=1718760923&hsa_kw=&hsa_ver=3&hsa_src=g&gclid=Cj0KCQjw0bunBhD9ARIsAAZl0E0tJzybmJJ0z7NTn_wTQ10Fz_H0nooNNWUuG7o7t0pnojQuP3VnOUaAjMIEALw_wcB | | | | |
| Social Skills Inventory | Riggio (2002) | 8th grade reading level + | • Interview format/or observational checklist<br>• Questionnaire | • Social and emotional skills (sensitivity, control and expressivity) |
| For more information: https://www.mindgarden.com/144-social-skills-inventory | | | | |
| Stress Index for Parents of Adolescents (SIPA) | Sheras & Abadin (1998) | 11–19 | • Questionnaire<br>• Standardized, norm referenced | • Assesses parent–adolescent interactions<br>• Parent assessment of life restrictions, relationship with spouse/partner, social alienation, and incompetence/guilt<br>• Adolescent assessment of moodiness/emotional lability, social isolation/withdrawal, delinquency/antisocial, and failure to achieve or persevere |
| For more information: https://www.parinc.com/Products/Pkey/412 | | | | |
| Structured Observation of Sensory Integration-Motor (SOSI-M) | Blanche, Reinoso, & Kiefer (2021) | 5–14 | • Standardized, norm referenced | • Gross motor/mobility<br>• Sensory processing/sensory integration |
| For more information: https://assessments.academictherapy.com/i/structured-observations-of-sensory-integration-motor-sosi-m | | | | |
| Supports Intensity Scale—Children's version (SIS–C) | Thompson, Wehmeyer, Hughes, Shogren, Seo, Little, Schalock, Realon, Copeland, Patton, Polloway, Shelden, Tanis, & Tassé (2016) | 5–16 | • Standardized, norm referenced | • Measures the pattern and intensity of supports that a child with intellectual and developmental disabilities (IDD) requires to be successful in age-appropriate community settings. |
| For more information: https://www.aaidd.org/sis/sis-c | | | | |
| Survey of Teenage Readiness and Neurodevelopmental Status (STRANDS) | Hooper & Leven (2001) | Teens | • Interview format<br>• Questionnaire | • Cognitive<br>• Assess learning problems in high school students |
| For more information: Hooper, S. & Levin, M. D. (2001). STRANDS manual: Survey of teenage readiness and neurodevelopment status, administration, scoring, and interpretation. Educators Pub. Service. | | | | |
| Teen Transition Inventory (TTI) | Dekker, van der Vegt, van der Ende, Tick, Louwerse, Maras, Verhulst, & Greaves-Lord (2017) | Teens | • Questionnaire (parent and teen self-report) | • Sexuality<br>• Psychosexual socialization, psychosexual self-hood and sexual and intimate behavior) |
| For more information: https://pubmed.ncbi.nlm.nih.gov/28299510/ | | | | |
| Temperament and Atypical Behavior Scale (TABS) | Bagnato, Neisworth, Salvia, & Hunt (1999) | .11–5.11 | • Standardized, norm referenced | • Temperament and self-regulation<br>• Behavioral/social emotional<br>• Mental health |

| Assessment | Authors | Age Range* | Type | Areas Assessed |
|---|---|---|---|---|
| For more information: https://products.brookespublishing.com/Temperament-and-Atypical-Behavior-Scale-TABS-Complete-Set-P527.aspx | | | | |
| Test of Environmental Supportiveness (Toes) | Bundy (1999) | All ages | • Interview format/or observational checklist | • Play/leisure<br>• Environment's influence on child's play |
| For more information: Bundy A.C. (1999). *Test of Environmental Supportiveness.* Ft Collins, CO: Colorado State University. https://journals.sagepub.com/doi/abs/10.1177/153944920102100403?journalCode=otja#:~:text=The%20TOES%20assesses%20the%20extent,administered%20simultaneously%20with%20the%20ToP | | | | |
| Test of Gross Motor Development (3rd ed.) (TGMD-3) | Ulrich (2013) | 3–11 | • Interview format/or observational checklist<br>• Standardized, norm referenced | • Gross motor/mobility (locomotor and ball skills) |
| For more information: https://www.kines.umich.edu/tgmd-3 and https://sites.google.com/view/tgmd-3/home | | | | |
| Test of Handwriting Skills, Revised (THS-R) | Milone (2017) | 6–18.11 | • Standardized, norm referenced | • Handwriting |
| For more information: https://www.wpspublish.com/ths-r-test-of-handwriting-skills-revised | | | | |
| Test of Playfulness (ToP) | Bundy (2010) | .6–18 | • Observational checklist | • Play/leisure<br>• Approach, style, and attitude towards play |
| For more information: Bundy, A. (2010). *Test of Playfulness Manual.* Boulder, CO: Colorado State University. https://journals.sagepub.com/doi/abs/10.1177/153944920102100405?journalCode=otja | | | | |
| Test of Visual Motor Skills (3rd ed.) (TVMS-3) | Martin (2015) | 3–90+ | • Standardized, norm referenced | • Visual motor |
| For more information: https://www.wpspublish.com/tvms-3-test-of-visual-motor-skills-third-edition | | | | |
| Test of Visual-Perceptual Skills (4th ed.) (TVPS-4) | Martin (2017) | 5–21 | • Standardized, norm referenced | • Visual perception (e.g., visualization, flexibility of closure, visual memory, memory span) |
| For more information: https://assessments.academictherapy.com/i/test-of-visual-perceptual-skills-4th-edition-tvps-4 | | | | |
| Toddler and Infant Motor Evaluation (TIME) | Miller, & Roid (1994) | 0–3.5 | • Standardized, norm referenced | • Fine motor<br>• Gross motor/mobility<br>• Social participation or social skills |
| For more information: https://psycnet.apa.org/doiLanding?doi=10.1037%2Ft15158-000 | | | | |
| Tolerance of Risk in Play Scale (TriPS) | Hill & Bundy (2014) | Parents and caregivers of children 3–13 | • Questionnaire | • Play/leisure<br>• Parents' tolerance to risk factors in play |
| For more information: https://pubmed.ncbi.nlm.nih.gov/22846064/ | | | | |
| Transdisciplinary Play-Based Assessment (2nd ed.) (TPBA-2) | Linder (2008) | 0–6 | • Interview format and observational checklist | • Behavioral/social emotional<br>• Cognitive<br>• Fine motor<br>• Gross motor/mobility<br>• Play/leisure<br>• Social participation or social skills |
| For more information: https://products.brookespublishing.com/Transdisciplinary-Play-Based-Assessment-Second-Edition-TPBA2-P215.aspx | | | | |
| Transition Assessment and Goal Generator (TAGG) | University of Oklahoma (2015) | Middle and high school | • Questionnaire | • IADL<br>• Social participation or social skills<br>• Work/transition |

*Continued*

| Assessment | Authors | Age Range* | Type | Areas Assessed |
|---|---|---|---|---|
| For more information: https://www.ou.edu/education/zarrow/tagg | | | | |
| Transition Behavior Scale (3rd ed.) (TBS-3) | McCarney & Arthaud (2012) | 12–18 | • Rating scales for child, teacher, parent<br>• Standardized, criterion referenced | • Provides assessment of child's predicted success of independent living and work<br>• Work/transition |
| For more information: https://www.hawthorne-ed.com/transition-behavior-scale-third-edition-complete-kit-details.html#:~:text=The%20TBS%2D3%20subscales%20measure,and%20readiness%20for%20transition%20activities | | | | |
| Transition Planning Inventory (TPI) | Patton & Clark | 14–22 | • Interview format/or observational checklist<br>• Questionnaire<br>• Not standardized | • ADL<br>• IADL<br>• Social participation or social skills<br>• Work/transition<br>• Other |
| For more information: https://www.proedinc.com/Products/14865/tpi3-transition-planning-inventorythird-edition-complete-kit.aspx | | | | |
| Transition Skills Inventory (2nd ed.) (TSI-2) | Brigance (2021) | Middle/high school | • Interview format/or observational checklist<br>• Questionnaire | • ADL<br>• IADL<br>• Social participation or social skills<br>• Work/transition |
| For more information: https://www.curriculumassociates.com/programs/brigance/special-education/transition-skills | | | | |
| Vineland Adaptive Behavior Scales (3rd ed.) (Vineland-3) | Sparrow, Cichettie, & Balla (2016) | 0–90 | • Standardized, norm referenced<br>• Telehealth | • ADL<br>• Behavioral/social emotional<br>• Cognitive<br>• Fine motor<br>• Gross motor/mobility<br>• Play/leisure<br>• Social participation or social skills |
| For more information: https://www.pearsonassessments.com/store/usassessments/en/Store/Professional-Assessments/Behavior/Adaptive/Vineland-Adaptive-Behavior-Scales-%7C-Third-Edition/p/100001622.html | | | | |
| Visual Skills Appraisal (2nd ed.) (VSA-2) | Richards | 5–14 | • Standardized, norm referenced | • Visual perception<br>• Pursuits<br>• Scanning<br>• Aligning<br>• Locating/Saccadic Eye Movements<br>• Eye-Hand Coordination |
| For more information: https://assessments.academictherapy.com/i/visual-skills-appraisal-2-vsa-2 | | | | |
| Vocational Fit Assessment (2nd ed.) (VocFit 2.0) | Persch & Cleary, (2024) | Teens–adults | • Interview format/or observational checklist<br>• Questionnaire | • IADL<br>• Work/transition<br>• Other |
| For more information: http://www.vocfit.com/and https://research.aota.org/ajot/article/69/6/6906180080p1/6054/Development-and-Psychometric-Evaluation-of-the | | | | |
| Volitional Questionnaire (VQ) | De las Heras, Geist, Kielhofner, & Li (2007) | 7+ | • Observational checklist | • Motivations, values, interests, perceived self-efficacy for occupational participation |
| For more information: https://moho-irm.uic.edu/productDetails.aspx?aid=8 | | | | |
| Waisman-ADL Scale | Maenner, Smith Hong, Makuch Greenberg, & Mailick (2013) | Teens–adults | • Observational scale | • ADL |

| Assessment | Authors | Age Range* | Type | Areas Assessed |
|---|---|---|---|---|
| For more information: http://www.waisman.wisc.edu/family/WADL/ and Maenner, M.J., Smith, L.E., Hong, J., Makuch, R., Greenberg, J., & Mailick, M.R. (2013). An evaluation of an activities of daily living scale for adolescents and adults with developmental disabilities. *Disability and Health Journal*, 6(1), 8–17. https://doi.org/10.1016/j.dhjo.2012.08.005 | | | | |
| WeeFIM Functional Independence Measure for children | Uniform Data System for Medical Rehabilitation | 3–8 | • Interview format/or observational checklist<br>• Standardized, criterion referenced | • ADL<br>• Cognitive<br>• Gross motor/mobility |
| For more information: https://www.scribd.com/document/327882673/WeeFIM-Score-Sheet-MS-Word | | | | |
| Worker Role Interview (WRI) | Braveman, Robson, Velozo, Kielhofner, Fisher, Forsyth, & Kerschbaum (2005) | | • Semi-structured interview | • Psychosocial and environmental factors that impact return to work<br>• Work/transition |
| For more information: https://moho-irm.uic.edu/productDetails.aspx?aid=11 | | | | |
| Young Children's Participation and Environment Measure (YC-PEM) | Khetani, Coster, Law & Bedell (2013) | Caregivers and parents of children 0–5 | • Questionnaire | • Child's participation in home, school, community (e.g., ADL, IADL, Play/leisure, social participation, education)<br>• Environmental factors that support or hinder participation in home, school, and community |
| For more information: https://www.canchild.ca/en/shop/23-yc-pem-young-children-s-participation-and-environment-measure | | | | |

B APPENDIX

# Online Learning Resources

Online learning resources can be accessed by visiting Elsevier eBooks+ at eBooks.Health.Elsevier.com. Chapter authors have added materials to support student learning so that students can be more prepared for class, perform better on exams, and succeed in the coursework. Some chapters include handouts and resources to support occupational therapy practice.

## EACH CHAPTER INCLUDES

- PowerPoint slide shows
- Handouts for practice
- Resources (such as evidence-based tables)
- Multiple choice questions with the rationales for answers
- Video clips that include written background and guiding questions to reinforce key concepts

APPENDIX C

# Matrix of Case Examples Included in Each Chapter

*Jarrett Wolske*

This matrix summarizes the case examples provided in each chapter to provide instructors and students with an overview of clinical examples for referring to cases throughout the book. The case examples represent a wealth of clinical experience and are designed to stimulate discussion while applying key occupational therapy concepts for evaluating and providing occupational therapy intervention to children and adolescents. Instructors and students may use cases to reinforce content from other chapters. Applying concepts using a variety of cases (from other chapters) promotes therapeutic reasoning, discussion, learning, and integration of the material.

**Matrix: Description of Case Examples included in Each Chapter**

| Case Example (Chapter and Number) | Age | Setting | Diagnosis or Occupational Challenge | Content Emphasis |
|---|---|---|---|---|
| 1.1 | 3-month-old | Early Intervention | Prematurity | Overview of the occupational therapy process |
| 1.2 | 3-year-old | Outpatient | Challenges with play | Focus on important family concerns when creating intervention |
| 1.3 | 10-year-old | School and community | Autism | Strength-based focus |
| 1.4 | 6-year-old | School | Behavior and play | Grading and adapting activities for the "just-right challenge" |
| 1.5 | 4-year-old | Outpatient | Food selectivity | Using evidence-based practice guidelines |
| 2.1 | 7-year-old | Outpatient clinic | Social play, playground safety, dressing skills | Creativity in practice |
| 2.2 | Toddler | Early Intervention | Activities of daily living (ADLs), including feeding and oral motor skills | Serendipity in practice |
| 2.3 | 9-year-old | School | Handwriting and written expression | Promoting imagination |
| 2.4 | 6-year-old | School | Challenges playing, pretending, and being creative | Improvisation (using the "Yes And" approach in therapy) |
| 3.1 | 5-year-old | Inpatient | Anoxic brain injury | AOTA code of ethics |
| 3.2 | Young adult | Community organization | Work-readiness skills | Teach-back method |
| 3.3 | 18-month-old | Early Intervention | Global developmental delays | Intentional Relationship Model: Interpersonal events, situational characteristics, and practitioners' communication |
| 4.1 | Occupational therapy practitioner | All settings | Client is a recent immigrant from a country the practitioner is unfamiliar with. | Cultural humility |
| 4.2 | Occupational therapist | Community setting | Parent is unable to make appointment due to her work schedule. | Cultural sensitivity |
| 4.3 | Occupational therapist | NICU | How to better support Indigenous women in the hospital for childbirth | Cultural safety |

*Continued*

## Matrix: Description of Case Examples included in Each Chapter —cont'd

| Case Example (Chapter and Number) | Age | Setting | Diagnosis or Occupational Challenge | Content Emphasis |
|---|---|---|---|---|
| 4.4 | 13-year-old | School | Learning disabilities | Use of capabilities approach during transition planning |
| 4.5 | Occupational therapy practitioner | All | Addressing professional issues in practice | Handling microaggressions in the workplace |
| 4.8 | 15-month-old | Early Intervention | Challenges walking and manipulating objects (right hemiplegia) | Applying bridging strategies with a child and family |
| 5.1 | 17-year-old | School | Anxiety disorder and attention-deficit hyperactivity disorder | Mental health challenges |
| 5.2 | 8-year-old | Progression from intensive care unit to outpatient rehabilitation | Traumatic brain injury | Adjusting intervention to support performance as the child makes progress |
| 5.3 | 3-year-old | Intensive care unit and acute care hospital | Spinal cord injuries and burns | Progression of intervention among settings for a child with SCI |
| 6.1 | 15-month-old | NICU, PICU, Early Intervention | Tetralogy of Fallot and an omphalocele | Variety of settings where children may receive services |
| 7.1 | Occupational therapy practitioner | All settings | | Implications of improper billing |
| 7.2 | 11-month-old | Early Intervention | Feeding | How to identify the appropriate evaluation codes |
| 7.3 | 3-year-old | Out-patient hospital | Evaluation | Differences between the CMS and AMA guidelines for billing |
| 8.1 | 4-year-old | Outpatient Occupational therapy through Head Start | Spastic cerebral palsy | Influence of context on occupational therapy intervention planning |
| 9. 1 | 10-month-old | Community clinic | Down Syndrome: referral to "evaluate and treat" | Evaluation planning process using the top-down approach |
| 9.2A | 12-month-old | Early intervention | Developmental delay and hydrocephalus | Applying two different models of practice to guide evaluation (1) Kielhofner's Model of Human Occupation and (2) Canadian Model of Occupational Performance |
| 9.2B | 6-year-old | School | Cerebral palsy: Right hemiplegia; challenges in school | |
| 9.3 | 6-year-old | Outpatient | Juvenile Rheumatoid Arthritis; pain and challenges with play and daily activities | Using an occupation-based model (person-environment-occupation-participation; PEOP) to organize the evaluation, along with a biomechanical frame of reference to understand the child's physical challenges |
| 9.4 | 5.5-year-old | School | Challenges learning to write, holding pencil, exerting pressure on paper, keeping up with her peers, falling frequently, being uncoordinated, being easily overwhelmed, and often having emotional outbursts | Norm-referenced testing, clinical observations, and interviews |
| 9.5 | 9-month-old | Outpatient | Developmental delay | Initial evaluation: Formal and informal assessment of body structures and function and development skills |
| 9.6 | 9-year-old | School | Bipolar disorder and attention deficit hyperactivity disorder (ADHD) experiencing behavioral difficulties (aggressive and refusing to do work) in the classroom | Evaluation of mental health and sensory-motor concerns |

**Matrix: Description of Case Examples included in Each Chapter —cont'd**

| Case Example (Chapter and Number) | Age | Setting | Diagnosis or Occupational Challenge | Content Emphasis |
|---|---|---|---|---|
| 10.1 | 14-year-old | School | Autism; challenges with poor personal hygiene and limited food range | Canadian Occupational Performance Measure to measure progress and practice outcomes |
| 10.2 | 4-year-old | School | Play, development, fine motor skills | Goal Attainment Scaling to create and measure client-centered meaningful goals for children |
| 10.3 | 1st grader | School | School performance challenges | Method to monitor a child's performance over time based on an expected rate of progress |
| 11.1 | 5-year-old | Outpatient hospital (feeding specialists) | Eosinophilic esophagitis; Feeding and eating challenges | Management of feeding challenges |
| 11.2 | 2-year-old | Early intervention | Feeding challenges: gagging, choking, food refusal | Occupational therapy intervention to transition from G-tube to oral feedings |
| 12.1 | 15-year-old | Outpatient | Challenges with sleep and rest. | Environmental factors affecting sleep and rest |
| 12.2 | 5-year-old | Outpatient | Challenges with sleep routine | Family intervention to address a child's sleep routine |
| 13.1 | 4-year-old | In-patient hospital | Complications due to muscular disorder; challenges with ADLs | Levels of participation in ADLs (e.g., independent, partial participation, directing others, dependent) |
| 13.2 | 12-year-old | Outpatient | Incoordination, poor memory, and limited judgment interfere with ADLs | Visual schedules and reminders (on phones or watches) to support ADL routines |
| 14.1 | 14-year-old | Outpatient | Hemiplegia: upper extremity weakness and mild cognitive deficit | Instrumental activity of daily living (IADL) intervention: Meal preparation |
| 14.2 | 17-year-old | School | Intellectual and Development Disability and B LE amputation | IADL Intervention: Grocery shopping |
| 14.3 | 6th grade | School | Autism, nonspeaking | IADL Intervention: Home management (clothing care) |
| 16.1 | 5-year-old | School | Mildly delayed motor skills, very limited pretend play | Promoting pretend play |
| 16.2 | 2.5-year-old | Early Intervention | Mild spastic diplegia, prematurity, shows fear of movement | Intervention session using directed or guided play |
| 16.3 | 9-year-old | School | Generalized anxiety disorder, bipolar disorder, and attention deficit disorder | Play as an occupation |
| 18.1 | 3-year-old | School | Spastic quadriplegia | Creating an inclusive environment for social participation in a preschool classroom |
| 18.2 | Students of low socio-economic status | School | Provided opportunities for physical activity and participatory learning about fitness and health | Self-determination skills |
| 18.3 | High school | School | Autism; challenges with group projects and social relationships | Peer-mediated intervention |
| 18.4 | High school | School | Two students (one with Menkes syndrome) | Programs to promote social relationships |

*Continued*

**Matrix: Description of Case Examples included in Each Chapter —cont'd**

| Case Example (Chapter and Number) | Age | Setting | Diagnosis or Occupational Challenge | Content Emphasis |
|---|---|---|---|---|
| 18.5 | 16–23 years of age | Community service and education program | Providing opportunities for children with disabilities to engage in community service | Community service: Empowering People for Inclusive Communities Service Warriors |
| 19.1 | 18-year-old | School | Intellectual disability; difficulty understanding different types of relationships and boundaries; wants to date | Addressing sexuality by tailoring the content to the child's needs |
| 19.2 | 14-year-old | Outpatient | Autism, challenges with socially appropriate behaviors | Social Stories to address behaviors |
| 20.1 | 18-year-old | Community: Driving specialist | Traumatic brain injury | Occupational therapy approach to driving |
| 20.2 | 17-year-old | Home health | Traumatic injuries | Role of generalist in driving |
| 20.3 | Occupational therapy practitioner | School | Need to consult with certified driving specialist | Referrals to certified Driving Rehabilitation Specialist (certified through ADED) |
| 21.1 | 21-year-old | Vocational Rehabilitation services | Autism; transition planning | Identifying the fit between the person's strengths and the environment of the job |
| 21.2 | 16-year-old | School | Spina bifida; transition planning | Concepts of universal design for learning and accessibility to support students in transition |
| 22.1 | 9-month-old | Outpatient occupational therapy | Congenital issues resulting in severe brain damage at birth | Caregiver-mediated approaches include family-centered practices, family capacity-building practices, and family and professional collaboration. |
| 22.2 | 30-month-old | Early Intervention | Developmental delays, behavioral challenges | Family-capacity building |
| 22.3 | 3-year-old | Outpatient | Unknown neurological condition interfering with his ability to sit, play, and feed himself | Professional and family collaboration |
| 23.1 | 24-month-old | Early Intervention - Telehealth | Concerns with gross and fine motor development, feeding, and suspected sensory processing problems | EI assessment with occupational therapy participation through telehealth, including the evaluation process, summary, interpretation, and sample goals and interventions |
| 23.2 | 5 years 8 months | School—Telehealth | Challenges with fine motor skills, sensory processing, and self-regulation | Telehealth occupational therapy assessment and intervention plan |
| 24.1 | Kindergarten Class | School | Social-emotional challenges | Promoting a child's interoception |
| 24.2 | 5th grade | School | History of trauma causing him to "shut down" | Neurosequential Model of Therapeutics to address the child's ability to self-regulate (e.g., provide strategies for the child to practice) using a bottom-up approach, later moving to top-down strategies that allow the child to reason and self-regulate |
| 24.3 | 25-month-old | Early Intervention | Aggressive against peers at the park | Promoting social interactions |
| 25.1 | 2.5-year old and 6-year-old | Early Intervention and School | Developmental Disabilities; challenging behaviors | Examples of challenging behaviors |
| 25.2 | 7-year-old | School | Uncontrollable aggressive outbursts | Functional behavioral analysis as part of occupational therapy intervention |

**Matrix: Description of Case Examples included in Each Chapter —cont'd**

| Case Example (Chapter and Number) | Age | Setting | Diagnosis or Occupational Challenge | Content Emphasis |
|---|---|---|---|---|
| 25.3 | 4-year-old | School | Autism; difficulty transitioning to new activities | Using a timer as a signal for transitions |
| 25.4 | 10-year-old | School | Challenges with attention to tasks, following directions, and completing assigned work | Behavioral approaches |
| 26.1 | 9-year-old | School | Challenges with printing skills, including placement, and spacing between words, which affect the overall legibility of written work and academic performance | CO-OP approach to support a child's handwriting performance in school |
| 26.2 | 16-year-old | School | Autism: challenges planning and preparing dinner on the days his father works late | Concept mapping |
| 26.3 | 10-year-old | School | Fine motor skills interfering with self-care activities such as tying her shoes, buttoning buttons, and zipping zippers | CO-OP approach to address self-care |
| 26.4 | 7-year-old | Private outpatient occupational therapy services | Developmental Coordination Disorder: learning to ride his new bike | CO-OP approach to address leisure and play. This example includes a description of the role of the environment in addressing occupational performance and includes home programs and parental support to reinforce learning. |
| 27.1 | 4-year-old | School | Somatodyspraxia: poor balance and bilateral integration, difficulties with specific gross and fine motor skills, and emerging concerns around socialization | Ayres Sensory Integration (ASI®) |
| 29.1 | 4-year-old | School or outpatient setting | Down syndrome with gross and fine motor delays | Kielhofner's Model of Human Occupation to plan occupational therapy intervention targeting motor control |
| 29.2 | 7-year-old | School | Difficulty using hands, completing schoolwork (e.g., coloring), and playing on the playground | Applies current motor control/motor learning principles and strategies to practice |
| 30.1 | 10-year-old | School | Dyspraxia and learning disability interfering with hand manipulation skills for school | Client-centered occupation-based intervention session to address in-hand manipulation skills (translation, shift, and rotation) |
| 30.2 | 9-year-old | School | Weak intrinsic hand muscle endurance | Intervention activities to build hand muscle endurance |
| 30.3 | 7-year-old | Outpatient Rehabilitation | Limited right upper extremity use resulting from a traumatic brain injury | Occupation-based fine motor goals |
| 30.4 | 2-year-old | Outpatient-based occupational therapy clinic | Cerebral palsy: right hemiplegia | Occupation-based intervention to address fine motor skills |
| 30.5 | 8-year-old | School | Difficulty handwriting and only writes one-to-two-word responses on open writing prompts | Addressing handwriting challenges |
| 31.1 | 4-year-old | School | Autism: Potential vision problems | Observations indicating potential visual problems |
| 31.2 | 11-year-old | School | Difficulty reading and working on a computer, blurred vision, and eyestrain after 10–15 minutes of reading, words start moving on the page, intermittent double vision, and headaches, all interfering with academic performance | Role of vision professionals |

*Continued*

**Matrix: Description of Case Examples included in Each Chapter —cont'd**

| Case Example (Chapter and Number) | Age | Setting | Diagnosis or Occupational Challenge | Content Emphasis |
|---|---|---|---|---|
| 31.3 | 6-year-old | School | Struggling in 1st grade. Difficulty with trouble with letter and number recognition; sight vocabulary; reversing and transposing letters, numbers, and words; and unable to copy off the board quickly enough. | Collaboration between an optometrist and occupational therapy practitioner |
| 32.1 | 8-month-old | Home | Neuro typical | Influence of movement and embodied cognition |
| 32.2 | 2-year-old | Early Intervention | Cerebral palsy, cannot ambulate but can bear weight | Mobility intervention process; equipment trial in power mobility |
| 32.3 | 16-year-old | School; Outpatient | Spastic diplegia cerebral palsy | Mobility intervention: power mobility |
| 33.1 | 7-year-old | Outpatient | Cerebral Palsy: Right hemiplegia | Kielhofner's Model of Human Occupation and the biomechanical frame of reference to address hand performance |
| 33.2 | 2-week-old | Inpatient | Arthrogryposis; upper extremity range of motion limitations | Addressing range of motion to promote development |
| 33.3 | 15-year-old | Outpatient rehabilitation | Cerebral palsy with a right-sided hemiplegia. Upper extremity tendon transfer | Orthotics as part of the occupational therapy intervention plan |
| 34.1 | 8-month-old | In-patient | Recent cardiac surgery; poor endurance and limited upper extremity strength | Assistive technology to support infant's development, endurance, and upper extremity functioning |
| 34.2 | 2-year-old | Early Intervention | Down syndrome | AT services to support occupational performance |
| 34.3 | 3rd grade | School | Spinal muscular atrophy: child reported their hands get tired when writing and handwriting looks "sloppy." | AT to support academic expression |
| 35 Blaise | 27 weeks gestation | Neonatal Intensive Care Unit and Early Intervention | Prematurity | Medical Model |
| 35 Connor | 3-year-old | Transition from early intervention to outpatient pediatric clinic | Cerebral Palsy | Motor Control and Motor Learning |
| 35 Julian | 4-year-old | Outpatient pediatric clinic | Mixed Expressive and Receptive Communication Delay | Person-Environment-Occupation-Performance Model |
| 35 Laura | 6-year-old | School | Somatodyspraxia | Model of Human Occupation; Ayres' Sensory Integration<br>Social and behavioral approaches |
| 35 Kevin | 7-year-old | Outpatient pediatric clinic | Duchenne Muscular Dystrophy | Model of Human Occupation; Biomechanical; Intentional Relationship Model |
| 35 Juana | 13-year-old | Secondary school therapy group | Attention-Deficit Hyperactivity Disorder | Occupational Analysis and Group Processes; Social Behavioral Approach |
| 35 Alessio | 16-year-old | Inpatient hospital setting | Cancer | Model of Human Occupation; Biomechanical |
| 35 Miriam | Transition-aged | Secondary to Post-Secondary Transition | Post-Secondary Transition Challenges (secondary COVID-19 Pandemic) | Person-Environment-Occupation |

# INDEX

*Note*: Page numbers followed by *f* indicate figures and *t* indicate tables.

## D